Office International des Epizooties

WORLD ORGANISATION FOR ANIMAL HEALTH

MANUAL OF STANDARDS
FOR DIAGNOSTIC TESTS AND VACCINES

Lists A and B diseases of mammals, birds and bees

2000

This *Manual* has been edited by the
OIE Standards Commission and adopted by the
International Committee of the OIE

OIE *Manual of Standards for Diagnostic Tests and Vaccines*
Fourth Edition, 2000

Manual of Recommended Diagnostic Techniques and Requirements for Biological Products:
Volume I, 1989; Volume II, 1990; Volume III, 1991.
Manual of Standards for Diagnostic Tests and Vaccines:
Second Edition, 1992
Third Edition, 1996

ISBN 92-9044-510-6

12 rue de Prony, 75017 Paris, France
Tel: 33-(0)1 44 15 18 88
Fax: 33-(0)1 42 67 09 87
E-mail: oie@oie.int

FOREWORD

The aims of this *Manual* are to facilitate the international trade in animals and animal products and to contribute to the improvement of animal health services world-wide. By describing internationally agreed laboratory methods for disease diagnosis and requirements for the production and control of biological products (mainly vaccines), its objective is to harmonise these important elements of animal disease prevention, surveillance and control.

This ambitious objective required the cooperation of animal health specialists from many countries. The Office International des Epizooties (OIE), the world organisation for animal health, is clearly one of the most appropriate organisations to undertake this task on a global level. The main activities of the organisation, which was established in 1924, are as follows:

1 To collect and disseminate to its Member Countries, information (including emergency information) on the occurrence, course and treatment of animal diseases

2 To provide guidelines and standards for health regulations applicable to international trade in animals

3 To promote and coordinate research on the pathology, diagnosis, treatment and prevention of animal diseases when international collaboration in such research is desirable.

In pursuing these activities (especially the second one), the OIE produced *the International Animal Health Code* (the first edition of which was published in 1968). This *Manual* is the companion volume to the *Code* and provides a wealth of internationally agreed essential scientific and technical information that complements the *Code's* trade provisions. The *Manual,* however, is not limited to those diseases for which the *Code* prescribes tests and biological products, but covers all of the OIE Lists A and B diseases, and some additional diseases of importance. Aquatic animal diseases important in trade are included in a separate Code and Manual.

The task of commissioning chapters and compiling the *Manual* was assigned to the OIE Standards Commission by the International Committee of the OIE. The first edition was published in 1989, the second edition in 1992, and the third edition in 1996. For this, the fourth edition, manuscripts were requested from specialists in each of the diseases or the other topics covered. After initial scrutiny by the Consultant Technical Editor, the chapters were sent to scientific reviewers, to the OIE Biotechnology Group, to experts at OIE Reference Laboratories and in some cases to wildlife experts. They were also circulated to all OIE Member Countries for review and comment. The Standards Commission and the Consultant Technical Editor took all the resulting comments into consideration, often referring back to the authors for further help, before finalising the chapters. The final text has the approval of the International Committee of the OIE.

In this edition, all chapters have been updated and considerable additional information has been included, especially with regard to recent advances in biotechnology. This has resulted in a larger volume than previous editions. As continual revision is required in such a dynamic field, the OIE intends to publish an updated edition of the *Manual* approximately once every four years.

Doctor Jean Blancou
Director General, OIE

Professor Marian Truszczynski
President, OIE Standards Commission

December 2000

ACKNOWLEDGEMENTS

I am most grateful to the many people whose combined efforts have gone into the preparation of this *Manual. In* particular, I would like to express my thanks to:

Dr J. Blancou, Director General of the OIE from 1990 to the present, who gave his encouragement and support to the project of preparing the new edition of this *Manual,*

The Members of the OIE Standards Commission, Prof. M. Truszczynski, Dr J.E. Pearson, Dr S. Edwards and Dr B. Schmitt, and observers at the Standards Commission's meeting, Dr Mark Robinson and Dr P. Wright, who were responsible for commissioning chapters and, with the Consultant Technical Editor, for editing all the contributions so as to finalise this edition of the *Manual,*

The contributors listed on pages xxii to xxxii who contributed their invaluable time and expertise to write the chapters,

The reviewers and OIE Reference Laboratory experts who also gave their time and expertise to scrutinising the chapters,

The OIE Biotechnology Group and representatives of the OIE Collaborating Centre for ELISA and Molecular Techniques, Vienna, Austria,

Those OIE Member Countries who submitted comments on the draft chapters that were circulated to them. These were essential in making the Manual internationally acceptable,

Dr G.A. Cullen, who acted as Consultant Technical Editor of the *Manual* and did a great deal, not only in editing and harmonising the contents, but also in providing missing information where required,

Ms Sara Linnane who, as Scientific Editor, organised this complex project and made major contributions to the quality of the text,

Members of both the OIE Scientific and Technical Department and the Publications Department, for their assistance.

Dr Romano Marabelli
President of the OIE International Committee

December 2000

CONTENTS

INTRODUCTION
(How to use this *Manual*)

• Arrangement of the *Manual* and numbering system

Part I, Section I.1., the beginning of this *Manual,* contains eight introductory chapters that deal with a variety of general subjects of interest to veterinary laboratory diagnosticians. These chapters are intended to give a brief introduction to their subjects. They are to be regarded as background information rather than standards.

The main part of the *Manual* (Part 2. Sections 2.1.–2.9.) covers standards for diagnostic tests and vaccines for the diseases listed in the OIE *International Animal Health Code.* They appear in the same order and use the same numbering system as that used in the *Code,* to facilitate cross-reference between the two books. List A contains the transmissible diseases that have the potential for very serious and rapid spread, irrespective of national borders. They have particularly serious socio-economic or public health consequences and are of major importance in the international trade of animals and animal products. List B contains the transmissible diseases that are considered to be of socio-economic and/or public health importance within countries and that are significant in the international trade of animals and animal products. List B is subdivided by animal host species.

Some additional diseases that may also be of importance in trade but that do not have a chapter in the *Code* are included in Part 3. Section X.

The contributors of all the chapters are listed on pages xxii–xxxii, but the final responsibility for the content of the *Manual* lies with the International Committee of the OIE.

There is an alphabetical index of the diseases at the back of the book.

• Format of chapters

Each disease chapter includes a summary intended to provide information for veterinary officials and other readers who need a general overview of the tests and vaccines available for the disease. This is followed by a text giving greater detail for laboratory workers. In each disease chapter, Part A deals with laboratory diagnosis of the disease, and Part B (where appropriate) with the requirements for vaccines or *in vivo* diagnostic biologicals. Bibliographic references that provide further information are listed at the end of each chapter.

• Explanation of the tests described and of the table on pages xii–xv

The table on pages xii–xv lists diagnostic tests in two categories: 'prescribed' and 'alternative'. Prescribed tests are those that are required by the *International Animal Health Code* for the testing of animals before they are moved internationally. In the *Manual* these tests are printed in blue. At present it is not possible to have prescribed tests for every disease of Lists A and B. 'Alternative tests' are those that are suitable for the diagnosis of disease within a local setting, and can also be used in the import/export of animals after bilateral agreement. There are often other tests described in the chapters, which may also be of some practical value in local situations or which may still be under development.

• List of OIE Reference Laboratories

A list of OIE Reference Laboratories is given in Part 4 of this *Manual.* These laboratories have been designated by the OIE as centres of excellence with expertise in their particular field. They are able to provide advice to other laboratories on methodology. In some cases standard strains of micro-organisms or reference reagents (e.g. antisera, antigens) can also be obtained from the reference laboratories.

The list of OIE Reference Laboratories will be updated by the International Committee of the OIE each year, and the revised list will be published in each May issue of the OIE *Bulletin* and on the OIE Web site.

LIST OF TESTS FOR INTERNATIONAL TRADE

The table below lists diagnostic tests in two categories: 'prescribed' and 'alternative'. Prescribed tests are those that are required by the *International Animal Health Code* for the testing of animals in connection with international trade. In the *Manual* these tests are printed in blue. At present it is not possible to have prescribed tests for every disease of Lists A and B. Alternative tests are those that are suitable for the diagnosis of disease within a local setting, and can also be used in the import/export of animals after bilateral agreement. There are often other tests described in the chapters that may also be of some practical value in local situations or that may still be under development.

Chapter No.	Disease name	Prescribed tests	Alternative tests
2.1.1.	Foot and mouth disease	ELISA, VN	CF
2.1.2.	Vesicular stomatitis	CF, ELISA, VN	–
2.1.3.	Swine vesicular disease	VN	ELISA
2.1.4.	Rinderpest	ELISA	VN
2.1.5.	Peste des petits ruminants	VN	ELISA
2.1.6.	Contagious bovine pleuropneumonia	CF	ELISA
2.1.7.	Lumpy skin disease	–	VN
2.1.8.	Rift Valley fever	–	HI, ELISA, PRN
2.1.9.	Bluetongue	Agent id., AGID, ELISA, PCR	VN
2.1.10.	Sheep pox and goat pox	–	VN
2.1.11.	African horse sickness	CF, ELISA	VN
2.1.12.	African swine fever	ELISA	IFA
2.1.13.	Classical swine fever (hog cholera)	NPLA, FAVN, ELISA	–
2.1.14.	Highly pathogenic avian influenza	–	AGID, HI
2.1.15.	Newcastle disease	–	HI
2.2.1.	Anthrax	–	–
2.2.2.	Aujeszky's disease	ELISA, VN	–
2.2.3.	Echinococcosis/Hydatidosis	–	–
2.2.4.	Leptospirosis	–	MAT
2.2.5.	Rabies	VN	–
2.2.6.	Paratuberculosis (Johne's disease)	–	DTH, ELISA
2.2.7.	Heartwater	–	ELISA, IFA
2.2.8.	New World screwworm *(Cochliomyia hominivorax* and Old World screwworm *Chrysomya bezziana)*	–	Agent id.
2.2.9.	Trichinellosis	Agent id.	ELISA
2.3.1.	Bovine brucellosis	BBAT, CF, ELISA	FPA

Chapter No.	Disease name	Prescribed tests	Alternative tests
2.3.2.	Bovine genital campylobacteriosis	Agent id.	–
2.3.3.	Bovine tuberculosis	Tuberculin test	–
2.3.4.	Enzootic bovine leukosis	AGID, ELISA	–
2.3.5.	Infectious bovine rhinotracheitis/ infectious pustular vulvovaginitis	VN, ELISA, Agent id. (semen only)	–
2.3.6.	Trichomonosis	Agent id.	Mucus agg.
2.3.7.	Bovine anaplasmosis	–	CF, Agg. card
2.3.8.	Bovine babesiosis	–	ELISA, IFA
2.3.9.	Cysticercosis	–	Agent id.
2.3.10.	Dermatophilosis	–	–
2.3.11.	Theileriosis	Agent id., IFA	–
2.3.12.	Haemorrhagic septicaemia	–	Agent id.
2.3.13.	Bovine spongiform encephalopathy	–	–
2.4.1.	Ovine epididymitis *(Brucella ovis)*	CF	ELISA
2.4.2.	Caprine and ovine brucellosis (excluding *Brucella ovis* infection)	BBAT, CF	Brucellin test
2.4.3.	Contagious agalactia	–	–
2.4.4/5.	Caprine arthritis/encephalitis & Maedi-visna	AGID	ELISA
2.4.6.	Contagious caprine pleuropneumonia	CF	–
2.4.7.	Enzootic abortion of ewes (ovine chlamydiosis)	–	CF
2.5.1.	Contagious equine metritis	Agent id.	–
2.5.2.	Dourine	CF	IFA, ELISA
2.5.3.	Equine encephalomyelitis (Eastern and Western)	–	HI, CF, PRN
2.5.4.	Equine infectious anaemia	AGID	ELISA
2.5.5.	Equine influenza	–	HI
2.5.6.	Equine piroplasmosis	CF, IFA	–
2.5.7.	Equine rhinopneumonitis	–	VN
2.5.8.	Glanders	Mallein test, CF	–
2.5.10.	Equine viral arteritis	VN, Agent id. (semen only)	–
2.5.12.	Venezuelan equine encephalomyelitis	–	HI, CF, PRN
2.5.13.	Epizootic lymphangitis	–	–
2.5.14.	Japanese encephalitis	–	–
2.6.1.	Atrophic rhinitis of swine	–	–
2.6.2.	Porcine brucellosis	BBAT	ELISA, FPA
2.6.3.	Enterovirus encephalomyelitis (previously Teschen/Talfan diseases)	–	VN
2.6.4.	Transmissible gastroenteritis	–	VN, ELISA
2.7.1.	Infectious bursal disease (Gumboro disease)	–	AGID, ELISA
2.7.2.	Marek's disease	–	AGID

Chapter No.	Disease name	Prescribed tests	Alternative tests
2.7.3.	Avian mycoplasmosis *(Mycoplasma gallisepticum)*	–	Agg., HI
2.7.4.	Avian chlamydiosis	–	–
2.7.5.	Fowl typhoid and Pullorum disease	–	Agg., Agent id.
2.7.6.	Avian infectious bronchitis	–	VN, HI, ELISA
2.7.7.	Avian infectious laryngotracheitis	–	AGID, VN, ELISA
2.7.8.	Avian tuberculosis	–	Tuberculin test, Agent id.,
2.7.9.	Duck virus hepatitis	–	–
2.7.10.	Duck virus enteritis	–	–
2.7.11.	Fowl cholera (avian pasteurellosis)	–	–
2.8.1.	Myxomatosis	–	AGID, CF, IFA
2.8.2.	Tularemia	–	Agent id.
2.8.3.	Rabbit haemorrhagic disease	–	HI
2.9.1.	Acariosis of bees	–	–
2.9.2.	American foulbrood	–	–
2.9.3.	European foulbrood	–	–
2.9.4.	Nosemosis of bees	–	–
2.9.5.	Varroosis	–	–
X.1	Leishmaniosis	–	Agent id.
X.2	Malignant catarrhal fever	–	VN, IFA, PCR
X.3	Q fever	–	CF
X.4.	Salmonellosis	–	Agent id.
X.5.	Bovine viral diarrhoea	Agent id.	–
X.6	Trypanosomosis (Tsetse-transmitted)	–	IFA
X.7	Ovine pulmonary adenomatosis	–	–
X.8.	Nairobi sheep disease	–	–
X.9.	Scrapie	–	–
X.10.	Border disease	Agent id.	–
X.11.	Surra *(Trypansoma evansi)*	–	–
X.12.	Porcine reproductive and respiratory syndrome	–	ELISA, IFA, IPMA
X.13	Fowl pox	–	–
X.14.	Mange	–	Agent id.
X.15	*Tropilaelaps* infestation of honey bees *(Tropilaelaps clareae, T. koenigerum)*	–	–

Note: The tests prescribed by the *International Animal Health Code* for the purposes of international trade are printed in blue in this *Manual*.

Abbreviations

Agent id.	Agent identification
Agg.	Agglutination test
AGID	Agar gel immunodiffusion
BBAT	Buffered *Brucella* antigen test
CF	Complement fixation
CIEP	Counter immunoelectrophoresis
DTH	Delayed-type hypersensitivity
ELISA	Enzyme-linked immunosorbent assay
FAVN	Fluorescent antibody virus neutralisation
FPA	Fluorescence polarisation assay
HI	Haemagglutination inhibition
IFA	Indirect fluorescent antibody
IPMA	Immunoperoxidase monolayer assay
MAT	Microscopic agglutination test
NPLA	Neutralising peroxidase-linked assay
PCR	Polymerase chain reaction
PRN	Plaque reduction neutralisation
VN	Virus neutralisation
–	No test designated yet

COMMON ABBREVIATIONS USED IN THIS *MANUAL*

ABTS	2,2'-Azino-di-(3-ethyl-benzthiazoline)-6-sulphonic acid
AGID	Agar gel immunodiffusion
ATCC[1]	American type culture collection
BBAT	Buffered *Brucella* antigen test
BFK	Bovine fetal kidney (cells)
BGPS	Beef extract-glucose-peptone-serum (medium)
BHK	Baby hamster kidney (cell line)
BLP	Buffered lactose peptone
BPAT	Buffered plate antigen test
BSA	Bovine serum albumin
BSF	Bovine serum factors
CAM	Chorioallantoic membrane
CEF	Chicken embryo fibroblast
CF	Complement fixation (test)
CFU	Colony-forming unit
CIEP	Counter immunoelectrophoresis
CK	Calf kidney (cells)
CNS	Central nervous system
CPE	Cytopathic effect
CPLM	Cysteine-peptone-liver infusion maltose (medium)
CSY	Casein-sucrose-yeast (agar)
DEPC	Diethyl pyrocarbonate
DEAE	Diethylaminoethyl
DMEM	Dulbecco's modified Eagle's medium
DMSO	Dimethyl sulphide
DTH	Delayed-type hypersensitivity
EDTA	Ethylene diamine tetra-acetic acid
EGTA	Ethylene glycol tetra-acetic acid
EID	Egg-infective dose
ELISA	Enzyme-linked immunosorbent assay
EMTM	Evans' modified Tobie's medium
EYL	Earle's yeast lactalbumin (balanced salt solution)
FAT	Fluorescent antibody test
FAVN	Fluorescent antibody virus neutralisation
FITC	Fluorescein isothiocyanate
FLK	Fetal lamb kidney (cells)
FPA	Fluorescence polarisation assay
g	Relative centrifugal force
GIT	Growth inhibition test
HA	Haemagglutination
HAD	Haemadsorption
HBSS	Hanks' balanced salt solution
HEP	High-egg-passage (virus)
HEPES	N-2-hydroxyethylpiperazine, N-2-ethanesulfonic acid [buffer]
HI	Haemagglutination inhibition
HRPO	Horseradish peroxidase
IB	Immunoblot test
ICFTU	International complement fixation test unit
ICPI	Intracerebral pathogenicity index
ID_{50}	Median infectious dose
IFA	Indirect fluorescent antibody (test)
IHA	Indirect haemagglutination
IPMA	Immunoperoxidase monolayer assay
IU	International units
IVPI	Intravenous pathogenicity index
LA	Latex agglutination
LD	Lethal dose
LEP	Low egg passage (virus)
MAb	Monoclonal antibody
MAT	Microscopic agglutination test
MCS	Master cell stock
MDT	Mean death time
MEM	Minimal essential medium
MSV	Master seed virus
NI	Neutralisation index
OGP	1-octyl-beta-D-glucopyranoside (buffer)
OPD	Orthophenyldiamine (buffer)
OPG	Oxalase-phenol-glycerin (preservative solution)
PAGE	Polyacrylamide gel electrophoresis
PAP	Peroxidase–antiperoxidase (staining procedure)
PAS	Periodic acid-Schiff (reaction)
PBS	Phosphate buffered saline
PCR	Polymerase chain reaction
PD	Protective dose
PFU	Plaque-forming unit
PHA	Passive haemagglutination (test)
PPD	Purified protein derivative
PPLO	Pleuropneumonia-like organisms
PRN	Plaque reduction neutralisation
PSG	Phosphate buffered saline glucose
RBC	Red blood cell
RFLP	Restriction fragment length polymorphism
RK	Rabbit kidney

RPM	Revolutions per minute
RSA	Rapid serum agglutination
RT-PCR	Reverse-transcription polymerase chain reaction
SAT	Serum agglutination test
SDS	Sodium dodecyl sulphate
SPF	Specific pathogen free
SPG	Sucrose phosphate glutamic acid
SRBC	Sheep red blood cells
$TCID_{50}$	Tissue culture infective dose
TMB	Tetramethyl benzidine
TSI	Triple sugar iron (medium)
VB	Veronal buffer
VBS	Veronal buffered saline
Vero	African green monkey kidney (cells)
VN	Virus neutralisation

1 American Type Culture Collection, 10801 University Boulevard, Manassas, Virginia 20110-2209, United States of America

GLOSSARY OF TERMS

The definitions given below have been selected and restricted to those that are likely to be useful to users of this OIE Manual.

A. DIAGNOSTICS

- **Cut-off/threshold**

The test result value selected for distinguishing between negative and positive results.

- **Incidence**

The number of new cases of a disease that occur per population at risk in a particular geographical area within a defined time interval, e.g. cases per 100,000 per year.

- **Laboratory**

Laboratory means a properly equipped institution staffed by technically competent personnel under the supervision of a specialist in veterinary diagnostic methods. The Veterinary Administration approves and monitors such laboratories in regard to tests for specific diseases for international trade.

- **Predictive value**

The probability that an animal with a positive test result does have the disease and one with a negative test result does not have the disease. This is determined by the prevalence of the condition and the sensitivity and specificity of the test. It can be expressed in two ways: the Positive Predictive Value and the Negative Predictive Value. These two values are not exact opposites.

- **Prevalence**

A measure of the prevalence of disease in a population at one given time, e.g. cases per 100,000.

- **Repeatability**

Agreement between replicates within and between runs of the same assay.

- **Reproducibility**

The ability of a test to provide consistent results when applied to aliquots of the same sample at different laboratories.

- **Sensitivity (analytical)**

This is the smallest detectable amount of the analyte in question.

- **Sensitivity (diagnostic)**

The proportion of known infected reference animals that test positive in the assay; infected animals that test negative are considered to have false-negative results.

- **Specificity (analytical)**

This is the degree to which the assay does not cross-react with other analytes.

- **Specificity (diagnostic)**

The proportion of uninfected reference animals that test negative in the assay; uninfected reference animals that test positive are considered to have false-positive results.

- **Standard (antisera and antigens)**

- **International Standard Reagent**

  This is the standard reagent by which all other reagents and assays are calibrated. A large batch is divided into aliquots and stored at an International Reference Laboratory, for issue to National Laboratories.

- **National Standard Reagents**

  These are calibrated by comparison with the International Standard Reagent.

- **Working Standards (reagents)**

  These are standard reagents which are included in routine diagnostic testing as controls. They are calibrated against National Standard Reagents.

  For most serological assays, three International Standard Sera are required: a strong positive, a weak positive, and a negative. In preparing the positive sera, it will often be necessary to make a one-time dilution of the hyperimmune serum in negative serum, in order to achieve a defined reactivity that is within the detection range of the diagnostic test.

- **Tests**

- **Prescribed**

  Tests which are required by the *International Animal Health Code* and are considered optimal for determining the health status of animals.

- **Alternative**

  Tests suitable for the diagnosis of disease in a local situation, and which can also be used for import/export with bilateral agreement.

- **Screening**

  Tests of high diagnostic sensitivity suitable for large-scale application.

- **Confirmatory**

  Tests of high diagnostic specificity used to confirm the results of previous tests performed with another method.

B. VACCINES

- **Batch**

All the vaccine derived from the same homogeneous bulk and identified by a unique code number.

- **Cell line**

A stably transformed line of cells that have a high capacity for multiplication *in vitro*.

- **Dose**

The amount of a biological product recommended on the label to be given to one animal of a specified age, at one time by a specified route of administration.

- **Efficacy**

Specific ability of the biological product to produce the result for which it is offered, when used under the conditions recommended by the manufacturer.

- **Final product (lot)**

All the sealed final containers that have been filled from the same homogenous batch of vaccine in one working session, freeze-dried together in one continuous operation (if applicable), sealed in one working session, and identified by a unique code number.

- **In-process control**

The test procedures carried out during manufacture of a biological product to ensure that the product will comply with the agreed quality standards.

- **Master cell (line, stock, seed)**

A collection of aliquots of cells of defined passage level, for use in the preparation or testing of a biological product, distributed into containers in a single operation, processed together and stored in such a manner as to ensure uniformity and stability and to prevent contamination.

- **Master seed (agent, strain)**

A collection of aliquots of an organism at a specific passage level, from which all other seed passages are derived, which are obtained from a single bulk, distributed into containers in a single operation and processed together and stored in such a manner as to ensure uniformity and stability and to prevent contamination.

- **Potency**

Relative strength of a biological product as determined by appropriate test methods. (Initially the potency is measured using an efficacy test in animals. Later this may be correlated with tests of antigen content, or antibody response, for routine batch potency tests.)

- **Primary cells**

A pool of original cells derived from normal tissue up to and including the tenth subculture.

- **Production seed**

An organism at a specified passage level that is used without further propagation for initiating preparation of a production bulk.

- **Purity**

Quality of a biological product prepared to a final form and:

a) Relatively free from any extraneous microorganisms and extraneous material (organic or inorganic) as determined by test methods appropriate to the product; and

b) Free from extraneous microorganisms or material which could adversely affect the safety, potency or efficacy of the product.

- **Safety**

Freedom from properties causing undue local or systemic reactions when used as recommended or suggested by the manufacturer and without known hazard to in-contact animals, humans and the environment.

- **Specific pathogen free (SPF)**

Refers to animals that have been shown by the use of appropriate tests to be free from specified pathogenic microorganisms, and also refers to eggs derived from SPF birds.

- **Sterility**

Freedom from viable contaminating microorganisms, as demonstrated by approved and appropriate tests.

- **Working seed**

An organism at a passage level between master seed and production seed.

C. TECHNIQUES

- **Absorbance/optical density**

Absorbance and optical density are terms used to indicate the strength of reaction, for example immunoassay, using a spectrophotometer. It has not been possible to standardise authors' use of these two terms which, for practical purposes, are generally regarded as synonymous. However, 'absorbance' is the preferred term.

- **Centrifugation**

Throughout the text, the rate of centrifugation has been expressed as the Relative Centrifugal Force, denoted by '*g*'. The formula is:

$$\frac{(\text{RPM} \times 0.10472)^2}{980} \times \text{Radius (cm)} = g$$

where RPM is the rotor speed in revolutions per minute, and where Radius (cm) is the radius of the rotor arm, to the bottom of the tube, in centimetres.

It may be necessary to calculate the RPM required to achieve a given value of g, with a particular rotor. The formula is:

$$\text{RPM} = \frac{\sqrt{g \times 980}\ /\text{Radius (cm)}}{0.10472}$$

- **Dilutions**

Where dilutions are given for making up liquid reagents, they are expressed as, for example, 1 to 4, meaning one part added to four parts, i.e. a 1 in 5 dilution or a 20% solution of A in B.

- v/v – This is volume to volume (two liquids).
- w/v – This is weight to volume (solid added to a liquid).

- **Dilutions used in virus neutralisation tests**

There are two different conventions used in expressing the dilution used in virus neutralisation (VN) tests. In Europe, it is customary to express the dilution before the addition of the antigen, but in the United States of America and elsewhere, it is usual to express dilutions after the addition of antigen.

These alternative conventions are expressed in the *Manual* as 'initial dilution' or 'final dilution', respectively.

- **Room temperature**

The term room temperature is intended to imply the temperature of a comfortable working environment. Precise limits for this cannot be set, but guiding figures are 18–25°C. Where a test specifies room temperature, this should be achieved, with air conditioning if necessary, otherwise the test parameters may be affected.

CONTRIBUTORS

CONTRIBUTORS AND PROFESSIONAL ADDRESS AT TIME OF WRITING

I.1.1. Sampling methods

Dr G.A. Cullen (retired)
Formerly VLA Weybridge, New Haw, Addlestone, Surrey KT15 3NB, UK.

I.1.2. Quality Management in veterinary diagnostic laboratories

Dr A. Wiegers
USDA, APHIS, VS, National Veterinary Services Laboratories and Center for Veterinary Biologics – Laboratory, P.O. Box 844, Ames, Iowa 50010, USA.

I.1.3. Principles of validation of diagnostic assays for infectious diseases

Dr R. Jacobson (retired)
Formerly Diagnostic Laboratory, College of Veterinary Medicine, Cornell University, Ithaca, New York 14850-5786, USA.

I.1.4. Tests for sterility and freedom from contamination of biological materials

Dr L. Elsken
USDA, APHIS, Center for Veterinary Biologics, Suite 104, 510 South 17th Street, Ames, Iowa 50010, USA.

I.1.5. Human safety in the veterinary microbiology laboratory

Dr G.A. Cullen (retired)
Formerly VLA Weybridge, New Haw, Addlestone, Surrey KT15 3NB, UK.

I.1.6. Principles of veterinary vaccine production

Dr D.A. Espeseth (retired)
Formerly Director, Center for Veterinary Biologics – Licensing and Policy Development, USDA, APHIS, 4700 River Road, Riverdale, Maryland 20737, USA.

I.1.7. Biotechnology in the diagnosis of infectious diseases and vaccine development

Dr J. Gorham
College of Veterinary Medicine, Department of Veterinary Microbiology and Pathology, Washington State University, Pullman, Washington 99164-7030, USA.

Dr D. Knowles
Animal Disease Research Unit, ARS, USDA, Washington State University, Pullman, Washington 99164-6630, USA.

I.1.8. The role of international bodies in the regulation of veterinary biologicals	**Dr Ph. Vannier** AFSSA Ploufragan, Laboratoire d'études et de recherches avicoles et porcines, Zoopôle des Côtes d'Armor-Les Croix, BP 53, 22440 Ploufragan, France.
	Dr P.-P. Pastoret Immunology–Vaccinology, Faculty of Veterinary Medicine B43B, University of Liège, B-4000 Liège, Belgium.
	Dr D.A. Espeseth (retired) Formerly Director, Center for Veterinary Biologics – Licensing and Policy Development, USDA, APHIS, 4700 River Road, Riverdale, Maryland 20737, USA.
	Dr O. Itoh National Veterinary Assay Laboratory, JMAFF, 1-15-1 Tokura, Kokubunji, Tokyo 185-8511, Japan.
2.1.1. Foot and mouth disease	**Dr R.P. Kitching, Dr P.V. Barnett & Dr A.I. Donaldson** Institute for Animal Health, Pirbright Laboratory, Ash Road, Pirbright, Surrey GU24 0NF, UK.
	Dr D.K.J. Mackay Veterinary Medicines Directorate, Woodham Lane, New Haw, Addlestone, Surrey KT12 3LJ, UK
2.1.2. Vesicular stomatitis	**Dr B. Schmitt** USDA, APHIS, National Veterinary Services Laboratories, P.O. Box 844, Ames, Iowa 50010, USA.
2.1.3. Swine vesicular disease	**Dr R.P. Kitching & Dr A.I. Donaldson** Institute for Animal Health, Pirbright Laboratory, Ash Road, Pirbright, Surrey GU24 0NF, UK.
	Dr D.K.J. Mackay Veterinary Medicines Directorate, Woodham Lane, New Haw, Addlestone, Surrey KT12 3LJ, UK
2.1.4. Rinderpest	**Dr W.P. Taylor** 14 Beach Crescent, Littlehampton, West Sussex BN17 5NT, UK.
	Dr P.L. Roeder FAO, Animal Production and Health Division, Viale delle Terme di Caracalla, 00100 Rome, Italy.
2.1.5. Peste des petits ruminants *2.1.6. Contagious bovine pleuropneumonia*	**Dr P.C. Lefèvre** Conseil Général Vétérinaire, Ministère de l'Agriculture et de la Pêche, 251 rue de Vaugirard, 75732 Paris Cedex 15, France.

2.1.7. Lumpy skin disease	**Dr R.P. Kitching** Institute for Animal Health, Pirbright Laboratory, Ash Road, Pirbright, Surrey GU24 0NF, UK. **Dr V. Carn** Highbury, Thornford, Sherborne, Dorset DT9 6QD, UK.
2.1.8. Rift Valley fever	**Dr B.J.H. Barnard (retired) & Dr G.H. Gerdes** Onderstepoort Veterinary Institute, Private Bag X05, Onderstepoort 0110, South Africa.
2.1.9. Bluetongue	**Dr B. Eaton** Australian Animal Health Laboratory, CSIRO, Livestock Industries, 5 Portarlington Road, Geeling, Victoria 3220, Australia.
2.1.10. Sheep pox and goat pox	**Dr R.P. Kitching** Institute for Animal Health, Pirbright Laboratory, Ash Road, Pirbright, Surrey GU24 0NF, UK. **Dr V. Carn** Highbury, Thornford, Sherborne, Dorset DT9 6QD, UK.
2.1.11. African horse sickness	**Dr J.M. Sánchez-Vizcaíno** Centro de Investigación en Sanidad Animal, Instituto Nacional de Investigación y Tecnología Agraria y Alimentaria, CISA-INIA, Valdeolmos 28130 Madrid, Spain.
2.1.12. African swine fever	**Dr P.J. Wilkinson** Institute for Animal Health, Pirbright Laboratory, Ash Road, Pirbright, Surrey GU24 0NF, UK.
2.1.13. Classical swine fever (hog cholera)	**Dr C. Terpstra** Institute for Animal Science and Health (ID-Lelystad), Research Branch Houtribweg, Houtribweg 39, P.O. Box 65, NL-8200 AB Lelystad, The Netherlands.
2.1.14. Highly pathogenic avian influenza *2.1.15. Newcastle disease*	**Dr D.J. Alexander** VLA Weybridge, New Haw, Addlestone, Surrey KT15 3NB, UK.
2.2.1. Anthrax	**Dr P.C.B. Turnbull** Formerly Centre for Applied Microbiology and Research, Porton Down, Salisbury, Wiltshire SP4 0JG, UK.
2.2.2. Aujeszky's disease	**Prof. B. Toma & Prof. M. Eloit** École nationale vétérinaire d'Alfort, 7 avenue du Général de Gaulle, 94704 Maisons-Alfort Cedex, France. **Dr Ph. Vannier** AFSSA Ploufragan, Laboratoire d'études et de recherches avicoles et porcines, Zoopôle des Côtes d'Armor-Les Croix, BP 53, 22440 Ploufragan, France.

2.2.3. Echinococcosis/Hydatidosis

Prof. P.S. Craig
Division of Biological Sciences, School of Environment & Life Sciences, University of Salford, Salford M5 4WT, UK.

Dr M.A. Gemmell (retired)
Formerly Department of Clinical Veterinary Medicine, University of Cambridge, Madingley Road, Cambridge CB3 OES, UK.

2.2.4. Leptospirosis

Prof. C.A. Bolin
Professor and Section Chief, Animal Health Diagnostic Laboratory, College of Veterinary Medicine, A3A Veterinary Medical Center, Michigan State University, East Lansing, Michigan 48824, USA.

2.2.5. Rabies

Dr M. Aubert (Formerly), Dr F. Cliquet & Dr J. Barrat
AFSSA Nancy, Domaine de Pixérécourt, BP 9, F-54220 Malzeville, France.

2.2.6. Paratuberculosis (Johne's disease)

Dr M.-F. Thorel
AFSSA Alfort, Laboratoire d'Études et de Recherches en Pathologie Animale et Zoonoses, 22 rue Pierre Curie, BP 67, 94703 Maisons-Alfort Cedex, France.

2.2.7. Heartwater

Dr E. Camus
CIRAD-EMVT, Programme santé animale, TA/30G, 34398 Montpellier Cedex 5, France.

Dr D. Martinez
CIRAD-EMVT, Domaine de Duclos, Prise d'Eau, 97170 Petit-Bourg, Guadeloupe.

Prof. F. Jongejan
Department of Parasitology & Tropical Veterinary Medicine, Faculty of Veterinary Medicine, Utrecht University, P.O. Box 80.165, 3508 TD Utrecht, The Netherlands
AND
Department of Veterinary Tropical Diseases, Faculty of Veterinary Science, University of Pretoria, Onderstepoort 0110, South Africa.

2.2.8. Old World screwworm (Cochliomyia hominivorax) *and* New World *screwworm* (Chrysomya bezziana)

Dr M.J.R. Hall
Department of Entomology, The Natural History Museum, Cromwell Road, London SW7 5BD, UK.

2.2.9. Trichinellosis

Dr H.R. Gamble (retired)
Formerly USDA, ARS, Parasite Biology and Epidemiology Laboratory, Beltsville, Maryland 20705, USA.

2.3.1. Bovine brucellosis

Dr A.P. MacMillan & Dr J. Stack
VLA Weybridge, New Haw, Addlestone, Surrey KT15 3NB, UK.

2.3.2. Bovine genital campylobacteriosis

Dr J.A. Wagenaar & M.A.P. Van Bergen, BSc
Institute for Animal Science and Health (ID-Lelystad), P.O. Box 65, 8200 AB Lelystad, The Netherlands.

Dr B. Guérin
Ministère de l'Agriculture, Laboratoire pour la Contrôle des Reproducteurs, 13 rue Jouët, 94703 Maisons-Alfort Cedex, France.

2.3.3. Bovine tuberculosis

Dr J. Haagsma
Meidoornsingel 144, 3052 BT Rotterdam, The Netherlands.

2.3.4. Enzootic bovine leukosis

Dr L. Renström
National Veterinary Institute, Department of Virology, SE-751 89 Uppsala, Sweden.

2.3.5. Infectious bovine rhinotracheitis/ infectious pustular vulvovaginitis

Prof. J.T. van Oirschot
Department of Mammalian Virology, Institute for Animal Science and Health, ID-Lelystad, Edelhertweg 15, P.O. Box 65, 8200 AB Lelystad, The Netherlands.

2.3.6. Trichomonosis

Prof. M. Taylor
VLA Weybridge, New Haw, Addlestone, Surrey KT15 3NB, UK.

2.3.7. Bovine anaplasmosis

Dr T.F. McElwain
Washington State University, Animal Disease Diagnostic Laboratory, 155 N Bustad Hall, Pullman, Washington 99164-7034, USA.

2.3.8. Bovine babesiosis

Dr A.J. de Vos
Queensland Department of Primary Industries, Animal and Plant Health Service, Tick Fever Research Centre, 280 Grindle Road, Wacol, Queensland 4076, Australia.

Dr W.K. Jorgensen & Dr J.B. Molloy
Queensland Department of Primary Industries, Agency for Food & Fibre Sciences, 665 Fairfield Rd, Yeerongpilly, Queensland 4105, Australia.

2.3.9. Cysticercosis

Dr S. Lloyd
Department of Clinical Veterinary Medicine, University of Cambridge, Madingley Road, Cambridge CB3 0ES, UK.

2.3.10. Dermatophilosis

Prof. D.H. Lloyd
Dept of Small Animal Medicine and Surgery, Royal Veterinary College, Hawkshead Lane, North Mymms, Hatfield, Hertfordshire AL9 7TA, UK.

2.3.11. Theileriosis

Prof. E. Pipano & Dr V. Shkap
Division of Parasitology, Kimron Veterinary Institute, P.O. Box 12, Beit Dagan, 50250 Israel.

2.3.12. Haemorrhagic septicaemia	**Dr S. Chandrasekaran** Veterinary Research Institute, P.O. Box 369, 30740 Ipoh, Malaysia.
	Dr K. Townsend Diagnostic Bacteriology Laboratory, Veterinary Pathology and Anatomy, School of Veterinary Science, The University of Queensland, Brisbane QLD 4072, Australia.
	Dr M.C.L. De Alwis (retired) Formerly Veterinary Research Institute, Department of Animal Production and Health, P.O. Box 28, Peradeniya, Sri Lanka.
2.3.13. Bovine spongiform encephalopathy	**Mr G.A.H. Wells, Mr R. Bradley* & Prof. J.W. Wilesmith** VLA Weybridge, New Haw, Addlestone, Surrey KT15 3NB, UK.
*2.4.1. Ovine epididymitis (*Brucella ovis*)* *2.4.2. Caprine and ovine brucellosis (excluding* Brucella ovis *infection)*	**Dr Bruno Garin-Bastuji** AFSSA Alfort, Laboratoire d'Études et de Recherches en Pathologie Animale et Zoonoses, BP 67, F94703 Maisons-Alfort Cedex, France.
	Dr J.M. Blasco Dpt Sanidad Animal, Servicio de Investigacion Agraria/DGA, Apartado 727, 50080 Zaragoza, Spain.
2.4.3. Contagious agalactia	**Dr P.C. Lefèvre** Conseil Général Vétérinaire, Ministère de l'Agriculture et de la Pêche, 251 rue de Vaugirard, 75732 Paris Cedex 15, France.
2.4.4/5. Caprine arthritis/encephalitis & Maedi-visna	**Dr D. Knowles** Animal Disease Research Unit, ARS, USDA, Washington State University, Pullman, Washington 99164-6630, USA.
2.4.6. Contagious caprine pleuropneumonia	**Dr F.R Rurangirwa** Department of Veterinary Microbiology and Pathology, Washington State University, Pullman, Washington 99164-7040, USA.
	Dr J.H. Kinyili Kenya Veterinary Vaccines Production Institute, P.O. Box 53260, Nairobi, Kenya.
2.4.7. Enzootic abortion of ewes (ovine chlamydiosis)	**Prof. I.D. Aitken** Edinburgh Centre for Rural Research, Pentlands Science Park, Bush Loan, Penicuik, Edinburgh EH26 0PZ, UK.
2.5.1. Contagious equine metritis	**Dr N. Chanter** Animal Health Trust, Lanwades Park, Kentford, Newmarket, Suffolk CB8 7UU, UK.

* VLA is contact address.

2.5.2. Dourine	**Dr C. Staak (retired)** Formerly Federal Institute for Health Protection of Consumers and Veterinary Medicine, Diedersdorfer Weg 1, 12277 Berlin, Germany.
2.5.3. Equine encephalomyelitis (Eastern and Western)	**Dr J.E. Pearson (retired)** Formerly USDA, APHIS, National Veterinary Services Laboratories, P.O. Box 844, Ames, Iowa 50010, USA.
2.5.4. Equine infectious anaemia	**Prof. L. Coggins (retired)** Emeritus Professor, Department of Microbiology, Pathology and Parasitology, North Carolina State University, 4700 Hillsborough Street at William Moore Drive, Raleigh, North Carolina 27606, USA.
2.5.5. Equine influenza	**Dr J.A. Mumford** Animal Health Trust, Lanwades Park, Kentford, Newmarket, Suffolk CB8 7UU, UK.
2.5.6. Equine piroplasmosis	**Dr D.T. de Waal** Onderstepoort Veterinary Institute, Private Bag X05, 0110 Onderstepoort, South Africa.
2.5.7. Equine rhinopneumonitis	**Dr G.P. Allen** University of Kentucky, College of Agriculture, Veterinary Science, 108 Gluck Equine Research Center, Lexington, Kentucky 40546-0099, USA.
2.5.8. Glanders	**Dr F.G.van Zijderveld & Dr J. Bongers** Institute for Animal Science and Health (ID-Lelystad), Department of Bacteriology, Edelhertweg 5, P.O. Box 65, 8200 AB Lelystad, The Netherlands.
2.5.10. Equine viral arteritis	**Dr P.J. Timoney** University of Kentucky, Department of Veterinary Science, 108 Gluck Equine Research Center, Lexington, Kentucky 40546-0099, USA.
2.5.12. Venezuelan equine encephalomyelitis	**Dr J.E. Pearson (retired)** Formerly USDA, APHIS, National Veterinary Services Laboratories, P.O. Box 844, Ames, Iowa 50010, USA.
2.5.13. Epizootic lymphangitis	**Dr J.A.W. Coetzer** Department of Veterinary Tropical Diseases, Faculty of Veterinary Science, University of Pretoria, Private Bag X04, Onderstepoort 0110, South Africa.
2.5.14. Japanese encephalitis	**Dr I. Takashima** Laboratory of Public Health, Department of Environmental Veterinary Sciences, Graduate School of Veterinary Medicine, Hokkaido University, Sapporo 060-0818, Japan.

2.6.1. Atrophic rhinitis of swine	**Dr N. Chanter** Animal Health Trust, Lanwades Park, Kentford, Newmarket, Suffolk CB8 7UU, UK.
	Dr P.W. Jones & Dr S. Barnard Institute for Animal Health, Compton Laboratory, Compton, Nr Newbury, Berkshire RG20 7NN, UK.
	Dr A. Pennings Intervet International, Wim de Körverstraat 35, P.O. Box 31, 5830 AA Boxmeer, The Netherlands.
2.6.2. Porcine brucellosis	**Dr A.P. MacMillan & Dr J. Stack** VLA Weybridge, New Haw, Addlestone, Surrey KT15 3NB, UK.
	Dr R.D. Angus Angus Associates, P.O. Box 156, Bancroft, Idaho, USA.
2.6.3. Enterovirus encephalomyelitis (previously Teschen/Talfan diseases)	**Dr V. Mádr** Hudcova 66, 62100 Brno, Czech Republic.
2.6.4. Transmissible gastroenteritis	**Dr D.J. Paton** VLA Weybridge, New Haw, Addlestone, Surrey KT15 3NB, UK.
	Dr L.J. Saif The Ohio State Universtiy, Ohio Agricultural Research and Development Center, Food Animal Health Research Program, 1680 Madison Avenue, Wooster, Ohio 44691-4096, USA.
	Dr R.L. Levings USDA, APHIS, National Veterinary Services Laboratories, Large Animal Biologics Virology Section, P.O. Box 844, Ames, Iowa 50010, USA.
2.7.1. Infectious bursal disease (Gumboro disease)	**Dr P.J. Wyeth** VLA Weybridge, New Haw, Addlestone, Surrey KT15 3NB, UK.
2.7.2. Marek's disease	**Dr J.M. Sharma** Veterinary PathoBiology, College of Veterinary Medicine, University of Minnesota, St Paul, Minnesota 55108, USA.
*2.7.3. Avian mycoplasmosis (*Mycoplasma gallisepticum*)*	**Dr S.H. Kleven** University of Georgia, College of Veterinary Medicine, Department of Avian Medicine, Athens, Georgia 30602-4875, USA.
	Dr F.T.W. Jordan & Dr J.M. Bradbury University of Liverpool, Department of Veterinary Pathology, Veterinary Field Station, Leahurst, Neston, South Wirral CH64 7TE, UK.
2.7.4. Avian chlamydiosis	**Dr A.A. Andersen** USDA, ARS, National Animal Disease Center, P.O. Box 70, Ames, Iowa 50010, USA.

2.7.5. Fowl typhoid and Pullorum disease	**Dr C. Wray (retired) & Dr R. Davies** VLA Weybridge, New Haw, Addlestone, Surrey KT15 3NB, UK.
2.7.6. Avian infectious bronchitis	**Dr R. Gough & Dr D.J. Alexander** VLA Weybridge, New Haw, Addlestone, Surrey KT15 3NB, UK.
2.7.7. Avian infectious laryngotracheitis	**Dr R.C. Jones** University of Liverpool, Department of Veterinary Pathology, Jordan Building, Veterinary Field Station, 'Leahurst', Neston, South Wirral CH64 7TE, UK.
2.7.8. Avian tuberculosis	**Dr J. Haagsma** Meidoornsingel 144, 3052 BT Rotterdam, The Netherlands.
2.7.9. Duck virus hepatitis *2.7.10. Duck virus enteritis*	**Dr P.R. Woolcock** California Animal Health and Food Safety Laboratory System – Fresno Branch, School of Veterinary Medicine, University of California, Davis, 2789 South Orange Avenue, Fresno, California 93725, USA.
2.7.11. Fowl cholera (avian pasteurellosis)	**Dr R.B. Rimler (deceased)** Formerly, Avian and Swine Respiratory Diseases Research USDA, ARS, Unit, National Animal Disease Center, P.O. Box 70, Ames, Iowa 50010, USA.
	Dr S.B. Houghton Intervet UK Ltd, Walton Manor, Walton, Milton Keynes, Bucks MK7 7AJ, UK.
2.8.1. Myxomatosis	**Dr J. Chantal** École Nationale Vétérinaire, 23 Chemin de Capelles, 31076 Toulouse Cedex 03, France.
2.8.2. Tularemia	**Dr T. Mörner** Department of Wildlife, The National Veterinary Institute, 751 89 Uppsala, Sweden
	Dr G. Sandström Department of Clinical Immunology, Infectious Diseases, Umeå University and National Defence Research Establishment, SE-901 82 Umeå, Sweden.
2.8.3. Rabbit haemorrhagic disease	**Dr A. Lavazza & Dr L. Capucci** Istituto Zooprofilattico Sperimentale della Lombardia e dell'Emilia Romagna, Via Bianchi 7/9, 25124 Brescia, Italy.
2.9.1. Acariosis of bees	**Dr W. Ritter** CVUA-Freiberg, Tierhygiene Fb,: Bienen, Am Moosweiher 2, D79018 Freiberg, Germany.
2.9.2. American foulbrood	**Dr H. Shimanuki (retired) & Dr D.A. Knox** USDA, ARS, Bee Research Laboratory, Bldg 476, BARC-East, Beltsville, Maryland 20705, USA.

2.9.3. European foulbrood	**Dr B. Ball** IACR-Rothamstead, Harpenden, Hertfordshire AL5 2JQ, UK.
2.9.4. Nosemosis of bees	**Dr A. de Ruijter** Research Centre for Insect Pollination and Beekeeping, Ambrosiusweg 1, 5081 NV Hilvarenbeek, The Netherlands.
2.9.5. Varroosis	**Dr W. Ritter** CVUA-Freiberg, Tierhygiene Fb,: Bienen, Am Moosweiher 2, D79018 Freiberg, Germany.
X.1. Leishmaniosis	**Dr L. Gradoni & Dr M. Gramiccia** Istituto Superiore di Sanità, Laboratorio di Parassitologia, Viale Regina Elena 299, I-00161 Rome, Italy.
X.2. Malignant catarrhal fever	**Dr H.W. Reid** Moredun Research Institute, International Research Centre, Pentlands Science Park, Bush Loan, Penicuik EH26 0PZ, Scotland, UK.
X.3. Q fever	**Dr M. Pépin, Dr P. Russo & Dr E. Rousset** AFSSA Sophia Antipolis, Laboratoire d'Études et de Recherches sure les Petits Ruminants et les Abeilles, BP 111, F-06902 Sophia Antipolis Cedex, France.
	Dr M.P. Durand 161 bis rue R. Salengro, 37000 Tours, France.
X.4. Salmonellosis	**Dr C. Wray (retired) & Dr R. Davies** VLA Weybridge, New Haw, Addlestone, Surrey KT15 3NB, UK.
X.5. Bovine viral diarrhoea	**Dr S. Edwards & Dr T. Drew** VLA Weybridge, New Haw, Addlestone, Surrey KT15 3NB, UK.
	Prof. J. Brownlie The Royal Veterinary College, Hawkshead Lane, North Mymms, Hatfield, Hertfordshire AL9 7TA, UK.
X.6. Trypanosomosis (Tsetse-transmitted)	**Dr J. Schlater** USDA, APHIS, National Veterinary Services Laboratories, P.O. Box 844, Ames, Iowa 50010, USA.
	Dr P. Van Den Bossche Regional Tsetse and Trypanosomosis Control Programme, P.O. Box A560, Avondale, Harare, Zimbabwe.
X.7. Ovine pulmonary adenomatosis	**Dr J.M. Sharp** Moredun Research Institute, International Research Centre, Pentlands Science Park, Bush Loan, Penicuik EH26 0PZ, Scotland, UK.
X.8. Nairobi sheep disease	**Dr F.G. Davies** The Whittery, Chirbury, Montgomery, Powys SY15 6DA, UK.

X.9. Scrapie	**Mr G.A.H. Wells** VLA Weybridge, New Haw, Addlestone, Surrey KT15 3NB, UK.
X.10. Border disease	**Dr P.F. Nettleton** Moredun Research Institute, International Research Centre, Pentlands Science Park, Bush Loan, Penicuik EH26 0PZ, Scotland, UK.
*X.11. Surra (*Trypanosoma evansi*)*	**Dr A.G. Luckins** Centre for Tropical Veterinary Medicine, Easter Bush Veterinary Centre, Roslin, Midlothian EH25 9RG, UK.
X.12. Porcine reproductive and respiratory syndrome	**Dr L.R. Ludemann** USDA, APHIS, Center for Veterinary Biologics, Laboratory, P.O. Box 844, Ames, Iowa 50010, USA. **Dr R. Magar** Agence canadienne d'inspection des aliments, Laboratoire d'hygiène vétérinaire et alimentaire, 3400 Casavant ouest, Saint-Hyacinthe, Québec J2S 8E3, Canada.
X.13. Fowl pox	**Dr D.N. Tripathy** University of Illinois at Urbana-Champaign, College of Veterinary Medicine, Department of Veterinary Pathbiology, 2001 South Lincoln Avenue, Urbana, Illinois 61802, USA.
X.14. Mange	**Dr P. Bates** VLA Weybridge, New Haw, Addlestone, Surrey KT15 3NB, UK.
X.15. Tropilaelaps *infestation of honey bees* (Tropilaelaps clareae, T. koenigerum)	**Dr D. Sammataro** Pennsylvania State University, Department of Entomology, 501 Agricultural Sciences and Industries Building, University Park, Pennsylvania 16802, USA. **Dr U. Gerson** Department of Entomology, Faculty of Agricultural, Food and Environmental Sciences, P.O. Box 12, Rehovot 76-100, Israel.

PART I

GENERAL INFORMATION

SECTION I.1

INTRODUCTORY CHAPTERS

CHAPTER I.1.1.

SAMPLING METHODS

INTRODUCTION

The starting point for the laboratory investigation of an animal disease is the taking of a sample. This first introductory chapter considers some of the general principles involved. Each of the disease chapters that follow contains specific information that is appropriate for that particular disease. Samples may be taken from animals, or their environment, for a variety of purposes. These may be for helping to establish a disease diagnosis, for health surveillance, for health certification or for monitoring the response to treatment or vaccination. A great variety of different combinations of samples and species of animal may occur. In all cases, the samples need to be appropriate for the purpose required, and adequate in number and amount to provide a statistically valid result. Samples must be taken with care, to avoid undue stress or damage to the animal or danger to the operator. It is usually important to adopt aseptic techniques, and care must be taken to avoid cross-contamination between samples.

Having obtained suitable material, it must be carefully packaged, labelled, and transmitted to the laboratory by the fastest practicable method, preferably with temperature control. Relevant shipping regulations must be obeyed. If material is sent to a laboratory in another country, this laboratory must be consulted in advance to ensure that it is willing to receive the material. An import licence may be required. All samples must be accompanied by a written note indicating the sender, the origin of the material, the relevant history, and the tests required. Suggestions for further reading are given at the end of the chapter.

A. COLLECTION OF SAMPLES

Before taking samples, careful consideration must be given to the purpose for which they are required. From this will follow the type and number of samples needed to provide valid results. When samples are taken from live animals, care must be taken to avoid injury or distress to the animal or danger to the operator and attendants. It may be necessary to use mechanical restraint or, in some cases, tranquillisation. Whenever handling biological material, from either live or dead animals, the risk of zoonotic disease must be kept in mind, and precautions taken to avoid human infection (see also Chapter I.5. Human safety in the veterinary microbiology laboratory). Post-mortem examinations must be carried out under conditions that are as hygienic as is practicable in the field, taking care to avoid environmental contamination by spillage of body fluids, or risk of spread of disease through dissemination by flies or other possible mechanical vectors. Disposal arrangements must also be satisfactory.

1. Tissues (general)

Samples of tissue from a variety of organs may be taken at post-mortem. In veterinary work it is unusual to take biopsy samples of tissues, but this can be done in certain circumstances, using appropriate surgical techniques.

Animal health personnel should be trained in the correct procedures for post-mortem examination of the species of animals with which they work. The equipment required will depend on the size and species of animal, but a knife, saw and cleaver will be required, and also scalpel, forceps and scissors, including scissors with a rounded tip on one blade, for opening intestines. A plentiful supply of containers appropriate to the nature of the sample required must be available, and also labels, and report forms. Special media may be required for transport of samples from the field. The operator should wear protective clothing: overalls, washable apron, rubber gloves and rubber boots. Additionally, if potential zoonotic diseases are being investigated, an efficient face mask and eye protection should be worn. If rabies or transmissible spongiform encephalopathies (TSEs) are suspected, it is usual to detach the animal's head.

Tissues may be collected for microbiological culture, parasitology, biochemistry, histopathology and/or immunohistochemistry and now also for detection of proteins or genome nucleic acids. The person removing the tissues should be experienced in post-mortem techniques and have a knowledge of anatomy and pathology sufficient to select the right organs and the most promising lesions for sampling. The skin of the dead animal may be removed with nonsterile instruments, but the body cavities should preferably be opened with sterile instruments, and a fresh set of sterile instruments should be used to collect pieces of the various organs required. Each piece of tissue should be placed in a separate sterile screw-capped jar or plastic bag, fully labelled with the date, tissue and animal identification. Care must be taken not to contaminate one tissue with another. Instruments can be sterilised in the field in a simple boiler, for 20 minutes, which can be heated on a burner with portable packs of liquid gas or by using local fuel to light a fire. Boiling water will not inactivate all pathogens; spore forms are resistant to heat. If it is not practicable to have several sets of sterile instruments, an alternative is to dip instruments in 100% ethanol, during the post-mortem examination, then burn of the alcohol by igniting in a flame. Disinfectants must not be used on or near tissues to be sampled for bacterial culture or virus isolation.

The fresh samples should be forwarded to the laboratory by the fastest direct route. If they can reach the laboratory within 24 hours tissues in containers should be forwarded in a wide-mouthed vacuum flask with wet ice. An alternative is to use polystyrene containers and chemical refrigeration bricks. Only if the samples are likely to take more than 24 hours to reach the laboratory is it necessary to cool the samples and send them on ice. Freezing at −20°C may be detrimental to virus isolation. The tissues may be sent to the laboratory dry or in bacterial or virus transport medium, depending on the examinations required. Formulations for making up different transport media are given in ref. 1. For histopathology, blocks of tissue not more than 0.5 cm thick and 1–2 cm^2 are cut and placed in neutral buffered 4–10% formalin, which should be at least ten times the volume of the tissue sample. Samples for histology should not be frozen. For certain suspected diseases, e.g. rabies, larger portions of brain are required; the brain is sectioned using a saggital cut, half is submitted fresh, on ice, and the other half in 10% buffered formalin. For scrapie, bovine spongiform encephalopathy and other TSEs, whole brains in formalin may be required. Store and pack formalin-fixed tissues separately from fresh tissues, blood and smears. Once fixed, tissues can be removed from formalin and, as long as they are kept moist and protected (e.g. by wrapping in formalin-soaked paper towels, then sealed in screw-capped jars), they can be forwarded to the laboratory without formalin.

2. Blood

Blood samples may be taken for haematology or for culture and/or direct examination for bacteria, viruses, or protozoa, in which case it is usual to use anticoagulants, such as heparin. They may also be taken for serology, in which case a clotted sample is required. Blood plasma is also used for some procedures. A blood sample is taken, as cleanly as possible, by venepuncture. In most large mammals, the jugular vein or a caudal vein are selected, but brachial veins and mammary veins are also used. In birds, a wing vein (brachial vein) is usually selected. Blood may be taken by syringe and needle, or by needle and vacuum tube (not easy in delicate veins but convenient in strong veins). Small quantities of blood are conveniently obtained by pricking with a triangular, solid-pointed needle. Ideally the skin at the site of venepuncture should first be shaved (plucked) and swabbed with 70% ethyl alcohol and allowed to dry.

Whole blood samples can have antibiotics added to reduce bacterial growth, taking care that the antibiotics are chosen so as to avoid interference with the growth of the pathogens concerned. For samples with anticoagulant and/or antibiotics, thorough mixing is necessary as soon as the sample has been taken. It may also be necessary to make a smear of fresh blood on a microscope slide; both thick and thin smears may be prepared. For serum samples, the blood should be left to stand at ambient temperature (but protected from excessive heat) for 1–2 hours until the clot begins to contract. The clot can then be ringed round with a sterile rod and the bottles placed in a refrigerator at 4°C. After several hours, or overnight, the serum can be decanted or removed with a pipette. This can be followed by centrifugation at about 1000 ***g*** for 10–15 minutes and removal of the clear serum to a fresh tube. Chemical preservatives, such as boric acid or thiomersal (Merthiolate), should be avoided in sera to be used in virus neutralisation tests. An alternative method is to transport a drop of dried blood on a filter paper disk that contains enough material for sensitive antibody assay systems.

3. Faeces

Freshly voided faeces of suitable quantity (about 5–10 g) should be selected, and sent with or without a transport medium. Faeces for parasitology should fill the container or be topped up with sterile water to reduce air and prevent hatching of parasite eggs. An alternative and sometimes preferable method is to take swabs from the rectum (or cloaca), taking care to swab the mucosal surface. The swabs should be visibly coated with faecal material, but even then may not be sufficient for parasitology. Care must be exercised when taking swabs from small, delicate animals or birds to avoid injuring them. Swabs may be transported either dry or in transport medium. Faeces are best stored and transported at 4°C.

4. Skin

In diseases producing vesicular rashes or where lesions are exclusively in the skin, samples are taken from the lesions themselves. Scrapings of the lesion may be taken; 2 g of affected epithelial tissue is taken as aseptically as possible and placed in 5 ml phosphate buffered glycerin virus transport medium at pH 7.6. Additionally, the vesicular fluid should be sampled where unruptured vesicles are present; if possible, vesicular fluid should be aspirated with a syringe and placed in a separate sterile tube. Plucked hair or wool samples may be useful and, in birds, feather follicle skin can be taken for culture for Marek's disease.

5. Genital tract and semen

Samples may be taken by vaginal or preputial washing, or by the use of suitable swabs. Sometimes the cervix or urethra are also sampled by swabbing. Samples of semen are best obtained using an artificial vagina or by artificial stimulation. The sperm-rich fraction should be present in the sample and contamination by antiseptic washing solutions must be avoided.

6. Eye

A swab of the surface of the conjunctiva may be taken gently, holding the palpebra apart. The swab is then broken off into transport medium. Scrapings may also be taken on to a microscope slide. The handles of metal-handled swabs are useful for this, to ensure that sufficient cells are removed for microscopic examination.

7. Nasal discharge (saliva, tears)

Samples may be taken with dacron, cotton or gauze swabs, preferably on wire handles as wood is inflexible and may snap. It may be helpful if they are first wetted with transport medium. They should be allowed to remain in contact with the secretions for up to 1 minute, then placed in transport medium and sent to the laboratory without delay at 4°C.

8. Milk

Samples of milk should be taken after cleansing and drying the tip of the teat, but antiseptics should be avoided at this time. The initial stream of milk should be discarded and a tube filled with the next stream(s). In severe mastitis, there may be little fluid present. A sample of bulk tank milk is used for some purposes. Milk for serological tests should not have been frozen, heated or subjected to violent shaking.

9. Environment and feed

Samples may be taken to monitor hygiene or as part of a disease enquiry. Environmental samples are commonly taken from litter or bedding and voided faeces or urine. Swabs may be taken from the surface of ventilation ducts (which are usually dusty), feed troughs and drains. This kind of sampling is particularly important in hatcheries, artificial insemination centres and slaughter houses in which specialised equipment is maintained. Samples may also be taken from animal feed, in troughs or bulk containers. Water may be sampled in troughs, drinkers, header tanks or from the natural or artificial supply.

10. Honey bees

Adult bees, either dead or moribund, may be collected in the vicinity of the colonies. Live bees should be killed by freezing. Brood samples are taken by removing a piece of brood comb that shows abnormalities. This should be wrapped in paper and placed in a box for transport to the laboratory.

B. SELECTION OF SAMPLES

Considerable skill and care are required to decide on the correct samples to be sent to the laboratory. It is helpful to follow the principle of sample collection based on species of animal. Frequently a combination of blood samples for serology and tissues from dead or culled animals for microbiological culture will be required. Also, it is usually important to collect tissues for fixation for histology. These matters are considered in detail in the chapters dealing with each disease and will not be discussed further here. For more information on sample selection, a recently published book will be found very useful (4). This also gives a lot of information about media and solutions used for transport and in laboratory tests. It describes a number of laboratory methods and gives definitions of terms used in cell culture.

C. SAMPLE SIZE

There are some general statistical rules that should be borne in mind, particularly when sampling herds or flocks for a health surveillance scheme. It is possible to calculate how many animals must be sampled from a herd/flock of a certain size, to achieve a 95% probability of detecting infection assumed to be present in a certain percentage of the animals. For example, if disease were present in 5% of a herd of 500 animals, it would be necessary to sample 56 animals to be 95% confident of finding one positive, assuming that both the sensitivity and specificity of the test were 100% (1) (see also Chapter I.3. Principles of validation of diagnostic assays for infectious diseases).

D. INFORMATION TO BE SENT WITH SAMPLES

It is essential that samples be clearly identified using appropriate methods. Marking instruments must be able to withstand the condition of use, i.e. being wet or frozen. Pencil has a tendency to rub off containers and labels attached to plastic will fall off when packs are stored at –70°C. Information and case history should always accompany the samples to the laboratory, and preferably should be placed in a plastic envelope. The information should include the following points:

1. Name and address of owner/occupier where disease occurred, with telephone and fax numbers and date of dispatch,
2. Disease(s) suspected,
3. Samples submitted, tests required (transport medium used) and date of sampling,
4. Different species on the farm and number, age and sex of each affected animal, identification numbers,
5. Length of time on the farm; if recent arrival, where from,
6. Date of first cases and of subsequent cases or losses, with any appropriate previous submission reference numbers,
7. Description of the spread of infection in the herd or flock,
8. Number of animals dead, the number showing clinical signs, and their age, sex and breed,
9. The clinical signs and their duration including the condition of mouth, eyes and feet, and milk or egg production data,
10. Type and standard of husbandry, including the type of feed available, possible contact with poison or poisonous plants,
11. A list and description of the samples examined post-mortem with date of examination and the observed findings,
12. Any medication already applied to the animals, and when given,
13. Any vaccination already given, and when given,
14. Name and address of the sender, with telephone and fax number, and date of submission.

E. TRANSPORT OF SAMPLES

Samples (referred to as Diagnostic Specimens in official regulations) must be carefully packed, to avoid any possibility of leakage or cross-contamination. They should be delivered within 48 hours and should usually be kept cool during transit. Some samples should not be frozen. Screw-capped bottles should be used and should be additionally sealed with adhesive tape or paraffin wax. Samples in individually identified containers should be placed in larger strong outer containers and packed with enough absorbent material to protect from damage. Official shipping regulations must be consulted (2). For air transport, parcels should be placed in the pressurised hold of the aircraft and comply with UN 602 packaging requirements. It is advisable to contact the laboratory in advance in the case of unusual requests. It is essential to do so where material is sent to a laboratory in another country. Many countries require a special import licence to be obtained in advance for any biological material, especially for tissues that could contain animal pathogens. This should accompany the package and be attached in an envelope to the outside of the parcel.

F. PRESERVATION OF SAMPLES FOR PROLONGED STORAGE

Sometimes it is desirable to maintain a collection of samples for a long period of time. This may be because it is useful to maintain a culture collection of isolates obtained locally. It may also be useful to maintain a collection of fixed tissues, or paraffin blocks, for future histological examination. Possibly the most useful collection is the storage of serum samples. All these stored samples may be found useful in the future, when a retrospective investigation is carried out to compare the present disease status with that of earlier times.

• Serum banks

Serum samples can give a lot of information about the animals from which the sera were taken. There are many different tests that can be done on sera, to assay a variety of constituents, such as immunoglobulins, trace elements, toxins, hormones and enzymes. When a sufficient number of serum samples have been collected at random from a population, valid comparisons can be made of sex, age, breed and geographical location. High risk groups can be identified, vaccination priorities established, and patterns and rates of disease determined (3).

A serum bank is a catalogued collection of sera that are stored so as to preserve their immunological and other biochemical properties. Both the catalogue and the storage conditions are essential for a successful serum bank. Each individual serum must be fully documented and identified. The database must contain all relevant information about the origin of the sample and test results obtained. Additional data that may be of interest, such as weather conditions and the animals productivity may also be included. Accurate records are essential. This begins in the field, when the blood samples are taken. The first essential is the identification of the animal. The amount of detail recorded must be appropriate to the abilities of the operator, accuracy being more important than quantity of information. Although pooling of sera reduces documentation and storage space, it is to be avoided if possible, because it greatly reduces the usefulness of the material. Care should be taken over asepsis, as far as possible, when taking the blood, and sterility should be maintained during separation of the serum and subsequent manipulations. The serum bank catalogue must be very well organised, and is likely to be maintained on a computer database. A suggested methodology has been described in detail (3).

Sera may be stored for issue as required over a period of time, or may be kept in long-term storage for historical purposes. These two types of function should be separated. Storage conditions should minimise loss of immunological and other biochemical properties of the sera. There are three methods: deep freezing, dry storage on paper disks at ambient temperature and lyophilisation (freeze-drying). For long-term storage of sera by deep freezing, a core temperature below –60°C should be maintained. The lower the temperature the better, but lower temperatures are more expensive to maintain. Liquid phase N_2 is at –196°C, vapour phase N_2 is at –100°C and an ultra-deep freezer will maintain –90°C. Deep-freeze machines must be carefully monitored for temperature in case of mechanical break down or power failure. A stand-by generator is essential together with alternative cold storage space in case the contents of a machine have to be transferred. Paper disk storage is a simple and inexpensive method, but it allows only a small quantity of serum to be stored. The disks must be kept in a cool, dry atmosphere. They can probably provide satisfactory results for up to about 5 years, but the particular test system to be used should be validated first. Lyophilisation is generally regarded as the best method for long-term storage of sera. It minimises loss of serum characteristics when freeze-drying conditions are optimised, but it requires expensive equipment and is a time-consuming process. Lyophilised vials should be stored at 4°C.

REFERENCES

1. AUSTRALIAN BUREAU OF ANIMAL HEALTH (1982). Livestock Disease Surveys: A Field Manual for Veterinarians. Australian Government Publishing Service.

2. INTERNATIONAL AIR TRANSPORT ASSOCIATION (1995). Dangerous Goods Regulations, 36th Edition. International Air Transport Association, 2000 Peel Building, Montreal, Quebec H3A 2R4, Canada.

3. MOORHOUSE P.D. & HUGH-JONES M.E. (1981). Serum banks. *Vet. Bull.*, 51, 277–290.

4. WORLD HEALTH ORGANIZATION/FOOD AND AGRICULTURE ORGANIZATION OF THE UNITED NATIONS (WHO/FAO) (1994). Basic Procedures for Diagnostic Veterinary Laboratories in Developing Countries, Pini A., Parodi P., Demeneghi D., Belemu U., Kabilika H. & Ghirotti M., eds. WHO/FAO Collaborating Centre, Viale Regina Elena 299, 00161 Rome, Italy, 142 pp.

*
* *

CHAPTER I.1.2.

QUALITY MANAGEMENT IN VETERINARY DIAGNOSTIC LABORATORIES

SUMMARY

In any testing work, the final expression of quality is a reliable result. This is the product of thought, planning, care, knowledge, skill, experience, and environment. Good laboratory practice, quality control, and quality assurance are inter-related and comprise one complex subject of increasing importance in the conduct of biological assays. In recent years this subject, including process control of laboratory work, has been increasingly implemented at the international level. The advent of widely recognised international standards, such as the International Standard ISO/IEC 17025 (1), and the increased application in laboratories of total quality management and the ISO/IEC 9000 series (2), have made it imperative that laboratories have a formal, visible, and appropriate quality system.

KEY ELEMENTS OF QUALITY IN TESTING

The activities and elements necessary to achieve quality in testing may be described in the following six categories.

1. The laboratory environment

Before developing any test or conducting a test, a laboratory must ensure it has appropriate facilities and resources. These are outlined in the two categories that follow.

a) Laboratory building and grounds

The laboratory must have:

i) Adequate funding for operation;

ii) Safety and security;

iii) Adequate space;

iv) Adequate lighting;

v) Appropriate and dependable environmental control, e.g. adequate and/or appropriately controlled ventilation, vibration levels, dust, sound, temperature, humidity, electromagnetic interference, and electrical power supply;

vi) Necessary and properly housed and maintained equipment, instruments, and materials, including both internal and applicable external equipment. Equipment must be traceable, calibrated, adequate for the job, capable of achieving the accuracy required, and otherwise fit for the intended purpose;

vii) Good housekeeping;

viii) Appropriate storage and archiving;

ix) Access to necessary literature references.

b) Personnel

There must be a sufficient number of staff to do the work. Staff must have the right combination of education, experience, and training to do the work to the required standard, and, where necessary, must have the appropriate scientific and technical credentials. All staff must have training specific to the activities required and the testing to be done, and this training must be verified as effective with dates and signatures. An up to date *curriculum vitae* must be maintained for each member of staff. Supervisory and managerial staff must also have appropriate credentials, experience, and training. In addition, for laboratory results to be of consistently high quality, the following are needed:

i) Defined and appropriate organisational structure and responsibilities;

ii) Encouragement of staff to be responsible, to take initiatives, and to ask questions;

iii) Visible involvement and commitment to quality by everyone, including management. Management must provide the resources necessary to implement the identified quality standards;

iv) Management must ensure that staff are free from influences that could adversely affect test results, and enforce compliance with the requirements of the quality standards and procedures of the laboratory;

v) Organised commitment to ongoing training for all staff, both to maintain expertise and to learn new processes.

2. The test design

No amount of quality control, supervision, or resources will compensate for a bad test design. The critical activities that are needed for a good test design must establish a clear understanding of what laboratory personnel and the client can expect from the test. These activities are addressed in the three categories that follow.

a) Selection of the test method

Quality may be defined as fitness for the intended use (3). The selection of an appropriate test method must be based on this and on the factors listed below.

- **Key elements in selection of the test method**

i) International acceptance;

ii) Scientific acceptance;

iii) Method not outdated;

iv) Performance characteristics, such as sensitivity, specificity, the isolation rate (if culture), and precision (repeatability, reproducibility and accuracy);

v) Behaviour in species and populations of interest;

vi) Money and time available for development or adaptation;

vii) Performance time/turnaround time;

viii) Type of sample (serum, tissue, etc.) and its quality;

ix) Analyte (antibody, antigen, etc.);

x) Resources and technology of the laboratory;

xi) Nature of the intended use (export, import, domestic control, field screening, confirmatory, etc.);

xii) User expectations;

xiii) Safety;

xiv) Number of tests to be done;

xv) Cost of test, per sample;

xvi) Existence of reference standards, including certified reference materials.

b) Optimisation of the test method

Once the method has been selected, it must be set up at the laboratory. Optimisation is a series of experiments and subsequent data analysis, and establishes critical specifications and performance standards for the test process and for use in monitoring the correct performance of the test. Optimisation should ensure that a method is brought under statistical control, and that it is performing optimally. Optimisation should also determine:

i) Critical specifications for equipment and instruments;

ii) Critical specifications for reagents (chemicals, biologicals);

iii) Ruggedness, critical control points and acceptable ranges, attributes or behaviour at critical control points, using statistically acceptable procedures;

iv) The quality control activities necessary to monitor these critical control points;

v) The type, number, range, frequency, and/or arrangement of controls needed;

vi) The requirements for control behaviour for nonsubjective acceptance or rejection of test results;

vii) The elements of a fixed procedure or a protocol for use by laboratory staff;

viii) The level of technical competence required for the staff that carry out the test.

c) Validation of the test method

Validation further evaluates the test for its fitness for a given use. Validation establishes performance characteristics for the method, such as sensitivity, specificity, and isolation rate, and for diagnostic parameters, such as positive/negative cut-off, and titre of interest or significance. Depending on logistical and risk factors, validation may involve any number of activities and amount of data, with subsequent data analysis using appropriate statistics. Validation activities might include:

i) Field and/or epidemiological studies;

ii) Comparison with other methods, preferably reference methods or methods approved by international bodies;

iii) Comparison with reference standards (if available);

iv) Collaborative studies with other laboratories using the same method or procedure, including the exchange of samples, preferably of undisclosed composition or titre. It is preferabe that these be issued by a qualified conducting laboratory that organises the study and evaluates the results provided by the participants;

v) Reproduction of data from an accepted standard method, or from a reputable publication;

vi) Experimental challenge studies.

3. Test control

No matter how well designed, a test must be well controlled to produce reliable results. The activities and materials needed to ensure and demonstrate control are as follows.

a) Techniques

Techniques should be correct and appropriate (for pipetting, weighing, use of instruments, etc.). Where indicated, these should be formally controlled and documented.

b) Test protocols

Protocols must be written, complete, current, on site, available, understood, and followed. They should include:

i) Relevant references, including the source of the method;

ii) A full description of the test method, using a high level of descriptive detail;

iii) An orderly and logical format;

iv) Scope (e.g. South American cattle);

v) Description of the type of item to be tested (e.g. bovine serum);

vi) Parameters or quantities of the analyte to be determined (e.g. presence or level of antibody);

vii) Objective criteria for acceptance or rejection of samples;

viii) Test-specific criteria for collection, identification, registration, handling, transporting, preparation, storage, and retention of samples and where relevant, procedures for animal slaughter and necropsy, and sample collection from carcasses;

ix) Critical specifications for equipment, instruments, software, and materials, including the quality control necessary and the criteria for acceptance or rejection of such materials as media or reagents used in the test;

x) Special environmental and safety conditions required;

xi) Reference materials or standards needed;

xii) Checks to be made before work is started, including verification that instruments and equipment (including computers and software if necessary for the test), are working properly and are calibrated or adjusted;

xiii) Critical control points and the criteria for acceptable performance or the acceptable range at each point, including the checks necessary and the action to be taken if criteria are not met;

xiv) A description of the controls used and the allowed limits on each;

xv) Criteria for acceptance or rejection of the test results (e.g. control results);

xvi) The data to be recorded and the method of recording, analysis and presentation;

xvii) A description of calculations and statistics, if used;

xviii) The method of diagnostic interpretation (e.g. titres of >1/4 are recorded as positive);

xix) Procedures for measuring the uncertainty of the result, if applicable.

c) Further activities

Other control items include procedures and activities that ensure:

i) Proper operation, verification, and calibration of instruments and equipment. Calibrations and verifications must be done by competent, qualified individuals, using suitable equipment and methods, at intervals that are appropriate for the uncertainty to be tolerated, and as equipment behaviour indicates. Computers and software (if required) must be fully validated and verified before use and on a continuing basis;

ii) Timely purchase, reception, storage, and availability of consumable materials of the proper specifications. The laboratory should have a system of procurement and inventory;

iii) Appropriate contingency and emergency plans of action, such as backup reagents and equipment, including emergency power;

iv) The verification of analyst capability to perform the test successfully, such as the use of blind proficiency panels or samples at planned, appropriate intervals;

v) Accurate sample tracking and reporting of results: There must be a continuous and traceable system of sample identification. There must be procedures for ensuring the confidentiality, security, integrity, and retrievability of test results, including access, entry, processing, transmission, storage, and amendment. A computerised and validated sample tracking system is recommended. ISO/IEC International Standard 17025 gives the requirements for information that must be on test reports;

vi) Adequate supervision, with sufficient skill, knowledge and experience to provide assistance and guidance, and with the capability to demonstrate hands-on techniques;

vii) Adequate checks on calculations and transpositions of data and results, and that interpretation and correlation of test results are done by authorised and qualified personnel;

vii) The use of devices, such as control charts for spotting present and potential problems and trends;

ix) The traceability of critical variables, including traceability of calibrations, to a national standard of measurement. Calibration records must contain sufficient information to ensure that this traceability is documented;

x) Security, integrity and retrievability of records and all data for a specified period of time, e.g. 7 years after completion of the test;

xi) The timeliness of reporting test results;

xii) That for each test run, the following information should be recorded:

Original observations directly concerning the test result (e.g. for an enzyme-linked immunosorbent assay, the absorbance),

Calculations and derived data,

Control results,

Critical parameters (e.g. pH, temperature),

Initials of the analyst,

Date,

Time (if applicable),

Identification of equipment (where applicable),

Reagent lot numbers (where applicable).

4. A formal quality management system

Each laboratory must have a quality management system appropriate to its scope of activities. Some laboratories, particularly those seeking accreditation from an outside body or a third party that is preferably recognised as a competent registrar or an accreditor at the national or international level, choose specific standards for the quality system. However, any laboratory quality system should include the following:

- **Requirements**

i) A quality policy, which must be endorsed by the chief executive of the laboratory and which should include:

A statement of the laboratory's intentions and commitment with respect to the level of service it will provide, including any quality standard used;

The purpose of the quality system;

The requirement that all staff be familiar with and implement all policies and procedures of the quality system and of the laboratory.

ii) A quality manager with documented authority and access to the highest level of management in the laboratory;

iii) A qualified person in charge of technical issues;

iv) A quality manual, which should contain:

The quality policy;

The scope of the quality system;

An overview of the laboratory organisation;

The roles and responsibilities of technical and quality personnel;

An outline of the structure of the quality system, including documentation.

The quality manual should contain or make reference to supporting operational and technical policies and procedures. The following areas should be addressed by policy and supporting procedures, that describe and/or ensure:

- Regular review and improvement of the quality system, including managerial and technical procedures;
- Conditions for acceptance of new testing work by the laboratory;
- Acquisition of test methods, including how methods are selected, verified as suitable for use, transferred into and approved for use by the laboratory. This should involve the clients of the laboratory;
- Document control, including the identification, approval, distribution, revision, archiving and disposal of documents;
- Data control, including traceability, collection (including experimental design), manipulation (including calculations and transpositions), handling, transmission, processing (including statistical methods), modification, storage, archiving, and approval for use;
- Records control, including assurance of legibility, completeness, security (including confidential and proprietary aspects), integrity, traceability and retrievability, and covering the creation, modification, retention, archiving and disposal of all records, including all data (in electronic or any other format),

documents, original observations relating to test results, and test results produced by the laboratory. All data affecting test results must be traceable to a particular test result;

- Control of supplied materials (reagents, animals, media, glassware, etc.), to ensure there are no adverse effects on test results. This may involve testing materials to ensure that they are fit for the purpose for which they will be used and that test results are not adversely affected by batch differences;
- Environmental safety, including disposal of waste, and emissions;
- An equipment monitoring, verification, calibration, and preventive maintenance programme, which includes how instruments and equipment are identified, commissioned, maintained, and serviced;
- A training programme that ensures that personnel can do their work safely and proficiently, including planning for ongoing training and the participation of each analyst in a planned continuing proficiency sample programme;
- A planned programme of interlaboratory sample exchanges to assess the performance of the tests and of the laboratory, including all aspects of the preparation and characterisation of such samples, if applicable;
- The proper care, use, and handling of reference materials and equipment;
- The traceability of laboratory measurements to national standards of measurement;
- An audit programme;
- Client complaint and problem resolution;
- Dealing with poor quality samples;
- Dealing with incorrect or questionable test results, including data entry errors;
- Corrective and preventive action;
- Authorisation of exclusions from policy and procedure;
- Sample management, including subsampling, population sampling schemes, obtaining test material, shipment, handling, storage, packaging, preservation, retention and disposal;
- Sample identification and traceability;
- Reporting and amending results including the limitations of their interpretation and use;
- Correlation and interpretation of results, including correlation of different test results for the same analyte, different analytes on the same sample, inconclusive test results, and complex correlations (e.g. testing of samples for multiple exotic diseases by multiple methods);
- If work is subcontracted, that the subcontractor complies with equal standards of quality so that there is no detrimental effect on test results.

5. Comparison of standards and future planning

Continuous improvement is essential. Comparison of standards used by different laboratories is a necessary activity towards improvement. This may be accomplished by:

i) Participation in conferences and in local and international organisations (Office International des Epizooties, Food and Agriculture Organization of the United Nations, Association of Official Analytical Chemists International, International Association of Veterinary Laboratory Diagnosticians, International Symposium of Veterinary Epidemiology and Economics, etc.);

ii) Participation in writing national and international standards (e.g. participation on ISO committees);

iii) Consulting publications and exchanging the latest information about developing technology by electronic means (e.g. on-line databases, file transfer by e-mail, and Internet discussion groups);

iv) Visits to other laboratories;

v) Cooperative programmes (e.g. Inter-American Institute for Cooperation in Agriculture, etc.);

vi) Exchange of procedures, protocols, methods, reagents, samples, personnel, and ideas;

vii) Wherever possible, accreditation or registration to a recognised quality standard by a third party that is itself certified or recognised as competent to perform the accreditation or registration.

6. Published standards

Several standards are available for, and can apply to, laboratories and quality assurance programmes. Such standards are best exemplified by the ISO Guides and Standards (1, 2). These are numerous, and include documents that address such aspects of laboratory quality assurance as quality systems, laboratory accreditation, competence of testing and calibration laboratories, and proficiency sample programmes. Formal and visible quality systems, good laboratory practices, and correct and appropriate quality control and quality assurance activities are necessary for any laboratory and for trade certification. Official schemes are available in many countries for monitoring good laboratory practice, for assessing the competence of laboratories, and for accrediting laboratories to a standard. Information on such schemes may be obtained from the national standards body of each country, or from the international Laboratory Accrediation Cooperation (ILAC).

REFERENCES

1. INTERNATIONAL STANDARD ISO/IEC 17025 (1999). General requirements for the competence of testing and calibration laboratories. International Organization for Standardization (ISO)/International Electrochemical Commission (IEC), Case postale 56, CH-1211, Geneva 20, Switzerland.

2. INTERNATIONAL ORGANIZATION FOR STANDARDIZATION (1998). ISO 9000 Compendium: ISO 9000 International Standards for Quality Management, Seventh Edition., *op. cit.*

3. JURAN J.M. & BLANTON GODFREY A. (1999). Juran's Quality Control Handbook, Fifth Edition. McGraw Hill, New York, USA.

*

* *

CHAPTER 1.1.3.

PRINCIPLES OF VALIDATION OF DIAGNOSTIC ASSAYS FOR INFECTIOUS DISEASES

INTRODUCTION

Validation is the evaluation of a process to determine its fitness for a particular use. A validated assay yields test results that identify the presence of a particular analyte (e.g. an antibody) and allows predictions to be made about the status of the test subject. However, for infectious disease diagnostic assays, the identity and definition of the criteria required for assay validation are elusive, and the process leading to a validated assay is not standardised.

By considering the variables that affect an assay's performance, the criteria that must be addressed in assay validation become clearer. The variables can be grouped into three categories: (a) the sample – host/organism interactions affecting the analyte composition and concentration in the serum sample; (b) the assay system – physical, chemical, biological and technician-related factors affecting the capacity of the assay to detect a specific analyte in the sample; and (c) the test result – the capacity of a test result, derived from the assay system, to predict accurately the status of the host relative to the analyte in question.

Factors that affect the concentration and composition of analyte in the serum sample are mainly attributable to the host and are either inherent (e.g. age, sex, breed, nutritional status, pregnancy, immunological responsiveness) or acquired (e.g. passively acquired antibody, active immunity elicited by vaccination or infection). Nonhost factors, such as contamination or deterioration of the sample, may also affect the analyte in the sample.

Factors that interfere with the analytical accuracy of the assay system include instrumentation, technician error, reagent choice (both chemical and biological) and calibration, accuracy and acceptance limits of controls, reaction vessels, water quality, pH and ionicity of buffers and diluents, incubation temperatures and durations, and error introduced by detection of closely related analytes, such as antibody to cross-reactive organisms, rheumatoid factor, or heterophile antibody.

Factors that influence the capacity of the test result to predict accurately the infection or analyte status of the host[1] are diagnostic sensitivity (D-SN), diagnostic specificity (D-SP), and prevalence of the disease in the population targeted by the assay. D-SN and D-SP are derived from test results on samples obtained from selected reference animals. The methods used to select the reference animals are critical to the accuracy of the estimates (4). The degree to which the reference animals represent all of the host and environmental variables in the population targeted by the assay has a major impact on the accuracy of test-result interpretation. For example, experienced diagnosticians are aware that an assay, validated by using samples from northern European cattle, may not give valid results for the distinctive populations of cattle in Africa.

The capacity of a positive or negative test result to predict accurately the infection status of the animal is the most important consideration of assay validation. This capacity is not only dependent on a highly precise and accurate assay and carefully derived estimates of D-SN and D-SP, but is heavily influenced by prevalence of the infection in the targeted population or the likelihood that an animal is infected based on clinical criteria. Without a current estimate of the disease prevalence in

---

1 *In this chapter, the terms 'positive' and 'negative' have been reserved for test results and never refer to infection or antibody/antigen status of the host. Whenever reference is made to 'infection' or 'analyte', any method of exposure to an infectious agent that could be detected directly (e.g. antigen) or indirectly (e.g. antibody) by an assay, should be inferred.*

that population or likelihood of infection in an individual animal, the interpretation of a positive or negative test result may be compromised.

Many variables obviously must be addressed before an assay can be considered to be 'validated' (4, 10). However, there is no consensus whether the concept of assay validation is a time-limited process during which only those factors intrinsic to the assay are optimised and standardised, or whether the concept includes an ongoing validation of assay performance for as long as the assay is used. Accordingly, the term 'validated assay' elicits various interpretations among laboratory diagnosticians and veterinary clinicians. Therefore, a working definition of assay validation is offered as a context for the guidelines outlined below. Ideally, all diagnostic assays would be fully validated, but in practice there are sometimes limitations to the completeness of validation.

A. DEFINITION OF ASSAY VALIDATION

A validated assay consistently provides test results that identify animals as positive or negative for an analyte or process (e.g. antibody, antigen, or induration at skin test site) and, by inference, accurately predicts the infection status of animals with a predetermined degree of statistical certainty. This chapter will focus on the principles underlying development and maintenance of a validated assay. Guidelines for the initial stages in assay development are included because they constitute part of the validation process. How this early process is carried out heavily influences the capacity of the eventual test result to provide diagnostic accuracy.

It must be emphasised that an assay, when applied to target populations, will minimise misclassifications of animals as false positive or false negative only to the extent that validity is assured for all stages of the assay validation process. This assumes that a well designed and documented test method and proper reagents, in combination with well trained technicians, will give a stable assay within the laboratory. It also assumes a thorough use of the most rigorous experimental design and epidemiological and statistical tools. These are required to reduce bias, random error, and false assumptions about the reference population of animals upon which the assay performance estimates are made (4).

The working definition of assay validation used in this paper generalises a process that takes on many different forms depending on the intended use of the assay being developed. No matter what the form of the assay, without scientific rigour in the validation process, the assay will not perform to expectations. However, there are many traditional techniques in widespread use that have not been subjected to the full validation process.

B. STAGES OF ASSAY VALIDATION

Development and validation of an assay is an incremental process consisting of at least five stages: 1) Determination of the feasibility of the method for a particular use; 2) Choice, optimisation, and standardisation of reagents, techniques and methods; 3) Determination of the assay's performance characteristics; 4) Continuous monitoring of assay performance; and 5) Maintenance and enhancement of validation criteria during routine use of the assay (Figure 1). Although some scientists may question the relevance of the fourth and fifth stages as validation criteria, they are included here because an assay can be considered to be valid only to the extent that test results are valid, i.e. whether they fall within statistically defined limits and provide accurate inferences. In practice, there are many traditional techniques in widespread use that have not been through the formal validation process given above. In such cases the process may appropriately be entered at stages 4 and 5, thus building up a data set of validation data for assays that lack the necessary information for stages 1–3.

An indirect enzyme-linked immunosorbent assay (ELISA) test for detection of antibody will be used in this chapter to illustrate the principles of assay validation. It is a test format that can be difficult to validate because of signal amplification of both specific and nonspecific components (2). This methodology serves to highlight the problems that need to be addressed in any assay validation process. The same basic principles are used in validation of other complex or simple assay formats.

Because of space limitations, this introductory chapter provides only basic guidelines for the principles concerned with assay validation. It is derived from a more detailed treatment of the subject (7).

STAGE 1. FEASIBILITY STUDIES

In the ELISA example, feasibility studies are the first stage in validating a new assay. They are carried out in order to determine if the selected reagents and protocol have the capacity to distinguish between a range of antibody concentrations to an infectious agent while providing minimal background activity. Feasibility studies also give initial estimates of repeatability, and of analytical sensitivity and specificity.

1. Control samples

It is useful to select four or five samples (serum in our example) that range from high to low levels of antibodies against the infectious agent in question. In addition, a sample containing no antibody is required. These samples will be used to optimise the assay reagents and protocol during feasibility studies, and later as control samples. The samples ideally should represent known infected and uninfected animals from the population that eventually will become the target of the validated assay. The samples should have given expected results in one or more serological assay(s) other than the one being validated. The samples are preferably derived from individual animals, but they may represent pools of samples from several animals. A good practice is to prepare a large volume (e.g. 10 ml) of each sample and divide it into 0.1 ml aliquots for storage at or below –20°C. One aliquot of each sample is thawed, used for experiments, and ideally then discarded. If it is impractical to discard the aliquot, it may be held at 4°C between experiments for up to approximately 2 weeks; however, there is a possibility of sample deterioration under these circumstances. Then, another is thawed for further experimentation. This method provides the same source of serum with the same number of freeze–thaw cycles for all experiments (repeated freezing and thawing of serum can denature antibodies so should be avoided). Also, variation is reduced when the experimenter uses the same source of serum for all experiments rather than switching among various sera between experiments. This approach has the added advantage of generating a data trail for the repeatedly run samples. After the initial stages of assay validation are completed, one or more of the samples can become the serum control(s) that are the basis for data expression and repeatability assessments both within and between runs of the assay. They may also serve as standards if their activity has been predetermined; such standards provide assurance that runs of the assay are producing accurate data (10).

It is highly desirable to include international standard sera if they are available. This may lead to harmonisation between the assay under development and a standard test method in which international standard sera are normally used (9).

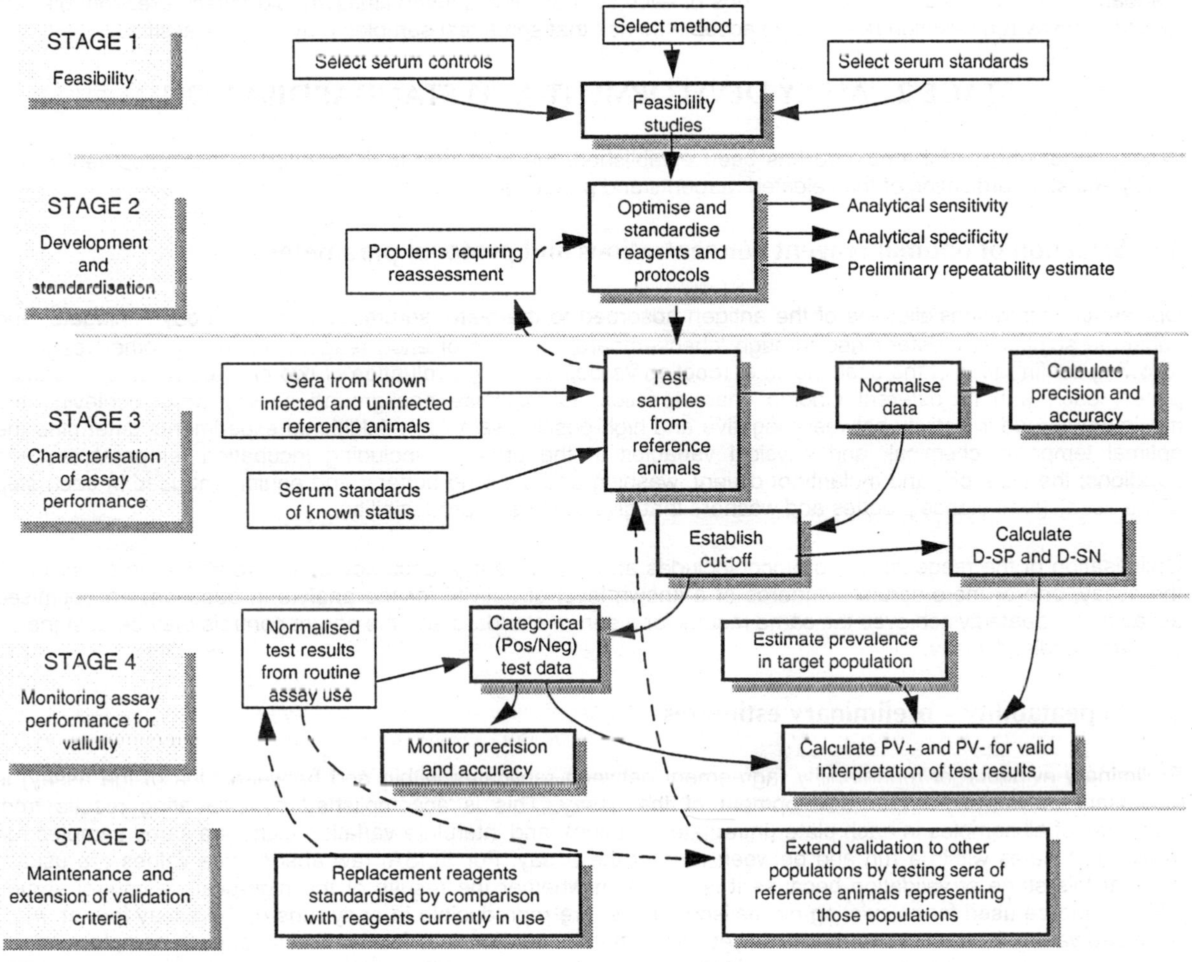

Fig. 1. Stages in the incremental process of assay validation.

2. Selection of method to achieve normalised results

Normalisation adjusts raw test results of all samples relative to values of controls included in each run of the assay (not to be confused with transformation of data to achieve a 'normal' [Gausian] distribution). The method of normalisation and expression of data should be determined, preferably no later than at the end of the feasibility studies. Comparisons of results from day to day and between laboratories are most accurate when normalised data are used. For example, in ELISA systems, raw optical density (absorbance) values are absolute measurements that are influenced by ambient temperatures, test parameters, and photometric instrumentation. To account for this variability, results are expressed as a function of the reactivity of one or more serum control samples that are included in each run of the assay. Data normalisation is accomplished in the indirect ELISA by expressing absorbance values in one of several ways (10). A simple and useful method is to express all absorbance values as a percentage of a single high-positive serum control that is included on each plate. This method is adequate for most applications. More rigour can be brought to the normalisation procedure by calculating results from a standard curve generated by several serum controls. It requires a more sophisticated algorithm, such as linear regression or log-logit analysis. This approach is more precise because it does not rely on only one high-positive control sample for data normalisation, but rather uses several serum controls, adjusted to expected values, to plot a standard curve from which the sample value is extrapolated. This method also allows for exclusion of a control value that may fall outside expected confidence limits.

For assays that are end-pointed by sample titration, such as serum (viral) neutralisation, each run of the assay is accepted or rejected based on whether control values fall within predetermined limits. Because sample values usually are not adjusted to a control value, the data are not normalised by the strict definition of the term.

Whatever method is used for normalisation of the data, it is essential to include additional controls for any reagent that may introduce variability and thus undermine attempts to achieve a validated assay. The normalised values for those controls need to fall within predetermined limits (e.g. within an appropriate multiple of the standard deviation of the mean of many runs of each control). The chosen limits should reflect a reasonable and tolerable assay run rejection rate and an acceptable risk that some test samples may be misclassified.

STAGE 2. ASSAY DEVELOPMENT AND STANDARDISATION

When the feasibility of the method has been established, the next step is to proceed with development of the assay and standardisation of the selected reagents and protocols.

1. Selection of optimal reagent concentrations and protocol parameters

Optimal concentrations/dilutions of the antigen adsorbed to the plate, serum, enzyme–antibody conjugate, and substrate solution are determined through 'checkerboard' titrations of each reagent against all other reagents, following confirmation of the best choice of reaction vessels (usually evaluation of two or three types of microtitre plates, each with its different binding characteristics, to minimise background activity while achieving the maximum spread in activity between negative and high-positive samples). Additional experiments determine the optimal temporal, chemical, and physical variables in the protocol, including incubation temperatures and durations; the type, pH, and molarity of diluent, washing and blocking buffers; and equipment used in each step of the assay (for instance pipettes and washers that give the best reproducibility).

Optimisation of the reagents and protocol includes an assessment of accuracy by incorporating, in each run of the assay, one or more serum standards of a known level of activity for the analyte in question. An optimised assay that repeatedly achieves the same results for a serum standard and the serum controls may be designated as a standardised assay.

2. Repeatability – preliminary estimates

Preliminary evidence of repeatability (agreement between replicates within and between runs of the assay) is necessary to warrant further development of the assay. This is accomplished by evaluating results from replicates of all samples in each plate (intraplate variation), and interplate variation using the same samples run in different plates within a run and between runs of the assay. For ELISA, raw absorbance values are usually used at this stage of validation because it is uncertain whether the results of the high-positive control serum, which could be used for calculating normalised values, are reproducible in early runs of the assay format. Also, expected values for the controls have not yet been established. Three-to-four replicates of each sample run in at least five plates on five separate occasions are sufficient to provide preliminary estimates of repeatability. Coefficients of variation (standard deviation of replicates/mean of replicates), generally less than 20% for raw absorbance values, indicates adequate repeatability at this stage of assay development. However, if evidence of excessive variation (>30%) is apparent for most samples within and/or between runs of the assay, more preliminary studies should be done to determine whether stabilisation of the assay is possible, or whether the test format should be abandoned. This is important because an assay that is inherently variable has a high probability of not withstanding the rigours of day-to-day testing on samples from the targeted population of animals.

3. Determination of analytical sensitivity and specificity

The analytical sensitivity of the assay is the smallest detectable amount of the analyte in question, and analytical specificity is the degree to which the assay does not cross-react with other analytes. These parameters are distinguished from diagnostic sensitivity and specificity as defined below. Analytical sensitivity can be assessed by end-point dilution analysis, which indicates the dilution of serum in which antibody is no longer detectable. Analytical specificity is assessed by use of a panel of sera derived from animals that have experienced related infections that may stimulate cross-reactive antibodies. If, for instance, the assay does not detect antibody in limiting dilutions of serum with the same efficiency as other assays, or cross-reactivity is common when sera from animals with closely related infections are tested, the reagents need to be recalibrated or replaced, or the assay should be abandoned. However, there is a place for a test with low specificity, providing the sensitivity is high, for use as a 'screening test' in situations where a large number of samples have to be screened and where there is a 'confirmatory test' that has high specificity.

STAGE 3. DETERMINING ASSAY PERFORMANCE CHARACTERISTICS

If the feasibility and initial development and standardisation studies indicate that the assay has potential for field application, the next step is to identify the assay's performance characteristics.

1. Diagnostic sensitivity and specificity

a) Principles and definitions

Estimates of diagnostic sensitivity (D-SN) and diagnostic specificity (D-SP) are the primary parameters obtained during validation of an assay. They are the basis for calculation of other parameters from which inferences are made about test results. Therefore, it is imperative that estimates of D-SN and D-SP be as accurate as possible. Ideally, they are derived from testing a series of samples from reference animals of known history and infection status relative to the disease/infection in question. Diagnostic sensitivity is the proportion of known infected reference animals that test positive in the assay; infected animals that test negative are considered to have false-negative results. Diagnostic specificity is the proportion of uninfected reference animals that test negative in the assay; uninfected reference animals that test positive are considered to have false-positive results. The number and source of reference samples used to derive D-SN and D-SP are of paramount importance if the assay is ever to be properly validated for use in the general population of animals targeted by the assay.

It is possible to calculate the number of reference samples, from animals of known infection/exposure status, required for determinations of D-SN and D-SP that will have statistically defined limits. Formulae for these calculations, their limitations, and a discussion of the selection criteria for standard sera are detailed elsewhere (4, 7). Because of the many variables that must be accounted for, it is desirable to include at least 300 reference samples from known-infected animals, and about 1000 samples from known-uninfected animals should be included to determine initial estimates of D-SN and D-SP, respectively. Such a large number of reference animals may be difficult to achieve. Starting with fewer animals followed by updating of D-SN and D-SP estimates as more reference animals become available may be the only practical way to get initial estimates of D-SN and D-SP (See Stage 5 below).

b) Standards of comparison for the new assay

In serology, the 'standard of comparison' is the results of a method or combination of methods with which the new assay is compared. Although the term 'gold standard' is commonly used to describe any standard of comparison, it should be limited to methods that unequivocally classify animals as infected or uninfected. Some isolation methods themselves have problems of repeatability and sensitivity. Gold standard methods include unequivocal isolation of the agent or pathognomonic histopathological criteria. Because a true gold standard is impossible to achieve, relative standards of comparison are often necessary; these include results from other serological assays and from experimentally infected or vaccinated animals. Calculations of D-SN and D-SP are most reliable when the gold standard of comparison is available. When only relative standards of comparison are available, estimates of D-SN and D-SP for the new assay may be compromised because the error in the estimates of D-SN and D-SP for the relative standard is carried over into those estimates for the new assay.

c) Precision, repeatability, reproducibility, and accuracy

Repeatability and reproducibility are estimates of precision in the assay. Precision is a measure of dispersion of results for a repeatedly tested sample; a precise assay has only a small amount of dispersion. Repeatability in a diagnostic assay has two elements: the amount of agreement between replicates (usually two or three) of each sample within a run of the assay, and the amount of between-run agreement for the normalised values of each control sample. Reproducibility is the amount of agreement between results of the same samples tested in different laboratories. Accuracy is the amount of agreement between a test value and the expected value for an analyte in a standard sample of known activity (e.g. titre or concentration). An assay system may be precise, but not accurate, if the test results do not agree with the expected value for the standard.

Reliable estimates of repeatability and accuracy, both within and between runs of the assay, can be obtained by use of normalised results from the many runs of the new assay that were required to assess the sera of reference animals (less reliable estimates were obtained from preliminary data using raw absorbance values). At least 10, and preferably 20 runs of the assay will give reasonable initial estimates of these parameters. Methods for evaluating these parameters have been described in detail (7).

Accuracy can be assessed by inclusion of one or more standards (samples of known titre, concentration, etc.) in each run of the assay. The standards may be control sera provided that the amount of analyte (e.g. titre, concentration) in each one has been previously determined by comparison with primary or secondary reference standards (10), and the control sera are not used in the data normalisation process.

Reproducibility of the assay is determined in several laboratories using the identical assay (protocol, reagents, and controls) on a group of at least 10 samples, preferably duplicated to a total of 20 samples. These samples need to represent the full range of expected analyte concentrations in samples from the target population. The extent to which the collective results for each sample deviate from expected values is a measure of assay reproducibility. The degree of concordance of between-laboratory data is one more basis for determining whether the assay's performance characteristics are adequate to constitute a validated assay.

2. Selection of the cut-off (positive/negative threshold)

To achieve estimates of D-SN and D-SP of the new assay, the test results first must be reduced to positive or negative categories. This is accomplished by insertion of a cut-off point (threshold or decision limit) on the continuous scale of test results. Although many methods have been described for this purpose, three examples will illustrate different approaches, together with their advantages and disadvantages. The first is a cut-off based on the frequency distributions (7) of test results from uninfected and infected reference animals. This cut-off can be established by visual inspection of the frequency distributions, by receiver-operator characteristics (ROC) analysis (5, 11), or by selection that favours either D-SN or D-SP, whichever is required for a given assay (8). A second approach is establishing a cut-off based only on uninfected reference animals; this provides an estimate of D-SP but not D-SN. The third method provides an 'intrinsic cut-off' based on test results from sera drawn randomly from within the target population with no prior knowledge of the animals' infection status (3). Although no estimates of D-SN and D-SP are obtained by this method, they can be determined as confirmatory data are accumulated.

If considerable overlap occurs in the distributions of test values from known infected and uninfected animals, it is difficult to select a cut-off that will accurately classify these animals according to their infection status. Rather than a single cut-off, two cut-offs can be selected that define a high D-SN (e.g. inclusion of 99% of the values from infected animals), and a high D-SP (e.g. 99% of the values from uninfected animals). The values that fall between these percentiles would then be classified as suspicious or equivocal, and would require testing by a confirmatory assay or retesting for detection of seroconversion.

3. Calculation of diagnostic sensitivity and specificity

The selection of a cut-off allows classification of test results into positive or negative categories. Calculation of D-SN and D-SP are aided by associating the positive/negative categorical data with the known infection status for each animal using a two-way (2 × 2) table (Table 1). After the cut-off is established, results of tests on standard sera can be classified as true positive (TP) or true negative (TN) if they are in agreement with those of the gold standard (or other standard of comparison). Alternatively, they are classified as false positive (FP) or false negative (FN) if they disagree with the standard. Diagnostic sensitivity is calculated as TP/(TP + FN) whereas diagnostic specificity is TN/(TN + FP); the results of both calculations are usually expressed as percentages (Table 1).

Table 1. *Calculations of D-SN and D-SP aided by a 2 x 2 table that associates infection status with test results from 2000 reference animals*

		Reference animals of known infection status	
		Infected (*n* = 600)	**Uninfected (*n* = 1400)**
Test result	**Positive**	570 (TP)	46 (FP)
	Negative	30 (FN)	1354 (TN)
		Diagnostic sensitivity	**Diagnostic specificity**
		$\frac{TP}{TP+FN} = \frac{570}{600} = 95.0\%$	$\frac{TN}{TN+FP} = \frac{1354}{1400} = 96.7\%$

4. Harmonisation of assays

When an international standard method (9) is available for detection of an analyte, it is possible to compare the performance of that method with the one under development. This process requires use of the same serum controls and/or standards in both assays. If international standard sera are available (preferably at least three: negative, weak positive and strong positive), they should be included in the assay-comparison study. This could lead to a new assay that is indexed to an international standard method and international standard sera (9). Harmonisation of the two assays may then be realised.

STAGE 4. MONITORING VALIDITY OF ASSAY PERFORMANCE

1. Interpretation of test results – factors affecting assay validity

An assay's test results are useful only if the inferences made from them are accurate. A common error is to assume that an assay with 99% D-SN and 99% D-SP will generate one false-positive and one false-negative result for approximately every 100 tests on animals from the target population. Such an assay may be precise and accurate, but produce test results that do not accurately predict infection status. For example, if the prevalence of disease in a population targeted by the assay is only 1 per 1000 animals, and the false-positive test rate is 1 per 100 animals (99% D-SP), for every 1000 tests on that population, ten will be false positive and one will be true positive. Hence, only approximately 9% of positive test results will accurately predict the infection status of the animal; the positive test results will misclassify the animal 91% of the time. This illustrates that the capacity of a positive or negative test result to predict infection status is dependent on the prevalence of the infection in the target population (6). Of course, the prevalence will probably have been determined by use of a serological test.

An estimate of prevalence in the target population is necessary for calculation of the predictive values of positive (PV+) or negative (PV–) test results. When test values are reported without providing estimates of the assay's D-SP and D-SN, it is not possible to make informed predictions of infection status from test results (6). It is, therefore, highly desirable to provide an interpretation statement with test results accompanied by a small table indicating PV+ and PV– for a range of expected prevalences of infection in the target population. Without provision of such information, test results from the assay may have failed to classify accurately the infection status of animals, and thus do not reflect a fully validated assay.

STAGE 5. MAINTENANCE AND ENHANCEMENT OF VALIDATION CRITERIA

A validated assay needs constant monitoring and maintenance to retain that designation. Once the assay is put into routine use, internal quality control is accomplished by consistently monitoring the assay for assessment of repeatability and accuracy (1).

Reproducibility between laboratories should be assessed at least twice each year. It is useful to volunteer membership in a consortium of laboratories that are interested in evaluating their output. In the near future, good laboratory practice, including implementation of a total quality assurance programme, will become essential for laboratories seeking to meet national and international certification requirements (see Chapter I.2.).

Proficiency testing is a form of external quality control for an assay. It is usually administered by a reference laboratory that distributes panels of samples, receives the results from the laboratories, analyses the data, and reports the results back to the laboratories. If results from an assay at a given laboratory remain within acceptable limits and show evidence of accuracy and reproducibility, the laboratory may be certified by government agencies or reference laboratories as an official laboratory for that assay. Panels of sera for proficiency testing should contain a full representation of an analyte's concentration in animals of the target population. If the panels only have high-positive and low-positive sera (with none near the assay's cut-off), the exercise will only give evidence of reproducibility at the extremes of analyte concentration, and will not clarify whether routine test results on the target population properly classify infection status of animals.

Because of the extraordinary set of variables that impact on the performance of serodiagnostic assays, it is highly desirability to expand the number of standard sera from animals of known infection status because of the principle that error in the estimates of D-SN and D-SP is reduced with increasing sample size. Furthermore, when the assay is to be transferred to a completely different geographical region, it is essential to re-validate the assay by subjecting it to sera from populations of animals that reside under local conditions.

When a serum control sample is nearing depletion, it is essential to prepare and repeatedly test a replacement before the serum control is depleted. The prospective control sample should be included in 10–20 runs of the assay before depletion of the original control to establish its proportional relationship to the nearly depleted control. If the depleted sample was a positive control in ELISAs where the normalised value is expressed as a per cent of that positive control, the proportional difference in ELISA activity between the original and replacement sera must be factored into the normalisation algorithm to retain the same cut-off, and thus the same D-SN and D-SP in the assay. When other reagents, such as antigen for capture of antibody, must be replaced, they should be produced using the same criteria as for the original reagents, and tested in at least five runs of the assay using a panel of sera that has been designed for this purpose. Whenever possible, it is important to change only one reagent at a time to avoid the compound problem of evaluating more than one variable at a time.

C. VALIDATION OF ASSAYS OTHER THAN ENZYME-LINKED IMMUNOSORBENT ASSAY

Although the example used has been an indirect ELISA test, the same principles apply to the validation of any diagnostic assay. It is of utmost importance not to stop after the first two stages of assay validation – that does not constitute a validated assay for diagnostic use. Although reagent and protocol refinement are important, the selection of the reference populations is probably the most critical factor. It is no surprise when reviewing the literature to find a wide range of estimates for D-SN and D-SP for the same basic assay. Although part of the variation may be attributed to the reagents chosen, it is likely that the variation in estimates of D-SN and D-SP is due to biased selection of sera on which the test was 'validated'. This stage in assay validation needs more attention than it has been given previously. This is particularly true in the current atmosphere of international trade agreements and all their implications with regard to the movement of animals and animal products.

REFERENCES

1. CEMBROWSKI G.S. & SULLIVAN A.M. (1992). Quality control and statistics. *In:* An Introduction to Clinical Chemistry, Bishop M.L., Duben-Engelkirk J.L. & Fody E.P., eds. Lippincott, Philadelphia, USA, 63–101.

2. CROWTHER J.R. (1995). ELISA theory and practice. *In:* Methods in Molecular Biology. Humana Press, Totowa, NJ, USA, 1–256.

3. GREINER M., FRANAKE C.R., BOHNING D. & SCHLATTMANN P. (1994). Construction of an intrinsic cut-off value for the sero-epidemiological study of *Trypanosoma evansi* infections in a canine population in Brazil: a new approach towards unbiased estimation of prevalence. *Acta Trop.*, **56**, 97–109.

4. GREINER M. & GARDNER I. (2000). Epidemiologic issues in the validation of veterinary diagnostic tests. *Vet. Prev. Med.*, **45**, 3–22.

5. GREINER M., PFEIFFER D. & SMITH R.D. (2000). Principles and practical application of the receiver operating characteristic (ROC) analysis for diagnostic tests. *Vet. Prev. Med.*, **45**, 23–41.

6. JACOBSON R.H. (1991). How well do serodiagnostic tests predict the infection of disease status of cats. *J. Am. Vet. Med. Assoc.*, **199**, 1343–1347.

7. JACOBSON R.H. (1998). Validation of serological assays for diagnosis of infectious diseases. *Rev. sci. tech. Off. int. Epiz.*, **17**, 469–486.

8. SMITH R.D. (1991). Clinical Veterinary Epidemiology. Butterworth-Heinemann, Stoneham, MA, USA, 1–223.

9. WRIGHT P.F. (1998). International standards for test methods and reference sera for diagnostic tests for antibody detection. *Rev. sci. tech. Off. int. Epiz.*, **17**, 527–533.

10. WRIGHT P.F., NILSSON E., VAN ROOIJ E.M.A., LELENTA M. & JEGGO M.H. (1993). Standardization and validation of enzyme-linked immunosorbent assay techniques for the detection of antibody in infectious disease diagnosis. *Rev. sci. tech. Off. int. Epiz.*, **12**, 435–450.

11. ZWEIG M.H. & CAMPBELL G. (1993). Receiver-operating characteristic (ROC) plots: a fundamental evaluation tool in clinical medicine. *Clin. Chem.*, **39**, 561–577.

*

* *

CHAPTER 1.1.4.

TESTS FOR STERILITY AND FREEDOM FROM CONTAMINATION OF BIOLOGICAL MATERIALS

INTRODUCTION

Sterility is defined as the absence of living organisms. It is achieved by heating, by filtration, by treatment with ethylene oxide or by ionising irradiation, and by conducting any subsequent processes aseptically. Freedom from contamination is defined as the absence of specified living organisms. This may be achieved by selecting materials from sources shown to be free from the specified organisms and by conducting subsequent procedures aseptically. Adequate assurance of sterility and freedom from contamination can only be achieved by proper control of the primary materials used and their subsequent processing and storage. Tests on the product are necessary to check that this control has been achieved.

A. GENERAL PROCEDURES

1. Primary materials must be collected from sources shown to be free from contamination and handled in such a way as to minimise contamination and the opportunities for any contaminants to multiply.

2. Materials that can be sterilised without their biological activities being affected unduly must be sterilised by a method effective for the materials concerned. The method must reduce the level of contamination to be undetectable, as determined by an appropriate sterility test (see paragraph B.3. below).

3. If a sterilisation process is used, it shall be validated to demonstrate its suitability and adequately controlled to show that it has functioned properly on each occasion.

4. Materials that are not sterilised and those that are to be processed further after sterilisation must be handled aseptically.

5. The environment in which any aseptic handling is carried out must be maintained in a clean state and protected from external sources of contamination, and must be controlled so as to reduce internal contamination to a minimum.

B. LIVING VIRAL VACCINES FOR ADMINISTRATION BY INJECTION

1 Materials of animal origin shall be (a) sterilised, or (b) obtained from healthy animals that, in so far as is possible, should be shown to be free from pathogens that can be transmitted from the species of origin to the species to be vaccinated, or any species in contact with them, or (c) the material shall be shown to be free from such pathogens.

2. Seed lots of virus and of any continuous line cell used for virus growth shall be shown to be free from bacteria, fungi, mycoplasmas, extraneous viruses and other pathogens that can be transmitted from the species of origin to the species to be vaccinated or any species in contact with them.

3. Each batch of vaccine shall pass a test for sterility that is similar to published methods (1–3, 5).

4. Each batch of vaccine shall pass tests appropriate to prove that the vaccine is free from extraneous viruses. (Such tests include tests in cell cultures susceptible to viruses of the species to be vaccinated, tests in embryonated eggs, and, where necessary, tests in animals.)

5. Some countries require that each batch of vaccine pass a test for freedom from mycoplasmas. Suitable test methods have been published (1–3, 5).

6. Tests for freedom from certain specific bacteria may be required, e.g. for *Salmonella pullorum*, *Mycobacterium tuberculosis* and *M. paratuberculosis*, *Brucella* spp. and *Leptospira* spp.

C. LIVING VIRAL VACCINES FOR ADMINISTRATION THROUGH DRINKING WATER, SPRAY, OR SKIN SCARIFICATION

1. Paragraphs B.1., 2., 4., 5., and 6. apply.

2. A limited number of contaminating, nonpathogenic bacteria and fungi may be permitted (see Section J.2.5. below).

D. INACTIVATED VIRAL VACCINES

1. Paragraphs B.2. and 3. apply.

2. Each batch of vaccine shall pass a test for inactivation of the vaccinal virus. This is done before addition of preservative. The inactivation process and the tests used to detect live virus after inactivation must be validated and shown to be suitable for their intended purpose.

3. Demonstration that the method of inactivation also inactivates representative pathogens may be required unless the vaccine satisfies the conditions of paragraphs B.1. and B.4.

E. LIVING BACTERIAL VACCINES

1. Paragraph B.1. applies.

2. Seed lots of bacteria shall be shown to be free from other bacteria as well as fungi and mycoplasmas.

3. Each batch of vaccine shall pass a test for purity carried out using solid media and ignoring the growth of the vaccinal bacterium.

4. Some countries require that each batch of vaccine passes a test for freedom from mycoplasmas. Suitable test methods have been published (ref. 5, and for avian mycoplasmas ref. 2).

F. INACTIVATED BACTERIAL VACCINES

1. Paragraphs B.1., B.3., and E.2. apply.

2. Each batch of vaccine shall pass a test for inactivation of the vaccinal bacterium. If appropriate, the test for sterility may be used for this purpose.

G. SERA FOR ADMINISTRATION TO ANIMALS

1. Paragraph B.1. applies.

2. Paragraph B.2. or E.2. applies, as appropriate, if a virus or a bacterium is used in serum production.

3. Each batch of serum shall pass a test for sterility that conforms to that found in ref. 5. Suitable test methods have been published (1–3).

4. Each batch of serum shall pass tests appropriate to prove that the serum is free from extraneous viruses. (Such tests include tests in cell cultures susceptible to viruses of the species to be treated, tests in embryonated eggs and, where necessary, tests in animals.)

5. Some countries require that each batch of serum passes a test for freedom from mycoplasmas. Suitable test methods have been published (ref. 5, and for avian mycoplasmas ref. 2).

H. DIAGNOSTIC AGENTS FOR ADMINISTRATION TO ANIMALS

1. Paragraphs B.1. and 3. apply.

2. Paragraphs B.2. and D.2. apply if a virus is used in the production of the diagnostic agent; E.2. and F.2. apply if a bacterium is used.

I. EMBRYOS, OVA, AND SEMEN

Special precautions must be taken with relation to the use of embryos, ova and semen (4).

J. PROTOCOL EXAMPLES

1. General procedures

Materials used in the production of biological products should be sterilised and/or tested to ensure the absence of contaminants before being used. Samples of the finished biological product should also be tested for bacterial, fungal, or mycoplasmal contaminants.

The assays for bacteria, mycoplasma, fungi, and viruses described here are derived from various sources and they are given as examples of methods that can be used with confidence.

2. Detection of bacteria and fungi

These assays describe the materials and methods that are used for the detection of bacteria and fungi by either the membrane filtration method, or the direct inoculation of fluid media method used for materials that are unsuitable for membrane filtration.

2.1. General procedure for detecting viable bacteria and fungi

Standard tests for detecting extraneous bacteria and fungi in raw materials, seed stocks, or final product are: the membrane filtration test or the direct inoculation sterility test.

For the membrane filtration technique, a filter having a nominal pore size not greater than 0.45 µm and a diameter of at least 47 mm should be used. Cellulose nitrate filters should be used if the material is aqueous or oily; cellulose acetate filters should be used if the material is strongly alcoholic, oily or oil-adjuvanted. Immediately before the contents of the container or containers to be tested are filtered, the filter is moistened with 20–25 ml of Diluent A or B.

Diluent A – for aqueous products or materials: Dissolve 1 g peptic digest of animal tissue in water to make 1 litre, filter or centrifuge to clarify, adjust the pH to 7.1±0.2, dispense into containers in 100 ml quantities, and sterilise by steam.

Diluent B – for oil-adjuvanted products or materials: Add 1 ml polysorbate 80 to 1 litre Diluent A, adjust the pH to 7.1±0.2, dispense into containers in 100 ml quantities, and sterilise by steam.

If the biological being tested has antimicrobial properties, the membrane is washed three times after sample application with approximately 100 ml of the appropriate diluent (A or B). The membrane is then transferred whole to culture media, aseptically cut into equal parts and placed in media, or the media is transferred to the membrane in the filter apparatus. If the test sample contains merthiolate as a preservative, fluid thioglycollate medium (FTM) is used and the membranes are incubated at both 30–35°C and 20–25°C. If the test sample is a killed biological without merthiolate preservative, FTM is used at 30–35°C and soybean casein digest medium (SCDM) at 20–25°C. If the sample tested is a live viral biological, SCDM is used at both incubation temperatures.

If direct inoculation of culture media is chosen, a sterile pipette or syringe and needle are used to aseptically transfer the biological material directly into liquid media. If the biological being tested has antimicrobial properties, the ratio of the inoculum to the volume of culture medium must be determined before the test is started. To determine the correct medium volume to negate antimicrobial activity, 100 colony-forming units (CFU) of the control microorganisms listed in Table 1 are used. If the test sample contains merthiolate as a preservative, FTM is used in test vessels incubated at both 30–35°C and 20–25°C. Growth should be clearly visible after an appropriate incubation time (see Section J.2.2.). If the test sample is a killed biological without merthiolate, or a live bacterial biological, FTM is used at 30–35°C and SCDM at 20–25°C. If the test sample is a live viral biological, SCDM is used at both incubation temperatures. If the inactivated bacterial vaccine is a clostridial biological, or contains a clostridial component, the use of FTM with 0.5% added beef extract (FTMB) in place of FTM is preferred.

Table 1. *Some American type culture collection*[1] *strains with their respective medium and incubation conditions*

		Incubation	
Medium	Test microorganism	Temperature (°C)	Conditions
FTM	*Bacillus subtilis* ATCC # 6633	30–35	Aerobic
FTM	*Candida krusei* ATCC # 6258	20–25	Aerobic
SCDM	*Bacillus subtilis* ATCC # 6633	30–35	Aerobic
SCDM	*Candida kursei* ATCC # 6258	20–25	Aerobic
FTMB	*Clostridium sporogenes* ATCC # 11437	30–35	Anaerobic

For both membrane filtration and direct inoculation sterility tests, all media are incubated for no fewer than 14 days. At intervals during incubation, and after 14 days' incubation, the test vessels are examined for evidence of microbial growth. Microbial growth should be confirmed by subculture and Gram stain.

2.2. Growth promotion and test interference

The sterility of the media should be confirmed by incubating representative containers at the appropriate temperature for the length of time specified for each test.

The ability of the culture media to support growth in the presence and absence of product, product components, cells, seeds, or other test material should be determined each time a test is performed.

To test for ability to support growth in the absence of the test material, media should be inoculated with 10–100 viable control organisms of the suggested American Type Culture Collection (ATCC) strains listed in Table 1 and incubated according to the conditions specified.

To test for ability of the culture media to support growth in the presence of the test material, containers should be inoculated simultaneously with both the test material (see Section J.2.3.) and 10–100 viable control organisms. The number of containers used should be at least one-half the number used to test the product or product component. The test media are satisfactory if clear evidence of growth of the control organisms appears in all inoculated media containers within 7 days. In the event that growth is evident, the organism should be identified to confirm that it is the organism originally added to the medium. The sterility test is considered invalid if any of the media show inadequate growth response, or if the organism recovered is not the organism used to inoculate the material.

2.3. Number of items to be tested

The number of items in a batch determines the number of containers that should be tested for sterility. If the batch size is not more than 100, then 10% or four containers, whichever is the greater, should be tested. If the batch contains between 100 and 500 containers, then ten containers should be tested. If the batch has more than 500 containers, then 2% or 20 containers, whichever is the lesser, should be tested. The amount of sterility test inoculum is dependent on the quantity of biological in each container. If the quantity is less than 1 ml, then the entire contents are divided among each medium. If the quantity is from 1 to 4 ml, then half the contents are used in each medium. If the quantity is from 4 to 20 ml, then 2 ml inoculum per medium is used. If the quantity in each container is from 20 to 100 ml, then 10% of the contents are used per medium. If the quantity per container is greater than 100 ml, then 10% or 50 ml, whichever is the greater, is used to inoculate each medium.

1 American Type Culture Collection, 10801 University Boulevard, Manassas, Virginia 20110-2209, USA.

2.4. Interpretation of sterility test results

If growth is found in any medium but it can be demonstrated by controls that the media or technique were faulty, then the first test is declared invalid and may be repeated. If microbial growth is found in any of the test vessels of the first test but there is no evidence invalidating it, then a retest may be conducted. The minimum number of biological containers, test vessels, and membrane filters in a retest is double the number used in the first test. If no growth is found in the first test or retest, the biological meets the requirements of the test and is considered satisfactory for sterility. If microbial growth is found in any of the retest vessels, the biological is considered unsatisfactory for sterility. If, however, it can be demonstrated by controls that the media or technique of the retest were faulty, then the retest may be repeated.

2.5. General procedure for testing live viral vaccines produced in eggs and administered through drinking water, spray, or skin scarification for the presence of bacteria and fungi

Each batch of final container biological should have an average contamination of not more than one bacterial or fungal colony per dose for vaccines recommended for poultry, or ten colonies per dose for other animals (see Section J.2.3. above to determine the number of samples to test). From each container sample, each of two Petri dishes are inoculated with vaccine equal to ten doses if the vaccine is recommended for poultry, or one dose if recommended for other animals. To each plate add 20 ml of brain–heart infusion agar containing 0.007 IU (International Units) of penicillinase per ml. One plate should be incubated at 30–35°C for 7 days and the other at 20–25°C for 14 days. Colony counts are made at the end of each incubation period. An average colony count of all the plates representing a batch should be made for each incubation condition. If the average count at either incubation condition exceeds one colony per dose for vaccines recommended for poultry, or ten colonies per dose for vaccines recommended for other animals in the initial test, one retest to rule out faulty technique may be conducted using double the number of unopened final containers. If the average count at either incubation condition of the final test for a batch exceeds one colony per dose for vaccines recommended for poultry, or ten colonies per dose for vaccines recommended for other animals, the batch of vaccine should be considered unsatisfactory.

2.6. General procedure for testing seed lots of bacteria and live bacterial biologicals for purity

Each seed lot of bacteria or batch of live bacterial biological should be tested for purity by inoculation of SCDM, which is incubated at 20–25°C for 14 days, and FTM, which is incubated at 30–35°C for 14 days (see Section J.2.3. above to determine the number of samples to be tested and the amount of test inoculum to be used). A sterile pipette or syringe and needle is used to aseptically transfer the quantity of biological directly into the two types of culture medium. The minimum ratio of inoculum to culture medium is 1/15.

If the inoculum or growth of the bacterial vaccine renders the medium turbid so that the absence of atypical microbial growth cannot be determined by visual examination, subcultures should be made from all turbid tubes on day 3 through to day 11. Subculturing is done by transferring 0.1–1.0 ml to differential broths and agar and incubating for the balance of the 14-day period. Microscopic examination by Gram stain should also be done.

If no atypical growth is found in any of the test vessels when compared with a positive control included in the test, the lot of biological may be considered satisfactory for purity. If atypical growth is found but it can be demonstrated by control that the media or technique were faulty, then the first test may be repeated. If atypical growth is found but there is no evidence invalidating the test, then a retest may be conducted. Twice the number of biological containers and test vessels of the first test are used in the retest. If no atypical growth is found in the retest, the biological is considered to be satisfactory for purity. If atypical growth is found in any of the retest vessels, the biological is considered to be unsatisfactory for purity. If, however, it can be demonstrated by controls that the media or technique of the retest were faulty, then the retest may be repeated.

3. Detection of *Mycoplasma* contamination

3.1. General procedure for detecting *Mycoplasma* contamination

Each batch of live viral vaccine, each lot of master seed virus (MSV), each lot of primary and master cell stock (MCS), and all ingredients of animal origin not steam sterilised should be tested for the absence of mycoplasmas. Solid and liquid media, such as Frey's mycoplasma media, that will support the growth of small numbers of test organisms, including *Acholeplasma laidlawii* (ATCC # 23206), *Mycoplasma arginini* (ATCC # 23838), *M. hyorhinis* (ATCC # 17981), and *M. orale* (ATCC # 23714), should be used. For avian biologicals, the test organism *M. synoviae* (ATCC # 25204) should also be used. Ideally, some recent low passage isolates of mycoplasma, identified by comparison with reference strains, should be included in the tests of media. The nutritive properties of the solid medium should be such that no fewer than 100 CFU should occur with each test organism when approximately 200 CFUs are inoculated per plate. An appropriate colour change should occur in the liquid media when approximately 20 CFUs of each test organism are inoculated.

One sample of each lot of vaccine, MSV, etc., should be tested. Inoculate each of four plates of solid medium with 0.25 ml of the sample being tested, and inoculate 100 ml of the liquid medium with 10 ml of the sample. Incubate two plates at 35–37°C aerobically (an atmosphere of air containing 5–10% CO_2 and adequate humidity) and two plates anaerobically (an atmosphere of nitrogen containing 5–10% CO_2 and adequate humidity) for 28 days. On day 3 or day 4 after inoculation, subculture 0.25 ml from the liquid media on to two plates of solid media. Incubate one plate aerobically and the second anaerobically at 35–37°C until day 28 of the test. Repeat the subculture procedure on day 6, 7, or 8 and again on day 13 or 14. Observe the liquid media daily and, if any colour change occurs, subculture immediately.

3.2. Interpretation of *Mycoplasma* test results

At the end of the incubation period (day 28), examine all the inoculated solid media microscopically for the presence of mycoplasma colonies. The test sample passes the test if the growth of mycoplasma colonies has not occurred on any of the inoculated solid media. If at any stage of the test, more than one plate is accidentally contaminated with bacteria or fungi, or is broken, the test is invalid and should be repeated. If mycoplasma colonies are found on any agar plate, the test should be repeated once to confirm the mycoplasma contamination. If mycoplasma colonies are found on any of the agar plates of the retest, the test sample should be considered unsatisfactory because of mycoplasma contamination. Some mycoplasmas cannot be cultivated, in which case the MSV and MCS have to be tested using DNA staining or polymerase chain reaction (PCR) methods.

4. Detection of *Salmonella* contamination

Each batch of live virus biological made in eggs should be free from contamination with *Salmonella*. Five samples of each batch should be tested; 5 ml or one-half of the container contents, whichever is the lesser, of the sample should be used to inoculate 100 ml of tryptose broth and tetrathionate broth. The inoculated broths should be incubated for 18–24 hours at 35–37°C. Transfers from these broths should be made on to MacConkey and salmonella–shigella agar, incubated for 18–24 hours, and examined. If no growth typical of *Salmonella* is noted, the agar plates should be incubated an additional 18–24 hours and again examined. If colonies typical of *Salmonella* are observed, further subculture on to suitable differential media should be made for positive identification. If *Salmonella* is found, the batch of biological is unsatisfactory.

5. Detection of viruses in biological materials

Biological materials subject to viral contamination that cannot be sterilised before use, such as ingredients of animal origin (for example, serum), primary cells, line cells or viral seed stocks, should be tested before they are used. Assays are described to detect viral contaminants by cytopathic effects, haemadsorption, haemagglutination, fluorescent antibody techniques and other suitable methods, e.g. PCR and enzyme-linked immunosorbent assay.

Cells shall be tested in the following manner. On day 0, primary or frozen cells to be tested are seeded on 75 cm^2 (or similar) flasks; 7 days later, at least two 75 cm^2 flasks are prepared. On day 14, one flask is used to test the cells for cytopathology, haemadsorption, and fluorescent antibody staining (procedures follow). The other flask is passaged a second time, and on day 21 is subjected to three freeze–thaw cycles. After the third freeze–thaw cycle, the cells are centrifuged at 2000 *g* for 10 minutes, and the supernatant is used to inoculate appropriate virus-sensitive cells, i.e. cells susceptible to viruses that may be present in the species of animal from which the cells were obtained, cells susceptible to viruses that may occur in the animals in which the material is going to be used and cells susceptible to pestiviruses. These cells are then passed twice at 7-day intervals, and tested for cytopathology, haemadsorption and by fluorescent antibody staining.

Ingredients of animal origin are tested on both African green monkey kidney (Vero) cells and on a cell line or primary cells derived from the same species as the ingredient under test. Cells are inoculated using 75 cm^2 flasks with 3.75 ml of test material in 25 ml of media or 15% of the test material, whichever is the lesser. The cells are passaged twice at 7-day intervals and tested for cytopathology, haemadsorption and fluorescent antibody staining.

MSV are tested on Vero cells, cell lines or primary cells of the species for which the product is intended, and cell lines or primary cells of the species in which the product is prepared (if different from the intended species).

For each cell type required for testing, 1 ml of the test MSV is thawed or reconstituted and neutralised with the addition of 1 ml monospecific antiserum. The serum must be shown to be free from antibodies against any of the contaminants for which the test is intended. At least two cell types are always required, so a minimum of 2 ml of MSV and 2 ml of antiserum are required. The antiserum is allowed to neutralise the MSV at room temperature for 1 hour. Of the MSV/antiserum mixture, 2 ml is then inoculated on to a 75 cm^2 flask of the appropriate cells. If the MSV is known to be high-titred or is a difficult agent to neutralise, or if the blocking serum is known to be low-titred, the blocking antiserum can be added to the growth medium at a final concentration of 1–5%. The cells should be passaged at least twice over a 14-day period, and the final culture is examined for cytopathology, haemadsorption and by fluorescent antibody staining.

The May–Grünwald–Giemsa staining procedure is usually used to detect cytopathology caused by extraneous viruses. Monolayers are usually prepared on two-chambered tissue culture slides and incubated for 7 days. The plastic wells of the slides are removed leaving the rubber gasket attached to the slide. The slides are rinsed in warm Dulbecco's phosphate buffered saline (PBS), fixed in alcohol and placed on a staining rack. The slides are stained for 15 minutes at room temperature with May–Grünwald stain diluted 1/5 with absolute methanol. The May–Grünwald stain is removed by inverting the slides. The slides are then stained for 20 minutes with Giemsa stain diluted 1/15 in deionised water. The Giemsa stain is removed by inverting the slides and rinsing them in deionised water for 10–20 seconds. The slides are air-dried, and paraffin oil and a cover-slip are applied. The May–Grünwald–Giemsa stain will differentially stain DNA and RNA nucleoproteins. DNA nucleoproteins stain red-purple, while RNA nucleoproteins stain blue. The monolayers are examined with a conventional microscope for the presence of inclusion bodies, an abnormal number of giant cells, or other cytopathology attributable to a viral contaminant. The inoculated monolayers are compared with the noninoculated monolayers. If specific cytopathology attributable to an extraneous virus is found, the test material should be considered unsatisfactory.

Testing to detect extraneous viruses that produce haemadsorption in infected cells is usually carried out on monolayers of the second passage of test-material-inoculated cell cultures and noninoculated cell cultures. The monolayers are usually on 25 cm^2 plastic flasks. Guinea-pig, chicken, and any other blood for use in this assay is collected in an equal volume of Alsever's solution. The blood may be stored at 4°C for up to 7 days if it is washed several times in Alsever's solution before storage in an equal volume of Alsever's. Just prior to use, the stored erythrocytes are again washed by adding 5 ml of blood in Alsever's solution to 45 ml of calcium- and magnesium-free PBS and centrifuging in a 50 ml centrifuge tube at 500 ***g*** for 10 minutes. The supernatant is removed by suction and the erythrocytes are suspended in PBS and recentrifuged. This washing procedure is repeated at least twice until the supernatant is clear. Erythrocytes from each species are combined by adding 0.1 ml of each type of packed blood cells to 100 ml of PBS. The erythrocytes from different species may be kept separate or combined, as desired. To each flask, add 5 ml of the erythrocyte suspension, and incubate the flasks at 4°C for 30 minutes. The monolayers are washed twice with PBS and examined for haemadsorption. If no haemadsorption is apparent, 5 ml of the erythrocyte suspension is added to each flask, the flasks are incubated at 20–25°C for 30 minutes, rinsed as before, and examined for haemadsorption. Separate flasks may be used for each incubation temperature if desired. Monolayers are examined for the presence of haemadsorbtion both grossly (using an illuminated glovebox) and microscopically at ×30–60. It is important to compare the noninoculated monolayers with the test monolayers to detect nonspecific haemadsorption that may occur with some cell types. The use of calcium- and magnesium-free PBS and fresh erythrocytes should prevent most nonspecific haemadsorption from occurring. If specific haemadsorption attributable to an extraneous agent is found, the test material should be considered to be unsatisfactory.

Tests to detect extraneous viruses by fluorescent antibody usually use monolayers of the second passage of test-material-inoculated cell cultures and noninoculated cell cultures. The monolayers are usually on eight-chamber tissue culture slides. One positive control slide (consisting of eight monolayers) is made for each antiviral conjugate by inoculating each monolayer with approximately 100 $TCID_{50}$ (50% tissue culture infective dose) of the appropriate virus. Three groups of monolayers are stained with each antiviral conjugate. They are Group 1 – the second passage of test-material-inoculated cell cultures; Group 2 – the second passage of the noninoculated cell cultures; and Group 3 – the second passage of noninoculated cell cultures (for the production of positive control cell cultures). At the time of staining, the plastic walls of the slides are removed, leaving the rubber gasket attached to the slide. The slides are rinsed in Dulbecco's PBS, fixed for at least 10 minutes in acetone at 4°C, and dried. Approximately 0.1 ml of each conjugate is placed on each well of one slide from Groups 1, 2, and the corresponding positive control slide from Group 3. The slides are incubated in a humidified chamber at 37°C for 30 minutes, rinsed once in Dulbecco's PBS, and placed in a container of Dulbecco's PBS for 10 minutes. The slides are rinsed thoroughly in deionised water and dried. All slides are examined for fluorescence attributable to each specific virus. The three slides from each group with the same conjugate are compared. If the slide prepared from cells inoculated with test material shows any evidence of specific viral fluorescence, the MSV should be considered unsatisfactory.

• Acknowledgement

Parts of this chapter were taken from or based on the chapter on Tests for sterility and freedom from contamination of biological materials in previous editions of the *Manual*.

REFERENCES

1. CODE OF FEDERAL REGULATIONS (1998). Animals and Animal Products, Title 9, Parts 1–199. The Office of the Federal Register, National Archives and Records Administration. US Government Printing Office, Washington DC, USA.

2. COUNCIL OF EUROPE (1997). European Pharmacopoeia, Third Edition. Editions of the Council of Europe, Strasbourg, France. ISBN 92-871-2990-8.

3. EUROPEAN UNION (1999). The Rules Governing Medicinal Products in the European Union. Eudralex, Vols 4–9. Office Publications of the European Communities, Luxembourg.

4. HARE W.C.D. (1985). Diseases transmissible by semen and embryo transfer techniques. OIE Technical Series No. 4. OIE, Paris, France.

5. WORLD HEALTH ORGANIZATION (WHO) (1998). WHO Expert Committee on Biological Standardization. World Health Organization Technical Report Series, Report No. 858. World Health Organization, Geneva, Switzerland. ISBN 92-4-120878-3.

FURTHER READING

Details of methods and culture media will be found in the following books, and also in commercial catalogues.

A. BARROW G.I. & FELTHAM R.K.A. (EDS) (1993). Cowan and Steel's Manual for the Identification of Medical Bacteria, Third Edition. Cambridge University Press, Cambridge, UK.

B. CODE OF FEDERAL REGULATIONS (1998). Subchapter E. Viruses, serums, toxins, and analogous products; organisms and vectors. *In:* Code of Federal Regulation, Animals and Animal Products, Title 9, Parts 101–124. The Office of the Federal Register, National Archives and Records Administration. U.S. Government Printing Office, Washington DC, USA, 501–676.

C. COLLINS C.H., LYNE P.M. & GRANGE J.M., eds. (1995). Collins and Lyne's Microbiological Methods, Seventh Edition. Butterworth Heinemann, Oxford, UK.

D. PINI A., PARODI P., DEMENEGHI D., BELEMU J., KABILIKA H. & GHIROTTI M., eds. (1994). Basic Procedures for Diagnostic Veterinary Laboratories in Developing Countries. World Health Organization/Food and Agriculture Organization of the United Nations (WHO/FAO) Collaborating Centre, Viale Regina Elena 299, 00161 Rome, Italy, 142 pp.

*

* *

CHAPTER I.1.5.

HUMAN SAFETY IN THE VETERINARY MICROBIOLOGY LABORATORY

INTRODUCTION

Laboratory work of the type described in this Manual *should be carried out with a minimum of risk to the health of the staff. This requires careful consideration of the risks involved in a particular procedure, followed by appropriate measures to minimise the risk of human disease. This is a complex subject that can only be considered in outline in an introductory chapter. This chapter is concerned almost exclusively with risks from infectious agents, but physical and chemical injuries in microbiology laboratories must also be prevented. Risks from infection are reduced by good laboratory techniques and secure facilities, which aid in the containment of pathogens. It is important to understand that containment of pathogens can be used for two purposes. One is to prevent disease in humans, the other is to prevent disease in animals. Often the same methods of containment are used for both preventing laboratory-acquired infection in humans and for preventing escape of pathogens that could cause an outbreak of animal disease. Although the methods, techniques and facilities required may be the same, the list of pathogens and categorisation into levels of risk will differ depending on whether it is human or animal disease control that is the primary objective.*

Existing national and international reference laboratories have considerable experience in the operation of safe working practices and provision of appropriate facilities. When new laboratories are being established, it would be prudent to seek advice from the competent authorities at established institutes. It is important to comply with legislative requirements.

A. ASSESSMENT OF RISK FROM PATHOGENS

It is necessary first to assess the risk from a pathogen, so that it can be assigned to a risk group. Work with it can then be assigned to an appropriate containment category. To assess the risk to humans from a particular pathogen it is necessary to know whether infection with that organism can cause death, disease or inconvenience to the people working with it, and whether it could then spread to cause disease in the general human population. (There are additional considerations relating to the containment of animal pathogens and preventing spread of infection to animals, which is a separate, though related, subject. Information on this may be found in the OIE *International Animal Health Code,* Chapter 1.4.6., which for convenience is reproduced at the end of this chapter as Appendix 1.) To assess this risk it is necessary to know the epidemiological background of the organism and also such attributes of the organism as infectivity for humans, stability in the environment, ability to infect by different routes, and susceptibility to specific treatments or prophylaxis (1, 2, 4, 5). It is relatively easy to obtain this information when working with a known pathogen, but the problem is more complex in a diagnostic laboratory receiving clinical material that may be infected with a variety of unknown pathogens, some of which could be extremely hazardous to human health. Some of the considerations to take into account when evaluating risk are:

1. Known occurrence of human infection with the organism or related organisms with similar characteristics, any history of laboratory-acquired infection, infective dose and disease severity. Production of toxins or allergens;

2. The volume of culture to be handled and the concentration of the organism likely to be present. (Procedures such as antigen or vaccine production that require large quantities of organisms usually carry a higher risk than attempted isolation procedures.);

3. The origin of the sample, for example samples from wildlife species may contain human pathogens not normally encountered;

4. The history of the isolate being handled. Pathogens on primary isolation or of low passage level are often more dangerous than pathogens of high passage level. In some cases, pathogenicity may be enhanced by passage or subculture using different media;

5. The possibility of aerosol formation should be especially taken into consideration when handling fluid samples or, for example, during grinding, homogenisation and centrifugation;

6. The threat that the organism may pose to food-producing or companion animals or to wildlife, irrespective of the threat to laboratory personnel. Additional precautions for handling and storage are required for animal disease agents from foreign countries;

7. The physical state of the employees. For example, in the case of pregnancy, immunodeficiency or allergy, special precautions may be required. Sometimes certain individuals have to be excluded from particular types of work that would be specially hazardous to them;

8. A higher level of risk may arise when agents such as *Brucella* or *Mycobacteria* are inoculated into animals.

B. GROUPING OF MICROORGANISMS

The considerations outlined above have been used by several National Authorities to designate microorganisms into four hazard groups (2, 3) representing increasing hazards to human health. Such categorisation of pathogens makes no allowance for people who are particularly susceptible, for example due to pre-existing disease, a compromised immune system or pregnancy. The four groups may be summarised thus:

Group 1 – Organisms that are unlikely to cause human disease;

Group 2 – Organisms that may cause human disease but are unlikely to be spread in the community and for which effective prophylaxis and treatment are available;

Group 3 – Organisms that can cause severe human disease and may spread in the community but for which there is usually effective prophylaxis and treatment;

Group 4 – Organisms that cause severe human disease, may represent a high risk of spread in the community and for which there is usually no effective prophylaxis or treatment.

Additional considerations apply to animal disease agents that are controlled by veterinary authorities, where it is necessary to prevent spread to domestic animals or wildlife. These aspects are dealt with in the OIE *International Animal Health Code*.

Infectious organisms that might be encountered in laboratory work have been assigned to hazard groups 1–4 by authorities in several countries (2, 3). Some examples of the dangerous pathogens that may be found in a veterinary laboratory are listed in Table I. Bovine spongiform encepthalopathy (BSE) has been placed in Hazard Group 3 by the European Union. Also, some very serious Group 4 agents, including Hendra and Nipah, have been isolated from diagnostic specimens in veterinary laboratories.

Table 1. *Examples of some of the microorganisms in Hazard Groups 2 and 3 that are capable of causing human disease and that may be present in a veterinary laboratory*

Group 2

Viruses: Influenza viruses types A, B, C; Newcastle disease virus; Orf (parapox virus)

Bacteria: *Alcaligenes* spp.; *Arizona* spp.; *Campylobacter* spp.; *Chlamydia psittaci* (nonavian); *Clostridium tetani; Clostridium botulinum; Corynebacterium* spp.; *Erysipelothrix rhusiopathiae; Escherichia coli; Haemophilus* spp.; *Leptospira* spp.; *Listeria monocytogenes; Moraxella* spp.; *Mycobacterium avium; Pasteurella* spp.; *Proteus* spp.; *Pseudomonas* spp.; *Salmonella* spp.; *Staphylococcus* spp.; *Yersinia enterocolitica; Yersinia pseudotuberculosis*

Fungi: *Aspergillus fumigatus; Microsporum* spp.; *Trichophyton* spp.

Group 3

Viruses: Rabies virus; Equine encephalomyelitis virus (Eastern, Western and Venezuelan); Japanese B encephalitis virus; Louping ill virus

Bacteria: *Bacillus anthracis; Burkholderia mallei (Pseudomonas mallei); Brucella* spp.; *Chlamydia psittaci* (avian strains only); *Coxiella burnetti; Mycobacterium bovis*

C. REQUIREMENTS FOR WORK WITH INFECTIOUS AGENTS

A. Known pathogens

Having decided the risk level of certain work it is then possible to decide the appropriate 'containment level' that is needed to minimise the risk of human disease. The containment level is defined by a combination of the physical facilities and working practices employed. Organisms of the four risk groups indicated above may be placed into containment levels appropriate for safe working, see below. Laboratories usually appoint a Safety Officer, responsible for ensuring that microorganisms are handled at the appropriate containment level. They should have sufficient expertise and be of sufficient seniority to oversee and advise on all safety matters. In large organisations with a network of laboratories, it is appropriate to appoint a central Safety Officer to advise on and coordinate safety matters of a corporate nature, which are implemented by local laboratory Safety Officers at each site. The working methods for a particular procedure or work station should be written out and readily available. Staff must be fully trained and fully aware of any health risks associated with their work. Staff should also be given a medical card indicating pathogens to which they might be exposed. In some cases staff can be specially vaccinated to give additional protection, e.g. when working with the rabies virus; this should also be recorded on the medical card. Such information is useful for a medical practitioner in the event of illness occurring. Regular medical examinations of employees are recommended and, as appropriate, monitoring tests of employees working with the organisms that cause certain serious human diseases, such as brucellosis and tuberculosis.

Much information is available on containment of pathogens, and sophisticated apparatus and buildings may be constructed for containment of the more hazardous organisms as required by the guidelines, standards and regulations of each country. The essential requirements for any work with infectious agents, however innocuous they may seem, are as follows:

1. The laboratory should be easy to clean, with surfaces that are impervious to water and resistant to chemicals. There must be a wash-hand basin and emergency shower, including an eye bath, in each laboratory. Procedures must be established for frequent cleaning and disinfection during and at the end of the work period;

2. Personnel access to the laboratory should be restricted;

3. Protective clothing, including gloves, masks (or better, respirators) and eyeshields as appropriate, must be worn in the laboratory and removed when leaving the laboratory;

4. The laboratory door should be closed when work is in progress and ventilation should be provided by extracting air from the room. (Where biohazard cabinets are used, care must be taken to balance ventilation systems.);

5. Food and/or drink must not be stored or consumed in laboratories;

6. Smoking and/or application of cosmetics must not take place in the laboratory;

7. Pipetting must not be done by mouth;

8. Care must be taken to minimise the production of aerosols;

9. In the event of spillage or contamination, effective disinfectant must be available for cleaning up, and contaminated protective clothing must be removed and decontaminated. Hands must be thoroughly washed immediately. Bench tops should be cleaned and disinfected after use. Safety showers must be immediately available;

10. Used laboratory glassware and other materials must be stored safely before disinfection. Materials for disposal must be transported without spillage in strong containers. Waste material should be autoclaved, incinerated or otherwise made safe before disposal. Reusable material must be decontaminated by appropriate means;

11. No infectious material shall be discarded down laboratory sinks or any other drain;

12. Any accidents or incidents must be recorded and reported to the Safety Officer.

At the Group 2 level of containment, in addition to the points given above, a microbiological safety cabinet should be used but can be operated in the open front mode (Class I cabinet). A class II cabinet provides less operator protection, but may be used when there is potential for generating aerosols or when handling large quantities of culture or where there is a real need to protect the biological product. Emergency protocols should be posted within the laboratory to advise personnel of procedures to follow in case of a pathogen spill or the need to evacuate the laboratory in the event of a fire or other emergency.

At the Group 3 level of containment, it is advisable to site the laboratory in some isolation and to restrict entry to named individuals. Appropriate signage is required at all entry doors to indicate the hazard present and the name and telephone number of the person(s) responsible. Emergency protocols should be posted within the laboratory to advise personnel of procedures to follow in case of a pathogen spill or the need to evacuate the laboratory in the event of a fire.

In addition to the previous requirements, a ventilation system is required that removes air from the laboratory through a high efficiency particulate air (HEPA) filter. Safety cabinets of either Class I or Class III must be provided. The laboratory should be under negative pressure to surrounding areas where less hazardous work is done. It may be necessary for staff to shower and they must change their clothes, before leaving the building.

Note. Because of the link between bovine spongiform encephalopathy (BSE) and new variant Creutzfeldt-Jakob disease in humans, BSE and related agents are now categorised with the human transmissible spongiform encephalopathies in hazard group 3. Consequently, veterinarians and laboratory workers conducting necropsies on BSE-suspect animals or handling tissues derived from such animals, must conduct the work under appropriately strict containment conditions, sometimes with derogations allowed by the nature of the work and the results of local risk assessment. It is important that appropriate protective clothing be worn and that a strict code of practice be followed to prevent exposure to the agent. Laboratories conducting work on BSE must comply with national biocontainment and biosafety regulations.

At the Group 4 level of containment, the most stringent precautions are required, including access to the building through a system of air locks, the building being maintained under negative air pressure. Inlet air to the laboratory must be filtered through a single HEPA filter and extract air through double HEPA filters. All work with infective materials must be conducted in a Class III microbiological safety cabinet. All sewage from the laboratory, laboratory effluent and autoclave drain effluent must be treated by appropriate means to ensure that all infectious material is destroyed before entering the public sewerage system. Staff must shower and change their clothing before leaving the building. Other precautions as described for Group 3 would also apply. There is an additional, internationally accepted way of providing containment at level 4. This is by the use of one-piece positive pressure suits.

B. Diagnostic specimens

Veterinary diagnostic centres readily receive specimens that are submitted because they are suspect for a variety of diseases. The infectious nature of the specimens is usually unknown, but they have the potential to contain biological agents that may cause disease in animals and humans. Practices and procedures need to be in place that will minimise the risk of occupational exposure of employees to such pathogens. It is therefore advisable that initial processing of all unknown specimens should be carried out as though the material contained a Group 2 pathogen. The most important aspects are to prevent percutaneous and mucous membrane exposure. Biological safety cabinets should be used for all manipulations that may generate aerosols. Class I or II are appropriate depending on the need for protection of the samples from contamination. Additionally, there should be no mouth pipetting, personal protective clothing should be worn with, in some cases, eye and respiratory protection, depending on the anticipated level of exposure. Although initial diagnostic procedures may be carried out at level 2, once a Group 3 organism has been isolated (or suspected) further work must be carried out at the higher containment level.

D. MICROBIOLOGICAL SAFETY CABINETS

These are used at the different containment levels, as described in Section C.A. above. They are of three types:

Class I: An open-fronted cabinet designed specifically to provide operator protection and not to give protection to the work being handled.

Class II: An open-fronted cabinet, sometimes referred to as a laminar flow recirculating cabinet. They are designed primarily to give product protection but also give some operator protection. The air flow is slower than in a Class I cabinet and operator protection is less, therefore a Class II cabinet should only be used where there is a real need to protect the biological materials being handled.

Class III: These cabinets are closed, with glove ports at the front, and provide the highest degree of containment by complete separation of work and worker. Some cabinets have a removable glove port and are known as Class III/I cabinets, i.e. they can be used in either mode.

Descriptions of safety cabinets and safe working practices have been published (6).

E. STORAGE OF PATHOGENS

Storage of live pathogens requires appropriate containment and security to avoid risks due to breakage or unauthorised use of material. Storage facilities should be appropriately labelled to indicate the nature of the pathogens (e.g. their group) and the person(s) responsible for them. A complete inventory of the pathogens in storage should be kept up to date and available. Special care must be taken when opening glass vials of freeze-dried pathogens, as these can sometimes shatter. Care must be taken when working with liquid nitrogen.

Many of the considerations given above relate not only to human safety but also to prevention of spread of infection to animals. In a veterinary laboratory an important responsibility is to minimise any risk of escape of pathogens to animals, either wild or domestic, in the outside community. Close communication must be maintained with the veterinary authorities. Special licences may be required to work with certain microorganisms.

F. PHYSICAL AND CHEMICAL HAZARDS

Laboratory work involves many manipulations that are potentially dangerous, such as pushing glass tubes through rubber stoppers, and work with needles or other sharp instruments. There must be special facilities for disposal of 'sharps'.

Laboratory staff risk receiving a burn from hot solids or liquids. Autoclaves must be fitted with safety devices to prevent accidental opening of doors when under pressure, and be regularly serviced and tested. Heat-protective gloves must be provided. Extreme cold can also be a risk, for example when working with liquid nitrogen; splashes on exposed skin can be very damaging. Gloves should be worn that provide insulation from cold and that are also waterproof, to prevent penetration of the liquid nitrogen. Face masks and boots should also be worn when working with liquid nitrogen.

Irradiation is a serious health risk that may be present due to the use of X-ray machines, or use of gamma-emitters or other sources. Equipment must be regularly serviced and tested. All use of radioactive material must be meticulously recorded. All staff must be provided with a radiation monitoring device and have annual health checks. Local and national regulations must be followed (7).

A wide range of chemicals is in use in veterinary laboratories, many of which may be toxic or mutagenic and some carcinogenic. It should be remembered that it is the dose that makes the poison (i.e. in sufficient quantities, even a 'harmless' substance can become toxic). Vapours are specially hazardous, and some chemicals can be absorbed by penetration of intact skin. Procedures sufficient to protect pregnant laboratory workers should be followed at all times. A list of hazardous chemicals must be maintained, and a file record kept of chemicals to which individual staff members could be exposed. This is now a legal requirement in some countries. Chemicals must be correctly stored in appropriate containers and at the correct temperature. Those that are very flammable must be kept in a fireproof chemical store. A record must be maintained of the purchase and use of hazardous chemicals: how much, when used, by whom and for what purpose. Disposal of some chemicals is subject to official regulation.

Further information on physical and chemical safety precautions can be found in the literature (8, 9).

G. LABORATORY ANIMAL FACILITIES

Work with pathogens in laboratory animals poses special hazards. Animal rooms have to be constructed to appropriate standards and containment levels, just as laboratories. Containment in animal houses is very important because of the large amount of infectious agents that they may generate. Similar considerations also apply regarding the training of staff, protective clothing and the recording of working procedures. Special care must be taken to avoid injury to staff, e.g. through animals biting and kicking. Any such incidents should be recorded and wounds appropriately treated. There must be provision for incineration or rendering of carcasses and for the thorough cleansing and disinfection of animal rooms. The animal rooms should not only provide a suitable environment for the animals themselves but should be constructed and ventilated in such a way as to ensure comfort for the attendants. This is a large subject that can only be referred to briefly here. An excellent book on health and safety in laboratory animal facilities has been published recently (12).

H. EMERGENCY PROVISIONS

First-aid equipment must be provided next to all work stations. This equipment must be appropriate to the work and properly maintained. An example is the provision of bottles of eye-wash. It is essential that these be kept clean, full of suitable sterile liquid, and ready to hand for immediate emergency use. Bandages, dressings and simple medicines should be available. Some staff should receive training in safety and first aid from recognised authorities and should possess a valid certificate as evidence of competence. Their names and locations should be known to everyone and posted on notice boards. All staff should be aware of the importance of safety. There must be suitable procedures and equipment for dealing with spillages and decontamination. A record must be kept of all accidents.

Many laboratories have a staff safety committee to increase safety awareness and to discuss safety issues with management. Managers should be responsible for safety in their area of command and should not allow consideration of speed or cost of work to come before the safety of their staff.

There should be an emergency procedure for calling medical assistance if required, and for hospitalisation when needed. Fire alarms must be fitted, and tested regularly. Each unit should designate a fire officer who conducts periodic fire drills to make staff aware of what to do and where to assemble in the event of fire. The fire officer is responsible for checking that everyone has left the building. Procedures for other natural disasters, such as hurricanes and earthquakes, should be in place where they present a risk. All these procedures should be written down and periodically reviewed.

I. TRANSPORT OF INFECTIOUS MATERIAL

Great care must be taken when preparing and packing diagnostic specimens for transport, to ensure that there is no breakage of containers or leakage of contents that could put at risk postal workers, couriers or staff at the receiving laboratory (see Chapter I.1. Sampling methods).

J. CONCLUSION

High standards of laboratory safety that will ensure healthy working conditions for laboratory staff must be of the greatest priority. They can only be achieved by careful study of the principles involved followed by practical application to premises, facilities, operating procedures and hygiene. Training of all laboratory personnel must be a high priority and no personnel should be allowed to work until appropriate training has been completed and documented. There is a large published literature on all aspects of the subject, and further reading is recommended (5, 10, 11).

REFERENCES

1. ACHA P.N. & SZYFRES B. (1987). Zoonoses and Communicable Diseases Common to Man and Animals, Second Edition. Pan American Health Organisation, Scientific Publication No. 503. PAHO, Washington DC, USA.

2. ADVISORY COMMITTEE ON DANGEROUS PATHOGENS (1995). Categorisation of Biological Agents According to Hazard and Categories of Containment, Fourth Edition. Health and Safety Executive Books, P.O. Box 1999, Sudbury, Suffolk, CO10 6FS, UK. ISBN 0-7176-1038-1.

3. BARBEITO M.S., ABRAHAM G., BEST M., CAIRNS P., LANGEVIN P., STERRITT W.G., BARR D., MEULEPAS W., SANCHEZ-VIZCAINO J.M., SARAZA M., REQUENA E., COLLADO M., MANI P., BREEZE R., BRUNNER H., MEBUS C.A., MORGAN R.L., RUSK S., SIEGFRIED L.M. & THOMPSON L.H. (1995). Recommended biocontainment features for research and diagnostic facilities where animal pathogens are used. *Rev. sci. tech. Off. int. Epiz.*, **14**, 873–887.

4. BELL J.C., PALMER S.R. & PAYNE J.M. (1988). The Zoonoses. Edward Arnold, London, UK.

5. BERAN G.W. & STEELE J.H. (EDS) (1994). Handbook of Zoonoses, Second Edition. Section A. (Bacterial, Rickettsial, Chlamydial and Mycotic Zoonoses) and Section B (Viral Zoonoses), CRC Press, USA.

6. COLLINS C.H. (1990). Health hazards in microbiology. *In:* Handbook of Laboratory Health and Safety Measures, Pal S.B., ed. Kluwer Academic Publications, Dordrecht, The Netherlands, 159–188.

7. INTERNATIONAL ATOMIC ENERGY AGENCY (IAEA) (1994). International Basic Safety Standards for Protection against Ionizing Radiation and for the Safety of Radiation Sources, Interim Edition. Safety Series No. 115-I. IAEA, Vienna, Austria.

8. OFFICE OF BIOSAFETY, LABORATORY CENTRE FOR DISEASE CONTROL, HEALTH AND WELFARE CANADA (1996). Laboratory Biosafety Guidelines, Second Edition. Ministry of Supply and Services Canada, Cat. No. MR 21-2/1996.

9. RAYBURN S.R. (1990). The Foundations of Laboratory Safety (a Guide for the Biomedical Laboratory). Springer-Verlag, New York, USA.

10. SEWELL D.L. (1995). Laboratory associated infections and biosafety. *Clin. Microbiol. Rev.*, **8**, 389–405.

11. US DEPARTMENT OF HEALTH AND HUMAN SERVICES, CENTRES FOR DISEASE CONTROL AND PREVENTION AND NATIONAL INSTITUTES OF HEALTH (1999). Biosafety in Microbiological and Biomedical Laboratories, Fourth Edition. Catalogue number 017-040-00547-4. United States Government Printing Office, Washington DC, USA.

12. WOOD M. & SMITH M.W. (EDS) (1999). Health and Safety in Laboratory Animal Facilities. Royal Society of Medicine Press, London, UK, pp. 249.

APPENDIX 1.1.5.1.

INTERNATIONAL TRANSFER AND LABORATORY CONTAINMENT OF ANIMAL PATHOGENS[1]

A. OBJECT

To prevent the introduction and spread of animal diseases caused by pathogens.

B. INTRODUCTION

1. The consequences of the introduction into a country of an infectious disease or an animal pathogen or new strain of animal pathogen from which it is currently free, are potentially very serious. This is because animal health, human health, the agricultural economy and trade may all be adversely affected to a greater or a lesser degree. Countries will already have in place a range of measures, such as requirements for pre-import testing and quarantine, to prevent such introductions through the importation of live animals or their products.

2. However, there is also the risk that disease may occur as a result of the accidental release of animal pathogens from laboratories that are using them for various purposes such as research, diagnosis or the manufacture of vaccines. Such pathogens may already occur in the country or they may have been imported deliberately or inadvertently. It is therefore necessary to have in place measures to prevent their accidental release. These measures may be applied (a) at national borders by prohibiting or controlling the importation of specified pathogens or their carriers (see G. Importation of animal pathogens) or (b) within national boundaries by specifying the conditions under which laboratories must handle them. In practice, a combination of external and internal controls is likely to be applied depending on the risk to animal health posed by the pathogen in question.

C. PURPOSE

1. To provide guidance on the laboratory containment of animal pathogens according to the risk they pose to animal health and the agricultural economy of a country, particularly when the disease they cause is not enzootic.

2. To provide guidance on the import conditions applicable to animal pathogens.

3. Where animal pathogens also pose a risk to human health, guidance on their laboratory containment should be sought from the *Manual* and other relevant published documents.

D. CLASSIFICATION OF ANIMAL PATHOGENS

1. Animal pathogens should be categorised on the risk they pose to animal health, should they be introduced into a country or accidentally released from a laboratory. In categorising pathogens into four groups according to containment requirements, the following factors should be taken into account: the organism's pathogenicity, the biohazard it presents, its ability to spread, the economic aspects and the availability of prophylactic and therapeutic treatments.

2. Some pathogens need to be transmitted by specific vectors or require intermediate hosts to complete their life cycles before they can infect animals and cause disease. In countries where such vectors or intermediate hosts do not occur, or where climatic or environmental factors mitigate against their survival, the pathogen poses a lower risk to animal health than in countries where such vectors or intermediate hosts occur naturally or could survive.

---

1 This Appendix is taken from Chapter 1.4.6. of the OIE *International Animal Health Code*, 2000.

3. When categorising animal pathogens into specific groups, the following criteria should be taken into account:

   a) **Group 1 animal pathogens**

   Disease-producing organisms that are enzootic but not subject to official control.

   b) **Group 2 animal pathogens**

   Disease-producing organisms that are either exotic or enzootic but subject to official control and that have a low risk of spread from the laboratory.

   i) They do not depend on vectors or intermediate hosts for transmission.
   ii) There is very limited or no transmission between different animal species.
   iii) Geographical spread if released from the laboratory is limited.
   iv) Direct animal to animal transmission is relatively limited.
   v) The need to confine diseased or infected nondiseased animals is minimal.
   vi) The disease is of limited economic and/or clinical significance.

   c) **Group 3 animal pathogens**

   Disease-producing organisms that are either exotic or enzootic but subject to official control and that have a moderate risk of spread from the laboratory.

   i) They may depend on vectors or intermediate hosts for transmission.
   ii) Transmission between different animal species may readily occur.
   iii) Geographical spread if released from the laboratory is moderate.
   iv) Direct animal to animal transmission occurs relatively easily.
   v) The statutory confinement of diseased, infected and in-contact animals is necessary.
   vi) The disease is of severe economic and/or clinical significance.
   vii) Prophylactic and/or therapeutic treatments are not readily available or of limited benefit.

   d) **Group 4 animal pathogens**

   Disease-producing organisms that are either exotic or enzootic but subject to official control and that have a high risk of spread from the laboratory.

   i) They may depend on vectors or intermediate hosts for transmission.
   ii) Transmission between different animal species may occur very readily.
   iii) Geographical spread if released from the laboratory is widespread.
   iv) Direct animal to animal transmission occurs very easily.
   v) The statutory confinement of diseased, infected and in-contact animals is necessary.
   vi) The statutory control of animal movements over a wide area is necessary.
   vii) The disease is of extremely severe economic and/or clinical significance.
   viii) No satisfactory prophylactic and/or therapeutic treatments are available.

E. CONTAINMENT LEVELS

1. The principal purpose of containment is to prevent the escape of the pathogen from the laboratory into the national animal population. Some animal pathogens can infect humans. In these instances the risk to human health may demand additional containment than would otherwise be considered necessary from purely animal health considerations.

2. The level of physical containment and biosecurity procedures and practices should be related to the group into which the pathogen has been placed and the detailed requirements should be appropriate to the type of organism (i.e. bacterium, virus, fungus or parasite). The lowest containment level will be required for

pathogens in group 1 and the highest level for those in group 4. Guidance on the containment requirements for groups 2, 3 and 4 is provided in Table 1.

3. Arthropods may be pathogens or vectors for pathogens. If they are a vector for a pathogen being used in the laboratory, the appropriate containment level for the pathogen will be necessary in addition to the containment facilities for the arthropod.

Table 1. *Guidance on the laboratory requirements for the different containment groups*

	Requirements of the laboratory	Containment group 2	Containment group 3	Containment group 4
A)	**Laboratory siting and structure**			
1.	Not next to known fire hazard	Yes	Yes	Yes
2.	Workplace separated from other activities	Yes	Yes	Yes
3.	Personnel access limited	Yes	Yes	Yes
4.	Protected against entry/exit of rodents and insects	Yes	Yes	Yes
5.	Liquid effluent must be sterilised		Yes and monitored	Yes and monitored
6.	Isolated by airlock. Continuous internal airflow		Yes	Yes
7.	Input and extract air to be filtered using HEPA or equivalent		Single on extract	Single for input, double for extract
8.	Mechanical air supply system with fail-safe system		Yes	Yes
9.	Laboratory sealable to permit fumigation		Yes	Yes
10.	Incinerator for disposal of carcasses and waste	Available	Yes	Yes on site
B)	**Laboratory facilities**			
11.	Class 1/2/3 exhaust protective cabinet available	Yes	Yes	Yes
12.	Direct access to autoclave	Yes	Yes with double doors	Yes with double doors
13.	Specified pathogens stored in laboratory	Yes	Yes	Yes
14.	Double-ended dunk tank required		Preferable	Yes
15.	Protective clothing not worn outside laboratory	Yes	Yes	Yes
16.	Showering required before exiting laboratory			Yes
17.	Safety Officer responsible for containment	Yes	Yes	Yes
18.	Staff receive special training in the requirements needed	Yes	Yes	Yes
C)	**Laboratory discipline**			
19.	Warning notices for containment area	Yes	Yes	Yes
20.	Laboratory must be lockable	Yes	Yes	Yes
21.	Authorised entry of personnel	Yes	Yes	Yes
22.	On entering all clothing removed and clean clothes put on		Yes	Yes
23.	On exiting all laboratory clothes removed, individual must wash and transfer to clean side		Yes	
24.	Individual must shower prior to transfer to clean side			Yes
25.	All accidents reported	Yes	Yes	Yes

Table 1. Guidance on the laboratory requirements for the different containment groups (cont.)

Requirements of the laboratory	Containment group 2	3	4
D) Handling of specimens			
26. Packaging requirements to be advised prior to submission	Yes	Yes	Yes
27. Incoming packages opened by trained staff	Yes	Yes	Yes
28. Movement of pathogens from an approved laboratory to another requires a licence	Yes	Yes	Yes
29. Standard Operating Procedures covering all areas must be available	Yes	Yes	Yes

F. POSSESSION AND HANDLING OF ANIMAL PATHOGENS

1. A laboratory should be allowed to possess and handle animal pathogens in group 3 or 4 only if it can satisfy the relevant authority that it can provide containment facilities appropriate to the group. However, depending on the particular circumstances of an individual country, the authority might decide that the possession and handling of certain pathogens in group 2 should also be controlled. The authority should first inspect the facilities to ensure they are adequate and then issue a licence specifying all relevant conditions. There should also be a requirement for appropriate records to be kept and for the authority to be notified if it is suspected that a material being handled contains a pathogen not covered by the licence. The authority should visit the laboratory periodically to ensure licence conditions are being complied with. It is important that authority staff carrying out the visit should not have any contact with species susceptible to the pathogens being handled at the laboratory for a specified period after visiting the laboratory. The length of this period will depend on the pathogen.

2. Licences should specify:

   a) how the pathogen is to be transported and the disposal of the packaging;

   b) the name of the person responsible for the work;

   c) whether the pathogen may be used *in vivo* (and if so whether in laboratory animals or other animals) and/or only *in vitro*;

   d) how the pathogen and any experimental animals should be disposed of when the work is completed;

   e) limitations on contact by laboratory staff with species susceptible to the pathogens being used;

   f) conditions for the transfer of pathogens to other laboratories;

   g) specific conditions relating to the appropriate containment level and biosecurity procedures and practices.

G. IMPORTATION OF ANIMAL PATHOGENS

1. The importation of any animal pathogen, pathological material or organisms carrying the pathogen should be permitted only under an import licence issued by the relevant authority. The import licence should contain conditions appropriate to the risk posed by the pathogen and, in relation to air transport, the appropriate standards of the International Air Transport Association concerning the packaging and transport of hazardous substances. The import licence for group 2, 3 or 4 should only be granted to a laboratory that is licensed to handle the particular pathogen as in F. Possession and handling of animal pathogens.

2. When considering applications to import pathological material from other countries, the authorities should have regard to the nature of the material, the animal from which it is derived, the susceptibility of that animal to various diseases and the animal health situation of the country of origin. It may be advisable to require that material is pretreated before import to minimise the risk of inadvertent introduction of a pathogen.

CHAPTER 1.1.6.

PRINCIPLES OF VETERINARY VACCINE PRODUCTION

SUMMARY

A reliable supply of pure, safe, potent, and effective vaccines is essential for maintenance of animal health and the successful operation of animal health programmes. Immunisation of animals with high quality vaccines is the primary means of control for many animal diseases. In other cases, vaccines are used in conjunction with national disease control or eradication programmes.

The requirements and procedures described here are intended to be general in nature and to be consistent with published standards that are generally available for guidance in the production of veterinary vaccines. The approach to ensuring the quality, safety, potency, and efficacy of veterinary vaccines may vary from country to country depending on local needs. However, proper standards and production controls are essential to ensure the availability of consistent, high quality products for use in animal health programmes.

As the pathogenesis and epidemiology of each disease varies, the role and efficacy of vaccination as a means of control also varies from one disease to another. Some vaccines may be highly efficacious, inducing an immunity that not only prevents clinical signs of the disease, but also prevents infection and replication of the disease-causing agent. Other vaccines may prevent clinical disease, but not prevent infection and/or the development of the carrier state. In other cases, immunisation may be completely ineffective or only able to reduce the severity of the disease. Thus the decision whether to recommend vaccination as part of an animal disease control strategy requires a thorough knowledge of the characteristics of the disease agent and its epidemiology, as well as the characteristics and capabilities of the various available vaccines. There is also growing public concern about the animal welfare implications of veterinary vaccine production and use. In any case, if vaccines are used, successful performance requires that they be produced in a manner that ensures a uniform and consistent product of high quality.

NOMENCLATURE

The nomenclature for veterinary biological products varies from country to country. For example, in the United States of America (USA) the term 'vaccine' is used for products containing live or inactivated viruses or protozoa, live bacteria, or nucleic acids. Products containing killed bacteria and other microorganisms are identified as bacterins, bacterial extracts, subunits, bacterintoxoids, or toxoids, depending on the type of antigen they contain. For example, products containing antigenic or immunising components of microorganisms may be called 'subunits' or 'bacterial extracts', and those produced from the inactivation of toxins are called 'toxoids'. In the European Union (EU), Veterinary Medicinal Products are defined as 'products administered to animals in order to produce active or passive immunity or to diagnose the state of immunity', see Directive 90/677/EEC. For this chapter, however, the term 'vaccine' will include all products designed to stimulate active immunisation of animals against disease, without regard to the type of microorganism or microbial toxin from which they may be derived or that they contain. This use is more consistent with international nomenclature. 'Vaccine' will not be used in this discussion in reference to biological products recommended for passive immunisation, immunostimulation, treatment of allergies, or diagnosis.

VACCINE TYPES OR FORMS

Vaccines may be prepared as live or inactivated (killed) products. Some live vaccines are prepared from low virulence, mild, field isolates of a disease-causing agent that have been found to be safe and effective when administered by an unnatural route or under other conditions where exposure to the microorganism will immunise rather than cause disease. Other live vaccines are prepared from isolates of disease-causing agents that have been modified by passage through laboratory animals, culture media, cell cultures, or avian embryos to select an isolate of reduced virulence. The development of recombinant DNA (rDNA) procedures has provided some unique opportunities for vaccine production. Modified live vaccines may now be specifically produced by deletion of virulence-related genes from a microorganism. Others are produced by the insertion of genes that code for specific immunising antigens from a disease-causing microorganism into a nonvirulent vector microorganism. Nucleic-acid-mediated vaccines containing plasmid DNA are being developed. This is usually in plasmid form and codes for immunising antigens from disease-causing microorganisms.

Killed products may contain: 1) Cultures of microorganisms that have been inactivated by chemical or other means; 2) Inactivated toxins; or 3) Subunits (antigenic parts of microorganisms) that have been extracted from cultures or that have been produced through rDNA procedures.

Both live and inactivated vaccines may be formulated with adjuvants designed to enhance their efficacy. These adjuvants are typically water-in-oil emulsions (either single or double), made with mineral or vegetable oil and an emulsifying agent. Other adjuvants, such as aluminium hydroxide gel, are also used.

QUALITY ASSURANCE

The consistent production of high quality, safe, potent, and efficacious vaccines requires quality assurance procedures to ensure the uniformity and consistency of the production process. As production processes for vaccines provide a great opportunity for variability, care must be taken to control variability to the greatest extent possible, preferably using validated procedures, and to protect the product from contamination through all stages of production.

Vaccine quality, safety, potency, and efficacy must be ensured by consistency in the production process. Consistent product quality (batch-to-batch uniformity) must be built in at each stage. Final product testing is used as a check to verify that the controls on the production procedures have remained intact and that the released product meets the specification previously agreed with the licensing authority.

Regulatory authorities in different countries have developed various approaches to ensuring the quality of vaccines. Although alike in their ultimate goal, these systems may vary in the emphasis given to control of the production process (process standards) in comparison with control through testing of the final product (performance standards). The control procedures selected should be those that best fit the conditions under which vaccines are being produced and should, where possible, comply with good manufacturing practice.

The control standards and procedures established for a product define the risk or possibility of producing and releasing a product that is worthless, contaminated, dangerous, or harmful. The acceptable degree of risk may depend on the benefits to be gained by having the product available to prevent disease losses. Thus standards may justifiably vary from country to country or product to product, depending on local animal health conditions. However, control authorities should strive to establish control standards and procedures that ensure a finished product of the highest quality, safety, potency and efficacy possible.

The optimal quality assurance system should address both production procedures and final product testing in proper balance. An absolutely fail-safe system that would result in no risk of releasing an unsatisfactory product would probably be too expensive with regard to cost of production as well as control. Thus regulatory officials and manufacturers of vaccines must select control procedures that are capable of ensuring an acceptable low level of risk in relation to hazard. Such procedures, however, must not be burdensome to the extent that they inhibit the development and availability of the products needed to provide proper preventative medical care at a cost that is acceptable to the consumer.

PRODUCTION FACILITIES

Facilities used for the production of vaccines should be designed to protect the purity of the product throughout the production process and to safeguard the health of the personnel. They must be constructed so that: 1) they can be readily and thoroughly cleaned; 2) they provide adequate separation of preparation rooms; 3) they have adequate ventilation; 4) they have ample clean hot and cold water and efficient drainage and plumbing; and 5) they have dressing rooms and other facilities for personnel that are accessible without passing through biological product preparation areas. Facilities must be adequate to provide for all applicable production functions, such as: storage of master seeds, ingredients, and other production materials; preparation of growth media and cell cultures; preparation of glassware and production equipment; inoculation, incubation, and harvest of cultures; storage of in-process materials; inactivation, centrifugation, addition of adjuvant, and formulation of product; filling, desiccation, sealing of containers, labelling and storage of final product; quality control testing of in-process materials and final product; and research and development.

Separate areas are generally required for different activities. All rooms and air-handling systems must be constructed so as to prevent cross-contamination from other products and to prevent contamination by people or equipment. Virulent or dangerous microorganisms must be prepared and stored in rooms separate from the remainder of the establishment. In particular, challenge organisms must be completely separated from vaccine strains. All equipment that comes into contact with product must be sterilised using validated procedures.

Production facilities have to be designed in such a way that contamination of the environment is prevented. Any material used during production has to be made safe before leaving the facility. If highly contagious microorganisms are propagated, the exhaust air must be treated to prevent escape of infectious agents. Personnel must follow safety procedures such as showering, and avoid contact with susceptible animals after leaving the production facilities.

Although the quality and design of production facilities may vary significantly, they must always meet standards considered to be appropriate for the vaccines that are to be produced. For example, the requirements for facilities for the production of chicken embryo vaccines administered by oral, intranasal or intraocular routes may not need to be quite as demanding as those for the production of cell culture vaccines administered subcutaneously or intramuscularly.

FACILITIES PLAN

For each vaccine made in a facility, there should be a detailed production plan that describes where each step in the production process will occur. This plan should be documented in a detailed standard operating procedure (SOP) or by a blueprint (building plan) and blueprint legend. Each room in the establishment should be uniquely identified, and all functions performed and all microorganisms involved should be specified for each room. Disinfection procedures, monitoring of equipment and other procedures used in the operation of the facilities to prevent contamination or errors during production should also be documented. This plan should be updated as new products are added to the facility, or other changes or improvements in procedures are developed.

DOCUMENTATION OF THE MANUFACTURING PROCESS

A detailed Outline of Production, a series of SOPs, or other documents should also be prepared to describe the protocol for the manufacture and testing of each product produced in an establishment. Criteria and standards for source materials should be clearly and accurately documented. Documentation should also address such things as: the source, isolation, and passage (subculturing) history of each strain of microorganism; methods for identifying the microorganisms and determining their virulence and purity; the medium or cell culture system used for seed and production cultures, including the methods used to demonstrate that media are free from contamination; the source of ingredients of animal origin; methods of media sterilisation; storage conditions of cell lines and seed cultures; size and types of containers used for growth of cultures; methods for preparing seed cultures and inoculating production cultures; time and conditions for incubation; observations during growth; criteria and specifications for satisfactory harvest material; and harvest techniques. It should also include: a description of all tests conducted to assess the purity and quality of the product as it proceeds through the production process; each step in the formulation of the final product; the tests used for assessing the quality, safety, potency, and other requirements of each batch of completed product; the specifications for finishing, including packaging and labelling with complete indications and recommendations for use; and the expiry date established for the product.

Guidelines for the preparation of such documents for veterinary vaccines are published by competent control authorities. This documentation is intended to define the product and to establish its specifications and standards. It should serve along with the blueprints and blueprint legends (or production plan and SOPs) as a uniform and consistent method of producing the product that should be followed in the preparation of each batch.

RECORD KEEPING

The producer should establish a detailed record-keeping system capable of tracking the performance of successive steps in the preparation of each biological product. Records kept should indicate the date that each essential step was taken, the name of the person who carried out the task, the identity and quantity of ingredients added or removed at each step, and any loss or gain in quantity in the course of the preparation. Records should be maintained of all tests conducted on each batch. All records relevant to a batch of product should be retained for at least 2 years after the expiry date on the label. In addition, a record should be maintained of all labels used on all products, with each label identified as to its name, product number, product licence number, package size, and label identification number. All labels printed should be accounted for. Records must be kept concerning sterilisation and pasteurisation procedures. These are usually made by means of automatic recording devices. The manufacturer must also keep complete records for all animals at the establishment, including results of tests performed, treatment administered, maintenance, necropsy, and disposal.

MASTER SEED

A master seed should be established for each microorganism used in the production of a product to serve as the source of seed for inoculation of all production cultures. Working seeds and production seeds may be prepared from the master seed by subculturing; generally the final production cultures should not be more than five (sometimes ten) passages from the master seed. The number of passages should be determined by data and designated in each case. Using a master seed and limiting the number of passages of seed microorganism in this manner assists in maintaining uniformity and consistency in production. The master seed should consist of a single uniform batch of seed that has been mixed and filled into containers as one batch. Master seed should be frozen or desiccated and stored at low temperatures such as –40°C or –70°C, or under other conditions found to be optimal for maintaining viability. Each master seed should be tested to ensure its identity, safety and efficacy. Purity should also be established by testing to ensure freedom from extraneous bacteria, fungi, mycoplasma, and viruses.

MASTER CELL STOCKS

When cell cultures are used to prepare a product, a master cell stock (MCS) should be established for each type of cell to be used. For each product, the highest and lowest passage levels of cells that may be used for production should be established and specified in the Outline of Production or SOP. Some control authorities do not permit more than 20–40 subcultivations. Each MCS should be characterised to ensure its identity, and its genetic stability should be demonstrated when subcultured from the lowest to the highest passage used for production. Purity of MCSs should be established by testing to ensure freedom from extraneous bacteria, fungi, mycoplasma, and viruses.

• Primary cells

These are defined as a pool of original cells derived from normal tissue up to and including the tenth subculture used in the production of biologicals. In the case of products for use in poultry, these cells are usually obtained from specific pathogen free embryonated chicken eggs that have originated in an unvaccinated flock subjected to intensive microbiological monitoring. Other primary cells are derived from normal tissue of healthy animals and are tested for contamination with a wide variety of microorganisms as appropriate, including bacteria, fungi, mycoplasmas, and cytopathic and/or haemadsorbing agents and other extraneous viruses. Some control authorities only allow the use of primary cells in exceptional cases.

• Embyronating eggs

These are also commonly used in the production of biologicals. In almost all cases they should be derived from specific pathogen free chicken flocks that have been intensively monitored for infectious agents and have not been vaccinated. The route of inoculation of the egg and the choice of egg material to be harvested are dependent on the particular organism that is being propagated.

INGREDIENTS

The specifications and source of all product ingredients should be defined in the Outline of Production, SOP, or other appropriate documents. All ingredients of animal origin that are not subject to sterilisation should also be tested to ensure freedom from extraneous bacteria, fungi, mycoplasma, and viruses. Their country of origin should be known. Some control authorities discourage the use of preservatives or (more importantly) antibiotics as a means of controlling adventitious contamination during production and prefer the use of strict aseptic techniques to ensure purity. However, they sometimes allow the use of preservatives in multidose containers to protect the product during use. These control authorities usually limit any addition of antibiotics in the manufacture of the product to cell culture fluids and other media, egg inocula, and material harvested from skin or possibly other tissues. They normally permit the use of no more than three antibiotics in the same product. Some control authorities also prohibit the use of penicillin or streptomycin in vaccines administered by aerosol or parenterally. If the antibiotics used are not recommended for use in the target species, they should be shown to have no harmful effects in the vaccinated animals and not result in the contamination of food derived from vaccinated animals.

EFFICACY TESTS

The efficacy of veterinary vaccines should be demonstrated by statistically valid vaccination-challenge studies in the host animal, using the youngest animals for which the product is to be recommended. Data should support the efficacy of the vaccine in each animal species by each vaccination regimen that is described in the product label recommendation, including studies on the duration of immunity. The tests should be performed under controlled conditions starting, wherever possible, with seronegative animals. Where validated potency tests are available, target species vaccination-challenge studies may not be required if predictive serological test results are available. The application of procedures to replace, reduce, and refine animal tests (the 'three Rs rule') should be encouraged whenever possible.

Efficacy studies should be conducted with final product vaccine that has been produced at the highest passage level from the master seed that is permitted in the Outline of Production, or other documentation of the manufacturing process. The Outline of Production or other documentation of the manufacturing process for a vaccine specifies the minimum amount of antigen per dose that must be in the final product throughout the entire authorised shelf-life. The antigen level per dose in the vaccine tested for efficacy must be at or below this minimum amount. The precise challenge method and the criteria for determining protection vary with the immunising agent and should be standardised whenever possible.

Field efficacy studies may be used to establish efficacy when meaningful vaccination-challenge studies are not feasible. However, it is generally more difficult to obtain statistically significant data to demonstrate efficacy under field conditions. Protocols for field studies are more complex, and care must be given to establish proper controls to ensure the validity of the data. Even when properly designed, field efficacy studies may be inconclusive because of uncontrollable outside influences. Some problems include: a highly variable level of challenge; a low incidence of disease in nonvaccinated controls; and exposure to other organisms causing a similar disease. Therefore, efficacy data from both laboratory and field studies may be required to establish the efficacy of some products.

INTERFERENCE TESTS

For products with two or more antigenic components, tests must confirm that there is no interference between individual components, that is, one component causing a decrease in the protective immunological response to another component. Interference testing should be conducted for each combination product prior to approval.

A loss of potency may also result when residual inactivating agent in a killed liquid product used as a diluent for a desiccated live fraction reduces the viability of the live organisms because of viricidal or bacteriocidal activity. Each batch of liquid killed vaccine that is to be used as a diluent for live vaccines must, therefore, be tested for viricidal or bacteriocidal activity prior to release.

Consideration must also be given to possible interference between two different vaccines from the same manufacturer recommended to be given to the same animal within a 2-week period.

REVERSION TO VIRULENCE TESTS

With live vaccines, there is concern that the organism might be shed from the host and transmitted to contact animals, causing disease if it retains residual virulence or reverts to virulence. Therefore, all live vaccines should be tested for reversion to virulence by means of passage studies. Vaccine organisms are propagated *in vivo* by inoculating a group of target animals with master seed, usually using the natural route of infection for that organism. The vaccine organism is recovered from tissues or excretions and is used directly to inoculate a further group of animals, and so on. After the fifth passage (more for poultry products), the isolate must be fully characterised, using the same procedures used to characterise the master seed. The vaccine organism must retain an acceptable level of attenuation after propagation in this way.

ASSESSING RISK TO THE ENVIRONMENT

The ability of each live vaccine to shed, to spread to contact target and nontarget animals, and to persist in the environment must be evaluated to provide information for assessing the risk of the vaccine to the environment.

In some cases this may be done in conjunction with the reversion to virulence tests.

CONSISTENCY OF PRODUCTION

Prior to marketing approval of any new product, each establishment should produce in its facilities three consecutive production batches of completed product to evaluate the consistency of production. These batches should be prepared according to the procedures described in the Outline of Production and blueprints and legends, SOPs or other documentation of the manufacturing process. The size of each of the three batches should be at least one-third the size of the average batch that will be produced once the product is in production.

The manufacturer should test each of these batches for quality, safety, and potency as provided in the Outline of Production or other documentation of the manufacturing process. Applicable Standard Requirements and test procedures, for example those described in CFR (Code of Federal Regulations) Title 9 part 113, in EU Directive 92/18/EEC, in the European Pharmacopoeia, or as described in this *Manual* may be used. Satisfactory test results should be demonstrated for all three batches prior to approving the production of the product in the facilities and its release for marketing. Each subsequent batch should be tested in the same manner with satisfactory results prior to release for marketing.

POTENCY TESTS

Potency tests, required for each batch prior to release, are designed to correlate with the host animal vaccination-challenge efficacy studies. For inactivated viral or bacterial products, potency tests may be conducted in laboratory or host animals, or by means of quantitative *in vitro* methods. The potency of live vaccines is generally measured by means of bacterial counts or virus titration.

When testing a live bacterial vaccine for release for marketing, the bacterial count must be sufficiently greater than that shown to be protective in the master seed immunogenicity (efficacy) test to ensure that at any time prior to the expiry date, the count will be at least equal to that used in the immunogenicity test. When testing a live viral vaccine for release, the virus titre must, as a rule, be sufficiently greater than that shown to be protective in the master seed immunogenicity test in order to ensure that at any time prior to the expiry date, the titre will be at least equal to that used in the immunogenicity test. Some control authorities specify higher bacterial or viral content than these. It is evident that the appropriate release titre is primarily dependent on the required potency and secondarily dependent on the rate of decay of the bacteria or viruses in the vaccine, as indicated by the stability test.

Standard Requirements have been developed and published by competent authorities for potency testing several vaccines. These tests can be found in CFR Title 9 part 113, in the European Pharmacopoeia, and in this *Manual.*

STABILITY TESTS

Stability studies (based on an acceptable potency test) are required to establish the validity of the expiry date that appears on the product package. For estimating stability to determine a provisional expiry date, a new product may be subjected to accelerated stability tests, e.g. incubating at 37°C for 1 week for each year of dating. Such estimates must be confirmed by periodic real-time potency tests on at least three different batches through the period of time indicated by the expiry date, and 3–6 months beyond. For products containing viable organisms, testing should be done at release and at the approximate expiry date until a statistically valid record has been established. For nonviable products, each batch presented for licensing is tested at release and at, or after, the requested expiry date. Some authorities also require an intermediate test. If at the end of the dating period (shelf life) specified, the product is tested and found still to be above the release quality, consideration can be given to extending the designated shelf life, by request to the control authority. Stability testing also provides the opportunity to test for residual moisture and for other important parameters, such as the stability of adjuvant emulsions.

SAFETY TESTS

The intrinsic safety of a vaccine should be demonstrated early in the development stage, using the master seed virus (MSV). These studies should include the safety of a single dose, of an overdose and of repeated single doses. Safety tests for release of a batch are described in CFR Title 9 part 113, in the European Pharmacopoeia, in this *Manual* and elsewhere. Standard procedures are given for mouse, guinea-pig, cat, dog, horse, pig, and sheep safety tests. Products may require more than one type of safety test. The required safety test for a poultry product is described in the specific Standard Requirement or the Outline of Production for that product. As a general rule, overdose studies are required for all vaccines: ×10 for live and ×2 for inactivated vaccines (if this is not practical, an indication of safety may be obtained from the results of the potency tests).

For inactivated virus products, where host animals are used for potency testing, safety may be determined by daily observation of the vaccinates during the prechallenge period of the potency tests. Further evidence concerning the safety of products is derived from reversion to virulence studies on modified live products (discussed above) and from field safety trials (discussed below), but these tests are not required for each batch.

PURITY TESTS

Purity is determined by testing for a variety of contaminants. Tests to detect contaminants are performed on: master seeds, primary cells, MCSs, ingredients of animal origin if not subjected to sterilisation (e.g. fetal bovine serum, bovine albumin, or trypsin), and each batch of final product prior to release.

Purity test procedures have been published, for example in CFR Title 9 part 113, in EU Directive 92/18/EEC, in the European Pharmacopoeia, or in this *Manual,* for the detection of extraneous viruses, bacteria, mycoplasma and fungi, including for example: *Salmonella, Brucella,* chlamydial agents, haemagglutinating viruses, avian lymphoid leukosis, pathogens detected by a chicken inoculation test, pathogens detected by a chicken embryo inoculation test, lymphocytic choriomeningitis, cytopathic and haemadsorbing agents, and pathogens detected by enzyme-linked immunosorbent assay, polymerase chain reaction, or the fluorescent antibody technique. Tests to be used vary with the nature of the product, and should be prescribed in the Outline of Production or other documentation of the manufacturing process.

OTHER TESTS

Depending on the form of vaccine being produced, certain tests may be indicated and should be provided as appropriate in the Outline of Production or other documentation of the manufacturing process. These tests may concern: the level of moisture contained in desiccated products, the level of residual inactivant in killed products, the complete inactivation of killed products, pH, the level of preservatives and permitted antibiotics, physical stability of adjuvants, retention of vacuum in desiccated products, and a general physical examination of the final vaccine. Tests for these purposes may also be found in CFR Title 9 part 113, in EU Directive 92/18/EEC, in the European Pharmacopoeia, or in this *Manual.*

SAMPLING

Samples should be selected from each batch of product. The selector should pick representative final containers from each batch and store these samples at the storage temperature recommended on the label. The producer should keep these reserve samples at the recommended storage temperature for 6 months after the expiry date shown on the label, so that they are available to assist in evaluating the cause of any field problems reported from the use of the vaccine.

LABELLING

Standards for labelling products will vary from country to country; however, the label indications and all claims that are made on the label should be supported by appropriate data that have been reviewed and approved by competent authorities. It is recommended that all labels for veterinary vaccines contain the following information, although for very small containers, the label may instead refer to the carton label or to an enclosed package insert for some of the less prominent information:

1. The true name of the product, prominently lettered and with equal emphasis on each word;
2. The name and address of the producer (and also the importer for imported products);
3. The recommended storage temperature;
4. A statement that the product is 'for veterinary (or animal) use only'. Full instructions for use, including all required warnings;
5. For food animals, a statement indicating that the animals should not be vaccinated within a specified number of day before slaughter. This will depend on the vaccine (e.g. type of adjuvant) and is not required for all products;
6. The expiry date;
7. The batch number by which to identify the product in the producer's record of preparation, and its licence number;
8. The recoverable quantity and number of doses;
9. A statement that the entire contents of a multidose container should be used when the container is first opened (or with appropriate holding time for certain products, as supported by data) and that any unused portions should be disposed of in a proper manner;
10. A safety warning to the operator, if appropriate, e.g. accidental self-injection with oil emulsion vaccines.

Labels may also include other factual statements that are not false or misleading. Special restrictions concerning the use or handling of the product, when applicable, should also be indicated.

Similar information should also be given in a Product Data Sheet that is provided as a package insert. This will also contain much more detail about method of use and possible adverse reactions.

FIELD TESTS (SAFETY AND EFFICACY)

All veterinary biological products administered to animals should be tested for safety and, if possible, for efficacy in the field, using good clinical practice, before being authorised for general use. Field studies are designed to demonstrate efficacy under working conditions and to detect unexpected reactions, including mortality, that may not have been observed during the development of the product. Under field conditions there are many uncontrollable variables that make it difficult to obtain good efficacy data, but demonstration of safety is more reliable. The tests should be done on the host animal, at a variety of geographical locations, using large numbers of susceptible animals. The test animals should represent all the ages and husbandry practices for which the product is indicated; unvaccinated controls must be included. The product tested should be one or more production batches. A protocol should be developed indicating the observation methods and the recording methods.

INSPECTION OF PRODUCTION FACILITIES

Establishments that are approved to produce veterinary biologicals should be subject to in-depth inspections of the entire premises by national competent authorities to ensure compliance with the Outline of Production and blueprints and legends, SOPs, or other documentation of the manufacturing process. These inspections may include such items as: personnel qualifications; record keeping; general sanitation and laboratory standards; research activities on products being developed; production procedures; operation of sterilisers, pasteurisers, incubators, and refrigerators; filling, desiccating, and finishing procedures; care and control of animals; testing procedures; distribution and marketing; and product destruction. It is desirable to have good manufacturing practice (for manufacturing) and good laboratory practice (for quality assurance testing). (See chapter I.2. for guidelines.)

The inspectors should prepare a comprehensive report documenting the findings of the inspection and stating the actions that the establishment must take to improve its production processes. The establishment should receive a copy of the report. When necessary a follow-up inspection should be conducted to determine whether appropriate action has been taken to correct deficiencies. Continued reassessment in this manner is needed to ensure that production facilities continue to be operated in an acceptable manner. Periodic inspections also encourage continual improvements in production procedures and facilities that are consistent with advances in technology.

TESTING PRIOR TO RELEASE FOR DISTRIBUTION

Prior to release, the manufacturer must test each batch for quality, safety, and potency, as well as perform any other tests described in the firm's Outline of Production or other documentation of the manufacturing process for that product. In countries that have national regulatory programmes that include check testing final product, samples of each batch should also be submitted for testing in government laboratories by competent authorities. If unsatisfactory results are obtained for tests conducted either by the firm or by competent authorities, the batch should not be released. In such cases, subsequent batches of the product should be given priority for check testing by competent authorities.

UPDATING THE OUTLINE OF PRODUCTION

Before production procedures are changed, the corresponding Outline of Production or other documentation of the manufacturing process should be changed. Establishments should have internal review procedures to evaluate all changes in production before they are initiated. Changes should also be reviewed and approved by competent authorities prior to their implementation. In cases where a significant production step is altered, revisions may require additional data to support the purity, safety, potency, and/or efficacy of the product. In countries with regulatory programmes that include check testing the final product at national laboratories, revisions should entail testing of the new product by competent authorities.

PERFORMANCE MONITORING

Manufacturers must be required to maintain an adverse reaction notification system and an effective mechanism for rapid product recall. These should both be subject to audit by regulatory bodies. The manufacturer must notify all adverse reactions immediately to the regulatory authority, along with any remedial action taken.

After release of a product, its performance under field conditions should continue to be monitored by competent authorities. Consumer complaints may serve as one source of information; however, such information needs to be investigated to determine whether or not the reported observations are related to the use of the product. Users of veterinary vaccines should be informed of the proper procedures for making their complaints. The manufacturer of the product should be informed of all complaints received by competent authorities. Competent authorities should also ascertain whether they have received other similar complaints for this product and, if so, whether the manufacturer has taken appropriate action. Control laboratories may test samples of the batch of product involved, if necessary.

When the investigation is complete, a final report should be prepared and a summary of the findings sent to the complainant and to the manufacturer. When it is determined that a product is causing serious problems, quick action should be taken to remove the product from the market and to notify animal health authorities.

ENFORCEMENT

National programmes established to ensure the quality, safety, potency, and efficacy of veterinary vaccines must have adequate legal authority to ensure compliance with product registration conditions and other programme requirements. The goal should be to obtain voluntary compliance with established regulatory requirements. However, when violations occur, competent authorities must have adequate legal authority to protect animal health. Authority for detention, seizure, and condemnation of products found to be worthless, contaminated, dangerous, or harmful may be valuable for this purpose. Under such authority, product may be detained for a period of time, and if during that time compliance cannot be achieved, competent authorities may seek a court order or decree for seizure and condemnation.

The authority to remove or suspend establishment and/or product licenses, obtain injunctions, and stop the sale of product are also needed. Civil penalties or criminal prosecution may also be necessary for serious or deliberate violations.

LICENSING OF PRODUCTS DERIVED THROUGH BIOTECHNOLOGY

Recent advances in biotechnology have made possible the development and commercialisation of new biological products with useful antigenic and diagnostic properties. Many such products have now been licensed or approved, and more are being developed. Products of rDNA technology do not differ fundamentally from conventional products. Therefore, existing laws and regulations are fully applicable to these new products.

CLASSIFICATION OF BIOTECHNOLOGY-DERIVED VACCINES

Each competent authority with power to regulate organisms and products derived from recombinant techniques should ensure that the public health and the environment are protected from any potentially harmful effects. For the purpose of evaluating licence applications, veterinary vaccines derived through rDNA technology may be divided into three broad categories. The division is based on the products' biological properties and on the safety concerns they present.

Category I consists of nonviable or killed products that pose no risk to the environment and present no new or unusual safety concerns. Such products include inactivated microorganisms, either whole or as subunits, created by using rDNA techniques.

Category II products contain live microorganisms modified by adding or deleting one or more gene(s). Added genes may code for marker antigens, enzymes, or other biochemical by-products. Deleted genes may code for virulence, oncogenicity, marker antigens, enzymes, or other biochemical by-products. The licence application must include a characterisation of the DNA segments added or deleted, as well as a phenotypic characterisation of the altered organism. The genetic modifications must not result in any increase in virulence, pathogenicity, or survivability in the altered organism in comparison with the wild-type form. It is important that the genetic modification does not cause a deterioration in the safety characteristics of the organism.

Category III products make use of live vectors to carry recombinant-derived foreign genes that code for immunising antigens. Live vectors may carry one or more foreign gene(s) that have been shown to be effective for immunising target host animals. The use of DNA vaccines containing recombinant-derived foreign genes that code for immunising antigens (plasmid DNA vaccines) constitutes a new approach to vaccine development. The proper categorisation of this type of rDNA-derived product will be established as biological properties and safety characteristics are determined. These new vaccines may find application in a wide variety of situations much as conventional products have. Guidelines for the development, production, characterisation, and control of these new products are still preliminary and subject to change as new data and knowledge are developed. Information concerning the current thinking on regulatory guidelines for plasmid DNA vaccines may be found on the Internet at the following addresses: http://www.fda.gov/cber/points.htm; http://www.cba.unige.it/VL/bio-info.html; http://www.orcbs.msu.edu/biological/biolsaf.htm; http://www.pestlaw.com/index.html.

RELEASE OF LIVE rDNA PRODUCTS

The release of live rDNA and plasmid DNA vaccines (Categories II and III) for field testing or general distributions as an approved or licensed product may have a significant effect on the quality of the human environment. Before release is authorised, the manufacturers of the vaccine should conduct a risk assessment to evaluate the impact on the human environment. In the USA, for example, a procedure is adopted that could be used as a model system in other countries. It is performed as follows:

A risk assessment is carried out that should contain the following information: the purpose and need for the proposed action; the alternatives considered; a list of the government agencies, organisations, and persons consulted; and the affected environment and the potential environmental consequences. The topics discussed should include: the characteristics of the vaccine organism, human health risks, animal health risks for both target and nontarget animals, persistence in the environment, and reversion to virulence.

If the risk assessment results in a finding by competent authorities that the proposed release of the recombinant vaccine into the environment for field trials or general distribution would not have a significant impact on the environment, a notice should be published and distributed to the public announcing this and that the risk assessment and findings are available for public review and comment. If no substantive comments are received to refute the findings, competent authorities may authorise the field testing or grant the license or approval for general distribution.

The preparation of a risk assessment and the findings made from the assessment may also include the scheduling of one or more public meetings if a proposed action has ecological or public health significance. Such meetings should be announced through a public notice. Interested persons should be invited to make presentations, along with presentations by the producer of the product, and government personnel. The transcripts of such meetings should become part of the public record.

If, in the course of preparing a risk assessment, competent authorities conclude that the proposed action may have a significant effect on the human environment, an Environmental Impact Statement (EIS) should be prepared. The EIS provides a full and fair discussion of the significant environmental impacts, and informs decision-makers and the public of any reasonable alternatives that would avoid or minimise the adverse impacts. (Environmental documents are considered in CFR Title 40 part 1508.) See also EU Directives 90/219/EEC and 90/220/EEC.

FURTHER READING

The following are some suggested texts that contain guidelines on aspects of vaccine production.

A. COMMISSION OF THE EUROPEAN COMMUNITIES (1999) The Rules Governing Medicinal Products in the European Union. Eudralex. Volumes IV–IX. Office Publications of the European Communities, 1999, Luxembourg. See also EU Directives: 90/219/EEC 90/220/EEC and 92/18/EEC.

B. COUNCIL OF EUROPE (1997). European Pharmacopoeia, Third edition. Editions of the Council of Europe, Strasbourg, France.

C. ESPESETH D.A. (1993). Licensing Veterinary Biologics in the United States. The First Steps Towards an International Harmonization of Veterinary Biologicals; and Free circulation of vaccines within the EEC. *Dev. Biol. Stand.*, **79**, 17–25.

D. ESPESETH D.A. & GOODMAN J.B. (1993). Chapter 13. *In:* Licensing and Regulation in the USA. Vaccines for Veterinary Application. Butterworth Heinemann, London, UK, 321–342.

E. GAY C.G. & ROTH H.J. (1994). Confirming the safety characteristics of recombinant vectors used in veterinary medicine: a regulatory perspective. Recombinant vectors in vaccine development. *Dev. Biol. Stand.*, **82**, 93–105.

F. ROTH H.J. & GAY C.G. (1996). Specific safety requirements for products derived from biotechnology. *In:* Veterinary Vaccinology, Pastoret P.-P., Blancou J., Vannier P. & Verschueren C., eds. Elseviers Science Publishers B.V. Amsterdam, The Netherlands.

G. UNITED STATES DEPARTMENT OF AGRICULTURE (USDA) (1998). Code Of Federal Regulations, Title 9, Parts 1–199. US Government Printing Office, Washington D.C., USA.

H. USDA-APHIS[1]-CENTER FOR VETERINARY BIOLOGICS (1984). Basic License Requirements for Applicants. Veterinary Biologics Memorandum No. 800.50. USDA-APHIS-Veterinary Biologics, 4700 River Road, Riverdale, MD 20737, USA.

I. USDA-APHIS-VETERINARY BIOLOGICS (1995). Guidelines for Submission of Materials in Support of Licensure. Veterinary Biologics Memorandum No. 800.84. USDA-APHIS-Veterinary Biologics, 4700 River Road, Riverdale, MD 20737, USA.

J. USDA-APHIS-VETERINARY BIOLOGICS (1995). Veterinary Biologics General Licensing Considerations No. 800.200, Efficacy Studies. USDA-APHIS-Veterinary Biologics, 4700 River Road, Riverdale, MD 20737, USA.

K. USDA-APHIS-VETERINARY BIOLOGICS (1995). Veterinary Biologics General Licensing Considerations No. 800.201, Back passage studies. USDA-APHIS-Veterinary Biologics, 4700 River Road, Riverdale, MD 20737, USA.

L. USDA-APHIS-VETERINARY SERVICES (1964–1994). Standard Assay Methods, Series 100–900. National Veterinary Services Laboratories, Ames, IA 50010, USA.

*

* *

1 United States Department of Agriculture (USDA), Animal and Plant Health Inspection Services (APHIS). USDA-APHIS-CENTER FOR VETERINARY BIOLOGICS HOME PAGE: http://www.aphis.usda.gov/vs/cvb/index.html

CHAPTER I.1.7.

BIOTECHNOLOGY IN THE DIAGNOSIS OF INFECTIOUS DISEASES AND VACCINE DEVELOPMENT

INTRODUCTION

Molecular biological methods have become increasingly applicable to the diagnosis of infectious disease and vaccine development. To become widely used the methods need to be easy, safe, sensitive, reproducible and eventually automated to facilitate the evaluation of large numbers of samples.

The purpose of this chapter is to provide general background information for the nonspecialist. Two issues of the OIE Scientific and Technical Review *are concerned with biotechnology and the diagnosis of animal disease, and may be consulted for a more detailed review (38, 39). The following is an outline of the topics briefly reviewed in this chapter.*

A. Detection of genome nucleic acids
1. Diagnosis by restriction fragment length polymorphisms
2. Polymerase chain reaction
3. Diagnosis by DNA probes

B. Detection of protein
1. Immunohistochemistry
2. Immunoblotting
3. Antigen-capture enzyme-linked immunosorbent assay (ELISA) (monoclonal-antibody-capture ELISA)

C. Antibody detection
1. Competitive ELISA (Blocking ELISA)
2. Production of antigens by recombinant DNA technology

D. Vaccines
1. Gene-deletion vaccines
2. Marker vaccines
3. Virus-vectored vaccines
4. DNA vaccines
5. New developments in vaccine technology

A. DETECTION OF GENOME NUCLEIC ACIDS

1. Diagnosis by restriction fragment length polymorphisms

The commonly employed serological tests to identify microorganisms are sometimes not sufficiently discriminatory to distinguish closely related bacterial or viral isolates. Restriction fragment length polymorphism analysis can detect differences in the genomes of closely related microbial species. If it is desired to map the genome of a microorganism, the DNA is extracted and enzymatically cleaved into fragments of specific nucleotide sequences with restriction endonucleases. The resultant DNA fragments are then separated in agarose gel by electrophoresis and stained with ethidium bromide. The resulting gel provides restriction fragment sizes that can be mapped; each strain exhibits a specific map, frequently referred to as a restriction fragment length polymorphism (RFLP), which may or may not differ from that of other strains. Selection of appropriate restriction enzymes may allow differentiation of different strains or different isolates. The fragments can be hybridised with a labelled probe to investigate further the differences or similarities in the genomes.

The RFLP analysis may be used, for example, in epidemiological studies. In this instance it might be employed to investigate the differences or similarities in the genomes of several closely related bacterial or viral isolates. In this way the involvement of a particular isolate in a disease outbreak can be defined and the epidemiological tracing of isolates within a country or between countries should be possible. Epidemiological investigations using RFLP analysis of Aujeszky's disease virus isolates shed light on the direct and indirect origin of the field isolates in Hungary (29). RFLP analysis was used by Holmberg *et. al* (14) to trace antibiotic-resistant *Salmonella newport* of animal origin to people who were seriously ill, particularly people on antibiotic therapy. Regional variants of the rabies virus in Canada were identified by RFLP analysis (after prior reverse transcription to DNA), demonstrating consistent differences in the viruses from distinct geographical regions (36).

Except for use in epidemiological studies, the potential diagnostic value of RFLPs is not clear. The diagnostic use or other interpretation of RFLP data involves the construction of databases where RFLP profiles are linked to factors such as virulence, host range and clinical significance. In practice it is usual not to rely on one restriction site but to use sites from several genes to classify the isolate. A question that veterinary diagnosticians will have to confront in the future will be: What level of difference between virus isolates or between bacterial isolates is significant? RFLP analysis can detect single base-pair substitutions in DNA based on the loss or acquisition of a restriction endonuclease site. However, the loss or acquisition of restriction endonuclease site(s) is not necessarily associated with differences in the ability of the viruses or bacteria to cause disease so the difference detected by RFLPs may not be significant, except as a distinguishing feature. Differences in DNA structure may not be reflected in differences in RFLP. If differences do not result in changes in restriction endonuclease site(s) and do not result in detectable changes in length of fragments, isolate differences may not be detected by this method, particularly if the changes do not affect the ability of the cDNA to hybridise with the target fragment. Also changes in the nucleotide sequence may be outside the site recognised by the restriction enzyme that has been used and therefore will not be detected. This method is suited to organisms that are easy to culture, but less practical for organisms such as *Cryptosporidium* where *in-vitro* culture is not available.

2. Polymerase chain reaction

The polymerase chain reaction (PCR) procedure exploits natural DNA replication, producing, *in vitro*, large quantities of a desired sequence of DNA from a complex mixture of heterogeneous sequences (9, 47). PCR can amplify copies of a selected region of 50 to several thousand base pairs into millions of copies.

The amplification of DNA by the PCR is accomplished via a cyclic succession of incubation steps at different temperatures. The target DNA is heat-denatured to separate the two complementary strands to provide a template. Specific primers (short synthetic molecules of DNA complementary to both strands of the DNA flanking the target sequences) are then annealed to the single-stranded template at low temperature and extended with DNA polymerase at an intermediate temperature. Once the polymerase has synthesised a new strand of DNA, the product is separated from the template by heating to a higher temperature. These steps, referred to as cycles, are repeated 20–40 times, yielding amplification of target DNA sequences. The key to geometric amplification of target DNA sequences by the PCR is selection of paired primers that, when extended, will create additional reciprocal primer-annealing sites for primer extension in subsequent cycles. An example is given in Chapter 2.1.12. African swine fever. A detailed discussion on the methodology and applications of PCR is given in reference 34.

With RNA viruses, a complementary DNA (cDNA) copy of the RNA must first be made using reverse transcriptase (RT), then the PCR can be used for amplification. This technique, referred to as RT-PCR, is used to detect RNA viruses. An example is given in Chapter 2.1.4. Rinderpest.

The PCR product has a characteristic size and its identity is generally confirmed using DNA probes (see below) or restriction (enzyme or endonuclease) digests. The advent of automated cycle sequencing techniques has allowed for rapid and detailed characterisation of PCR products. Such techniques have been used in the virulence typing of avian influenza A virus, in which virulence-associated structural motifs at the haemagglutinin (HA) gene cleavage site have been shown to be reliable indicators of high pathogenicity in chickens (15). The sensitivity of PCR may be enhanced by the use of a second set of primers to amplify a subfragment from the PCR product of the first reaction. This increases the sensitivity of the procedure, and is commonly referred to as 'nested PCR'. The nested PCR is a test to detect low levels of *Anaplasma marginale* in persistently infected cattle (7). However, some investigators have found that the use of nested PCR increased the rate of false-positive results.

PCR is a highly sensitive procedure for detecting infectious agents in host tissues and vectors, even when only a small number of host cells are infected. It does not differentiate between viable and nonviable organisms. PCR can target and amplify a gene sequence that has become integrated into the DNA of infected host cells. It can also target and amplify unintegrated viral gene sequences. It is clear that PCR may have a role in the testing of vaccines to detect contamination. However, the ability to detect nonviable agents as well as incomplete pieces of genomic DNA may complicate interpretation of results and affect the applicability of PCR in this role.

The PCR may prove to be very useful in the diagnosis of chronic-persistent infections such as those caused by retroviruses (bovine leukaemia virus, caprine arthritis/encephalitis virus, etc.) and latent infections caused by herpesviruses (e.g. infectious bovine rhinotracheitis and Aujeszky's disease). These diseases present serious problems in terms of diagnosis and prevention as infected animals often do not demonstrate clinical signs until there is advanced disease, and infected animals appear to be a constant potential source for transmission.

When PCR is used for diagnosis, a great deal of care is required to avoid contamination of the samples because the exquisite sensitivity of PCR can easily lead to false-positive results. Some multicentre studies have shown that positive samples are detected consistently between laboratories, but that with known negative samples, several false positives are frequently obtained, indicating the continuing presence of contamination problems (49). Systems have been developed to deal with this problem, for example the uDTP-UNG system (d-uracil triphosphate and uracil-N-glycosylase), and kits are available (Perkin Elmer). This system uses an enzymatic reaction to specifically degrade PCR products from previous PCR amplification (in which uDTP has been incorporated) without degrading native nucleic acid templates (4). This, of course, does not deal with contamination of the sample with extraneous virus. A new generation of robotic workstations is now available where PCR reactions may be set up with only a single tube open at any one time. This greatly reduces the risk of contamination. It is also important to control for potential 'negative' results caused by the presence of interfering substances in the PCR reaction mixture or patient's sample by the inclusion of a template that is known to produce a PCR product (4). Use of these precautions will allow the PCR to become a realistic option for the diagnostician.

3. Diagnosis by DNA probes

Probes used alone may not be very sensitive. The use of DNA hybridisation procedures when combined with PCR provides a powerful tool in the diagnosis of protozoal, bacterial and viral diseases through the use of highly conserved DNA sequences. DNA probes can exhibit remarkable specificity (45). Two examples can be given. *Anaplasma marginale* was detected in infected tick vectors using cloned DNA probes (11); and *Babesia equi* was identified in red blood cells of experimentally infected horses by hybridisation to *B. equi* (43). Alternatively, DNA probes may be designed to cross-react with a range of organisms.

To make a probe, which is usually based on a cloned segment of the genome of the particular pathogen, DNA is heated or treated chemically until the two strands separate. Each strand will recognise and bind to a strand of DNA that has complementary nucleotide bases. A DNA probe will 'search' for the complementary nucleotide sequence of the pathogen. To determine whether binding (hybridisation) has occurred, the single strand of the DNA was traditionally labelled with radioactive ^{32}P, but now it is more usual to use a chemiluminescent detectable marker. Nonradioactive labels are safer and have now replaced ^{32}P in most diagnostic applications.

Denatured DNA is freed from clinical samples (blood, saliva, urine, exudates) and applied to a solid support system such as nylon or nitrocellulose membranes. If the DNA sequence of the probe and the target DNA of the clinical sample are complementary, they will hybridise. After washing to move the unbound probe, the membrane is placed in contact with X-ray film. The X-ray film is then examined for the presence of the radioactive ^{32}P label of the probe. The sample is positive for the pathogen if the label is detected. If the specimen is negative, the labelled probe will not bind to the sample and will be washed away in the procedure. Although radioactive probes are very sensitive, they have some disadvantages. The ^{32}P isotope has a short half-life and is a radiation hazard.

To facilitate the practical use of DNA probes, sensitive long shelf-life nonradiolabelled tags have been developed and these are replacing radioactive labels. There are probes that use the tenacious attraction between biotin and avidin or streptavidin. In this instance, the DNA probe is labelled with biotin and is detected by streptavidin that is linked to horseradish peroxidase or alkaline phosphate, both of which yield conspicuous colour in the presence of their substrates and can be assayed. These systems can also be used with chemiluminescent substrates that use X-ray film for detection and a permanent record. Such nonradioactive probes have a long shelf-life, and the assay time can be reduced to a couple of hours, whereas the radiolabelling procedure may require an overnight radiograph. Some investigators using biotinylated probes have encountered sensitivity problems.

B. DETECTION OF PROTEIN

1. Immunohistochemistry

As an adjunct to the isolation of causative organisms from tissue, immunohistochemistry is rapidly becoming a standard tool in diagnostic laboratories for the identification of antigens associated with viral, bacterial and protozoal microorganisms. Immunohistochemistry is used for the demonstration of prion proteins (PrP) in the lymphoid tissue of the nictitating membrane for the preclinical diagnosis of scrapie (40). It is also used for the detection of prion protein in brain tissue to confirm bovine spongiform encephalopathy and other transmissible spongiform encephalopathies. The detection of antigens in fixed tissues offers a number of advantages over other diagnostic techniques. These advantages are: (a) convenience of sample submission; (b) safe handling of potential human pathogens; (c) retrospective studies of stored specimens are possible; (d) the technique is rapid; and (e) immunohistochemistry allows the detection of nonviable organisms (12). As the number of monoclonal antibodies (MAbs) to defined antigens increases, the use of immunohistochemistry for the identification of organisms and other specific markers for autoimmunity and neoplasia will increase. The limiting step in the process of immunohistochemistry is identifying a MAb/antigen combination that will bind in formalin-fixed tissues. This may be overcome by using frozen sections or employing antigen retrieval techniques (e.g. proteolytic enzyme digestion, microwaving) before immunostaining.

2. Immunoblotting

Immunoblotting is often the first step in identifying immunodominant proteins recognised in antibodies from infected animals. Proteins are detected with a polyclonal or a MAb after separation, for example, by sodium dodecyl sulphate/polyacrylamide gel electrophoresis (SDS/PAGE) and transfer on to nitrocellulose paper. After incubation with an antibody, the protein bands (immune complexes) are visualised with peroxidase-conjugated anti-species detection antisera and a colour reagent. A colour develops in the bands where antibody binds to the antigen. Immunoblotting is performed chiefly in diagnostic laboratories to identify and/or characterise infectious agents based on antigen specificity or to use known antigens to look for a specific serological response. False-positive and false-negative results in other diagnostic assays can often be resolved by immunoblotting (33). SDS/PAGE is particularly useful for resolving interpretation of samples tested with techniques of low specificity. In some applications, monospecific polyclonal antibodies are preferable to MAbs. When using SDS/PAGE or reducing conditions, the user has to be aware that diagnostic epitopes may be denatured.

3. Antigen-capture enzyme-linked immunosorbent assay

The antigen-capture enzyme-linked immunosorbent assay (ELISA) facilitates detection of antigen from pathogens directly from an animal prior to or during clinical disease. The main component of the antigen-capture ELISA is a specific MAb, although polyclonal antibodies can also be used effectively for antigen capture. Antigens from the test sample are first captured by a specific MAb or polyclonal antibody bound to a solid-phase support and their presence is detected through the use of a second radio- or enzyme-labelled MAb or polyclonal antibody. The desired characteristics of the capture MAb are strong binding to the pathogen, recognition of a conserved epitope highly specific for the target agent and the ability to attach to an ELISA plate without loss of reactivity. In addition, a second MAb recognising an epitope other than that recognised by the capture MAb that is bound to the ELISA plate is often used as part of the indicator system. Examples of antigen-capture ELISAs are the system for detection of *Anaplasma marginale* in the blood of preclinical cattle (52), the use of antigen-capture ELISA on cattle blood samples for the detection of BVD virus (48), and the rapid detection of rinderpest and peste des petits ruminants virus antigens in clinical samples (27). Respiratory syncytial antigen in nasal secretions was captured using ELISA with MAbs directed against epitopes of the viral capsid (37). Related antigen-capture methods using immunomagnetic beads are now important and well accepted methods for detecting certain bacterial infections, including *Listeria, Salmonella,* and *Escherichia coli.*

Immuno-PCR is a promising method for detection of antigen that combines the principles of ELISA diagnostics with the amplification power of PCR. This involves the conjugation of a DNA fragment (as opposed to enzymes used in traditional ELISAs) to the antibody, which then, in the presence of the appropriate antigen, undergoes subsequent amplification by PCR for the purposes of detection. Several studies have shown this procedure to increase the sensitivity of ELISA techniques significantly, by as much as tenfold in the case of BHV-1 (35).

C. ANTIBODY DETECTION

This section is concerned with infectious diseases where antibodies are produced and can be detected. There are, of course, infections such as tuberculosis and leishmaniosis that do not usually generate a sufficient antibody response. In such cases the organisms themselves or cell-mediated reactions/products must be detected.

1. Competitive enzyme-linked immunosorbent assay

The competitive ELISA (blocking ELISA) was first described for use in detecting anti-bluetongue virus antibody (1). The competitive ELISA has largely replaced the indirect ELISA and the virus neutralisation test for serological studies following rinderpest vaccination campaigns. The procedure has been used in the screening of large numbers of pig sera for classical swine fever antibodies (54). Competitive ELISA detected malignant catarrhal fever virus antibody in inapparently infected sheep, deer and bison (26), and anti-*Babesia equi* and *B. caballi* antibodies in persistently infected horses (18, 24). Recently the procedure was employed to detect persistent *Anaplasma marginale,* suggesting its use in epidemiological studies and eradication programmes (7, 23).

Components of the competitive ELISA include an MAb or polyclonal monospecific antiserum and the corresponding epitope. The MAb must possess an appropriate binding affinity such that polyclonal antibody can replace it in the competitive reaction. Desirable epitope characteristics include a linear peptide composition, immunodominance, and conservation among isolates. The latter is an important characteristic in cases where production of the epitope by molecular cloning and expression is required. As the specificity of the competitive ELISA depends entirely on the antibody used, the competitive ELISA is well suited for use with recombinant antigens. If the recombinant antigen is expressed in sufficient quantity to provide an appropriate signal:noise ratio after application to the ELISA plate as a bacterial lysate, additional purification of the recombinant antigen is not necessary.

In summary, MAb-based ELISAs have tremendous potential for use in the diagnosis of infectious diseases of animals. The antigen-capture ELISA can directly detect the presence of pathogens during the clinical stages of disease when treatment is most efficacious, and the competitive ELISA format can be used to detect carriers of persistent infections and animals previously exposed or immune to disease. A very important attribute of the competitive ELISA is the ease with which it can be used with recombinant antigens. This is especially important in those diseases for which diagnostic antigen cannot yet be produced in cell culture. Furthermore, the production of recombinant antigen in *Eschericha coli* or in eukaryotic or yeast expression systems, precludes the need to infect animals for antigen production when *in-vitro* culture systems are not available.

2. Production of antigens by recombinant DNA technology

A problem that is encountered using some current diagnostic tests is that the test antigens must be continuously produced from cell culture or harvested from an infected animal. These antigen preparations are expensive, often have a short shelf-life, need to be standardised with each new batch, and potentially contain additional antigens that may be recognised by animals immunised with vaccines prepared from cell culture systems and may cause false-positive results. Production of antigens for diagnostic tests by molecular cloning potentially overcomes these problems, as does the use of competition for a particular epitope. Furthermore, when recombinant antigens are used in combination with the competitive ELISA format, purification of the recombinant antigen from the lysate may not be necessary as the specificity of the competitive ELISA resides mainly in the MAb used. An example of the procedure is the cloning of the envelope genes of caprine arthritis/encephalitis lentivirus in a vaccinia expression vector (28). Recombinant baculoviruses have been employed to produce bluetongue virus proteins for immunisation (42).

A general procedure for the preparation of an antigen by recombinant DNA technology is as follows. An antigen of potential diagnostic significance is identified by studying the antibody response of the host to the proteins of the organism in question. For example, immunodominant antigens may be defined as those organism proteins against which the host responds with the highest potential diagnostic titre. Following identification of proteins of potential diagnostic significance, specific reagents such as MAbs or monospecific polyvalent sera may be generated for use in screening recombinant gene libraries for genes encoding the protein(s) of interest. Recombinant libraries can be produced from the genomic DNA of the organism or by cDNA synthesis using organism messenger RNA (mRNA) as a template. Fragments of the genomic DNA or cDNA are molecularly cloned into a prokaryotic or eukaryotic expression system, and the gene library screened for expression of the desired protein. The use and applications of recombinant antigens in diagnostic assays are discussed in refs 10 and 13. A specific example of recombinant antigens used in diagnostic tests are the ELISA tests developed for lyme borreliosis (30). Current trends in this area involve the development of synthetic peptide antigens which may be superior to recombinants in the area of quality control (32).

D. VACCINES

Molecular biology procedures have and will continue to have major impact on the preparation of veterinary vaccines. Products of recombinant technology may be easier to monitor because they may have specific markers introduced into or deleted from the vaccine.

Even though genetic information is often manipulated in live recombinant vaccines, there are significant safety concerns surrounding their usage. In general, safety and potency requirements should be consistent with those for other live vaccines. A potential always exists for adverse reactions to the vector agent being used, although this potential can be diminished by the inactivation or deletion of virulence factor genes in the vector virus (41). Other risks include adverse recombination events with wild-type infectious agents, changes in cell tropism or virulence due to genomic alterations, and potential undesired ecological effects (21). The latter can be of particular concern when spread occurs to a species in which the vector agent may differ in degree of attenuation (21).

1. Gene-deleted vaccines

Virus genes coding for virulence can be deleted, leaving a virion that can be used in live virus vaccines with reduced virulence. The virulence of the BUK vaccine strain of Aujeszky's disease was reduced by engineering a mutation of the thymidine kinase (TK) gene, so that the vaccine has no detectable TK activity. More recently, the emphasis in Aujesky's disease vaccines has been on the deletion of glycoprotein genes. Deletion of the glycoprotein E gene has been used successfully to develop attenuated PRV virus isolates that lack neurotropism and can also be used as markers to distinguish the vaccine strain from wild-type strains in serological testing (16) (see discussion on marker vaccines below). In addition to a TK deletion, a second deletion removed a gene coding for viral glycoprotein that prevents antibodies being produced against the glycoprotein (22). This second deletion allows vaccinated pigs to be identified by ELISA from naturally infected pigs. Diagnostic kits for Aujeszky's disease diagnostics are discussed in the chapter on this disease. Other constructs may have deletions in global genes such as aroA, cya or crp. These deletion mutants are frequently unable to replicate without the addition of specifically required nutrients. The vaccine agent undergoes restricted replication in the vaccinate but is unable to continue replication cycles. This results in a vaccine that is capable of inducing an immune response in a similar way to other live vaccines, but which has greater safety because it will not persist in the animal or in the environment.

2. Marker vaccines

During the development of both conventional vaccines and those produced using recombinant technology, consideration must be given to the development of appropriate tests to differentiate vaccinated from infected animals. This has lead to the development of marker vaccines. A marker vaccine uses a specific deletion or an added microbial protein code into the genome in order to distinguish between vaccinated and infected individuals (53). A series of successful marker vaccines have been created for BHV-1 in cattle. The most efficacious of these have been shown to involve a deletion of the glycoprotein E or G gene (17). The presence or absence of this glycoprotein can then be tested for using an immunoperoxidase assay with a specific MAb to the glycoprotein (17).

3. Virus-vectored vaccines

The most discussed vectored vaccines are the vaccinia-vectored viruses of rinderpest vaccine and the oral rabies vaccines. A plasmid is constructed containing the DNA of the donor rinderpest virus. Then the rinderpest cDNA segments in the plasmid are inserted into the TK locus of the vaccinia virus genome (58). The haemagglutinin (H) gene of rinderpest can be inserted into the haemagglutinin region of the vaccinia vector, thus inactivating the corresponding H gene of the vaccinia. The lack of haemagglutinating activity in the recombinant vaccine gene can be used as a biological marker. The recombinant vaccinia virus grown in cell culture produces the rinderpest virus haemaglutinin protein that serves as a protective antigen (57). A recombinant vaccinia rabies vaccine was constructed by inserting a plasmid bearing a cDNA copy of the rabies glycoprotein gene into vaccinia-virus-infected cells. Subsequent recombination between the TK locus of the vaccinia virus and the plasmid resulted in a live recombinant vaccinia including a gene for the rabies glycoprotein (19). This vaccine when fed to foxes, raccoons and skunks produced high levels of neutralising antibody and conferred long-term protection (3). Safety concerns about the use of some vaccinia strains (e.g. Copenhagen) have led to other viruses being used, including non-pox viruses.

A single capripox recombinant vaccine was effective in protecting cattle against rinderpest and lumpy skin disease (46). Fowl pox has been used as the vector for a recently approved Newcastle disease/fowl pox vaccine in the United States of America (51). Yamanouchi *et al.*, have recently reviewed vector vaccines for veterinary use. The vector and the inserted genes are given in ref. 56.

4. DNA vaccines

DNA vaccination is the direct introduction into host cells of a bacterial plasmid DNA that is able to cause expression of an antigenic protein. Several DNA vaccines for veterinary use are currently being developed (56). Such genetic immunisation is a very promising new approach to vaccination (44). For this, a plasmid DNA, carrying a gene of the immunising protein under the control of a eukaryotic promoter, is inoculated into the host animal. The foreign antigen is expressed within the host and will stimulate the host's immune system. It has been demonstrated that such a vaccine can be produced at a low cost and can provoke strong humoral and cellular immunity. An example is the protection of cattle against bovine herpesvirus 1 by plasmid DNA (6). The immune response can be further improved by simultaneous inoculation of immunostimulators such as CpG motif sequences and plasmids expressing cytokines (20, 55).

5. New developments in vaccine technology

Subunit vaccines contain purified protein or glycoprotein components of a pathogen that have been identified as carrying critical epitopes involved in inducing a protective immune response (2). These vaccines have distinct advantages in the realm of safety, and recent improvements in their production using recombinant DNA technology may facilitate more widespread usage (8).

Synthetic peptide vaccines have been engineered with distinct advantages in handling properties and safety, and they are relatively inexpensive to produce (31). A synthetic peptide vaccine for foot and mouth disease virus has been developed, but only limited protection has been observed in host animals (50). There may be many reasons why a synthetic peptide may not induce full immunogenicity, including polymorphism of class II MHC (major histocompatibility complex) molecules, inadequate antigen presentation of peptides, and the high variability of RNA viruses (50). In order to address this problem, researchers have recently engineered parvovirus-like particles that express foreign polypeptides in certain positions, which in turn results in large-scale production of the foreign peptides and an enhanced cell-mediated immunity (5). Other virus-like particle vaccines that involve self-assembling proteins that can be used to carry foreign antigens have been made from particles produced from the TYA gene of the yeast retrotransposon Ty (25).

REFERENCES

1. ANDERSON J. (1984). Use of monoclonal antibody in a blocking ELISA to detect group specific antibodies to bluetongue virus. *J. Immunol. Methods*, **74**, 139–149.

2. BABIUK L.A. (1997). Subunit Vaccines. *In:* Veterinary Vaccinology, Pastoret P.-P., Blancou J., Vannier P. & Verschueren C., eds. Elsevier Science BV, Amsterdam, The Netherlands, 262–264.

3. BLANCOU J., KIENY M.P., LATHE R., LECOCQ J.P. & PASTORET P., SOULEBOT J.P. & DESMETTRE P. (1986). Oral vaccination of the fox against rabies using a live recombinant vaccinia virus. *Nature*, **332**, 373–375.

4. BURKHARDT H.J. (2000). Standardisation and Quality control of PCR analyses. *Clin. Chem. Lab. Med.*, **38**, 87–91.

5. CASAL G.I., RUEDA P. & HURTADO A. (1999). Parvovirus-like particles as vaccine vectors. *Methods*, **19**, 174–186.

6. COX G.J., ZAMB T.J. & BABIUK L.A. (1993). Bovine herpesvirus 1: immune responses in mice and cattle injected with plasmid DNA. *J. Virol.*, **67**, 5664–5667.

7. DEECHAIDE S.T., KNOWLES D., MCGUIRE T., PALMER G., SUAREZ C. & MCELWAIN T. (1998). Detection of cattle naturally infected with *Anaplasma marginale* in a region of endemicity by nested PCR and a competitive enzyme-linked immunosorbent assay using recombinant surface protein 5. *J. Clin. Microbiol.*, **36**, 777–782.

8. DESMETTRE P. (1999). Diagnosis and prevention of equine infectious diseases: present states, potential, and challenges for the future. *Adv. Vet. Med.*, **41**, 359–377.

9. ERLICH H.A., GELFAND D.H. & SAIKI, R.S. (1988). Specific DNA amplification. *Nature*, **331**, 461–462.

10. FOX J. & KLASS M. (1989). Antigens produced by recombinant DNA technology. *Clin. Chem.*, **35**, 1838–1842.

11. GOFF W., BARBET A., STILLER D., PALMER G., KNOWLES D., KOCAN K.M., GORHAM J.R. & MCGUIRE T.C. (1988). Detection of *Anaplasma marginale* infected tick vectors by using cloned DNA probes. *Proc. Natl. Acad. Sci. USA*, **85**, 919–923.

12. HAINES D.M. & CLARK E.G. (1991). Enzyme immunohistochemical staining of formalin-fixed tissues for diagnosis in veterinary pathology. *Can. Vet. J.*, **32**, 295–302.

13. HARPER D.R. (1994). Medical Applications – Molecular Diagnostics. *In:* Molecular Virology. BIOS Scientific Publishers, Oxford, UK, 127–140.

14. HOLMBERG S.D., OSTERHOLM, M.T. & SENGER K.A. (1984). Drug-resistant salmonella from animals fed antimocrobials. *N. Engl. J. Med.*, **311**, 617–622.

15. HORIMOTO T. & KAWAOKA Y. (1995). Direct reverse transcriptase PCR to determine virulence potential of influenza A virus in birds. *J. Clin. Microbiol.*, **33**, 748–75.1.

16. JACOBS L. (1994). Glycoprotein E of pseudorabies virus and homologous proteins in other alphaherpesvirinae. *Arch. Virol.*, **137**, 209–228.

17. KAASHOEK M.J., RIJSEWIJK F.A.M., RUULS R.C., KEIL G.M., THIRY E., PASTORET P.P. & VAN OIRSCHOT J.T. (1998). Virulence, immunogenicity, and reactivation of bovine herpesvirus 1 mutants with a deletion in the gC, gG, gI, gE, or in both the gI and gE gene. *Vaccine*, **16**, 802–809.

18. KAPPMEYER L.S., PERRYMAN L.E., HINES S.A., BASZLER T.V., KATZ J.B., HENNAGER S.G. & KNOWLES D.P. (1999). Detection of equine antibodies to *Babesia caballi* by recombinant B. Caballi rhoptry-associated protein 1 in a complete inhibition enzyme-linked immunosorbent assay. *J. Clin. Microbiol.*, **37**, 2285–2290.

19. KIENY M.P., LATHE R., DRILLIEN R., SPEHNER D., SKORY S., SCHMITT D., WIKTOR, T, KOPROWSKI H. & LECOCQ J.P. (1984). Expression of rabies virus glycoprotein from a recombinant vaccinia virus. *Nature*, **312**, 163–166.

20. KIM J.J., TRIVEDI N.N., NOTTINGHAM L.K., MORRISON L., TSAI A., HU Y., MAHALINGAM S., DANG K., AHN L., DOYLE N.K., WILSON D.M., CHATTERGOON M.A., CHALIAN A.A., BOYER J.D., AGADJANYAN M.G. & WEINER D.B. (1998). Modulation of amplitude and direction of *in vivo* immune responses by co-administration of cytokine gene expression cassettes with DNA immunogens. *Eur. J. Immunol.*, **28.**, 1089–1103.

21. KIMMAN T.G. (1992). Risks connected with the use of conventional and genetically engineered vaccines. *Vet. Q.*, **14**, 110–118.

22. KIT S., SHEPPARD M., ICHIMURA H. & KIT M. (1987). Second generation pseudorabies vaccine with deletions in thymidine kinase and glycoprotein genes. *Am. J. Vet. Res.*, **48**, 780–793.

23. KNOWLES D., DEECHAIDE S.T., PALMER G., MCGUIRE T., STILLER D. & MCELWAIN T. (1996). Antibody against an *Anaplasma marginale* MSP5 epitope common to tick and erythrocyte stages identifies persistently infected cattle. *J. Clin. Microbiol.*, **34**, 2225–2230.

24. KNOWLES D.P., KAPPMEYER L.S., STILLER D., HENNAGER S.G. & PERRYMAN L.E. (1992). Antibody to a recombinant merozoite protein epitope identifies horses infected with *Babesia equi. J. Clin. Microbiol.*, **30**, 3122–3126.

25. LAYTON GT. (1997). Ty virus-like particles as an antigen delivery system. *In:* New Generation Vaccines, Levine M.M., Woodrow G.C., Kaper J.B. & Cobon G.S., eds. Marcel Dekker, New York, USA, 239–245

26. LI H., SHEN D.T., KNOWLES D.P., GORHAM J.R. & CRAWFORD T.B. (1994). Competitive inhibition enzyme-linked immunosorbent assay for antibody in sheep and other ruminants to a conserved epitope of malignant catarrhal fever virus. *J. Clin. Microbiol.*, **32**, 1674–1679.

27. LIBEAU G., DIALLO A., COLAS F. & GUERRE L. (1994). Rapid differential diagnosis of rinderpest and peste des petits ruminants using an immunocapture ELISA. *Vet. Rec.*, **134**, 300–304.

28. LICHTENSTEIGER C.A., KNOWLES D.P., MCGUIRE T.C. & CHEEVERS W.P. (1991). Recombinant gp135 envelope glycoproteins of caprine arthritis-encephalitis lentivirus variants inhibit homologous and heterologous variant-specific neutralizing antibodies. *Virology*, **185**, 2–9.

29. LOMNICZI B., NAGY E., KUKEDI A. & ZSAK L. (1988). Molecular epidemiology of Aujeszky's disease virus in Hungary. *Curr. Top. Vet. Med. Anim. Sci.*, **30**, 3–14.

30. MAGNARELLI L.A., FIKRIG E., PADULA S.J., ANDERSON J.F. & FLAVELL R.A. (1996). Use of recombinant antigens of *Borrelia burgdorferi* in serologic tests for diagnosis of lyme borreliosis. *J. Clin. Microbiol.*, **34**, 237–240.

31. MELOEN R.H. (1997). Synthetic Peptide Vaccines. *In:* Veterinary Vaccinology, Pasturet P.-P., Blancou J., Vannier P. & Verschueren C., eds. Elsevier Science BV, Amsterdam, The Netherlands, 272–276.

32. MELOEN R.H., LANGEDIJK J.P.M. & LANGEVELD J.P.M. (1997). Synthetic peptides for diagnostic use. *Vet. Q.*, **19**, 114–118.

33. MOLINA CABALLERO J.M., ANGUIANO A., FERRER O., SERRANO E. & UCEDA A. (1993). Use of an enzyme-linked immunosorbent assay for serodiagnosis of clinical paratuberculosis in goats. Study by Western blotting of false-positive reactions. *Rev. sci. tech. Off. int. Epiz.*, **12**, 629–638.

34. Mullis K.B., Ferre F. & Gibbs R.A., eds (1994). PCR: The Polymerase Chain Reaction. Birkhäuser Boston, Cambridge, USA.

35. Mweene A.S., Ito T., Okazaki K., Ono E., Shimizu Y. & Kida H. (1996). Development of immuno-PCR for diagnosis of bovine herpesvirus 1 infection. *J. Clin. Microbiol.*, **34**, 745–750.

36. Nadin-Davis S.A., Casey G.A. & Wandeler A. (1993). Identification of regional variants of the rabies virus within the Canadian province of Ontario. *J. Gen. Virol.*, **74**, 829–837.

37. Obert G. & Beyer C. (1988). An enzyme-linked immunosorbent assay using monoclonal antibodies for the detection of respiratory syncytial virus in clinical specimens. *Arch. Virol.*, **100**, 37–49.

38. Office International des Epizooties (1990). Biotechnology and Veterinary Science (theme of entire issue). *Rev. sci. tech. Off. int. Epiz.*, **9**, 611–916.

39. Office International des Epizooties (1993). Biotechnology Applied to the Diagnosis of Animal Diseases (theme of entire issue). *Rev. sci. tech. Off. int. Epiz.*, **12**, 313–672.

40. O'Rourke K., Baszler T., Parish S. & Knowles D. (1998). Preclinical selection of PrP^{SC} in nictitating membrane lymphoid tissue of sheep. *Vet. Rec.*, **142**, 489–491.

41. Paoletti E., Taylor J., Meignier B., Meric C. & Tartaglia J. (1995). Highly attenuated poxvirus vectors: NYVAC, ALVAC and TROVAC. *Dev. Biol. Stand.*, **84**, 159–163.

42. Pearson L.D. & Roy P. (1993). Genetically engineered multi-component virus-like particles as veterinary vaccines. *Immunol. Cell Biol.*, **71**, 381–389.

43. Posnett E.S. & Ambrosio R.E. (1989). Repetitive DNA probes for the detection of *Babesia equi. Molec. Biochem. Parasitol.*, **34**, 75–78.

44. Robinson H.L. (1997). Nucleic acid vaccines: an overview. *Vaccine*, **15**, 785–787.

45. Rodriguez M. & Schudel A.A. (1993). Nucleic acid hybridization and polymerase chain reaction in the diagnosis of infectious animal diseases. *Rev. sci. tech. Off. int. Epiz.*, **12**, 405–423.

46. Romero C.H., Barrett T., Evans S.A., Kitching R.P., Gershon P.D., Bostock C. & Black D.N. (1993). Single capripoxvirus recombinant vaccine for the protection of cattle against rinderpest and lumpy skin disease. *Vaccine*, **11**, 737–742.

47. Saiki R., Gefland D., Stoffel S., Schanf S., Higuchi R., Horn G., Mullis K. & Erlich H. (1988). Primer-directed enzymatic amplification of DNA with thermostable DNA polymerase. *Science*, **293**, 487–491.

48. Sandvik T. & Krogsrud J. (1995). Evaluation of an antigen-capture ELISA for detection of bovine viral diarrhea virus in cattle blood samples. *J. Vet. Diagn. Invest.*, **7**, 65–71.

49. Schweiger B., Pauli G., Zeichhardt H. & Kucherer C. (1997). A multicentre quality assessment study to monitor the performance of HIV-1 PCR. *J. Virol. Methods*, **67**, 45–55.

50. Sobrino F., Blanco E., Garcia-Briones M. & Ley V. (1999). Synthetic peptide vaccines: foot-and-mouth disease virus as a model. *Dev. Biol. Stand.*, **101**, 39–43.

51. Taylor J., Edbaur C., Rex-Senelonge A., Boquet J.F., Norton E., Goebel S., Desmettre P. & Paoletti E. (1990). Newcastle disease virus fusion protein expressed in a fowl pox virus recombinant confers protection in chickens. *J. Virol.*, **64**, 1441–1450.

52. Trueblood E.S., McGuire T.C. & Palmer G.H. (1991). Detection of *Anaplasma marginale* rickettsemia prior to onset of clinical signs by using an antigen capture enzyme-linked immunosorbent assay. *J. Clin. Microbiol.*, **29**, 1542–1544.

53. Van Oirschot J.T. (1999). Bovine Viral Vaccines, Diagnostics, and Eradication. *In:* Veterinary Vaccines and Diagnostics, Schultz R.O., ed. Academic Press, London, UK, 197–213

54. WENSVOORT G., BLOEMRAAD M. & TERPSTRA C. (1988). An enzyme immunoassay employing monoclonal antibodies and detecting specifically antibodies to classical swine fever virus. *Vet. Micriobiol.*, **17**, 129–140.

55. XIANG Z. & ERTL H.C. (1995). Manipulation of the immune response to a plasmid-encoded viral antigen by coinoculation with plasmids expressing cytokines. *Immunity*, **2**, 129–135.

56. YAMANOUCHI K., BARRETT T. & KAI C. (1998).New approaches to the development of virus vaccines for veterinary use. *Rev. sci. tech. Off. int. Epiz.*, **17**, 641–653.

57. YAMANOUCHI K., INUI K., SUGIMOTO M., ASANO K., NISHIMAKI F., KITCHING R.P., TAKAMATSU H. & BARRETT T. (1993). Immunization of cattle with a recombinant vaccinia vector expressing the haemagglutinin gene of rinderpest virus. *Vet. Rec.*, **132**, 152–156.

58. YILMA T., HSU D., JONES L., OWENS S., GRUBMAN M., MEBUS C., YAMANAKA M. & DALE B. (1988). Protection of cattle against rinderpest with vaccinia virus recombinants expressing the HA or F gene. *Science*, **242**, 1058–1061.

*
* *

CHAPTER I.1.8.

THE ROLE OF OFFICIAL BODIES IN THE INTERNATIONAL REGULATION OF VETERINARY BIOLOGICALS

SUMMARY

The official control of veterinary biologicals is vested in various national and regional organisations that differ in their approach to ensuring the quality, safety and efficacy of the products. International harmonisation of regulations concerning biological products did not begin until well after those concerning chemically defined products. The first biological products for veterinary use were not manufactured and distributed until the end of the nineteenth century. They were often produced under unsophisticated conditions, and distributed or sold without any control other than those of their manufacturers. Later, each manufacturer developed their own standards. In Europe, these were subject to State controls as early as 1895 for certain diagnostic products (e.g. mallein, tuberculin) or vaccines. Gradually the conditions for international harmonisation of standards evolved, beginning with the comparative testing of products being issued by different European laboratories. It was only in the second half of the twentieth century that national laws covering veterinary biologicals were imposed. These demanded that precisely defined techniques be followed before biological products for veterinary use could be licensed. This was followed by considerable efforts to harmonise these national regulations, first at the regional level (notably in Europe and the Americas) then at the global level, notably by the Office International des Épizooties (OIE) with the publication of the first edition of the OIE Manual of Standards for Diagnostic Tests and Vaccines *in 1989.*

World-wide harmonisation of standards for veterinary biologicals will be of help to Chief Veterinary Officers who must follow the instructions given in the OIE International Animal Health Code, *as they apply to all biological products for use in international trade. It will also be of assistance to vaccine producers, who have expressed their wish for world-wide harmonisation of registration rules so as to simplify and facilitate marketing of their products. Evidently, it will also be of interest to farmers and to consumers, who would benefit from the fact that the safety and efficacy of the products that they use would have been assured to a uniformly high level.*

The different sections of this chapter will review and compare regulations from the regions of the world that have made most progress in this field and will describe current attempts at harmonising these regulations on an international scale.

***Note:** In this chapter the term 'veterinary biological' will be taken to include vaccines for use in animals, antisera for use in animals, and* in-vivo *diagnostic preparations.*

A. REGULATION OF VETERINARY BIOLOGICALS: PRESENT SITUATION

1. In Japan

1.1. Introduction

Medicinal products that are exclusively used for animals, including veterinary biologicals, are under the jurisdiction of the Ministry of Agriculture, Forestry and Fisheries, and securing their quality, efficacy and safety is stipulated in the Pharmaceutical Affairs Law (1). Since 1972, registration procedures have been developed with the aim of rationalising the examination procedure and facilitating the acquisition of approval. These procedures are stipulated in the Pharmaceutical Affairs Law and other related regulations. Consequently, a speedy and simple examination procedure has been achieved with emphasis on the assurance of quality, safety and efficacy.

1.2. Regulations governing the approval and quality assurance of veterinary biologicals

a) Application for approval and licence

Those who intend to manufacture or import veterinary biologicals must prepare an application using the designated format for each product, and obtain approval from the Minister of Agriculture, Forestry and Fisheries. The application should be submitted with designated appended documents, such as those on clinical studies. Of the latter, the safety studies and clinical studies using the target species should have been performed in compliance with GLP (Good Laboratory Practice) and GCP (Good Clinical Practice).

A licence to manufacture, import and sell veterinary biologicals is issued by the Minister of Agriculture, Forestry and Fisheries to each applicant and the licence must be renewed every 5 years. Conformity to GMP (Good Manufacturing Practice) is stipulated as one of the conditions for obtaining a licence to manufacture.

b) National assay

After receiving a licence, each batch of the veterinary biological must be examined by the National Veterinary Assay Laboratory according to the procedures of the Assay Standard for Veterinary Biological Products (3, 9). Each product for marketing must include an official identification stamp on the container or the package as a seal.

c) Re-examination and re-evaluation

Re-examination is performed on newly approved veterinary biologicals. Usually a field assessment of the drug is conducted, over a period of 6 years following initial approval of the vaccine. During this investigation, efficacy and safety are re-examined.

Re-evaluation is performed on approved products available on the market by order of the Minister of Agriculture, Forestry and Fisheries. This may happen when it is suspected that a veterinary biological does not conform with the latest standards.

d) Minimum requirement of veterinary biological products

The examinations provide information about the consistency of the manufacturing process and the quality of the product: manufacturing methods, properties of strains used for manufacturing, methods of quality control, methods of storage and shelf life, according to the standards given in the 'Minimum Requirement of Veterinary Biological Products' (2). Any product that does not conform to these product standards cannot be manufactured, imported or marketed.

e) Cases of rejection of approval

When the quality of the veterinary biological that has been submitted for approval is found to be unsatisfactory, or its adverse effects are marked as compared with its indications, the product is judged to be of little value and approval is not given.

f) Cancellation of approvals

At the time of granting approval to manufacture or import, the quality, safety and efficacy of the product are carefully examined with reference to the latest available technology. However, if scientific knowledge acquired since the granting of approval indicates that there could be a health hazard associated with the product, re-examination and re-evaluation are performed and an order of 'cancellation of approval' may be made.

1.3. Procedure for approval to manufacture (import)

The quality, safety and efficacy of the product as a veterinary vaccine are the most important criteria when manufacturing (importing) is intended. A licence is not required for each manufacturing facility. One approval for each product is sufficient even if the manufacturer intends to manufacture (import) in more that one facility. It is also possible to apply simultaneously for approval of the quality of the product and for a licence to manufacture.

When a manufacturer (importer, distributor) manufactures (imports) veterinary biologicals, an application for approval to manufacture (import) the veterinary drug must be submitted on a designated form to an official in charge of veterinary drugs at the Department of Livestock Industry of each Prefecture. If the documentation is satisfactory, the application for approval to manufacture (import), together with appended documents, are sent to and reviewed by the Office of the Ministry of Agriculture, Forestry and Fisheries. At that time, a hearing may be conducted if necessary. The application is then discussed in the Central Pharmaceutical Affairs Council, and if no problems are found, notice of approval to manufacture (import) the veterinary product is sent to the applicant.

2. In the European Union

2.1. Introduction

The pharmaceutical legislation of the European Community, which has evolved over a 30-year period, covers both medicinal products for human and veterinary use. Harmonisation of requirements in the area of veterinary medicines began in 1981 with the adoption of Directives 81/851/EEC and 81/852/EEC, laying down common requirements for manufacturing and marketing authorisation, based on the evaluation of the quality, safety, and efficacy of the product. A series of detailed guidelines were first published in 1994 entitled 'Rules Governing Medicinal Products in the EU' (7). These have since been updated and describe in detail the legal basis for obtaining marketing authorisations, how dossiers should be compiled and how they should be assessed. These rules serve as extremely useful reference publications for any authority that is setting up a system for authorisation of veterinary biologicals. The rules were formally adopted and applied specifically to veterinary biologicals from 1993. Many additional measures were taken to further harmonise the procedures and the criteria for the evaluation of veterinary medicinal products, such as framework requirements and interpretive guidelines for their testing, principles and guidelines of GMP, and a Community procedure for the evaluation of high-technology products. However, granting of authorisations remained at the national level. As a consequence, although applications were evaluated on the basis of these harmonised criteria and procedures, and in some cases simultaneously by the authorities of the Member States, there were differences in the decisions reached by the Member States on individual products. This was why in 1990 the Commission proposed a new system for marketing authorisation for medicinal products, which was adopted by the Council of Ministers in 1993 and entered into force on 1 January 1995.

One of the first consequence was the creation of the European Medicines Evaluation Agency (EMEA) in London, United Kingdom (UK).

2.2. The role of the European Medicines Evaluation Agency

In 1995, a new European system for the authorisation of medicinal products came into force. After 10 years of cooperation between national registration authorities at the European Union (EU) level and 4 years of negotiations, the Council of the EU adopted, in June 1993, three directives and one regulation, which together form the legal basis of the system (5).

The EMEA was established by Council Regulation (EEC) 2309/93 of 22 July 1993. (OJ No. L 214, 24.8.1993), and London, UK, was chosen as its location by decision made by the Heads of State and Government on 29 October 1993. This agency formulates opinions and, apart from the administrative staff and the management board, is composed of two scientific committees, the CPMP (Committee for Proprietary Medicinal Products) in charge of medicinal products for humans and the CVMP (Committee for Veterinary Medicinal Products) in charge of medicinal and other products for use in animals.

The CVMP is responsible for the evaluation of applications for marketing authorisation for products derived from biotechnology, for productivity enhancers, new chemical entities and other innovative new products. In addition, the CVMP makes recommendations regarding MRLs (maximum residue limits) for substances used in food-producing animals. To support its activities, the CVMP relies on a pool of 400 experts put at the disposal of the agency by the EU Member States. These experts may participate in any of the CVMP working parties. Among the working parties, the Immunologicals Working Party (CVMP/IWP) has a double mandate: to assist the CVMP, if necessary examining on behalf of the Scientific Advice Coordinator of the CVMP, in part or in whole any request for scientific advice made by a company during the development of a new vaccine, and to advise the CVMP on more general policy issues such as the elaboration and revision of guidelines on immunological products. The guidelines for the testing of veterinary medicinal products are contained within 'The Rules Governing Medicinal Products in the EU', last published by the European Union in 1999 (7).

2.3. Present European procedures for marketing authorisation

Since 1995, two new registration procedures for human and veterinary medicinal products have become available through the EU: the *centralised* and the *decentralised* procedures (12).

a) **The centralised procedure**

This applies to high technology products defined in the Annex to Council Regulation 2309/93. It is compulsory for some products ('Part A' – certain biotechnological products and novel growth promoters), and optional for others ('Part B' – other innovatory products). The assessment is co-ordinated by one of the members of the CVMP, known as the 'rapporteur', under contract to the EMEA. Data requirements and criteria are the same as those for national procedures. The authorisation subsequently issued by the Commission is valid in all Community Member States. However, in the case of veterinary vaccines, one or more Member States may prohibit the use of a vaccine either because of the absence of the infection in their territory or because an eradication programme is being implemented there, as certified by Competent Authorities.

b) **The decentralised procedure**

Applications for authorisation of a product may still be obtained in a single Member State (the 'Reference Member State') by means of a national procedure. The same 'Rules Governing Medicinal Products in the EU' apply. Following approval in the Reference Member State, applications may be made, if desired, to other 'Concerned' Member States for identical authorisations to be granted on the basis of '*mutual recognition*'. If another Member State has grounds for considering that the product, as authorised, constitutes a 'risk to animal or public health or to the environment', it may refer the dossier to the EMEA for arbitration. The Commission then issues a binding decision based on the opinion of the CVMP.

2.4. Manufacturing authorisation and batch release control

In accordance with Directive 81/851/EEC, authorisation is also required for the manufacture of veterinary medicinal products, including immunologicals. This directive provides for regular inspections and stipulates that manufacture must be supervised by a 'qualified person', who certifies that each batch is in conformity with the approved specifications for the product. For the implementation of these requirements, the commission has adopted Directive 91/412/EEC relating to the principle and guidelines of GMP, and published a detailed guide on GMP developed by a group of pharmaceutical inspectors from the Member States.

Manufacturers are required to have the services of a qualified person at their disposal to certify that each batch of product has been manufactured and checked in accordance with the conditions for marketing authorisation. This is a basic requirement of the pharmaceutical legislation. In the case of batches imported from third countries, each batch has to undergo a full qualitative and a quantitative analysis of at least the active ingredients in the first Member State of import into the EU, under the supervision of a qualified person. Not until this control by the qualified person has been carried out can a batch circulate within the EU without further control. In the special case of immunological veterinary medicinal products, an additional step may be introduced. Directive 90/677/EEC allows those Member States that consider it necessary to ask for the submission of samples of each production batch of the bulk and/or finished product for examination by a control laboratory before that batch is placed on the market. This official batch release does not relinquish the requirement of batch control by the qualified person. Except in specially justified circumstances, batch release carried out by one national control laboratory must be recognised without repetition by the other Member States. To ensure the smooth operation of this provision, an administrative information exchange procedure has been agreed between the Competent Authorities. Although all Member States do not require official batch release for veterinary immunologicals, it was felt by all that they had to be involved in this information exchange scheme. Discussions are currently in progress (year 2000) to establish a harmonised system of batch release in all Member States of the EU. Although the system has yet to be finalised, it is likely to combine testing of some veterinary biologicals by official laboratories with more stringent monitoring of the testing carried out by the manufacturers themselves.

2.5. The role of the European Pharmacopoeia

The past 30 years have seen profound changes in the organisation of European countries and the regulation of medicinal products (4). Thirty years ago, each country had its own regulations, and among them the European countries had two-thirds of the world's pharmacopoeias. The European Pharmacopoeia Convention has now been signed by 24 parties: 23 countries[1], and just recently by the Commission of the European Communities; moreover 10 European and non-European countries[2], and the World Health Organisation (WHO) have observer

---

1 Austria, Belgium, Cyprus, Croatia, Denmark, Finland, France, Germany, Greece, Iceland, Ireland, Italy, Luxembourg, the Netherlands, Norway, Portugal, Slovenia, Spain, Sweden, Switzerland, Turkey, the United Kingdom, and the Former Yugoslav Republic of Macedonia; Member States must apply the standards of the European Pharmacopoeia.

2 Albania, Australia, Bulgaria, Canada, Hungary, the Czech Republic, the People's Republic of China, Lithuania, Slovakia, and Poland; Observer States do not have to apply the European Pharmacopoeia standards. Some of them apply the standards on a voluntary basis.

status. Close relations are maintained with the licensing authorities of the European Economic Area, where integration is developing through contact with the EMEA and the implementation of common directives and guidelines on medicines for human and veterinary use. In 1990, the European Pharmacopoeia co-founded, with the Japanese Pharmacopoeia and the United States (US) Pharmacopoeia, the Pharmacopoeial Discussion Group (PDG); this group is working assiduously for harmonisation at the world level, and it participates in the International Conference on Harmonisation of Technical Requirements for Registration of Pharmaceuticals for Human Use (ICH) programme. Unfortunately this will have no consequences in the field of veterinary vaccines as there are no monographs on these preparations in the US and Japanese pharmacopoeias.

The European Pharmacopoeia also contains a department called the 'European Department for the Quality of Medicines' (EDQM). This creates, maintains and distributes the international standard reagents referred to in monographs of the European Pharmacopoeia. To date there are few standards for veterinary biologicals, but there are indications that the EDQM intends to become increasingly active in this area.

3. In the United States of America

3.1. Introduction

In the United States of America (USA), veterinary biologics or veterinary biological products are defined as all viruses, sera, toxins (excluding substances that are selectively toxic to microorganisms, e.g. antibiotics), or analogous products at any stage of production, shipment, distribution, or sale, that are intended for use in the treatment (prevention, diagnosis, management, or cure) of diseases of animals and that act primarily through the direct stimulation, supplementation, enhancement, or modulation of the immune system or immune response. The term biological products includes, but is not limited to, vaccines, bacterins, allergens, antibodies, antitoxins, toxoids, immunostimulants, certain cytokines, antigenic or immunising components of live organisms, and diagnostic components that are of natural or synthetic origin or that are derived from synthesising or altering various substances or components of substances such as microorganisms, genes or genetic sequences, carbohydrates, proteins, antigens, allergens, or antibodies.

3.2. Legal basis

The Virus/Serum/Toxin Act of 1913 (the 'VST Act'), as amended, 21 U.S.C. Sections 151 to 159, provides the legal authority for the regulation of immunologicals and biologicals for animal use in the USA. The regulatory programme implementing the requirements of the VST Act is administered by the Center for Veterinary Biologics (CVB), Animal and Plant Health Inspection Service (APHIS) of the United States Department of Agriculture (USDA). Administrative regulations, duly promulgated and with effect of law, are published in Title 9, Code of Federal Regulations Parts 101 to 118 (6). In addition, APHIS has issued programme guidance in CVB Notices, Veterinary Services Memoranda, Veterinary Biologics General Licensing Considerations, and the Veterinary Biologics Program Manual.

The VST Act requires that products governed by the Act that enter channels of commerce be 'not worthless, contaminated, dangerous or harmful'. The regulatory scheme implementing these standards is structured to require manufacturers of these products to apply for licences prior to marketing, and to place certain evidentiary burdens on those applicants, i.e. manufacturers are required to demonstrate through the submission of certain information, research data, and test results that their products are 'pure, safe, potent and efficacious'. The APHIS programme for immunologicals and biologicals for animal use regulates the manufacture and release of products on to the market through a system of licensing, inspection, testing and post-marketing surveillance that ensures that the statutory and regulatory standards are met.

3.3. Licensing and initial inspection

Any person or firm seeking to manufacture in the USA an immunological or biological for animal use must obtain from APHIS both a licence to manufacture at a specified facility (Establishment Licence), and a licence for every particular product to be manufactured (Product Licence). These licence requirements apply whether the product is to be released on to the US market or is to be exported to markets abroad. Typically, an applicant will request a facility licence at the same time as the licence for the first product. Once the facility licence and one product licence have been obtained, a firm that seeks to manufacture and market new products needs only to apply for additional product licences. A person or firm located overseas that seeks to market its product in the USA must also apply for marketing authorisation. In the case of an imported product, however, the authorisation is termed a 'permit' rather than a 'licence'.

To obtain a facility licence, the applicant must submit for approval the blueprint (that is, the architects plan of the buildings) and blueprint legends for the facility. APHIS reviews these blueprints and legends to ensure that the facility will operate in a manner consistent with GMP. If the applicant subsequently makes any physical or operational changes to the facility, revised blueprints and legends must be submitted immediately.

To obtain a product licence, the applicant must establish the purity and identity of all master seeds and master cell stocks that will be used in the manufacture of the product, and must submit for approval a detailed outline of production. The outline of production includes not only the details of the method of product manufacture, but also a description of the procedures for collecting and submitting samples and for releasing batches. The applicant must also provide information regarding the professional and technical credentials of company personnel, and must identify a qualified individual (termed under US regulations as the 'government liaison') who acts as the official contact with CVB during the licensing process, and who is subsequently responsible for the submission of the firm's test reports in conjunction with the release of the product on to the market. The applicant is required to submit test data that demonstrate that the product produced in accordance with the outline is pure, safe, potent and efficacious. The applicant must submit to CVB laboratories samples of three consecutive batches of the product so that the results of the applicant's tests of the product can be confirmed.

Finally, before the facility or product licences are issued, the applicant's premises are subject to a comprehensive inspection by APHIS examiners. The inspection ensures that the facility is operating in a manner consistent with GMP by confirming that the establishment is configured in the manner set out in the approved blueprints and legends, that the production line is set up and operating in accordance with the approved outline of production, and that records are adequately kept and maintained for each step in production. The inspection also confirms that the applicant follows GLPs, that the in-process and final product testing programme is conducted properly and appropriately documented, that the sampling is conducted properly, and that adequate procedures for determining and documenting the release of the product on to the market are in place.

3.4. Post-licensing inspection

Once a firm has been issued facility and product licences, APHIS will routinely conduct thorough follow-up inspections of the facility to ensure that the licensee continues to operate the establishment in accordance with the programme regulations and in the manner represented at the time of licensing. Post-licensing inspections are conducted unannounced, and ordinarily within 12–18 months after the last inspection. If the licensee proposes any significant changes to the facility or to the method of production of a licensed product, APHIS retains the right to conduct a special inspection prior to approving the changes.

3.5. Testing

Each licensee is responsible for thoroughly testing all of its production processes and products prior to release on to the market. The type and amount of testing required depends on the particular product, but is determined and approved by the regulatory authority prior to the issuing of the product licence. A qualified individual employed by the licensee ('government liaison') is responsible for selecting the samples to be tested, for monitoring the licensee's testing programme, and for certifying the test results to the regulatory authority.

At the same time that the firm selects its samples for its own in-house testing, it also selects samples to be submitted to the CVB laboratories. Using a programme for random selection, CVB then selects and tests approximately 10% of the samples submitted as a way of testing the accuracy and proficiency of the company tests. By regulation, CVB is required to put its selected samples on test within 14 days of the date on which the samples are received; ordinarily, samples are put on test sooner than the 14-day limit so that the testing of production by the firm and the CVB proficiency testing programme are effectively being conducted at the same time.

When the firm receives the results of its own tests, the government liaison submits those results to the regulatory authority along with a batch release form, initiating the release procedure. If the batch has not been selected as part of the proficiency testing programme, or if it has been selected but the CVB tests confirm the company's test results, the release form is countersigned by the regulatory authority completing the release procedure. If either the company tests or the proficiency tests indicate that the batch may be unsatisfactory, the batch is not eligible for release.

If the licensee makes a proposal to modify its facility or its operation in any way that could affect the purity, safety, potency or efficacy of the product, the regulatory authority may require the licensee to provide data demonstrating the purity, safety, potency and efficacy of the product as well as to submit samples of the product to CVB's laboratories for confirmatory testing.

3.6. Post-marketing surveillance

CVB operates a post-marketing surveillance programme to monitor the performance of products on the market. Under this programme, CVB typically learns of any problems relating to product quality through consumer reports or complaints, although the programme regulations also place an obligation on the licensee to inform CVB of any problem that comes to its attention regarding the purity, safety or potency of the product. CVB has the legal authority to intervene in the marketplace where there are serious concerns with respect to the purity, safety, potency or efficacy of the product.

B. COMPARISON OF EUROPEAN UNION AND UNITED STATES REGULATIONS

Veterinary biologicals must meet certain basic criteria, regardless of the Regulatory Agency overseeing their production. These criteria include:

- Safety: the product must be safe in the target species and, if live, in species exposed to shed organisms;
- Efficacy: the product should be effective according to claims indicated on the label;
- Quality: (includes purity, potency and consistency)
- Purity: the product must be free from contaminating agents;
- Potency: each batch of product should be formulated, and tested, to ensure effectiveness and reproducibility of activity as demonstrated in the registration data.

Although, on a global basis, agencies and regulations differ, all strive to ensure that products offered to the end-consumer conform to these basic standards.

The EU uses a complete system that is a combination of GMP, including validated processes and specifications of materials, together with production methods that ensure the quality of the final product. In-process and batch controls (tests) constitute additional guarantees of the quality of IVMPs. The safety tests are conducted under GLP and the efficacy tests under GCP. The USA defines acceptable manufacturing processes in the Outline of Production and detailed facility description (blueprints and blueprint legends), and relies on inspection and confirmatory testing to achieve the same goal. Although different, both systems are designed to allow only pure, safe, potent, and effective biologicals to be released to the consumer.

In addition to the data provided by the applicant, expert reports have to be included in the EU marketing authorisation application file (dossier). Each main section of the EU dossier, including analytical, safety and efficacy, must be reviewed by an independent expert. The assessment of the expert is included in the marketing authorisation file. No such system of third-party review exists under the USDA registration system.

There are many procedural differences between the EU and the USA. Harmonisation between the two systems should be established where possible, on the recognition of equivalence for tests and procedures that are performed to assess a vaccine and that ensure quality, safety and efficacy of the product. Mutual recognition agreements (MRAs) covering veterinary biologicals have been signed between the EU and Australia and between the EU and New Zealand. Implementation of these MRAs is at a transitional stage. Progress on MRAs between the EU and the USA, regarding veterinary biologicals, is likely to take longer to achieve.

C. THE ROLE OF INTERNATIONAL ORGANISATIONS

Most nations have a range of official acts that regulate the sale and use of veterinary biologicals. Almost all of these acts stipulate 'minimum requirements' for quality, safety and efficacy of veterinary biologicals (mostly vaccines), to be tested at independent laboratories, usually under State supervision. These acts and tests may differ from one country to another, and they involve costs and restrictions for producers, users and testers.

Many of the vaccines described in this *Manual* are produced and/or used in countries that do not currently apply regimens of authorisation and testing as stringent as those described in this chapter. Nevertheless, it is useful to be aware of the regulations operating in different regions and, therefore, the testing and inspection that is likely to have been carried out there on a veterinary biological.

The idea of harmonising this testing to simplify and reduce costs on a regional, or even world scale, is not new, and much has been accomplished during the past 20 years. The purpose of this section is to review the current situation by describing the role of international organisations in the regulation of veterinary vaccines.

In this section the term 'international organisation' refers to those concerned with animal health on a world-wide scale (OIE, the Food and Agriculture Organization of the United Nations [FAO] and the WHO]).

1. The role of the Office International des Epizooties

The OIE was founded in Paris in 1924 as the world organisation for animal health, and comprises 155 Member Countries in the year 2000. The three principal aims of the OIE are to provide information on animal health world-wide, to promote international coordination of research into and control of certain animal diseases, and to harmonise import and export regulations for animals and animal products at an international level (13).

Within the OIE there are four Specialist Commissions: the International Animal Health Commission, which deals with the *International Animal Health Code,* the Standards Commission, the Foot and Mouth Disease and Other Epizootics Commission and the Fish Diseases Commission (including diseases of molluscs and crustaceans). In addition, there are four Working Groups that deal with animal health information systems, wildlife diseases, veterinary drug registration, and biotechnology. The latter two groups are involved in the activities of the OIE with regard to vaccine registration, harmonisation and control.

Among the Specialist Commissions, the one most closely connected with standardisation is the Standards Commission. This Commission establishes standards for diagnostic methods (including diagnostic preparations) and for vaccines. Its terms of reference reflect the Commission's obligation to participate in the standardisation of biological products, including vaccines used for prophylactic purposes. The Standards Commission is responsible for the preparation of the *OIE Manual of Standards for Diagnostic Tests and Vaccines* (11), and the organisation of Reference Laboratories for many of the diseases contained in OIE Lists A and B.

However, full standardisation of vaccine testing can be achieved only when the necessary standards have been devised. It is hoped to reach the goal of standardisation and wide availability of standards through the participation of OIE Reference Laboratories. The functions and responsibilities of experts at the 138 OIE Reference Laboratories include the provision of a centre of excellence in a designated activity; standardisation of methods; preparation, storage and distribution of standard antisera, antigens and other reagents.

Among the nine OIE Collaborating Centres, three may be involved at some stage in veterinary vaccine control and/or harmonisation: the Collaborating Centre for Veterinary Medicinal Products in Fougères (France), the Collaborating Centre for ELISA (enzyme-linked immunosorbent assay) and Molecular Techniques in Animal Disease Diagnosis in Vienna (Austria), and the Collaborating Centre for the Diagnosis of Animal Diseases and Vaccine Evaluation in the Americas in Ames (USA).

In 1994, following discussions with the International Technical Consultation on Veterinary Drug Registration (ITCVDR), the OIE set up an Ad hoc Group on the Harmonisation of Veterinary Medicines, which was the first step towards the creation of the 'Veterinary International Cooperation on Harmonisation' (VICH) (see Section C.4. below).

2. The role of the Food and Agriculture Organization of the United Nations

FAO, established in 1945, is responsible for agricultural development and food production. The Animal Production and Health Division ('AGA') within the Agriculture Department is concerned with livestock development, and it includes the Animal Health Service ('AGAH'), the main role of which is to assist Member Countries in the control of animal diseases, with the aim of improving livestock production as an integral component of general social, economic and agricultural development. FAO's involvement in testing veterinary biologicals is primarily through its technical assistance system to Member Countries to set up and even execute independent quality control of vaccines and other biologicals. One example is FAO's assistance to the OAU (Organization of African Unity) in setting up a system for continental testing of veterinary vaccines, especially against rinderpest and contagious bovine pleuropneumonia, by the Pan African Veterinary Vaccine Center (PANVAC). FAO also commissions, at the request of Member Countries, initiatives for either quality assurance of vaccines and other biologicals or expert consultations on this subject, or publication of manuals on the production and quality control of vaccines. Furthermore, two auxiliary services can be asked to intervene on matters concerning these products, namely Codex Alimentarius and the Division of Nuclear Techniques in Food and Agriculture. The latter is operated jointly by FAO and the International Atomic Energy Agency (IAEA) based in Vienna (Austria). It has an Animal Production and Health Section, which assists veterinary services and research institutes in developing countries to establish radio-immunoassay (RIA) and ELISA techniques. Linked to this activity is a quality assurance scheme under which laboratories in receipt of FAO/IAEA ELISA kits are required to routinely monitor internal quality controls and to periodically (once or twice a year) test a batch of unknown samples, and to forward the results to IAEA. The overall aim is to provide assurance to all concerned that the results being generated through the use of such internationally standardised and validated kits can be relied upon as correct.

3. The role of the World Health Organization

Currently WHO is not directly involved in preparing international reference preparations (i.e. antigens or antibodies) for purely veterinary use, but has developed and still retains in the National Institute for Biological Standards and Control (London) some materials related to purely veterinary diseases (e.g. Newcastle disease live vaccine, anti-swine fever serum). WHO wishes to retain a role in this area in instances where the veterinary reference preparations and guidance documents have a direct relevance to human health (8, 10, 15, 16). This involves zoonotic and potentially zoonotic agents and other infectious agents of animal origin that are potential contaminants of biological products, whether these are vaccines produced in cell cultures or organs for xenotransplantation. At the meeting of the Expert Committee on Biological Standardization in October 1998, a review of currently retained international standards and reference preparations for veterinary medicine was carried out and a list of candidates for discontinuation, replacement and revision was suggested (8). The Expert Committee however decided to defer taking action on preparation of veterinary reference materials pending an evaluation by WHO with its partners in the veterinary field of the need for these various biological products. In addition, the present day topicality of certain preparations, especially veterinary vaccines against known zoonoses (e.g. anthrax, brucellosis) adopted and/or revised in the 1960s and 1970s, also needs to be evaluated.

The format of the list of Requirements for Biological Substances published as an annex to each report of the Expert Committee on Biological Standardization has been revised in 1998 and should facilitate retrieving information and achieve the aim of improved transparency.

4. The role of VICH

4.1. The terms of reference

The objectives of the VICH are to:

- Provide a forum for a constructive dialogue between regulatory authorities and the veterinary medicinal products industry on the real and perceived differences in the technical requirements for product registration in the EU, Japan and the USA, with the expectation that such a process may serve as a catalyst for wider international harmonisation;

- Identify areas where modifications in technical requirements or greater mutual acceptance of research and development procedures could lead to a more economical use of human, animal and material resources, without compromising safety;

- Make recommendations on practical ways to achieve harmonisation of technical requirements affecting registration of veterinary products and to implement these recommendations in the three regions. Once adopted, VICH recommendations should replace corresponding regional requirements. These recommendations should focus on the essential scientific requirements needed to address a topic and should eliminate unnecessary or redundant requirements;

- VICH should be conducted in a transparent and cost-effective manner and should provide the opportunity for public comment on recommendations at the draft stage.

VICH will focus on harmonising registration requirements for veterinary medicinal products in the EU, USA and Japan. Countries not involved in VICH will be kept informed of its progress through the OIE. Consideration will be given to biologicals but not, for the time being, to feed additive growth promoters.

4.2. The Steering Committee

Fundamental to the existence of VICH is the Steering Committee that is empowered to drive the harmonisation process. The Steering Committee comprises two delegates from each of the regulatory authorities and industry associations in the three regions. Australia/New Zealand and South America will have observer status with one delegate from each regional government and each industry association.

4.3. The Working Groups

In order to achieve harmonisation on the selected topics, the VICH Steering Committee will appoint working groups to draft recommendations. Each working group will normally comprise six experts – one representing each VICH full member. Additional experts from observer countries – or even other countries – may be appointed by the Steering Committee if deemed appropriate.

A topic leader will be appointed by the Steering Committee for each topic. The topic leader is responsible for initiating the working group and guiding its work. He/she will normally chair the working group and be accountable to the Steering Committee for delivering the draft.

The Steering Committee has established a specific Working Group to deal with harmonisation of tests used for the control of veterinary vaccines. This is the Working Group on Biologicals Quality Monitoring.

4.4. VICH and the role of industry federations

COMISA[3], the 'industry motor' in the VICH process, is responsible for the entire VICH secretariat. This will entail the preparation of documents for meetings of VICH members, publishing Press releases, distributing working group documents and publishing recommendations adopted by the Steering Committee. COMISA will also

3 Confédération Mondiale de l'Industrie de la Santé Animale (World Animal Health Industry Confederation).

coordinate the positions of the three regional industry federations. The AHI[4], FEDESA[5] and JVPA[6] have responsibility for ensuring that their regional views are properly represented. They send industry experts to each working group, liaise with their regional authorities and are responsible for organising local conferences to discuss and publicise VICH recommendations.

CONCLUSION

At the moment, there is a clear intention to achieve greater international harmonisation of regulatory requirements for veterinary biologicals (14). Progress has already been achieved through international organisations to allow fair competition in the marketing of veterinary products. Although past efforts by international organisations have not resulted in a level of harmonisation sufficient to facilitate international trade, they have laid the groundwork for current efforts. National authorities recognise the advantages of harmonisation and are now committed to working toward this goal.

The efforts of international organisations have made the goal of harmonisation possible and have resulted in an organisation and process for proceeding toward this goal. Success in achieving this goal will depend on the willingness of participating national authorities to work together and accept the compromises that will be necessary to resolve the difficult scientific and policy issues.

REFERENCES

1. ANON (1960). The Pharmaceutical Affairs Law. Japan Law No. 145 in 1960, as amended on 26 June 1996. Pharmaceutical Affairs Law, Enforcement Ordinance and Enforcement Regulations, Yakugyo Jiho, Japan, 2–91 (in Japanese and English).

2. ANON (1993). The Minimum Requirements for Biological Products for Animal Use. Ministry of Agriculture, Forestry and Fisheries Notice No. 599 in 1987, as amended ON 3 May 1993. Japan Association of Veterinary Biologics, Tokyo, Japan, 1–435 (in Japanese).

3. ANON (1995). The Assay Standard for Biological Products for Animal Use. Ministry of agriculture, Forestry and Fisheries Notice No. 1542 in 1995, as amended at 25 September 1997. Japan Association of Veterinary Biologics, Tokyo, Japan, 1–309 (in Japanese).

4. ARTIGES A. (1997). The role of the pharmacopoeias. *In:* Veterinary Vaccinology, Pastoret P.P., Blancou J., Vannier P. & Verschueren C., eds. Elsevier Science, Amsterdam, the Netherlands, 674–679.

5. BRUNKO P. (1997). Procedures and technical requirements in the European Union. *In:* Veterinary Vaccinology, Pastoret P.P., Blancou J., Vannier P. & Verschueren C., eds. Elsevier Science, Amsterdam, the Netherlands, 705–717.

6. CODE OF FEDERAL REGULATIONS (1998). Animals and Animal Products, Title 9, Parts 1–199. The Office of the Federal Register, National Archives and Records Administration. US Government Printing Office, Washington DC, USA.

7. EUROPEAN UNION (1999). The Rules Governing Medicinal Products in the European Union. Eudralex, Vols 4–9. Office Publications of the European Communities, Luxembourg.

8. JOINT FOOD AND AGRICULTURE ORGANIZATION OF THE UNITED NATIONS (FAO)/WORLD HEALTH ORGANIZATION (WHO) EXPERT COMMITTEE ON BRUCELLOSIS (1986). Sixth Report. WHO Technical Report Series No. 740, World Health Organization, Geneva, Switzerland, 132 pp.

9. MAKIE H. (1998). The activities of veterinary vaccine control laboratories. *Rev. sci. tech. Off. Int. Epiz.*, 17, 578–584.

10. MESLIN F.-X., KAPLAN M.M. & KOPROWSKI H. (1996). Laboratory Techniques in Rabies. World Health Organization, Geneva, Switzerland, 476 pp.

11. OFFICE INTERNATIONAL DES EPIZOOTIES (OIE) (2000). Manual of Standards for Diagnostic Tests and Vaccines, Fourth Edition. Office International des Epizooties, Paris, France.

4 Animal Health Institute (USA)
5 Fédération Européenne de la Santé Animale
6 Japanese Veterinary Pharmaceutical Association

12. PASTORET P.P. & FALIZE F. (1998). Licensing procedures for immunological veterinary medicinal products in the European Union. *Adv. Vet. Med.*, **41**, 595–607.

13. TRUSZCZYNSKI M. & BLANCOU J (1992). The role of the Office International des Epizooties in the standardisation of biologicals. *In:* Symposium on the First Steps Towards an International Harmonization of Veterinary Biologicals and Free Circulation of Vaccines within the EEC, Ploufragan, 1992. *Dev. Biol. Stand.*, **79**, 95–98.

14. VANNIER P., TRUSZCYNSKI M. & ESPESETH D. (1997). Implementing International harmonisation. *In:* Veterinary Vaccinology, Pastoret P.P., Blancou J., Vannier P. & Verschueren C., eds. Elsevier Science, Amsterdam, the Netherlands, 712-717.

15. WORLD HEALTH ORGANIZATION (WHO) EXPERT COMMITTEE ON BIOLOGICAL STANDARDISATION (1992). Forty-second Report. WHO Technical Report Series No. 822, World Health Organization, Geneva, Switzerland, 84 pp.

16. WORLD HEALTH ORGANIZATION (WHO) EXPERT COMMITTEE ON RABIES (1992). Eighth Report. WHO Technical Report Series No. 824, World Health Organization, Geneva, Switzerland, 75 pp.

*

* *

PART 2

OIE LISTED DISEASES

SECTION 2.1.

LIST A DISEASES

CHAPTER 2.1.1.

FOOT AND MOUTH DISEASE

SUMMARY

Foot and mouth disease (FMD) is the most contagious disease of mammals and has a great potential for causing severe economic loss in susceptible cloven-hoofed animals. There are seven serotypes of FMD virus, namely, O, A, C, SAT 1, SAT 2, SAT 3 and Asia 1. Infection with one serotype does not confer immunity against another. FMD cannot be differentiated clinically from other vesicular diseases, including swine vesicular disease, vesicular stomatitis, and vesicular exanthema. Laboratory diagnosis of any suspected FMD case is therefore a matter of urgency.

Typical cases of FMD are characterised by a vesicular condition of the feet, buccal mucosa and, in females, the mammary glands. Clinical signs can vary from mild to severe and fatalities may occur, especially in young animals. In some species the infection may usually be subclinical, e.g. African buffalo (Syncerus caffer). *The preferred tissue for diagnosis is epithelium from unruptured or freshly ruptured vesicles. Where this is not possible, blood and/or oesophageal–pharyngeal fluid samples taken by probang cup in ruminants or throat swabs from pigs provide an alternative source of virus. Myocardial tissue or blood can be submitted from fatal cases, but vesicles are again preferable if present.*

It is vital that samples from suspected cases be transported under secure conditions and according to international regulations. They should only be dispatched to authorised laboratories.

Diagnosis of FMD is by the demonstration of FMD viral antigen or nucleic acid in samples of tissue or fluid. Detection of specific humoral antibody can also be used for diagnosis, especially in wildlife, but this requires the absence of any history of vaccination, as it is not always possible to differentiate a serological response to natural infection from that due to vaccination. Diagnosis based on serological response may also be problematical in endemic areas due to the possibility of previous infection.

***Identification of the agent:** The demonstration of FMD viral antigen is sufficient for a positive diagnosis.*

Complement fixation (CF) has been the traditional test for diagnosis, but has been replaced in many laboratories by the enzyme-linked immunosorbent assay (ELISA), as this is more specific and sensitive and is not affected by pro- or anti-complementary factors. If the sample is inadequate or the test result inconclusive, it will be necessary to grow the virus in cell cultures or in 2–7-day old unweaned mice. The cultures should preferably be of primary bovine thyroid, but pig, lamb or calf kidney cells, or cell lines of comparable sensitivity may be used. When a cytopathic effect (CPE) appears in the cultures, the fluids can be used in CF tests or ELISAs. Similar tests can be performed on homogenised suspensions of the dissected musculo-skeletal tissues of any mice that die. In the absence of CPE or any dead mice, a further passage should be made at a 48-hour interval, with freeze–thawing of the cells, before the sample is declared to be negative.

Nucleic acid recognition tests, such as the polymerase chain reaction and in situ *hybridisation, are being used increasingly as rapid and sensitive diagnostic methods. Electron microscopic examination of lesion material is sometimes useful to differentiate FMD from disease caused by pox or other viruses.*

Serological tests: *The demonstration of specific antibody titres in nonvaccinated animals, where a vesicular condition is present, is sufficient for a positive diagnosis. This is particularly useful in mild cases or where epithelial tissue cannot be collected.*

Virus neutralisation (VN) tests and ELISAs are used as serotype-specific serological tests. VN tests depend on tissue cultures and are therefore more prone to variability than ELISAs; they are also slower and subject to contamination. ELISAs for antibodies have the advantage of being faster, and are not dependent on cell cultures. The ELISA can be performed with inactivated antigens, thus requiring less restrictive biocontainment facilities.

Requirements for vaccines and diagnostic biologicals: *Inactivated virus vaccines of varying composition are available commercially. Typically, virus is used to infect a suspension or monolayer cell culture and the resulting preparation is clarified, inactivated with ethyleneimine and blended with adjuvant. Many FMD vaccines are multivalent to provide cover against the different serotypes likely to be encountered in a given field situation.*

The finished vaccine must be shown to be free from residual live virus. This is usually done using a combination of in-vitro *tests on the inactivated virus preparation and* in-vivo *tests on the finished vaccine. Challenge tests are also conducted in vaccinated cattle to establish a PD_{50} (50% protective dose) value, although a serological test is considered to be satisfactory where the vaccine producer has established a statistically significant correlation between protection and specific antibody response.*

Diagnostic and reference reagents are available from the OIE/FAO (Food and Agriculture Organization of the United Nations) World Reference Laboratory for FMD[1], or from Regional Reference Laboratories for FMD.

A. DIAGNOSTIC TECHNIQUES

Foot and mouth disease (FMD) is caused by a virus of the genus Aphthovirus, family Picornaviridae. There are seven serotypes of FMD virus, namely O, A, C, SAT 1, SAT 2, SAT 3, and Asia 1, that infect cloven hoofed animals. Infection with any one serotype does not confer immunity against another. Within serotypes, many subtypes can be identified by biochemical and immunological tests.

In Africa, FMD viruses are maintained by cattle and African buffalo *(Syncerus caffer).* Available evidence indicates that although other domestic and wild species become infected, they are unable to maintain the infection for more than a few months in the absence of cattle or African buffalo. Elsewhere in the world cattle are usually the main reservoir, although in some instances the viruses involved appear to be specifically adapted to domestic pigs or sheep and goats. It is probable that these adapted viruses are able to modify their adaptation and affect other species if given the opportunity. Wildlife outside Africa have not, so far, been shown to be able to maintain FMD viruses. The evidence indicates that infection of deer in the past was derived from contact, direct or indirect, with infected domestic animals.

Of the domesticated species, cattle, pigs, sheep, goats and buffalo are susceptible to FMD (21). In addition, many species of cloven-hoofed wildlife, such as deer, antelope and wild pigs may become infected, although, apart from the African buffalo their involvement in the epidemiology of FMD in the domesticated species is not certain. Strains of FMD virus that infect cattle have been isolated from wild pigs and deer. For the diagnosis of FMD in wild species, procedures similar to those described for farm animals can be applied.

Infection of susceptible animals with FMD virus leads to the appearance of vesicles on the feet, in and around the oral cavity, and on the mammary glands of females. Vesicles can also occur at other sites, such as inside the nostrils and at pressure points on the limbs – especially in pigs. The severity of clinical signs varies with the strain of virus, the exposure dose, the age and breed of animal, the host species and its degree of immunity (29). The signs can range from a mild or inapparent infection to one that is severe. Death may result in some cases. Mortality from a multifocal myocarditis is most commonly seen in young animals: myositis may also occur in other sites. Adult animals may occasionally succumb.

1 OIE/FAO (Food and Agriculture Organization of the United Nations) World Reference Laboratory for FMD, Pirbright Laboratory, Ash Road, Pirbright, Woking, Surrey GU24 ONF, United Kingdom.

On premises with a history of sudden death in young cloven-hoofed livestock, close examination of adult animals may often reveal the presence of vesicular lesions if FMD is involved. The presence of vesicles in fatal cases is variable.

In animals with a history of vesicular disease, the detection of FMD virus in samples of vesicular fluid, epithelial tissue, milk, or blood is sufficient to establish a diagnosis. Diagnosis may also be established by the isolation of FMD virus from the blood, heart or other organs of fatal cases. A myocarditis may be seen macroscopically in a proportion of fatal cases.

FMD virus can replicate and be excreted from the respiratory tract of animals. Airborne excretion of virus occurs during the acute phase of infection. FMD viruses may occur in all the secretions and excretions of acutely infected animals including expired air. Transmission is generally effected by contact between infected and susceptible animals or, more rarely, exposure of susceptible animals to the excretions and secretions of acutely infected animals. Following recovery from the acute stage of infection, infectious virus disappears from all secretions and excretions with the exception, in the case of ruminants, of those of oesophageal–pharyngeal (OP) origin. Animals in which the virus persists in the OP for more than 28 days after infection are referred to as carriers. Pigs do not become carriers. Circumstantial evidence indicates that carriers are able, on rare occasions, to transmit the infection to susceptible animals with which they come in close contact: the mechanism involved is unknown. The carrier state in cattle usually does not persist for more than 6 months, although in a small proportion it may last up to 3 years. In African buffalo individual animals have been shown to harbour the virus for at least 5 years, but it is probably not a lifelong phenomenon. Within a herd of buffalo, the virus may be maintained for 24 years or longer. Domestic buffalo, sheep and goats do not usually carry FMD viruses for more than a few months.

Due to the highly contagious nature and economic importance of FMD for many countries, the laboratory diagnosis and serotype identification of the virus should be done in a virus-secure laboratory. Countries lacking access to such a specialised national or regional laboratory should send specimens to the OIE/FAO World Reference Laboratory (WRL) for FMD (26).

Diagnostic and standard reagents are available in kit form or as individual items from the OIE/FAO WRL for FMD. The use of inactivated antigens in the enzyme-linked immunosorbent assay (ELISA), as controls in the antigen-detection test or to react with test sera in the liquid-phase blocking ELISA, reduces the disease security risk involved in the use of live virus. Reagents are supplied freeze-dried and can remain stable at 4°C in this state for many years. The International Atomic Energy Agency[2] has produced a manual that includes a recommended test and quality control protocols.

For laboratory diagnosis, the tissue of choice is epithelium. Ideally, at least 1 g of epithelial tissue should be collected from an unruptured or recently ruptured vesicle. To avoid injury to personnel collecting the samples, as well as for animal welfare reasons, it is recommended that animals be sedated before any samples are obtained.

Epithelial samples should be placed in a transport medium composed of equal amounts of glycerol and 0.04 M phosphate buffer pH 7.2–7.6, preferably with added antibiotics (penicillin [1000 international units (IU)], neomycin sulphate [100 IU], polymyxin B sulphate [50 IU], mycostatin [100 IU]). If 0.04 M phosphate buffer is not available, tissue culture medium or phosphate buffered saline (PBS) can be used instead, but it is important that the final pH of the glycerol/buffer mixture be in the range pH 7.2–7.6. Samples should be kept refrigerated or on ice until received by the laboratory.

Where epithelial tissue is not available from ruminant animals, for example in advanced or convalescent cases, or where infection is suspected in the absence of clinical signs, samples of OP fluid can be collected by means of a probang (sputum) cup (or in pigs by swabbing the throat[3]) for submission to a laboratory for virus isolation.

Before the collection of OP samples from cattle or large ruminants (e.g. buffaloes), 2 ml transport fluid (composed of 0.08 M phosphate buffer containing 0.01% bovine serum albumin, 0.002% phenol red, antibiotics (1000 units/ml penicillin, 100 units/ml mycostatin, 100 units/ml neomycin, and 50 units/ml polymyxin), and adjusted to pH 7.2) should be added to a container of around 5 ml capacity capable of withstanding freezing above solid carbon dioxide (dry ice) or liquid nitrogen.

After collection of OP fluid by probang, the contents of the cup should be poured into a wide-necked transparent bottle of around 20 ml capacity. The fluid is examined, and should contain some visible cellular material. Of this, 2 ml is then added to the 2 ml of transport fluid, ensuring that cellular material is transferred; the mixture is shaken gently and should have a final pH of around pH 7.6. Samples contaminated with ruminal contents may be unsuitable for culture. Samples seen to contain blood are not entirely satisfactory. Repeat sampling can be done after the mouth and throat of the animal have been rinsed with water or PBS.

---

2 International Atomic Energy Agency, Wagramerstrasse 5, P.O. Box 100, A-1400 Vienna, Austria.

3 The pig should be properly restrained, ideally held on its back in a wooden cradle with its neck extended. Holding a swab in a suitable instrument, such as an artery forceps, the swab is pushed to the back of the mouth into the pharynx.

OP samples from small ruminants are collected by putting 2 ml of transport fluid into a wide-necked bottle of about 20 ml capacity and, after collection, rinsing the probang cup in this transport fluid to discharge the OP sample. This is then transferred to a container of about 5 ml capacity for transport. The small container should be capable of withstanding freezing above solid carbon dioxide or liquid nitrogen (26).

Samples of OP fluid should be refrigerated or frozen immediately after collection. If they are to remain in transit for more than a few hours, they should be frozen by being placed either above solid carbon dioxide or liquid nitrogen. Before freezing, the containers should be carefully sealed using airtight screw caps or silicone. This is particularly important when using solid carbon dioxide, as introduction of CO_2 into the OP sample will lower its pH, inactivating any FMD virus that may be in the samples. Glass containers should not be used because there is a risk that they will explode on defrosting in the event of liquid nitrogen leaking into them. Samples should reach the laboratory in a frozen state.

Special precautions are required when sending perishable suspect FMD material both within and between countries. These regulations are mainly designed to prevent leakage and consequent contamination, but are also important in ensuring that the specimens arrive in a satisfactory state. If wet ice is put inside a package, escape of water must be prevented. The receiving laboratory must be notified in advance of the despatch.

1. Identification of the agent

a) Virus isolation

The epithelium sample should be taken from the PBS/glycerol, blotted dry on absorbent paper to reduce the glycerol content, which is toxic for cell cultures, and weighed. A suspension should be prepared by grinding the sample in sterile sand in a sterile pestle and mortar with a small volume of tissue culture media and antibiotics. Further media should be added until a final volume of ten times that of the epithelial sample has been added, giving a 10% suspension. This is clarified on a bench centrifuge at 2000 ***g*** for 10 minutes. Such suspensions of field samples suspected to contain FMD virus once clarified are inoculated into cell cultures or unweaned mice. Sensitive cell culture systems include primary bovine thyroid cells and primary pig, calf or lamb kidney cells. Established cell lines, such as baby hamster kidney BHK-21 and IB-RS-2 cells, may be used but are less sensitive than primary cells for detecting low amounts of infectivity (9). The cell cultures should be examined for cytopathic effect (CPE) for 48 hours. If no CPE is detected, the cells should be frozen and thawed, used to inoculate fresh cultures and examined for CPE for another 48 hours. Unweaned mice are an alternative to cell cultures and should be 2–7 days of age and of selected inbred strains. Some field viruses may require several passages before they become adapted to mice (33).

b) Immunological methods

- **Enzyme-linked immunosorbent assay**

At the OIE/FAO WRL for FMD (see footnote 1), the preferred procedure for the detection of FMD viral antigen and identification of viral serotype is the ELISA (20, 31). This is an indirect sandwich test in which different rows in multiwell plates are coated with rabbit antisera to each of the seven serotypes of FMD virus. These are the 'capture' sera. Test sample suspensions are added to each of the rows, and appropriate controls are also included. Guinea-pig antisera to each of the serotypes of FMD virus are added next, followed by rabbit anti-guinea-pig serum conjugated to an enzyme. Extensive washing is carried out between each stage to remove unbound reagents. A colour reaction on the addition of enzyme substrate, indicates a positive reaction. With strong positive reactions this will be evident to the naked eye, but results can also be read spectrophotometrically at an appropriate wavelength. In this case, an absorbance reading greater than 0.1 above background indicates a positive reaction; the serotype of FMD virus can also be identified. Values close to 0.1 should be confirmed by retesting or by amplification of the antigen by tissue culture passage and testing the supernatant once a CPE has developed. A suitable protocol is given below.

Depending on the species affected and the geographical origin of samples, it may be appropriate to simultaneously test for swine vesicular disease (SVD) virus or vesicular stomatitis (VS) virus. Ideally a complete differential diagnosis should be undertaken in all vesicular conditions.

Rabbit antiserum to the 146S antigen of each of the seven serotypes of FMD virus (plus SVD virus if required) is used as a trapping antibody at a predetermined optimal concentration in carbonate/bicarbonate buffer, pH 9.6.

Control antigens are prepared from selected strains of each of the seven types of FMD virus (plus SVD virus if appropriate) grown on monolayer cultures of BHK-21 cells (IB-RS-2 cells for SVD virus). The unpurified supernatants are used and pretitrated on ELISA plates. The final dilution chosen is that which gives an absorbance at the top of the linear region of the titration curve (optimal density approximately 2.0), so that the five-fold dilutions of the control antigens used in the test give two additional lower optimal density readings from which the titration curve can be derived. PBS containing 0.05% Tween 20 and phenol red indicator is used as a diluent (PBST).

Guinea-pig antisera prepared by inoculating guinea-pigs with 146S antigen of one of the seven serotypes of FMD virus (plus SVD virus if required) and preblocked with normal bovine serum (NBS) is used as the detecting antibody. Predetermined optimal concentrations are prepared in PBS containing 0.05% Tween 20, and 5% dried, nonfat skimmed milk (PBITM).

Rabbit (or sheep) anti-guinea-pig immunoglobulin conjugated to horseradish peroxidase and preblocked with NBS is used at a predetermined optimum concentration in PBITM.

- **Test procedure**

i) ELISA plates are coated with 50 µl/well rabbit antiviral sera in carbonate/bicarbonate buffer, pH 9.6. Rows A to H receive, respectively, antisera to serotypes O, A, C, SAT 1, SAT 2, SAT 3, Asia 1 and SVD virus (optional).

ii) Leave overnight at 4°C in a stationary position or place on an orbital shaker set at 100–120 revolutions per minute in a 37°C incubator for 1 hour.

iii) Prepare test sample suspension (with 10% original sample suspension or undiluted clarified cell culture supernatant fluid).

iv) The ELISA plates are washed five times in PBS.

v) On each plate, load wells of columns 4, 8 and 12 with 50 µl PBST. Additionally, add 50 µl of PBST to wells 2 and 3 of rows A to H on plate 1. To well 1 of row A of plate 1 add 50 µl of control antigen type O, and to well 2 of row A add 12.5 µl of control antigen type O. Mix antigen and diluent in well 2 and transfer 12.5 µl from well 2 to well 3 of row A. Mix and discard 12.5 µl from well 3 (this gives a five-fold dilution series of antigen O). Similarly repeat with antigen A, adding 50 µl of antigen type A to well 1 of row B, and 12.5 µl of antigen type A to well 2, and then mix and transfer 12.5 µl to well 3 (as done before with antigen type O), and continue for types C, SAT 1, SAT 2, SAT 3, Asia 1 and SVD (if appropriate). It is only necessary to change pipette tips on the micropipette between antigens. The remainder of the plate can be loaded with the test sample(s). Add 50 µl of sample one to wells 5, 6 and 7 of rows A to H, the second sample is placed similarly in columns 9, 10 and 11, rows A to H.

If more than two samples are to be tested at the same time, the other ELISA plates should be used as follows:

Dispense 50 µl of the PBST to the wells (rows A to H) of columns 4, 8 and 12 (buffer control columns). Note that the control antigens are not required on these plates. These test samples may be added in 50 µl volumes in rows A to H to columns 1, 2, 3; 5, 6, 7; 9, 10, 11, respectively.

vi) Cover with lids and place on an orbital shaker at 37°C for 1 hour.

vii) Wash the plates by flooding with PBS – wash three times as before and empty residual wash fluid. Blot the plates dry.

viii) Transfer 50 µl volumes of each guinea-pig serum dilution to each plate well in the appropriate order, e.g. rows A to H receive, respectively, antisera to serotypes O, A, C, SAT 1, SAT 2, SAT 3, Asia 1 and SVD virus (optional).

ix) Cover plates with lids and replace on the orbital shaker. Incubate at 37°C for 1 hour.

x) The plates are washed again three times and 50 µl of rabbit anti-guinea-pig immunoglobulin conjugated to horseradish peroxidase is added to each well. The plates are incubated at 37°C for 1 hour on a rotary shaker.

xi) The plates are washed again three times and 50 µl of orthophenylene diamine containing 0.05% H_2O_2 (30% w/v) is added to each well.

xii) The reaction is stopped after 15 minutes by the addition of 50 µl of 1.25 M sulphuric acid. The plates are read at 492 nm on a spectrophotometer linked to a computer.

- **Complement fixation test**

The ELISA is preferable to the complement fixation (CF) test because it is more sensitive and specific, and it is not affected by pro- or anti-complementary factors. If ELISA reagents are not available, however, the CF test may be performed as follows:

Antisera to each of the seven types of FMD virus are diluted in veronal buffer diluent (VBD) in 1.5-fold dilution steps from an initial 1/16 dilution to leave 25 µl of successive antiserum dilutions in U-shaped wells across a microtitre plate or appropriate volumes in test tubes. To these are added 50 µl of 3 units of complement, followed by 25 µl of test sample suspension(s). The test system is incubated at 37°C for 1 hour prior to the addition of 25 µl of 1.4% standardised sheep red blood cells (SRBC) in VBD sensitised with 5 units of rabbit anti-SRBC. The reagents are incubated at 37°C for a further 30 minutes and the plates are subsequently centrifuged and read. Appropriate controls for the test suspension(s), antisera, cells and complement are included. CF titres are expressed as the reciprocal of the serum dilution producing 50% haemolysis. A CF titre ≥36 is considered to be a positive reaction. Titre values of 24 should be confirmed by retesting an antigen that has been amplified through tissue culture passage.

c) Nucleic acid recognition methods

The polymerase chain reaction (PCR) can be used to amplify the genome fragments of FMD virus in diagnostic material (2, 7). Specific primers have been designed to distinguish between each of the seven serotypes. *In situ* hybridisation techniques have been developed for investigating the presence of FMD virus RNA in tissue samples (39). These techniques are only in use in specialised laboratories.

The molecular epidemiology of FMD is based on the comparison of genetic differences between virus isolates. Dendrograms showing the genomic relationship between vaccine and field strains for all seven serotypes have been published based on sequences derived from the 1D gene. Reverse-transcription polymerase chain reaction (RT-PCR) amplification of FMD virus RNA, followed by nucleotide sequencing, is the current preferred option for generating the sequence data to perform these comparisons. The WRL and other laboratories have developed techniques for performing these studies, and a database of over 2000 sequences is currently held.

The recommended method is to:

i) Extract FMD virus RNA directly from epithelial suspensions, or from a low cell culture passage.

ii) Perform an RT-PCR of the complete VP1 gene (or if only part of the VP1 gene, then the 3' end of the gene is more useful).

iii) Determine the nucleotide sequence of the PCR product (or at least 170 nucleotides [preferably 420 for the SAT types] at the 3' end of the gene).

A protocol, complete with primer sequences is available from the WRL on request or can be downloaded from the following World Wide Web URL:

http://www.iah.bbsrc.ac.uk/virus/picornaviridae/aphthovirus/fmdv.htm

Research on monoclonal antibodies (MAbs) that identify individual antigenic sites on the surface of the FMD virus may have future potential. Panels of neutralising antibodies are being developed for each serotype and characterised by nucleotide sequencing of escape mutant virus. The neutralising site against which each MAb acts can be deduced by identifying the sequence change in the mutant virus that allowed it to escape neutralisation.

2. Serological tests

FMD virus infection can be diagnosed by the detection of a specific antibody response. The tests generally used are virus neutralisation (VN) and ELISA (23, 24, 36). These are also the prescribed tests for trade. The VN test is serotype specific, requires cell culture facilities and takes 2–3 days to provide results. The ELISA is also serotype specific, sensitive and quantitative, and has the advantage that it is quicker to perform, is less variable, and is not dependent on tissue culture systems. Low titre false-positive reactions can be expected in a small proportion of the sera in either test. An approach combining screening by ELISA and confirming the positives by the VN test minimises the occurrence of false-positive results.

The detection of antibody to the nonstructural (NS) proteins of FMD virus has been used to identify past or present infection with any of the seven serotypes of the virus, whether or not the animal has also been vaccinated. Conventionally this has been carried out by measuring antibody to the virus infection-associated antigen (VIAA; the viral RNA polymerase protein 3D) using agar gel immunodiffusion (AGID) (28). Although relatively insensitive, the test is inexpensive, easy to perform and has been used extensively in South America to detect viral activity on a population basis during FMD eradication campaigns. The VIAA test has now largely been superseded by assays that measure antibody to FMD virus NS proteins produced by recombinant techniques in a variety of *in-vitro* expression systems. Antibody to the polyproteins 3AB or 3ABC are the single most reliable indicator of infection (10, 27, 34). In animals seropositive for antibody to 3AB or 3ABC, antibody to one or more of the other NS proteins including the L, 2C, 3A or 3D protein is further confirmation of infection (8, 27, 34). The test can be used on a herd basis to detect FMD virus infection in vaccinated and unvaccinated populations. Care must be taken when interpreting results from single animals as some repeatedly vaccinated animals produce antibody to 3ABC. It has not yet been established whether or not all animals that have been both vaccinated and infected seroconvert to this protein. A negative result for antibody to NS proteins cannot therefore be taken as definitive proof that an individual animal has not been exposed to FMD virus. This must be taken into account if NS protein antibody tests are used for assessment of risks for animals involved in international trade.

a) **Virus neutralisation (a prescribed test for international trade)**

The quantitative VN microtest for FMD antibody is performed with IB-RS-2, BHK-21, lamb or pig kidney cells in flat-bottomed tissue-culture grade microtitre plates.

Stock virus is grown in cell monolayers and stored at –20°C after the addition of 50% glycerol. (Virus has been found to be stable under these conditions for at least 1 year.) The sera are inactivated at 56°C for 30 minutes before testing. The control standard serum is 21-day convalescent serum (usually pig). A suitable medium is Eagle's complete medium/LYH (Hank's balanced salt solution with yeast lactalbumin hydrolysate) with antibiotics.

The test is an equal volume test in 50 µl amounts.

- **Test procedure**

i) Starting from a 1/4 dilution; sera are diluted in a twofold dilution series across the plate, using at least two rows of wells per serum, preferably four rows, and a volume of 50 µl.

ii) Previously titrated virus is added; each 50 µl unit volume of virus suspension should contain about 100 $TCID_{50}$ (50% tissue culture infective dose) within an accepted range (e.g. 35–350 $TCID_{50}$).

iii) Controls include a standard antiserum of known titre, a negative serum, a cell control, a medium control, and a virus titration used to calculate the actual virus titre used in the test.

iv) Incubate at 37°C for 1 hour with the plates covered.

v) A cell suspension at 10^6 cells/ml is made up in medium containing 10% bovine serum (specific antibody negative) for cell growth. A volume of 50 µl of cell suspension is added to each well.

vi) Plates are sealed with pressure-sensitive tape and incubated at 37°C for 2–3 days. Alternatively, the plates may be covered with loosely fitting lids and incubated in an atmosphere of 3–5% carbon dioxide at 37°C for 2–3 days.

vii) Microscope readings may be feasible after 48 hours, the plates are finally fixed and stained routinely on the third day. Fixation is effected with 10% formol/saline for 30 minutes. For staining, the plates are immersed in 0.05% methylene blue in 10% formalin for 30 minutes. An alternative fixative/stain solution is naphthalene blue black solution (0.4% [w/v] naphthalene blue black, 8% [w/v] citric acid in saline) (22). The plates are rinsed in tap water.

viii) Positive wells (where the virus has been neutralised and the cells remain intact) are seen to contain blue-stained cells sheets; the negative wells (where virus has not been neutralised) are empty. Titres are expressed as the final dilution of serum present in the serum/virus mixture at the 50% end-point, i.e. a well where there is an incomplete cell sheet (Kärber). The test is considered to be valid when the amount of virus used per well is in the range $\log_{10}$ 1.5–2.5 $TCID_{50}$, and the positive standard serum is within twofold of its expected titre.

ix) Interpretation of tests can vary between laboratories in regard to end-points taken. Laboratories should establish their own criteria by reference to standard reagents that can be obtained from the OIE/FAO WRL for FMD (see footnote 1). At the WRL, a titre of 1/45 or more of the final serum dilution in the serum/virus mixture is regarded as positive. Titres of 1/16 to 1/32 are considered to be doubtful, and further serum samples are requested for testing. Animals are considered to be positive if the second sample has a titre of 1/16 or greater. A titre of 1/8 or less is considered to be negative.

b) **Liquid-phase blocking enzyme-linked immunosorbent assay (a prescribed test for international trade)**

Rabbit antiserum to the 146S antigen of one of the seven types of FMD virus is used as the trapping antibody at a predetermined[4] optimal concentration in carbonate/bicarbonate buffer, pH 9.6.

Antigens are prepared from selected strains of FMD virus grown on monolayers of BHK-21 cells. The unpurified supernatants are used and pretitrated according to the VN protocol but without serum. The final dilution chosen is that which, after addition of an equal volume of diluent (see below), gives an absorbance on the upper part of the linear region of the titration curve (optical density approximately 1.5). PBS containing 0.05% Tween 20 and phenol red indicator is used as a diluent (PBST).

4 A chequerboard titration of the rabbit-trapping antiserum, the guinea-pig antiserum and the anti-guinea-pig antiserum is performed. Before using the antigen-trapping ELISA or the liquid-phase blocking ELISA, each of these reagents is titrated one against another, keeping the third reagent at a fixed concentration. In this way the optimal dilutions (for positive colour and low background colour) can be determined. These 'predetermined' dilutions are then used for all future tests using these particular batches of reagents.

Guinea-pig antisera prepared by inoculating guinea-pigs with 146S antigen of one of the seven serotypes and preblocked with NBS is used as the detecting antibody. Predetermined optimal concentrations are prepared in PBS containing 0.05% Tween 20, and 5% dried, nonfat skimmed milk (PBSTM).

Rabbit (or sheep) anti-guinea-pig immunoglobulin conjugated to horseradish peroxidase and preblocked with NBS is used at a predetermined optimum concentration in PBSTM.

Test sera are diluted in PBST.

- **Test procedure**

i) ELISA plates are coated with 50 µl/well rabbit antiviral sera and left overnight in a humid chamber at room temperature.

ii) The ELISA plates are washed five times with PBS.

iii) In U-bottomed multiwell plates (carrier plates) 50 µl of a duplicate, twofold series of each test serum are prepared, starting at 1/4. To each well, 50 µl of a constant dose of homologous viral antigen is added and the mixtures are left overnight at 4°C, or incubated at 37°C for 1 hour. The addition of the antigen increases the starting serum dilution to 1/8.

iv) Then 50 µl of serum/antigen mixtures are transferred from the carrier plates to the rabbit-serum coated ELISA plates and incubated at 37°C for 1 hour on a rotary shaker.

v) After washing, 50 µl of guinea-pig antiserum homologous to the viral antigen used in the previous step (iv) is added to each well. The plates are then incubated at 37°C for 1 hour on a rotary shaker.

vi) The plates are washed and 50 µl of rabbit anti-guinea-pig immunoglobulin conjugated to horseradish peroxidase is added to each well. The plates are incubated at 37°C for 1 hour on a rotary shaker.

vii) The plates are washed again and 50 µl of orthophenylene diamine containing 0.05% H_2O_2 (30%, w/v) is added to each well.

viii) The reaction is stopped after 15 minutes by the addition of 50 µl of 1.25 M sulphuric acid. The plates are read at 492 nm on a spectrophotometer linked to a microcomputer.

ix) *Controls:* A minimum of four wells each of strong positive, weak positive and negative bovine reference sera at a final dilution of 1/32 should be included on each plate together with an equivalent number of reaction (antigen) control wells containing antigen in diluent alone without serum. For end-point titration tests, duplicate twofold dilution series of positive and negative homologous bovine reference sera should be included on at least one plate of every run.

x) *Interpretation of the results:* Antibody titres are expressed as the 50% end-point titre, i.e. the dilution at which 50% of the wells show greater than 50% inhibition of the median OD of the reaction (antigen) control wells (Kärber). Titres greater than 1/40 are considered to be positive. Titres close to 1/40 should be retested using the VN test.

c) Nonstructural protein antibody tests

Antibody to VIAA is conventionally detected by AGID. The test is based on immunoprecipitation lines formed in the agar between the FMD antigen (concentrated cell-culture fluids rich in FMD virus RNA-dependent RNA polymerase or 3D) located in a centre well, and hexagonally arranged adjacent wells containing standard positive sera or unknown test sera. Precipitation lines forming between the test sera and the control antigen well that show identity with the lines of precipitation formed by the reference sera, confirm the specificity of the reactions (28).

Antibody to expressed, recombinant FMD virus NS proteins can be measured by ELISA or immunoblotting. No single test format has yet been conclusively demonstrated to be optimal. An MAb trapping (MAT) ELISA for detecting antibody to 3ABC (10) and blocking ELISAs for detecting antibody to 3AB or 3ABC (34) have been shown to be sensitive, specific and reliable in a number of laboratories. The simultaneous detection of antibody to several NS proteins in a single test by ELISA (27, 34) or by enzyme-linked immuno-electrotransfer blot (EITB), a type of Western blot, (8) is useful for confirmation of animals positive for antibody to 3AB or 3ABC. There are currently no internationally recognised standards for antibody to FMD virus NS proteins, but an application for these tests is described in detail below.

- **Indirect enzyme-linked immunosorbent assay**

- **Test procedure**

i) Microplates are coated overnight at 4°C with 1 µg/ml of the fusion antigen 3ABC in carbonate/ bicarbonate buffer, pH 9.6 (100 µl per well). Antigen 3ABC was expressed and purified as indicated for the EITB tests (30).

ii) The plates are washed six times with PBS, pH 7.2, supplemented with 0.05% Tween 20.

iii) Test sera (100 µl per well) are added in a 1/20 dilution in blocking buffer consisting of PBS, 0.05% Tween 20, 5% nonfat dry milk, 10% equine sera and 0.1% *Escherichia coli* lysate. Each plate includes a set of reference standards as defined for the EITB assay.

iv) The plates are incubated for 30 minutes at 37°C and washed six times in PBS–Tween.

v) Horseradish-peroxidase-conjugated rabbit anti-species IgG is diluted optimally in the blocking buffer, added at 100 µl per well and the plate incubated for 30 minutes at 37°C.

vi) After six washings, each well is filled with 100 µl of 3.3', 5.5'-tetramethylbenzidine plus 0.004% (w/v) H_2O_2 in phosphate/citrate buffer, pH 5.5.

vii) The reaction is stopped after 15 minutes of incubation at room temperature by adding 100 µl of 0.5 M H_2SO_4. Absorbance is read at 450 nm and at 620 nm for background correction.

• **Interpreting the results**

For the test system to be valid the following performance criteria are applied: the absorbance of negative controls should be <0.10 after correction for absorbance of blank wells. The cut-off serum, obtained as described in the EITB test, should give absorbance values of 0.15–0.40. Results are expressed as an index derived by dividing the absorbance value of the serum tested by that of the cut-off control. The ratio of the weak positive/cut-off controls should be 2.5 with a coefficient of variation <20%. Test sera with ratios >0.8 are considered to be suspect or positive and are retested by EITB. Coated plates and secondary standards are available from the PANAFTOSA[5] on request.

• **Enzyme-linked immunoelectrotransfer blot assay**

The FMD situation in South America is complex and includes a variety of ecosystems and animal populations of varying immune status immunised with vaccines of different formulation. Tests for serological diagnosis therefore must accommodate many variables. To date, the EITB assay has been widely applied in South America for serosurveillance and risk assessment associated with animal movement. Currently, the procedure is to perform an initial screening test using an indirect ELISA for antibody to 3ABC, and to follow that by a confirmatory EITB assay if samples give positive or suspect results. This combination of tests is particularly recommended when serosurveillance involves a large number of samples. Further information is available from the OIE Reference Laboratory in Brazil (see Table given in Part 4 of this *Manual*).

• **Preparation of test strips containing the recombinant antigens**

The five bioengineered FMD virus NS proteins 3A, 3B, 2C, 3D and 3ABC are expressed in *E. coli* C600 by thermo-induction. The 3D polypeptide is expressed in its complete form (30), whereas the rest of the proteins are obtained as fusions to the N-terminal part of the MS-2 polymerase gene (35).

The expressed polymerase is purified over phosphocellulose, followed by poly(U) Sepharose columns. The fused proteins 3A, 3B, 2C and 3ABC are purified by sequential extraction of the bacterial extracts with increasing concentrations of urea. The 7M fraction containing the fusion proteins is further purified on a preparative 10% SDS/PAGE (sodium dodecyl sulphate/polyacrylamide gel electrophoresis). The fusion protein band is excised from the gel and electroeluted (30).

A mixture containing 20 ng/ml of each one of the purified recombinant polypeptides is separated on 12.5% SDS/PAGE and electrophoretically transferred to nitrocellulose (30).

• **Test procedure**

i) The required amount of test strips should be assessed, taking into account that for each nitrocellulose sheet, which defines one transferred gel, a positive, a weakly positive, a cut-off and a negative control serum should be assayed. In general, 24 nitrocellulose strips, each 3 mm wide, should result from a gel.

ii) A volume of 0.8 ml of saturation buffer (50 mM Tris-HCl, pH 7.5; 150 mM NaCl; 0.2% Tween 20; 5% nonfat dry milk; and 0.05% bacterial *E. coli* lysate) is added to each well. The antigen-coated strips are blocked by placing the trays on a rocker and agitating for 30 minutes at room temperature (20–22°C).

iii) A dilution of 1/200 of test sera and of each of the controls is added to the appropriate trough. The strips must be completely submerged and facing upwards, and maintained in that position during the whole process.

iv) Strips are incubated for 60 minutes on a rocker at room temperature.

5 Centre Panamericano de Fiebre Aftosa, Caixa Postal 589, 20001-970 Rio de Janeiro, Brazil. (dir@aftosa.ops-oms.org)

v) Liquid is removed from the trays, and each test strip is washed three times with washing solution (50 mM Tris-HCl, pH 7.5; 150 mM NaCl; and 0.2% Tween 20) by agitation for 5 minutes.

vi) The alkaline-phosphatase-conjugated rabbit anti-bovine solution is added to each test well, and the strips are incubated with shaking for 60 minutes at room temperature.

vii) The liquid is removed from the trays and each test strip is washed three times with washing solution as above.

viii) Substrate solution (0.015% bromochloroindolylphosphate/0.03% nitroblue tetrazolium) is prepared in substrate buffer (100 mM NaCl; 5 mM $MgCl_2$; and 100 mM Tris-HCl, pH 9.3), and is added to each test well.

ix) Strips are incubated by placing the test tray on the orbital mixer and agitating until the cut-off control shows five distinct, discernible bands. Strips are washed with running deionised water and air-dried.

- **Reading the results**

A sample is nonreactive if all the bands are below the reactivity of the cut-off control, or a maximum of two bands are above the reactivity of the cut-off control. A sample is reactive if all four antigens (3ABC, 3A, 3B and 3D) ± 2C have a reactivity equal to or higher than the cut-off control. A sample has indeterminate reactivity if the above-mentioned criteria for reactive or nonreactive samples are not met. Densitometric reading is possible, but visual reading is recommended not only because it is less expensive, but also because borderline reactions rarely occur. The cut-off control serum is derived from a pool of sera and/or dilution of positive sera, representing background EITB reactivities observed individually for the different antigens in nonvaccinated animals from FMD-free regions. These controls are secondary standards, validated against a primary standard corresponding to a serum from an animal at 714 days after experimental infection from which no virus had been recovered from OP fluid for the past 364 days (8) This primary standard is diluted 1/2 when the test is used as an input for evaluation of risk analysis during selection of animals for import/export testing.

Sensitised strips and secondary standards are available on request from the PANAFTOSA (see footnote 5).

B. REQUIREMENTS FOR VACCINES AND DIAGNOSTIC BIOLOGICALS

The control of FMD is usually a national responsibility and, in many countries, the vaccine may be used only when authorised.

Routine vaccination against FMD is used in many countries where the disease is endemic. In contrast, a number of disease-free countries have never vaccinated their livestock but have preferred the use of strict movement controls and slaughter of infected and contact animals when outbreaks have occurred. Nevertheless, many disease-free countries maintain the option to vaccinate and have their own strategic reserves of highly concentrated inactivated virus preparations. Such antigen reserves offer the potential of supplying formulated vaccine in an 'emergency' at short notice (16).

FMD vaccines are chemically inactivated cell-culture-derived preparations of the virus that have been blended with a suitable adjuvant. In the case of vaccines destined for use in swine, oil adjuvants are preferred.

Because of the presence of multiple serotypes of the virus, many FMD vaccines are multivalent and it is common practice to prepare vaccines from two or more different virus strains. In areas where the disease is maintained by free-living buffalo, it is necessary to include more than one virus per serotype to ensure broad antigenic coverage against prevailing viruses.

1. Seed management

a) Characteristics of the seed

Selection of seed viruses should ideally be based on their ease of growth in cell culture, virus yield, stability and broad antigenic spectrum (32). The production strains should be characterised and distributed by the official control laboratories; they should be selected in accordance with the epidemiological importance of each variant.

b) Method of culture

Many manufacturers of FMD vaccines derive their vaccine strains from local field isolates and, for those grown in cell culture, adapt them for growth in suspension or monolayer cells by serial passage. The number of passages in cell culture should be kept to a minimum as there is evidence of antigenic 'drift' of FMD virus during this procedure.

c) **Validation as a vaccine**

Seed viruses must be antigenically characterised and proven to be free from contaminating microorganisms, to establish homology to the original candidate isolates, purity and effectiveness against the circulating strains for which they were developed. This often encompasses a number of methods, but to establish applicability to field strains a virus neutralisation is often used. Seed viruses may be stored at –20°C if glycerinated or at a lower temperature (e.g. –70°C) if not glycerinated. Working seed viruses may be expanded in one or a few more passages from the mother seed stock and used to infect the final cell culture at an approximate rate of 1 PFU (plaque-forming unit) per 100 cells.

2. Method of manufacture

FMD virus is usually produced in either large-scale monolayer or suspension cell systems under aseptic conditions. It is essential that all pipework and vessels be thoroughly sterilised ensuring that no areas in the system harbour microorganisms. In addition to general considerations of sterility, it is important to note that the virus is vulnerable to attack by proteolytic enzymes, such as those produced by microorganisms (12). Control of pH and temperature are also critical because of the acid and temperature lability of the virus (11). Optimum temperature for cell, virus growth and inactivation, normally around 37°C, should be precisely controlled. During other stages of manufacture, the temperature should be reduced to 4–6°C. Virus should be maintained at approximately pH 7.6 and should never be below pH 7.0.

A suitable strain of the virus is used to infect a suspension or monolayer of a transformed cell line, such as BHK. Such cell cultures should be free from contaminating microorganisms. It is common practice to keep stocks of BHK cells over liquid nitrogen and revive as necessary. On revival, they are expanded in nutrient medium to a volume and cell density appropriate to seeding the main culture. As an approximation, the main culture is seeded to give an initial density of 0.2–0.5 × 10^6 cells/ml, which is allowed to multiply to 2–3 × 10^6 cells/ml before being infected with virus.

When the virus has reached its maximum titre, which is variously determined by infectivity, CF or other tests, the culture is clarified and filtered, often with centrifugation. The virus is subsequently inactivated by addition of ethyleneimine (EI), usually in the form of binary ethyleneimine (BEI). This is usually prepared by dissolving, to a concentration of 0.1 M, 2-bromoethylamine hydrobromide in 0.2 N sodium hydroxide solution, and incubating at 37°C for 1 hour (4). The BEI formed is then added to a virus suspension held at 20–37°C, to give a final concentration of 0.001 M. Inactivation is usually continued for 24 hours, followed by a second dose of EI for a further 24 hours. After inactivation any residual BEI in the harvest can be neutralised by adding sodium thiosulphate solution to a final concentration of 2%. To decrease the likelihood of live virus failing to contact the EI at the second application, it is essential to transfer the vessel contents immediately to a second sterile vessel where inactivation is allowed to go to completion at 48 hours.

The inactivated virus may be concentrated by ultrafiltration, polyethylene glycol precipition or polyethylene oxide adsorption (1, 38). These concentrated antigens can be kept at –70°C or lower temperatures for many years, if necessary, and made into vaccine when required by dilution in a suitable buffer and addition of adjuvants (14).

Conventional FMD vaccines are usually formulated in one of two ways. The vaccine most commonly used for cattle is prepared by adsorbing the virus on to aluminium hydroxide gel, one of the adjuvant constituents of the final vaccine blend. Other components of the final blend include antifoam, phenol red dye (if permitted by the country requiring vaccine), lactalbumin hydrolysate, tryptose phosphate broth, antibiotics, amino acids, vitamins and buffer salts. A second adjuvant, saponin, derived from the South American tree *Quillaja saponaria mollina*, is also incorporated, as well as merthiolate/chloroform as a preservative.

An alternative formulation uses mineral oils, such as Marcol and Drakeol, as adjuvants. These preparations offer a number of advantages over the standard aluminium hydroxide/saponin vaccine, not least of which is their efficacy in pigs. They are widely used for vaccinating cattle in South America because of the longer duration of immunity obtained. The mineral oil is usually premixed with an emulsifying agent, such as mannide monooleate, before the addition of an equal volume of the aqueous phase of the vaccine, and emulsified by use of a colloid mill or continuous mechanical or flow ultrasonic emulsifier. More complex double emulsions (water/oil/water) may be produced by emulsifying once more in an aqueous phase containing a small amount of Tween 80 (25).

Significant advances made in recent years have seen the introduction of alternative 'ready-to-use' oil adjuvants. Oils containing esters of octadecenoic acid and 2,5 anhydro-d-mannitol, for example, readily form double or mixed emulsions (water/oil/water), that are both stable and of low viscosity, without the requirement of sophisticated emulsification equipment (5, 16).

3. In-process control

In general, virus titres reach optimum levels within about 24 hours of the cell culture being infected. The time chosen to harvest the culture may be based on a number of assays; for instance cell death. Virus concentration may be assessed by plaque assay, sucrose density gradient (13) or serological techniques. It is preferable to use a method for measuring antigenic mass, such as sucrose density gradient analysis, as well as one that measures infectivity, as the two properties do not necessarily coincide and the different methods may complement one another.

During inactivation of the virus, timed samples should be taken at regular intervals for the purpose of monitoring the rate and linearity of the inactivation process. Virus titres in the samples are determined by inoculation of cell cultures proven to be highly susceptible to FMD virus, e.g. BHK or bovine thyroid cells. Such cultures permit the testing of statistically meaningful samples under reproducible conditions. The $\log_{10}$ infectivities of the timed samples are plotted against time, and the inactivation procedure is not considered to be satisfactory unless at least the latter part of the slope of the line is linear and extrapolation indicates that there would be less than one infectious particle per 10^4 litres of liquid preparation at the end of the inactivation period.

4. Batch control

a) Sterility

The bulk inactivated antigen, the adjuvants, the dilution buffers and the final formulated product should all undergo sterility testing. This may be carried out directly with components of the vaccine or the final product, but the preferred method is to collect any contaminating microorganisms by membrane filtration of the material to be examined and to detect them by incubation of the membranes with culture media. The latter procedure allows the removal of preservatives, etc., which may inhibit the detection of microorganisms. Guidelines on techniques and culture media, which allow the detection of a wide range of organisms, are described in the European Pharmacopoeia 1997 (ref. 19; also refer to Chapter 1.4.).

b) Safety

Following inactivation, a sample of each batch of inactivated antigen representing at least 200 doses should be tested for freedom from infectious virus by inoculation of sensitive monolayer cell cultures, preferably of the same origin as those used for the production of antigen. It may be preferable to concentrate the antigen to do this, in which case it must be shown that the concentrated material does not interfere with the sensitivity or reading of the assay. The cell sheets are examined daily over a period of 3 days, after which the spent medium is transferred to fresh monolayers and the original monolayers replenished with fresh medium. Using this method, traces of live virus can be amplified by the passage procedure and detected on the basis of CPE observed. Two to three passages of the original virus preparation are commonly used. A variant on this method is to freeze–thaw the old monolayers to release intracellular virus, which can be detected by further passage.

c) Potency

Potency is only examined on the final formulated product (see Section B.5.b.).

d) Duration of immunity

In order to establish a satisfactory level of immunity it is usual to give a primary course of two inoculations, 2–4 weeks apart, followed by revaccination every 4–12 months. The frequency of revaccination will depend on the epidemiological situation and the type and quality of vaccine used. Where access to the animals is difficult, it is preferable to use oil adjuvanted vaccine at 4 months and 1 year of age, followed by annual revaccination.

For calves born of vaccinated dams, the first vaccination should be delayed as long as possible to allow decline of maternal antibody, but not beyond 4 months, as at that time a high proportion can be expected to respond effectively to vaccination. For calves born of nonvaccinated dams, the first vaccination may be at 1 week of age (3).

e) Stability

The shelf life of conventional FMD vaccines is usually 1–2 years at 4°C, but they are temperature labile and should neither be frozen nor stored above 4°C.

f) Preservatives

The most commonly used preservatives are chloroform and merthiolate. The latter is used at a final concentration of 1/30,000 (w/v).

g) Precautions (hazards)

Current FMD vaccines are innocuous and present no toxic hazard to the user. Care must be taken to avoid self-injection with oil-emulsion vaccines.

5. Tests on the final product

a) Safety

It is necessary to test FMD vaccines to ensure that the final product is noninfectious and is not unduly toxic. Some laboratories determine noninfectivity by eluting the virus from the vaccine, but this is not universally applicable to all formulations. For example, saponin influences greatly the elution of FMD from aluminium hydroxide/saponin vaccines (15). If the elution procedure is appropriate to a particular formulation, then it may be validated by seeding parallel samples of vaccine with trace amounts of live virus (6).

Toxicity and noninfectivity may be assessed simultaneously in an *in-vivo* test in cattle (18). Each of three healthy seronegative cattle are inoculated intradermally on the dorsal surface of the tongue with 0.1 ml of vaccine at 20 sites (four rows with five inoculation sites each). The animals are observed for no fewer than 4 days, after which three full bovine doses of vaccine are administered by the manufacturer's recommended route to each animal. The animals are observed for a further 6 days. Should any of the animals develop signs of FMD, the vaccine will fail the safety test. Equally, any undue toxicity attributable to the vaccine should be assessed and may prevent its acceptance. Ideally, vaccines prepared for species other than cattle should be safety tested in the species for which they are intended, administering a double dose of vaccine according to the manufacturer's recommended route and dose volume. The animals should be examined daily for a minimum of 7 days for evidence of toxicity or signs of FMD.

Provided that laboratory rodents have been shown to be a satisfactory alternative to the target species for toxicity testing of FMD vaccines, these may be used to assess toxicity (17). The test involves the subcutaneous inoculation of two guinea-pigs and five mice with 2 ml each and 0.5 ml each of vaccine, respectively. The animals are observed for 7 days and the test is considered to be satisfactory if none of the animals dies or shows significant local or systemic reaction.

b) Potency

Cattle of at least 6 months of age, obtained from areas free from FMD, that have not previously been vaccinated against FMD and are free from antibodies neutralising the different types of FMD virus should be used. Three groups of no fewer than five cattle per group should be vaccinated by the route recommended by the manufacturer. The vaccine should be administered at different doses per group by injecting different volumes of the vaccine. For example, if the label states that the injection of 2 ml corresponds to the administration of 1 dose of vaccine, a 1/4 dose of vaccine would be obtained by injecting 0.5 ml, and a 1/10 dose would be obtained by injecting 0.2 ml. These animals and a control group of two nonvaccinated animals are challenged 3 weeks after vaccination with a suspension of bovine virus that is fully virulent and appropriate to the virus types in the vaccine under test by inoculating 10,000 ID_{50} intradermally into two sites on the upper surface of the tongue (0.1 ml per site). Animals are observed for 8–10 days. Unprotected animals show lesions at sites other than the tongue. Control animals must develop lesions on at least three feet. From the number of animals protected in each group, the PD_{50} (50% protective dose) content of the vaccine is calculated. The vaccine should contain at least 3 PD_{50} per dose for cattle, when employed for routine prophylactic use, or 6 PD_{50} per dose when used for emergency ('ring') vaccination. In some cases, vaccine of high potency will prevent the development of local tongue lesions at the site of challenge. In South American countries a variation of the potency test is performed, the PGP test (percentage of protection against generalised foot infection).

Potency tests in other target species, such as sheep, goats or buffalo are not common, as a successful test in cattle is considered sufficient to endorse its use in other species. Under circumstances where a vaccine is produced for use primarily in one particular species, it may be more appropriate to potency test the vaccine in that same species. However, in respect to the limited data for African buffalo or Asiatic buffalo *(Bubalus bubalis)* and sheep, and the often inapparent nature of the disease in these species, potency results from a cattle test should be a good indicator of the vaccines applicability in these other species.

A similar protocol to the cattle test can be adopted for potency testing FMD vaccines in pigs. Using three groups of five pigs, one group is vaccinated with the full pig dose recommended by the manufacturer, one group receives a 1/4 dose, and a third group receives a 1/16 dose of vaccine. Traditionally, the response to oil vaccine is allowed longer to develop, and not until day 28 after vaccination are the three groups, plus two unvaccinated control pigs challenged. Challenge is by intradermal injection into the heel bulbs of one foot with 10,000 $TCID_{50}$ (0.2 ml) of a virulent challenge virus homologous to a strain used in the vaccine. The animals are observed daily for 10 days after challenge for clinical signs of FMD, but animals are removed as soon as they develop generalised FMD to avoid excessive challenge to those remaining. Both control animals should develop clinical signs on more than one foot. Probit tables are used to determine the potency of the vaccine under test. The vaccine should contain at least 3 PD_{50} per dose for pigs.

Other tests, including measurement following vaccination of virus neutralising antibodies in cell culture, or ELISA antibodies, or serum-protecting antibodies in suckling mice, may be used to assess the potency of a vaccine provided that a statistical evaluation has established a satisfactory correlation between the results obtained by the test on the relevant vaccine serotype and the potency test in cattle (37). For example, the expected percentage of protection is used to analyse the sera of a group of at least 16 vaccinated cattle and to express the probability of an animal being protected by measuring neutralising, ELISA or protecting antibodies. In a single group of animals given a half dose of vaccine, the expected percentage protection should be equal to or greater than 80%.

The presence of more than one serotype in a vaccine does not interfere with the induction of antibodies against another serotype or the correlation of antibody titre with protection.

REFERENCES

1. ADAMOWICZ PH., LEGRAND B., GUERCHE J. & PRUNET P. (1974). Un nouveau procedé de concentration et de purification du virus. Application du virus de la fièvre aphteuse produit sur cellules BHK21 pour l'obtention des vaccins hautement purifiés. *Bull. OIE*, **81**, 1125–1150.

2. AMAREL-DOEL C.M.F., OWEN N.E., FERRIS N.P., KITCHING R.P. & DOEL T.R. (1993). Detection of foot-and-mouth disease viral sequences in clinical specimens and ethyleneimine-inacctivated preparations by the polymerase chain reaction. *Vaccine*, **11**, 415–421.

3. AUGE DE MELLO P., GOMES I. & BAHNEMANN H.G. (1989). The vaccination of young cattle with an oil adjuvant foot-and-mouth disease vaccine. *Bol. Centr. Panam. Fiebre. Aftosa*, **55**, 3–14.

4. BAHNEMANN H.G. (1975). Binary ethyleneimine as an inactivant for foot-and-mouth disease virus and its application for vaccine production. *Arch. Virol.*, **47**, 47–56.

5. BARNETT P.V., PULLEN L., WILLIAMS L. & DOEL T.R. (1996). International bank for foot-and-mouth disease vaccine: assessment of Montanide ISA 25 and ISA 206, two commercially available oil adjuvants. *Vaccine*, **14**, 1187–1198.

6. BARTELING S.Z. & VREESWIJK Z. (1991). Developments in foot-and-mouth disease vaccines. *Vaccine*, **9**, 75–88.

7. BASTOS A.D.S. (1998). Detection and characterization of foot-and-mouth disease virus in sub-Saharan Africa. *Onderstepoort J. Vet. Res.*, **65**, 37–47.

8. BERGMANN I.E., DE MELLO P.A., NEITZERT E., BECK & GOMEZ, I. (1993). Diagnosis of persistent aphthovirus infection and its differentiation from vaccination response in cattle by use of enzyme-linked immunoelectrotransfer blot analysis with bioengineered non-structural viral antigens. *Am. J. Vet. Res.*, **54**, 825–831.

9. CLARKE J.B. & SPIER R.E. (1980). Variation in the susceptibility of BHK populations and cloned cell lines to three strains of foot-and-mouth disease virus. *Arch. Virol.*, **63**, 1–9.

10. DE DIEGO M., BROCCHI E., MACKAY D. & DE SIMONE F. (1997). The use of the non-structural polyprotein 3ABC of FMD virus as a diagnostic antigen in ELISA to differentiate infected from vaccinated cattle. *Arch. Virol.*, **142**, 2021–2033.

11. DOEL T.R. & BACCARINI P.J. (1981). Thermal stability of FMDV. *Arch. Virol.*, **70**, 21–32.

12. DOEL T.R. & COLLEN T. (1982). Qualitative assessment of 146S particles of FMDV in preparations destined for vaccines. *J. Biol. Stand.*, **10**, 69–81.

13. DOEL T.R., FLETTON B. & STAPLE R.F. (1982). Further developments in the quantification of small RNA viruses by UV photometry of sucrose density gradients. *Dev. Biol. Stand.*, **50**, 209–219.

14. DOEL T.R. & PULLEN L. (1990). International bank for foot-and-mouth disease vaccines: stability studies with virus concentrates and vaccines prepared from them. *Vaccine*, **8**, 473–478.

15. DOEL T.R. & STAPLE R.F. (1982). The elution of FMDV from vaccines adjuvanted with aluminium hydroxide and with saponin. *J. Biol. Stand.*, **10**, 185–195.

16. DOEL T.R., WILLIAMS L. & BARNETT P.V. (1994). Emergency vaccination against foot-and-mouth disease. The rate of development of immunity and its implications for the carrier state. *Vaccine*, **12**, 592–600.

17. EUROPEAN PHARMACOPOEIA (1986). Second Edition. Editions of the Council of Europe, Strasbourg, France.

18. EUROPEAN PHARMACOPOEIA (1993). Second Edition. Monograph No. 63. Editions of the Council of Europe, Strasbourg, France.

19. EUROPEAN PHARMACOPOEIA (1997). Third Edition. Section 5: 5.1.1. and 5.1.2. Editions of the Council of Europe, Strasbourg, France.

20. FERRIS N.P. & DAWSON M. (1988). Routine application of enzyme-linked immunosorbent assay in comparison with complement fixation for the diagnosis of foot-and-mouth and swine vesicular disease. *Vet. Microbiol.*, **16**, 201–209.

21. FOOD AND AGRICULTURAL ORGANIZATION OF THE UNITED NATIONS (FAO) (1984). Emerging Diseases of Livestock. Vol. 1. The Diseases and their Diagnosis, Geering W.A., ed. FAO, Rome, Italy, 43–51.

22. GOLDING S.M., HEDGER R.S., TALBOT P. & WATSON J. (1976). Radial immunodiffusions and serum neutralisation techniques for the assay of antibodies to swine vesicular disease. *Res. Vet. Sci.*, **20**, 142–147.

23. HAMBLIN C., BARNETT I.T.R. & HEDGER R.S. (1986). A new enzyme-linked immunosorbent assay (ELISA) for the detection of antibodies against foot-and-mouth disease virus. I. Development and method of ELISA. *J. Immunol. Methods*, **93**, 115–121.

24. HAMBLIN C., KITCHING R.P., DONALDSON A.I., CROWTHER J.R. & BARNETT I.T.R. (1987). Enzyme-linked immunosorbent assay (ELISA) for the detection of antibodies against foot-and-mouth disease virus. 3. Evaluation of antibodies after infection and vaccination. *Epidemiol. Infect.*, **99**, 733–744

25. HERBERT W.J. (1965). Multiple emulsions. A new form of mineral-oil antigen adjuvant. *Lancet*, **II**. 771.

26. KITCHING R.P. & DONALDSON A.I. (1987). Collection and transportation of specimens for vesicular virus investigation. *Rev. sci. Tech. Off. int. Epiz.*, **6**, 263–272.

27. MACKAY D.K.J, FORSYTH M.A., DAVIES P.R., BERLINZANI, A., BELSHAM G.J., FLINT M. & RYAN M.D. (1997). Differentiating infection from vaccination in foot-and-mouth disease using a panel of recombinant, non-structural proteins in ELISA. *Vaccine,* **16**, 446–459.

28. MCVICAR J.W. & SUTMOLLER P. (1970). Foot-and-mouth disease: the agar gel immunodiffusion precipitin test for antibody to virus-infection-associated (VIA) antigen as a tool for epizootiologic surveys. *Am. J. Epidemiol.*, **92**, 273–278.

29. MINISTRY OF AGRICULTURE, FISHERIES AND FOOD (1986). Foot-and-mouth disease. Ageing of lesions. Her Majesty's Stationery Office, London, UK.

30. NEITZERT E., BECK E., AUGE DE MELLO P., GOMES I. & BERGMANN I.E. (1991). Expression of the aphthovirus RNA polymerase gene in *Escherichia coli* and its use together with other bioengineered non-structural antigens in detection of late persistent infections. *Virology*, **184**, 799–804.

31. ROEDER P.L. & LE BLANC SMITH P.M. (1987). The detection and typing of foot-and-mouth disease virus by enzyme-linked immunosorbent assay: a sensitive, rapid and reliable technique for primary diagnosis. *Res. Vet. Sci.*, **43**, 225–232.

32. SAMUEL A.R., OULDRIDGE E.J., ARROWSMITH A.E.M., KITCHING R.P. & KNOWLES N.J. (1990). Serological analysis of type O isolates of FMD from the Middle East 1981–88. *Vaccine*, **8**, 390–395.

33. SKINNER H.H. (1960). Some techniques for producing and studying attenuated strains of the virus of foot and mouth disease. *Bull. OIE*, **53**, 634–650.

34. SORENSEN K.J., MADSEN K.G., MADSEN E.S., SALT J.S., NQUINDI J. & MACKAY D.K.J. (1998). Differentiation of infection from vaccination in foot-and-mouth disease by the detection of antibodies to the non-structural proteins 3D, 3AB and 3ABC in ELISA using antigens expressed in baculovirus. *Arch. Virol.*, **143**, 1461–1476.

35. STREBEL K., BECK E., STROHMAIER D. & SCHALLER H. (1986). Characterisation of foot-and-mouth disease virus gene products with antisera against bacterially synthesised fusion proteins. *J. Virol.*, **57**, 983–991.

36. VAN MAANEN C. (1990). A complex-trapping-blocking (CTB) ELISA, using monoclonal antibodies and detecting specifically antibodies directed against foot and mouth disease types A, O and C. 1. Method and characteristics. *Vet. Microbiol.*, **24**, 171–178.

37. VIANNA FILHO Y.L., ASTUDILLO V., GOMES I., FERNANDEZ G., ROZAS C.E.E., RAVISON J.A. & ALONSO A. (1993). Potency control of foot-and-mouth disease vaccine in cattle. Comparison of the 50% protective dose and protection against generalisation. *Vaccine*, **11–14**, 1424–1428.

38. WAGNER G.G., CARD J.L. & COWAN K.M. (1970). Immunochemical studies of foot-and-mouth disease virus. VII. Characterization of foot-and-mouth disease virus concentrated by polyethylene glycol precipitation. *Arch. Ges. Virusforsch.*, **30**, 343–352.

39. WOODBURY E.L., ILOTT M.C., BROWN C.C. & SALT J.S. (1995). Optimization of an *in situ* hybridization technique for the detection of foot-and-mouth disease virus in bovine tissues using the digoxigenin system. *J. Virol. Methods*, **51**, 89–94.

*

* *

CHAPTER 2.1.2.

VESICULAR STOMATITIS

SUMMARY

Vesicular stomatitis (VS) is a vesicular disease of horses, cattle and pigs caused by a vesiculovirus of the family Rhabdoviridae. This disease is clinically indistinguishable from foot and mouth disease (FMD), vesicular exanthema (VE), or swine vesicular disease (SVD) when horses are not involved. Sheep, goats and many other wild species can be infected. Humans are also susceptible. The disease is limited to the Americas; however, it was previously described in France and in South Africa.

Although VS is transmitted directly by the transcutaneous or transmucosal route, the VS virus has been isolated from sandflies and mosquitoes, suggesting that it could be insect-borne. There is, therefore, seasonal variation in the occurrence of VS: it disappears at the end of the rainy season in tropical areas, and at the first frosts in temperate zones. There is also some evidence that VS virus could be a plant virus and that animals are the end of the epidemiological chain. The pathogenesis of the disease is unclear, and it has been observed that the humoral-specific antibodies do not always prevent infection with VS virus.

Although VS may be suspected when horses are involved as well as pigs and cattle, prompt differential diagnosis is essential because the clinical signs of VS are indistinguishable from FMD when cattle and pigs are affected, and from SVD or VE when only pigs are affected.

***Identification of the agent:** VS virus can be readily isolated by the inoculation of several tissue culture systems, unweaned mice or embryonated chicken eggs. Viral antigen can be identified by an indirect sandwich enzyme-linked immunosorbent assay (IS-ELISA) – this is the least expensive and most rapid test. The complement fixation (CF) test is also a good alternative. The virus neutralisation (VN) test may be used, but it is elaborate and time-consuming.*

***Serological tests:** Convalescent animals develop serotype-specific antibodies within 4–8 days of infection that are demonstrated by a liquid-phase blocking ELISA (LP-ELISA) and VN. Other described tests are CF, agar gel immunodiffusion, counter immunoelectrophoresis and a competitive ELISA.*

***Requirements for vaccines and diagnostic biologicals:** Inactivated virus vaccines with aluminium hydroxide or oil as adjuvants have been tested in the United States of America and in Colombia, respectively. Both vaccines generated high levels of specific antibodies in the sera of vaccinated cattle. However, it is not yet clear if serum antibodies would prevent the disease. An attenuated virus vaccine has been used in the field with unknown efficacy.*

A. DIAGNOSTIC TECHNIQUES

Vesicular stomatitis (VS) was described in the United States of America (USA) in 1926 (17) and 1927 (7) as a vesicular disease of horses, and subsequently of cattle and pigs. Vesicles are caused by the VS virus on the tongue, lips, buccal mucosa, teats and in the epithelium of the coronary band of the feet of cattle, horses, pigs, and many other species of domestic and wild animals. Many species of laboratory animals are also susceptible. The disease is limited to the Americas; however, it was described in France (1915 and 1917) and in South Africa (1886 and 1897) (11).

Influenza-like signs, normally without vesicles, have been observed in humans who are in contact with animals with VS or who handle infective VS virus. This indicates that all manipulations involving VS virus, including infective materials from animals, should be undertaken with adequate biohazard containment.

There are two major immunological types of VS virus, New Jersey (NJ) and Indiana (IND). Both viruses are members of the genus *Vesiculovirus*, family Rhabdoviridae and have been extensively studied at the molecular level. Several other closely related rhabdoviruses have been isolated from sick animals over the past decades. These VS viruses are represented by the Salto-Argentina/63 and Alagoas-Brazil/64 strains, which are considered to be subtypes 2 and 3, respectively, of the IND serotype (8). Strains of the serotype NJ and subtype IND-1 are identified in the endemic areas of the disease: south-eastern USA, Mexico, Central America, Panama, Venezuela, Colombia, Ecuador and Peru. The IND-2 Salto-Argentina/63 strain was isolated from horses in Argentina in 1963. This strain, along with the IND-2 Maipú-Argentina/86 and two other strains isolated in 1966 and 1979 in Brazil, and classified in the same subtype, only affected horses (2, 3). Cattle living together with the affected horses did not present antibody conversion (2). The IND-3 subtype, represented by the strain IND-3 Alagoas-Brazil/64, has been identified, sporadically, in Brazil only. Until 1977, strains of the IND-3 subtype were isolated from horses only. However, the IND-3 Espinosa-Brazil/77 was the first strain isolated from cattle. The known IND-3 strains affect cattle to a lesser degree than horses (2, 3). This finding confirms the first descriptions, in 1926 and 1927 (7, 17), of the NJ and IND serotypes in horses, and subsequently in cattle and pigs.

The mechanism of transmission of VS virus is unclear. The fact that the virus has been isolated from sandflies, mosquitoes, and other insects tends to substantiate the hypothesis that it could be transmitted by insects (6, 10, 16). There are also hypotheses that the VS virus is a plant virus present in pasture (16), and that animals are the end of the epidemiological chain. In special circumstances, the virus could undergo an adaptational process to infect animals, followed by direct transmission between susceptible animals. The 1982 epizootic in western USA showed direct transmission in many cases (19). While VS is not diagnosed in livestock every year in the USA, it is considered to be endemic in feral pigs on Ossabaw Island, Georgia (5).

The incidence of disease can vary widely among affected herds. Usually 10–15% of the animals show clinical signs. Clinical cases are mainly seen in adult animals. Cattle and horses under 1 year of age are rarely affected. Mortality is close to zero in both species. However, high mortality rates in pigs affected by the NJ virus have been observed. Sick animals recover in about 2 weeks. The most common complications of economic importance are mastitis and loss of production in dairy herds (15). Both NJ and IND-1 serotypes in the 1995, 1997 and 1998 US outbreaks primarily caused clinical disease in horses, although seroconversion was seen in cattle.

VS cannot be reliably clinically differentiated from the other vesicular diseases, such as foot and mouth disease (FMD), vesicular exanthema (VE) and swine vesicular disease (SVD), when horses are not involved. An early laboratory diagnosis of any suspected VS case is therefore a matter of urgency.

The sample collection and technology used for the diagnosis of VS must be in concordance with the methodology used for the diagnosis of FMD, VE and SVD, in order to facilitate the differential diagnosis of these vesicular diseases.

Vesicle fluid, epithelium covering unruptured vesicles or epithelial flaps of freshly ruptured vesicles are the best diagnostic samples. These samples can be collected from mouth lesions, as well as from the feet and any other sites of vesicle development. It is recommended that animals should be sedated before samples are collected to avoid injury to helpers and for reasons of animal welfare. Epithelial samples should be placed in bottles of Tris-buffered tryptose broth with phenol red, pH 7.6. Samples must be kept at 4°C if shipped within 24 hours. If Tris-buffered tryptose broth is not available, the epithelial samples can be frozen and shipped on dry ice in securely closed bottles. Leakage of carbon dioxide (CO_2) into bottles must be prevented because it will destroy the virus. If complement fixation (CF) is to be carried out for antigen, the sample can be collected in glycerol/phosphate buffer, pH 7.2–7.6 (Note: glycerol is toxic to VS virus and decreases the sensitivity of virus isolation; it is therefore only recommended for collection of samples for CF test).

When epithelial tissue is not available from cattle, samples of oesophageal–pharyngeal (OP) fluid can be collected by means of a probang (sputum) cup. In pigs, throat swabs can be taken for submission to a laboratory for virus isolation. This material should be sent to the laboratory in Tris-buffered tryptose broth. OP fluids must be transported on wet ice (<24 hours in transport) or dry ice (>24 hours in transport).

When it is not possible to collect samples for identification of the agent, serum samples from recovered animals can be used for detecting and quantifying specific antibodies. Pairs of sera from the same animals, collected 2 weeks apart, are preferred for checking the change in antibody titre.

Specific diagnostic reagents for VS virus are not commercially available and each laboratory produces its own. The two OIE Reference Laboratories for vesicular stomatitis (see Table given in Part 4 of this *Manual*), and the Institute for Animal Health[1], produce and distribute diagnostic reagents on request.

1 Institute for Animal Health, Pirbright Laboratory, Ash Road, Pirbright, Woking, Surrey GU24 0NF, United Kingdom.

1. Identification of the agent

For identification of VS virus and the differential diagnosis of vesicular diseases, clarified suspensions of field samples suspected to contain VS virus should be submitted for immunological testing. For virus isolation, the same samples are inoculated into appropriate cell cultures. The inoculation of African green monkey kidney (Vero), baby hamster kidney (BHK-21) and IB-RS-2 cell cultures with the same sample permits differentiation of the vesicular diseases: VS virus causes a cytopathic effect (CPE) in all three cell lines; FMD virus causes a CPE in BHK-21 and in IB-RS-2, while SVD virus causes a CPE in IB-RS-2 only. Many other cell lines, as well as most primary cell cultures of animal origin, are susceptible to VS virus.

The VS virus replicates and can be isolated in 8–10-day-old chicken embryos by inoculation into the allantoic sac, in 2–7-day-old unweaned mice by inoculation by any route, or in 3-week-old mice by intracerebral inoculation. In all three cases, VS virus causes death in between 2 and 5 days after inoculation.

The most susceptible route for horses and cattle is intradermalingual administration. Pigs are inoculated in the coronary band of the foot or on the snout. Vesicular lesions may be observed in the epithelial tissues of the mouth, teats and feet, 2–4 days after inoculation. The presence of secondary vesicles after inoculation of cattle and horses depends mainly on the VS virus strain used. The snout is normally affected in pigs.

If a CPE develops in the cultures, the suspension fluids can be used for identification of the agent by different immunological tests and the cell culture can be stained with VS-specific fluorescent antibody conjugate. Similar tests can be performed on homogenate suspensions of the dissected musculo-skeletal tissues of any dead mice and chicken embryos and with suspensions of epithelial samples. The brain tissue from mice is an excellent source of virus.

Due to the different morphological characteristics of the rhabdovirus (VS virus), picornavirus (FMD virus and SVD virus), calicivirus (VE) and the large number of virus particles present in vesicular fluids and epithelial tissues, electron microscopy can be a useful diagnostic tool for differentiating the virus family involved.

The preferred procedures for the identification of the viral antigens at the laboratory by immunological methods are the enzyme-linked immunosorbent assay (ELISA) (2, 9), the CF test (2, 13) and fluorescent antibody staining. The virus neutralisation (VN) test with known positive antisera of VS virus NJ and IND serotypes may be used in tissue cultures, unweaned mice or embryonated eggs, but it is more time-consuming.

a) Enzyme-linked immunosorbent assay

The indirect sandwich ELISA (IS-ELISA) (2, 9) is currently the diagnostic method of choice for identification of viral serotypes of VS and other vesicular diseases. Specifically, the ELISA procedure with a set of polyvalent rabbit/guinea-pig antisera, prepared against virions of the representative strains of the three subtypes of the IND serotype, identifies all strains of the VS virus IND serotype (2). For detection of VS virus NJ strains, a monovalent set of rabbit/guinea-pig antisera is suitable (2, 9).

- **Test procedure**

i) *Solid phase:* ELISA plates are coated either for 1 hour at 37°C or overnight at 4°C with rabbit antisera and normal rabbit serum (as described in refs 2 and 4), and optimally diluted in carbonate/bicarbonate buffer, pH 9.6. Subsequently, the plates are washed once with phosphate buffered saline (PBS) and blocked for 1 hour at room temperature with 1% ovalbumin in PBS. The plates are used immediately or are washed three times and stored at –20°C for future use.

ii) *Test samples:* Antigen suspensions of test samples (10–20% epithelial tissue suspension, musculo-skeletal tissue of chicken embryo or mice in PBS or undiluted clarified cell culture supernatant fluid) are deposited in the corresponding wells and the plates are incubated for 30 minutes at 37°C on an orbital shaker.

iii) *Detector:* Monovalent and polyvalent guinea-pig antisera to VS virus NJ and IND serotypes, respectively, that are homologous to coated rabbit serum and that have been diluted appropriately in PBS containing 0.05% Tween 20, 1% ovalbumin, 2% normal rabbit serum, and 2% normal bovine serum (PBSTB) are added to the corresponding wells and left to react for 30 minutes at 37°C on an orbital shaker.

iv) *Conjugate:* Peroxidase/rabbit or goat IgG anti-guinea-pig Ig conjugate, diluted in PBSTB, is added and left to react for 30 minutes at 37°C on an orbital shaker.

v) *Substrate:* H_2O_2-activated substrate is added and left to react at room temperature for 15 minutes, followed by the addition of sulphuric acid to stop the reaction. Absorbance values are measured using an ELISA reader.

Throughout the test, 50 µl reagent volumes are used. The plates are washed five times between each stage with PBS containing 0.05% Tween 20. Controls for the reagents used are included.

vi) *Interpretation of the results:* An antiserum giving an absorbance more than 20% greater than the other antisera, negative serum and controls is considered to be positive for the corresponding virus subtype.

b) Complement fixation test

The ELISA is preferable to the CF test because it is more sensitive and it is not affected by pro- or anti-complementary factors. When ELISA reagents are not available, however, the CF test may be performed. The CF test in U-bottomed microtitre plates, using the reagents titrated by CF50% test, will be described.

- **Test procedure**

i) *Antisera:* Guinea-pig monovalent anti-NJ VS virus and polyvalent anti-IND VS virus, diluted in veronal buffer (VB) at a dilution containing 2.5 CFU_{50} (50% complement fixation units) against homologous virus, are deposited in plate wells. Those antisera are the detectors used in ELISA.

ii) *Test samples:* The same antigen suspension of test samples used for IS-ELISA are added to the wells with serum.

iii) *Complement:* 4 CHU_{50} (50% complement haemolytic units) are added over the serum and antigen. The mixture of antisera, test samples and complement is incubated at 37°C for 30 minutes.

iv) *Haemolytic system:* A suspension of sheep red blood cells (SRBC) in VB, sensitised with 10 HU_{50} (50% haemolytic units) of rabbit anti-SRBC serum, is added to the wells. The haemolytic system has an absorbance of 0.66 read at 545 nm, in the proportion of two volumes of haemolytic system + three volumes of distilled water. The mixture is incubated for 30 minutes at 37°C. Subsequently, the plates are centrifuged and the reaction is observed visually.

Volumes of 25 µl for antisera, test samples and complement, and 50 µl of haemolytic system, are required. Appropriate controls for the antisera, antigens, complement and haemolytic system are included.

It is possible to perform the CF50% test in tubes (2) using reagent volumes eight times greater than those indicated for the CF in microtitre plates. With the CF50% test, the reaction can be expressed as absorbance read spectrophotometrically at 545 nm.

v) *Interpretation of the results:* When controls are as expected, samples with haemolysis <20% for one antiserum in comparison with the other antiserum and controls are considered to be positive for the corresponding type.

Negative results of field samples by ELISA or CF test are inoculated into cell culture or unweaned mice. If at the third passage they continue to be negative, the specimen is considered to be negative for VS virus.

c) Nucleic acid recognition methods

The polymerase chain reaction (PCR) can be used to amplify small genomic areas of the vesicular stomatitis virus (12, 18). This technique will detect the presence of VS virus RNA in tissue and vesicular fluid samples and cell culture, but cannot determine if the virus is infectious. In general, PCR techniques are not routinely used for screening diagnostic cases for vesicular stomatitis virus.

2. Serological tests

For the identification and quantification of specific antibodies in serum, the ELISA and the VN test are preferable. The CF test may be used for quantification of early antibodies.

a) Enzyme-linked immunosorbent assay (a prescribed test for international trade)

The liquid-phase blocking ELISA (LP-ELISA) is the method of choice for the detection and quantification of antibodies to VS virus. The use of viral glycoproteins as antigen is recommended because they are not infectious, detect neutralising antibodies and give fewer false-positive results than the VN (4).

- **Test procedure**

i) *Solid phase:* As described above in Section A.1.a. for the IS-ELISA.

ii) *Liquid phase:* Duplicate, twofold dilution series of each test serum, starting at 1/4, are prepared in U-bottomed microtitre plates. An equal volume of VS virus NJ or IND glycoprotein, in a dilution providing 70% of reaction, is added to each well and the plates are incubated for 1 hour at 37°C. 50 µl of these mixtures is then transferred to the ELISA plates with the solid phase and left to react for 30 minutes at 37°C on an orbital shaker.

iii) *Detector, conjugate and substrate:* The same reagents and methods are used as those indicated for the IS-ELISA.

iv) *Interpretation of the results:* 50% end-point titres are expressed in log_{10} in reference to the 50% reduction of negative serum control, according to the Spearmann–Kärber method. Titres of >1.3 (1/20) are considered to be positive.

- **Competitive enzyme-linked immunosorbent assay (a prescribed test for international trade)**

A competitive ELISA for detection of antibodies has also been developed. The procedure described here is based on a procedure described by Afshar *et al.* (1). It uses vesicular stomatitis NJ and IND-1 recombinant antigens as described by Katz *et al.* (14).

- **Test procedure**

i) *Solid phase:* Antigens are diluted in carbonate/bicarbonate buffer, pH 9.6, and 50 µl is added to each well of a 96-well ELISA plate. Plates are incubated overnight at 4°C; coated plates can be frozen at –70°C for up to 30 days. Plates are thawed, antigen is decanted, and 100 µl of blocking solution is added. Plates are then incubated at 25°C for 30 minutes and blocking solution is decanted. Plates are washed three times with PBS/0.05% Tween 20 solution.

ii) *Liquid phase:* 50 µl of serum diluted 1/8 in 1% nonfat dry milk in PBS is added to each of the duplicate wells for each sample. Plates are incubated at 37°C for 30 minutes. Without washing, 50 µl of polyclonal ascites fluid is added to each well and plates are incubated at 37°C for 30 minutes.

iii) *Detector:* Plates are washed three times, and 50 µl of goat anti-mouse horseradish-peroxidase conjugate diluted in 1% nonfat drymilk is added to each well. Plates are incubated at 37°C for 30 minutes, washed three times, and 50 µl of tetramethyl-benzidine (TMB) substrate solution is added to each well. Plates are incubated at 25°C for 20 minutes or until diluent control wells reach approximately 1.0 optical density. Then 50 µl of 0.05 M sulphuric acid is added to each well and plates are read at 450 nm.

iv) *Interpretation of the results:* A sample is positive if the absorbance is ≤50% of the absorbance of the diluent control.

b) Virus neutralisation (a prescribed test for international trade)

The VN test is carried out in tissue culture microtitre plates with flat-bottomed wells using inactivated serum as test sample, 1000 $TCID_{50}$ (50% tissue culture infective dose) of NJ or IND VS virus and Vero M cells, and preformed monolayer (4) or suspension IB-RS-2 cells to test for the presence of unneutralised virus.

- **Test procedure**

i) *Virus:* NJ or IND VS virus are grown in Vero cell monolayers and stored in liquid nitrogen or frozen at –70°C.

ii) *Test samples:* Sera are inactivated at 56°C for 30 minutes before testing. Positive and negative control standard sera are included in the test.

iii) *Virus neutralisation:* Sera are diluted in a twofold dilution series across the plates, starting from 1/4 dilution. Two rows of wells are used per serum. The same volume of NJ or IND VS virus suspension containing about 1000 $TCID_{50}$/25 µl is added and incubated at 37°C for 60 minutes to allow neutralisation to take place. Subsequently, 50 µl of the mixtures is deposited on preformed cell monolayers in microtitre plates, and 150 µl of 300,000/ml IB-RS-2 or Vero cell suspension is added to each well with the serum/virus mixtures. The plates are covered with loosely fitting lids and incubated for 48 hours at 37°C in an atmosphere of 5% CO_2 or sealed with pressure-sensitive tape and incubated in a normal atmosphere.

iv) *Interpretation of the results:* Wells without CPE are considered to be protected. End-point titres are determined by the Spearmann–Kärber method when the 1000 $TCID_{50}$ are between 500 and 1330 $TCID_{50}$ and when titres of positive and negative standard sera are within twofold of their mean values as estimated from previous titration. The 50% neutralisation titres of each serum are expressed at log 10. Sera with values >1.6 (1/40) are considered to be positive for VS.

c) Complement fixation (a prescribed test for international trade)

A detailed description of this test is given in Section A.1.b. This is modified as follows. The CF test may be used for quantification of early antibodies. For this purpose, twofold serum dilutions are mixed with 2 CFU_{50} of known antigen and with 5% normal bovine or calf sera included in 4 CHU_{50} of complement. The mixture is incubated for 3 hours at 37°C or overnight at 4°C. Subsequently, the haemolytic system is added followed by incubation for 30 minutes at 37°C. The serum titre is the highest dilution in which no haemolysis is observed. Titres of 1/5 or greater are considered to be positive. This CF has low sensitivity and is frequently affected by anticomplementary or nonspecific factors.

B. REQUIREMENTS FOR VACCINES AND DIAGNOSTIC BIOLOGICALS

Attenuated virus vaccines have been tested in the field in the USA, Panama, Guatemala, Peru and Venezuela (15, 16) with unknown efficacy. At present, live or inactivated virus vaccines are not yet available commercially.

• **Acknowledgement**

Parts of this chapter were taken from or based on the chapter on vesicular stomatitis in previous editions of the *Manual*.

REFERENCES

1. AFSHAR A., SHAKARCHI N.H. & DULAC G.C. (1993). Development of a competitive enzyme linked immunosorbent assay for detection of bovine, equine, ovine and porcine antibodies to vesicular stomatitis virus. *J. Clin. Microbiol.*, **31**, 1860–1865.

2. ALONSO A., MARTINS M., GOMES M.P.D., ALLENDE R. & SONDAHL M.S. (1991). Development and evaluation of an enzyme-linked immunosorbent assay for detection, typing and subtyping of vesicular stomatitis virus. *J. Vet. Diagn. Invest.*, **3**, 287–292.

3. ALONSO FERNANDEZ A. & SONDAHL M.S. (1985). Antigenic and immunogenic characterisation of various strains of the Indiana serotype of vesicular stomatitis isolated in Brazil. *Bol. Cen. Panam. Fiebre Aftosa,* **51**, 25–30.

4. ALLENDE R., SEPULVEDA L., MENDES DA SILVA A., MARTINS M., SONDAHL M.S. & ALONSO FERNANDEZ A. (1992). An enzyme-linked immunosorbent assay for the detection of vesicular stomatitis virus antibodies. *Prev. Vet. Med.,* **14**, 293–301.

5. BORING W. & SMITH D. (1962). Vesicular Stomatitis Virus: A Survey and Analysis of the Literature. Technical Study No. 43, US Army Biological Laboratories, Fort Detrick, USA.

6. COMER S.A., CORN J.L., STALLKNECHT D.E., LANDGRAF J.G. & NETTLES V.F. (1992). Titers of vesicular stomatitis virus New Jersey serotype in naturally infected male and female *Lutzomyia shannoni* (Diptera: Psychodidae) in Georgia. *J. Med. Entomol.,* **29**, 368–370.

7. COTTON W.E. (1927). Vesicular stomatitis. *Vet. Med.,* **22**, 169–175.

8. FEDERER K.E., BURROWS R. & BROOKSBY J.B. (1967). Vesicular stomatitis virus – the relation between some strains of the Indiana serotype. *Res. Vet. Sci.*, **8**, 103–117.

9. FERRIS N.P. & DONALDSON A.I. (1988). An enzyme-linked immunosorbent assay for the detection of VSV antigen. *Vet. Microbiol.*, **18**, 243–258.

10. FRANCY D.B., MOORE C.G., SMITH G.C., TAYLOR S.A. & CALISER C.H. (1988). Epizootic vesicular stomatitis in Colorado, 1982: isolation of virus from insects collected along the northern Colorado Rocky Mountain Front Range. *J. Med. Entomol.,* **25**, 343–347.

11. HANSON R.P. (1952). The natural history of vesicular stomatitis. *Bacteriol. Rev.*, **16**, 179–204.

12. HOFNER M.C., CARPENTER W.C., FERRIS N.P., KITCHING R.P. & BOTERO F.A. (1994). A hemi-nested PCR assay for the detection and identification of vesicular stomatitis virus nucleic acid. *J. Virol. Methods*, **50**, 11–20.

13. JENNY E.W., MOTT L.O. & TRAUB E. (1958). Serological studies with the virus of vesicular stomatitis. I. Typing of vesicular stomatitis by complement fixation. *Am. J. Vet. Res.*, **19**, 993–998.

14. KATZ J.B., SHAFER A.L. & EERNISSE K.A. (1995). Construction and insect larval expression of recombinant vesicular stomatitis nucleocapsid protein and its use in competitive ELISA. *J. Virol. Methods*, **54**, 145–157.

15. LAUERMAN L.H., KUNS M.L. & HANSON R.S. (1962). Field trial of live virus vaccination procedure for prevention of vesicular stomatitis in dairy cattle. I: Preliminary immune response. Proceedings of the 66th Annual Meeting of the United States Animal Health Association, 365–369.

16. MASON J. (1978). The epidemiology of vesicular stomatitis. *Bol. Cen. Panam. Fiebre Aftosa*, **29–30**, 35–53.

17. OLTSKY P.K., TRAUM J. & SCHOENING H.W. (1926). Comparative studies on vesicular stomatitis and foot and mouth disease. *J. Am. Vet. Med. Assoc.*, **70**, 147–167.

18. RODRIQUEZ L.L., LETCHWORTH G.J., SPIROPOULOU C.F. & NICHOL S.T. (1993). Rapid detection of vesicular stomatitis virus New Jersey serotype in clinical samples by using polymerase chain reaction. *J. Clin. Microbiol.*, **31**, 2016–2020.

19. SELLERS R.F. & MAAROUF A.R. (1990). Trajectory analysis of winds in vesicular stomatitis in North America. *Epidemiol. Infect.*, **104**, 313–328.

*
* *

CHAPTER 2.1.3.

SWINE VESICULAR DISEASE

SUMMARY

Swine vesicular disease (SVD) is a contagious disease of pigs, caused by an enterovirus and characterised by vesicles on the coronary bands, heels of the feet and occasionally on the lips, tongue, snout and teats. Strains of SVD virus (SVDV) vary in virulence, and the disease may be subclinical, mild or severe, the latter usually only being seen when pigs are housed on abrasive floors in damp conditions. The main importance of SVD is that it is clinically indistinguishable from foot and mouth disease (FMD), and any outbreaks of vesicular disease in pigs must be assumed to be FMD until investigated by laboratory tests and proven otherwise.

***Identification of the agent:** Where a vesicular condition is seen in pigs, the demonstration by enzyme-linked immunosorbent assay (ELISA) of SVD viral antigen in a sample of lesion material or vesicular fluid is sufficient for a positive diagnosis. If the quantity of lesion material submitted is not sufficient (less than 0.5 g), or if the test results are negative or inconclusive, isolation of virus may be carried out by the inoculation of porcine cell cultures. If any cultures subsequently develop a cytopathic effect, the demonstration of SVD viral antigen by ELISA will suffice to make a positive diagnosis.*

***Serological tests:** Specific antibody to SVDV can be identified using the microneutralisation test or ELISA. Although the microneutralisation test requires 2–3 days to complete, it remains the definitive test for antibody to SVDV. A small proportion (up to 0.1%) of normal, uninfected pigs will react positively in serological tests for SVD. These singleton reactors can only be differentiated from infected pigs by resampling of the positive animal and its cohorts.*

***Requirements for vaccines and diagnostic biologicals:** There are currently no commercial vaccines available against SVD. Diagnostic and standard reagents are available from regional reference laboratories.*

A. DIAGNOSTIC TECHNIQUES

Swine vesicular disease (SVD) can be a subclinical, mild or severe vesicular condition depending on the strain of virus involved, the route and dose of infection, and the husbandry conditions under which the pigs are kept. Clinically, SVD is indistinguishable from foot and mouth disease (FMD) and this is its main importance. It is therefore urgent that cases of SVD be distinguished from FMD by laboratory investigation.

The incubation period for SVD is between 2 and 7 days, after which a transient fever of up to 41°C may occur. Vesicles then develop on the coronary band, typically at the junction with the heel. These may affect the whole coronary band resulting in loss of the hoof. More rarely, vesicles may also appear on the snout, particularly on the dorsal surface, on the lips, tongue and teats, and shallow erosions may be seen on the knees. Affected pigs may be lame and off their feed for a few days. Abortion is not a typical feature of SVD. Recovery is usually complete in 2–3 weeks, with the only evidence of infection being a dark, horizontal line on the hoof where growth has been temporarily interrupted. The clinical signs vary according to the age of pigs affected, the conditions under which they are kept and the strain of SVD virus (SVDV) involved (7). Disease caused by mild strains may remain unobserved, particularly in pigs kept on grass or housed on deep straw. Younger animals are more severely affected, although mortality due to SVD is very rare, in contrast with FMD in young stock. Nervous signs have been reported, but are unusual. Affected pigs may excrete virus from the nose and mouth and in the faeces up to 48 hours before the onset of clinical signs. Most virus is produced in the first 7 days after infection, and virus excretion from the nose and mouth normally stops within 2 weeks. Virus may continue to be shed for up to 3 months in the faeces. The SVDV is extremely resistant to inactivation in the environment, and is stable in the pH range 2.5–12.0 (8). This is in contrast to the FMD virus, which is very labile outside the pH range 6.0–8.0.

Because SVD may be mild or subclinical, it is essential when submitting samples from suspect clinical cases that serum samples from both the suspect pigs and other apparently unaffected animals in the group be included. It is possible for SVD to circulate unnoticed until it affects a particularly susceptible group, and therefore, in order to ascertain how long infection has been present, it is necessary to look for seroconversion to SVDV in apparently healthy animals.

SVD is clinically indistinguishable from FMD. Samples for virus isolation or antigen detection must be handled and submitted as though they contained FMD virus and must be transported in phosphate buffered saline (PBS) mixed with glycerol (1/1), pH 7.2–7.6, with antibiotics such as (final concentration per ml) penicillin (1000 international units [IU]), neomycin sulphate (100 IU), polymyxin B sulphate (50 IU), and mycostatin (100 IU) (5).

SVDV has been classified as a pig enterovirus, in the family Picornaviridae. Antigenically it is related to the human virus coxsackievirus B5. There are reports of seroconversion to SVDV in laboratory workers handling the agent. Clinical disease was reported to be mild with the exception of a single case of meningitis associated with SVDV infection. However, there have been no reported cases of serconversion or disease in farmers or veterinarians working with infected pigs. Under experimental conditions, it has not been possible to show transmission of coxsackievirus B5 between pigs.

1. Identification of the agent

Any vesicular condition in pigs may be FMD. If FMD has been eliminated, the diagnosis of SVD requires the facilities of a specialised laboratory. Countries that lack such a facility should send samples for investigation to the OIE/FAO World Reference Laboratory (WRL) for Foot and Mouth Disease[1]. In the Americas, parallel testing for vesicular stomatitis viral antigen should also be conducted.

Investigation should start with the examination of a 10% suspension of lesion material in PBS by enzyme-linked immunosorbent assay (ELISA) using antisera specific for SVD and FMD viruses. This suspension should also be inoculated on to monolayers of IB-RS-2 cells (or other susceptible porcine cells), primary calf thyroid cells, and primary (or secondary) calf kidney cells. FMD virus will grow in all three tissue culture systems; SVD will grow in cells of porcine origin only.

a) Culture

A portion of the clarified epithelial suspension is inoculated on to monolayers of IB-RS-2 cells or other susceptible porcine cells. For differential diagnosis (e.g. FMD) bovine cell culture systems should also be employed. A culture medium found to be satisfactory is 50/50 Eagle's complete medium/yeast lactalbumin hydrolysate (LYH). For cell growth, add 10% bovine serum; for maintenance, add 3% bovine serum; and for virus isolation, add antibiotics only, i.e. do not add serum.

Cultures are examined twice daily. If a cytopathic effect (CPE) is observed, the supernatant fluid is harvested and used as antigen in the ELISA for virus identification. Negative cultures are blind-passaged after 48 or 72 hours, and observed for a further 3 days. When isolating virus from faeces in which the amount of virus present may be low, a third tissue culture passage may be required.

b) Immunological methods

- **Enzyme-linked immunosorbent assay**

The detection of SVD viral antigen by an indirect sandwich ELISA has replaced the complement fixation test as the method of choice. The test is the same as that used for FMD diagnosis. Duplicate rows in multiwell ELISA plates are coated with rabbit antiserum to SVDV. This is the trapping serum. Test sample suspensions are added to each of the rows. Appropriate controls are also included. Guinea-pig detection serum is added at the next stage followed by rabbit anti-guinea-pig serum conjugated to horseradish peroxidase. Extensive washing is carried out between each stage to remove unbound reagents. A positive reaction is indicated if there is a colour reaction on the addition of chromogen (orthophenylenediamine) and substrate (H_2O_2). With strong positive reactions this will be evident to the naked eye, but results can also be read spectrophotometrically at 492 nm, in which case an absorbance reading ≥0.1 above background indicates a positive reaction. As an alternative to guinea-pig and rabbit antisera, suitable monoclonal antibodies (MAbs) can be used, coated to the ELISA plate as catching antibody, or peroxidase conjugated as tracing antibody.

An MAb-based ELISA can also be used to study antigenic variation among strains of SVDV. Tissue-culture grown viral antigens are trapped by a rabbit hyperimmune antiserum to SVDV adsorbed to the solid phase.

1 OIE/FAO (Food and Agriculture Organization of the United Nations) World Reference Laboratory for FMD, Institute for Animal Health, Pirbright, Woking, Surrey GU24 ONF, United Kingdom.

Appropriate panels of MAbs are then reacted and the binding of MAbs to field strains is compared with the binding of MAbs to the parental strains. Strong binding indicates the presence of epitopes shared between the parental and the field strains (1).

c) Nucleic acid recognition methods

Nucleic acid recognition methods can be used to detect SVD viral genome in clinical material using the polymerase chain reaction (PCR) and to establish relationships between isolates of SVDV by determining the nucleotide sequence of part of the genome. By sequencing approximately 200 nucleotides within the *1D* gene, which codes for the major structural protein VP1, it has been possible to group strains of SVDV according to their sequence homology, and to relate epidemiologically strains causing disease in different regions or at different times (2). Techniques using the PCR have been developed to improve the sensitivity of diagnosis. A PCR has been described that combines extraction of RNA using commercially available silica gel columns with a reverse-transcription PCR (RT-PCR) using primers corresponding to highly conserved regions in the *1C* and *1D* genes (6). The technique is rapid, detects all genotypes of SVDV, and is sufficiently sensitive for use on samples collected from cases of suspect clinical disease. Where subclinical infection is suspected, or when samples are collected after the resolution of clinical disease, a more sensitive nested RT-PCR can be combined with a more elaborate RNA extraction method to produce a detection system at least as sensitive, and considerably more rapid, than multiple passage on tissue culture. At the time of writing, several laboratories are developing alternative PCRs using a variety of protocols.

2. Serological tests

SVD is often diagnosed solely on the evidence of serological tests. Because of the subclinical or mild nature of the disease, it is often first suspected following routine serology for disease surveillance or export certification. The virus neutralisation (VN) test, the double immunodiffusion test, the radial immunodiffusion test, the counter immunoelectrophoresis test and the ELISA have all been used for the detection of antibodies to SVDV (1, 3, 4). The VN test and the ELISA are used most frequently. The VN test is the accepted standard test, but has the disadvantage that it takes 2–3 days to complete and requires tissue culture facilities. The ELISA is more rapid and can be more easily standardised. A small proportion of sera from animals with no previous exposure to SVDV will react positively in serological tests for antibody to SVDV. The 5B7 MAb competition ELISA (MAC-ELISA) is the most reliable SVD antibody ELISA described to date (1). Results from up to approximately 1% of sera from normal pigs are borderline or positive by the MAC-ELISA and should be retested by the VN test. Up to approximately 10% of these sera will also be positive by the VN test (i.e. 0.1% of the original population). Animals positive by ELISA, but negative by VN test can be regarded as uninfected. Repeat samples should be collected from animals positive in both tests and from cohorts. A constant or declining titre in the positive animal and the absence of antibody to SVDV in cohorts confirms the status of the positive animal as a 'singleton reactor'. The factors responsible for 'singleton reactors' are unknown. Serological cross-reactivity with SVDV might arise due to infection with another, as yet unidentified, picornavirus or may be due to other nonspecific factors present in the serum. Identification of the isotype of antibody present in positive sera (1) can be helpful as sera from infected pigs usually contain specific IgG alone or both IgG and IgM, whereas sera from 'singleton' reactors contain exclusively IgM.

a) Virus neutralisation (the prescribed test for international trade)

The quantitative VN microtest for antibody to SVDV is performed using IB-RS-2 cells (or suitable susceptible porcine cells) in flat-bottomed tissue-culture grade microtitre plates.

Virus is grown on IB-RS-2 cell monolayers and stored at –20°C after the addition of an equal volume of glycerol. SVDV has been found to be stable under these conditions for at least 1 year. The sera are inactivated at 56°C for 30 minutes before testing. A suitable medium is Eagle's complete medium/LYH with antibiotics.

The test is an equal volume test in 50 µl volumes:

i) Starting from a 1/4 dilution, sera are diluted in a twofold dilution series across the plate, two rows of wells per serum.

ii) Previously titrated virus is added; each 50 µl unit volume of virus suspension contains about 100 $TCID_{50}$ (50% tissue culture infective dose).

iii) Controls include a strong positive serum, a weak positive serum and a negative serum, a cell control, a medium control and a virus titration used to calculate the actual virus titre used in the test.

iv) Incubate at 37°C for 1 hour with the plates covered.

v) A cell suspension at 10^6 cells/ml is prepared in medium containing 10% bovine serum for cell growth. 50 µl of cell suspension is added to each well.

vi) Plates are sealed with pressure-sensitive tape and incubated at 37°C for 2–3 days. Alternatively, the plates may be covered with loosely fitting lids and incubated in an atmosphere of 5% carbon dioxide at 37°C for 2–3 days.

vii) Microscopic readings may be feasible after 48 hours; the plates are finally fixed and stained routinely on the third day. Fixation is effected with 10% formol/saline for 30 minutes; staining is done by immersion in 0.05% methylene blue in 10% formalin for 30 minutes. The plates are rinsed in tapwater.

viii) Positive results are blue-stained cell sheets; the negative wells are empty. Titres are expressed as the final dilution of serum present in the serum–virus mixture at the 50% end-point. The test is considered to be valid when the amount of virus actually used per well is between $10^{1.5}$ and $10^{2.5}$ $TCID_{50}$, and the positive standard sera are within twofold of their expected titre.

ix) *Interpretation of the results:* At the OIE/FAO WRL for FMD (see footnote 1), VN titres less than or equal to 1/11 are considered to be negative. Titres of 1/16 to 1/32 are doubtful and VN titres of 1/45 or more are regarded as positive. However, as titres depend on the cell system used, laboratories should establish their own criteria by reference to standard reagents available from the OIE/FAO WRL for FMD.

b) Enzyme-linked immunosorbent assay

In the ELISA developed by Brocchi *et al.* (1), the SVD viral antigen is trapped to the solid phase using the MAb 5B7. The ability of test sera to inhibit the binding of peroxidase-conjugated MAb 5B7 to the trapped antigen is then evaluated. Finally, the amount of conjugated MAb bound is detected by the addition of substrate and chromogen.

i) ELISA plates are coated with 50 µl/well of MAb 5B7 at a dilution of 10 µg/ml in carbonate/bicarbonate buffer, pH 9.6, by overnight incubation at 4°C.

ii) The plates are washed three times with PBS containing 0.05% Tween 20, and 50 µl of SVD antigen (SVDV grown in IB-RS-2 cells, clarified, filtered and inactivated) at a predetermined optimal dilution, is added to each well. The optimal dilution of antigen is determined by checkerboard titrations of antigen and conjugated MAb that define the working dilution giving an absorbance on the upper part of the linear region of the antigen titration curve (between 1.5 and 2.0 optical density units). Plates are then incubated for 1 hour at 37°C.

iii) After three additional washes, 50 µl of diluted test sera (not inactivated) and control sera are incubated with the trapped antigen for 1 hour at 37°C. Three-fold dilution series of sera are obtained directly in ELISA wells by adding 10 µl of serum to 65 µl of buffer (1/7.5 dilution) then transferring 25 µl to sequential wells containing 50 µl of buffer, mixing, and finally discarding 25 µl.

iv) After incubation, 25 µl of an optimal dilution of peroxidase-conjugated MAb 5B7 (see ii above) is added to each well and the plates are incubated at 37°C for a further 1 hour.

v) After a final series of washes, the colorimetric reaction is developed by distributing 50 µl per well of the substrate solution (0.5 mg/ml orthophenylene-diamine [OPD] in phosphate-citrate buffer, pH 5, containing 0.02% H_2O_2).

vi) The reaction is stopped after 10 minutes by adding 50 µl of 2 N H_2SO_4. The absorbance is read at 492 nm using a microplate reader.

Antigen, sera and conjugate are diluted in PBS, pH 7.4, containing 0.05% Tween 20 and 1% yeast extract; the dilution buffer for sera contains, in addition, 1.0% mouse serum to prevent nonspecific binding of pig serum to MAb 5B7 either coated to the plate or conjugated to peroxidase.

vii) *Controls:* Four wells on each plate containing all reactants except test serum confirm the maximum absorbance reading for the antigen; convalescent pig serum at four selected dilutions; negative pig serum; a low positive standard pig serum.

viii) *Interpretation of the results:* Reactions are expressed as the percentage inhibition by each test serum of the MAb reaction with the SVD antigen. Sera are positive if percentage inhibition values are greater than 80% at the 1/7.5 serum dilution. All doubtful or positive results are retested by VN test.

STANDARD REFERENCE SERA FOR SVD SEROLOGY

The FAO/OIE WRL for FMD maintains a panel of reference sera that have been extensively validated by the National SVD Reference Laboratories of the Member States of the European Union.

B. REQUIREMENTS FOR VACCINES AND DIAGNOSTIC BIOLOGICALS

No commercial SVD vaccines are currently available. Standard sera can be obtained from the OIE/FAO WRL for FMD (see footnote 1). MAb 5B7 is available from the OIE Reference Laboratory for Swine Vesicular Disease in Italy (see Table given in Part 4 of this *Manual*).

REFERENCES

1. BROCCHI E., BERLINZANI A., GAMBA D. & DE SIMONE F. (1995). Development of two novel monoclonal antibody-based ELISAs for the detection of antibodies and the identification of swine isotypes against swine vesicular disease virus. *J. Virol. Methods*, **52**, 155–167.

2. BROCCHI E., ZHANG G., KNOWLES N.J., WILSDEN G., MCCAWLEY J.W., MARQUARDT O., OHLINGER V.F. & DE SIMONE F. (1997). Molecular epidemiology of recent outbreaks of swine vesicular disease: two genetically and antigenically distinct variants in Europe, 1987–1994. *Epidemiol. Infect.*, **118**, 51–61.

3. DONALDSON A.I., FERRIS N.P., KNOWLES N.J. & BARNETT I.T.R. (1983). Comparative studies of United Kingdom isolates of swine vesicular disease virus. *Res. Vet. Sci.*, **35**, 295–300.

4. GOLDING S.M., HEDGER R.S., TALBOT P. & WATSON J. (1976). Radial immunodiffusion and serum neutralisation techniques for the assay of antibodies to swine vesicular disease. *Res. Vet. Sci.*, **20**, 142–147.

5. KITCHING R.P. & DONALDSON A.I. (1987). Collection and transportation of specimens for vesicular virus investigation. *Rev. sci. tech. Off. int. Epiz.*, **6**, 263–272.

6. LIN F., MACKAY D.K.J. & KNOWLES N.J. (1997). Detection of swine vesicular disease virus RNA by reverse transcription-polymerase chain reaction. *J. Virol. Methods*, **65**, 111–121.

7. LOXAM J.R. & HEDGER R.S. (1983). Swine vesicular disease: clinical signs, diagnosis, epidemiology and control. *Rec. sci. tech. Off. int. Epiz.*, **2**, 11–24.

8. MANN J.A. (1981). Swine vesicular disease. *In:* Virus Diseases of Farm Animals, Vol. 2, Gibbs E.P.J., ed. Academic Press, London, UK, 365–381.

*

* *

CHAPTER 2.1.4.

RINDERPEST

SUMMARY

Rinderpest is an acute, fatal disease of domestic cattle, buffaloes and yaks caused by a morbillivirus. Sheep, goats, pigs and wild ungulates may also be affected. Clinically the disease is characterised by pyrexia, the progressive development of shallow erosions on the gums, tongue, cheeks and hard palate together with serous or mucopurulent ocular and nasal discharges. Alimentary tract involvement is marked by the development of severe diarrhoea and dysentery.

Two lineages of the virus still occur in eastern Africa and a third lineage occurs in Asia. Except for part of the Arabian Peninsula, West Asia is probably rinderpest-free, but periodic outbreaks could continue to occur until the virus is eradicated from Pakistan, the only South Asian country in which the disease remains endemic. The Food and Agriculture Organization of the United Nations (FAO) has launched a Global Rinderpest Eradication Programme (GREP) calling for eradication of the virus by the year 2010.

***Identification of the agent:** Laboratory confirmation is based on demonstrating the presence of the virus, virus-specific RNA or (group specific) precipitating antigens in samples from the spleen, lymph nodes, or ocular or nasal secretions of acutely infected animals. It is particularly important to isolate the virus if a geographical extension or significant zoosanitary deterioration has occurred. In countries reporting peste des petits ruminants (PPR), rinderpest cannot be confirmed in sheep or goats on the basis of precipitating antigens because they will be common to both viruses. Under these circumstances, differentiation must be made on the basis of an enzyme-linked immunosorbent assay (ELISA) reaction following specific antigen capture or by viral-specific RNA detection methods including molecular techniques such as* in situ *nucleic acid probe hybridisation and reverse-transcription polymerase chain reaction.*

Post-mortem examinations should pay particular attention to the abomasum, which may be highly engorged or show a grey discoloration; to the Peyer's patches, which may show lymphoid necrosis; and to the development of linear engorgement and blackening of the crests of the folds of the caecum, colon and rectum. The principal differential diagnoses are PPR in sheep and goats, and bovine viral diarrhoea/mucosal disease and malignant catarrhal fever in cattle; differentiation of these diseases requires the use of appropriate laboratory methods.

***Serological tests:** The OIE has drawn up a set of Recommended Standards for Epidemiological Surveillance for Rinderpest (commonly referred to as the 'OIE Pathway') that govern the actions of Member Countries wishing to demonstrate that they have achieved freedom from infection. To this end, a competitive ELISA test is available that will determine the presence of rinderpest antibodies in animals that have been infected with field virus or with rinderpest vaccine. Neutralising antibody estimations may be used for the same purpose. The possible occurrence of PPR must be considered.*

***Requirements for vaccines and diagnostic biologicals:** A live attenuated cell culture vaccine is available that confers lifelong immunity in cattle after a single inoculation. In countries undertaking serosurveillance for the presence of wild virus, if protection against PPR is required, a homologous vaccine should be used to avoid the creation of rinderpest-immune small ruminant populations.*

A. DIAGNOSTIC TECHNIQUES

Rinderpest is a highly fatal disease of domestic cattle, buffaloes and yaks caused by a morbillivirus of the family Paramyxoviridae. The virus also affects sheep, goats and some breeds of pigs and a large variety of wildlife species within the order Artiodactyla, although not always in a clinically apparent form.

Historically the virus was widely distributed throughout Europe, Africa, Asia and West Asia, but never became established in either the Americas or Australia/New Zealand. The Food and Agriculture Organization of the United Nations (FAO) has launched a Global Rinderpest Eradication Programme (GREP); the application of which will probably result in a rapid change in the list of countries in which endemic rinderpest still occurs. In Africa and Asia gene sequencing analysis places both historical and contemporary virus isolates into three nonoverlapping lineages. In Africa there have been no reports of rinderpest in any Central or West African country for over 10 years, but in southern Sudan lineage 1 remains endemic and a constant and immediate threat to Ethiopia, Kenya and Uganda. Of similar concern is the fact that lineage 2 virus, isolated in central Kenya in 1952, reappeared in southern Kenya in 1994, drawing attention to the possibility of long-term cryptic persistence; this virus subsequently spread to neighbouring Tanzania. Rinderpest has not been found in Ethiopia since 1995. In Pakistan, the Asian lineage virus remains endemic, but the Indian subcontinent and Sri Lanka are free from the virus. In West Asia it is still too early to be confident that rinderpest has died out in the Yemen and Saudi Arabia.

Following an incubation period of between 1 and 2 weeks, the ensuing clinical disease is characterised by an acute febrile attack within which prodromal and erosive phases can be distinguished. The prodromal period lasts approximately 3 days, during which affected animals develop a pyrexia of between 40 and 41.5°C with partial anorexia, constipation, congestion of visible mucosae, serous ocular and nasal discharges, depression and drying of the muzzle. However, it is not until the onset of the erosive phase, and the development of necrotic mouth lesions, that a tentative clinical diagnosis of rinderpest can be made. Still at the height of fever, small pin-head sized flecks of raised, whitish, necrotic epithelium appear on the lower lip and gum and in rapid succession may also appear on the margin between the upper gum and dental pad, on the underside of the tongue, on the cheeks and cheek papillae and on the hard palate. Through the enlargement of existing lesions and the development of new foci, the extent of the oral necrosis can increase dramatically over the following 2–3 days. Much of the necrotic material works loose giving rise to shallow, nonhaemorrhagic mucosal erosions.

Diarrhoea is another characteristic feature of rinderpest and develops 1–2 days after the onset of mouth lesions. The diarrhoea is usually copious and watery at first, but later on may contain mucus, blood and shreds of epithelium, and it may be accompanied by tenesmus. During the erosive phase, necrosis may be observed in the nares, in the vulva and vagina, and on the preputial sheath. Anorexia becomes absolute, the muzzle dries out completely, the animal is profoundly depressed, and mucopurulent ocular and nasal discharges develop. The breath is fetid and, in the terminal stages of the disease, the animal may become recumbent for 24–48 hours; during this period a characteristic delayed, grunted exhalation may be noted.

Animals may die while showing severe necrotic lesions, high fever and diarrhoea or while similarly affected but after a precipitous fall in body temperature, often to subnormal values. Alternatively, the pyrexia may remit slightly in the middle of the erosive period and then, 2–3 days later, return rapidly to normal accompanied by a rapid resolution of the mouth lesions, a halt to the diarrhoea and an uncomplicated convalescence.

Most virus strains circulating in Africa or Asia produce a disease picture that more or less conforms to the above description. On the Arabian Peninsula, however, and in association with highly susceptible imported cattle, peracute disease has been seen in which deaths occurred at the end of the prodromal period. Mild strains, which may be difficult to diagnose clinically because of the fleeting and greatly reduced number of mouth lesions, still occur in parts of Africa.

Typically, the carcass is dehydrated, emaciated and soiled. The nose and cheeks bear evidence of mucopurulent discharges, the eye is sunken and the conjunctiva congested. In the oral cavity, there is often extensive desquamation of necrotic epithelium, which always appears sharply demarcated from adjacent areas of healthy mucosa. The lesions frequently extend on to the soft palate and may also involve the pharynx and the upper portion of the oesophagus; the rumen, reticulum and omasum are usually unaffected, although necrotic plaques are occasionally encountered on the pillars of the rumen. The abomasum, especially the pyloric region, is severely affected and shows congestion, petechiation and oedema of the submucosa. Epithelial necrosis gives the mucous membrane a slate-like colour. The small intestine is not commonly involved except for striking changes in the Peyer's patches where lymphoid necrosis and sloughing leave the supporting architecture engorged or blackened. In the large intestine, changes involve the ileocaecal valve, the caecal tonsil and the crests of the longitudinal folds of the caecal, colonic and rectal mucosae. The folds appear highly engorged in acute deaths or darkly discoloured in long-standing cases; in either event, the lesions are referred to as 'zebra striping'.

1. Identification of the agent

A variety of laboratory tests are available for the identification of rinderpest, but it is important to understand the limitations of some of the older methods and the complexity of diagnosing rinderpest in small ruminants in countries with a history of concurrent infection with both rinderpest and peste des petits ruminants (PPR). In view of the efforts now being directed towards the global eradication of rinderpest, any outbreak assumes a high level of epidemiological significance, even in countries where the disease is still regarded as endemic. Consequently, samples from all outbreaks diagnosed as rinderpest on clinical or pathological grounds must be routinely submitted for laboratory confirmation.

Although rapid diagnostic procedures will become increasingly common, the future availability of virus isolates for epidemiological studies or pathogenicity trials makes it absolutely essential to retain virus isolation routines within the diagnostic process (1).

Rinderpest virus can be cultured from the leukocyte fraction of whole blood that has been collected into heparin or EDTA (ethylene diamine tetra-acetic acid) anticoagulants at a final concentration of 10 International Units [IU]/ml and 0.5 mg/ml, respectively. Samples should be thoroughly mixed and transferred to the laboratory on ice, but not frozen. Virus may also be isolated in samples obtained from the spleen, or the prescapular or mesenteric lymph nodes of dead animals; these samples may be chilled to subzero temperatures.

To isolate the virus from blood, uncoagulated blood is centrifuged at 2500 ***g*** for 15 minutes to produce a buffy coat layer at the boundary between the plasma and red blood cells. This is removed as cleanly as possible, mixed in 20 ml physiological saline and recentrifuged in a washing procedure designed to remove any neutralising antibody present in the plasma. The resulting cell pellet is suspended in cell culture maintenance medium, and 2 ml aliquots are distributed on to established monolayers of B95a Marmoset lymphoblastoid cells, primary calf kidney cells or African green monkey kidney (Vero) cells. The monolayers should be re-fed periodically and observed microscopically for the development of cytopathic effects (CPE) characterised by refractility, cell rounding, cell retraction with elongated cytoplasmic bridges (stellate cells) or syncytial formation. Isolates of virus can be partially identified by the demonstration of morbillivirus-specific precipitinogens in infected cell debris, or completely identified by the demonstration of specific immunofluorescence using a conjugated monoclonal antibody (MAb).

Alternatively, 20% suspensions (w/v) of lymph node or spleen may be used for virus isolation. These should be made by macerating the solid tissues in serum-free culture maintenance medium using standard grinding or shearing techniques[1] and inoculating monolayers as before.

In bovines only, either an agar gel immunodiffusion (AGID) or a counter immunoelectrophoresis (CIEP) test can be used as a rapid diagnostic test to demonstrate the presence of precipitinogens in the ocular secretions of infected animals. Secretions should be collected during either the prodromal or erosive phases using cotton wool buds manoeuvred beneath both the upper and lower eyelids.

a) Agar gel immunodiffusion

The AGID tests may be conducted in Petri dishes or on glass microscope slides (1, 6). In either instance the surface should be covered with agar to a depth of about 4 mm using a 1% aqueous solution of any high quality agar or agarose. Wells are usually cut in a hexagonal pattern of six peripheral wells around a single central well. For slides, wells should be 3 mm in diameter and 2 mm periphery to periphery. For Petri dishes, the wells can be increased to 4 mm in diameter and the distance between wells to 3 mm. The closer the wells are placed, the shorter will be the reaction time.

Using a Pasteur pipette, rinderpest hyperimmune rabbit serum should be placed in the central well. Similarly, control positive antigen prepared from rinderpest-infected cell debris or from the macerated mesenteric lymph nodes of a rabbit infected with the Nakamura III strain of lapinised virus, should be placed in peripheral wells one, three and five. Negative control antigen is placed in well four. Test antigens are obtained as exudates from the cut surface of spleen or lymph nodes submitted for testing; if no exudate can be obtained, a small portion of the sample should be ground with a minimum of saline. Ocular exudates may be squeezed directly from the swabs or, alternatively, by compression in a microtip (the cotton wool should be cut off the swab and placed into the wide end of a plastic 50–250 µl pipette tip; the stem of the

1 The release of virus from solid tissue can be achieved in several ways. Perhaps the easiest is with a pestle and mortar, but this technique requires the use of sterile sand as an abrasive. Alternatively, tissues may be ground without an abrasive using all-glass grinders, for example, a Ten Broeck grinder. Shearing techniques are equally applicable using, for example, Silverson or Waring blenders. Virus-containing suspensions are clarified by low speed centrifugation. The volume of the inoculum is not critical; a working answer would be a volume of between 1 and 2 ml. Commonly used antibiotics are penicillin and streptomycin in combination, each at a concentration of 100 IU/ml. A similar broad-spectrum cover can be obtained using neomycin at 50 µl/ml. Fungizone should be included at 2.5 µg/ml.

swab may then be used to compress the cotton wool and force a small volume of exudate out of the narrow end of the tip). Test samples are added to wells two and six. Tests are best developed at 4°C or low ambient temperatures. The reaction area should be inspected from 2 hours onwards for the appearance of clean, sharp lines of precipitation. The result is not acceptable unless precipitation reactions are also obtained giving a line of identity with the control positive antigen preparation.

b) Counter immunoelectrophoresis

CIEP tests may yield a positive reaction slightly ahead of the AGID test (1, 6). Reactions are carried out on standard microscope slides coated to a depth of 2.0 mm with 1% agar or agarose in 0.025% veronal acetate buffer, pH 8.6. Wells are cut in pairs at an interperipheral distance of 6 mm, the left-hand side is anodal and is filled with rinderpest hyperimmune serum; the right-hand side is cathodal and the wells are filled with test samples or positive and negative antigen preparations. Samples are run for 40–60 minutes at a constant current of 10 mAmp/slide or a constant voltage of 6 volts/cm, after which the reaction area is examined for precipitation.

At post-mortem examination, tissues should be collected and placed in 10% buffered formalin for histopathology and immunohistochemistry; the base of the tongue, retropharyngeal lymph node and eyelid are suitable tissues. Sections stained with haematoxylin and eosin should be examined for the presence of syncytial cell formation, and cells with intranuclear viral inclusions. The presence of rinderpest antigens can be demonstrated in the same formalin-fixed tissues by immunoperoxidase staining following the quenching of endogenous peroxidase activity. If a polyclonal antiserum is used, this test will fail to differentiate between rinderpest and PPR. However, this problem can be circumvented by using a negative-sense RNA probe to the rinderpest N protein gene (3).

• Differentiation between rinderpest and peste des petits ruminants

a) Differential immunocapture

Given the inability of clinical observations or precipitinogen detection tests to differentiate between rinderpest and PPR, in countries where both diseases occur, tests capable of differentiating the two diseases are mandatory for all rinderpest-like outbreaks in sheep or goats. Although such differentiation can follow the inoculation of experimental animals, it can be undertaken more rapidly and cost-effectively using a differential immunocapture enzyme-linked immunosorbent assay (ELISA) (8). This test employs MAb directed against the N protein of the two viruses. One MAb, with a reactivity against both viruses, is used as a capture antibody, while a second biotinylated MAb specific for a nonoverlapping antigenic N protein site, and specific against either rinderpest or PPR, is used to determine which N protein has been captured.

High protein binding ELISA plates (or strips) are coated with 100 µl/well of capture antibody. After three washes, the wells are loaded with 50 µl of test sample diluted 1/10 in a lysis buffer, 25 µl of the manufacturer's recommended dilution of the virus-specific MAb and 25 µl of streptavidin–peroxidase at a final dilution of 1/3000. The wells are then placed on an orbital shaker for 1 hour at 37°C, after which time they are again washed; following the addition of 100 µl of ortho-phenylenediamine (OPD), the wells are reincubated at room temperature for 10 minutes. Reactions are halted by the addition of 100 µl of 1 N sulphuric acid, and the results, measured at 492 nm with an automated ELISA reader, are expressed as absorbance values. The test can be used to confirm the identity of rinderpest or PPR viruses in field samples (11) or those grown in tissue culture.

b) Polymerase chain reaction

The reverse-transcription polymerase chain reaction (RT-PCR) provides a method for the differential diagnosis of rinderpest from PPR (7); it also produces DNA suitable for gene sequence analysis. The viral RNA used in the test can be purified from any of the following: tissues (spleen [but not ideal due to its high blood content], lymph node and tonsil [ideal], and gum scrapings and eye swabs [contingent], peripheral blood lymphocytes (PBLs), or swabs from eyes or mouth lesions. RNA is extracted using the acid guanidinium thiocyanate-phenol-chloroform method of Chomczynski & Sacchi (4). Solid tissues (0.5–1.0 g) are minced and homogenised with 4.0 ml denaturing solution[2], eye and mouth swabs are treated with

---

2 Solution D (disruption solution): the procedure is that recommended by Chomczynski & Sacchi (4) to minimise the hazard of handling the poisonous guanidium thiocyanate. It should be carried out in a chemical safety hood. The following are the amounts of guanidium thiocyanate for a 250 g bottle, but the volumes can be adjusted for the other quantities available from Fluka, the supplier. Do not attempt to weigh out the guanidium thiocyanate, but dissolve it in the manufacturer's bottle by adding 293 ml sterile distilled water, 17.6 ml 0.75 M sodium citrate, pH 7.0, and 26.4 ml 10% sarcosyl. Heat to 65°C in a water bath to dissolve. This solution can be kept for several months in the dark at room temperature in a chemical safety cabinet. The final solution D is made by the addition of 0.36 ml 2-mercaptoethanol to 50 ml of the stock solution. This solution should not be kept for more than 1 month.

1.0 ml, and purified PBLs (from 5 to 10 ml whole blood) are treated with 0.4 ml according to the published procedure. The resulting RNA is precipitated with 2.5 volumes of ethanol, washed in 70% ethanol, dissolved in sterile water or TE buffer (Tris/EDTA, 10 mM, pH 7.5, 1 mM EDTA), and stored at –70°C or –20°C until required. The cDNA synthesis is carried out using random hexanucleotide primers to enable several different specific primer sets to be used in the PCR amplification step. Aliquots of the resulting cDNA are amplified using at least three primer sets that can detect and differentiate between the two morbilliviruses. These primer sets include two 'universal' sets based on highly conserved regions in the phosphoprotein and nucleoprotein genes that should detect all morbilliviruses, and rinderpest virus-specific and PPR virus-specific sets based on sequences in the fusion protein genes of each virus. The PCR products are analysed on a 1.5% agarose gel along with a suitable DNA marker to identify the specific DNA product. A positive control such as measles or canine distemper virus RNA, and a negative control using sterile distilled water instead of RNA, must be included in each RT-PCR. Positive reactions should be confirmed either by using 'nested' primer sets based on the F gene sequences or by sequence analysis of the DNA product. It is important to use more than one set of primers for the PCR step when testing for the presence of RNA viruses, as their nucleotide sequences can vary significantly and one change at the 3'-end of the primer sequence may result in failure of the primers to amplify the DNA. The FAO World Reference Laboratory in the United Kingdom (UK), which is also an OIE Reference Laboratory for rinderpest, and the OIE Reference Laboratory in France (see Table given in Part 4 of this *Manual*), can advise on the use of the technique for field sample analysis.

2. Serological tests

a) Competitive enzyme-linked immunosorbent assay (the prescribed test for international trade)

A competitive ELISA test is available for the detection of rinderpest antibodies in the serum of animals of any species previously exposed to the virus. The test is based on the ability of positive test sera to compete with a rinderpest anti-H protein MAb for binding to rinderpest antigen. The presence of such antibodies in the test sample will block binding of the MAb, producing a reduction in the expected colour reaction following the addition of enzyme-labelled anti-mouse IgG conjugate and a substrate/chromogen solution. As this is a solid-phase assay, wash steps are required to ensure the removal of any unbound reagents.

The rinderpest antigen is prepared from Madin–Darby bovine kidney cell cultures infected with the attenuated Kabete 'O' strain of rinderpest virus. The antigen is concentrated from the infected cell culture supernate by ammonium sulphate precipitation. The MAb was obtained by fusing the splenocytes of hyperimmunised mice with the NS0 myeloma cell line, and then shown to be rinderpest specific (2); this MAb has now been designated as C1. Both C1 and standardised rinderpest antigen are directly available from the OIE Reference Laboratory for Rinderpest in the UK (see Table given in Part 4 of this *Manual*). Kits are available commercially.

- **Test procedure**

i) Reconstitute the freeze-dried rinderpest antigen with 1 ml of sterile water and further dilute it to the manufacturer's recommended working dilution using 0.01 M phosphate buffered saline (PBS), pH 7.4.

ii) Immediately dispense 50 µl volumes of the diluted antigen into an appropriate number of wells of a flat-bottomed, high protein-binding ELISA microplate using two wells per test serum. Tap the sides of the microplate to ensure that the antigen is evenly distributed over the bottom of each well and, having sealed the plate, incubate it on an orbital shaker for 1 hour at 37°C. Wash the wells three times with 0.002 M PBS, pH 7.4.

iii) Add 40 µl of blocking buffer (0.01 M PBS, 0.1% [v/v] Tween 20 and 0.3% [v/v] normal bovine serum) to each test well followed by 10 µl volumes of all test sera.

iv) Follow the manufacturer's recommendations to prepare a working dilution of the MAb in blocking buffer, and add 50 µl of this to each test well. Seal the plates and reincubate on an orbital shaker for 1 hour at 37°C.

v) Follow the manufacturer's recommendations to prepare a working dilution of rabbit anti-mouse immunoglobulin horseradish-peroxidase conjugate in blocking buffer and add 50 µl to each test well. Seal the plates and reincubate on an orbital shaker for 1 hour at 37°C.

vi) At the end of this period, the plates are washed as before and immediately refilled with 50 µl volumes of substrate/chromogen mixture (1 part 3% H_2O_2 to 250 parts OPD), and incubate at room temperature for 10 minutes without shaking. Add 50 µl of a stopping solution consisting of 1 M sulphuric acid.

vii) The test system must include known rinderpest positive and negative serum samples, an MAb control and a conjugate control.

viii) Measure the resulting absorbance values on an ELISA reader with a 492 nm interference filter and express the test results as percentage inhibition values compared with the value obtained using the MAb control. Inhibition values of 50% or more are considered to be positive and values below 50% are considered to be negative.

b) Virus neutralisation

The standard virus neutralisation test is undertaken in roller-tube cultures of calf kidney or Vero cells. Inactivated sera are diluted at intervals of 1 in 2 or 1 in 10 and, starting with neat serum, mixed with approximately $10^{3.0}$ $TCID_{50}$ (50% tissue culture infective dose) per ml of the vaccine strain of the virus. Mixtures containing equal volumes of virus and serum are held overnight at 4°C, after which 0.2 ml volumes are inoculated into each of five roller tubes, immediately followed by 1 ml of dispersed indicator cells suspended in growth medium at a rate of 2×10^5 per ml. Tubes are sloped for 3 days at 37°C, after which those showing virus-specific cytopathology are discarded; the medium in the remaining tubes is changed to a maintenance formulation, after which they are rolled pending final examination at 10 days.

For calculating end-points, the virus dose is regarded as satisfactory if it falls within the range $10^{1.8}$–$10^{2.8}$ $TCID_{50}$/tube; serum dilutions are considered to double after mixing with the virus dose. This test can be used to measure the antibody levels present in individual sera or to qualify susceptible cattle for vaccine testing or for export. Under these circumstances, the presence of any detectable antibody in the 1/2 final serum dilution is considered to be positive.

In the microplate method, 50 µl volumes of serum are incubated with 50 µl volumes of virus diluted to contain between $10^{1.8}$ and $10^{2.8}$ $TCID_{50}$ (15). Following a 45-minute or an overnight incubation period at 4°C, between 1 and 2×10^5 calf kidney, lamb kidney or Vero cells are added as indicators. Tests are terminated after 6 or 7 days. Such tests may give indications of nonspecific neutralisation at high serum concentrations. (There appear to be factors is some normal [with respect to prior rinderpest exposure] sera that bring about the failure of the virus to penetrate and replicate in the indicator cells. In the older tube test method these factors were probably removed during changes of the maintenance medium; in the microplate they remain present the whole time. The result is that a serum that fails to neutralise the virus in the more sensitive tube test apparently neutralises it in the microwell test. If the most concentrated final serum dilution is limited to 1/10, the effect disappears. The nature of the factors involved have not been investigated.)

B. REQUIREMENTS FOR VACCINES AND DIAGNOSTIC BIOLOGICALS

Susceptible animals may be immunised with a live attenuated tissue culture rinderpest vaccine (TCRV), which induces a lifelong immunity. TCRV was developed at the former East African Veterinary Research Organisation by serial passage of the virulent bovine rinderpest strain Kabete 'O' (RBOK). It is safe for use in cattle, buffalo, sheep and goats of all ages and in zoological collections. If vaccinated animals are fully susceptible, immunologically competent and correctly vaccinated by the subcutaneous route, they will develop a long-lived immunity. In the past TCRV has been used in conjunction within annual vaccination programmes designed to protect the national bovine population of countries with endemically infected regions. Due to individual variations in the duration of passive immunity, animals were not regarded to be fully immunised until they were vaccinated once when over 1 year of age; such animals were generally marked by branding or ear notching. Although younger animals were often included in such campaigns in case they had not developed an adequate maternal immunity, such animals were not marked.

Where the regional eradication of rinderpest has been attempted, vaccine has been the principal tool for endeavouring to create a large pool of bovines in which the prevalence of immunity exceeds 85%. Although such campaigns have made considerable contributions to reducing the global incidence of rinderpest, eliminating the final pockets of infection probably requires a somewhat different approach based on a careful preliminary investigation to establish the extent of the infected area. When this is known, TCRV should be employed in a manner designed to produce a very high level of coverage in the shortest possible period. The effectiveness of such campaigns should be assessed serologically immediately the campaign ends as a campaign quality control procedure. Any short-falls should be rectified immediately.

1. Seed management

a) Characteristics of the seed

Seed lots used in the manufacture of TCRV must produce a cell culture vaccine that is safe, that confers an immunity in cattle lasting at least 5 years, that retains its attenuated characteristics during at least five back passages in cattle, and that lacks the ability to spread by contact. Substrains of RBOK used in the manufacture of TCRV must be identifiable by written historical records, which must include information on the origin of the strain and of its subsequent manipulations.

b) Method of culture

Vaccine seed must be maintained in a seed-lot system between passage levels 90 and 120. Seed-lot virus must be preserved in a freeze-dried state at a temperature of –20°C or lower. The virus must be cultured in Vero cells or primary or serially cultivated kidney cells derived from a normal bovine fetus or a very young calf. Serially cultivated cells may not be more than ten passages removed from the primary cultivation.

c) Validation as a vaccine

Seed lots must be shown to be:

i) *Pure:* Free from contamination with viruses, bacteria, fungi or mycoplasmas.

ii) *Safe:* Inducing no abnormal clinical reaction on inoculation into rinderpest-susceptible cattle.

iii) *Efficacious:* Inducing an immunity to rinderpest in rinderpest-susceptible cattle.

2. Method of manufacture

Individual vaccine batches are prepared by infecting cell cultures and, after an appropriate incubation period, harvesting the overlying media into which large numbers of live virus particles have been released. To facilitate long-term storage and cold-chain distribution, this fluid is freeze-dried in the presence of a cryoprotectant consisting of 5% lactalbumin hydrolysate and 10% sucrose. Virus may be grown in primary kidney cells from bovine embryos or calves, or cells derived in a homogeneous manner by up to ten serial subcultures from either of these sources. In addition, vaccine may be manufactured in approved continuous cell lines provided the cells are known to be noninfected with bovine viral diarrhoea (BVD) virus and are maintained in a seed-lot system; Vero cells have been used for this purpose. To constitute a batch, infected cultures must have been inoculated with the same seed virus and incubated and harvested together. Two harvests are permissible from the same set of cultures and may be pooled to form a bulk suspension. Written records must accompany all stages of vaccine manufacture.

3. In-process control

Cells: Primary cells, serially cultivated primary cells or continuous cell lines must have been derived from normal-looking animals or embryos, and must retain a normal morphology during cultivation. They must be shown to be free from contamination with adventitious viruses, particularly BVD virus. Whatever cells are committed for vaccine production, uninfected control cultures must be maintained using the same media and incubation conditions as the rinderpest-infected cells. They must be subjected to frequent microscopic examinations. After harvesting the vaccine, the control cultures should be washed to remove ox serum and reincubated for 10 days in media containing ox serum substitutes. They are again subject to frequent microscopic examinations for evidence of cytopathic change. Simultaneously a sample of the cultures should be examined for the presence of noncytopathic BVD virus using an immunofluorescence or immunoperoxidase test or RT-PCR. The serum used in the culture media must come from rinderpest-susceptible animals.

Virus: A virus titration must be undertaken on the seed lot using tenfold virus dilutions in a microplate or roller tube system and employing ten replicates per dilution. A similar titration must be undertaken on the final bulk. Virus should be derived from cultures maintained in roller bottles and may not be harvested more than 10 days after the date that these cultures were infected. The harvest should be clarified by low-speed centrifugation before mixing with cryoprotectant. Prior to lyophilisation it may be held for not more than 5 days at 4°C, but for considerably longer if frozen at between –20°C and –60°C. As adventitious viral contamination may arise during a manufacturer's manipulations or from the use of contaminated media, rabbit hyperimmune rinderpest antiserum should be used to neutralise the rinderpest content of a sample of the bulk suspension, after which the mixture should be used to infect calf kidney or Vero cells, which are handled as described above. The final bulk must be tested for freedom from bacteria, fungi and mycoplasmas.

4. Batch control

a) Identity

The contents of one container from each filling lot must be exposed to neutralisation by rabbit hyperimmune rinderpest antiserum, using a varying virus/constant serum method, and inoculated into bovine kidney cells. The identity of the product is established if no rinderpest-specific CPE develop.

b) Sterility

Tests for sterility and freedom from contamination of biological materials may be found in Chapter I.4.

c) Safety and efficacy

Using rinderpest-susceptible cattle, the contents of five randomly selected vials are pooled and used to inoculate one ox with a volume equivalent to 100 cattle field doses and one ox with a volume equivalent to 1/10 of a cattle field dose. These animals are maintained in close contact with an uninoculated ox for the following 3 weeks. During this period the animals are subjected to daily temperature recording and frequent clinical inspections. At the end of the 3 weeks, the cattle are examined for rinderpest neutralising antibodies and challenged with a strain of rinderpest capable of inducing a pyrexia. The vaccine is considered to be safe and efficacious if it does not induce any abnormal clinical reaction, if both animals receiving vaccine are protected, and if there is no evidence that the vaccine virus has been transmitted. This test is not a potency test. Each vaccine lot must also be tested for innocuity in small animals.

d) Potency

The close relationship between immunising potency and infectivity allows the latter to be used as the basis for potency estimations. Three infectivity titrations are undertaken using cells of an approved continuous line or cells grown from each of three different bovine calf or embryonic kidneys. For the first titration, the pool of vials used for the safety test may be employed. The second and third estimates are made on further pools, each of three final containers. The sensitivity of the cells used in each working session must be measured using a standard laboratory rinderpest virus preparation. The final titre is the geometric mean of the three estimates, each undertaken using tenfold dilutions and ten observations per dilution.

For field use, the minimum dose of vaccine is defined as $10^{2.5}$ $TCID_{50}$.

e) Duration of immunity

It is unnecessary to routinely establish the duration of immunity to TCRV. The reported results (12) indicate that lifelong immunity can be expected following the successful vaccination of cattle free of all vestiges of maternal immunity.

f) Stability

TCRV is highly stable when correctly freeze-dried and will keep for long periods at either 4°C or –20°C (14) provided the product is stored under vacuum. Recent evidence indicates that the rate of degradation of lyophilised TCRV can be altered by the choice of stabiliser and by variations in the drying cycle. The most advantageous results were associated with the use of a 5% lactalbumin hydrolysate/10% sucrose stabiliser, a 72–74-hour drying cycle under reduced vacuum (100 milliTorr), initial drying for 16 hours at –30°C, and a final shelf temperature of 35°C (9, 10). With high release titres, such vaccine can be used in the field for 30 days without refrigeration. Following reconstitution in either normal saline or 1 M magnesium sulphate, the virus becomes much more thermolabile (13). The period for field distribution of reconstituted vaccine should not exceed its half-life, but as this parameter is temperature dependent and varies between 8 and 24 hours over a range from 4°C to 37°C, a common-sense limit must be applied; this can be determined by National Control Authorities, but a universal period of 4 hours can be recommended.

g) Preservatives

TCRV contains lactalbumin hydrolysate and sucrose, which are added as cryoprotectants; otherwise it contains no specific chemical preservative.

h) Precautions (hazards)

There are no known hazards associated with the manufacture or field use of TCRV.

5. Tests on the final product

a) Safety

As in Section B.4.c.

b) **Potency**

As in Section B.4.d.

Quality control procedures have been documented (5).

REFERENCES

1. ANDERSON J., BARRETT T. & SCOTT G.R. (1996). Manual on the Diagnosis of Rinderpest, Second Edition. FAO Animal Health Manual No. 1. The Food and Agriculture Organization of the United Nations (FAO), Rome, Italy, 143 pp.

2. ANDERSON J., MCKAY J.A. & BUTCHER R.N. (1991). The use of monoclonal antibodies in competitive ELISA for detection of antibodies to rinderpest and peste des petits ruminants. *In:* The Seromonitoring of Rinderpest throughout Africa. Phase One. Proceedings of Final Research Coordination Meeting. Joint FAO/IAEA Division, Vienna, Austria, 43–53.

3. BROWN C.C. (1997). A review of three pathology-based techniques for retrospective diagnosis of rinderpest, with comparison to virus isolation. *Res. Vet. Sci.,* **63,** 103–106.

4. CHOMCZYNSKI P. & SACCHI N. (1987). Single-step method of RNA isolation by acid guanidinium thiocyanate-phenol-chloroform extraction. *Anal. Biochem.*, **162**, 156–159.

5. FOOD AND AGRICULTURE ORGANIZATION OF THE UNITED NATIONS (FAO) (1994). Quality control testing of rinderpest cell culture vaccine: standard operating procedures. FAO Animal Production and Health Paper 118. FAO, Rome, Italy.

6. FOREMAN A.J., ROWE L.W. & TAYLOR W.P. (1983). The detection of rinderpest antigen by agar gel diffusion and counter immunoelectrophoresis. *Trop. Anim. Health Prod.,* **15**, 83–85.

7. FORSYTH M.A. & BARRETT T. (1995). Evaluation of polymerase chain reaction for the detection and charecterisation of rinderpest and peste des petits ruminants viruses for epidemiological studies. *Virus Res.*, **39**, 151–163.

8. LIBEAU G., DIALLO A., COLAS F. & GUERRE L. (1994). Rapid differential diagnosis of rinderpest and peste des petits ruminants using an immunocapture ELISA. *Vet. Rec.,* **134**, 300–304.

9. MARINER J.C., HOUSE J.A., MEBUS C.A., SOLLOD A. & STEM C. (1991). Production of a thermostable Vero cell-adapted rinderpest vaccine. *J. Tissue Culture Methods,* **13**, 253–256.

10. MARINER J.C., HOUSE J.A., SOLLOD A.E., STEM C., VAN DEN ENDE M. & MEBUS C.A. (1990). Comparison of the effects of various chemical stabilizers and lyophilization cycles on the thermostability of a Vero cell-adapted rinderpest vaccine. *Vet. Microbiol.,* **21**, 195–209.

11. NANDA Y.P., CHATTERJEE A., PUROHIT A.K., DIALLO A., INNUI K., SHARMA R.N., LIBEAU G., THEVASAGAYAM J.A., BRUNING A., KITCHING R.P., ANDERSON J., BARRETT T. & TAYLOR W.P. (1996). The isolation of peste des petite ruminants virus from northern India. *Vet. Microbiol.,* **51**, 207–216.

12. PLOWRIGHT W. (1984). The duration of immunity in cattle following inoculation of rinderpest cell culture vaccine. *J. Hyg.,* **92**, 285–296.

13. PLOWRIGHT W., HERNIMAN K.A.J. & RAMPTON C.S. (1971). Studies on rinderpest culture vaccine. IV. The stability of the reconstituted product. *Res. Vet. Sci.,* **12**, 40–46.

14. PLOWRIGHT W., RAMPTON C.S., TAYLOR W.P. & HERNIMAN K.A.J. (1970). Studies on rinderpest culture vaccine. III. Stability of the lyophilised product. *Res. Vet. Sci.,* **11**, 71–81.

15. TAYLOR W.P. & ROWE L.W. (1984). A microneutralisation test for the detection of rinderpest virus antibodies. *Rev. Elev. Med. Vet. Pays Trop.*, **37,** 155–159.

*
* *

CHAPTER 2.1.5.

PESTE DES PETITS RUMINANTS

SUMMARY

Peste des petits ruminants (PPR), is an acute contagious disease caused by a Morbillivirus in the family Paramyxoviridae. It affects small ruminants, especially goats, which are highly susceptible, and occasionally wild animals. It occurs in Africa (south of the Sahara), the Arabian Peninsula, throughout most of the Middle Eastern countries, and south-west Asia.

The clinical disease resembles rinderpest in cattle. It is usually acute and characterised by serous ocular and nasal discharges. PPR is characterised by severe pyrexia, which can last for 3–5 days, erosive lesions, which occur in the mouth, diarrhoea and pneumonia. At necropsy, characteristic zebra markings occur in the large intestine. Lesions also occur in the lungs showing congestion or bronchopneumonia when associated with bacterial infection.

The disease must be differentiated from rinderpest, bluetongue, foot and mouth disease and other exanthemous conditions.

***Identification of the agent:** The collection of samples at the correct time is important to achieve a diagnosis by virus isolation. Samples should be obtained in the acute phase of the disease when clinical signs are still apparent. Swabs can be made of the conjuctival sac, nasal secretions, and buccal and rectal mucosae. Unclotted blood is also taken.*

Rapid diagnosis can be made by immunocapture enzyme-linked immunosorbent assay (ELISA), counter immunoelectrophoresis and agar gel immunodiffusion. As specific primers are available, polymerase chain reaction may also be used. The OIE and FAO[1] Reference Laboratory for PPR in France (see Table given in Part 4 of this Manual*) can advise on the use of this technique for virus identification in field samples.*

***Serological tests:** Serological tests that are routinely used include a virus neutralisation test and competitive ELISA. Other tests, such as counter immunoelectrophoresis, indirect fluorescent antibody tests and a precipitinogen inhibition test, may be employed.*

***Requirements for vaccines and diagnostic biologicals:** Vaccination has been carried out using rinderpest tissue culture vaccine based on the principle that an antigenic relationship exists between PPR and rinderpest viruses. A homologous vaccine has been developed and tested in field trials. The use of this PPR vaccine is strongly recommended to avoid confusion with rinderpest during serological surveys. It is now commercially available.*

A. DIAGNOSTIC TECHNIQUES

Peste des petits ruminants (PPR) is an acute viral disease of small ruminants characterised by fever, oculonasal discharges, stomatitis, diarrhoea and pneumonia. Infected animals present clinical signs similar to those of rinderpest in cattle, from which it must be differentiated. PPR virus causes clinical disease in sheep and goats but, whereas it will infect cattle, it produces no clinical signs. It is transmitted by aerosols between animals living in close contact (14).

On the basis of its similarities to the viruses of rinderpest, canine distemper and measles, the PPR virus has been classified within the genus Morbillivirus in the family Paramyxoviridae (12).

1 Food and Agriculture Organization of the United Nations

PPR was first described in Côte d'Ivoire (11), but it occurs in most African countries south of the Sahara and north of the equator (14), the Arabian Peninsula (10, 24), and in most of the Middle Eastern countries such as Jordan, Israel, and Lebanon (15, 19). PPR is also wide-spread in India and south-west Asia (21).

The natural disease affects mainly goats and sheep, but it is usually more severe in goats where it causes heavy losses, and is only occasionally severe in sheep. A case of clinical disease has been reported in wildlife resulting in deaths of gazelles *(Gazella dorcas)*, ibex *(Capra ibex nubiana)*, gemsbok *(Oryx gazella)* and Laristan sheep *(Ovis orientalis laristanica)* (10). The American white-tailed deer *(Odocoileus virginianus)* is readily infected experimentally (13). In Ethiopia, a disease thought to be caused by PPR virus in one-humped camels has been reported and is under investigation.

The incubation period is 4–6 days, but may range between 3 and 10 days. The clinical disease is acute, with a pyrexia up to 41°C that can last for 3–5 days; the animals become depressed, anorexic and develop a dry muzzle. The serous oculonasal discharges become progressively mucopurulent and, if death does not ensue, persist for around 14 days. Within 4 days of the onset of fever, the gums become hyperaemic, and erosive lesions develop in the oral cavity with excessive salivation. These lesions may become necrotic. A watery bloodstained diarrhoea is common in the later stage. Pneumonia, coughing, pleural rales and abdominal breathing also occur. The morbidity rate can be up to 100% and, in severe outbreaks, with 100% mortality. In milder outbreaks, the mortality rate may not exceed 50%. A tentative diagnosis of PPR is made on these clinical signs, but where rinderpest exists in cattle, laboratory confirmation is required.

At necropsy, the lesions are very similar to those observed in cattle affected with rinderpest. Erosive lesions may extend from the mouth to the reticulo–rumen junction. Characteristic linear haemorrhages or zebra stripes occur in the large intestine, commonly at the caeco–colic junction. Lymph nodes are enlarged, the spleen may show necrotic lesions, and there is an apical pneumonia.

There are no known health risks to humans working with PPR virus as no report of human infection with the virus exists.

1. Identification of the agent

a) Collection of samples

In live animals, swabs are made of the conjuctival discharges from the nasal and buccal mucosae. Whole blood is also collected in anticoagulant for virus isolation, polymerase chain reaction (PCR) and haematology. At necropsy (two to three animals), lymph nodes, especially the mesenteric and bronchial nodes, lungs, spleen and intestinal mucosae should also be collected aseptically, chilled on ice and transported under refrigeration. Fragments of organs collected for histopathology are placed in 10% formalin. At the end of the outbreak, blood can be collected for serological diagnosis.

b) Agar gel immunodiffusion

Agar gel immunodiffusion (AGID) is a very simple and cheap test that can be performed in any laboratory and even in the field. Standard PPR viral antigen is prepared from mesenteric or bronchial lymph nodes, spleen or lung material and ground up as 1/3 suspensions in buffered saline. These are centrifuged at 500 ***g*** for 10–20 minutes, and the supernatant fluids are stored in aliquots at -20°C. They may be retained for 1–3 years. Control antigen is prepared similarly from normal tissues. Standard antiserum is made by hyperimmunising sheep with 5 ml of PPR virus with a titre of 10^4 $TCID_{50}$ (50% tissue culture infective dose) per ml given at weekly intervals for 4 weeks. The animals are bled 5–7 days after the last injection (5). Standard rinderpest hyperimmune antiserum is also effective in detecting PPR antigen.

i) Dispense 1% agar in normal saline, containing thiomersal (0.4 g/litre) or sodium azide (1.25 g/litre) as a bacteriostatic agent, into Petri dishes (6 ml/5 cm dish),

ii) Wells are punched in the agar following an hexagonal pattern with a central well. The wells are 5 mm in diameter and 5 mm apart.

iii) The central well is filled with positive antiserum, three peripheral wells with positive antigen, and one well with negative antigen. The two remaining peripheral wells are filled with test antigen, such that the test and negative control antigens alternate with the positive control antigens.

iv) Usually, 1–3 lines will develop between the serum and antigens within 18–24 hours (7, 22). These are intensified by washing the agar with 5% glacial acetic acid for 5 minutes (this procedure should be carried out with all apparently negative tests before recording a negative result). Positive reactions show lines of identity with the positive control antigen.

Results are obtained in 1 day, but the test is not sensitive enough to detect mild forms of PPR due to the low quantity of viral antigen that is excreted.

c) Immunocapture enzyme-linked immunosorbent assay

The immunocapture enzyme-linked immunosorbent assay (ELISA) (16), using several anti-N monoclonal antibodies (MAb), allows a rapid differential identification of PPR or rinderpest viruses, and this is of great importance as the two diseases have a similar geographical distribution and may affect the same animal species.

i) Microtitre ELISA plates are coated with 100 µl of a capture MAb solution (diluted according to the instructions of the Reference Laboratory providing the kit). This MAb reacts with both rinderpest and PPR viruses.

ii) After washing, 50 µl of the sample suspension is added to four wells, and control wells are filled with buffer.

iii) Immediately, 25 µl of a detection biotinylated MAb for PPR and 25 µl of streptavidin–peroxidase are added to two wells, and 25 µl of a detection MAb for rinderpest and 25 µl of streptavidin–peroxidase are added to the two other wells.

iv) The plates are incubated at 37°C for 1 hour with constant agitation.

v) After three vigorous washes, 100 µl of ortho-phenylenediamine (OPD) in hydrogen peroxide is added, and the plates are incubated for 10 more minutes at room temperature.

vi) The reaction is stopped by the addition of 100 µl of 1 N sulphuric acid, and the absorbance is measured at 492 nm on a spectophotometer/ELISA reader.

The cut-off above which samples are considered to be positive is calculated from each blank (PPR blank and rinderpest blank) as three times the mean absorbance values.

A sandwich ELISA can also be performed: the sample is first allowed to react with the detection MAb and the immunocomplex is then captured by the second MAb adsorbed on to the ELISA plate.

The test is very specific and sensitive (it can detect $10^{0.6}$ $TCID_{50}$/well for the PPR virus and $10^{2.2}$ $TCID_{50}$ for the rinderpest virus). The results are obtained in 2 hours.

d) Nucleic acid recognition methods

cDNA ^{32}P labelled clones have been used to differentiate PPR and rinderpest (3), but their use in routine diagnosis is not recommended due to the short half-life of the ^{32}P and the need for special equipment to protect the users.

A PCR technique based on the amplification of the NP and F protein genes has been developed for the specific diagnosis of PPR (2, 9). This technique is very sensitive compared with other tests and results are obtained in 5 hours, including the RNA extraction. The OIE and FAO Reference Laboratory for PPR in France (see Table given in Part 4 of this *Manual*) can advise on the use of this technique.

e) Counter immunoelectrophoresis

Counter immunoelectrophoresis (CIEP) is the most rapid test for viral antigen detection (7, 18). It is carried out on a horizontal surface using a suitable electrophoresis bath, which consists of two compartments connected through a bridge. The apparatus is connected to a high-voltage source. Agar or agarose (1–2%, [w/v]) dissolved in 0.025 M barbitone acetate buffer is dispensed on to microscope slides in 3 ml volumes From six to nine pairs of wells are punched in the solidified agar. The reagents are the same as those used for the AGID test. The electrophoresis bath is filled with 0.1 M barbitone acetate buffer. The pairs of wells in the agar are filled with the reactants: sera in the anodal wells and antigen in the cathodal wells. The slide is placed on the connecting bridge and the ends are connected to the buffer in the troughs by wetted porous paper. The apparatus is covered, and a current of 10–12 milliamps per slide is applied for 30–60 minutes. The current is switched off and the slides are viewed by intense light: the presence of 1–3 precipitation lines between pairs of wells is a positive reaction. There should be no reactions between wells containing the negative controls.

f) Culture and isolation methods

Even when diagnosis has been carried out by rapid techniques, the virus should always be isolated from field samples in tissue cultures for further studies (7, 14).

PPR virus may be isolated in primary lamb kidney or in African green monkey kidney (Vero) cell tissue cultures. Monolayer cultures are inoculated with suspect material (swab material, buffy coat or 10% tissue suspensions) and examined daily for evidence of cytopathic effect (CPE). The CPE produced by PPR virus can develop within 5 days and consists of cell rounding and aggregation culminating in syncytia formation in lamb kidney cells. In Vero cells, it is sometimes difficult to see the syncytia. If they exist, they are very small. However, in stained, infected Vero cells, small syncytia are always seen. Syncytia are recognised by a circular arrangement of nuclei giving a 'clock face' appearance. Cover-slip cultures may give a CPE earlier than day 5. There are also intracytoplasmic and intranuclear inclusions. Some cells are vacuolated. Similar cellular changes may be seen in stained histopathological sections of infected tissues. After 5–6 days, blind passages should always be carried out as CPE may take time to appear.

2. Serological tests

Goats and sheep infected with PPR virus develop antibodies that may be demonstrated to support a diagnosis by the antigen-detection tests. Tests that are routinely used are the virus neutralisation (VN) test and the competitive ELISA. Other tests, such as CIEP (8), AGID (24), precipitinogen inhibition and indirect fluorescent antibody test (6), have been described, but remain of little interest compared with the VN and ELISA.

a) Virus neutralisation (the prescribed test for international trade)

This test is sensitive and specific, but it is time-consuming. The standard neutralisation test is carried out in roller-tube cultures of primary lamb kidney cells, or Vero cells when primary cells are not available.

i) Dilute 1 ml of inactivated serum in a twofold dilution series and mix with a stock virus suspension containing approximately 10^3 $TCID_{50}$/ml.

ii) Incubate the virus/serum mixtures either for 1 hour at 37°C or overnight at 4°C.

iii) Inoculate 0.2 ml of the mixture into each of five roller tubes, followed immediately by 1 ml of Vero cell suspension in growth medium at a rate of 2×10^5 cells/ml.

iv) Incubate the sloped tubes for 3 days at 37°C.

v) Discard the tubes showing virus-specific CPE; replace the medium in the remaining tubes with maintenance medium, and roll the tubes for a further 7 days. The virus-challenge dose is acceptable if it falls between $10^{1.8}$ and $10^{2.8}$ $TCID_{50}$/ tube. Any detectable antibody at a dilution of 1/8 is considered to be positive.

Usually, a cross-neutralisation test is carried out with rinderpest virus and a serum is considered to be positive for PPR when the neutralisation titre is at least twofold higher for PPR than for rinderpest.

b) Competitive enzyme-linked immunosorbent assay

Competitive ELISAs using anti-N or anti-H MAbs have been described (1, 15) and are specific and sensitive (relative specificity: 99.4% and relative sensitivity: 94.5%) (15, 17, 20).

i) Coat microtitre plates with 50 µl of a predetermined dilution of N-PPR protein (produced by a recombinant baculovirus) for 1 hour at 37°C with constant agitation.

ii) Wash the plates three times and blot dry.

iii) Distribute 45 µl of blocking buffer (PBS + 0.5% Tween 20 + 0.5 fetal calf serum) to all wells, and then add 5 µl of test sera to test wells (at a final dilution of 1/20) and 5 µl of the different control sera (strong positive, weak positive and negative serum) to control wells.

iv) Add 50 µl of MAb diluted 1/100 in blocking buffer, and incubate at 37°C for 1 hour.

v) Wash the plates three times and blot dry.

vi) Add 50 µl of anti-mouse conjugate diluted 1/1000, and incubate at 37°C for 1 hour.

vii) Wash the plates three times.

viii) Prepare OPD in hydrogen peroxide solution. Add 50 µl of substrate/conjugate mixture to each well. Stop the reaction after 10 minutes with 50 µl of 1 M sulphuric acid.

ix) Read on an ELISA reader at 492 nm.

The absorbance is converted to percentage of inhibition (PI) using the formula:

PI = 100 – (absorbance of the test wells/absorbance of the MAb control wells) × 100

Sera showing PI greater than 50% are positive.

B. REQUIREMENTS FOR VACCINES AND DIAGNOSTIC BIOLOGICALS

Sheep and goats that recover from PPR develop an active immunity against the disease. Antibodies have been demonstrated 4 years after infection (6), but immunity is probably life long. A homologous PPR vaccine is available. In 1998, the OIE International Committee endorsed the use of this vaccine in countries that have decided to follow the 'OIE pathway' for epidemiological surveillance for rinderpest in order to avoid confusion when serological surveys are performed.

1. Seed management

a) Characteristics of the seed

Homologous vaccine against PPR is a live vaccine cultured in Vero cells. The original strain of virus for the homologous vaccine against PPR is strain PPR 75/1, isolated in Nigeria in 1975 (23). This is attenuated by passage in Vero cell cultures (4). The strain provided for vaccine production is the 70th passage in Vero cells (PPRV 75/1 I.K6 BK2 Vero 70). It is stored in freeze-dried form at –20°C and may be obtained from Reference Laboratories (see Table given in Part 4 of this *Manual*). Tests of vaccine activity show that it retained the ability to protect (at a dose of 10^3 $TCID_{50}$) up to the 120th passage in Vero cells, the latest passage tested so far.

b) Method of culture

- **Cells**

PPR vaccine is produced in Vero cells, which must be free from all bacterial, fungal and viral contamination.

- **Culture medium**

Minimal essential medium (MEM) supplemented with antibiotics (for example penicillin + streptomycin at final concentrations of 100 IU [International Units]/ml and 100 µg/ml, respectively), and an antifungal agent (nystatin [Mycostatin] at a final concentration of 50 µg/ml). The medium is enriched with 10% fetal calf serum (complete medium) for cell growth. This proportion of serum is reduced to 2% for maintenance medium once the cell monolayer is complete.

- **Primary seed batch of vaccine virus**

This consists of virus in its 70th passage in Vero cells (PPRV 75/1 LK6 BK2 Vero 70). The freeze-dried contents of a flask from the seed bank is reconstituted with 2 ml of sterile water (or cell culture medium without serum). This liquid is mixed with Vero cells suspended in complete culture medium to provide at least 0.001 $TCID_{50}$ per cell. Cell culture dishes are filled with this virus/cell mixture (around 2×10^7 Vero cells in a 175 cm^2 dish). They are incubated at 37°C. The cultured cells are examined regularly to detect a CPE. The medium is renewed every 2 days, reducing the proportion of serum to 2% once the cell monolayer is complete. Virus is first harvested when there is 40–50% CPE. This viral suspension is stored at –70°C. Successive harvesting is made every 2 days until the CPE reaches 70–80%, which is the time for final freezing of the culture dishes (in general, at least two further harvestings can be made before final freezing of the culture dishes). All suspensions of virus collected are submitted to two freeze–thaw cycles, then added to form a single batch, which serves as the primary seed batch. This is divided into small volumes in bottles and stored at –70°C. The contents of five flasks are thawed and titrated (minimum titre required: 10^5 $TCID_{50}$/ml). It is best to freeze-dry this seed in order to store it at –20°C. In this case it will be necessary to titrate the freeze-dried virus (five bottles). A batch made up in this way must pass all tests for sterility.

When preparing seed batches, it is important to avoid infecting the cells with too strong a dose of virus (high mutiplicity of infection), as this will lead to accumulation of defective particles in the viral suspension produced, which will diminish the titre of subsequent products. On the other hand, very weak multiplicity of infection (e.g. 0.0001) will prolong the culture time.

- **Preparation of the working seed batch**

This is done under the same conditions as for the primary seed batch. A large stock of virus is formed, from which the final vaccine will be produced. This batch is distributed into receptacles and stored at –70°C. It must satisfy tests for sterility. Five samples are titrated (minimum titre required: 10^6 $TCID_{50}$/ml).

c) Validation as a vaccine

It is necessary to confirm or rule out the presence of PPR virus in the product under test. For this purpose, anti-PPR serum is used to neutralise the virus in cell culture.

- **Test procedure**

i) Mix the contents of two vaccine bottles with sterile double-distilled water to provide a volume equal to the volume before freeze-drying.

ii) Make tenfold dilutions of the reconstituted vaccine in serum-free culture medium (0.5 ml of viral suspension + 4.5 ml of medium).

iii) Make two series of mixtures for virus dilutions from each bottle on a 96-well plate as follows:

Series 1:	Dilutions of viral suspension:	–1	–2	–3	–4
	Viral suspension (in µl)	50	50	50	50
	Culture medium (in µl)	50	50	50	50
Series 2:	Dilutions of viral suspension:	–1	–2	–3	–4
	Viral suspension (in µl)	50	50	50	50
	PPR antiserum (in µl)	50	50	50	50

(Note: PPR antiserum used for this purpose is prepared in goats and freeze-dried. It is reconstituted with 1 ml of sterile double-distilled water in a dilution of 1/10).

iv) Incubate the mixtures at 37°C for 1 hour

v) Add to each well 100 µl of cells suspended in complete culture medium (30,000 cells/well).

vi) Incubate the microplate at 37°C in the presence of CO_2.

vii) Read the plate after 10–15 hours of incubation.

Normally a CPE is present only in the wells containing cells infected with the mixture of virus and culture medium. If it is detected in the wells of Series 2, it will be necessary to identify PPR virus by immunofluorescence, using a PPR MAb, or by immunocapture (specific PPR MAb, and the immunocapture test kit are available from the OIE Reference Laboratory for PPR in France [see Table given in Part 4 of this *Manual*]). If this identification confirms the presence of PPR virus, the PPR antiserum used must have been too weak, or the batch must be changed. If immunofluorescence or immunocapture is negative, a viral contaminant must be present, and the material under test must be destroyed.

2. Method of manufacture

a) Vaccine production

This operation is performed on a larger scale. Cells can be infected with virus at a multiplicity of infection as before or with high doses, e.g. up to 0.01. Products of the various harvests, after two freeze–thaw cycles, are brought together (to form the final product) and stored at –70°C pending the results of titration and tests for sterility. If these results are satisfactory, the vaccine is freeze-dried.

b) Freeze-drying

The freeze-drying medium (Weybridge medium) is composed of 2.5% (w/v) lactalbumin, 5% (w/v) sucrose and 1% (w/v) sodium glutamate, pH 7.2.

This medium is added to an equal volume of viral suspension for freeze-drying (which may have been diluted beforehand to provide the desired number of vaccine doses per bottle). The resulting mixture is kept cool, homogenised, then distributed into bottles and freeze-dried. At the end of a freeze-drying cycle, the probe is adjusted and kept at 35°C for 4 hours. Once this operation has been completed, the bottles are capped under vacuum. Randomly selected samples (e.g. 5%) of this final batch are submitted to tests for innocuity, efficacy and sterility, and residual moisture is estimated by the Karl Fisher method (optimum ≤3.5%). If the tests give unsatisfactory results, the entire batch is destroyed.

3. In-process control

Cells used in cultures must be checked for normal appearance and shown to be free from contaminating viruses, especially bovine viral diarrhoea virus. A virus titration must be undertaken on the seed lot: using MEM (serum-free) medium, a series of tenfold dilutions is made (0.5 ml virus + 4.5 ml diluent) down to 10^{-6} of the product to be titrated. Vero cells from one flask are trypsinised and suspended in complete culture medium at 300,000/ml. They are distributed on a 96-well plate (30,000 cells per well, equivalent to 100 µl of cell suspension). Then, 100 µl of virus diluted tenfold is added to the cells (dilutions ranging from 10^{-2} to 10^{-6}). One row of wells serves as a control for uninfected cells to which virus-free culture medium (100 µl) is added. The plate is incubated at 37°C in the presence of CO_2. The plates are read (by examining for CPE) 10–15 days after infection.

Virus titre is determined by the Spearman–Kärber method. The minimum titre per dose is $10^{2.5}$.

4. Batch control

a) Identity

The contents of one container from each filling lot must be checked for identity by culture after neutralisation with specific antiserum.

b) Sterility

This consists of testing for viral, bacterial or fungal contaminants. It is done on cells and sera before their use in vaccine production, the seed stock and the vaccine before and after freeze-drying. Any product that fails this test for sterility is destroyed.

Tests for sterility and freedom from contamination of biological materials may be found in Chapter I.4.

c) Safety

This test is done in rodents in order to detect any nonspecific toxicity associated with the product. The test requires reconstituted vaccine in solvent (mixed contents of five bottles), six guinea-pigs, each weighing 200–250 g; ten unweaned mice (17–22 g., Swiss line or similar).

Vaccine, 0.5 ml, is injected intramuscularly into a hind limb of two guinea-pigs, 0.5 ml into the peritoneal cavity of two guinea-pigs, and 0.1 ml into the peritoneal cavity of six mice. Two guinea-pigs and four mice are kept as uninoculated controls. The animals are observed for 3 weeks. If one guinea-pig or two mice die, the test must be repeated. Dead animals undergo post-mortem examination to ascertain the cause of death. At the end of 3 weeks of observation, all animals are killed for post-mortem examination. All the results are recorded. The vaccine is considered to be satisfactory if, during the first or second test, at least 80% of animals remain in good health during the period of observation, and no significant post-mortem lesion is found.

d) Potency and efficacy in small ruminants

This test requires the following: vaccine reconstituted with normal saline (the mixed contents of five bottles) to provide 100 doses and 0.1 dose/ml; six goats and six sheep, all approximately 1-year old and free from antibodies to rinderpest or PPR; sterile syringes and needles; and pathogenic PPR virus previously titrated in goats, diluted with sterile normal saline to provide 10^3 of the 50% infectious dose for goats (GID_{50}).

Vaccinate two goats and two sheep subcutaneously with 100 doses per animal; vaccinate two goats and two sheep subcutaneously with 0.1 dose per animal; keep the remaining animals as in-contact controls. The animals are observed and temperature measurements are recorded daily for 3 weeks. At the end of this period, blood is taken from all animals for the preparation of sera. All animals are challenged by subcutaneous injection of a 1 ml suspension of pathogenic PPR virus (10^3 GID_{50} per animal). The animals are observed and their body temperature measurements are recorded daily for 2 weeks.

The vaccine is considered to be satisfactory if all vaccinated animals resist the challenge infection, while at least half of the in-contact controls develop signs of PPR. The serum neutralisation test must be positive for PPR antibody (in serum diluted at least 1/10) in vaccinated animals only in samples taken 3 weeks after vaccination. If any of the controls are also positive, the experiment must be repeated, using another batch of pathogenic PPR virus. The batch of vaccine is destroyed if vaccinated animals react to the virulent challenge.

- **Titration of neutralising PPR antibody**

This test requires the following: cell suspensions at 600,000/ml; 96-well cell culture plates; sera to be titrated (inactivated by heating to 56°C for 30 minutes); complete cell culture medium; PPR virus diluted to give 1000, 100, 10 and 1 $TCID_{50}$/ml.

Dilute the sera at 1/5, then make a twofold dilution in cell culture medium. Mix 100 µl of virus at 1000 $TCID_{50}$/ml (to give 100 $TCID_{50}$ in each well) and 100 µl of a given dilution of serum (using six wells per dilution) in the wells of the cell culture plate. Arrange a series of control wells for virus and uninfected cells as follows: six wells with 100 $TCID_{50}$ (100 µl) per well; six wells with 10 $TCID_{50}$ (100 µl) per well; six wells with 1 $TCID_{50}$ (100 µl) per well; six wells with 0.1 $TCID_{50}$ (100 µl) per well; and six wells with 200 µl of virus-free culture (control cells) per well.

Make the wells containing the virus controls up to 100 µl with complete culture medium, and incubate the plates for 1 hour at 37°C. Add 50 µl of cell suspension to each well. Incubate the plates at 37°C in the presence of CO_2. Read the plates after 1 and 2 weeks of incubation. The results should be as follows: 100% CPE in virus control wells of 100 and 10 $TCID_{50}$, 50% CPE for the 1 $TCID_{50}$ dilution, no CPE for the 0.1 $TCID_{50}$ dilution, no CPE in wells where the virus had been neutralised by serum during the test, and CPE in wells where the virus had not been neutralised by serum during the test.

e) Duration of immunity

Duration of immunity is at least 3 years.

f) Stability

Freeze-dried vaccine can be kept for at least 2 years at 2–8°C (although storage at –20°C is better), provided it is stored under vacuum and protected from light.

5. Tests on the final product

a) Safety

See Section B.4.c.

c) Potency

See Section B.4.d.

REFERENCES

1. ANDERSON J. & MCKAY J.A. (1994). The detection of antibodies against peste des petits ruminants virus in cattle, sheep and goats and the possible implication to rinderpest control programmes. *Epidem. Infect.*, **112**, 225–234.

2. COUACY-HYMANN E. (1994). La Lutte contre la Peste Bovine en Côte-d'Ivoire – Coûts et Bénéfices des Campagnes de Prophylaxie – Problèmes Posés pour son Éradication. Thèse Doctorat es-Sciences, Université Paris XII, France.

3. DIALLO A., BARRETT T., BARBRON M., SUBBARAO S.M. & TAYLOR W.P. (1988). Differentiation of rinderpest and peste des petits ruminants viruses using specific cDNA clones. *J. Virol. Methods*, **23**, 127–136.

4. DIALLO A., TAYLOR W.P., LEFEVRE P.C. & PROVOST A. (1989). Atténuation d'une souche de virus de la peste des petits ruminants: candidat pour un vaccin homologue vivant. *Rev. Elev. Med. Vet. Pays Trop.*, **42**, 311–319.

5. DUROJAIYE O.A. (1982). Precipitating antibody in sera of goats naturally affected with peste des petits ruminants. *Trop. Anim. Health Prod.*, **14**, 98–100.

6. DUROJAIYE O.A. (1984). Detection of the antigen of peste des petits ruminants virus in tissues by indirect immunofluorescence technique. *Niger. Vet. J.*, **13**, 77–80.

7. DUROJAIYE O.A., OBI T.U. & OJO O. (1983). Virological and serological diagnosis of peste des petits ruminants. *Trop. Vet.*, **1**, 13–17.

8. DUROJAIYE O.A. & TAYLOR W.P. (1984). Application of counter current immunoelectro-osmophoresis to the serology of peste des petits ruminants. *Rev. Elev. Med. Vet. Pays Trop.*, **37**, 272–276.

9. FORSYTH M.A. & BARRETT T. (1995). Evaluation of polymerase chain reaction for the detection and characterisation of rinderpest and peste de petit ruminants viruses for epidemiological studies. *Virus Res.*, **39**, 151–163.

10. FURLEY C.W., TAYLOR W.P. & OBI T.U. (1987). An outbreak of peste des petits ruminants in a zoological collection. *Vet. Rec.*, **121**, 443–447.

11. GARGADENNEC L. & LALANNE A. (1942). La peste des petits ruminants. *Bull. Serv. Zoo. A.O.F.*, **5**, 15–21.

12. GIBBS E.P.J., TAYLOR W.P., LAWMAN M.J.P. & BRYANT J. (1979). Classification of peste des petits ruminants virus as the fourth member of the genus *Morbillivirus*. *Intervirology*, **II**, 268–274.

13. HAMDY F.M. & DARDIRI A.H. (1976). Response of white-tailed deer to infection with peste des petits ruminants virus. *J. Wildl. Dis.*, **12**, 516–522.

14. LEFEVRE P.C. & DIALLO A. (1990). Peste des petits ruminants. *Rev. sci. tech. Off. int. Epiz.*, **9**, 951–965.

15. LEFEVRE P.C., DIALLO A., SCHENKEL F., HUSSEIN S. & STAAK G. (1991). Serological evidence of peste des petits ruminants in Jordan. *Vet. Rec.*, **128**, 110.

16. LIBEAU G., DIALLO A., COLAS F. & GUERRE L. (1994). Rapid differential diagnosis of rinderpest and peste des petits ruminants using an immunocapture ELISA. *Vet. Rec.*, **134**, 300–304.

17. LIBEAU G., PREHAUD C., LANCELOT R., COLAS F., GUERRE L., BISHOP D.H.L. & DIALLO A. (1995). Development of a competitive ELISA for detecting antibodies to the peste des petits ruminants virus using a recombinant nucleoprotein. *Res. Vet. Sci.*, **58**, 50–55.

18. MAJIYAGBE K.A., NAWATHE D.R. & ABEGUNDE A. (1984). Rapid diagnosis of PPR infection, application of immuno-electro-osmophoresis (IEOP) technique. *Rev. Elev. Med. Vet. Pays Trop.*, **37**, 11–15.

19. PERL S., ALEXANDER A., YAKOBSON B., NYSKA A., HARMELIN A., SHEIKHAT N., SHIMSHONY A., DAVIDSON N., ABRAMSON M. & RAPOPORT E. (1994). Peste des petits ruminants (PPR) of sheep in Israel: case report. *Israel J. Vet. Med.*, **49**, 59–62.

20. SALIKI J.T., LIBEAU G., HOUSE J.A., MEBUS C.A. & DUBOVI E.J. (1993). Monoclonal antibody-based blocking enzyme-linked immunosorbent assay for specific detection and titration of peste-des-petits ruminants virus antibody in caprine and ovine sera. *J. Clin. Microbiol.*, **31**, 1075–1082.

21. SHAILA M.S., PURUSHOTHAMAN V., BHASAVAR D., VENUGOPAL K. & VENKATESAN R.A. (1989). Peste des petits ruminants in India. *Vet. Rec.*, **125**, 602.

22. TAYLOR W.P. (1979). Serological studies with the virus of peste des petits ruminants in Nigeria. *Res. Vet. Sci.*, **26**, 236–242.

23. TAYLOR W.P. & ABEGUNDE A. (1975). The isolation of peste des petits ruminants virus from Nigerian sheep and goats. *Res. Vet. Sci.*, **26**, 94–96

24. TAYLOR W.P., ALBUSAIDY S. & BARRETT T. (1990). The epidemiology of peste des petits ruminants in the Sultanate of Oman. *Vet. Microbiol.*, **22**, 341–352.

*

* *

CHAPTER 2.1.6.

CONTAGIOUS BOVINE PLEUROPNEUMONIA

SUMMARY

Contagious bovine pleuropneumonia (CBPP) is a disease of cattle caused by Mycoplasma mycoides *subsp.* mycoides *SC (bovine biotype) (SC: small colonies). It is manifested by anorexia, fever and respiratory signs such as dyspnoea, polypnoea, cough and nasal discharges. Diagnosis depends on the isolation of the aetiological agent. The main problems for control or eradication are the frequent occurrence of subacute or asymptomatic infections and the persistence of chronic carriers after the clinical phase.*

Identification of the agent: *Samples to be taken from live animals are nasal swabs and/or broncho-alveolar washings or pleural fluid obtained by puncture. Samples to be taken at necropsy are lung lesions, lymph nodes, pleural fluid and synovial fluid from those animals with arthritis. Direct examination of the exudate or smears is possible, but requires great skill.*

For cultivation of the pathogen, the tissues are ground in medium with antibiotics and inoculated into media that contain inhibitors to prevent the growth of contaminating bacteria. As the growth of M. m. *subsp.* m. SC *takes several days, desiccation of the solid medium should be limited by closing the Petri dishes hermetically or by using controlled humidity incubators.*

In broth, growth is visible within 3–10 days as a homogeneous cloudiness with whirls when shaken; on agar, small colonies develop, 1 mm in diameter, with the classical 'fried-egg' appearance. The biochemical characteristics to be checked are the following: sensitivity to digitonin, reduction of tetrazolium salts, breakdown of glucose, absence of arginine hydrolysis, and the absence of phosphatase and proteolytic activities. Special media have been described that are recommended for these tests. Diagnosis is confirmed by immunological tests, such as the growth inhibition and immunofluorescence tests (both use hyperimmune sera). The polymerase chain reaction has now been brought into use as a rapid, specific, sensitive and easy to use test.

Serological tests: *For diagnosis, the modified Campbell & Turner complement fixation test remains the prescribed test for international trade. However, it has significant limitations regarding sensitivity and specificity. A competitive enzyme-linked immunosorbent assay and an immunoblotting test have undergone evaluation and are regarded as highly specific and sensitive tests.*

Requirements for vaccines and diagnostic biologicals: *One attenuated strain is now recommended for vaccine production: the T_1-44. The minimal recommended titre is 10^7 viable mycoplasmas per vaccinal dose.*

A. DIAGNOSTIC TECHNIQUES

Contagious bovine pleuropneumonia (CBPP) is a contagious disease of cattle caused by *Mycoplasma mycoides* subsp. *mycoides* SC (bovine biotype) (SC: small colonies). Members of the *M. mycoides* group, *M. capricolum* group, and Leach's group 7 form the so-called *M. mycoides* cluster, which consists of six mycoplasma species, subspecies or groups of strains, originating from bovines and goats (6). These six mycoplasmas share serological and genetic characteristics, and this causes taxonomic and diagnostic problems (6). In natural conditions, *Mycoplasma mycoides* subsp. *mycoides* SC *(MmmSC)* affects only the ruminants of the *Bos* genus, i.e. mainly bovine and zebu cattle. *MmmSC* (bovine biotype) has been isolated from buffaloes in Italy (23) and sheep and goats in Portugal. Among wild animals, one single case has been reported in American buffaloes *(Bison bison)* and none in African buffaloes *(Syncerus caffer)* or other wild ruminants. CBPP is manifested by anorexia, fever and respiratory signs, such as dyspnoea, polypnoea, cough and nasal discharges. However, clinical signs are not always evident. Subacute or asymptomatic forms occur frequently.

1. Identification of the agent

The causal organism can be isolated from samples taken either from live animals or at necropsy. Samples are taken from live animals as nasal swabs or nasal discharges, broncho-alveolar lavage or transtracheal washing and pleural fluid collected aseptically by puncture made in the lower part of the thoracic cavity between the seventh and eighth ribs. Blood may also be cultured (13). Samples taken at necropsy are lungs with lesions, pleural fluid ('lymph'), lymph nodes of the broncho-pulmonary tract, and synovial fluid from those animals with arthritis.

The presence of pathogens varies greatly with the development of the lesions, and a negative result is not conclusive, particularly after treatment with an antibiotic.

When dispatching the samples to the laboratory, it is advisable to use a transport medium that will protect the mycoplasmas and prevent proliferation of other bacteria (heart-infusion broth without peptone and glucose, 10% yeast extract, 20% serum, 0.3% agar, 500 International Units (IU)/ml penicillin, thallium acetate 1/7000).

The samples must be kept cool at 4°C if stored for a few days or frozen at or below –25°C for a longer period. For laboratory-to-laboratory transfer, lung fragments or pleural fluid can also be freeze-dried. Samples should be frozen if they cannot be processed on the day that they are collected.

a) Culture

MmmSC needs appropriate media to grow (19). In attempting isolation, 2–3 blind passages may be required. Many attempts to isolate fail because the organism is labile, is often present in small quantities, and is demanding in its growth requirements. The media should contain a basic medium (such as heart-infusion or peptone), yeast extract (preferably fresh), and horse serum (10%). Several other components can be added, such as glucose, glycerol, DNA, and fatty acids, but the effects vary with the strains. To avoid growth of other bacteria, inhibitors, such as penicillin, colistin or thallium acetate, are necessary. The media can be used as broth or solid medium with 1.0–1.2% agar.

After grinding in broth with antibiotics, the lung samples are diluted tenfold to minimise contaminating bacteria and are inoculated into five tubes of broth and on to solid medium. The pleural fluid can be inoculated directly without previous dilution. Hermetic sealing of the Petri dishes or the use of incubators with a controlled humid atmosphere is recommended in order to avoid desiccation. CO_2 incubators. The tubes and Petri dishes are inspected every day for 10 days. In fluid medium, a homogeneous cloudiness usually appears within 3–5 days, frequently with a silky, fragile filament called a 'comet', which is characteristic of *MmmSC* (or *M. capricolum* subsp. *capripneumoniae*, the cause of caprine contagious pleuropneumonia). During the following days a uniform opacity develops with whirls when shaken. On agar media, the colonies are small (1 mm in diameter) and have the classical appearance of 'fried eggs' with a dense centre. At this stage, the indirect fluorescent antibody (IFA) test can be performed.

b) Biochemical tests

Biochemical tests are to be regarded as confirmatory tests, to be carried out by reference laboratories. For routine field use, the immunological tests are sufficient, but where these give dubious results and in all cases of identification of first isolates, biochemical tests should be confirmed by a reference laboratory. For this purpose, after two or three subcultures, antibiotics should be omitted from the medium to check if the isolate is a mycoplasma or an L-form of a bacterium that will regain its original shape in the medium without inhibitors. Once this test is done and after cloning (at least three colonies should be selected), the organism can be identified using biochemical tests (1).

MmmSC is sensitive to digitonin (like all members of the order Mycoplasmatales), does not produce 'film and spots', ferments glucose, reduces tetrazolium salts (aerobically or anaerobically), does not hydrolyse arginine, has no phosphatase activity, and has no or weak proteolytic properties.

For these tests, special media have been developed that include the same basic ingredients (heart-infusion broth or Bacto PPLO [pleuropneumonia-like organisms] broth, horse serum, 25% yeast extract solution, 0.2% DNA solution), to which is added 1% of a 50% glucose solution for glucose hydrolysis, 4% of a 38% arginine HCl solution for arginine hydrolysis, and 1% of a 2% triphenyl tetrazolium chloride solution for tetrazolium reduction. For demonstration of proteolysis, growth is carried out on casein agar and/or coagulated serum agar.

Once the biochemical characteristics have been checked, immunological tests are necessary to confirm the identification: disk growth inhibition test (DGIT), fluorescent antibody test (FAT), and the dot immunobinding on membrane filtration (MF-dot) test.

The isolation and identification of the CBPP agent can be difficult and time consuming and depends on careful use of the appropriate procedures and media. When possible, classical bacteriology laboratories should set up a special section for handling mycoplasmas only.

c) Nucleic acid recognition methods

Radiolabelled or enzyme probes have been developed, but their use is restricted due to their many drawbacks.

On the other hand, the polymerase chain reaction (PCR) is very sensitive, highly specific, rapid, and easy to perform. Primers specific for the *M. mycoides* cluster (24) and for *MmmSC* (7) have been prepared, and PCR assays have been developed (2, 3, 7, 15). Using samples such as lung exudate, the PCR can be applied directly after denaturation in boiling water, without any DNA extraction. It can even be applied to dry samples on filter paper. Lung fragments have first to be ground and submitted to a low speed centrifugation before denaturation and PCR. The PCR can also be performed with urine or blood. The main advantage of the PCR technique is that it can be applied to poorly conserved samples (contaminated or without any viable mycoplasmas as may occur following antibiotic treatment). If direct extraction of DNA from the organ under test fails, specimens should be enriched by culturing them in an appropriate medium for 24–48 hours, followed by DNA extraction attempted from culture.

d) Immunological tests

The aetiological agent or its antigens can be demonstrated by immunochemical tests in infected tissues, organic fluids and/or in culture. However, as some of these tests are dependent on a minimum number of organisms being present in the sample, only positive results are taken into account.

i) *Indirect fluorescent antibody test*

The IFA test can be performed on smears from clinical material using hyperimmune cattle serum against *MmmSC* and labelled anti-bovine IgG. The test is satisfactory when applied to pleural fluid smears, but is less satisfactory with lung smears due to considerable nonspecific fluorescence. However, good results can be obtained using lung smears counterstained with Erichrome black.

ii) *Fluorescent antibody test*

The FAT is commonly performed on broth and agar cultures. It is slightly less specific than the IFA test.

Broth culture: Place two drops on a microscope slide. Fix for 15 minutes with methyl alcohol, and leave in contact with the labelled hyperimmune serum for 30 minutes at 37°C in a humid chamber. Rinse three times with phosphate buffered saline (PBS) and examine under an epifluorescence microscope (×80).

Colonies grown on solid medium: Cut a block of agar supporting a number of young colonies and place on a slide with the colonies facing upwards. Place one or two drops of the labelled hyperimmune serum on the block and leave it in a humid chamber for 30 minutes. Place the block into a tube and wash twice for 10 minutes with PBS. Place the block on a slide with the colonies facing upwards and examine as before.

Petri dish culture: The gel should not be too thick (no more than 3 mm) and should contain as little horse serum as possible. Rinse the gel three times with PBS, flood the surface with 1 ml of labelled serum and incubate for 30 minutes in a humid chamber. Rinse four times with PBS and examine directly under the microscope. The FAT in a Petri dish is used mainly just after isolation and before cloning, as it is very useful in the case of mixed infection with several mycoplasma species.

In the FAT with broth culture, the mycoplasmas appear bright green on a dark background. However, experience is required for the FAT carried out with colonies on agar, because the background appears dark green.

iii) *Disk growth inhibition test*

The DGIT is based on the direct inhibition of the growth of the agent on a solid medium by a specific hyperimmune serum (10). It is a specific and simple test to perform, but some results require experience to be interpreted: small inhibition zones (less than 2 mm wide), partial inhibition with 'breakthrough colonies', false-negative and false-positive reactions (very rare). The quality of the hyperimmune serum used in this test is critical for good results. Cross-reactions within the mycoides cluster are common and great care should be taken to differentiate *MmmSC* (bovine biotype) from *MmmLC* (caprine biotype; LC: large colonies).

iv) *Agar gel immunodiffusion test*

The agar gel immunodiffusion (AGID) test can detect the specific antigen present at the surface of *MmmSC* and the circulating galactan invading the haemolymph system of sick animals (12). Pleural fluid, ground lung fragments or even sequestrae can be tested against a hyperimmune serum in two wells cut 5 mm apart in the gel. The gel is composed of Noble agar (12 g) and thallium acetate (1/7000) in PBS, pH 7.2 (1000 ml). The results are better when the plate is incubated at 37°C and can be read within 24 hours, but only positive reactions should be taken into account. A simpler field test has been developed using impregnated paper discs instead of wells (18).

v) *Interfacial precipitation test*

The interfacial precipitation test is a quicker test based on the same principle as the AGID, but is performed in liquid medium. Ideally in this test, the samples should be centrifuged in order to be absolutely transparent (27).

vi) *Dot immunobinding on membrane filtration*

The MF-dot test can be used for routine testing in the laboratory. This technique may be performed both with polyclonal antisera, adopting a quantitative procedure, or by using monoclonal antibodies (MAbs) (17).

vii) *Immunohistochemistry*

MmmSC immunoreactive sites can be detected in lung lesions using the peroxidase–antiperoxidase method on sections of paraffin-embedded material (9). Because the isolation of the agent is not always achieved from chronic cases and after treatment with antimicrobial drugs, this test is only supplementary to the diagnosis of CBPP (8); a negative result is not conclusive.

2. Serological tests

a) Complement fixation (the prescribed test for international trade)

The Campbell & Turner complement fixation (CF) test remains the recommended procedure (although the current method is slightly different from the original one), and it is widely used in all countries where infection occurs (18). The CF test, as a micromethod, has been harmonised in the European Union (11). For antigen titration and harmonisation purposes, internal standard positive sera were prepared (840 and 845, PS1 and PS2, respectively) and are available from the Laboratório Nacional de Investigação Veterinária, Lisboa, Portugal (11). However, the CF test is still difficult to perform, requiring well-trained personnel.

- **Reagents**

i) Veronal buffer (VB), pH 7.3. A concentrated stock solution is used diluted 1/5 in sterilised double-distilled water.

ii) The serum samples, free from erythrocytes, must be inactivated at 56°C for 30 minutes and diluted 1/10 in VB.

iii) The antigen is a suspension of *MmmSC*, previously checkerboard titrated and used at a dose of 2 complement fixing units (CF units). It must be kept at 4°C and not frozen. It is produced, tested and delivered by Internationally recognised laboratories.

iv) The complement (C') is a guinea-pig normal serum. It is freeze-dried and reconstituted with double-distilled water. It must be kept at –20°C after reconstitution.

v) The haemolysin is a hyperimmune rabbit serum to sheep red blood cells (SRBC). The quantity used is 12 haemolytic doses read at 50% end-point (HD_{50} [50% haemolysing dose]).

vi) The SRBC are obtained by aseptic puncture of the jugular vein. They can be preserved in Alsever's solution or with sodium citrate. They are used in a 6% suspension.

vii) The haemolytic system (HS) is prepared by diluting haemolysin in VB to give a dose of 12 HD_{50}. An equal volume of 6% SRBC suspension is added, and the system is sensitised in a water bath at 37°C for 30 minutes with periodic shaking.

viii) The two positive standard sera, PS_1 and PS_2, are bovine sera from naturally infected animals with a low and a high titre, respectively, for CF test harmonisation and control, and antigen titration (PS_2). They are negative to *Brucella, Mycobacterium paratuberculosis, Chlamydia, Coxiella burnetii, Leptospira,* infectious bovine rhinotracheitis/infectious pustular vulvovaginitis and bovine leukosis virus antibodies.

ix) The negative control serum (NS) is a healthy bovine serum, negative to the above microrganisms.

- **Test procedure (using microplates)**

i) Dispense 25 µl of the test serum samples (already diluted 1/10). Add 25 µl of antigen at a dose of 2 CF units.

ii) Add 25 µl of C' at a dose of 2.5 units. Shake and incubate at 37°C for 30 minutes with periodic shaking.

iii) Add 25 µl of HS. Shake and incubate at 37°C for 30 minutes with periodic shaking.

It is necessary to set up the following controls:

Complement: 0.5 units, 1 unit and 2.5 units.

Haemolytic system: 75 µl of VB + 25 µl of HS.

Antigen: 25 µl of 2 CF units of antigen + 25 µl of C' at 2.5 units + 25 µl of HS.

Note: the microplates must be shaken twice during the incubation period. The above-mentioned controls, the PS and the NS are always used in each microplate or in a series of microplates where the same batches of reagents are used.

iv) *Reading and interpreting the results:* After centrifugation of the microplates at 125 ***g*** for 2 minutes, the reading is carried out based on the percentage of complement fixation observed.

Positive result : ++++ at 1/10;

Doubtful result : +; ++; +++ at 1/10.

It is recommended that any fixation of complement, even partial (+, ++, +++), at a serum dilution of 1/10 should be followed by additional investigations.

The limitations of the CF test are well known. With a specificity of 99.5%, the CF test can detect nearly all sick animals with acute lesions, but a rather smaller proportion of animals in the early stages of the disease or of animals with chronic lesions. In addition, therapeutic interventions and improperly conducted prophylactic operations (partial slaughter) may increase the number of false-negative reactions. However, for groups of animals (herd or epidemiological unit) the CF test is capable of detecting practically 100% of infected groups.

The nature of the pathogenesis of the disease is such that the incubation period, during which antibodies are undetectable by the CF test, may last for several months.

Despite the high specificity of the CF test, false-positive results can occur (less than 0.5%) of which an important cause is serological cross-reactions with other mycoplasmas, particularly other members of the *M. mycoides* cluster.

The validity of the results has to be confirmed by post-mortem and bacteriological examination, and serological tests on blood taken at the time of slaughter.

b) Competitive enzyme-linked immunosorbent assay

A competitive enzyme-linked immunosorbent assay (C-ELISA) developed by the OIE Collaborating Centre for the diagnosis and control of animal diseases in tropical countries (see Table given in Part 4 of this *Manual*) (14), has undergone evaluation (26). Compared with the CF test, the C-ELISA has equal sensitivity and greater specificity. The C-ELISA is a herd test that is easier to perform than the CF test, but its performance characteristics have not yet been fully assessed (14). The reagents for the ELISA can be obtained as kits[1].

Validation tests (1, 14) have been carried in several African and European countries that show i) that the true specificity of the C-ELISA is at least 99.5%; ii) that the sensitivity of the C-ELISA and the CF test are similar; and iii) that the C-ELISA can detect infected animals as quickly as the CF test.

- **Reagents**

i) Stock antigen is prepared by washing a concentrated suspension of mycoplasma (2 mg/ml) and lysis with sodium dodecyl sulphate at 0.1%. The stock is kept at –20°C until use.

ii) MAbs are available from the OIE Collaborating Centre for the Diagnosis and Control of Animal Diseases in Tropical Regions (see Table given in Part 4 of this *Manual*).

iii) *Conjugate:* DAKO P260 diluted 1/1500 in PBS with 0.5% horse serum and 0.05% Tween 20.

iv) Substrate is made of 1 mM ABTS (2,2'-Azino-bis-[3-ethylbenzothiazoline-6-sulphonic acid]) and H_2O_2 in citrate buffer.

- **Test procedure**

i) ELISA plates are coated with a lysed antigen solution in PBS, pH 7.4 (100 µl/well) and incubated overnight at 4°C.

ii) The plates are washed once in PBS diluted 1/5 with 0.05% Tween 20.

iii) Nondecomplemented sera (diluted 1/10) and MAb diluted in PBS with 0.5% horse serum and 0.05% Tween 20 are left in contact with the antigen for 1 hour at 37°C under moderate agitation in a humid chamber.

iv) The plates are washed twice and conjugate is added to all the wells (100 µl); the wells are then incubated for 1 hour at 37°C.

v) The plates are washed three times and the substrate is added to all the wells (100 µl).

vi) Reading is performed at 405 nm when the absorbance in the control MAb has reached 0.8–1.6.

c) Immunoblotting test

An immunoenzymatic test designated the immunoblotting test (IB test) has been developed and is considered to be of diagnostic value. A field evaluation indicated a higher sensitivity and specificity than the CF test (21, 22). A core profile of antigenic bands, present both in experimentally and naturally infected cattle, was considered to be immunodominant. The more accurate picture of the immune status of animals given by this test is due to the possibility of a more precise analysis of the host's immune response in relation to the electrophoretic profile of *MmmSC* antigens; thus the test overcomes problems related to nonspecific binding. It should be used primarily as a confirmatory test, after other tests and should be used in all cases in which the CF test has given a suspected false result. It is of particular value where disease control or eradication policies are being implemented.

- **Preparation of antigen strips**

i) The antigen is prepared by harvesting and washing a suspension of mycoplasma cells obtained from a 48-hour culture.

ii) A 4% stacking/5–15% gradient-resolving SDS/PAGE (sodium dodecyl sulphate/polyacrylamide gel) is prepared and used to perform electrophoresis of the sample with appropriate molecular weight standards.

iii) The separated proteins are transferred to a 14 × 14 cm 0.45 µm nitrocellulose membrane at 70 V constant voltage in transfer buffer (20% methanol in 193 mM glycine, 25 mM Tris-HCl, pH 8.3).

iv) The membrane is dried and labelled on the side on which the proteins were electrophoresed. The nitrocellulose membrane is incubated in blocking buffer (PBS containing 5% skim milk, 1 M glycine and 1% egg albumin) for 2 hours at room temperature. After washing at room temperature for three 15-minute washes in 0.1% (v/v) Tween 20 in PBS, the nitrocellulose membrane is then washed again in PBS alone. The sheet is then dried and one strip cut and tested from the edge of the membrane. Specific bands are identified at 110, 98, 95, 62/60 and 48 kDa.

---

1 International Atomic Energy Agency, Wagramerstrasse 5, P.O. Box 100, A-1400 Vienna, Austria or CIRAD/EMVT, Campus international de Baillarguet, Montferriez-sur-Lez, B.P. 5035, 34032 Montpellier Cedex 01, France.

v) The nitrocellulose membrane sheet is cut into strips, 0.4 cm wide and each strip is labelled. These strips are the antigen used for blotting.

- **Test procedure**

NB: The strips must be kept with the antigen side up during the procedure.

i) Serum samples for testing are diluted 1/3 and positive and negative control sera are prepared using dilution buffer (PBS containing 0.1% skim milk and 0.1% egg albumin).

ii) An antigen strip is placed in each test sample (and controls) and incubated at 37°C for 2 hours with continuous agitation. Strips are then washed, as above.

iii) Strips are incubated for 1 hour at room temperature in an appropriate dilution of peroxidase-conjugated anti-bovine IgG (H + L chains) in dilution buffer, with continuous agitation. Wash as above.

iv) Substrate is made by adding 30 mg 4-chloro-1-naphtol dissolved in 10 ml methanol to 50 ml PBS and 30 µl H_2O_2. Substrate is added to the strips, which are then left in the dark with continuous agitation and examined periodically until the protein bands are suitably dark. The reaction is stopped with distilled water.

v) *Reading the results:* The strips are dried and examined for the presence of the core IgG immunoblot profile of five specific antigenic bands of 110, 98, 95, 62/60 and 48 kDa. Sera giving a similar immunological profile are considered to be positive.

d) Other tests

MAbs have been prepared and ELISA systems have been developed (4, 13, 14, 16).

The passive haemagglutination test (5, 20) may be used as a screening test due to its higher sensitivity.

A rapid field slide agglutination test with either whole blood or serum (28) has been developed to detect specific agglutinins: the antigen is a dense suspension of stained mycoplasmas that is mixed with a drop of blood or serum. Due to a lack of sensitivity, the test detects only animals in the early stages (i.e. acute phase) of the disease and therefore should be used only on a herd basis.

B. REQUIREMENTS FOR VACCINES AND DIAGNOSTIC BIOLOGICALS

Since the beginning of the 20th century, many vaccines against CBPP have been described (e.g. killed vaccines, and heterologous vaccines), but none of them has proven to be really satisfactory. Today, the only vaccines commonly used are produced with attenuated *MmmSC* strains.

1. Seed management

a) Characteristics of the seed

Only one strain is recommended for preparing CBPP vaccines: strain T_1/44 is a naturally mild strain isolated in 1951 by Sheriff & Piercy in Tanzania. The 44th egg-passage is sufficiently attenuated to protect cattle without post-vaccinal severe reactions. Post-vaccination reactions may occur at the inoculation site. Cattle breeds should be assessed for their sensitivity before mass vaccination.

The identity of the strain can be verified with the insertion sequence profile (29).

The vaccinal strain is kept in freeze-dried form at –20°C.

b) Method of culture

For vaccine production, a system of freeze-dried seed lots originating from vaccinal cultures is used. These seed lots are kept at –20°C.

The media used for seed cultures are either Gourlay's medium or F_{66} medium: they both contain the same basic ingredients, but F_{66} medium is more complex (19). The media are sterilised by filtration, have a pH of 7.8–8.0, and should be used within a few days of preparation. Samples of medium should be distributed in tubes and incubated at 37°C for 48 hours to check sterility before use.

For vaccine bulk cultures, in order to avoid the risk of inadvertent cloning of vaccine seed, the whole content of a vaccine seed vial should be inoculated directly into 100 ml of medium.

2. Method of manufacture

The media used for vaccine production, either Gourlay's medium or F_{66} medium, are described above in Section B.1.b. They should be distributed in 1 litre flasks (500 ml per flask) and 10 litre flasks (5 litres per flask), and incubated at 37°C for 48 hours to check sterility before use.

To obtain high bacterial counts, the culture should be harvested just before the end of the logarithmic growth phase before the peak is reached, as the number of viable mycoplasmas will decrease quickly afterwards. Therefore, a kinetic curve should be drawn in each production laboratory. The contents of a vial of the working seed is used in a tenfold dilution series, in tubes. If no contamination occurs after incubation, the second tube is used, when the culture is still in the exponential rate of growth, to inoculate 1 litre flasks. The 10 litre flasks are heavily inoculated with a 48-hour-old culture of the 1 litre flasks (10 ml/litre of medium) and incubated at 37°C. After 24 hours of incubation, slow magnetic stirring is recommended. Just before the peak is reached (between 60 and 70 hours after incubation), the culture is prepared for freeze-drying.

All the following steps should be carried out on melting ice:

- Addition of the freeze-drying protective medium: dried skimmed milk (4.5% i.e. 225 g per 5 litres).
- Distribution into vials (the volume depends on the number of doses required per vial and on the steps of lyophilisation).

For freeze-drying, shelf freeze-driers are recommended so that the different steps can be controlled and monitored. The vials must be sealed in the freeze-drying machine in order to avoid leakage.

3. In-process control

Microscopic examination of Gram-stained preparations of the broth or blood agar plate cultures of the broth must be performed at every step to check for the absence of bacterial contamination.

A rapid examination should also be carried out to check for the presence of *MmmSC* by phase-contrast microscopic examination of the harvested medium, FAT examination with a labelled hyperimmune antiserum, or an interfacial precipitation test in tubes.

Samples of the freeze-dried vaccine are inoculated into mycoplasma agar or into broth to carry out growth-inhibition tests (9).

4. Batch control

a) Sterility

Bacteriological broths are inoculated, together with blood agar, and incubated at 37°C. All media should remain sterile (19). Tests for sterility may be found in Chapter I.4.

b) Titration

The minimum titre is 10^7 colony-forming units per vaccinal dose, but higher titres, at least 10^8, are recommended. Titration is performed after reconstitution of the freeze-dried vaccine in the diluent recommended for vaccination. Titrations should be performed on at least five vials per batch.

Classic technique: Tenfold dilutions are made in Gourlay's medium. The use of an agitator (vortex type) is useful to homogenise the suspension in each tube. First, 5 ml from the tubes with dilutions from 10^{-6} to 10^{-12} are inoculated in five further tubes of medium (1 ml per tube, five tubes per dilution). All the tubes are then incubated for 4 days at 37°C and growth is detected by colour change of the indicator. The titre is obtained using MacCrady's 'Most Probable Number' table or by modification of the Reed & Muench method. This technique is simple and easy to perform, but lacks precision (±0.5 log).

A microtitration method that is more accurate has been described (25) and should be used when possible.

c) Safety

After reconstitution in cold buffer, the vaccine is inoculated subcutaneously into two mice, intraperitoneally into two mice and intraperitoneally into two male guinea-pigs. None of the animals should die within the following month, and the guinea-pigs should not show signs of orchitis. Safety tests should be carried out on (at least two) cattle or zebu cattle. These are inoculated with ten vaccinal doses each, and observed for adverse effects for at least 4 weeks.

d) **Potency**

At least ten cattle are injected subcutaneously at the recommended site with one dose of vaccine, as stated on the label. At least ten similar animals are kept as unvaccinated controls. After no fewer than 2 months, all the cattle are challenged by placing them in contact with experimentally infected donor cattle, in an enclosed space, using at least one donor for every three cattle being challenged. The cattle are kept in contact for 3 months. After this time, all animals are killed and post-mortem examinations are carried out. The vaccinated cattle should show no more than mild clinical signs of disease, and no post-mortem lesions of pleuropneumonia. At least 80% of the control animals must show typical lesions at post-mortem.

e) **Duration of immunity**

Strain T_1/44 confers protection for approximately 1 year (13). Serological conversion (CF test) takes place in some animals. The antibodies disappear 2 months after vaccination.

f) **Stability**

Periodic titration of the stored vaccine allows the shelf life to be calculated. Freeze-dried vaccine must be stored at –20°C. At this temperature its storage life is at least 1 year (19).

g) **Preservatives**

For lyophilisation, dried skimmed milk is added: 45 g/litre of culture medium. For reconstitution of a freeze-dried vaccine normal saline is used. Alternatively, a molar solution of magnesium sulphate (248 g per litre) is used at room temperature. This molar solution protects mycoplasmas against inactivation by heat (19). The purity of the salts used is important.

h) **Precautions (hazards)**

Procedures for use in the field and reconstitution of freeze-dried vaccines have been described by Provost *et al.* (19). Regarding post-vaccinal reactions, mycoplasmas appear briefly in the blood.

Local reactions can be severe, but they should not be an obstacle to vaccination. Local reactions vary in incidence, intensity, species (cattle or zebu cattle) and vaccination site (19)

The general sensitivity of a given bovine population should be first tested by vaccinating sample groups (19).

5. Tests on the final product

These tests should be performed after reconstitution of a pool of at least five vials of the freeze-dried vaccine in the recommended diluent.

a) **Safety**

Safety tests should be carried out on cattle or zebu cattle, according to Section B.4.c.

b) **Potency**

The test is carried out according to the protocol described in Section B.4.d. Because CBPP cannot be easily reproduced experimentally, and due to its cost, only one potency test need be performed on each seed lot.

REFERENCES

1. AL-AUBAIDI J.M. & FABRICANT J. (1971). Characterization and classification of bovine mycoplasma. *Cornell Vet.*, **61**, 490–518.

2. AMANFU W., SEDIADIE S., MASUPU K.V., BENKIRANE A., GEIGER R. & THIAUCOURT F. (1998). Field validation of a competitive ELISA for the detection of contagious bovine pleuropneumonia in Botswana. *Rev. Elev. Med. Vet. Pays Trop.*, **51**, 189–193.

3. BASHIRUDDIN J. B., NICHOLAS R. A. J., SANTINI F. G., READY R. A., WOODWARD M.J. & TAYLOR T. K. (1994). Use of the polymerase chain reaction to detect *Mycoplasma* DNA in cattle with contagious pleuropneumonia. *Vet. Rec.*, **134**, 240–241.

4. BROCCHI E., GAMBA D., POUMARAT F., MARTEL J.L. & DE SIMONE F. (1993). Improvements in the diagnosis of contagious bovine pleuropneumonia through the use of monoclonal antibodies. *Rev. sci. tech. Off. int. Epiz.*, **12**, 559–570.

5. CHIMA J.C. & ONOVIRAN O. (1982). A passive haemagglutination test for detection of antibodies against *Mycoplasma mycoides* subsp. *mycoides* using glutaraldehyde-fixed sheep erythrocytes. *Vet. Microb.*, **7**, 343–349.

6. COTTEW G.S., BREARD A., DAMASSA A.J., ERNO H., LEACH R.H., LEFEVRE P.C., RODWELL A.W. & SMITH G.R. (1987). Taxonomy of the *Mycoplasma mycoides* cluster. *Israel J. Med. Sci.*, **23**, 632–635.

7. DEDIEU L., MADY V. & LEFEVRE P.C. (1994). Development of a selevtive polymerase chain reaction assay for the detection of *Mycoplasma mycoides* subsp. *mycoides* SC (contagious bovine pleuropneumonia agent). *Vet. Microbiol.*, **42**, 327–339.

8. FERRONHA M.H., CORREIA I., SOUSA FERREIRA H. & REGALLA J. (1992). Immunohistochemistry as a contribution to the diagnosis of contagious bovine pleuropneumonia. VIth International Symposium of WAVLD, Lyon, France, 9–12 June, 207.

9. FERRONHA M.H., NUNES PETISCA J.L., SOUSA FERREIRA H., MACHADO M., REGALLA J. & PENHA GONCALVES A. (1990). Detection of *Mycoplasma mycoides* subsp. *mycoides* immunoreactive sites in pulmonary tissue and sequestra of bovines with contagious pleuropneumonia. *In:* Contagious Bovine Pleuropneumonia. Regalla J., ed. Doc. No. EUR 12065 EN of the Commission of the European Communities, Luxembourg, 17–25.

10. FREUNDT E.A., ERNO H. & LEMCKE R.M. (1979). Identification of mycoplasmas. *In:* Methods in Microbiology, Vol. 13, Bergen T. & Norris J.R., eds. Academic Press, London, UK, 377–434.

11. GARRIDO ABELLAN F., LEGOFF C., MARTEL J., REGALLA J. & SANTINI F.G. (1993). Report of the Expert Subcommittee of the Veterinary Scientific Committee on the Epidemiology and Methods of Diagnosis of Contagious Bovine Pleuropneumonia (CBPP) Standardised at Community Level. Commission of the European Community, DGVI 3152/93.

12. GRIFFIN R.M. (1965). A gel diffusion test for contagious bovine pleuropneumonia. *J. Comp. Pathol.*, **75**, 223–231.

13. HUDSON J.R. (1971). Contagious Bovine Pleuropneumonia. Food and Agriculture Organization of the United Nations (FAO) Agricultural Studies No. 86. FAO, Rome, Italy.

14. LE GOFF C. & THIAUCOURT F. (1998). A competitive ELISA for the specific diagnosis of contagious bovine pleuropneumonia (CBPP). *Vet. Microbiol.*, **60**, 179–191.

15 MISEREZ R., PILLOUD T., CHENG., NICOLET J., GRIOT C. & FREY J. (1997). Development of a sensitive nested PCR method for the specific detection of *Mycoplasma mycoides* subsp. *mycoides* SC. *Mol. Cell. Probe*, **11**, 103–111.

16. ONOVIRAN O. & TAYLOR-ROBINSON D. (1979). Detection of antibody against *Mycoplasma mycoides* subsp. *mycoides* in cattle by an enzyme-linked immunosorbent assay. *Vet. Rec.*, **105**, 165–167.

17. POUMARAT F., LONGCHAMBON D. & MARTEL J.L. (1992). Application of dot immunobinding on membrane filtration (MF dot) to the study of relationships within '*M. mycoides* cluster' and within 'glucose and arginine-negative cluster' of ruminant mycoplasmas. *Vet. Microbiol.*, **32**, 375–390.

18. PROVOST A. (1972). Recherches immunologiques sur la péripneumonie. XIV. Description de deux techniques applicables sur le terrain pour le diagnostic de la maladie. *Rev. Elev. Med. Vet. Pays Trop.*, **25**, 475–496.

19. PROVOST A., PERREAU P., BREARD A., LE GOFF C., MARTEL J.L. & COTTEW G.S. (1987). Péripneumonie contagieuse bovine. *Rev. sci. tech. Off. int. Epiz.*, **6**, 565–624.

20. REGALLA J., CORREIA I., FERREIRA H. & PENHA GONCALVES A. (1992). The importance of the passive haemagglutination test in the serodiagnosis of contagious bovine pleuropneumonia. VIth International Symposium of WAVLD, Lyon, France, 9–12 June, 206.

21. REGALLA J., GONCALVES R., NIZA RIBEIRO J., DUARTE L., NICHOLAS R., BASHIRUDDIN J.B., DE SANTIS P., GARRIDO ABELLAN F. & PENHA GONCALVES A. (1999). Development of immunoblotting as a diagnostic tool for contagious bovine pleuropneumonia. International Symposium - COST Action 826: Mycoplasmas of Ruminants: Pathogenicity, Diagnostics, Epidemiology and Molecular Genetics. Joint Workshops of E.U. Projects. Toulouse, France, June 2–4, 1999.

22. REGALLA J., GONCALVES A., NIZA RIBEIRO J., DUARTE L. & PENHA GONCALVES A. (1996). Use of immunoblotting test for carrier state definition in contagious bovine pleuropneumonia. *In:* Proceedings of Thessaloniki Workshop, Frey J., ed. COST (European Cooperation in the Field of Scientific and Technical Research) Programme: Action 826 - Mycoplasmosis of Ruminants.

23. SANTINI F.G., VISAGGIO M., FARINELLI G., DI FRANCESCO G., GUARDUCCI M., D'ANGELO A.R., SCACCHIA M. & DI GIANNATALE E. (1992). Pulmonary sequestrum from *Mycoplasma mycoides* var. *mycoides* SC in a domestic buffalo; isolation, anatamo-histopathology and immuno-histochemistry. *Veterinaria Italiana*, **4**, 4–10.

24. TAYLOR T.K., BASHIRUDDIN J.B. & GOULD A.R. (1992). Relationships between members of the *Mycoplasma mycoides* cluster as shown by DNA probes and sequence analysis. *Int. J. Syst. Bact.*, **42**, 593–601.

25. THIAUCOURT F. & DI MARIA A. (1992). A new microtitration method for the enumeration of contagious bovine pleuropneumonia (CBPP) vaccines. *Biologicals*, **20**, 11–13.

26. THIAUCOURT F., GEIGER R., NICOLET J., PINI A., PROZESKY L., REGALLA J., ROGER F. & YAYA A. (1998). Validation of a competitive ELISA for contagious bovine pleuropneumonia. Third Workshop on Mycoplasma of Ruminants; Pathogenicity, Diagnostics, Epidemiology, and Molecular genetics. COST Action 826. Budapest, Hungary, May 5–8, 1998.

27. TURNER A.W. (1962). Detection of *Mycoplasma mycoides* antigens and antibody by means of precipitin tests as aids to diagnosis of bovine contagious pleuropneumonia. *Aust. Vet. J.*, **38**, 335–337.

28. TURNER A.W. & ETHERIDGE J.R. (1963). Slide agglutination tests in the diagnosis of contagious bovine pleuropneumonia. *Aust. Vet. J.*, **39**, 445–451.

29. VILEI E.M., NICOLET J. & FREY J. (1999). IS1634, a novel insertion element creating long, variable-length direct repeats which is specific for *Mycoplasma mycoides* subsp. *mycoides* small colony type. *J. Bacteriol.*, **181**, 1319–1323.

*

* *

CHAPTER 2.1.7.

LUMPY SKIN DISEASE

SUMMARY

Lumpy skin disease (LSD, knopvelsiekte) is a pox disease of cattle characterised by fever, nodules on the skin, mucous membranes and internal organs, emaciation, enlarged lymph nodes, oedema of the skin, and sometimes death. The disease is of economic importance because it causes reduced production, particularly in dairy herds. It also causes damage to the hide. LSD is caused by strains of capripoxvirus disease that are antigenically indistinguishable from strains causing sheep pox and goat pox. However, LSD has a different geographical distribution to sheep and goat pox, suggesting that cattle strains of capripoxvirus do not infect and transmit between sheep and goats. Transmission of LSD virus is thought to be predominantly by insects, natural contact transmission in the absence of insect vectors being inefficient. Until 1988 LSD was confined to sub-Saharan Africa, but then spread into Egypt. There has been only one laboratory-confirmed outbreak of LSD outside Africa, in Israel in 1989, which was eliminated by slaughter of all infected and in-contact cattle, and vaccination. Outbreaks reported in Bahrain and Reunion in 1993 were not confirmed by virus isolation.

Identification of the agent: *Laboratory confirmation of LSD is most rapid by the demonstration of typical capripox virions in biopsy material or dessicated crusts using the transmission electron microscope in combination with a clinical history of a generalised nodular skin disease and enlarged superficial lymph glands in cattle. Capripoxvirus is distinct from parapoxvirus, which causes bovine papular stomatitis and pseudocowpox, but cannot be distinguished morphologically from cowpox and vaccinia virus, both orthopoxvirus infections of cattle; however, neither causes generalised infection and both are uncommon in cattle. LSD virus will grow in tissue culture of bovine, ovine or caprine origin, although maximum yield is obtained using lamb testis cells. Capripoxvirus causes a characteristic cytopathic effect and intracytoplasmic inclusion bodies, and is distinct from the virus of pseudo-LSD (Allerton – herpes mammillitis), which is a herpesvirus producing syncytia and intranuclear inclusion bodies. The antigen of capripoxvirus can be demonstrated in tissue culture using immunoperoxidase or immunofluorescent staining and the virus can be neutralised using specific antisera.*

An antigen detection enzyme-linked immunosorbent assay (ELISA) using a polyclonal detection serum raised against a recombinant immunodominant antigen of capripoxvirus has been developed. Genome detection using capripoxvirus-specific primers for the fusion protein gene and attachment protein gene has also been reported.

Serological tests: *The virus neutralisation test is the most specific serological test, but because immunity to LSD infection is predominantly cell mediated, the test is not sufficiently sensitive to identify animals that have had contact with LSD virus and developed only low levels of neutralising antibody. The agar gel immunodiffusion test and indirect immunofluorescent antibody test are less specific due to cross-reactions with antibody to other poxviruses. Western blotting using the reaction between the P32 antigen of LSD virus with test sera is both sensitive and specific, but is difficult and expensive to carry out. The use of this antigen, expressed by a suitable vector, in an ELISA offers the prospect of an acceptable and standardised serological test.*

Requirements for vaccines and diagnostic biologicals: *All strains of capripoxvirus examined so far, whether derived from cattle, sheep or goats, share immunising antigens. Attenuated cattle strains, and strains derived from sheep and goats have been used as live vaccines.*

A. DIAGNOSTIC TECHNIQUES

Lumpy skin disease (LSD) was first seen in Zambia in 1929, spreading into Botswana by 1943 (14), and then into South Africa, where it affected over eight million cattle causing major economic loss. In 1957 it entered Kenya, associated with an outbreak of sheep pox (22). In 1970 LSD spread north into the Sudan, by 1974 it had spread west as far as Nigeria, and in 1977 was reported from Mauritania, Mali, Ghana and Liberia. Another epidemic of LSD between 1981 and 1986 affected Tanzania, Kenya, Zimbabwe, Somalia and the Cameroon, with reported mortality rates in affected cattle of 20%. However, the true extent of this epidemic was not clear, and it probably affected a considerable area of central Africa. In 1988 LSD became established in Egypt, and in 1989 a single outbreak was reported in Israel. LSD must be considered to have the potential to become established outside Africa. The principle method of transmission is mechanical by arthropod vector (6).

The severity of clinical signs of LSD, (Neethling or knopvelsiekte), depends on the strain of capripoxvirus and the breed of host. *Bos taurus* is more susceptible to clinical disease than *Bos indicus;* the Asian buffalo has also been reported to be susceptible. Within *Bos taurus,* the fine skin Channel Island breeds develop more severe disease, with lactating cows appearing to be the most at risk. However, even among groups of cattle of the same breed kept together under the same conditions, there is a large variation in the clinical signs presented, ranging from subclinical infection to death (7). There may be failure of the virus to infect the whole group, depending on vector prevalence.

In the acutely infected animal, there is an initial pyrexia, which may exceed 41°C and persist for 1 week. The incubation period under field conditions has not been reported, but following inoculation is 6–9 days until the onset of fever. A rhinitis and conjunctivitis develop, and in lactating cattle there is a marked reduction in milk yield. Nodules of 2–5 cm in diameter develop over the body, particularly on the head, neck, udder and perineum. These nodules involve the dermis and epidermis and may initially exude serum, but over the following 2 weeks may become necrotic plugs that penetrate the full thickness of the hide. All the superficial lymph nodes are enlarged, the limbs may be oedematous and the animal is reluctant to move. The nodules on the mucous membranes of the eyes, nose, mouth, rectum, udder and genitalia quickly ulcerate, and by then all secretions contain LSD virus. On the appearance of clinical signs, the discharge from the eyes and nose becomes mucopurulent, and keratitis may develop. Nodules may also develop in the mouth, subcutis and muscle, in the trachea and alimentary tract, particularly the abomasum, and in the lungs, resulting in primary and secondary pneumonia. Pregnant cattle may abort, and there are reports of aborted fetuses being covered in nodules. Bulls may become permanently or temporarily infertile. Recovery from severe infection is slow; the animal is emaciated, may have pneumonia and mastitis, and the necrotic plugs of skin, which may have been subject to fly strike, are shed leaving deep holes in the hide (20).

LSD virus is not transmissible to humans.

1. Identification of the agent

• Sample collection, submission and preparation

Material for virus isolation and antigen detection should be collected by biopsy or on post-mortem from skin nodules, lung lesions or lymph nodes. Samples for virus isolation and antigen-detection enzyme-linked immunosorbent assay (ELISA) should be collected within the first week of the occurrence of clinical signs, before the development of neutralising antibodies (11). Samples for genome detection by polymerase chain reaction (PCR) may be collected when neutralising antibody is present. However, the virus can be demonstrated for up to 35 days in old lesions. Buffy coat from blood collected into heparin or EDTA (ethylene diamine tetra-acetic acid) during the viraemic stage of LSD (before generalisation of lesions or within 4 days of generalisation), can also be used for virus isolation. Samples for histology should include tissue from the surrounding area and should be placed immediately following collection into ten times the sample volume of 10% formalin.

Tissues in formalin have no special transportation requirements. Blood samples with anticoagulant for virus isolation from the buffy coat should be placed immediately on ice and processed as soon as possible. In practice, the samples may be kept at 4°C for up to 2 days prior to processing, but should not be frozen or kept at ambient temperatures. Tissues for virus isolation and antigen detection should be kept at 4°C, on ice or at -20°C. If it is necessary to transport samples over long distances without refrigeration, the medium should contain 10% glycerol; the samples should be of sufficient size that the transport medium does not penetrate the central part of the biopsy, which should be used for virus isolation.

Material for histology should be prepared by standard techniques and stained with haematoxylin and eosin (H&E) (2). Lesion material for virus isolation and antigen detection is minced using sterile scissors and forceps and then ground in a sterile pestle and mortar with sterile sand and an equal volume of sterile phosphate buffered saline (PBS) containing sodium penicillin (1000 international units [IU]/ml), streptomycin sulphate (1 mg/ml), mycostatin (100 IU/ml) or fungizone (2.5 µg/ml) and neomycin (200 IU/ml). The suspension is freeze–thawed three times and then partially clarified by centrifugation using a bench centrifuge at 600 ***g*** for 10 minutes. Buffy coats may be prepared from unclotted blood by centrifugation at 600 ***g*** for 15 minutes, and the buffy coat carefully removed into 5 ml of cold double distilled water using a sterile Pasteur pipette. After 30 seconds, 5 ml of cold double strength growth medium is added and mixed. The mixture is centrifuged at 600 ***g*** for 15 minutes, the supernatant is discarded and the cell pellet is suspended in 5 ml growth medium, such as Glasgow's modified Eagle's medium (GMEM). After centrifugation at 600 ***g*** for a further 15 minutes, the resulting pellet is suspended in 5 ml of fresh GMEM. Alternatively, the buffy coat may be separated from a heparinised sample by using a Ficoll gradient.

a) Culture

LSD virus will grow in tissue culture of bovine, ovine or caprine origin, although primary or secondary culture of lamb testis (LT) cells are considered to be the most susceptible, particularly those derived from a breed of wool sheep. First 1 ml of clarified supernatant is inoculated on to a 25 cm^2 culture flask at 37°C and allowed to absorb for 1 hour. The culture is then washed with warm PBS and covered with 10 ml of a suitable medium, such as GMEM, containing antibiotics and 2% fetal calf serum. If available, tissue culture tubes containing LT cells and a flying cover-slip, or tissue culture microscope slides, are also infected.

The flasks are examined daily for 14 days for evidence of cytopathic effect (CPE) and the medium is replaced if it appears to be cloudy. Infected cells develop a characteristic CPE consisting of retraction of the cell membrane from surrounding cells, and eventually rounding of cells and margination of the nuclear chromatin. At first only small areas of CPE can be seen, sometimes as soon as 2 days after infection; over the following 4–6 days these expand to involve the whole cell sheet. If no CPE is apparent by day 14, the culture should be freeze–thawed three times, and clarified supernatant inoculated on to fresh LT culture. At the first sign of CPE in the flasks, or earlier if a number of infected cover-slips are being used, a cover-slip should be removed, fixed in acetone and stained using H&E. Eosinophillic intracytoplasmic inclusion bodies, which are variable in size but up to half the size of the nucleus and surrounded by a clear halo, are diagnostic for poxvirus infection. The CPE can be prevented or delayed by inclusion in the medium of specific anti-LSD serum. The herpesvirus of pseudo-LSD produces a Cowdry type A intranuclear inclusion body. Syncytia formation is not a feature of capripoxvirus infection, unlike the herpesvirus causing pseudo-LSD.

Strains of capripoxvirus that cause LSD have been adapted to grow on the chorioallantoic membrane of embryonated chicken eggs and African green monkey kidney (Vero) cells. This is not recommended for primary isolation.

- **Electron microscopy**

Before centrifugation, material from the original biopsy suspension is prepared for examination under the transmission electron microscope by floating a 400-mesh hexagon electron microscope grid, with pileoform-carbon substrate activated by glow discharge in pentylamine vapour, on to a drop of the suspension placed on parafilm or a wax plate. After 1 minute, the grid is transferred to a drop of Tris/EDTA buffer, pH 7.8, for 20 seconds and then to a drop of 1% phosphotungstic acid, pH 7.2, for 10 seconds. The grid is drained using filter paper, air-dried and placed in the electron microscope. The capripox virion is brick shaped, covered in short tubular elements and measures approximately 290 × 270 nm. A host-cell-derived membrane may surround some of the virions, and as many as possible should be examined to confirm their appearance (18).

The virions of capripoxvirus are indistinguishable from those of orthopoxvirus, but, apart from vaccinia virus and cowpox virus, which are both uncommon in cattle and do not cause generalised infection, no other orthopoxvirus causes lesions in cattle. However, vaccinia virus may cause generalised infection in young immunocompromised calves. In contrast, orthopoxviruses are a common cause of skin disease in domestic buffalo causing buffalo pox, a disease that usually manifests as pock lesions on the teats, but may cause skin lesions at other sites, such as the perineum, the medial aspects of the thighs and the head. Orthopoxviruses that cause buffalo pox cannot be readily distinguished from capripoxvirus by electron microscopy. The virions of parapoxvirus that cause bovine papular stomatitis and pseudocowpox are smaller, oval in shape and each is covered in a single continuous tubular element that appears as striations over the virion. The capripoxvirus is also distinct from the herpesvirus that causes pseudo-LSD (Allerton – herpes mammillitis).

b) Immunological methods

- **Fluoresent antibody tests**

Capripoxvirus antigen can also be identified on the infected cover-slips or tissue culture slides using fluorescent antibody tests. Cover-slips or slides should be washed and air-dried and fixed in cold acetone for 10 minutes. The indirect test using immune cattle sera is subject to high background colour and nonspecific reactions. However, a direct conjugate can be prepared from sera from convalescent cattle (or from sheep or goats convalescing from capripox) or from rabbits hyperimmunised with purified capripoxvirus. Uninfected tissue culture should be included as a negative control as cross-reactions, due to antibodies to cell culture, can cause problems.

- **Agar gel immunodiffusion**

An agar gel immunodiffusion (AGID) test has been used for detecting the precipitating antigen of capripoxvirus, but has the disadvantage that this antigen is shared by parapoxvirus. Agarose (1%) is prepared in borate buffer, pH 8.6, dissolved by heating, and 2 ml is poured on to a glass microscope slide (76 × 26 mm). When the agar has solidified, wells are cut to give a six-well rosette around a central well. Each well is 5 mm in diameter, with a distance of 7 mm between the middle of the central well and the middle of each peripheral well. The wells are filled as follows: 18 µl of the 10% lesion suspension is added to three of the peripheral wells, alternately with positive control antigen, and 18 µl of positive capripoxvirus control serum is added to the central well. The slides are placed in a humid chamber at room temperature for 48 hours, and examined for visible precipitation lines using a light box. The test material is positive if a precipitation line develops with the control serum that is confluent with that produced by the positive control antigen.

To prepare antigen for the AGID, one of two 125 cm^2 flasks of LT cells is infected with capripoxvirus, and harvested when there is 90% CPE (8–12 days). The flask is freeze–thawed twice, and the cells are shaken free of the flask. The contents are centrifuged at 4000 ***g*** for 15 minutes, most of the supernatant is decanted and stored, and the pellet is resuspended in the remaining supernatant. The cells should be lysed using an ultrasonic probe for approximately 60 seconds. This homogenate is then centrifuged as before, the resulting supernatant being pooled with that already collected. The pooled supernatant is then added to an equal volume of saturated ammonium sulphate at pH 7.4 and left at 4°C for 1 hour. This solution is centrifuged at 4000 ***g*** for 15 minutes, and the precipitate is collected and resuspended in a small volume of 0.8% saline for use in the AGID test. The uninfected flask is processed in an identical manner throughout, to produce a tissue culture control antigen (17).

- **Enzyme-linked immunosorbent assay**

Following the cloning of the highly antigenic capripoxvirus structural protein P32, it is possible to use expressed recombinant antigen for the production of diagnostic reagents, including the raising of P32 monospecific polyclonal antiserum and the production of monoclonal antibodies (MAbs). These reagents have facilitated the development of a highly specific ELISA (5). Using hyperimmune rabbit antiserum, raised by inoculation of rabbits with purified capripoxvirus, capripox antigen from biopsy suspensions or tissue culture supernatant can be trapped on an ELISA plate. The presence of the antigen can then be indicated using guinea-pig serum, raised against the group-specific structural protein P32, commercial horseradish-peroxidase-conjugated rabbit anti-guinea-pig immunoglobulin and a chromogen/substrate solution.

c) Nucleic acid recognition methods

It is not possible to distinguish between strains of capripoxvirus from cattle, sheep or goats using serological techniques. However, strains can be characterised by comparing the genome fragments generated by *Hin*dIII digestion of their purified DNA (1, 12, 16). This technique has identified differences between isolates from the different species, but these are not consistent and there is evidence of the movement of strains between species and recombination between strains in the field (13).

The PCR can be used to detect the capripoxvirus genome in biopsy or tissue culture samples. Primers for the viral attachment protein gene and the viral fusion protein gene are specific for capripoxvirus, and the nature of the PCR products can be confirmed using restriction enzyme recognition sites (15).

2. Serological tests

a) Virus neutralisation

Either a test serum can be titrated against a constant titre of capripoxvirus (100 $TCID_{50}$ [50% tissue culture infective dose]) or a standard virus strain can be titrated against a constant dilution of test serum in order to calculate a neutralisation index. Because of the variable sensitivity of tissue culture to capripoxvirus, and the consequent difficulty of ensuring the use of 100 $TCID_{50}$, the neutralisation index is the preferred method. The test is described using 96-well flat-bottomed tissue-culture grade microtitre plates, but it can be performed equally well in tissue culture tubes with the appropriate changes to the volumes used, although it is more difficult to read an end-point in tubes. The use of Vero cells in the virus neutralisation test has been reported to give more consistent results.

- **Test procedure**

i) Test sera including a negative and a positive control are diluted 1/5 in Eagle's/HEPES (N-2-hydroxyethylpiperazine, N-2-ethanesulphonic acid) and inactivated at 56°C for 30 minutes.

ii) Next, 50 ml of the first inactivated serum is added to columns 1 and 2, rows A to H of the microtitre plate. The second serum is placed in columns 3 and 4, the third in columns 5 and 6, the positive control serum is placed in columns 7 and 8, the negative control serum is placed in columns 9 and 10, and 50 µl of Eagle's/HEPES without serum is placed in columns 11 and 12 and to all wells in row H.

iii) A reference strain of capripoxvirus, usually a vaccine strain known to grow well in tissue culture, with a titre of over $\log_{10}$ 6 $TCID_{50}$ per ml is diluted in Eagle's/HEPES in bijoux bottles to give a log dilution series of $\log_{10}$ 5.0; 4.0; 3.5; 3.0; 2.5; 2.0; 1.5 $TCID_{50}$ per ml (equivalent to $\log_{10}$ 3.7; 2.7; 2.2; 1.7; 1.2; 0.7; 0.2 $TCID_{50}$ per 50 µl).

iv) Starting with row G and the most diluted virus preparation, 50 µl of virus is added to each well in that row. This is repeated with each virus dilution, the highest titre virus dilution being placed in row A.

v) The plates are covered and incubated for 1 hour at 37°C.

vi) LT cells are prepared from pregrown monolayers as a suspension of 10^5 cells/ml in Eagle's medium containing antibiotics and 2% fetal calf serum. Following incubation of the microtitre plates, 100 µl of cell suspension is added to all the wells, except wells H11 and H12, which serve as control wells for the medium. The remaining wells of row H are cell and serum controls.

vii) The microtitre plates are covered and incubated at 37°C for 9 days.

viii) Using an inverted microscope, the monolayers are examined daily from day 4 for evidence of CPE. There should be no CPE in the cells of row H. Using the 0240 KSGP vaccine strain of capripoxvirus, the final reading is taken on day 9, and the titre of virus in each duplicate titration is calculated according to Kärber (1931). If left longer, there is invariably a 'breakthrough' of virus in which virus that was at first neutralised appears to disassociate from the antibody.

ix) *Interpretation of the results:* The neutralisation index is the log titre difference between the titre of the virus in the negative serum and in the test serum. An index of ≥1.5 is positive. The test can be made more sensitive if serum from the same animal is examined before and after infection. Because the immunity to capripox is predominantly cell mediated, a negative result, particularly following vaccination in which the response is necessarily mild, does not imply that the animal from which the serum was taken is not protected.

A constant virus-varying serum method has been described using serum dilutions in the range 1/5 to 1/500 and fetal calf muscle cells. Because these cells have a lower sensitivity to capripoxvirus than LT cells, the problem of virus 'breakthrough' is overcome.

Antibodies to capripoxvirus can be detected from day 2 after the onset of clinical signs. These remain detectable for about 7 months, but a significant rise in titre is usually seen between days 21 and 42.

b) Agar gel immunodiffusion

The AGID test cannot be recommended as a serological test for the diagnosis of LSD because of the cross-reaction with antibody to bovine papular stomatitis and pseudocowpox virus. A consequence of this cross-reaction is false-positive results. Lack of sensitivity of the test can also lead to false-negative results.

c) Indirect fluorescent antibody test

Capripoxvirus-infected tissue culture grown on flying cover-slips or tissue culture microscope slides can be used for the indirect fluorescent antibody test. Uninfected tissue culture control, and positive and negative control sera, should be included in the test. The infected and control cultures are fixed in acetone at –20°C for 10 minutes and stored at 4°C. Dilutions of test sera are made in PBS, starting at 1/20 or 1/40, and positives are identified using an anti-bovine gamma-globulin conjugated with fluorescein isothiocyanate. Antibody titres may exceed 1/1000 after infection. Sera may be screened at 1/50 and 1/500. Cross-reactions can occur with orf, bovine papular stomatitis and perhaps other poxviruses.

d) Western blot analysis

Western blotting of test sera against capripoxvirus-infected cell lysate provides a sensitive and specific system for the detection of antibody to capripoxvirus structural proteins, although the test is expensive and difficult to carry out.

Capripoxvirus-infected LT cells should be harvested when 90% CPE is seen, freeze–thawed three times, and the cellular debris pelleted by centrifugation. The supernatant should be decanted, and the proteins should be separated by SDS/PAGE (sodium dodecyl sulphate/polyacrylamide gel electrophoresis). A vertical discontinuous gel system, using a stacking gel made up of acrylamide 5% in Tris (125 mM), pH 6.8, and SDS (0.1%), and a resolving gel made up of acrylamide (10–12.5%) in Tris (560 mM), pH 8.7, and SDS (0.1%), is recommended for use with a glycine running buffer containing Tris (250 mM), glycine (2 M), and SDS (0.1%). Samples of supernatant should be prepared by boiling for 5 minutes with an appropriate lysis buffer prior to loading. Alternatively, purified virus or recombinant antigens may replace tissue-culture-derived antigen.

Molecular weight markers should be run concurrently with the protein samples. The separated proteins in the SDS/PAGE gel should be transferred electrophoretically to a nitrocellulose membrane (NCM). After transfer, the NCM is rinsed thoroughly in PBS and blocked in 3% bovine serum albumin (BSA) in PBS, or 5% skimmed milk powder in PBS, on a rotating shaker at 4°C overnight. The NCM can then be separated into strips by employing a commercial apparatus to allow the concurrent testing of multiple serum samples, or may be cut into strips and each strip incubated separately thereafter. The NCM is washed thoroughly with five changes of PBS for 5 minutes on a rotating shaker, and then incubated at room temperature on the shaker for 1.5 hours, with the appropriate serum at a dilution of 1/50 in blocking buffer (3% BSA and 0.05% Tween 20 in PBS; or 5% milk powder and 0.05% Tween 20 in PBS). The membrane is again thoroughly washed and incubated (in blocking buffer) with anti-species immunoglobulin horseradish-peroxidase-conjugated immunoglobulins at a dilution determined by titration. After further incubation at room temperature for 1.5 hours, the membrane is washed and a solution of diaminobenzidin tetrahydrochloride (10 mg in 50 ml of 50 mm Tris-HCl, pH 7.5, and 20 µl of 30% [v/v] hydrogen peroxide) is added. This is then incubated for approximately 3–7 minutes at room temperature on a shaker with constant observation, and the reaction is stopped by washing in PBS before excessive background colour is seen. A positive and negative control serum should be used on each occasion.

Positive test samples and the positive control will produce a pattern consistent with reaction to proteins of molecular weights 67, 32, 26, 19 and 17 kDa – the major structural proteins of capripoxvirus – whereas negative serum samples will not react with this pattern. Hyperimmune serum prepared against parapoxvirus (bovine papular stomatitis, pseudocowpox) will react with some of the capripoxvirus proteins, but not the 32 kDa protein that is specific for capripoxvirus.

e) Enzyme-linked immunosorbent assay

A capripoxvirus antibody ELISA has been developed using the expressed structural protein P32 of capripoxvirus and MAbs raised against the P32 protein (8).

B. REQUIREMENTS FOR VACCINES AND DIAGNOSTIC BIOLOGICALS

Two live attenuated strains of capripoxvirus have been used as vaccines specifically for the control of LSD (3, 4): a strain of Kenya sheep and goat pox virus passaged 18 times in LT or fetal calf muscle cells, and a strain from South Africa, passaged 60 times in lamb kidney cells and 20 times on the chorioallantoic membrane of embryonated chicken eggs. All strains of capripoxvirus examined so far, whether of bovine, ovine or caprine origin, share a major neutralising site, so that animals recovered from infection with one strain are resistant to infection with any other strain. Consequently, it is possible to protect cattle against LSD using strains of capripoxvirus derived from sheep or goats (9). In 1989 and 1990 the Romanian strain of sheep pox vaccine was used to help control the LSD outbreak in Egypt (19). However, it is essential to carry out controlled trials, particularly using the most susceptible breeds in peak lactation, prior to introducing a vaccine strain not usually used in cattle. Protection following vaccination is probably lifelong, although as immunity wanes, local capripoxvirus replication will occur at the site of inoculation, but the virus will not become generalised. Both strains of capripoxvirus used routinely as vaccines can produce large local reaction at the site of inoculation in *Bos taurus* breeds, which some stock owners find unacceptable. This has discouraged the use of vaccine even though the consequences of an outbreak of LSD are invariably more severe.

A new generation of capripox vaccines is being developed that uses the capripoxvirus genome as a vector for the genes of other ruminant pathogens, for instance genes of rinderpest and peste des petits ruminants viruses. The recombinant vaccine will provide protection against LSD and rinderpest in a single vaccination (21).

1. Seed management

a) Characteristics of the seed

A strain of capripoxvirus used for vaccine production must be accompanied by a history describing its origin and tissue culture or animal passage. It must be safe to use in all breeds of cattle for which it is intended, including pregnant animals. It must also be nontransmissible, remain attenuated after further tissue culture passage, and provide complete protection against challenge with virulent field strains for a minimum of

1 year. A quantity of master seed vaccine virus should be prepared and stored in order to provide a consistent working seed for regular vaccine production.

b) Method of culture

Vaccine seed should be lyophilised and stored in 2 ml vials at –20°C. It may be stored wet at –20°C, but when wet, it is more stable at –70°C or lower. The virus should be cultured in primary or secondary LT cells of wool sheep origin for maximum yield. Vero cells may also be used.

c) Validation as a vaccine

Seed lots must be shown to be :

i) *Pure:* Free from adventitious viruses, in particular pestiviruses, such as border disease and bovine viral diarrhoea virus, and free from contamination with bacteria, fungi and/or mycoplasmas.

ii) *Safe:* Produce minimum clinical reaction in all breeds of cattle when given by the recommended route.

iii) *Efficacious:* Stimulate complete immunity to LSD in all breeds of cattle for at least 1 year.

The necessary tests are described in Section B.4.

2. Method of manufacture

Vaccine batches are produced on fresh monolayers of secondary LT cells. A vial of seed virus is reconstituted with GMEM and inoculated on to an LT monolayer that has been previously washed with warm PBS, and allowed to absorb for 15 minutes at 37°C before being overlaid with additional GMEM. After 4–6 days, there will be extensive (50–70%) CPE. The culture is freeze–thawed three times, and the suspension is removed and centrifuged at 600 *g* for 20 minutes. Before harvest, the culture should be examined for any evidence of nonspecific CPE, medium cloudiness or change in medium pH. A second passage may be required to produce sufficient virus for a batch production (to produce enough for 10^6 doses, the yield from five 175 cm^2 flasks is required).

The procedure is repeated and the harvests from individually numbered flasks are each mixed separately with an equal volume of sterile, chilled 5% lactalbumin hydrolysate and 10% sucrose, and transferred to individually numbered bottles for storage at –20°C. Prior to storage, 0.2 ml is removed from each bottle for sterility control. An additional 0.2 ml is removed; 2 ml pools composed of 0.2 ml samples taken from ten bottles are used for virus titration. A written record of all the procedures must be kept for all vaccine batches.

3. In-process control

Cells: Cells should be obtained from the testis of a healthy young lamb from a scrapie-free flock of a wool sheep breed. During cultivation, cells must be observed for any evidence of CPE, and for normal morphology (predominantly fibroblastic). They can usually be passaged successfully up to ten times. When used for vaccine production, uninfected control cultures should be grown in parallel and maintained for at least one additional passage for further observation. They should be checked for the presence of noncytopathic strains of bovine viral diarrhoea or border disease viruses by immunofluorescence or immunoperoxidase techniques. If possible, cells should be prepared and screened prior to vaccine production, and a stock stored in sterile DMSO (dimethyl sulphoxide) in liquid nitrogen (1–2 ml aliquots containing 20×10^6 cells/ml). Serum used in the growth medium must be free from antibody to capripoxvirus and contamination with pestivirus.

Virus: Seed virus and final vaccine must be titrated in tissue culture tubes or microtitre plates. The minimum recommended field dose of the Kenyan and South African vaccines is $\log_{10}$ 3.5 $TCID_{50}$, although the minimum protective dose is $\log_{10}$ 2.0 $TCID_{50}$. Capripoxvirus is highly susceptible to inactivation by sunlight, and allowance should be made for loss of activity in the field. The recommended field dose of the Romanian sheep pox vaccine for cattle is $\log_{10}$ 2.5 sheep infective doses (SID_{50}), and the recommended dose for cattle of the RM65-adapted strain of Romanian sheep pox vaccine is $\log_{10}$ 3 $TCID_{50}$ (10). Vaccine samples must be examined for the presence of adventitious viruses including cytopathic and noncytopathic strains of pestivirus, and should be mixed with a high-titre capripoxvirus-immune serum that has previously tested negative for antibodies to pestiviruses to prevent the vaccine virus itself interfering with the test. The vaccine can be held at –20°C until all sterility tests and titrations have been completed, at which time it should be freeze-dried. A further titration is carried out on five randomly chosen vials of the freeze-dried preparation to confirm the titre.

4. Batch control

a) Sterility

Tests for sterility and freedom from contamination with biological materials may be found in Chapter I.4.

b) Safety and efficacy

Six cattle of known susceptibility to LSD are placed in a high containment level large animal unit and serum samples are collected. Five randomly chosen vials of the freeze-dried vaccine are reconstituted in sterile PBS and pooled. Two cattle are inoculated with 100 times the field dose of the vaccine, the remaining vaccine is diluted with sterile PBS and two cattle are inoculated subcutaneously with the recommended field dose. The remaining two cattle are control animals. The animals are clinically examined daily and rectal temperatures are recorded. On day 21 after vaccination, the six animals are again serum sampled and challenged with a known virulent capripoxvirus strain by intradermal inoculation. The clinical response is recorded during the following 14 days. Control animals should develop the typical clinical signs of LSD, whereas there should be no local or systemic reaction in the vaccinates other than a delayed-type hypersensitivity reaction, which should disappear after 4 days. Serum samples are again collected on day 30 after vaccination. The day 21 serum samples are examined for seroconversion to selected viral diseases that could have contaminated the vaccine, and the days 0 and 30 samples are compared to confirm the absence of antibody to pestivirus. Because of the variable response in cattle to LSD challenge, generalised disease may not be seen in the control animals, although there should be a large local reaction.

The fully reconstituted vaccine is also tested in mice and guinea-pigs. Two guinea-pigs are inoculated intramuscularly with 0.5 ml into the hind leg, and two guinea-pigs and six mice are inoculated intraperitoneally with 0.5 ml and 0.1 ml, respectively. Two guinea-pigs and four mice are kept as uninoculated controls. The animals are observed for 3 weeks, humanely killed and a post-mortem examination is carried out. There should be no evidence of pathology due to the vaccine.

c) Potency tests

Potency tests in cattle must be undertaken for vaccine strains of capripoxvirus if the minimum immunising dose is not known. This is usually carried out by comparing the titre of a virulent challenge virus on the flanks of vaccinated and control animals. Following vaccination, the flanks of at least three animals and three controls are shaved of hair. Log_{10} dilutions of the challenge virus are prepared in sterile PBS and six dilutions are inoculated intradermally (0.1 ml per inoculum) along the length of the flank; four replicates of each dilution are inoculated down the flank. An oedematous swelling will develop at possibly all 24 inoculation sites on the control animals, although preferably there will be little or no reaction at the four sites of the most dilute inocula. The vaccinated animals should develop an initial hypersensitivy reaction at sites of inoculation within 24 hours, which should quickly subside. Small areas of necrosis may develop at the inoculation site of the most concentrated challenge virus. The titre of the challenge virus is calculated for the vaccinated and control animals; a difference of log titre $>\log_{10} 2.5$ is taken as evidence of protection.

d) Duration of immunity

Immunity to virulent field virus following vaccination lasts 2 years with the Kenyan strain and 3 years with the South African vaccine, and protection against generalised infection following intradermal challenge is effectively lifelong. The duration of immunity produced by other vaccine strains should be ascertained in cattle by undertaking controlled trials in an environment in which there is no possibility of field strains of capripoxvirus confusing the results.

e) Stability

Properly freeze-dried preparations of LSD vaccine, particularly those that include a protectant, such as sucrose and lactalbumin hydrolysate, are stable for over 25 years when stored at –20°C and for 2–4 years when stored at 4°C. There is evidence that they are stable at higher temperatures, but no long-term controlled experiments have been reported.

f) Preservatives

No preservatives other than a protectant, such as sucrose and lactalbumin hydrolysate, are required for the freeze-dried preparation.

g) Precautions (hazards)

There are no precautions other than those described above for sterility and freedom from adventitious agents. Strains of LSD virus are not a hazard to human health.

5. Tests on the final product

a) Safety

Safety tests should be carried out on the final product of each batch as described in Section B.4.b.

b) Potency

Once the potency of the particular strain being used for vaccine production has been determined in terms of minimum dose required to provide immunity, it is not necessary to repeat this on the final product of each batch, provided the titre of virus present has been ascertained.

REFERENCES

1. BLACK D.N., HAMMOND J.M. & KITCHING R.P. (1986). Genomic relationship between capripoxviruses. *Virus Res.*, **5**, 277–292.

2. BURDIN M.L. (1959). The use of histopathological examination of skin material for the diagnosis of lumpy skin disease in Kenya. *Bull. Epizoot. Dis. Afr.*, **7**, 27–36.

3. CAPSTICK P.B. & COAKLEY W. (1961). Protection of cattle against lumpy skin disease. Trials with a vaccine against Neethling type infection. *Res. Vet. Sci.*, **2**, 362–368

4. CARN V.M. (1993). Control of capripoxvirus infections. *Vaccine*, **11**, 1275–1279.

5. CARN V.M. (1995). An antigen trapping ELISA for the detection of capripoxvirus in tissue culture supernatant and biopsy samples. *J. Virol. Methods*, **51**, 95–102.

6. CARN V.M. & KITCHING R.P. (1995). An investigation of possible routes of transmission of lumpy skin disease virus (Neethling). *Epidemiol. Infect.*, **114**, 219–226.

7. CARN V.M. & KITCHING, R.P. (1995). The clinical response of cattle following infection with lumpy skin disease (Neethling) virus. *Arch. Virol.*, **140**, 503–513.

8. CARN V.M., KITCHING R.P., HAMMOND J.M., CHAND P., ANDERSON J. & BLACK D.N. (1994). Use of a recombinant antigen in an indirect ELISA for detecting bovine antibody to capripoxvirus. *J. Virol. Methods*, **49**, 285–294.

9. COAKLEY W. & CAPSTICK P.B. (1961). Protection of cattle against lumpy skin disease. Factors affecting small scale production of tissue culture propagated virus vaccine. *Res. Vet. Sci.*, **2**, 369–371.

10. DAVIES F.G. (1991). Lumpy Skin Disease, a Capripox Virus Infection of Cattle in Africa. FAO, Rome, Italy.

11. DAVIES F.G., KRAUSS H., LUND L.J. & TAYLOR M. (1971). The laboratory diagnosis of lumpy skin disease. *Res. Vet. Sci.*, **12**, 123–127.

12. GERSHON P.D. & BLACK D.N. (1987). Physical characterization of the genome of a cattle isolate of capripoxvirus. *Virology*, **160**, 473–476.

13. GERSHON P.D., KITCHING R.P., HAMMOND J.M. & BLACK D.N. (1989). Poxvirus genetic recombination during natural virus transmission. *J. Gen. Virol.*, **70**, 485–489.

14. HAIG D. (1957). Lumpy skin disease. *Bull. Epizoot. Dis. Afr.*, **5**, 421–430.

15. IRELAND D.C. & BINEPAL Y.S. (1998). Improved detection of capripoxvirus in biopsy samples by PCR. *J. Virol. Methods*, **74**, 1–7.

16. KITCHING R.P., BHAT P.P. & BLACK D.N. (1989). The characterization of African strains of capripoxvirus. *Epidemiol. Infect.*, **102**, 335–343.

17. KITCHING R.P., HAMMOND J.M. & BLACK D.N. (1986). Studies on the major precipitating antigen of capripoxvirus. *J. Gen. Virol.*, **70**, 485–489.

18. KITCHING R.P. & SMALE C. (1986). Comparison of the external dimensions of capripoxvirus isolates. *Res. Vet. Sci.*, **41**, 425–427.

19. MICHAEL A., SABER M.S., SOOLIMAN S.M., MOUSA A.A., SALAMA S.A., FAYED A.A., NASSAR M.I. & HOUSE J. (1996). Control of lumpy skin disease in Egypt with Romanian sheep pox vaccine. *Assiut. Vet. Med. J.*, **36**, 173–180.

20. PROZESKY L. & BARNARD B.J.H. (1982). A study of the pathology of lumpy skin disease in cattle. *Onderstepoort J. Vet. Res.*, **49**, 167–175.

21. ROMERO C.H., BARRETT T., EVANS S.A., KITCHING R.P., GERSHON P.D., BOSTOCK C. & BLACK D.N. (1993). Single capripoxvirus recombinant vaccine for the protection of cattle against rinderpest and lumpy skin disease. *Vaccine*, **11**, 737–742.

22. WEISS K.E. (1968). Lumpy skin disease. *Virol. Monogr.*, **3**, 111–131.

*

* *

CHAPTER 2.1.8.

RIFT VALLEY FEVER

SUMMARY

Rift Valley fever (RVF) is a peracute or acute zoonotic disease of domestic ruminants in Africa. It is caused by a single serotype of a mosquito-borne bunyavirus of the genus Phlebovirus. *The disease occurs in climatic conditions favouring the breeding of mosquito vectors and is characterised by liver damage. The disease is most severe in sheep, goats and cattle, in which it produces abortions in pregnant animals and a high mortality rate in the newborn. Older nonpregnant animals, although susceptible to infection, are more resistant to clinical disease. There is considerable variation in the susceptibility to RVF of animals of different genotypes. Those breeds or strains that are exotic to Africa or are from areas where RVF is not endemic, tend to be more susceptible. Camels suffer an inapparent infection with RVF, but abortion rates can be as high as in cattle.*

Humans are susceptible to infection by handling infected material and through transmission by mosquito vectors. Infection of humans by vectors is a striking feature in countries with a relatively small population of animal hosts. In such areas, RVF may be recognised first in humans. It has caused serious disease in laboratory workers and must be handled with high level biosecurity (11, 13).

***Identification of the agent:** RVF virus consists of a single serotype of a bunyavirus of the genus* Phlebovirus *and has morphological and physicochemical properties typical of bunyaviruses. The virus has a three-segmented, single-stranded, negative-sense RNA genome and consists of the three segments, L (large), M (medium) and S (small), which are contained in a separate nucleocapsid within the virion. The S segment is ambisense RNA, i.e. has bi-directional coding (9).*

The virus can be isolated from blood collected, preferably in an anticoagulant, during the febrile stage of the disease, or from liver, spleen and brain of animals that have died and from the organs of aborted fetuses. Primary isolations are usually made on cell cultures of various types, such as African green monkey kidney (Vero) cells, baby hamster kidney cells, chicken embryo reticulum (CER: cells developed by Tsunemasa Motohashi at the Nippon Institute for Biological Science, Tokyo, Japan), or primary cells of sheep or cattle origin. Alternatively, hamsters, adult or suckling mice, embryonated chicken eggs or 2-day-old lambs may be used for primary virus isolation.

A rapid diagnosis can be achieved by using the supernatant of homogenised samples as antigen in virus neutralisation (VN) tests; immunofluorescent staining of impression smears of liver, spleen, brain or infected cell cultures; or by the demonstration of virus in serum, taken during the febrile stage of the disease, by enzyme immunoassay or immunodiffusion.

The presence of characteristic histopathological lesions in the liver assists in the diagnosis.

***Serological tests:** Infected animals develop specific antibodies that may become demonstratable by VN as early as 3 days following infection and after 6–7 days by enzyme-linked immunosorbent assay, and by haemagglutination inhibition. Serological tests used less often include immunofluorescence, complement fixation and immunodiffusion.*

***Requirements for vaccines and diagnostic biologicals:** Live virus vaccines and antigens for use either in countries where RVF is endemic or during outbreaks, should be prepared from nonpathogenic mouse- or mutagen-attenuated strains of RVF virus grown in cell cultures. The mutagen-attenuated strain of RVF is not yet at a stage where it can be recommended for use.*

In RVF-free countries, vaccines and diagnostic tests should be limited to those using inactivated virus. Suitable virus strains can be obtained from the OIE Reference Laboratory for RVF (see Table given in Part 4 of this Manual*).*

A. DIAGNOSTIC TECHNIQUES

Rift Valley fever (RVF) is a peracute or acute, febrile, mosquito-borne, zoonotic disease caused by a virus of the family Bunyaviridae, genus *Phlebovirus.* It usually presents in epizootic form over large areas of a country and is characterised by high rates of abortion and neonatal mortality, and occurs primarily in sheep, goats and cattle. The susceptibility of different breeds to RVF varies considerably. Some indigenous African animals may have only inapparent infections, while exotic or other breeds suffer severe clinical disease with mortality and abortion. Although susceptible, older nonpregnant animals and some other species usually do not show signs of disease. Camels have been regularly involved in the RVF epidemics in East Africa and Egypt. Clinical disease is not seen in adult camels, but abortion occurs and some early post-natal deaths have been observed.

Signs of the disease tend to be nonspecific, rendering it difficult to recognise individual cases (5–8, 14, 20). During epidemics, however, the occurrence of numerous abortions and mortalities among young animals, together with disease in humans, is characteristic. Rift Valley fever has a short incubation period: 12–36 hours in lambs. A biphasic fever of up to 41°C may develop, and the fever remains high until shortly before death. Affected animals are listless, disinclined to move or feed, and may show enlarged superficial lymph nodes and abdominal pain. Lambs rarely survive longer than 36 hours after the onset of signs of illness. Animals older than 2 weeks may die peracutely, acutely or may develop an inapparent infection. Some animals may regurgitate ingesta and may show melaena or bloody, foul-smelling diarrhoea and bloodstained mucopurulent nasal discharge. Icterus may sometimes be observed, particularly in cattle. In addition to these signs, adult cattle may show lachrymation, salivation and dysgalactia. In pregnant sheep, the mortality and abortion rates vary from 5% to almost 100% in different outbreaks and between different flocks. The death rate in cattle is usually less than 10%.

The hepatic lesions of RVF are very similar in all species, varying mainly with the age of the infected individual (6). The most severe lesion occurring in aborted fetuses and newborn lambs is a moderately to greatly enlarged, soft, friable liver with a yellowish-brown to dark reddish-brown colour with irregular congested patches. Numerous greyish-white necrotic foci are invariably present in the parenchyma, but may not be clearly discernible. In adult sheep, the lesions are less severe and pinpoint reddish to greyish-white necrotic foci are distributed throughout the parenchyma. Haemorrhage and oedema of the wall of the gallbladder are common. Hepatic lesions in lambs are almost invariably accompanied by numerous small haemorrhages in the mucosa of the abomasum. The contents of the small intestine and abomasum are dark chocolate-brown as a result of the presence of partially digested blood. In all animals, the spleen and peripheral lymph nodes are enlarged, oedematous and may have petechiae.

Microscopically, hepatic necrosis is the most obvious lesion of RVF in both animals and humans. In fetuses and neonates of cattle and sheep, foci of necrosis consist of dense aggregates of cellular and nuclear debris, some fibrin and a few inflammatory cells. There is a severe lytic necrosis of most hepatocytes and the normal architecture of the liver is lost. In about 50% of affected livers, intranuclear inclusion bodies that are eosinophilic and oval or rod-shaped are found. Mineralisation of necrotic hepatocytes is also seen. In adult animals, hepatic necrosis is less diffuse and in sheep, icterus is more common than in lambs (18).

In humans, RVF infections are usually inapparent or associated with a moderate to severe, nonfatal, influenza-like illness (13). A minority of patients may develop ocular lesions, encephalitis, or severe hepatic disease with haemorrhagic manifestations, which is generally fatal. RVF virus is a biosafety level III agent and has caused serious human infection in laboratory workers. Staff should either be vaccinated, work under biosafety level III conditions, or wear respiratory protection. Particular care needs to be exercised when working with infected animals or when performing post-mortem examinations.

No significant antigenic differences have been demonstrated between RVF isolates and laboratory-passaged strains from many countries, but differences in pathogenicity have been demonstrated (19).

Infection of humans by mosquito vectors is a striking feature in countries, such as Egypt, with a relatively small population of animal hosts and a large population of mosquitoes. In such areas, RVF may be recognised first in humans and more cases may be recognised in humans than in livestock, which may suffer only inapparent infections.

RVF usually occurs in epizootics in Africa, which may involve several countries in a region at one and the same time. These follow the periodic cycles of exceptionally heavy rain, which may occur very rarely in semi-arid zones (30–35-year cycles), or more frequently (3–10-year cycles) in higher rainfall grasslands. RVF should be suspected when unusually heavy rains are followed by the occurrence of abortions together with fatal disease marked by necrosis and haemorrhages in the liver that particularly affect newborn lambs, kids and calves, concurrent with the occurrence of an influenza-like illness in farm workers and people handling raw meat.

Preventative measures to protect workers from infection should be employed when there are suspicions that RVF-virus-infected meat and tissue samples are to be handled.

1. Identification of the agent

RVF virus may be isolated from blood collected in an anticoagulant during the febrile stage of the disease, from liver, spleen and brain of animals that have died, or from aborted fetuses. Primary isolation is usually performed in hamsters, infant or adult mice, or on cell cultures of various types.

a) Culture

Approximately 5 ml of blood collected during the febrile stage of the disease or approximately 5 g of liver, spleen and brain collected after death should be presented for virus isolation. The samples should be kept at 0–4°C during transit. If transport to the laboratory is likely to take more than 24 hours, the samples should be frozen and sent on dry ice.

Approximately 1 g of homogenised tissue is suspended 1/10 in cell culture medium or buffered saline, pH 7.5, containing sodium penicillin (1000 International Units [IU]/ml), streptomycin sulphate (1 mg/ml), mycostatin, (100 IU/ml) or fungizone (2.5 µg/ml). The suspension is centrifuged at 1000 ***g*** for 10 minutes and the supernatant fluid is injected intracerebrally into 1–5-day-old mice or intraperitoneally into hamsters or adult mice. Infant mice will either die or be obviously ill by day 2. Adult mice are affected 1–3 days later. Although mice or hamsters are the laboratory animal of choice, lambs and embryonated chicken eggs may also be used.

A variety of cell monolayers including African green monkey kidney (Vero), baby hamster kidney (BHK), chicken embryo reticulum (CER: cells developed by Tsunemasa Motohashi at the Nippon Institute for Biological Science, Tokyo, Japan; recharacterised as a hamster line) (3) and primary kidney or testis cells of calves and lambs may be inoculated with 1 ml of clarified sample supernates and incubated at 37°C for 1 hour. It is advisable to also inoculate some cultures with a further 1/100 dilution of the inoculum. This is to avoid the production of defective particles, which follows the use of very high virus inocula. Some tubes containing flying cover-slips should also be prepared. The cultures are washed with phosphate buffered saline at room temperature and covered with medium containing 2% serum free from antibodies against RVF. The cultures are observed microscopically for 5–6 days. RVF virus induces a cytopathic effect (CPE) characterised by slight rounding of cells followed by destruction of the whole cell sheet within 12–24 hours. Specific identification of RVF virus antigen may be made 18–24 hours after infection by immunofluorescent staining of the cover-slip preparations.

The virus can also be identified by neutralisation with a known positive serum. Plaque reduction neutralisation (PRN) or microneutralisation using Vero or CER cells, or neutralisation in mice can be performed. Mice are injected intraperitoneally.

The virus may also be detected by direct or indirect immunofluorescence carried out on impression smears or on cryostat sections of liver, spleen and brain. A rapid diagnosis can sometimes be made by demonstrating viral antigen in tissues or in serum of febrile animals by agar gel immunodiffusion (AGID). A rapid diagnosis can also be made by detection of viral RNA using a reverse-transcription polymerase chain reaction (RT-PCR).

The PCR was used, among other techniques, for antigen detection in two recent RVF virus outbreaks in Africa – one in Kenya in 1998 and one in South Africa in 1999. RT-PCR followed by sequencing of the NS(S) protein-coding region has been used in phylogenetic analysis to characterise two distinct lineages of RVF viurs – one Egyptian and the other sub-Saharan – making this technique a powerful molecular epidemiological tool (17).

Histopathological examination of the liver of affected animals will reveal characteristic cytopathology, and immunostaining will allow the specific identification of the RVF viral antigen in infected cells. This is an important diagnostic tool, for liver or other tissue may be placed in formol saline in the field for diagnostic purposes, which facilitates handling and transport in areas remote from the laboratory.

2. Serological tests

Neutralisation tests including microneutralisation (VN – virus neutralisation), PRN and neutralisation in mice have been used to detect antibodies against RVF virus in the serum of a variety of species. Neutralisation tests are highly specific and will record the earliest response, but these tests can only be performed with live virus and are not recommended for use outside endemic areas.

Other available tests include enzyme-linked immunosorbent assay (ELISA), haemagglutination inhibition (HI), AGID, immunofluorescence, radioimmunoassay and complement fixation. In these tests, however, cross-reactions may occur between RVF virus and other members of the Phlebotomus fever serogroup. An advantage of these tests is the fact that they can be performed with inactivated antigen and can therefore be used in RVF-free countries.

The ELISA is a reliable and sensitive test that may be employed with several species to detect antibodies against RVF virus (16). Details and reagents are available from the OIE Reference Laboratory for RVF (see Table given in Part 4 of this *Manual*).

The HI test can be employed with great confidence in nonendemic areas. However, sera from individuals that have had previous infections with viruses of the Phlebotomus fever serogroup other than RVF may react with RVF antigen to titres as high as 40 and, rarely, to titres of 320 (19). In suspected cases, the OIE Reference Laboratory for RVF (see Table given in Part 4 of this *Manual*) can be of assistance in carrying out neutralisation tests for specificity. The HI antibody titre after vaccination with RVF virus vaccine may be as high as 640 or, rarely, 1280, whereas titres following natural infections with RVF virus are usually significantly higher.

a) Virus neutralisation

The VN test may be employed to determine the presence of antibodies in naturally infected animals and in animals vaccinated with RVF vaccine. The test is highly specific and can be used to test serum of any species. The test is generally used to measure vaccine efficacy and usually gives reliable results, even though it is not very sensitive and factors other than neutralising antibodies may play a part in resistance to RVF. The mouse-adapted Smithburn strain of highly attenuated RVF virus, also referred to as modified live virus and adapted to cell culture, is used as antigen. The antigen is stored at 4°C in freeze-dried form. The stock is titrated to determine the dilution that will give 100 $TCID_{50}$ (50% tissue culture infective dose) in 25 µl under the conditions of the test.

- **Test procedure**

i) Inactivate the test sera for 30 minutes in a water bath at 56°C.

ii) Add 25 µl of cell culture medium with 5% RVF-negative serum and antibiotics to each well of a 96-well cell culture plate.

iii) Add 25 µl of test serum to the first well of each row and make twofold dilutions using either a multichannel pipette or microdiluters. Titrate each serum in duplicate from 1/10 to 1/80 for screening purposes or in quadruplet and to higher dilutions for determination of end point titres. Include known positive and negative control sera.

iv) Add 25 µl per well of RVF virus antigen (diluted in cell culture medium and calculated to provide 100 $TCID_{50}$ per well) to each well that contains diluted test serum and to wells in rows containing negative and positive control serum. In addition, make twofold dilutions of antigen in at least two rows each containing cell culture medium only.

v) Incubate for 30 minutes at 37°C.

vi) Add 50 µl per well of Vero, CER or any other susceptible cell suspension at 3×10^5 cells/ml or at a dilution known to produce a confluent monolayer within 12 hours.

vii) Incubate the plates in an atmosphere of 3–5% CO_2 for 3–5 days.

viii) Using an inverted microscope, the monolayers are examined daily for evidence of CPE. There should be no CPE in rows containing positive control serum and clear evidence of CPE in rows containing negative control serum indicating the presence of virus. Determine the results by the Spearman–Kärber method.

b) Enzyme-linked immunosorbent assay

An indirect ELISA employing an inactivated, cell-culture-produced antigen and Protein G-peroxidase conjugate has been developed by the OIE Reference Laboratory (see Table given in Part 4 of this *Manual*). This test has been shown to be sensitive and provides confirmation of RVF antibodies within hours. Antigen, standard serum and test protocols can be obtained from this Reference Laboratory. An IgM-capture ELISA allows diagnosis of a recent infection to be made on a single serum sample.

c) Haemagglutination inhibition

Stocks of antigen are prepared and stored either frozen or, if lyophilised, at 4°C. An inactivated mouse liver antigen as described by Clarke & Casals (4) is used. This is diluted so that the amount used in each haem-agglutinating unit (HAU) is four or eight times that which agglutinates 50% of the red blood cells (RBCs) in the test system. Sera are first inactivated at 56°C for 30 minutes. Kaolin or acetone treatment may be used to remove nonspecific serum inhibitors. The RBCs should be derived from normal white male geese. The cells are washed three times by centrifugation, and a 0.3% suspension is prepared in isotonic saline. Sera should be absorbed before use by incubation with an equal volume of packed RBCs for 1 hour at 4°C.

Positive and negative control sera are incorporated into each test. A test is considered to be valid only if the control sera give the expected results. Sera with titres below 1/40 are considered to be negative; titres between 1/40 and 1/320 are considered to be doubtful. Titres above 1/320 are regarded as positive.

HI is an appropriate screening test for surveys although it is not specific. Marked cross-reactions do occur between the Phleboviruses, but homologous titres exceed heterologous titres. Experimentally, African Phleboviruses other than RVF have been shown to be nonpathogenic for ruminants, and antibodies that they might induce are unlikely to cause confusion in RVF diagnosis (19).

B. REQUIREMENTS FOR VACCINES AND DIAGNOSTIC BIOLOGICALS

A live vaccine prepared from Smithburn's attenuated strain of RVF virus has been used for the control of RVF in nonpregnant cattle in endemic areas and during outbreaks, while inactivated vaccines for use in pregnant animals and in RVF-free countries are prepared from virulent strains (1, 2). Inactivated virus vaccines should be prepared from highly immunogenic strains of RVF virus produced in cell culture. The virus should be inactivated with formaldehyde, beta-propiolactone or by any other suitable method. Adjuvants should be used to enhance immunogenicity.

In humans, an inactivated experimental RVF vaccine has been used with considerable success for 25 years to protect persons at risk. This vaccine is currently produced on diploid cells. However, the limited availability of the vaccine precludes its use in the general population. The only alternative for human application is a live mutagen-attenuated RVF vaccine (RVF MP-12) (10, 12, 15). In animals, it has been shown to be immunogenic, avirulent and protective. In limited tests it appears to be nonabortogenic, but additional field trials in animals are needed to provide definite information on its lack of abortogenic effect when administered at specific times during pregnancy, its effectiveness in different breeds and the effects of prior infection with other Phleboviruses. This vaccine is not yet available for commercial use. In the following description of vaccine production, information is given on live vaccine production adjacent to information on inactivated vaccine production. It must be stressed that live and inactivated vaccines must never be produced in the same facility at the same time, because of the risk of contaminating the attenuated live vaccine with a virulent strain of virus before it is inactivated. Staff handling live RVF virus should be vaccinated and work at biosafety level III to minimise the risk of self infection.

1. Seed management

a) Characteristics of the seed virus

Live vaccine: The stock antigen is derived from Smithburn's original neurotropic strain. This strain is not lethal to adult mice inoculated intraperitoneally and is safe for use in all breeds of cattle, sheep and goats. However, it may cause fetal abnormalities or abortion in pregnant animals.

Inactivated vaccine: For seed virus, a highly immunogenic strain of RVF virus adapted to growth in cell culture may be used. It differs from the attenuated strain in that it is lethal to adult mice when injected intraperitoneally.

b) Method of culture

Both attenuated and inactivated virus strains are produced on BHK, Vero or CER cell cultures. The viruses are stored in a lyophilised form in vials containing 1 ml of a cell culture suspension. The virus titre should be at least $10^{6.5}$ mouse LD_{50} (50% lethal dose) per ml.

c) Validation as a vaccine

Seed virus must be shown to be free from adventitious agents, safe for use and able to stimulate effective immunity in species and breeds for which it is intended.

- **Tests**

The lyophilised seed virus is reconstituted in sterile cell culture medium without antibiotics and tested for freedom from bacteria and fungi. The contents of a reconstituted vial are inoculated into two tubes of thioglycollate and two tubes of soybean casein digest medium. The thioglycollate cultures are incubated at 37°C for 7 days and the soybean casein digest medium cultures at 20°C for 14 days. The cultures should remain negative.

In addition, 5 ml of reconstituted seed virus is mixed with an equal volume of specific RVF antiserum produced in rabbits. After incubation of the serum/virus mixture at 37°C for 30 minutes, the virus suspensions are tested before and after neutralisation on cell cultures, as well as in adult and infant mice, embryonated eggs, and guinea-pigs. The neutralised virus is:

i) Seeded on to six roller tube cultures of primary lamb kidney cells and six roller tube cultures of BHK cells. The cell cultures are incubated at 37°C and observed daily for 7 days for CPE, after which they are subjected to the haemadsorption test with guinea-pig RBCs at 4°C and 37°C. There should be no evidence of CPE or haemadsorption. If cultures degenerate or show suspicious CPE, the material from these cultures should again be mixed with antiserum and subinoculated into new cell cultures, which are observed for a further period of 14 days. The presence of specific CPE or haemadsorption disqualifies the seed virus pool.

ii) Inoculated intraperitoneally (0.2 ml) into groups of at least six adult and six 2–5-day-old mice. The mice should remain healthy for 14 days. If any mice should die, appropriate tissue should be emulsified, mixed with antiserum and subinoculated into further groups of mice, which should again be observed for a further period of 14 days. If there is any evidence of specific mortality, the seed virus pool is disqualified.

iii) Inoculated into at least ten 8-day-old embryonated chicken eggs by means of the 'stab' method (combination of chorioallantoic membrane and allantoic sac route). The eggs are incubated at 37°C for 8 days and are candled daily. Embryos that die within 24 hours are discarded. However, the test should be repeated if <70% of the embryos are alive after 24 hours. The cause of embryo mortality during the subsequent observation period should be determined by setting up appropriate sterility and HI tests, and by examination of yolk-sac smears. If these tests are negative, subinoculation of embryo suspensions mixed with antiserum should be set up as before. On day 4 of incubation, at least four eggs are opened and allantoic fluid is collected. The remaining eggs are opened on day 8 of incubation. The membranes of both groups are examined for lesions and abnormalities of the embryos. The allantoic fluids are subjected to the HI test with guinea-pig and chicken RBCs at 4°C and 37°C. Specific embryo mortality, haemagglutinating activity of the allantoic fluids or any lesions on the membranes or embryo abnormalities disqualify the seed virus pool.

iv) Injected intraperitoneally with 1.0 ml of seed virus into each of two guinea-pigs. The guinea-pigs should remain healthy over an observation period of 14 days.

Failure to pass any test disqualifies the antigen for use as seed virus.

2. Method of manufacture

A vial of lyophilised seed virus is reconstituted and diluted 1/100 to 1/1000 with sterile Eagle's medium for the attenuated vaccine and 1/1000 for the inactivated vaccine. To prepare a working suspension, the diluted virus is seeded on to confluent BHK cell cultures in roller bottles and incubated at 37°C. When 70% of cells are affected (CPE), the medium and cells are harvested and the material is diluted 1/100 to 1/1000, after which 10 ml is again seeded on to roller bottles with confluent BHK cells and again incubated. As soon as 70% CPE is observed, the medium and cells are harvested and pooled.

Virus suspensions for both attenuated and inactivated vaccines are titrated intracerebrally in infant mice and should have a titre of at least $10^{6.5}$ mouse LD_{50}/ml. Alternatively, a plaque titration on CER cells may be performed.

Attenuated vaccine is lyophilised immediately after completion of titration and sterility testing.

A stabiliser should be used, such as 5% peptone in 0.3 M phosphate buffer. The volume of inactivated vaccine is adjusted so that the final vaccine will contain at least $10^{6.5}$ mouse LD_{50}/ml. The adjusted virus suspension is then inactivated at 37°C for 24 hours with formaldehyde at a final concentration of 0.2%. After inactivation, an equal volume of aluminium hydroxide gel is added to the cell suspension. The vaccine should have a final pH of 7–7.5.

3. In-process control

Prior to inoculation of cell cultures, seed virus is subjected to sterility tests in thioglycollate and soybean casein digest medium (see Section B.1.).

A representative sample from each batch of vaccine is selected and the contents of each are reconstituted with 5 ml sterile distilled water and tested for freedom from bacteria and fungi.

4. Batch control

a) Sterility

Prior to freeze-drying or inactivation, each container of pooled vaccine, and thereafter representative samples of both vaccines, are tested for sterility in thioglycollate and soybean casein digest medium.

b) Safety

Live vaccine: Final containers of lyophilised attenuated vaccine are selected at random, and each is reconstituted in distilled water as for vaccination. Four susceptible sheep are injected subcutaneously with one dose of vaccine. The sheep are observed daily for 14 days and the rectal temperatures are recorded. The sheep must remain healthy.

Vaccine is also injected intraperitoneally into six adult mice (0.25 ml each), two hamsters and two guinea-pigs (1 ml each). The animals are observed for a period of 14 days during which they should remain healthy. Mortality attributed to the vaccine disqualifies the batch.

Inactivated vaccine: In the case of inactivated RVF vaccine, each of four susceptible sheep are injected subcutaneously with 2.0 ml of vaccine, observed daily for 3 weeks and rectal temperatures are recorded. The sheep should remain healthy.

In addition, safety is also determined by intracerebral injection of six adult mice and two families of infant mice, and by intraperitoneal injection of two guinea-pigs and two hamsters. The mice, hamsters and guinea-pigs are observed for a period of 14 days. They should remain healthy. Mortality attributed to the vaccine disqualifies the batch.

c) Potency

Live vaccine: Lyophilised attenuated vaccine from two final containers is reconstituted and titrated intracerebrally in infant mice. The final vaccine should contain at least $10^{4.4}$ mouse LD_{50}/dose. Alternatively, titrations may be done on cell cultures.

Two final containers are kept at 37°C for 1 week, reconstituted and titrated as before. Each should contain at least $10^{3.4}$ mouse LD_{50}/dose. Alternatively, titrations may be done on cell cultures.

Inoculated sheep (see Section B.4.b.) are bled 2 and 3 weeks after vaccination, and their antibody response is determined by PRN. A virus neutralising antibody titre of 100 or more is regarded as satisfactory.

Inactivated vaccine: The sheep, injected subcutaneously to determine safety (Section B.4.b.), are bled after 3 weeks and their antibody response is determined by PRN. A virus neutralising antibody titre of 100 or more is regarded as satisfactory.

d) Duration of immunity

Both the live attenuated and the inactivated vaccines have had extensive field use. The live vaccine is considered to induce lifelong immunity against clinical disease, although controversy exists over the immunogenicity of the Smithburn vaccine. Nevertheless, cattle can be immunised with the live virus vaccine using this strain. Experience of the field efficacy of inactivated vaccines is limited because they are used in areas where RVF is not endemic, consequently natural field challenge of the vaccine does not occur. However, in South Africa, during the outbreak of RVF in 1976–1978, observations by State Veterinarians supported the efficacy of the vaccine. In more recent epizootics elsewhere, the inactivated vaccine failed to protect animals against abortion, following two vaccinations. When using the inactivated vaccine, a booster dose should be given 3–6 months after the initial vaccination and thereafter vaccination should be repeated yearly (1, 2).

e) **Stability**

When stored at 4°C, lyophilised attenuated vaccines are stable for at least 4 years, while inactivated vaccine may be stored for many years. Storage at higher temperatures is not recommended.

f) **Preservatives**

No preservatives are used.

g) **Precautions (hazards)**

Although humans can be infected by handling infected material, no case of disease is known to have occurred in humans infected with attenuated vaccine virus, but seroconversion often occurs. However, the strains used to prepare inactivated vaccine may cause disease. Therefore, all staff likely to be exposed to vaccine virus should be vaccinated with the human formalin-inactivated vaccine.

5. Tests on the final product

a) **Sterility**

Representative samples of the final product are collected and tested as in Section B.4.a.

b) **Moisture content**

The moisture content of the lyophilised attenuated vaccine should not exceed 3%.

• Acknowledgement

Parts of this chapter were taken from or based on the chapter on RVF in the previous editions of the *Manual*.

REFERENCES

1. BARNARD B.J.H. (1979). Rift Valley fever vaccine – antibody and immune response in cattle to a live and an inactivated vaccine. *J. S. Afr. Vet. Assoc.*, **50**, 155–157.

2. BARNARD B.J.H. & BOTHA M.J. (1977). An inactivated Rift Valley fever vaccine. *J. S. Afr. Vet. Assoc.*, **48**, 45–48.

3. BARNARD B.J.H. & VOGES S.F. (1986). Flaviviruses in South Africa: Diagnostic procedures. *Onderstepoort J. Vet. Res.*, **53**, 181–185.

4. CLARKE D.H. & CASALS J. (1958). Techniques for hemagglutination and hemagglutination inhibition with arthropod bovine viruses. *Am. J. Trop. Med. Hyg.*, **7**, 561–573.

5. COACKLEY W., PINI A. & GOSDIN D. (1967). Experimental infection of cattle with pantropic Rift Valley fever virus. *Res. Vet. Sci.*, **8**, 399–405.

6. COETZER J.A.W. (1982). The pathology of Rift Valley fever. 11. Lesions occurring in field cases in adult cattle, calves and aborted fetuses. *Onderstepoort J. Vet. Res.*, **49**, 11–17.

7. COETZER J.A.W. & BARNARD B.J.H. (1977). *Hydrops amnii* in sheep associated with hydranencephaly and arthrogryposis with Wesselsbron disease and Rift Valley fever viruses as ethological agents. *Onderstepoort J. Vet. Res.*, **44**, 119–126.

8. EASTERDAY B.C. (1965). Rift Valley fever. *Adv. Vet. Sci.*, **10**, 65–127.

9. GENTSCH J.R. & BISHOP D.L. (1979). M viral RNA segment of bunyaviruses codes for two glycoproteins, G1 and G2. *J. Virol.*, **39**, 767–770.

10. HUBBARD K.A., BASKERVILLE A. & STEPHENSON J.R. (1991). Ability of a mutagenised virus variant to protect young lambs from Rift Valley fever. *Am. J. Vet. Res.*, **52**, 50–55.

11. MCINTOSH B.M., RUSSEL D., DOS SANTOS I. & GEAR J.H.S. (1980). Rift Valley fever in humans in South Africa. *S. Afr. Med. J.*, **58**, 803–806.

12. MEADORS G.F., GIBBS P.H., & PETERS C.J. (1986). Evaluations of a new Rift Valley fever vaccine: Safety and immunogenicity trials. *Vaccine*, **4** 179–184.

13. MEEGAN J.M. (1981). Rift Valley fever in Egypt: An overview of the epizootics in 1977 and 1978. *Contrib. Epidemiol. Biostat.*, **3**, 100–103.

14. MEEGAN J.M. & BAILEY C.L. (1989). Rift Valley fever. *In:* The Arboviruses: Epidemiology and Ecology, Vol. IV, Monath T.P., ed. CRC Press, Boca Raton, Florida, USA, 52–76.

15. MORRILL J.C, JENNINGS.G.B., CAPLAN H., TURREL M.J., JOHNSON A.J. & PETERS C.J. (1987). Pathogenicity and immunogenicity of a mutagen-attenuated Rift Valley fever virus immunogen in pregnant ewes. *Am. J. Vet. Res.*, **48**, 1042–1047.

16. PAWESKA J.T., BARNARD B.J.H. & WILLIAMS R. (1995). The use of sucrose-acetone-extracted Rift Valley fever virus antigen from cell culture in an indirect enzyme-linked immunosorbent assay and haemagglutination-inhibition tests. *Onderstepoort J. Vet. Res.*, **62**, 227–233.

17. SALL A.A., DE AZANOTTO P.M., ZELLER H.G., DIGOUTTE J.P., THIONGANE Y. & BOULOY M. (1997). Variability of the NS(S) protein among Rift Valley fever virus isolates. *J. Gen. Virol.*, **78**, 2853–2858.

18. SWANEPOEL R. & COETZER J.A.W. (1994). Rift Valley fever. *In:* Infectious Diseases of Livestock with Special Reference to Southern Africa. Vol. 1, Coetzer J.A.W., Thomson G.R. & Tustin R.C., eds. Oxford University Press, UK.

19. SWANEPOEL R., STUTHERS J.K., ERASMUS M.J., SHEPHERD S.P., MCGILLIVRAY G.M., SHEPHERD A.J., ERASMUS B.J. & BARNARD B.J.H. (1986). Comparative pathogenicity and antigenic cross-reactivity of Rift Valley fever and other African phleboviruses in sheep. *J. Hyg. (Camb.)*, **97**, 331–346.

20. WEISS K.E. (1957). Rift Valley fever – a review. *Bull. Epizoot. Dis. Afr.*, **5**, 431–458.

*

* *

CHAPTER 2.1.9.

BLUETONGUE

SUMMARY

Bluetongue (BT) is an infectious, noncontagious, insect-borne viral disease of sheep and domestic and wild ruminants, such as goats, cattle, deer, bighorn sheep, most species of African antelope and various other artiodactyla. The outcome of infection ranges from inapparent in the vast majority of infected animals to fatal in a proportion of infected sheep, deer and wild ruminants. Clinical signs of disease, when they appear in domestic and wild ruminants, include a febrile response characterised by inflammation and congestion, facial oedema and haemorrhages, and ulceration of the mucous membranes. In severe cases the tongue may show intense hyperaemia, become swollen and oedematous and protrude from the mouth. Hyperaemia may extend to other parts of the body, particularly the groin, axilla and perineum. There is often severe muscle degeneration. Dermatitis may cause wool breaks. Sheep may become lame as a result of coronitis, inflammation of the coronary band of the hoof, or skeletal myopathy. A similar severe disease of wild ruminants is caused by epizootic haemorrhagic disease virus (EHDV), which, like BT virus (BTV), is a member of the Orbivirus *genus, but is classified in a separate serogroup. EHD may occasionally cause clinical signs in cattle that appear to be similar to bluetongue.*

Identification of the agent: *BTV is a member of the* Orbivirus *genus of the family Reoviridae. Within the genus there are 14 serogroups. The BT serogroup contains 24 serotypes. The former are differentiated by immunological tests that detect viral proteins that are conserved within each serogroup. Most serogroups appear to be immunologically distinct, but there is considerable cross-reaction between members of the BT and EHD serogroups. The serotype of individual viruses in each serogroup is identified on the basis of neutralisation tests. Complete BTV particles are double-shelled and the outer layer contains two proteins, one of which is the major determinant of serotype specificity. The inner icosahedral core contains two major and three minor proteins and ten species of double-stranded RNA. VP7 is a major core protein possessing the serogroup-definitive antigens. Virus identification traditionally requires isolation and amplification of the virus in tissue culture, and the subsequent application of serogroup- and serotype-specific tests. Recently, the application of polymerase chain reaction (PCR) technology has permitted very rapid amplification of BTV RNA in clinical samples, and PCR-based procedures are now available to provide information on virus serogroup and serotype.*

Serological tests: *Serological responses in ruminants appear some 7–14 days after BTV infection and are generally long-lasting. Until recently, tests such as agar gel immunodiffusion and indirect enzyme-linked immunosorbent assay (ELISA) were used to detect BT serogroup-specific antibody, although these tests had the major drawback of being unable to consistently distinguish between antibodies to viruses in the BT and EHD serogroups. The advent of monoclonal-antibody-based competitive ELISA has solved this problem, and competitive ELISAs to specifically detect anti-BTV antibodies are now available and recommended. Current procedures to determine the serotype specificity of antibodies in sera are cumbersome because they require determination of the capacity of test sera to inhibit the infectivity of panels of known virus serotypes in time-consuming neutralisation tests.*

Requirements for vaccines and diagnostic biologicals: *Live attenuated vaccines that are serotype specific are used in several countries, such as South Africa, where nonvaccination may lead to outbreaks of disease. Attenuated viruses are prepared by serial passage of field virus in embryonated chicken eggs or cultured cells. Following serial passage, virulence is attenuated and concomitantly, viruses replicate to lower titres in sheep. Attenuated virus vaccines are teratogenic and should not be administered to pregnant sheep during the first-half of pregnancy, as this may* *cause fetal death and abnormalities. In determining an appropriate degree of attenuation for vaccine purposes, a compromise is sought between a level of replication sufficient to reduce virulence but stimulate protective immunity in sheep, and a need to reduce the titre of virus in the blood in an attempt to prevent infection of feeding insects. Procedures to test vaccine efficacy and teratogenic potential in sheep are easily performed. In contrast, few studies have been carried out to determine whether or not attenuated virus can be transmitted by insects from vaccinated sheep to other animals. The fact that attenuated viruses are teratogenic makes determination of transmissibility very important, especially if live virus vaccines are used in countries for the first time.*

A. DIAGNOSTIC TECHNIQUES

Midges of the genus *Culicoides* transmit bluetongue virus (BTV) to and from susceptible animals, having become infected by feeding on viraemic vertebrates. After a replication period of 6–8 days, and following its appearance in the salivary gland, the virus can be transmitted to a vertebrate host during a blood meal. Infected midges remain infective for life. The central role of the insect in BT epidemiology ensures that prevalence of the disease is governed by ecological factors, such as high rainfall, temperature and humidity, which favour insect survival. In many parts of the world, therefore, the disease has a seasonal occurrence (9).

BT is an infectious, noncontagious disease of sheep and domestic and wild ruminants, such as goats, cattle, deer, bighorn sheep, most species of African antelope and various other artiodactyla. The outcome of infection ranges from inapparent in the vast majority of infected animals to fatal in a proportion of infected sheep, deer and some wild ruminants. Although the frequency of BTV infection of cattle is generally higher than in sheep, overt disease in cattle is rare and the signs, when they occur, are much milder than those observed in sheep. In nondomestic ruminants, the disease can vary from an acute haemorrhagic disease with high mortality, as observed in white-tailed deer *(Odocoilus virginianus)*, to an inapparent disease as seen in the North American elk *(Cervus canadensis)*. Epizootic haemorrhagic disease virus (EHDV) can produce a disease in wild ruminants with clinical manifestations identical to those observed in response to BTV infection.

Clinical signs of disease in domestic and wild ruminants range from subclinical in the vast majority of cases to an acute, febrile response characterised by inflammation and congestion leading to oedema of the face, eyelids and ears, and haemorrhages and ulceration of the mucous membranes. Extensive erosions can develop in the cheeks and on the tongue opposite molar teeth. The tongue may show intense hyperaemia and become swollen and oedematous, protrude from the mouth and, in severe cases, become cyanotic. Hyperaemia may extend to other parts of the body, particularly the groin, axilla and perineum. There is often severe muscle degeneration. Dermatitis may cause wool breaks. Coronitis with haemorrhage of the coronary band of the hoof is common and may cause lameness. When sheep die as a result of acute BT disease, the lungs may show interalveolar hyperaemia, severe alveolar oedema and the bronchial tree may be filled with froth. The thoracic cavity may contain several litres of plasma-like fluid and the pericardial sac may show many petechial haemorrhages. Most cases show a distinctive haemorrhage near the base of the pulmonary artery (8, 9).

BTV is a member of the *Orbivirus* genus, one of nine genera in the family Reoviridae. Family members are characterised by a segmented, double-stranded RNA genome and an icosahedral, double-shelled capsid. Orbiviruses differ from viruses in the other genera (except Coltiviruses) by virtue of the structure of their outer capsid layer, the number of genomic double-stranded RNA segments and the fact that they are insect borne. Within the *Orbivirus* genus, 14 groups are differentiated on serological grounds. The best studied orbiviruses are in the BT and EHD serogroups. Within the serogroups, individual members are differentiated on the basis of neutralisation tests, and 24 serotypes of BTV have been described to date. There is significant immunological cross-reactivity between members of the BT and EHD serogroups (11). Details of EHD-specific tests will not be provided in this chapter.

The surface topography of BTV and that of the underlying core particle has been determined by cryoelectron microscopy (14) and the structure of the core particle determined by X-ray crystallography at a resolution approaching 3.5 Å (13). The outer layer contains two proteins, VP2 and VP5. The former is the major determinant of serotype specificity and contains neutralising epitopes and haemagglutination sites. The inner icosahedral core contains two major proteins – VP3 and VP7 – three minor proteins, and ten species of double-stranded RNA. Trimers of VP7 are arranged on the surface of the core particle (13). All of the double-stranded RNA segments code for a single protein with the exception of one segment, which has been shown to code for two small, closely related minor proteins.

1. Identification of the agent (a prescribed test for international trade)

a) Virus isolation

The same diagnostic procedures are used for domestic and wild ruminants. A number of virus isolation systems are in common use, but two of the most efficient are embryonated chicken eggs (ECE) and sheep. Identification of BTV following inoculation of sheep may still be a useful approach if the titre of virus in the sample blood is very low, as may be the case several weeks after virus infection. Attempts to isolate virus in cultured cells *in vitro* may be more convenient, but the success rate is frequently much lower than that achieved with *in-vivo* systems. It is important to remember that within a virus population, not all BTV particles are identical at the genetic and amino acid level, and only a small, perhaps minute, proportion of the viruses present in the blood of infected animals may have appropriate amino acid sequences in key viral proteins to bind to and replicate in cells in culture. This may be the reason why direct inoculation into cultured cells of viraemic blood that contains a relatively small number of virus particles is an inefficient way to isolate BTV. A high-titre virus preparation, and one more likely to contain virus that has the ability to replicate in tissue culture, is most readily generated by one, or at most two, passages in ECE. Cell culture has proven to be a more sensitive technique for isolation of EHD virus.

- **Isolation in embryonated chicken eggs**

i) Blood is collected from febrile animals into an anticoagulant, such as heparin, EDTA (ethylene diamine tetra-acetic acid) or sodium citrate, and blood cells are washed three times with sterile phosphate buffered saline (PBS). Washed cells are resuspended in PBS or isotonic sodium chloride and either stored at 4°C or used immediately for attempted virus isolation.

ii) For long-term storage where refrigeration is not possible, blood samples are collected in oxalate-phenol-glycerin (OPG). If samples can be frozen, they should be collected in buffered lactose peptone and stored at –70°C or colder. The virus is not stable for long periods at –20°C.

iii) In fatal cases, spleen and lymph nodes are the preferred organs for virus isolation attempts. Organs and tissues should be kept and transported at 4°C to a laboratory where they are homogenised in PBS or isotonic saline, and used as described below, for blood cells.

iv) Washed blood cells are resuspended in distilled water or sonicated in PBS, and 0.1 ml volumes are inoculated intravascularly into 6–12 ECE that are 9–12 days old. This procedure is difficult to perform and requires practice.

v) The eggs are incubated in a humid chamber at 33.5°C and candled daily. Any embryo deaths within the first 24 hours post-inoculation are regarded as nonspecific.

vi) Embryos that die between days 2 and 7 are retained at 4°C, and embryos remaining alive at 7 days are killed. Infected embryos often have a haemorrhagic appearance. After removal of the heads, embryos are homogenised (dead embryos and those that live to 7 days are homogenised as two separate pools), and debris is removed by centrifugation.

vii) Virus in the supernatant may be identified either directly by antigen-capture enzyme-linked immunosorbent assay (ELISA), or indirectly by antigen-detection methods, such as immunofluorescence or immunoperoxidase, after further amplification in culture.

viii) Virus in the brain and liver of infected embryos may also be detected by antigen-capture ELISA.

ix) If no embryos are killed following inoculation of sample material, an inoculum made from the first egg passage material may be repassaged in ECE or in cell culture.

- **Isolation in cell culture**

Virus may also be added to mouse L, baby hamster kidney (BHK)-21, African green monkey kidney (Vero) or *Aedes albopictus* (AA) cells in culture. The efficiency of isolation is often significantly lower following direct addition to cultured cells compared with that achieved in ECE. Greatest efficiency of isolation in cell culture is achieved by first passaging ECE homongenates in AA cells, followed by either antigen detection procedures or additional passages in mammalian cell lines, such as BHK-21 or Vero. A cytopathic effect (CPE) is not necessarily observed in AA cells. Cell monolayers are monitored for the appearance of a CPE for 5 days at 37°C in 5% CO_2 with humidity. If no CPE appears, a second passage is made in cell culture. The identity of BTV in the culture medium of cells manifesting a CPE may be confirmed by antigen-capture ELISA, immunofluorescence, immunoperoxidase or virus neutralisation (VN) tests.

- **Isolation in sheep**

i) Sheep are inoculated with washed cells from 10 ml up to approximately 500 ml of blood, or 10–50 ml of tissue suspension. Inocula are administered subcutaneously in 10–20 ml aliquots. Large volumes may aid in the virus isolation attempts and should be administered intravenously.

ii) The sheep are held for 28 days and checked for antibody using the agar gel immunodiffusion (AGID) test or competitive ELISA as described below.

b) Immunological methods

- **Serogrouping of viruses**

Orbivirus isolates are typically serogrouped on the basis of their reactivity with specific standard antisera that detect proteins, such as VP7, that are conserved within each serogroup. The cross-reactivity between members of the BT and EHD serogroups raises the possibility that an isolate of EHD virus could be mistaken for BTV on the basis of a weak immunofluorescence reaction with a polyclonal anti-BTV antiserum. For this reason, a BT serogroup-specific monoclonal antibody (MAb) can be used. A number of laboratories have generated such serogroup-specific reagents (3, 17). In contrast to serogrouping, the usual method of serotyping is by virus neutralisation testing using methods described later. Commonly used methods for the identification of viruses to serogroup level are as follows.

i) *Immunofluorescence*

Monolayers of BHK or bovine fetal kidney cells on glass cover-slips are infected with either tissue-culture-adapted virus or virus in ECE lysates. After 24–48 hours at 37°C, or after the appearance of a mild CPE, infected cells are fixed with agents such as paraformaldehyde, acetone or methanol, dried and viral antigen is detected using anti-BTV antiserum and standard immunofluorescent procedures.

ii) *Antigen-capture enzyme-linked immunosorbent assay* (22)

Virus in ECE lysates, culture media and infected insects may be detected directly. In this technique, virus and/or core particles are trapped by antibody adsorbed to an ELISA plate and bound virus is detected using a second antibody. A serogroup-specific MAb may be used to either capture virus particles or detect particles trapped by bound polyclonal antibodies.

iii) *Immunospot test* (10)

Small volumes (2 µl) of infected cell culture supernatant or lysed or sonicated infected cells are adsorbed to nitrocellulose and air-dried. Nonspecific binding sites are blocked by incubation with a solution containing skim milk protein. After incubation with a BT serogroup-reactive MAb, bound antibody is detected using horseradish-peroxidase-conjugated anit-mouse IgG.

iv) *Indirect peroxidase–antiperoxidase identification* (6)

This test is now rarely used, having been replaced by an immunoperoxidase test using an MAb to VP7 and an anti-mouse conjugate. This has several advantages over immunofluorescence because it can be performed in microplates, does not require a UV microscope, and the results, as stained plates, can be stored indefinitely for later reference.

- **Serotyping by virus neutralisation**

Neutralisation tests are type-specific for the currently recognised 24 BTV serotypes and can be used to serotype a virus isolate, or can be modified to determine the specificity of antibody in sera. In the case of an untyped isolate, the characteristic regional localisation of BTV serotypes should generally obviate the need to attempt neutralisation by all 24 antisera, particularly when endemic serotypes have been identified.

There is a variety of tissue-culture-based methods available to detect the presence of neutralising anti-BTV antibody. Cell lines commonly used are BHK, Vero and L929. Four methods to serotype BTV are outlined briefly below. BTV serotype-specific antisera generated in guinea-pigs or rabbits have been reported to have less serotype cross-reactivity than those made in cattle or sheep. It is important that antiserum controls be included to ensure that an effective level of standard antiserum is used against comparable and standardised titres of standard and untyped virus.

i) *Plaque reduction*

The virus to be serotyped is diluted to contain approximately 100 plaque-forming units (PFU), and incubated with either no antiserum or with individual standard antisera to a panel of BTV serotypes. Virus/antiserum mixtures are added to monolayers of cells and the virus titre is determined by plaque assay. The unidentified virus is considered to be serologically identical to a standard serotype if the latter is run in parallel with the untyped virus in the test, and is similarly neutralised.

ii) *Plaque inhibition*

Tests are performed in 90 mm diameter Petri dishes containing confluent cell monolayers that are infected with approximately 5×10^4 PFU standard or untyped virus. After adsorption and removal of inoculum, monolayers are overlaid with agarose. Standard anti-BTV antisera are added to individual filter-paper discs and placed on the agarose surface. Dishes are incubated for at least 4 days. A zone of virus neutralisation, with concomitant survival of the cell monolayer, will surround the disc containing the homologous antiserum.

iii) *Microtitre neutralisation*

Approximately 100 $TCID_{50}$ (50% tissue culture infective dose) of the standard or untyped virus is added in 50 µl volumes to test wells of a flat-bottomed microtitre plate and mixed with an equal volume of standard antiserum diluted in tissue culture medium (24). Approximately 10^4 cells are added per well in a volume of 100 µl, and after incubation for 4–6 days, the test is read using an inverted microscope. Wells are scored for the degree of CPE observed. Those wells that contain cells only or cells and antiserum, should show no CPE. In contrast, wells containing cells and virus should show convincing CPE. The unidentified virus is considered to be serologically identical to a standard BTV serotype if both are neutralised in the test to a similar extent.

iv) *Fluorescence inhibition test* (5)

This simple neutralisation assay requires varying concentrations of an unknown virus and standard concentrations of reference antisera. Virus isolates grown in cell culture are serially diluted and mixed with individual reference antisera in the wells of a Lab-Tek slide for 1 hour prior to the addition of cells. After incubation for 16 hours, cells are fixed and probed by an immunofluorescent procedure using a BT serogroup-specific MAb. The serotype of the virus is indicated by the specificity of the antiserum causing the largest reduction in the number of fluorescent cells.

c) Polymerase chain reaction (a prescribed test for international trade)

Primer-directed amplification of viral nucleic acid has revolutionised BT diagnosis (7, 15, 20, 30). Results to date indicate that polymerase chain reaction (PCR) techniques may be used, not only to detect the presence of viral nucleic acid, but also to 'serogroup' orbiviruses and provide information on the serotype and possible geographical source (topotype or genotype) of BTV isolates within a few days of receipt of a clinical sample such as infected sheep blood. Traditional approaches, which rely on virus isolation followed by virus identification, may require at least 3–4 weeks to generate information on serogroup and serotype and yield no data on the possible geographical origin of the isolated virus.

Oligonucleotide primers used to date have been derived from RNA 7 (VP7 gene) (30), RNA 6 (NS1 gene) (7, 15), RNA 3 (VP3 gene) and RNA 2 (VP2 gene) (20). The size of the amplified transcripts is usually small – in the order of several hundred nucleotides – but can also be a full-length gene. In the procedure described in detail below, a 101 nucleotide stretch of RNA 6 is amplified (15). Primers derived from the highly conserved genes, such as VP3, VP6, VP7, NS1 and NS3 may be used for serogrouping (i.e. will react with all members of the BT serogroup) and topotyping (i.e. will react with BTV isolates from the same geographical area), while primers whose sequence was determined from VP2 gene sequences provide information on virus serotype.

Recognition that the nucleic acid sequence of known BTV genes appears to differ with the geographical area of isolation (12) has provided a unique opportunity to complement studies of BTV epidemiology. Thus, determination of the nucleic acid sequence of portions of RNA 3 and RNA 6 may provide information on whether the virus came from Australia, North America or South Africa. It appears likely that sequencing of BTV isolates from other parts of the world may permit finer discrimination of geographical origin.

It has been observed that BTV nucleic acid can be detected by PCR from the blood of infected calves and sheep at least 30 days, and sometimes over 90 days, after the virus can be isolated. When blood that was positive for virus isolation (infectious) and blood that was negative for virus isolation but positive by PCR (PCR-detectable only) were inoculated into or fed to the vector, *Culicoides variipennis*, it was shown that the virus was amplified and transmitted only by vectors exposed to infectious blood. Vectors exposed to PCR-detectable only blood did not amplify or transmit the BTV (18). Because of this, PCR-based diagnostics should be interpreted with caution. The PCR procedure will detect virus-specific nucleic acid, but this does not necessarily indicate the presence of infectious virus.

The capacity of PCR assays to detect single molecules of nucleic acid means that such tests are exquisitely sensitive to contamination by extraneous nucleic acids. The latter may include any primers in use in the laboratory or previously amplified polynucleotides. It is critical therefore to have a 'clean' area containing all equipment necessary for reagent and test preparation and a separate area with its own equipment for amplification. Latex gloves should be worn and changed frequently at all stages of the procedure, particularly after working with sample RNA or amplified DNA. This will help protect reagents and samples from contamination by ubiquitous RNases and other agents and from cross-contamination by DNA.

The PCR assay described here involves three separate procedures. In the first, BTV RNA is extracted from blood using a chaotropic agent such as guanidine thiocyanate (GuSCN) to denature protein and release viral RNA. A number of commercial kits are available for this purpose and the protocol below describes the use of one such kit, IsoQuick[1]. The reagents provided with the kit are numbered and their use is indicated in the protocol below. Other kits are available and one, TRIZOL[2], is particularly useful for the extraction of viral nucleic acid from spleen or blood clots. Operators should follow the procedures specified in each kit and use reagent solutions either provided or recommended for the kit of their choice. The second procedure is the denaturation of viral double-stranded RNA and reverse transcription (RT) to generate DNA, which is amplified by PCR. In the procedure described below, the Superscript™ Preamplification System (Life Technologies) is used to transcribe viral RNA and reagents from Perkin-Elmer are used for the PCR. Equivalent kits and reagents are available from other sources. The final step of the process is the analysis of the PCR product by electrophoresis.

- **Extraction of viral RNA**

i) Whole blood is collected from test and uninfected control animals in EDTA tubes and centrifuged at 800–1000 *g* for 10 minutes. The plasma is aspirated and the red blood cells (RBCs) are gently resuspended in sterile PBS. RBCs are pelleted by centrifugation at 1000 *g* for 10 minutes and the supernatant is removed.

ii) Next, 400 µl of test RBCs is added to each of four 1.7 ml microcentrifuge tubes and 400 µl of control RBCs is added to each of two microcentrifuge tubes. An equal volume of RNase-free water is added to each tube and the tubes are vortexed briefly to mix and lyse the cells. Two tubes containing test RBCs are frozen at –70°C for repository purposes and the extraction is continued in duplicate.

iii) Lysed test and control RBCs are centrifuged at 12,000–16,000 *g* for 10 minutes and the supernatant is discarded. Next, 800 µl RNase-free water is added and the tubes are vortexed and centrifuged again at the same speed for 10 minutes. The supernatant is removed and the RBC pellet is drained.

iv) A small volume of BTV (e.g. 5 µl containing from 10^3 to 10^7 PFU) is added to one of two control RBC pellets. This is the positive control. The other control RBC pellet remains as the negative control.

v) Next, 75 µl of sample buffer (IsoQuick reagent A) is added to each pellet, and the pellets are then vortexed vigorously, followed by the addition of 125 µl of the GuSCN-containing lysis solution (IsoQuick reagent 1). The mixture is vortexed vigorously for 30 seconds.

vi) Before use the extraction matrix provided with the kit (IsoQuick reagent 2 plus dye 2A) is shaken vigorously and 500 µl is added to the sample lysates. Then, 400 µl extraction buffer (IsoQuick reagent 3) is added and the tubes are vortexed for 10 seconds.

vii) The tubes are incubated at 65°C for 10 minutes, vortexed briefly after 5 minutes and centrifuged at 12,000 *g* for 5 minutes.

viii) The aqueous phase (500 µl) is transferred to a new microcentrifuge tube and an equal volume of extraction matrix (IsoQuick reagent 2) is added. The tubes are vortexed for 10 seconds and centrifuged at 12,000 *g* for 5 minutes.

ix) The aqueous phase (330 µl) is transferred to a new microcentrifuge tube and a 10% volume (33 µl) of sodium acetate (IsoQuick reagent 4) and 365 µl isopropanol are added. After gentle mixing, the tubes are placed at –20°C for from 20 minutes to 1 hour.

x) The RNA is pelleted by centrifugation at 12,000 *g* for 10 minutes. The supernatant is decanted and 1.0 ml 70% ethanol is added and mixed gently. After centrifugation at 12,000 *g* for 5 minutes, the supernatant is decanted and 1.0 ml 100% ethanol is added. The tubes are stored at –70°C until ready for use in the RT-PCR.

- **Reverse-transcription polymerase chain reaction**

i) RNA in ethanol is centrifuged at 12,000 *g* for 5 minutes. The ethanol is decanted and the tubes are inverted and allowed to drain. The pellet, which may not be obvious, must not be allowed to dry out because this makes resuspension difficult. A dry pellet is also likely to fall out of the inverted tube.

---

1 IsoQuick, Orca Research, Bothell, Washington, United States of America (USA).
2 TRIZOL, Life Technologies, Grand Island, New York, USA.

ii) Next, 12 µl RNase-free water is added to each tube, mixed and heated at 65°C for 5–10 minutes. The samples are placed in ice.

iii) In a 'clean' biohazard hood, stock solutions containing 200 pmol/µl of primers A, B, C and D are prepared in RNase-free water and stored at –70°C.

First stage PCR primers (to amplify RNA 6 from nucleotide 11 to 284)
Primer A: 5'-GTT-CTC-TAG-TTG-GCA-ACC-ACC-3'
Primer B: 5'-AAG-CCA-GAC-TGT-TTC-CCG-AT-3'

Nested PCR primers (to amplify RNA 6 from nucleotide 170 to 270)
Primer C: 5'-GCA-GCA-TTT-TGA-GAG-AGC-GA-3'
Primer D: 5'-CCC-GAT-CAT-ACA-TTG-CTT-CCT-3'

iv) Primer stock solutions are diluted to a concentration of 15–20 pmol/µl. Primers for the first stage PCR reaction are prepared by mixing equal volumes of A and B. Primers for the nested PCR reaction are prepared by mixing equal volumes of C and D. Small aliquots of pooled primer mixes are frozen at -20°C.

v) PCR reaction tubes are labelled and, for first stage synthesis, 4.0 µl of primer (A + B) mix is added to each tube. The tubes are held on ice.

vi) In a 'clean' fume hood methylmercuric hydroxide is diluted to 50 mM (1/20 dilution) and 2-mercaptoethanol is diluted to 350 mM (1/40 dilution) in RNase-free water. Methylmercuric hydroxide and 2-mercaptoethanol are considered to be extremely and highly toxic, respectively. Use both chemicals with extreme care and dispose of them and pipette tips as required by safety regulations.

vii) Next, 4 µl of test and positive and negative control RNA samples (step ii) are added to 4 µl of the primer mix in PCR tubes (step v).

viii) To each PCR tube 2.0 µl of the 1/20 dilution of methylmercuric hydroxide is added with gentle mixing and allowed to sit at room temperature for 10 minutes prior to adding 2.0 µl of the 1/40 dilution of 2-mercaptoethanol. For safety reasons, some laboratories use formamide instead of methylmercuric hydroxide for double-stranded RNA denaturation. However, for optimum sensitivity, methylmercuric hydroxide is preferred.

ix) In a 'clean' hood a cDNA mix is prepared containing the following reagents in sufficient volume for the number of samples being tested. The amount given is per sample and the reagents are contained in the Superscript™ Preamplification System (Life Technologies).

10 × Superscript™ buffer (200 mM Tris-HCl, pH 8.4, and 500 mM KCl)	2.0 µl
$MgCl_2$ (25 mM)	2.0 µl
dNTP mix (10 mM each dATP, dCTP, dGTP, dTTP)	1.25 µl
Dithiothreitol (DTT) (0.1 M)	2.0 µl
Reverse transcriptase (200 units/µl)	0.75 µl

x) Then, 8.0 µl of the mix is added to each PCR tube to a final volume of 20.0 µl.

xi) The PCR tubes are placed in a thermal cycler, such as GeneAmp™ PCR System 9600, which is programmed for reverse transcription as follows:

Hold 44°C 50 minutes
Hold 4°C Forever

xii) The tubes are removed from the thermal cycler and 1.0 µl RNase H and a wax bead are added to each tube. The cycler is programmed as follows:

Hold 37°C	20 minutes
Hold 08°C	4 minutes
Hold 4°C	Forever

xiii) In a 'clean' hood a first stage amplification mix is prepared containing the following reagents and in a volume sufficient for the number of samples being tested. All these reagents except water are available from Perkin-Elmer. The amount given is per sample.

RNase-free water	62.0 µl
10 × PCR Perkin-Elmer buffer (100 mM Tris HCl, pH 8.3, and 500 mM KCl)	7.0 µl
$MgCl_2$ (25 mM)	7.0 µl
dNTP mix (2.5 mM each dATP, dCTP, dGTP, dTTP)	4.0 µl
Taq DNA polmerase (5 units/µl)	0.85 µl

xiv) The first stage mix is removed from the 'clean' area to the thermal cycling area and 80 µl is overlaid in each sample tube. The wax layer must not be pierced. Each tube should now contain 101 µl.

xv) The tubes are placed in the thermal cycler, which is programmed as follows (correct for GeneAmp PCR System 9600 – programmes for other thermocyclers would need to be determined) for first stage amplification:

One cycle:	Hold 95°C	3 minutes
	Hold 58°C	20 seconds
	Hold 74°C	30 seconds
40 cycles:	Hold 95°C	25 seconds
	Hold 58°C	20 seconds
	Hold 74°C	25 seconds
One cycle:	Hold 95°C	25 seconds
	Hold 58°C	20 seconds
	Hold 74°C	5 minutes
	Hold 4°C	Forever

xvi) PCR reaction tubes are prepared for the nested reaction in a 'clean' hood 15 minutes before cycling is complete, and held on ice:

RNase-free water	17 µl per tube
Nested primer mix (C + D)	4.0 µl per tube
Wax bead	

xvii) When first stage amplification is complete, the tubes are removed from the thermal cycler and placed in a biological safety cabinet (not the 'clean' hood). Then, 1.5 µl of the first stage product is transferred to the corresponding nested PCR tube containing primer, water and a wax bead.

xviii) The tubes are placed in the thermal cycler, which is programmed as follows for wax layer formation:

Hold 98°C	4 minutes
Hold 4°C	Forever

xix) In a 'clean' hood the nested mix of the following reagents is prepared in sufficient volume for the number of samples being tested. The reagents used are the same as in the first stage (step xiii). The amount given is per sample.

RNase-free water	17.0 µl
10 × PCR buffer	5.0 µl
$MgCl_2$	3.5 µl
dNTP mix	4.5 µl
Taq DNA polmerase	0.5 µl

xx) The nested mix is removed from the 'clean' hood to the thermal cycler and 30 µl is overlaid into each sample tube. Each tube should now contain 52 µl.

xxi) The tubes are placed in the thermal cycler, which is programmed as follows for nested amplification. After completion, the tubes are held at 4°C or –20°C until electrophoresis:

One cycle:	Hold 95°C	3 minutes
	Hold 58°C	20 seconds
	Hold 72°C	30 seconds
40 cycles:	Hold 95°C	20 seconds
	Hold 58°C	20 seconds
	Hold 72°C	20 seconds
One cycle:	Hold 95°C	20 seconds
	Hold 58°C	20 seconds
	Hold 72°C	5 minutes
	Hold 4°C	Forever

- **Electrophoretic analysis of PCR product**

i) First, 1 × TBE buffer (0.045 mM Tris-borate, pH 8.6, and 1.5 mM EDTA) is prepared from a × 10 stock solution. For the Bio-Rad Wide Mini-Sub cell system, 700 ml buffer is prepared (100 ml for the gel and 600 ml for the tank buffer).

ii) A 3% solution of NuSieve 3/1 agarose[3] or an equivalent is prepared in TBE buffer. The solution is boiled until the agarose is completely dissolved, and then allowed to cool to 40°C. Ethidium bromide is added to a concentration of 0.5 µg/ml to both the agarose and the tank buffer. Ethidium bromide is a mutagen and is toxic. Gloves, protective clothing, and eye-wear must always be worn.

iii) The ends of the electrophoresis tray are taped and the agarose solution is poured. The comb is inserted and the agarose is allowed to solidify on a level surface for 30–60 minutes. The comb and the tape are gently removed from the electrophoresis tray.

iv) Pour the tank buffer into the electrophoresis apparatus and insert the tray with the agarose so that the buffer covers the agarose.

v) Test and positive and negative control samples are prepared for electrophoresis in 0.65 ml microcentrifuge tubes as follows:

Gel-loading solution[4]	5.0 µl
Amplified DNA from each of the PCR tubes and an extra tube is set up for a DNA ladder:	15.0 µl
Gel-loading solution[4]	5.0 µl
100 base-pair ladder[5]	1.0 µl

vi) Samples are loaded into the appropriate wells in the gel and run at 65–75 volts for 1–1.5 hours or until the dye has travelled about half the length of the gel. The gel is transferred to a transilluminator and photographed for a permanent record. Use protective eye-wear to visualise the gel bands.

vii) BT-positive samples will have a band of 101 base pairs. For the test to be valid, the positive control must show a band of the correct size, and the negative and 'no RNA' controls show no band. Samples are considered to be positive if there is a band of the same size as the positive control. Duplicate samples should show the same reaction. If there is disparity, the test should be repeated.

viii) A destaining bag[6] is placed in the tank buffer overnight to remove the ethidium bromide. The buffer can then be poured down the drain and the destaining bag, after reuse 10–15 times, should be placed in a properly identified ethidium bromide waste container and ultimately incinerated.

Kits and reagents for two prescribed serological tests, AGID and competitive ELISA, are available for three licensed manufacturers in the USA[7] and from the European Union 'Community Reference Laboratory' for BTV[8].

2. Serological tests

Anti-BTV antibody generated in infected animals can be detected in a variety of ways that depend on the sensitivity and type of test used. Both serogroup-specific and serotype-specific antibodies are elicited and if the animal was not previously exposed to BTV, the neutralising antibodies generated are specific for the infecting virus. Multiple infections with different BTV serotypes lead to the production of antibodies capable of neutralising serotypes to which the animal has not been exposed. There are two explanations for this phenomenon. First, several serotypes share MAb-defined neutralisation epitopes. Secondly, serotypes also share a large number of epitopes that are present in a neutralising conformation in one serotype, but in non-neutralising conformations in other serotypes.

a) Complement fixation

A complement fixation (CF) test to detect BTV antibodies was widely used until 1982, when it was largely replaced by the AGID test although the CF test is still in use in some countries.

b) Agar gel immunodiffusion (a prescribed test for international trade)

The AGID test to detect anti-BTV antibodies is simple to perform and the antigen used in the assay is relatively easy to generate. Since 1982, the test has been the standard testing procedure for the international movement of ruminants. However, one of the disadvantages of the AGID used for BT is its lack of specificity in that it can detect antibodies to other orbiviruses, particularly those in the EHD serogroup.

3 FMC Bioproducts, Rockland, Maine, USA.
4 Cat. G-2526, Sigma, St Louis, Missouri, USA.
5 Cat. 15268-019, Life Technologies, Grand Island, New York, USA.
6 Ameresco, Solon, Ohio, USA.
7 VMRD, P.O. Box 502, Pullman, Washington 99163, USA; or Veterinary Diagnostic Technology, 4980 Van Gordon Street, Suite 101, Wheat Ridge, Colorado 80033, USA; or Diagxotics, 27 Cannon Road, Wilton, Conneticut 06897, USA.
8 Pirbright Laboratory, Ash Road, Pirbright, Woking GU24 0NF, United Kingdom.

This fact and the subjectivity exercised in reading the results have encouraged the development of ELISA-based procedures for the specific detection of anti-BTV antibodies. The preferred format, a competitive ELISA, is described in Section A.2.c.

- **Test procedure**

i) A 2.8 mm thick layer of 0.9% agarose in 0.85% NaCl is prepared and circular wells 4.0 mm in diameter and 2.4 mm apart are cut out with six wells arranged around a central well.

ii) Viral antigen is prepared by generating a crude soluble preparation from BHK or Vero cells infected with a single BTV serotype 24–48 hours previously. Antigen can be concentrated by precipitation or ultrafiltration.

iii) Three positive and three test sera are placed in alternate wells surrounding antigen in the central well and the plates are incubated at 20–25°C in a humid environment for 24 hours.

iv) A series of precipitin lines form between the antigen and known positive sera and lines generated by strong positive test sera will join up with those of the positive controls. With weak positive samples, the control lines bend toward the antigen and away from the test sample well, but may not form a continuous line between the control test wells. With negative samples, the precipitin lines will continue into the sample wells without bending toward the antigen.

v) All weak positive samples and other samples that produce questionable results should be repeated using wells that are 5.3 mm in diameter placed 2.4 mm apart or retested using the competitive ELISA as described below.

c) Competitive enzyme linked immunosorbent assay (a prescribed test for international trade)

The BT competitive or blocking ELISA was developed to measure BTV-specific antibody without detecting cross-reacting antibody to other orbiviruses (1, 3, 17, 25). The specificity is the result of using one of a number of BT serogroup-reactive MAbs, such as MAb 3-17-A3 (3) or MAb 20E9 (17). The antibodies were derived in a number of laboratories, and although different, all appear to bind to the amino-terminal region of the major core protein VP7. In the competitive ELISA, antibodies in test sera compete with the MAbs for binding to antigen. The following procedure for the competitive ELISA has been standardised after comparative studies in a number of international laboratories.

- **Test procedure**

i) First, 96-well microtitre plates are coated at 4°C overnight or 37°C for 1 hour with 50–100 µl of either tissue-culture-derived sonicated cell culture antigen (3), baculovirus-expressed VP7 (23) or yeast-expressed viral VP7 antigen (19) diluted in 0.05 M carbonate buffer, pH 9.6.

ii) The plates are washed five times with PBST (0.01 M phosphate buffered saline containing 0.05% or 0.1% Tween 20, pH 7.2).

iii) Next, 50 µl of test sera is added in duplicate at a single dilution, either 1/5 (1) or 1/10 (17) in PBST containing 3% bovine serum albumin (BSA).

iv) Immediately 50 µl of a predetermined dilution of MAb diluted in PBST containing 3% BSA is added to each well. MAb control wells contain diluent buffer in place of test serum.

v) Plates are incubated for 1 hour at 37°C or 3 hours at 25°C, with continuous shaking.

vi) After washing as described above, wells are filled with 100 µl of an appropriate dilution of horseradish-peroxidase-labelled rabbit anti-mouse IgG (H+L) in PBST containing 2% normal bovine serum.

vii) Following incubation for 1 hour at 37°C, the conjugate solution is discarded and plates are washed five times using PBS or PBST. Wells are filled with 100 µl substrate solution containing 1.0 mM ABTS (2,2'-Azino-bis-[3-ethylbenzothiazoline-6-sulphonic acid]) – 4 mM H_2O_2 in 50 mM sodium citrate, pH 4.0, and plates are shaken at 25°C for 30 minutes. (Other substrates may be used and the reaction continued with shaking for an appropriate length of time to permit colour development.)

viii) The reaction is stopped by addition of a stopping reagent, such as sodium azide.

ix) After blanking the ELISA reader on wells containing substrate and stopping reagent, the absorbance values are measured at 414 nm. Results are expressed as percentage inhibition and are derived from the mean absorbance values for each sample by the following formula.

$$\%\text{ inhibition} = 100 - \left[\frac{\text{Mean absorbance test sample}}{\text{Mean absorbance MAb control}} \times 100\right]$$

NB: Some laboratories prefer to use a negative control serum that has previously been shown to have a percentage inhibition of zero, as an alternative to the MAb control.

x) Percentage inhibition values >50% are considered to be positive. Inhibition between 40% and 50% is considered to be suspicious. The results of the duplicates of test sera can vary as long as they do not lie either side of the chosen inhibition value.

xi) Strong and weak positive sera and a negative serum should be included on each plate. The weak positive should give 60–80% inhibition and the negative should give less than 40% inhibition.

B. REQUIREMENTS FOR VACCINES AND DIAGNOSTIC BIOLOGICALS

Of several vaccine options available, namely live attenuated, killed or recombinant, only attenuated virus vaccines are in current use in several countries. In South Africa, for example, they have been used for over 40 years and are known to induce an effective and lasting immunity (9). Although the efficacy of inactivated virus vaccines has been investigated in some laboratory studies (4), they do not appear to have been used in the field. There are several options for the development of recombinant BTV vaccines, including live virus delivery of BTV neutralisation antigens and the virus-like particles (VLP) generated in infected insect cells by recombinant baculoviruses expressing the four major BTV coat proteins, VP2, 3, 5 and 7. Only the latter has shown significant promise (27). However there is still much to determine, such as the longevity of the neutralising response generated to VLP, the need for multiple VLPs for different serotypes, and the commercial scale-up of VLP production in a cost-effective and efficient process. The following description applies to attenuated virus vaccines.

1. Seed management

a) Characteristics of the seed

The master or primary virus seed is prepared from a single plaque of serially passaged, attenuated BTV. Secondary seed lots, which are used as inocula for vaccine production, are usually not more than three passages beyond the primary seed lot. Primary seed virus must be free from contaminating bacteria, viruses, fungi and mycoplasma, and must be shown to have the desired serotype specificity. Each primary seed virus lot should also be tested for transmissibility and reversion to virulence prior to vaccine manufacture. Samples of vaccine prepared from secondary seed virus at the maximum permitted passage level should be tested in sheep for avirulence, safety and immunogenicity.

b) Method of culture

The first BT vaccines were propagated in ECE (2, 21). More recently, several different cells have been used for tissue culture adaptation and serial passage. These include primary bovine embryo (16), lamb and fetal lamb kidney cells, and the continuous BHK cells. Cells used for attenuation must be thoroughly checked for the presence of contaminating viruses. Not only may continuous cell lines harbour oncogenic viruses, but primary cells may contain a number of latent virus infections. Vaccine viruses have been attenuated by either passage in ECE, tissue culture cells or a combination of both.

c) Validation as a vaccine

Attenuated BT vaccines must be safe and efficacious, and a brief description of appropriate tests for these parameters is given below. In addition, attenuated viruses should not revert to virulence during replication in vaccinated animals or be transmitted from such animals by insect vectors. The latter criterion is very important because insect-mediated transmission of attenuated virus from vaccinated to nonimmune animals, with the subsequent replicative steps in each host species, increases the possibility of reversion to virulence. Although tests for reversion to virulence and transmissibility are rarely, if ever, performed, a brief description of what may be necessary is outlined.

i) *Avirulence*

A number of sheep, seronegative by BT competitive ELISA, are inoculated with either the primary seed stock virus or an equal volume of tissue culture medium. Temperatures are noted twice daily. The animals are monitored at regular intervals over a period of 28 days for clinical signs and any local or systemic reactions to ensure avirulence and innocuity. Blood samples removed at regular intervals can be used to measure viraemia and antibody responses. The test shall be valid if all of the sheep inoculated with vaccine show evidence of virus growth and do not display signs of disease other than mild transient illness. In South Africa, a clinical reaction index (27) is calculated for each animal between days 4 and 14 and must be below a specific standard value.

ii) *Safety*

Safety tests for attenuated vaccines do not address the issue of their teratogenicity (9, 28). Attenuated virus vaccines are teratogenic and should not be administered to pregnant sheep during the first-half of pregnancy, as this may cause fetal abnormalities and death.

iii) *Efficacy*

Vaccinated and unvaccinated sheep are challenged with virulent virus of the same serotype and animals are monitored for clinical signs of BT. Rectal temperatures are taken twice daily. Unvaccinated control sheep should show clinical signs of BT. However, it is difficult to be certain of the appearance of clinical disease following inoculation of sheep with certain BTV serotypes and isolates, and consequently, evidence of infection of unvaccinated control sheep may rest on the appearance of a temperature rise of at least 1.7°C over the prechallenge mean. Pre- and post-vaccination sera are checked for the presence of neutralising antibody.

iv) *Transmissibility*

Procedures to determine if attenuated virus can be transmitted by insects that feed on vaccinated, viraemic sheep are difficult to perform and analyse statistically, and consequently, this criterion of vaccine validation is rarely sought. Laboratory data indicate that laboratory-adapted viruses can be transmitted by insect vectors (29). A suitable procedure to determine attenuated virus transmissibility requires that sheep be vaccinated and, during viraemia, that they be exposed to competent, uninfected *Culicoides*, which are then permitted to feed on uninfected animals that are monitored for the presence of BTV and anti-BTV antibody. Due to the fact that the titre of attenuated virus in the blood of vaccinated sheep is low, very large numbers of *Culicoides* would be needed and only a small proportion of these would become infected and live long enough to feed on and potentially transmit the virus to other uninfected sheep. It is difficult to design a laboratory experiment that takes account of the large numbers of vaccinated sheep and insects that would be present in field situations. However, in South Africa it is estimated that the minimum titre of virus circulating in the bloodstream of an animal must be at least 10^3 before feeding *Culicoides* become infected, although it has also been suggested that a lower titre may sometimes be infective. Consequently, to select a suitable attenuated virus strain, whole blood is collected between days 4 and 14 after vaccination, and the virus titre is determined. Only attenuated viruses that generate titres under 10^3 are deemed to be acceptable as vaccines.

Current data indicate that during viraemia and in contrast to wild-type virus, laboratory-adapted strains of BTV may be found in the semen of bulls and rams (26). The implications of these observations for virus transmissibility are unclear.

v) *Reversion to virulence*

Validation studies confirm that attenuated viruses do not revert to virulence in vaccinated sheep. Consequently, if attenuated viruses are not transmitted by insects from vaccinated to unvaccinated animals, reversion to virulence becomes a theoretical possibility only. However, if attenuated viruses can be transmitted from vaccinated animals, reversion to virulence during a number of sheep–insect replication cycles becomes a distinct prospect. The most appropriate way to monitor reversion to virulence under these circumstances is to compare the virulence of the vaccine virus with that which had been subject to several sheep–insect replication cycles as described above. As indicated, this is exceedingly difficult to achieve. Consequently, the effect of a number of sheep–insect passages on the virulence of attenuated viruses has not been determined. It should be possible to examine the *in-vitro* correlate of this process using *Aedes albopictus* or *Culicoides* cell lines, although it is recognised that this may not exactly duplicate the situation in the intact insect. In South Africa it is accepted that if blood from vaccinated animals during the viraemic stages is serially passaged three times in sheep without reversion to virulence, the chances of reversion in the field will be infinitely small.

2. Method of manufacture

Attenuation of field isolates of BTV was first achieved by serial passage in ECE. More recently, it is clear that passage in cultured cells will also result in attenuation of virulence. No studies have been done to relate precisely passage number and extent of attenuation for individual virus isolates or serotypes. To prepare attenuated virus, field isolates are adapted to cell culture and passaged *in vitro* up to 40 times or more. Ideally, a number of plaque-purified viruses are picked at this stage and each is examined to determine the level of viraemia they generate and their ability to elicit a protective immune response in vaccinated sheep. The most suitable virus is one that replicates to low titre but generates a protective immune response, and this may represent the source of vaccine primary seed stock virus.

3. In-process control

All ingredients of animal origin, including serum and cells, must be checked for contamination by viable bacteria, viruses, fungi or mycoplasmas.

4. Batch control

a) Sterility

Every batch of vaccine should be tested for the presence of viable bacteria, extraneous viruses, fungi or mycoplasmas. For example, in South Africa a pool of ten randomly selected ampoules are inoculated into soya broth and thioglycollate broth, and incubated at room temperature and 37°C, respectively, for 14 days. If contaminated, the batch is disqualified.

b) Safety

Every batch is safety tested in newborn and adult mice, guinea-pigs and sheep. If any adverse reactions or significant signs are noted, the test is repeated. Any increase in the body temperature of the target animal that is above the level expected for the particular strain of attenuated virus under test should be regarded as symptomatic. If the results are unsatisfactory, the batch is disqualified.

c) Potency

Each batch is tested by inoculating susceptible sheep. Prevaccination, and 21- and 28-day post-vaccination sera are tested by VN assay to determine neutralising antibody levels. In order to be passed, the antibody titre must be equal to or higher than a set standard based on International vaccine standards.

d) Duration of immunity

Studies with live attenuated BTV vaccine have shown that antibodies in sheep may appear before day 10 post-vaccination, reach a maximum approximately 4 weeks later, and persist for well over a year. There is a temporal relationship between the increase in neutralising antibody titre and clearance of virus from the peripheral circulation. Live attenuated BTV vaccines have been in use for over 40 years and are known to induce an effective and lasting immunity (9). Many serotypes of BTV are present in endemic areas of South Africa, and polyvalent vaccines are used. The inclusion of 15 serotypes in the vaccine means that an effective immune response is not generated to all serotypes, presumably because the antigenic mass of individual serotype-specific antigens is small. In an attempt to broaden the response, vaccination is repeated annually (8).

e) Stability

Stability should be tested over a period of 2 years. Vaccines in liquid and lyophilised forms are deemed to have shelf lives of 1 and 2 years, respectively. Each batch of vaccine is subjected to an accelerated shelf-life test by storing it at 37°C for 7 days. It is then titrated and evaluated according to a set standard, as determined in the initial testing of the vaccine.

f) Precautions (hazards)

The polyvalent vaccine is safe except if used in ewes during the first-half of pregnancy. Lambs possessing colostral immunity cannot be effectively vaccinated before 6 months of age.

5. Tests on the final product

a) Safety

See B.4.b

b) Potency

See B.4.c

• Acknowledgement

I wish to thank Dr H. Aitchison for providing information relating to BT vaccine production and testing, particularly vaccine validation and batch control at Onderstepoort Biological Products, South Africa and Dr J.E. Pearson, National Veterinary Services Laboratories, Ames, Iowa, USA for providing the detailed bluetongue PCR protocol.

REFERENCES

1. AFSHAR A., THOMAS F.C., WRIGHT P.F., SHAPIRO J.L. & ANDERSON J. (1989). Comparison of competitive ELISA, indirect ELISA and standard AGID tests for detecting bluetongue virus antibodies in cattle and sheep. *Vet. Rec.*, **124**, 136–141.

2. ALEXANDER R.A. & HAIG D.A. (1951). The use of egg attenuated bluetongue in the production of a polyvalent vaccine for sheep. A. Propagation of the virus in sheep. *Onderstepoort J. Vet. Res.*, **25**, 3–15.

3. ANDERSON J. (1984). Use of monoclonal antibody in a blocking ELISA to detect group specific antibodies to bluetongue virus. *J. Immunol. Methods*, **74**, 139–149.

4. BARBER T.L. & CAMPBELL C.H. (1984). Experimental bluetongue vaccine inactivated by gamma irradiation. *Proc. U. S. Anim. Health Assoc.*, 131–142.

5. BLACKSELL S.D. & LUNT R.A. (1993). Serotype identification of Australian bluetongue viruses using a rapid fluorescence inhibition test. *J. Virol. Methods*, **44**, 241–250.

6. CHERRINGTON J.M., GHALIB H.W., SAWYER M.M. & OSBURN B.I. (1985). Detection of viral antigens in bluetongue virus-infected ovine tissues using the peroxidase-antiperoxidase technique. *Am. J. Vet. Res.*, **46**, 2356–2359.

7. DANGLER C.A., DE MATTOS C.A., DE MATTOS C.C. & OSBURN B.I. (1990). Identifying bluetongue virus ribonucleic acid sequences by the polymerase chain reaction. *J. Virol. Methods*, **28**, 281–292.

8. ERASMUS B.J. (1975). Bluetongue in sheep and goats. *Aust. Vet. J.*, **51**, 165–170.

9. ERASMUS B.J. (1990). Bluetongue virus. *In:* Virus Infections of Ruminants, Dinter Z. & Morein B., eds. Elsevier, New York, USA, 227–237.

10. GARD G.P. & KIRKLAND P.D. (1993). Bluetongue virology and serology. *In:* Australian Standard Diagnostic Techniques for Animal Diseases, Corner L.A. & Bagust T.J., eds. CSIRO Information Services, PO Box 89, East Melbourne, Victoria 3002, Australia.

11. GORMAN B.M. (1990). The bluetongue viruses. *Curr. Top. Microbiol. Immunol.*, **162**, 1–19.

12. GOULD A.R. (1987). The complete nucleotide sequence of bluetongue virus serotype 1 RNA3 and a comparison with other geographic serotypes from Australia, South Africa and the United States of America, and with other orbivirus isolates. *Virus Res.*, **7**, 169–183.

13. GRIMES J.M., BURROUGHS J.N., GOUET P., DIPROSE J.M., MALBY R., ZIENTARA S., MERTENS P.P. & STUART D.I. (1998). The atomic structure of the bluetongue virus core. *Nature*, **395**, 470–478.

14. HEWAT E.A., BOOTH T.F. & ROY P. (1992). Structure of bluetongue virus particles by cryoelectron microscopy. *J. Struct. Biol.*, **109**, 61–69.

15. KATZ J.B., ALSTAD, A.D., GUSTAFSON, G.A. & MOSER K.M. (1993). Sensitive Identification of bluetongue virus serogroup by a colorimetric dual oligonucleotide sorbent assay of amplified viral nucleic acid. *J. Clin. Microbiol.*, **31**, 3028–3030.

16. KEMENY L. & DREHLE L.E. (1961). The use of tissue culture propagated bluetongue virus for vaccine production. *Am. J. Vet. Res.*, **22**, 921–925.

17. LUNT R.A., WHITE J.R. & BLACKSELL S.D. (1988). Evaluation of a monoclonal antibody blocking ELISA for the detection of group-specific antibodies to bluetongue virus in experimental and field sera. *J. Gen. Virol.*, **69**, 2729–2740.

18. MacLachlan N.J., Nunamaker R.A., Katz J.B., Sawyer M.M., Akita G.Y., Osburn B.I. & Taberchnick W.J. (1994). Detection of bluetongue virus in the blood of inoculated calves: comparison of virus isolation, PCR assay and *in vitro* feeding of *Culicoides variipennis*. *Arch. Virol.*, **136**, 1–8.

19. Martyn C.J., Gould A.R. & Eaton B.T. (1990). High level expression of the major core protein VP7 and the non-structural protein NS3 of bluetongue virus in yeast. Use of expressed VP7 as a diagnostic group-reactive antigen in a blocking ELISA. *Virus Res.*, **18**, 165–178.

20. McColl K.A. & Gould A.R. (1991). Detection and characterisation of bluetongue virus using the polymerase chain reaction. *Virus Res.*, **21**, 19–34.

21. McKercher D.G., McGowan B., Cabasso V.J., Roberts G.I. & Saito J.K. (1957). Studies on bluetongue. III. The development of a modified live virus vaccine employing American strains of bluetongue virus. *Am. J. Vet. Res.*, **28**, 310–316.

22. Meecham J.O., Dean V.C., Wigington J.G. & Nunamaker R.A. (1990). Detection of bluetongue virus in *Culicoides variipennis* (Diptera: Ceratopogonidae) by an antigen capture enzyme-linked immunosorbent assay. *J. Med. Entomol.*, **27**, 602–606.

23. Oldfield S., Adachi A., Urakawa T., Hirasawa T. & Roy P. (1990). Purification and characterization of the major group-specific core antigen VP7 of bluetongue virus synthesized by a recombinant baculovirus. *J. Gen. Virol.*, **71**, 2649–2656.

24. Parker J., Herniman K.A.J., Gibbs E.P.J. & Sellers R.F. (1975). An experimental inactivated vaccine against bluetongue. *Vet. Rec.*, **96**, 284–287.

25. Reddington J.J., Reddington G.M. & MacLachlan N.J. (1991). A competitive ELISA for detection of antibodies to the group antigen of bluetongue virus. *J. Vet. Diagn. Invest.*, **3**, 144–147.

26. Roberts D.H., Lucus M.H. & Bell R.A. (1992). Animal and animal product importation and the assessment of risk. *In:* Bluetongue, African Horse Sickness and Related Orbiviruses, Walton T.E. & Osburn B.I., eds. CRC Press, Boca Raton, Florida, USA, 916–923.

27. Roy P., Bishop D.H.L., Leblois H. & Erasmus B.J. (1994). Long-lasting protection of sheep against bluetongue challenge after vaccination with virus-like particles: evidence for homologous and partial heterologous protection. *Vaccine*, **12**, 802–811.

28. Shultz G. & Delay P.D. (1955). Losses in newborn lambs associated with bluetongue vaccination of pregnant ewes. *J. Am. Vet. Med. Assoc.*, **128**, 224–226.

29. Standfast H.A., Dyce A.L. & Muller M.J. (1985). Vectors of BT virus in Australia. *In:* Bluetongue and Related Orbiviruses, Barber T.L. & Jochim M.M., eds. Alan R. Liss, New York, USA, 177–186.

30. Wade-Evans A.M., Mertens P.P.C. & Bostock C.J. (1990). Development of the polymerase chain reaction for the detection of bluetongue virus in tissue samples. *J. Virol. Methods*, **30**, 15–24.

*

* *

CHAPTER 2.1.10.

SHEEP POX AND GOAT POX

SUMMARY

Sheep pox and goat pox are viral diseases of sheep and goats characterised by fever, generalised papules or nodules, vesicles (rarely), internal lesions (particularly in the lungs), and death. Both diseases are caused by strains of capripoxvirus, all of which can infect sheep and goats, and although most of the strains examined cause more severe clinical disease in either sheep or goats, some strains have been isolated that are equally pathogenic in both species. It has been proposed that the malignant pox diseases of sheep and goats caused by capripoxvirus and including Kenyan sheep and goat pox, Indian goat dermatitis and north African stone pox of sheep and goats be referred to as capripox.

Capripox is endemic in Africa north of the Equator, the Middle East, Turkey, Iran, Afghanistan, Pakistan, India, Nepal, parts of the people's Republic of China and, since 1984, Bangladesh. Recently, it has made frequent incursions into southern Europe.

Identification of the agent: *Laboratory confirmation of capripox is most rapid by the demonstration of typical capripox virions using the transmission electron microscope in combination with a clinical history of generalised capripox infection. The capripox virion is distinct from the other poxvirus commonly infecting sheep and goats – a parapoxvirus that causes orf or contagious pustular dermatitis. A precipitating antigen can be identified by an agar gel immunodiffusion test (AGID) using lymph gland biopsy material taken from an early case of capripox and specific immune sera; however, there is a cross-reaction with parapoxvirus. Capripoxvirus will grow on tissue culture of ovine, caprine or bovine origin, although field isolates may require up to 14 days to grow or require one or more additional tissue culture passages. The virus causes intracytoplasmic inclusions, clearly seen using haemotoxylin and eosin staining. The antigen can also be detected in tissue culture using specific sera and immunoperoxidase or immunofluorescence techniques. Capripoxvirus antigen and inclusion bodies may be seen in stained cryostat or paraffin sections of biopsy or post-mortem lesion material.*

An antigen-detection enzyme-linked immunosorbent assay (ELISA) using a polyclonal detection serum raised against a recombinant immunodominant antigen of capripoxvirus has been developed. Genome detection using capripoxvirus-specific primers for the fusion protein gene and attachment protein gene has also been reported.

Serological tests: *The virus neutralisation test is the most specific serological test, but because immunity to capripox infection is predominantly cell mediated, the test is not sufficiently sensitive to identify animals that have had contact with the virus and developed only low levels of neutralising antibody. The AGID and indirect immunofluorescence test are less specific due to cross-reactions with antibody to other poxviruses. Western blotting using the reaction between the P32 antigen of capripoxvirus with test sera is both sensitive and specific, but is expensive and difficult to carry out. The use of this antigen, expressed by a suitable vector, in an ELISA offers the prospect of an acceptable and standardised serological test.*

Requirements for vaccines and diagnostic biologicals: *Live and inactivated vaccines have been used for the control of capripox. All strains of capripoxvirus so far examined share a major neutralisation site and will cross protect. Inactivated vaccines give, at best, only short-term immunity.*

A. DIAGNOSTIC TECHNIQUES

Sheep pox and goat pox (capripox) are endemic in central and north Africa, the Middle East and India. Capripox is caused by strains of capripoxvirus and produces a characteristic clinical disease in fully susceptible breeds of sheep and goats that cannot be confused with any other disease. In indigenous animals, generalised disease and mortality are less common, although they are seen where disease has been absent from an area or village for a period of time, when intensive husbandry methods are introduced, or in association with other disease agents, such as peste des petits ruminants virus or foot and mouth disease virus.

Capripox is a major constraint to the introduction of exotic breeds of sheep and goats, and to the development of intensive livestock production. Strains of capripoxvirus that cause lumpy skin disease (such as Neethling), are also found in cattle, but there is no evidence that these strains will naturally cause disease in sheep and goats. The geographical distribution of lumpy skin disease differs from that of sheep pox and goat pox.

Strains of capripoxvirus do pass between sheep and goats, although most cause more severe clinical disease in only one species; recombination also occurs between these strains, producing a spectrum showing intermediate host preferences and a range of virulence. Some strains are equally pathogenic in both sheep and goats. Capripox has the potential to spread and become established in countries outside its normal distribution. In 1983 it spread into Italy, in 1985 and 1989 into Cyprus, and in 1988 into Greece, but did not become established in these countries. In 1984, however, it spread into Bangladesh where it has persisted. During the past decade there have been further frequent incursions into Greece and Bulgaria.

The incubation period is between 8 and 13 days following contact between an infected and susceptible animals. It may be as short as 4 days following experimental infection by intradermal inoculation or mechanical transmission by insects. Some breeds of European sheep, such as Soay, may die of acute infection before the development of skin lesions. In other breeds there is an initial rise in rectal temperature to above 40°C, followed in 2–5 days by the development of, at first, macules – small circumscribed areas of hyperaemia, which are most obvious on unpigmented skin, and then of papules – hard swellings of between 0.5 and 1 cm in diameter, which may cover the body or be restricted to the groin, axilla and perineum. Papules may be covered by fluid-filled vesicles, but this is rare. A flat haemorrhagic form of capripox has been observed in some breeds of European goat, in which all the papules appear to coalesce over the body; this form is always fatal.

Within 24 hours of the appearance of generalised papules, affected animals develop rhinitis, conjunctivitis and enlargement of all the superficial lymph glands, in particular the prescapular lymph glands. Papules on the eyelids cause blepharitis of varying severity. As the papules on the mucous membranes of the eyes and nose ulcerate, so the discharge becomes mucopurulent, and the mucosae of the mouth, anus, and prepuce or vagina become necrotic. Breathing may become laboured and noisy due to pressure on the upper respiratory tract from the swollen retropharyngeal lymph glands and to the developing lung lesions.

If the affected animal does not die in this acute phase of the disease, the papules start to become necrotic from ischaemic necrosis following thrombi formation in the blood vessels at the base of the papule. In the following 5–10 days the papules form scabs, which persist for up to 6 weeks, leaving small scars. The skin lesions are susceptible to fly strike, and secondary pneumonia is common. Anorexia is not usual unless the mouth lesions physically interfere with feeding. Abortion is rare.

On post-mortem examination of the acutely infected animal, the skin lesions are often less obvious than on the live animal. The mucous membranes are necrotic and all the body lymph nodes are enlarged and oedematous. Papules, which may be ulcerated, can usually be found on the abomasal mucosa, and sometimes on the wall of the rumen and large intestine, on the tongue, hard and soft palate, trachea and oesophagus. Pale areas of approximately 2 cm in diameter may occasionally be seen on the surface of the kidney and liver, and have been reported to be present in the testicles. Throughout the lungs, but particularly in the diaphragmatic lobes, there are numerous hard lesions of up to 5 cm in diameter

The clinical signs and post-mortem lesions vary considerably with breed of host and strain of capripoxvirus. Indigenous breeds are less susceptible and frequently show only a few lesions, which could be confused with insect bites or contagious pustular dermatitis. However, lambs that have lost their maternally derived immunity, animals that have been kept isolated and animals brought into endemic areas from isolated villages, particularly if they have been subjected to the stress of moving long distances and mixing with other sheep and goats and their pathogens, can often be seen with generalised and sometimes fatal capripox. Invariably there is high mortality in unprotected imported breeds of sheep and goats following capripoxvirus infection. Capripox is not infectious to humans.

1. Identification of the agent

• Sample collection, submission and preparation

Material for virus isolation and antigen detection should be collected by biopsy or on post-mortem from skin papules, lung lesions or lymph nodes. Samples for virus isolation and antigen-detection enzyme-linked immunosorbent assay (ELISA) should be collected within the first week of the occurrence of clinical signs, before the development of neutralising antibodies. Samples for genome detection by polymerase chain reaction (PCR) may be collected when neutralising antibody is present. Buffy coat from blood collected into heparin or EDTA (ethylene diamine tetra-acetic acid) during the viraemic stage of capripox (before generalisation of lesions or within 4 days of generalisation), can also be used for virus isolation. Samples for histology should include tissue from the surrounding area and should be placed immediately following collection into ten times the sample volume of 10% formalin.

Tissues in formalin have no special transportation requirements. Blood samples with anticoagulant for virus isolation from the buffy coat should be placed immediately on ice and processed as soon as possible. In practice, the samples may be kept at 4°C for up to 2 days prior to processing, but should not be frozen or kept at ambient temperatures. Tissues for virus isolation, antigen detection and genome detection should be kept at 4°C, on ice or at -20°C. If it is necessary to transport samples over long distances without refrigeration, the medium should contain 10% glycerol; the samples should be of sufficient size that the transport medium does not penetrate the central part of the biopsy, which should be used for virus isolation/detection.

Material for histology should be prepared by standard techniques and stained with haematoxylin and eosin (H&E). Lesion material for virus isolation and antigen detection is minced using sterile scissors and forceps and then ground in a sterile pestle and mortar with sterile sand and an equal volume of sterile phosphate buffered saline (PBS) containing sodium penicillin (1000 international units [IU]/ml), streptomycin sulphate (1 mg/ml), mycostatin (100 IU/ml) or fungizone (2.5 µg/ml) and neomycin (200 IU/ml). The suspension is freeze–thawed three times and then partially clarified by centrifugation using a bench centrifuge at 600 ***g*** for 10 minutes. Buffy coats may be prepared from unclotted blood by centrifugation at 600 ***g*** for 15 minutes, and the buffy coat carefully removed into 5 ml of cold double distilled water using a sterile Pasteur pipette. After 30 seconds, 5 ml of cold double strength growth medium is added and mixed. The mixture is centrifuged at 600 ***g*** for 15 minutes, the supernatant is discarded and the cell pellet is suspended in 5 ml of growth medium, such as Glasgow's modified Eagle's medium (GMEM). After centrifugation at 600 ***g*** for a further 15 minutes, the resulting pellet is suspended in 5 ml of fresh GMEM. Alternatively, the buffy coat may be separated from a heparinised sample using a Ficoll gradient.

a) Culture

Capripoxvirus will grow in tissue culture of bovine, ovine or caprine origin, although primary or secondary cultures of lamb testis (LT) or lamb kidney (LK) cells are considered to be the most susceptible, particularly those derived from a wool sheep breed. Either 1 ml of buffy coat cell suspension or 1 ml of clarified biopsy preparation supernatant is inoculated on to a 25 cm^2 tissue culture flask of 90% confluent LT or LK cells, and allowed to absorb for 1 hour at 37°C. The culture is then washed with warm PBS and covered with 10 ml of a suitable medium, such as GMEM, containing antibiotics and 2% fetal calf serum. If available, tissue culture tubes containing LT or LK cells and a flying cover-slip, or tissue culture microscope slides, are also infected.

The flasks should be examined daily for 14 days for evidence of cytopathic effect (CPE), and the medium is replaced if it appears to be cloudy. Infected cells develop a characteristic CPE consisting of retraction of the cell membrane from surrounding cells, and eventually rounding of cells and margination of the nuclear chromatin. At first only small areas of CPE can be seen, sometimes as soon as 4 days after infection; over the following 4–6 days these expand to involve the whole cell sheet. If no CPE is apparent by day 14, the culture should be freeze–thawed three times, and clarified supernatant inoculated on to fresh LT or LK culture. At the first sign of CPE in the flasks, or earlier if a number of infected cover-slips are being used, a cover-slip should be removed, fixed in acetone and stained using H&E. Eosinophilic intracytoplasmic inclusion bodies, which are variable in size but up to half the size of the nucleus and surrounded by a clear halo, are diagnostic for poxvirus infection. Syncytia formation is not a feature of capripoxvirus infection. The CPE can be prevented or delayed by inclusion in the medium of specific anti-capripoxvirus serum. Some strains of capripoxvirus have been adapted to grow on African green monkey kidney (Vero) cells, but these are not recommended for primary isolation.

- **Electron microscopy**

Before centrifugation, material from the original suspension is prepared for examination under the transmission electron microscope by floating a 400-mesh hexagon electron microscope grid, with pileoform-carbon substrate activated by glow discharge in pentylamine vapour, on to a drop of the suspension placed on parafilm or a wax plate. After 1 minute, the grid is transferred to a drop of Tris/EDTA buffer, pH 7.8, for 20 seconds and then to a drop of 1% phosphotungstic acid, pH 7.2, for 10 seconds. The grid is drained using filter paper, air-dried and placed in the electron microscope. The capripox virion is brick shaped, covered in short tubular elements and measures approximately 290 × 270 nm. A host-cell-derived membrane may surround some of the virions, and as many as possible should be examined to confirm their appearance (15).

The virions of capripoxvirus are indistinguishable from those of orthopoxvirus, but, apart from vaccinia virus, no orthopoxvirus causes lesions in sheep and goats. The virions of parapoxvirus that cause contagious pustular dermatitis are smaller, oval in shape, and each is covered in a single continuous tubular element, which appears as striations over the virion.

- **Histology**

Following preparation, staining with H&E, and mounting of the formalin-fixed biopsy material, a number of sections should be examined by light microscopy. On histological examination, the most striking aspects of acute-stage skin lesions are a massive cellular infiltrate, vasculitis and oedema. Early lesions are characterised by marked perivascular cuffing. Initially infiltration is by macrophages, neutrophils and occasionally eosinophils, and as the lesion progresses, by more macrophages, lymphocytes and plasma cells. A characteristic feature of all capripoxvirus infections is the presence of variable numbers of 'sheep pox cells' in the dermis. These sheep pox cells can also occur in other organs where microscopic lesions of sheep and goat pox are present. These cells are large, stellate cells with eosinophillic, poorly defined intracytoplasmic inclusions and vacuolated nuclei. Vasculitis is accompanied by thrombosis and infarction, causing oedema and necrosis. Epidermal changes consist of acanthosis, parakeratosis and hyperkeratosis. Changes in other organs are similar, with a predominant cellular infiltration and vasculitis. Lesions in the upper respiratory tract are characterised by ulceration.

- **Animal inoculation**

Clarified biopsy preparation supernatant (see Section A.1.a. Culture), may also be used for intradermal inoculation into susceptible lambs. These lambs should be examined daily for evidence of a skin reaction.

b) Immunological methods

- **Fluorescent antibody tests**

Capripoxvirus antigen can also be identified on the infected cover-slips or tissue culture slides using fluorescent antibody tests. Cover-slips or slides should be washed and air-dried and fixed in cold acetone for 10 minutes. The indirect test using immune sheep or goat sera is subject to high background colour and nonspecific reactions. However, a direct conjugate can be prepared from sera from convalescent sheep or goats or from rabbits hyperimmunised with purified capripoxvirus. Uninfected tissue culture should be included as a negative control as cross-reactions, due to antibodies to cell culture antigens, can cause problems.

- **Agar gel immunodiffusion**

An agar gel immunodiffusion (AGID) test has been used for detecting the precipitating antigen of capripoxvirus, but has the disadvantage that this antigen is shared by parapoxvirus. Agarose (1%) is prepared in borate buffer, pH 8.6, dissolved by heating, and 2 ml is poured on to a glass microscope slide (76 × 26 mm). When the agar has solidified, wells are cut to give a six-well rosette around a central well. Each well is 5 mm in diameter, with a distance of 7 mm between the middle of the central well and the middle of each peripheral well. The wells are filled as follows: 18 µl of the lesion suspension is added to three of the peripheral wells, alternatively with positive control antigen, and 18 µl of positive capripoxvirus control serum is added to the central well. The slides are placed in a humidified chamber at room temperature for 48 hours, and examined for visible precipitation lines using a light box. The test material is positive if a precipitation line develops with the control serum that is confluent with that produced by the positive control antigen. This test will not, however, distinguish between capripox infection and contagious pustular dermatitis (orf).

To prepare antigen for the AGID, one of two 125 cm^2 flasks of LT or LK cells is infected with capripoxvirus, and harvested when there is 90% CPE (8–12 days). The flask is freeze–thawed twice, and the cells are shaken free of the flask. The contents are centrifuged at 4000 ***g*** for 15 minutes, most of the supernatant is decanted and stored, and the pellet is resuspended in the remaining supernatant. The cells should be lysed using an ultrasonic probe for approximately 60 seconds. This homogenate is then centrifuged as before, the resulting supernatant being pooled with that already collected. The pooled supernatant is added to an equal volume of saturated ammonium sulphate at pH 7.4 and left at 4°C for 1 hour. This solution is centrifuged at 4000 ***g*** for 15 minutes, and the precipitate is collected and resuspended in a small volume of 0.8% saline for use in the AGID test. The uninfected flask is processed in an identical manner throughout, to produce a tissue culture control antigen (13).

- **Enzyme-linked immunosorbent assay**

Following the cloning of the highly antigenic capripoxvirus structural protein P32, it is possible to use expressed recombinant antigen for the production of diagnostic reagents, including the raising of P32 monospecific polyclonal antiserum and the production of monoclonal antibodies (MAbs). These reagents have facilitated the development of a highly specific ELISA (4). Using hyperimmune rabbit antiserum raised by inoculation of rabbits with purified capripoxvirus, capripox antigen from biopsy suspensions or tissue culture supernatant can be trapped on an ELISA plate. The presence of the trapped antigen can then be indicated using guinea-pig serum raised against the group-specific structural protein P32, commercial horseradish-peroxidase-conjugated rabbit anti-guinea-pig immunoglobulin and a chromogen/substrate solution.

c) Nucleic acid recognition methods

It is not possible to distinguish between strains of capripoxvirus from cattle, sheep or goats using serological techniques. However, strains can be characterised by comparing the genome fragments generated by *Hin*dIII digestion of their purified DNA (1, 12). This technique has identified differences between isolates from the different species, but these are not consistent and there is evidence for the movement of strains between species and recombination between strains in the field (9).

The PCR can be used to detect the capripoxvirus genome in biopsy or tissue culture samples. Primers for the viral attachment protein gene and the viral fusion protein gene are specific for capripoxvirus, and the nature of the PCR products can be confirmed using restriction enzyme recognition sites (10).

2. Serological tests

a) Virus neutralisation

Either a test serum can be titrated against a constant titre of capripoxvirus (100 $TCID_{50}$ [50% tissue culture infective dose]) or a standard virus strain can be titrated against a constant dilution of test serum in order to calculate a neutralisation index. Because of the variable sensitivity of tissue culture to capripoxvirus, and the consequent difficulty of ensuring the use of 100 $TCID_{50}$, the neutralisation index is the preferred method. The test is described using 96-well flat-bottomed tissue-culture grade microtitre plates, but it can be performed equally well in tissue culture tubes with the appropriate changes to the volumes used, although it is more difficult to read an end-point in tubes. The use of Vero cells in the virus neutralisation test has been reported to give more consistent results.

- **Test procedure**

i) Test sera including a negative and a positive control are diluted 1/5 in Eagle's/HEPES (N-2-hydroxyethylpiperazine, N-2-ethanesulphonic acid) and inactivated at 56°C for 30 minutes.

ii) Next, 50 µl of the first inactivated serum is added to columns 1 and 2, rows A to H of the microtitre plate. The second serum is placed in columns 3 and 4, the third in columns 5 and 6, the positive control serum is placed in columns 7 and 8, the negative control serum is placed in columns 9 and 10, and 50 µl of Eagle's/HEPES without serum is placed in columns 11 and 12 and to all wells of row H.

iii) A reference strain of capripoxvirus, usually a vaccine strain known to grow well in tissue culture, with a titre of over $\log_{10}$ 6 $TCID_{50}$ per ml is diluted in Eagle's/HEPES in bijoux bottles to give a log dilution series of $\log_{10}$ 5.0; 4.0; 3.5; 3.0; 2.5; 2.0; 1.5 $TCID_{50}$ per ml (equivalent to $\log_{10}$ 3.7; 2.7; 2.2; 1.7; 1.2; 0.7; 0.2 $TCID_{50}$ per 50 µl).

iv) Starting with row G and the most diluted virus preparation, 50 µl of virus is added to each well in that row. This is repeated with each virus dilution, the highest titre virus dilution being placed in row A.

v) The plates are covered and incubated for 1 hour at 37°C.

vi) LT cells are prepared from pregrown monolayers as a suspension of 10^5 cells/ml in Eagle's medium containing antibiotics and 2% fetal calf serum. Following incubation of the microtitre plates, 100 µl of cell suspension is added to all the wells, except wells H11 and H12, which serve as control wells for the medium. The remaining wells of row H are cell and serum toxicity controls.

vii) The microtitre plates are covered and incubated at 37°C for 9 days.

viii) Using an inverted microscope, the monolayers are examined daily from day 4 for evidence of CPE. There should be no CPE in the cells of row H. Using the 0240 KSGP vaccine strain of capripoxvirus, the final reading is taken on day 9, and the titre of virus in each duplicate titration is calculated according to Kärber (1931). If left longer, there is invariably a 'breakthrough' of virus in which virus that was at first neutralised appears to disassociate from the antibody.

ix) *Interpretation of the results:* The neutralisation index is the log titre difference between the titre of the virus in the negative serum and in the test serum. An index of ≥1.5 is positive. The test can be made more sensitive if serum from the same animal is examined before and after infection. Because immunity to capripox is predominantly cell mediated, a negative result, particularly following vaccination in which the response is necessarily mild, does not imply that the animal from which the serum was taken is not protected.

A constant virus-varying serum method has been described using serum dilutions in the range 1/5 to 1/500 and fetal calf muscle cells. Because these cells have a lower sensitivity to capripoxvirus than LT cells, the problem of virus 'breakthrough' is overcome.

b) Agar gel immunodiffusion

The AGID test cannot be recommended as a serological test for the diagnosis of capripox because of the cross-reaction with antibody to contagious pustular dermatitis virus, which is the main differential diagnosis. A consequence of this cross-reaction is many false-positive results.

c) Indirect fluorescent antibody test

Capripoxvirus-infected tissue culture grown on flying cover-slips or tissue culture microscope slides can be used for the indirect fluorescent antibody test. Uninfected tissue culture control, and positive and negative control sera, should be included in the test. The infected and control cultures are fixed in acetone at –20°C for 10 minutes and stored at 4°C. Dilutions of test sera are made in PBS, starting at 1/5, and positives are identified using an anti-sheep gamma-globulin conjugated with fluorescein isothiocyanate (7). Cross-reactions can occur with orf, bovine papular stomatitis virus and perhaps other poxviruses.

d) Western blot analysis

Western blotting of test sera against capripoxvirus-infected cell lysate provides a sensitive and specific system for the detection of antibody to capripoxvirus structural proteins, although the test is expensive and difficult to carry out (6).

Capripoxvirus-infected LT cells should be harvested when 90% CPE is seen, freeze–thawed three times, and the cellular debris pelleted by centrifugation. The supernatant should be decanted, and the proteins should then be separated by SDS/PAGE (sodium dodecyl sulphate/polyacrylamide gel electrophoresis). A vertical discontinuous gel system, using a stacking gel made up of acrylamide (5%) in Tris (125 mM), pH 6.8, and SDS (0.1%), and a resolving gel made up of acrylamide (10–12.5%) in Tris (560 mM), pH 8.7, and SDS (0.1%), is recommended for use with a glycine running buffer containing Tris (250 mM), glycine (2 M), and SDS (0.1%). Samples of supernatant should be prepared by boiling for 5 minutes with an appropriate lysis buffer prior to loading. As an alternative to tissue culture antigen, it is possible to use purified virus or expressed recombinant P32.

Molecular weight markers should be run concurrently with the protein samples. The separated proteins in the SDS/PAGE gel should then be transferred by electroblotting to a nitrocellulose membrane (NCM). After blotting, the NCM is rinsed thoroughly in PBS and blocked in 3% bovine serum albumin (BSA) in PBS, or 5% skimmed milk powder in PBS, on a rotating shaker at 4°C overnight. The NCM can then be separated into strips by employing a commercial apparatus to allow the concurrent testing of multiple serum samples, or may be cut into strips and each strip can be incubated separately thereafter. The NCM is washed thoroughly with five changes of PBS for 5 minutes on a rotating shaker, and then incubated at room temperature on the shaker for 1.5 hours, with the appropriate serum at a dilution of 1/50 in blocking buffer (3% BSA and 0.05% Tween 20 in PBS; or 5% milk powder and 0.05% Tween 20 in PBS). The membrane is again thoroughly washed and incubated (in blocking buffer) with anti-species immunoglobulin horseradish-peroxidase-conjugated immunoglobulins at a dilution predetermined by titration. After further incubation at room temperature for 1.5 hours, the membrane is washed and a solution of diaminobenzidin tetrahydrochloride (10 mg in 50 ml of 50 mM Tris-HCl, pH 7.6, and 20 µl of 30% [v/v] hydrogen peroxide) is added. This is then incubated for approximately 3–7 minutes at room temperature on a shaker with constant observation, and the reaction is stopped by washing in PBS before excessive background colour is seen. A positive and negative control serum should be used on each occasion.

Positive test samples and the positive control will produce a pattern consistent with reaction to proteins of molecular weights 67, 32, 26, 19, and 17 kDa – the major structural proteins of capripoxvirus – whereas negative serum samples will not react with this pattern. Hyperimmune serum prepared against parapoxvirus (orf virus) will react with some of the capripoxvirus proteins, but not the 32 kDa protein that is specific for capripoxvirus.

e) Enzyme-linked immunosorbent assay

A capripoxvirus antibody ELISA has been developed using the expressed structural protein P32 of capripoxvirus and MAbs raised against the P32 protein (5).

B. REQUIREMENTS FOR VACCINES AND DIAGNOSTIC BIOLOGICALS

A variety of attenuated live and inactivated capripoxvirus vaccines has been used to provide protection to sheep and goats against capripox (see refs 3 and 11 for reviews). All strains of capripoxvirus of ovine, caprine or bovine origin examined so far share a major neutralising site, so that animals recovered from infection with one strain are resistant to infection with any other strain (2). Consequently, it is possible to use a single strain of capripoxvirus to protect both sheep and goats against all field strains of virus, regardless of whether their origin was in Asia or Africa (14, 16).

There are two antigenic forms of capripoxvirus, the intact virion covered in short tubular elements, and the intact virion additionally covered in a host-cell-derived membrane. The latter is the form usually produced by the infected animal, whereas the former is that seen when virus is produced by freeze–thawing infected tissue culture. Dead vaccines produced from tissue culture are almost entirely naked virions, and when used as a vaccine do not stimulate immunity to the membrane-bound virion. This in part explains the poor success of inactivated vaccines. An additional factor is that inactivated vaccines are less effective than live, replicating vaccine virus in stimulating the cell-mediated immune response, which is the predominant protective response to poxvirus infection. Dead capripox vaccines provide, at best, only temporary protection. A number of strains of capripoxvirus have had widespread use as live vaccines (8), for example the 0240 Kenya sheep and goat pox strain used in sheep and goats, the Romanian and RM-65 strains used mainly in sheep, and the Mysore and Gorgan strains used in goats. Immunity in sheep and goats against capripox following vaccination with the 0240 strain lasts over a year, and will probably provide lifelong protection against lethal challenge. The 0240 strain should not be used in *Bos taurus* breeds of cattle.

A new generation of capripox vaccines is being developed that uses the capripoxvirus genome as a vector for the genes of other ruminant pathogens, for instance genes of rinderpest and peste des petits ruminants (PPR) viruses. The recombinant vaccine will provide protection against capripox, rinderpest and PPR in a single vaccination (17).

1. Seed management

a) Characteristics of the seed

A strain of capripoxvirus used for vaccine production must be accompanied by a history describing its origin and tissue culture or animal passage. It must be safe to use in all breeds of sheep and goats for which it is intended, including pregnant animals. It must be nontransmissible, remain attenuated after further tissue culture passage, and provide complete protection against challenge with virulent field strains for a minimum of 1 year. A quantity of master seed vaccine virus should be prepared and stored in order to provide a consistent working seed for regular vaccine production.

b) Method of culture

Vaccine seed should be lyophilised and stored in 2 ml vials at –20°C. It may be stored wet at –20°C, but when wet, is more stable at –70°C or lower. The virus should be cultured in primary or secondary LT or LK cells of wool sheep origin for maximum yield. Vero cells may also be used.

c) Validation as a vaccine

Seed lots must be shown to be:

i) *Pure:* Free from adventitious viruses, in particular pestiviruses, such as border disease and bovine viral diarrhoea virus, and free from contamination with bacteria, fungi and/or mycoplasmas.

ii) *Safe:* Produce no clinical reaction in all breeds of sheep or goats when given by the recommended route.

iii) *Efficacious:* Stimulate complete immunity to capripox in all breeds of sheep and goats for at least 1 year.

The necessary tests are described in Section B.4.

2. Method of manufacture

Vaccine batches are produced on fresh monolayers of secondary LT or primary LK cells. A vial of seed virus is reconstituted with GMEM and inoculated on to an LT or LK monolayer that has been previously washed with warm PBS, and allowed to absorb for 15 minutes at 37°C before being overlaid with additional GMEM. After 4–

6 days, there will be extensive (50–70%) CPE. The culture should be examined for any evidence of nonspecific CPE, medium cloudiness or change in medium pH. The culture is freeze–thawed three times, the suspension removed and centrifuged at 600 ***g*** for 20 minutes. A second passage may be required to produce sufficient virus for a production batch (to produce enough for 10^6 doses, the yield from five 175 cm^2 flasks is required).

The procedure is repeated and the harvests from individually numbered flasks are each mixed separately with an equal volume of sterile and chilled 5% lactalbumin hydrolysate and 10% sucrose, and transferred to individually numbered bottles for storage at –20°C. Prior to storage, 0.2 ml is removed from each bottle for sterility control. An additional 0.2 ml is removed; 2 ml pools composed of 0.2 ml samples taken from ten bottles are used for virus titration. A written record of all the procedures must be kept for all vaccine batches.

Inactivated vaccines are produced, usually from unattenuated field strains of capripoxvirus, grown in tissue culture as described above, inactivated with 0.03% formaldehyde, and mixed with an equal volume of alhydrogel as adjuvant. Formaldehyde is no longer considered to be a suitable inactivant for certain other viral vaccines because its mode of action cannot be guaranteed to be totally effective in inactivating all the live virus. This has not been fully investigated for capripoxvirus.

3. In-process control

Cells: Cells should be obtained from the testis or kidney of a healthy young lamb from a scrapie-free flock of a wool sheep breed. During cultivation, cells must be observed for any evidence of CPE, and for normal morphology (predominantly fibroblastic). They can usually be passaged successfully up to ten times. When used for vaccine production, uninfected control cultures should be grown in parallel and maintained for at least one additional passage for further observation. They should be checked for the presence of noncytopathic strains of bovine virus diarrhoea or border disease viruses by immunofluorescence or immunoperoxidase techniques. If possible, cells should be prepared and screened prior to vaccine production, and a stock stored in sterile DMSO (dimethyl sulphoxide) in liquid nitrogen (1–2 ml aliquots containing 20×10^6 cells/ml). Serum used in the growth media must be free from antibody to capripoxvirus or contamination with pestivirus.

Virus: Seed virus and final vaccine must be titrated in tissue culture tubes or microtitre plates. Vaccine samples must be examined for the presence of adventitious viruses including cytopathic and noncytopathic strains of pestivirus, and should be mixed with a high-titre capripoxvirus-immune serum that has tested negative for antibody to pestivirus to prevent the vaccine virus itself interfering with the test. The vaccine can be held at –20°C until all sterility tests and titrations have been completed, at which time it should be freeze-dried in 1 ml aliquots in vials sufficient for 100 doses. The vaccine harvest diluted with lactalbumin hydrolysate and sucrose should have a minimum titre $\log_{10}$ 4.5 $TCID_{50}$ per ml after freeze-drying, equivalent to a field dose of $\log_{10}$ 2.5 $TCID_{50}$. A further titration is carried out on five randomly chosen vials of the freeze-dried preparation to confirm the titre.

4. Batch control

a) Sterility

Tests for sterility and freedom from contamination of biological materials may be found in Chapter I.4.

b) Safety and efficacy

Four sheep and four goats of known susceptibility to capripox are placed in a high containment level animal unit and serum samples are collected. Five randomly chosen vials of the freeze-dried vaccine are reconstituted in 1 ml of sterile PBS each, and pooled. One sheep and one goat are inoculated intradermally with 0.2 ml of the concentrated vaccine. The remaining vaccine is diluted 20 times with sterile PBS and two sheep and two goats are inoculated subcutaneously with 0.2 ml – the recommended field dose. The remaining sheep and goat are control animals. The animals are clinically examined daily and rectal temperatures are recorded. On day 21 after vaccination, the eight animals are again serum sampled and challenged with a known virulent capripoxvirus strain by intradermal inoculation. The clinical response is recorded during the following 14 days. Control animals should develop the typical clinical signs of capripox, whereas there should be no local or systemic reaction in the vaccinates other than a delayed-type hypersensitivity reaction, which will disappear within 4 days. Serum samples are again collected on day 30 after vaccination. The day 21 serum samples are examined for seroconversion to selected viral diseases that could have contaminated the vaccine, and the day 0 and 30 samples are compared to confirm the absence of antibody to pestivirus.

The fully reconstituted vaccine is also tested in mice and guinea-pigs. Two guinea-pigs are inoculated intramuscularly with 0.5 ml into the hind leg, and two guinea-pigs and six mice are inoculated intraperitoneally with 0.5 ml and 0.1 ml, respectively. Two guinea-pigs and four mice are kept as uninoculated controls. The animals are observed for 3 weeks, humanely killed and a post-mortem examination is carried out. There should be no evidence of pathology due to the vaccine.

c) **Potency tests**

Less than 1 $TCID_{50}$ of the 0240 strain is sufficient to immunise a sheep or goat. However potency tests must be undertaken for other strains of capripoxvirus if the minimum immunising dose is not known. This is usually carried out by comparing the titre of a virulent challenge virus on the flanks of vaccinated and control animals. Following vaccination, the flanks of at least three animals and three controls are shaved of wool or hair. Log_{10} dilutions of the challenge virus are prepared in sterile PBS and six dilutions are inoculated intradermally (0.1 ml per inoculum) along the length of the flank; four replicates of each dilution are inoculated down the flank. An oedematous swelling will develop at possibly all 24 inoculation sites on the control animals, although preferably there will be little or no reaction at the four sites of the most dilute inocula. The vaccinated animals should develop an initial hypersensitivy reaction at sites of inoculation within 24 hours, which should quickly subside. Small areas of necrosis may develop at the inoculation site of the most concentrated challenge virus. The titre of the challenge virus is calculated for the vaccinated and control animals; a difference of log titre $>log_{10}$ 2.5 is taken as evidence of protection.

d) **Duration of immunity**

Immunity to virulent field virus following vaccination of sheep or goats with the 0240 strain lasts over 1 year, and protection against generalised infection following intradermal challenge lasts at least 3 years and is effectively lifelong. The duration of immunity produced by other vaccine strains should be ascertained in both sheep and goats by undertaking controlled trials in an environment in which there is no possibility of field strains of capripoxvirus confusing the results.

The inactivated vaccines provide immunity for under 1 year, and for the reasons given at the beginning of this section, may not give immunity to the form of capripoxvirus usually associated with natural transmission.

e) **Stability**

Properly freeze-dried preparations of capripox vaccine, particularly those that include a protectant, such as sucrose and lactalbumin hydrolystate, are stable for over 25 years when stored at –20°C and for 2–4 years stored at 4°C. There is evidence that they are stable at higher temperatures, but no long-term controlled experiments have been reported.

The inactivated vaccines must be stored at 4°C, and their shelf life is usually given as 1 year.

f) **Preservatives**

No preservatives other than a protectant, such as sucrose and lactalbumin hydrolysate, are required for the freeze-dried preparation.

g) **Precautions (hazards)**

There are no precautions other than those described above for sterility and freedom from adventitious agents. The 0240 vaccine strain should not be used in *Bos taurus* breeds of cattle.

Capripoxvirus is not infectious to humans.

5. Tests on the final product

a) **Safety**

Safety tests should be carried out on the final product of each batch as described in Section B.4.b.

b) **Potency**

Once the potency of the particular strain being used for vaccine production has been determined in terms of minimum dose required to provide immunity, it is not necessary to repeat this on the final product of each batch, provided the titre of virus present has been ascertained.

REFERENCES

1. BLACK D.N., HAMMOND J.M. & KITCHING R.P. (1986). Genomic relationship between capripoxviruses. *Virus Res.*, **5**, 277–292.
2. CAPSTICK P.B. (1961). Annual Report. Kenya Veterinary Department, Kenya, 45–47.
3. CARN V.M. (1993). Control of capripoxvirus infections. *Vaccine,* **11**, 1275–1279.
4. CARN V.M. (1995). An antigen trapping ELISA for the detection of capripoxvirus in tissue culture supernatant and biopsy samples. *J. Virol. Methods,* **51**, 95–102.
5. CARN V.M., KITCHING R.P., HAMMOND J.M., CHAND P., ANDERSON J. & BLACK D.N. (1994). Use of a recombinant antigen in an indirect ELISA for detecting bovine antibody to capripoxvirus. *J. Virol. Methods,* **49**, 285–294.
6. CHAND P., KITCHING R.P. & BLACK D.N. (1994). Western blot analysis of virus-specific antibody responses to capripoxvirus and contagious pustular dermatitis infections in sheep. *Epidemiol. Infect.,* **113**, 377–385.
7. DAVIES F.G. & ATEMA C. (1978). The antibody response in sheep infected with a Kenyan sheep and goat pox virus. *J. Comp. Pathol.*, **88**, 205–210.
8. DAVIES F.G. & MBUGWA G. (1985). The alterations in pathogenicity and immunogenicity of a Kenya sheep and goat pox virus on serial passage in bovine foetal muscle cell cultures. *J. Comp. Pathol.*, **95,** 565–576.
9. GERSHON P.D., KITCHING R.P., HAMMOND J.M. & BLACK D.N. (1989). Poxvirus genetic recombination during natural virus transmission. *J. Gen. Virol.*, **70**, 485–489.
10. IRELAND D.C. & BINEPAL Y.S. (1998). Improved detection of capripoxvirus in biopsy samples by PCR. *J. Virol. Methods,* **74**, 1–7.
11. KITCHING R.P. (1983). Progress towards sheep and goat pox vaccines. *Vaccine*, **1**, 4–9.
12. KITCHING R.P., BHAT P.P. & BLACK D.N. (1989). The characterization of African strains of capripoxvirus. *Epidemiol. Infect.*, **102,** 335–343.
13. KITCHING R.P., HAMMOND J.M. & BLACK D.N. (1986). Studies on the major precipitating antigen of capripoxvirus. *J. Gen. Virol.*, **67**, 139–148.
14. KITCHING R.P., HAMMOND J.M. & TAYLOR W.P. (1986). A single vaccine for the control of capripox infection in sheep and goats. *Res. Vet. Sci.*, **42**, 53–60.
15. KITCHING R.P. & SMALE C. (1986). Comparison of the external dimensions of capripoxvirus isolates. *Res. Vet. Sci.*, **41**, 425–427.
16. KITCHING R.P. & TAYLOR W.P. (1985). Clinical and antigenic relationship between isolates of sheep and goat pox viruses. *Trop. Anim. Health Prod.*, **17**, 64–74.
17. ROMERO C.H., BARRETT T., EVANS S.A., KITCHING R.P., GERSHON P.D. & BLACK D.N. (1993). Single capripoxvirus recombinant vaccine for the protection of cattle against rinderpest and lumpy skin disease. *Vaccine,* **11**, 737–742.

*

* *

CHAPTER 2.1.11.

AFRICAN HORSE SICKNESS

SUMMARY

African horse sickness (AHS) is an infectious but noncontagious viral disease affecting all species of equidae. It is caused by an orbivirus of the family Reoviridae and is characterised by alterations in respiratory and circulatory functions. AHS is transmitted by at least two species of Culicoides. *Nine different serotypes of the virus have been described.*

All serotypes of AHS virus occur in eastern and southern Africa; this distribution reflects that of zebra, which cycle the virus asymptomatically. Only AHS serotype 9 is found in West Africa from where it occasionally spreads into countries surrounding the Mediterranean. Examples of outbreaks that have occurred outside Africa are: in the Middle East (1959–1961), in Spain (serotype 9, 1966; serotype 4, 1987–1990), and in Portugal (serotype 4, 1989).

Laboratory diagnosis of AHS is of great importance. Although the clinical signs and lesions are characteristic, they can be confused with those of other diseases.

As a viral disease, the laboratory diagnosis of AHS can be based on the identification of infectious virus, virus nucleic acid, viral antigens or specific antibodies. Over the past few years, a wide variety of laboratory tests have been adapted to the detection of both AHS virus and specific antibodies.

***Identification of the agent:** It is important to perform virus isolation and serotyping whenever outbreaks occur outside the enzootic regions.*

AHS virus can be isolated from blood collected during the early febrile stage. For virus isolation, the other tissues of choice for diagnosis are spleen, lung, and lymph nodes, collected at necropsy. Sample preparations can be inoculated in cell cultures, such as baby hamster kidney (BHK-21), monkey stable (MS) or African green monkey kidney (Vero), intravenously in embryonated eggs, and intracerebrally in newborn mice. Several enzyme-linked immunosorbent assays (ELISAs) for the rapid detection of AHS virus antigen in spleen tissues and supernatant from infected cells have been developed. Identification of AHS virus RNA has also been achieved using a reverse-transcription polymerase chain reaction method. Virus isolates can be serotyped by a type-specific serological test, such as virus neutralisation (VN).

***Serological tests:** Horses that survive natural infection develop antibodies against the infecting serotype of AHS virus within 8–12 days post-infection. This may be demonstrated by several serological methods, such as complement fixation test, ELISA, immunoblotting and VN. The latter test is used for serotyping. Other tests that have been described are immunodiffusion and haemagglutination inhibition.*

***Requirements for vaccines and diagnostic biologicals:** Attenuated (monovalent and polyvalent) live vaccines for use in horses, mules and donkeys, are currently available. A monovalent inactivated vaccine has been produced commercially, but is no longer available. New vaccines, including a subunit vaccine, have been evaluated experimentally.*

A. DIAGNOSTIC TECHNIQUES

African horse sickness (AHS) (Peste equina africana, Peste equine) is an infectious, noncontagious arthropod-transmitted disease of equidae, caused by a double-stranded RNA orbivirus belonging to the family Reoviridae. The genus *Orbivirus* also includes bluetongue (BT) virus and epizootic haemorrhagic disease (EHD) virus, which have similar morphological and biochemical properties but distinctive pathological and antigenic properties as well as host ranges. The genome of AHS virus is composed of ten double-stranded RNA segments, which encode seven structural proteins (VP1–7), most of which have been completely sequenced for AHS virus serotypes 4 and 6 (18, 24), and four nonstructural proteins (NS1, NS2, NS3, NS3A) (6, 13, 18). Proteins VP2 and VP5 form the outer capsid of the virion, and proteins VP3 and VP7 are the major inner capsid proteins. All four are highly conserved among the nine AHS virus serotypes, VP7 being the most conserved and VP2/5 the least. Proteins VP1, VP4 and VP6 constitute minor inner capsid proteins. Nine antigenically distinct serotypes of AHS virus have been identified by virus neutralisation (VP2 and VP5 are used for serotype specificity), but no cross-reactions with other known orbiviruses have been observed.

The disease is enzootic in sub-Saharan Africa, although occasional outbreaks have occurred in northern Africa (1965, 1989–1991), the Middle East (1959–1961), and in Europe (Spain, 1966, 1987–1990 and Portugal, 1989).

AHS has both a seasonal (late summer/autumn) and a cyclical incidence, with major epizootics in southern Africa during warm-phase events. Mortality due to AHS is related to the type of equidae affected and the vector population present. At least two field vectors are involved: *Culicoides imicola* and *C. bolitinos*. Among the equidae family, horses are the most susceptible to AHS with a mortality rate of 50–95%, followed by mules with a mortality rate around 50%. In enzootic regions of Africa, donkeys are very resistant to AHS and experience only subclinical infection. In European and Asian countries, however, donkeys are moderately susceptible and have a mortality rate of 10%. Zebras are also markedly resistant exhibiting no clinical signs, and may have extended viraemia (up to 40 days).

Laboratory diagnosis is essential. Although the clinical signs and lesions are characteristic, they can be confused with those of other diseases. For example, the supraorbital swellings, which are often present in horses with subacute AHS, are, in combination with an appropriate history, sufficient for a tentative diagnosis. The other signs and lesions are less specific for AHS and other diseases such as equine encephalosis, equine infectious anaemia, equine morbillivirus pneumonia, equine viral arteritis, babesiosis and purpura haemorrhagica should be excluded. There are four classical forms of AHS: pulmonary, cardiac, mixed, and horse sickness fever (4).

The peracute or pulmonary form, which has a short incubation period (3–5 days), is characterised by very marked and progressive respiratory involvement. An acute febrile reaction, lasting 1–2 days and reaching a maximum of approximately 40–41°C, may be the only clinical sign. This is followed by various degrees of respiratory distress – respiratory rate may increase to 60 or even 75 breaths/minute. The animal may be observed to stand with its forelegs spread apart, its head extended and its nostrils fully dilated. Profuse sweating is common and spasmodic coughing may be observed terminally, with frothy fluid exuding from the nostrils. Death usually occurs within a few hours after the first clinical signs are observed, the animal having literally drowned in its own serous fluid. The pulmonary form is usually observed in completely susceptible animals, animals infected with a highly virulent strain of virus, or animals that are worked during the febrile stage of the disease. Recovery from this form is very rare, occurring in <5% of cases.

The incubation period of the *subacute, oedematous or cardiac form* varies from about 7 to 14 days, and the onset of clinical disease is marked by a febrile reaction (39–41°C), which lasts for 3–6 days. Shortly before the decline of the fever, characteristic oedematous swellings may appear. These initially involve the temporal or supraorbital fossae and the eyelids, and later extend to the lips, cheeks, tongue, intermandibular space and laryngeal region. Subcutaneous oedema sometimes extends a variable distance down the neck towards the chest and, in severe cases, may involve the chest and shoulders. Terminally, petechial haemorrhages may be observed in the conjunctivae and under the ventral surface of the tongue. The animal finally becomes restless and may show signs of colic before death from cardiac failure. The mortality rate is about 50% and death usually occurs within 4–8 days after the onset of the febrile reaction. In recovering cases, swelling gradually subsides within a period of 3–8 days. This clinical form of AHS is usually associated with infection by virus strains of low virulence or is encountered in immune animals infected by heterologous virus strains, or may be a function of biological variation in the infected animal.

The acute or mixed form represents a mixture of the pulmonary and cardiac forms. Although seldom diagnosed clinically, it is seen at post-mortem examination in most fatal cases of AHS in horses and mules. The incubation period varies from 5 to 7 days, and the disease may manifest itself in the following ways:

- Initial pulmonary signs of a relatively mild degree are followed by marked oedematous swellings of the head and neck, with death resulting from heart failure.

- Oedematous swelling, typical of the subacute form, is followed by the sudden onset of dyspnoea and other clinical signs typical of the peracute pulmonary form.

The mortality rate in the mixed form is >80% and death usually follows within 3–6 days after the onset of the febrile reaction.

Horse sickness fever is the mildest form and is frequently overlooked in natural outbreaks. The incubation period varies from 5 to 14 days, and is followed by a febrile reaction (39–40°C) of the remittent type, with morning remissions and afternoon exacerbations, lasting for 5–8 days. Apart from the febrile reaction, other clinical signs are rare. The conjunctivae may be slightly congested, the pulse rate may be increased, and a certain degree of anorexia and depression may be present. This form of the disease is usually observed in immune animals infected with a heterologous virus type or in resistant species, such as the donkey and zebra.

There is no evidence that humans can become infected with any field strain of AHS virus, either through contact with naturally or experimentally infected animals or by virus manipulation in laboratories. However, it has been described that certain neurotropic vaccine strains may cause encephalitis and retinitis in humans following transnasal infections (22). Experimental and natural transmission of AHS virus to dogs has been reported through ingestion of infected horse meat (1). However, there is little evidence that dogs become infected by insect bites (21).

1. Identification of the agent

Several techniques are already available for AHS virus identification ranging from the rapid enzyme-linked immunosorbent assay (ELISA), using either polyclonal antibodies (PAbs) or monoclonal antibodies (MAbs), to the polymerase chain reaction (PCR) test or cell culture and inoculation of newborn mice. More than one test should be performed to diagnose an outbreak of AHS, starting with a quick test such as ELISA or PCR. Virus isolation by tissue culture followed by virus neutralisation (VN) for serotyping are necessary at the beginning of an outbreak. Subsequently, the ELISA may be very useful in laboratory diagnosis.

At present, there are no international standards for virus antigens or diagnostic reagents, and there is no standard methodology for the determination of AHS virus or specific antibodies. However, an international standard serum has been evaluated recently, and a comparative study of different ELISAs (using MAbs or PAbs) for AHS virus antigen and antibody determination has been carried out in different laboratories. The results have demonstrated a high level of correlation for either antigen or antibody detection (19) using the indirect sandwich ELISA for antigen studies (8, 12) or the indirect or competitive ELISA for antibody detection (7, 14).

A very important aspect of diagnosis is the selection of samples and their transportation to the laboratory.

a) Samples for virus isolation

Unclotted whole blood collected during the early febrile stage of the disease from sick animals, as well as small pieces (2–4 g) of spleen, lung and lymph nodes from animals that have died, are the selected samples for diagnosis. Samples should be kept at 4°C during transportation and storage.

b) Cell culture

Direct isolation of AHS virus in baby hamster kidney (BHK-21), monkey stable (MS) and African green monkey kidney (Vero) cell lines has been used successfully. Blood samples collected in heparin can be used undiluted. After 60 minutes of adsorption, the cell cultures are washed and maintenance medium is added. When tissue samples, such as spleen, lung, etc., are used, a 10% tissue suspension is prepared in phosphate buffered saline (PBS), pH 7.2, or cell culture medium, containing antibiotics.

A cytopathic effect (CPE) may appear between 2 and 8 days post-infection. Three blind passages should be performed before the samples are considered to be negative.

c) Newborn mice

In this method, isolation of AHS virus is by intracerebral inoculation into two families of 1–3-day-old mice (BALB/c, CD-1 swiss). In positive cases, animals develop nervous signs between 3 and 15 days post-inoculation. The brains from sick animals must be collected, homogenised and reinoculated intracerebrally into at least six newborn mice. This second passage should present a shortened incubation period (2–5 days) and 100% infectivity.

d) Sandwich enzyme-linked immunosorbent assay

At least two sandwich ELISAs have been developed and field tested for detection of AHS virus antigen from both field samples and laboratory-infected tissue cultures (8, 12).

One technique (8) uses PAbs to the AHS virus and the other (12) uses MAbs against one of the major proteins that is more conserved among serotypes – protein VP7. Both methods have been demonstrated to be adequate for the diagnosis of AHS due to their high sensitivity and specificity and the availability of results in only 2–4 hours (19).

Reagents for the ELISA may be obtained from the OIE Reference Laboratories for African horse sickness (see Table given in Part 4 of this *Manual*).

- **Test procedure: Monoclonal antibody enzyme-linked immunosorbent assay**

i) *Solid phase:* Coat ELISA plates with a mixture of MAb 5G5 and MAb 3D2 diluted in PBS, pH 7.2 (10 µg/ml each). Incubate overnight at 4°C.

ii) Wash the plates five times with distilled water containing 0.05% (v/v) Tween 20 (washing solution). Gently tap the plates on to absorbent material to remove any residual wash.

iii) Block the plates with PBS + 1% bovine serum albumin (BSA), pH 7.2, 200 µl/well, for 1 hour at 37°C.

iv) Remove the blocking solution and gently tap the plates on to absorbent material.

v) *Test samples:* Add the samples to be tested (twofold dilutions starting with undiluted spleen homogenates, or AHS virus cell culture supernatant) diluted in PBS + 1% BSA, pH 7.2, 100 µl/well. Incubate for 1 hour at 37°C. (Spleen homogenate: homogenise approximately 2 cm^3 [1 g] of spleen with 3 ml of MEM [minimal essential medium] culture medium. Centrifuge at 600 ***g*** for 10 minutes and save the supernatant.)

vi) Wash the plates as described in step ii.

vii) *Conjugate:* Dispense 100 µl/well of biotin-labelled MAb 5G5 diluted 1/500 in PBS + 1% BSA, pH 7.2. Incubate for 1 hour at 37°C. Wash the plates as described in step ii. Add 100 µl/well of avidin–peroxidase at optimal dilution in PBS + 1% BSA, pH 7.2. Incubate for 45 minutes at room temperature.

viii) Wash the plates as described in step ii.

ix) *Substrate:* Add 200 µl/well of substrate solution (10 ml of 80.6 mM DMAB [dimethyl aminobenzaldehyde] + 10 ml of 1.56 mM MBTH [3-methyl-2-benzo-thiazolinone hydrazone hydro-chloride] + 5 µl H_2O_2). Colour development is stopped by adding 50 µl of 3 M H_2SO_4 after approximately 5–10 minutes (before the negative control begins to be coloured).

x) Read the plates at 600 nm (or 620 nm).

xi) *Interpretation of the results:* Calculate the cut-off value as follows: C ± 0.6 = cut-off (where C is the absorbance value obtained with the negative control). Test samples giving absorbance values lower than the cut-off are regarded as negative. Test samples giving absorbance values greater than the cut-off + 0.20 are regarded as positive. Test samples giving intermediate absorbance values are doubtful and a second technique must be employed to confirm the result.

e) Polymerase chain reaction

PCR assays for the specific detection of AHS virus serotype 4 RNA have been developed. Primers correspond to the 5'-end (nucleotides 1–21) and 3'-end (nucleotides 1160–1179) of RNA segment 8 (16, 20, 25).

- **Test procedure**

Extraction of nucleic acids from spleen samples is carried out as follows: 1 g of tissue sample is homogenised in 1 ml of denaturing solution (4 M guanidium thiocyanate, 25 mM sodium citrate, pH 7; 0.1 M 2-mercaptoethanol, 0.5% [w/v] sarcosyl). After centrifugation, 1 µg of yeast RNA, 0.1 ml of 2 M sodium acetate pH 4, 1 ml of phenol (water equilibrated) and 0.2 ml of chloroform/isoamyl alcohol mixture (49/1) are added to the supernatant. The suspension is vigorously shaken and cooled on ice for 15 minutes. After centrifugation, the RNA present in the aqueous phase is phenol extracted, ethanol precipitated and resuspended in sterile water. The methods for cDNA synthesis and PCR amplification are performed using, in all cases, 37°C as renaturing temperature. The sequences of the PCR primers used are 5'-GTT-AAA-ATT-CGG-TTA-GGA-TG-3', which corresponds to the messenger RNA polarity, and 5'-GTA-AGT-GTA-TTC-GGT-ATT-G-3', which is complementary to the messenger RNA polarity. The PCR procedure itself involves 40 cycles (94°C for 1 minute, 55°C for 1.5 minutes, 72°C for 2.5 minutes and 70°C for 7 minutes) and then the PCR tubes are kept at 4°C. Analysis of the PCR products is carried out by electrophoresis in 1.2% (w/v) agarose gels containing ethidium bromide. AHS-positive samples will resolve in a 1179 base-pair band.

2. Serological tests

An indirect ELISA using either soluble AHS virus antigen or a recombinant protein VP7 (14) and a competitive ELISA using soluble AHS virus antigen (7) have proved to be good methods for the detection of anti-AHS virus group-reactive antibodies, especially for large-scale investigations. One of these tests (7) could also be used for testing wildlife as species-specific anti-globulin is not required with this method. An immunoblotting test has also been adapted for anti-AHS antibody determination (13). It is especially suitable for small numbers of sera. An indirect ELISA is also available that uses the AHS virus serotype 4 nonstructural protein NS3 as antigen, and could be used for the differentiation of animals infected or vaccinated with the live vaccine from those vaccinated with the inactivated vaccine made with purified virions (15). The complement fixation (CF) test has been widely used, but some sera are anticomplementary.

a) Indirect enzyme-linked immunosorbent assay (a prescribed test for international trade)

The recombinant VP7 protein has been used as antigen for anti-AHS virus antibody determination with a high index of sensitivity and specificity (14, 23). Other advantages of this antigen are its stability and its lack of infectivity.

- **Test procedure**

i) *Solid phase:* Coat ELISA plates with recombinant AHSV-4 VP7 diluted in carbonate/bicarbonate buffer, pH 9.6. Incubate overnight at 4°C.

ii) Wash the plates five times with distilled water containing 0.01% (v/v) Tween 20 (washing solution). Gently tap the plates on to absorbent material to remove any residual wash.

iii) Block the plates with PBS, pH 7.2, + 5% (w/v) skimmed milk (dry skim milk from Nestlé™), 200 µl/well, for 1 hour at 37°C.

iv) Remove the blocking solution and gently tap the plates on to absorbent material.

v) *Test samples:* Serum samples to be tested, and positive and negative control sera, are diluted 1/25 in PBS + 5% (w/v) skimmed milk + 0.05% (v/v) Tween 20, 100 µl per well. Incubate for 1 hour at 37°C. For titration, make a twofold dilution series from 1/25 (100 µl/well), one serum per plate column, and do the same with positive and negative controls. Incubate for 1 hour at 37°C.

vi) Wash the plates as described in step ii.

vii) *Conjugate:* Dispense 100 µl/well of horseradish-peroxidase-conjugated anti-horse gamma-globulin diluted in PBS + 5% milk + 0.05% Tween 20, pH 7.2. Incubate for 1 hour at 37°C.

viii) Wash the plates as described in step ii.

ix) *Substrate:* Add 200 µl/well of substrate solution (10 ml of 80.6 mM DMAB + 10 ml of 1.56 mM MBTH + 5 µl H_2O_2). Colour development is stopped by adding 50 µl of 3 M H_2SO_4 after approximately 5–10 minutes (before the negative control begins to be coloured). Other substrates such as ABTS (2,2'-Azino-bis-[3-ethylbenzothiazoline-6-sulphonic acid]), TMB (tetramethyl benzidine), or OPD (ortho-phenyldiamine) can also be used.

x) Read the plates at 600 nm (or 620 nm).

xi) *Interpretation of results:* Calculate the cut-off value by adding 0.6 to the value of the negative control. (0.06 is the standard deviation derived with a group of 30 negative sera.) Test samples giving absorbance values lower than the cut-off are regarded as negative. Test samples giving absorbance values greater than the cut-off + 0.15 are regarded as positive. Test samples giving intermediate absorbance values are doubtful and a second technique must be employed to confirm the result.

b) Immunoblotting

The binding of antibodies to viral proteins separated by electrophoresis and transferred to nitrocellulose paper has been used for the determination of anti-AHS virus antibodies (13).

- **Test procedure**

Semipurified proteins of AHS virus are separated by SDS/PAGE (sodium dodecyl sulphate/polyacrylamide gel electrophoresis) in 15% (w/v) acrylamide-N,N'-diallyltartar-diamide (DATD) gels. Separated proteins are transferred to a nitrocellulose membrane filter at a constant current of 280 mA for 6 hours at 4°C. Immunoblotting of a nitrocellulose membrane cut into strips is carried out using the sera at 1/20 dilution, peroxidase-conjugated rabbit-anti-horse immunoglobulin at 1/500 dilution and incubation time of 1 hour at 37°C. The bands recognised by the sera are developed by the 4-chloro-naphthol technique.

Interpretation of results: The comparison between the band pattern of a positive control and a negative control serum permits the identification of the specific viral bands. The appearance of two or more of these specific bands in a problem serum allows it to be classified as positive anti-AHS virus serum.

c) NS3 enzyme-linked immunosorbent assay

An indirect ELISA to distinguish between infected horses and horses vaccinated with the inactivated purified AHS virus serotype 4 vaccine, using a recombinant NS3 protein as antigen, has been adapted and evaluated. The results obtained (15) indicate that recombinant NS3 can indeed differentiate between infected and vaccinated animals implying that this recombinant could be an important diagnostic reagent, which would allow the transportation of vaccinated horses. To ensure the reliability of results it is essential that the selected AHS virus inactivated vaccine is a purified vaccine. This is to exclude with certainty any traces of NS3 that, if present, would stimulate the production of anti-NS3 antibodies in vaccinated horses, thus mimicking the response to a natural infection.

d) Complement fixation (a prescribed test for international trade)

The CF test has been extensively used, but due to the anticomplementary effect of some sera, as well as the good results obtained with the ELISA, its use is decreasing. The CF test is frequently used for the demonstration of group-specific antibodies against AHS virus. A sucrose–acetone mouse-brain extract is commonly used as antigen.

- **Reagents**

i) Veronal buffered saline containing 1% gelatin (VBSG).

ii) Serum samples, free from erythrocytes, must be heat inactivated: horse serum at 56°C, zebra serum at 60°C and donkey serum at 62°C, for 30 minutes.

iii) The antigen is a sucrose–acetone extract of AHS virus-infected mouse brain. The control antigen is uninfected mouse brain, extracted in the same way. In the absence of an international standard serum, the antigen should be titrated against a locally prepared positive control serum. In the test, 4–8 units are used.

iv) The complement (C') is a normal guinea-pig serum.

v) The haemolysin is a hyperimmune rabbit serum against sheep red blood cells (SRBCs).

vi) The SRBCs are obtained by aseptic puncture of the jugular vein and preserved in Alsever's solution[1] or sodium citrate.

vii) The haemolytic system (HS) is prepared by diluting the haemolysin to contain two haemolytic doses and using this to sensitise washed SRBCs. The SRBCs are standardised to a 3% concentration.

viii) Control sera. A positive control serum is obtained locally and validated. Serum from a healthy antibody-negative horse is used as the negative control serum.

- **Test procedure**

i) Sera, complement and antigen are reacted in 96-well round-bottom microtitre plates, or in tubes if the macro-technique is used, at 4°C for 18 hours.

ii) Sensitised SRBCs (3%) are added to all wells on the microtitre plate.

iii) The test plate is incubated for 30 minutes at 37°C.

iv) Plates are then centrifuged at 200 *g*, and the wells are scored for the presence of haemolysis.

v) The following controls are used: (a) serum and complement; (b) serum and SRBCs; (c) CF antigen and control antigen each with 4 CH_{50} (50% complement haemolytic units), 2 CH_{50}, and 1 CH_{50} of complement; (d) CF antigen and SRBCs; (e) control antigen and SRBCs; (f) complement dilutions of 4 CH_{50}, 2 CH_{50}, and 1 CH_{50}, and (g) SRBCs.

vi) Results are read using 50% haemolysis as the end point. The inverse of the highest dilution of serum specifically fixing complement with the CF antigen is called the titre.

vii) A titre of 1/10 or more is positive, under 1/10 is negative.

1 20.5 g dextrose (114 mM), 7.9 g sodium citrate $2H_2O$ (27 mM), 4.2 g NaCl (71 mM), H_2O to 1 litre. Adjust to pH 6.1 with 1 M citric acid.

e) Virus neutralisation

VN is the method of choice for serotyping. The test may be performed as follows (9, 10).

i) Stock virus is diluted to yield 30–100 $TCID_{50}$ (50% tissue culture infective dose) per 25 µl, and 25 µl is added to each of four microtitre wells containing 25 µl serum dilutions. For screening, a final serum dilution of 1/10 is used. Doubling dilutions are used for titrations.

ii) Serum/virus mixtures are incubated for 60 minutes at 37°C prior to the addition of 0.1 ml of Vero cell suspension (200,000 cells/ml) to each test well.

iii) A back titration of virus stock is prepared for each test using four wells per tenfold dilution, 25 µl per well. Test plates are incubated at 37°C, 5% CO_2, 95% humidity for 4–5 days, until the back titration indicates that the stock virus contains 30–100 $TCID_{50}$.

iv) The plates are then fixed and stained in a solution of 0.15% (w/v) crystal violet in 2% (v/v) glutaraldehyde and rinsed.

v) The 50% end-point titre of the serum is calculated by the Spearman–Kärber method and expressed as the negative $\log_{10}$.

B. REQUIREMENTS FOR VACCINES AND DIAGNOSTIC BIOLOGICALS

With respect to AHS vaccine, polyvalent or monovalent live attentuated vaccines based on the selection in Vero cell culture of genetically stable macroplaques are in general use (5). An inactivated monovalent (serotype 4) AHS virus vaccine based on virus purification and inactivation with formalin has been produced commercially, but is not available at the present time (2, 11). Requirements for both attenuated and inactivated vaccines are summarised below.

B1. Attenuated African horse sickness vaccine

1. Seed management

a) Characteristics of the seed

The seed virus is prepared by selection in Vero cells of genetically stable large plaques from low passage levels of AHS virus. The plaque mutants are then further multiplied by three passages in Vero cells. A large quantity of this antigen is lyophilised and stored at –20°C as master seed stock antigen.

b) Method of culture

The seed virus is grown in roller cultures of Vero cells.

c) Validation as a vaccine

The seed virus must be shown to be free from contaminating viruses, bacteria and mycoplasmas by the appropriate techniques. The serotype identity of the seed virus is confirmed.

2. Method of manufacture

At the onset of a production run, working antigens are produced from the master seed stock antigen in either BHK-21 or Vero cell cultures. The working antigens are tested for sterility, purity and identity and should contain at least 1×10^6 plaque-forming units (PFU)/ml of infectious virus.

Roller bottle cultures of Vero or BHK-21 cells are grown using gamma-irradiated bovine serum in the growth medium. Once the cultures are confluent, the medium is poured off and the cells are seeded with the working antigens. After 1 hour, maintenance medium is added to the cultures. Incubation is continued at 37°C for 2–3 days. When the CPE is advanced, both cells and supernatant medium are harvested. The products from the same serotype are pooled and stored at 4°C.

3. In-process control

The pooled harvests of the individual serotypes are tested for sterility and assayed for infectivity by plaque titration on Vero cell cultures. The minimum acceptable titre is 1×10^6 PFU/ml.

Finally, two quadrivalent vaccines are constituted by mixing equal volumes of serotypes 1, 3, 4, 5 and 2, 6, 7, 8, respectively. A monovalent type can also be prepared. After addition of suitable stabiliser, the vaccine is distributed in 1.0 ml volumes into glass vials and freeze-dried.

4. Batch control

a) Sterility

Following lyophilisation, five bottles of vaccine are selected at random and tested for sterility by internationally accepted methods. Tests for sterility and freedom from contamination of biological products are given in Chapter I.4.

b) Safety

Innocuity of a vaccine is determined by the inoculation of reconstituted vaccine into mice (0.25 ml intraperitoneally), guinea-pig (1.0 ml intraperitoneally), and a horse (5.0 ml subcutaneously). All the animals are observed daily for 14 days. The rectal temperature of the horse is taken twice daily for 14 days and should never exceed 39°C.

c) Potency

Potency is based on virus concentration in the vaccine and serological response to vaccination.

The minimum immunising dose for each serotype is about 1×10^3 PFU/dose. The infectivity titre of the final product is assayed by plaque titration in Vero cell cultures and should contain at least 1×10^5 PFU/dose. The horse used for safety testing is also used for determining the immunogenicity of a vaccine.

Serum samples are collected on the day of vaccination and 21 days later, and are tested for neutralising antibodies against each serotype by the plaque-reduction test using twofold serum dilutions and about 100 PFU of virus. The horse should develop a neutralising antibody titre of at least 20 against at least three of the four serotypes in the quadrivalent vaccine.

d) Duration of immunity

Duration of immunity is not assessed with every batch of vaccine, but immunity is known to persist for at least 4 years. However, in the light of possible interference between the individual serotypes in each quadrivalent vaccine, annual revaccination is advocated in enzootic regions. Vaccination with monovalent vaccine stimulates a practically lifelong immunity.

e) Stability

In the lyophilised state, the vaccine is known to retain its potency for many years when stored at 4–8°C. However, an expiry date of 2 years is normally given.

B2. Inactivated African horse sickness vaccine

1. Seed management

a) Characteristics of the seed

The seed virus is the attenuated vaccine strain (AHS virus serotype 4) used widely in the field in Africa and southern Europe (seed stocks are available from the OIE Reference Laboratory [Onderstepoort]). The virus was passaged ten times in the brains of newborn mice for attenuation, and then passaged a further ten times in roller tube cultures of BHK-21 cells. This material was plaque-purified three times in Vero cell cultures by selection of a large plaque (4–6 mm) at terminal dilutions. The final plaque material was passaged once in the brain of newborn mice and four times in Vero cell cultures. This material was lyophilised and constitutes the master seed virus.

b) Method of culture

The attenuated virus is propagated by passage in BHK-21 cells in roller bottles.

c) Validation as a vaccine

The seed virus must be shown to be free from contaminating viruses, bacteria and mycoplasmas by the appropriate techniques. The serotype identification is confirmed by a double-sandwich ELISA using MAbs.

2. Method of manufacture

Virus is harvested when characteristic CPE is fully developed. Cultivation thereafter is carried out in cell suspensions with serum-free Stoker's medium (MEM) at 37°C. Virus growth is checked by cell viability (CPE), and when optimum conditions are reached, the fermentor culture temperature is lowered to 4°C. The virus suspension is aseptically harvested.

The filtered suspension of attenuated virus is inactivated with formaldehyde at a final concentration of 1/1000. The suspension is transferred to another tank and kept at 4°C under mild agitation for at least 10 days to ensure that all virus is inactivated. Inactivation controls are also performed.

After inactivation, the antigen suspension is concentrated by ultrafiltration, then purified by selective precipitation by a complex of ethylene oxide and bivalent cations according to a patented process.

3. In-process control

Control of virus identity by double-sandwich ELISA, titration of virus before inactivation in Vero cell lines, sucrose gradient analysis to estimate the viral particle concentration, and sterility tests are performed.

4. Batch control

a) Sterility

Tests for sterility and freedom from contamination of biological products are given in Chapter I.4.

b) Safety

AHS virus-susceptible horses are inoculated intramuscularly or subcutaneously with a single or double dose of vaccine. Temperatures are recorded daily for 14 days, and horses are observed for signs of abnormality. Five guinea-pigs receive a horse vaccine dose by the intramuscular route. Sera collected at day 21 are tested for antibodies by VN.

c) Potency

The potency control is performed by challenge of vaccinated horses. Some animals are vaccinated with one dose, and others with two doses, of vaccine. The challenge is made by the intravenous route at 77 days after the first vaccine inoculation. Where two vaccinations are used, the second dose is given 21 days after the first dose.

Serum samples are collected on the day of vaccination and 21 days later, and are tested for neutralising antibodies and virus isolation.

d) Duration of immunity

No challenges have been performed on horses, only serological studies have been carried out. If the level of antibodies after two injections (recommended field protocol) and at 12 months post-vaccination are equivalent to the levels conferred by a single vaccination at 28 days post-vaccination, the horses are considered to be protected. With this standard, the duration of immunity is 1 year, starting 7–10 days after the first injection. One booster every year is sufficient to confer a protective level in the following years. The protocol for vaccination recommended by the manufacturer is two vaccinations (given 21 days apart) and one booster given at 365 days after the first vaccination.

e) **Stability**

Due to the fact that the inactivated vaccine is a relatively new product, not much data are available on the duration of its stability. Results have been obtained that demonstrate vaccine stability in excess of 3 years.

B3. AHS subunit vaccine

AHS virus serotype 4 outer capsid protein VP2 and VP5 plus inner capsid protein VP7, derived from single and dual recombinant baculovirus expression vectors were used in different combinations to immunise horses (17). The crude cell extracts containing the three structural proteins were sufficient to obtain a protective immune response in horses challenged with AHS virulent virus (10^6 $TCID_{50}$). Viraemia was not detectable in vaccinated horses (17). Further analysis of partially protective crude lysates revealed that only soluble VP2 was capable of inducing neutralising antibodies. More investigations are needed to find a way of limiting the formation of insoluble aggregates and optimise conditions for producing VP2 in a form capable of inducing protective immunity (3).

Although further experiments need to be performed to estimate the duration of the immunity induced by these proteins, the data indicate the effectiveness of this candidate vaccine.

• **Acknowledgement**

Parts of this chapter were taken from or based on the chapter on African horse sickness in previous editions of the *Manual.*

REFERENCES

1. BEVAN L.E.W. (1911). The transmission of African horse sickness in the dog by feeding. *Vet. J.*, **67**, 402–408.

2. DUBOURGET P., PREAUD J., DETRAZ F., LACOSTE F., FABRI A., ERASMUS B. & LOMBARD M. (1992). Development, production, and quality control of an industrial inactivated vaccine against African horse sickness virus serotype 4. *In:* Bluetongue, African Horse Sickness and Related Orbiviruses: Proceedings of the Second International Symposium, Walton T.E. & Osburn B.I., eds. CRC Press, Boca Raton, Florida, USA, 874–886.

3. DU PLESSIS M., CLOETE M., AITCHISON H. & VAN DIJK A.A. (1998). Protein aggregation complicates the development of baculovirus-expressed African horsesickness virus serotype 5 VP2 subunit vaccines. *Onderstepoort J. Vet. Res.*, **48**, 51–58.

4. ERASMUS B.J. (1973). The pathogenesis of African horse sickness. *In:* Conference on Equine Infectious Diseases, Bryans J.T. & Gerber H., eds. Karger, Basle, Switzerland, 1–11.

5. ERASMUS B.J. (1976). A new approach to polyvalent immunisation against African horse sickness. Proceedings of the Fourth International Conference on Equine Infectious Diseases, Lyon, France, September 1976, 401–403.

6. GRUBMAN M. & LEWIS S. (1992). Identification and characterisation of the structural and non-structural proteins of African horse sickness virus and determination of the genome coding assignments. *Virology*, **186**, 444–451.

7. HAMBLIN, G., GRAHAM S.D., ANDERSON E.C. & CROWTHER J.R. (1990). A competitive ELISA for the detection of group-specific antibodies to African horse sickness virus. *Epidemiol. Infect.*, **104**, 303–312.

8. HAMBLIN C., MERTENS P.P., MELLOR C., BURROUGHS J. & CROWTHER J. (1991). A serogroup specific enzyme-linked immunosorbent assay for the detection and identification of African horse sickness viruses. *J. Virol. Methods,* **31**, 285–292.

9. HAZRATI A. & OZAWA Y. (1965). Serologic studies of African horse sickness virus with emphasis on neutralisation in tissue culture. *Can. J. Comp. Med.*, **29**, 173–178.

10. HOUSE C., MIKICIUK P.E. & BERNINGER M.L. (1990). Laboratory diagnosis of African horse sickness: comparison of serological techniques and evaluation of storage methods of samples for virus isolation. *J. Vet. Diagn. Invest.,* **2**, 44–50.

11. HOUSE J., LOMBARD M., HOUSE C., DUBOURGET P. & MEBUS C. (1992). Efficacy of an inactivated vaccine for African horse sickness serotype 4. *In:* Bluetongue, African Horse Sickness and Related Orbiviruses: Proceedings of the Second International Symposium, Walton T.E. & Osburn B.I., eds. CRC Press, Boca Raton, Florida, USA, 891–895.

12. LAVIADA M.D., ARIAS M., DOMINGUEA J. & SANCHEZ-VIZCAINO J.M. (1992). Detection of African horse sickness virus in infected spleen by sandwich ELISA using two monoclonal antibodies specific for VP7. *J. Virol. Methods,* **38**, 229–242.

13. LAVIADA M., ARIAS M. & SANCHEZ-VIZCAINO J.M. (1993). Characterisation of African horse sickness virus serotype 4-induced polypeptides in Vero cells and their reactivity in Western blotting. *J. Gen. Virol.*, **74**, 81–87.

14. LAVIADA M., ROY P. & SANCHEZ-VIZCAINO J.M. (1992). Adaptation and evaluation of an indirect ELISA and immunoblotting test for African horse sickness antibody detection. *In:* Bluetongue, African Horse Sickness and Related Orbiviruses: Proceedings of the Second International Symposium, Walton T.E. & Osburn B.I., eds. CRC Press, Boca Raton, Florida, USA, 646–650.

15. LAVIADA, M., ROY P., SANCHEZ-VIZCAINO J.M. & CASAL I. (1995). The use of African horse sickness virus NS3 protein, expressed in bacteria, as a marker to differentiate infected from vaccinated horses. *Virus Res.*, **38**, 205–218.

16. LAVIADA M., SANCHEZ-VIZCAINO JM., ROY P., SOBRINO F. (1997). Detection of African horsesickness virus by the polymerase chain reaction. *Invest. Agr. S.A.*, **12**, 97–102.

17. MARTINEZ J., DIAZ-LAVIADA M., ROY P., SANCHEZ C., VELA C., SANCHEZ-VIZCAINO J.M. & CASAL I. (1996). Full protection against AHSV in horses induced by baculovirus-derived AHS virus serotype 4 VP2, VP5 and VP7. *J. Gen. Virol.*, **77**, 1211–1221.

18. ROY P., HIRASAWA T., FERNANDEZ M., BLINOV V.M. & SANCHEZ-VIZCAINO RODRIGUEZ J.M. (1991). The complete sequence of the group-specific relationship to bluetongue virus. *J. Gen. Virol.*, **72**, 1237–1241.

19. RUBIO C., CUBILLO M.A., HOOGHUIS H., SANCHEZ-VIZCAINO JM., DIAZ-LAVIADA M., PLATEAU E., ZIENTARA S., CRUCIERE C. & HAMBLIN C. (1998). Validation of ELISA for the detection of African horse sickness virus antigens and antibodies. *Arch. Virol* (Suppl.), **14**, 311–315.

20. STONE-MARSCHAT M., CARVILLE A., SKOWRONEK A. & LAEGREID W.W. (1994). Detection of African horse sickness virus by reverse transcription PCR. *J. Clin. Microbiol.*, **32**, 697–700.

21. THEILER A. (1906). Transmission of horse sickness into dogs. *Rep. Govt Vet. Bact.*, 160–162.

22. VAN DER MEYDEN C.H., ERASMUS B., SWANEPOEL R. & PROZESKY O. (1992). Encephalitis and chorioretinitis associated with neurotropic African horse sickness virus infection in laboratory workers. *S. Afr. Med. J.*, **81**, 451–454.

23. WADE-EVANS A., WOOLHOUSE T., O'HARA R. & HAMBLIN C. (1993). The use of African horse sickness virus VP7 antigen, synthesised in bacteria, and anti-VP7 monoclonal antibodies in a competitive ELISA. *J. Virol. Methods*, **45**, 179–188.

24. WILLIAMS C.F., INOUE T., LUCUS A.M., ZANOTTO P.M. & ROY Y.P. (1998). The complete sequence of four major structural proteins of African horse sickness virus serotype 6: evolutionary relationship within and between the orbivirus. *Virus Res.*, **53**, 53–73.

25. ZIENTARA S., SAILLEAU C., MOULAY S. & CRUCIERE C. (1994). Diagnosis of the African horse sickness virus serotype 4 by a one-tube, one manipulation RT-PCR reaction from infected organs. *J. Virol. Methods*, **46**, 179–188.

*

* *

CHAPTER 2.1.12.

AFRICAN SWINE FEVER

SUMMARY

African swine fever (ASF) is an infectious disease of domestic and wild pigs, which affects animals of all breeds and ages, caused by a virus that produces a range of syndromes. Acute disease is characterised by high fever, haemorrhages in the reticuloendothelial system, and a high mortality rate. Infectious virus can survive for several months in fresh and salted dried-meat products.

ASF virus is the only member of a family called ASF-like viruses.

Laboratory diagnostic procedures for ASF fall into two groups: the first contains the tests for virus isolation and the detection of virus antigens and genome DNA, while the second contains the tests for antibody detection. The selection of the tests to be carried out depends on the disease situation in the area or country.

In countries free from ASF but suspecting its presence, the laboratory diagnosis must be directed towards isolation of the virus by simultaneously carrying out the inoculation of pig leukocyte or bone marrow cultures, the detection of antigen in smears or cryostat sections of tissues by fluorescent antibody test (FAT) and, where possible, the detection of genome DNA by the polymerase chain reaction (PCR). The detection of antibodies in tissue fluids by the indirect fluorescent antibody test should also be carried out at the same time.

Identification of the agent: *Tissues submitted from pigs suspected of disease in the field should be examined for specific antigen by the FAT on smears or cryostat sections, and for the presence of virus by inoculation of primary pig leukocyte cultures, which are examined daily for haemadsorption and cytopathic effects. The cells from negative cultures are examined for antigen by FAT and subinoculation into fresh leukocyte cultures.*

The PCR can be used to detect virus genome in tissues and is especially useful if these are unsuitable for virus isolation and antigen detection.

In doubtful cases, the material is passaged and the procedures described above are repeated.

Serological tests: *Where the disease is endemic, or where a primary outbreak is caused by a strain of low virulence, the investigation of new outbreaks should start with the detection, using the enzyme-linked immunosorbent assay, of specific antibodies in serum or extracts of the tissues submitted.*

Requirements for vaccines and diagnostic biologicals: *At present, there is no vaccine for ASF.*

A. DIAGNOSTIC TECHNIQUES

African swine fever virus (ASFV) was originally classified as a member of the family Iridoviridae, but the structure of the genome and the replication strategy of the virus have been shown to have many features in common with members of the Poxviridae (13). The proposal that ASFV be placed in a family separate from the Iridoviridae was accepted at the Sixth Meeting of the International Committee on the Taxonomy of Viruses (ICTV) in Sendai (Japan) in 1984. This virus is currently classified as the only member of a family called ASF-like viruses.

ASF viruses produce a range of syndromes varying from peracute to chronic disease, and apparently healthy virus carriers. The more virulent strains produce peracute or acute haemorrhagic disease characterised by high fever, loss of appetite, haemorrhages in the skin and internal organs, and death in 2–10 days. Mortality rates may be as high as 100%. Less virulent strains produce mild clinical signs – slight fever, reduced appetite and depression – which can be readily confused with many other conditions in pigs and may not lead to suspicion of

ASF. Avirulent, nonhaemadsorbing strains produce mainly subclinical nonhaemorrhagic infection and seroconversion, but some animals may develop discrete lesions in the lungs or in the skin in areas over bony protrusions and other areas subject to trauma.

ASF cannot be differentiated from classical swine fever (hog cholera) by either clinical or post-mortem examination, and both diseases should be considered in the differential diagnosis of any acute febrile haemorrhagic syndrome of pigs. Bacterial septicaemias may also be confused with ASF and classical swine fever. Laboratory tests are essential to distinguish between these diseases.

In countries free from ASF but suspecting its presence, the laboratory diagnosis must be directed towards isolation of the virus by simultaneously carrying out the inoculation of pigs and pig leukocyte or bone marrow cultures, and detection of antigen in smears or cryostat sections of tissues by the fluorescent antibody test (FAT). However, the detection of antibodies in serum or tissue fluids by the enzyme-linked immunosorbent assay (ELISA), immunoblotting or indirect fluorescent antibody (IFA) test should also be carried out at the same time in order to avoid a delay in detecting infection by an unexpected virus of low virulence.

An additional technique now available is the polymerase chain reaction (PCR), which can be used to detect the virus genome in blood or tissues and is particularly useful if samples submitted are unsuitable for virus isolation and antigen detection because they have undergone putrefaction.

1. Identification of the agent

Where ASF is suspected, the following samples should be sent to the laboratory: blood in anticoagulant (heparin or ethylene diamine tetra-acetic acid [EDTA]), spleen, tonsil, kidney, lymph nodes. These should be kept as cold as possible, without freezing, during transit.

- **Sample preparation for haemadsorption and pig inoculation**

i) Prepare suspensions of tissues by grinding small pieces with a pestle and mortar containing sterile sand, then add 5–10 ml of a buffered salt solution or tissue culture medium containing antibiotics.

ii) Clarify the suspensions by centrifugation at 1000 ***g*** for 5 minutes.

Use the supernatant for haemadsorption (Section A.1.a. below) and pig inoculation (Section A.1.d. below), although pig inoculation is not recommended.

a) Haemadsorption test

The haemadsorption (HAD) test (5) is definitive for ASF and depends on the fact that pig erythrocytes will adhere to the surface of pig monocyte or macrophage cells infected with ASFV, and that most virus isolates produce this phenomenon of haemadsorption. A very small number of 'nonhaemadsorbing' viruses have been isolated, most of which are avirulent, but some do produce typical acute ASF. The test is carried out by inoculating blood or tissue suspensions from suspect pigs into primary leukocyte cultures (Procedure 1 below) or by preparing leukocyte cultures from the blood of pigs inoculated at the laboratory or from the blood of suspect pigs collected in the field (Procedure 2 below). Up to 300 cultures can be prepared from each 100 ml of defibrinated or heparinised blood collected. It is essential to carry out all procedures in such a way as to prevent contamination of the cultures.

- **Procedure 1: Haemadsorption test in primary leukocyte cultures**

i) Collect the required volume of fresh pig blood in heparin (100 International Units [IU]/ml blood).

ii) Centrifuge at 700 ***g*** for 30 minutes, remove the buffy coat cells and wash in medium.

iii) Resuspend the cells at a concentration of 10^7 cells/ml in tissue culture medium containing 10–30% pig serum and antibiotics. In order to prevent nonspecific haemadsorption, the medium should contain serum or plasma from the same pig from which the leukocytes were obtained.

iv) Dispense the cell suspension in aliquots of 1.5 ml in 160 × 16 mm tubes and incubate in a sloping position (5–10° from the horizontal) at 37°C.

Note: For routine diagnosis, only 2–4-day-old cultures are sufficiently sensitive.

v) Inoculate three tubes of cells by adding 0.2 ml of prepared samples of tissue per tube. It is advisable to inoculate tenfold and hundred-fold dilutions into cultures, and this is especially important when the field material submitted is in poor condition.

vi) Inoculate positive control cultures with haemadsorbing virus. Uninoculated negative controls are essential to monitor the possibility of nonspecific haemadsorption.

vii) After 3 days, add 0.2 ml of a fresh preparation of 1% pig erythrocytes in buffered saline to each tube.

viii) Examine the cultures daily for 7–10 days under a microscope for cytopathic effect (CPE) and haemadsorption.

ix) *Reading the results:* Haemadsorption consists of the attachment of large numbers of pig erythrocytes to the surface of infected cells. A CPE consisting of a reduction in the number of adherent cells in the absence of haemadsorption may be due to the cytotoxicity of the inoculum, Aujeszky's disease virus or nonhaemadsorbing ASFV, which can be detected by the FAT on the cell sediment or by use of PCR (see below). If no change is observed, or if the results of the immunofluorescence and PCR tests are negative, subinoculate the supernatant into fresh leukocyte cultures.

- **Procedure 2: Haemadsorption 'autorosette' test with peripheral blood leukocytes from infected pigs**

This procedure is quicker than the preparation and inoculation of primary pig leukocyte cultures (described in Procedure 1 above) and will give more rapid results in positive cases. It can be performed in laboratories that are not equipped for routine virological examinations; the minimum requirements are slides and cover-slips, a microscope and sterile medium, tubes or bottles and pipettes. Blood from suspect pigs in the field, or those inoculated in the laboratory, is collected in heparin and leukocyte cultures are prepared for direct examination for haemadsorption.

i) Collect 20 ml of whole blood in a syringe containing 2000 IU heparin in 2 ml of saline, mix and transfer to a glass tube or narrow bottle.

ii) Place the tube/bottle vertically in an incubator or water bath at 37°C, and allow the cells to settle. Sedimentation is improved by the addition of 2 ml of a plasma volume expander, such as 'Dextravan 150' which is a solution of Dextran 150 in 0.9% NaCl for injection (Fisons, United Kingdom).

iii) Incubate the cultures for 6–8 hours at 37°C, and then examine the cultures at 2–3-hour intervals by transferring small aliquots of the white-cell-rich supernatant, together with some erythrocytes, on to a glass slide and identify haemadsorbing cells under a microscope.

b) Antigen detection by fluorescent antibody test

The FAT (2) can be used to detect antigen in tissues of suspect pigs in the field or those inoculated at the laboratory. In addition, it can be used to detect ASFV antigen in leukocyte cultures in which no HAD is observed and can thus identify nonhaemadsorbing strains of virus. It also distinguishes between the CPE produced by ASFV and that produced by other viruses, such as Aujeszky's disease virus or a cytotoxic inoculum.

- **Test procedure**

i) Prepare cryostat sections or impression smears of test tissues, or spreads of cell sediment from inoculated leukocyte cultures on slides, air dry and fix with acetone for 10 minutes at room temperature.

ii) Stain with fluorescein isothiocyanate (FITC)-conjugated anti-ASFV immunoglobulin at the recommended or pretitrated dilution for 1 hour at 37°C in a humid chamber.

iii) Fix and stain positive and negative control preparations similarly.

iv) Wash in phosphate buffered saline (PBS), mount stained tissues in PBS/glycerol, and examine under an ultraviolet light microscope with suitable barrier and exciter filters.

v) *Reading the results:* Tissues are positive if specific granular cytoplasmic fluorescence is observed in paracortical tissue of lymphoid organs or in fixed macrophages in other organs.

c) Detection of virus genome by the polymerase chain reaction

The PCR technique has been developed, using primers from a highly conserved region of the genome, to detect and identify a wide range of isolates belonging to all the known virus genotypes, including both nonhaemadsorbing viruses and isolates of low virulence. It is particularly useful for identifying virus DNA in pig tissues that are unsuitable for virus isolation or antigen detection because they have undergone putrefaction, or when there is good reason to believe that virus may have been inactivated before samples are received in the laboratory. A suitable technique is as follows:

- **Sample preparation**

i) Prepare suspensions of tissue by grinding up small pieces of tissue with a pestle and mortar containing sterile sand, and make a 1/10 dilution by adding 5–10 ml of PBS containing 1% ox serum and antibiotics.

ii) Centrifuge at 500 ***g*** for 5 minutes.

iii) Extraction for control samples: 1/10 tissue homogenates (same tissue as the samples to be analysed): (a) a negative control: use 500 µl of a homogenate of ASFV-negative tissue; (b) a positive control: use 500 µl of a homogenate of ASFV-positive tissue.

iv) Transfer 500 µl to a screw-capped Eppendorf tube and boil for 10 minutes.

v) Centrifuge at 13,000 ***g*** in a microfuge for 5 minutes.

The tissue supernatant is used in the PCR test.

The sample preparation procedure given above is simple and inexpensive, but may produce false-negative results due to the presence of PCR inhibitors. An improved method, suitable for Reference Laboratories, is given below.

- **Alternative procedure for sample preparation**

In this procedure, use is made of commercially available products, the NucleoSpin Virus Kit (Macherey Nagel). This kit includes the reagents RAV1, RAV3 and NucleoSpin filter columns.

Working procedure for fluid samples: plasma, serum, cell culture medium.

(Note that for organ and tissue samples, first prepare a 1/10 homogenate of the material in PBS, then centrifuge to clarify at 12,000 ***g*** for 5 minutes. Use the supernatant fluid.)

Extraction for control samples: 1/10 tissue homogenates (same tissue as samples to be analysed): (a) a negative control: use 150 µl of a homogenate of ASFV-negative tissue; (b) a positive control: use 150 µl of a homogenate of ASVF-positive tissue.

i) Add 600 µl of RAV1 (carrier RNA included) to 150 µl of sample. Pipette up and down several times and vortex well. Incubate for 5–10 minutes at room temperature.

ii) Optional: If the resulting solution is turbid, centrifuge the mixture for 1 minute to clarify. Transfer supernatant to a new tube.

iii) Add 600 µl ethanol to the clear solution and mix by vortexing.

iv) Load 700 µl of the sample on to a NucleoSpin column, placed in a 2 ml centrifuge tube.

v) Centrifuge for 60 seconds at 6000 ***g*** at room temperature. Discard the flowthrough.

vi) Load the remaining sample (about 600 µl) on to the same NucleoSpin column and centrifuge as above. Discard the flowthrough.

vii) Add 500 µl of buffer RAV3 to the NucleoSpin column.

viii) Centrifuge for 30 seconds at 6000–8000 ***g***. Discard the flowthrough and repeat this washing step.

ix) Discard the flowthrough, then place the NucleoSpin column in a fresh 2 ml tube and centrifuge for 5 minutes at maximum speed to completely remove buffer RAV3.

x) Elution of nucleic acids: Place the NucleoSpin column in a sterile 1.5 ml centrifuge tube, add 50 µl of elution buffer (5 mM Tris/HCl, pH 8.5, preheated to 70°C), and incubate for 2 minutes.

xi) Centrifuge for 60 seconds at 8000 ***g***.

xii) Keep the 50 µl of eluted DNA at –20°C until use.

- **Stock solutions**

i) Taq DNA polymerase and PCR amplification buffer (10×) are commercially available.

ii) *Stock 1.25 mM dNTP:* Prepare 50 mM stock solutions of each of the following nucleotides: dATP, dCTP, dGTP and dTTP. Add 10 µl of each of these stock solutions to 360 µl sterile distilled water.

iii) *Primers at a concentration of 20 pmol/µl:* Primer 1 sequence 5'-ATGGA-TACCG-AGGGA-ATAGC-3' (positive strand); Primer 2 sequence 5'-CTTAC-CGATG-AAAAT-GATAC-3' (negative strand).

iv) *Loading buffer:* 0.25% Orange G in an aqueous solution of 30% glycerol.

v) *TAE buffer (50×) for agarose gel:* Tris base (242 g); glacial acetic acid (57.1 ml); 0.5 M EDTA, pH 8.0 (100 ml); distilled water (to 1 litre).

vi) *Marker DNA:* 100 base-pair ladder is commercially available.

- **Test procedure**

i) Add the following reagents to the required number of 0.75 ml polypropyl Eppendorf tubes:

Sterile distilled water (24.5 µl); (10× conc.) PCR amplification buffer (5 µl); magnesium chloride 25 mM (4 µl); 1.25 mM stock dNTP solution (8 µl); primer 1, 20 µM (1 µl); primer 2 (1 µl); tissue supernatant (10 µl); Taq DNA polymerase 5 U/µl (0.25 µl).

ii) Control tubes contain no tissue supernatant.

Negative control (no DNA): Add 10 µl of distilled water.

Positive control: Add 2 µl of ASFV DNA and 8 µl of distilled water.

iii) Overlay the mixture with 60 µl of mineral oil.

iv) Place all the tubes in an automated DNA thermal cycler and run the following programme:

One cycle at 94°C for 5 minutes.

Thirty-five cycles at 94°C for 1 minute, 50°C for 1 minute and 72°C for 1 minute.

One cycle at 72°C for 10 minutes.

Hold at 4°C.

v) At the end of the programme, carefully remove 20 µl of each reaction mixture from below the mineral oil, transfer to a clean tube and add 2 µl of loading buffer.

vi) Load all the samples in a 2% agarose gel in TAE buffer containing ethidium bromide at a final concentration of 0.5 µg/ml.

Add marker DNA to one lane on each side of the gel.

vii) Run the gel at a constant voltage of 150 volts for 2 hours.

viii) *Reading the results:* Examine the gel over a UV light source. In a positive sample, a discrete band will be present that should co-migrate with the PCR product of the positive control. Calculate the size of the PCR products in the test samples and the positive control by reference to the standard markers. The PCR product of the positive control has a size of 278 base pairs. No bands should be seen in the negative control.

d) Pig inoculation

In the past, pig inoculation has been used to differentiate between classical and African swine fever, which produce indistinguishable clinical signs. Samples were inoculated into two groups of pigs, one of which had been vaccinated against classical swine fever (hog cholera), the other remaining unvaccinated. This test is now unlikely to be necessary, because there are alternative laboratory tests that give reliable results for both ASF and classical swine fever. The pig inoculation test is slow, expensive and difficult to perform and results in acute distress for the animals involved. It can no longer be recommended.

2. Serological tests

Antibodies persist in recovered pigs for long periods after infection, sometimes for life, and a number of tests are available for detecting these antibodies, although only a few of them have been developed for routine use in diagnostic laboratories (1, 3, 7, 8, 11). The most commonly used is the ELISA (12, 14), which is suitable for examining either serum or fluid from the tissues. Confirmatory testing of ELISA-positive samples should be carried out in critical cases using an alternative test, such as the IFA test (10), immunoperoxidase staining or immunoblotting (3, 9). Antibody is usually not produced in pigs infected with virulent ASFV. High levels of antibody are produced in pigs infected with low or moderately virulent ASF viruses, but these are not neutralising antibodies.

Where ASF is endemic, confirmation of suspected cases of disease is best done using a standard serological test (ELISA), combined with an alternative serological test (IFA) or an antigen-detection test (FAT). In some countries, over 95% of positive cases have been identified using a combination of IFA tests and FAT (11).

It should be noted that when pigs have been infected with avirulent isolates or those of low virulence, serological tests may be the only way of detecting infected animals.

Both the counter immunoelectrophoresis test and ELISA can be used for the large-scale screening of sera, although the ELISA is more sensitive for detecting individual positive sera and has been used extensively as part of eradication programmes.

The method used depends on the staff and facilities available.

a) Enzyme-linked immunosorbent assay (the prescribed test for international trade)

The ELISA (1, 8) is a direct test that can detect antibodies to ASFV in pigs that have been infected by viruses of low or moderate virulence.

- **Antigen preparation**

The ELISA antigen is prepared from infected cells grown in the presence of pig serum (4).

i) Infect MS (monkey stable) cells at multiplicity of infection of 10 with adapted virus, and incubate in medium containing 2% pig serum.

ii) Harvest the cells at 36–48 hours post-infection, when the CPE is extensive. Wash in PBS, sediment at 650 *g* for 5 minutes, wash the cell pellet in 0.34 M sucrose in 5 mM Tris-HCl, pH 8.0, and centrifuge to pellet cells.

Carry out steps (iii) to (v) on ice:

iii) Resuspend the cell pellet in 67 mM sucrose in 5 mM Tris-HCl, pH 8.0 (1.8 ml per 175 cm^2 flask), and leave for 10 minutes with agitation after 5 minutes.

iv) Add nonionic detergent Nonidet P-40 to a final concentration of 1% (w/v), and leave for 10 minutes (with agitation after 5 minutes) to lyse the cells.

v) Add sucrose to a final concentration of 64% (w/w) in 0.4 M Tris-HCl, pH 8.0, and centrifuge at 1000 *g* for 10 minutes to pellet nuclei.

vi) Collect the supernatant and add EDTA (2 mM final concentration), beta-mercaptoethanol (50 mM final concentration) and NaCl (0.5 M final concentration) in 0.25 mM Tris-HCl, pH 8.0, and incubate for 15 minutes at 25°C.

vii) Centrifuge at 100,000 *g* for 1 hour at 4°C over a layer of 20% (w/w) sucrose in 50 mM Tris-HCl, pH 8.0.

Remove the band immediately above the sucrose layer and use as the ELISA antigen. Store at –20°C.

- **Test procedure (12)**

i) Coat ELISA microtitre plate(s) with antigen by adding 100 µl of the recommended or pretitrated dilution of antigen in 0.05 M carbonate/bicarbonate buffer, pH 9.6, to each well.

ii) Incubate at 4°C for 16 hours (overnight) and then wash five times with 0.05% Tween 20 in PBS, pH 7.2.

iii) Dilute the test sera and positive and negative control sera 1/30 in 0.05% Tween 20 in PBS, pH 7.2, and add 100 µl of each diluted serum to duplicate wells of the antigen-coated plate(s).

If four pairs of each positive and negative control serum are added to wells in different parts of the plate, 40 sera can be tested in duplicate on one plate, as shown on the plate plan below.

	1	2	3	4	5	6	7	8	9	10	11	12
A	+											–
B	+											–
C				+					–			
D				+					–			
E				–					+			
F				–					+			
G	–											+
H	–											+

iv) Incubate plates at 37°C for 1 hour (optionally on a plate shaker), and then wash five times with 0.05% Tween 20 in PBS.

v) To each well add 100 µl of protein-A/horseradish-peroxidase conjugate at the recommended or pretitrated dilution in 0.05% Tween 20 in PBS.

vi) Incubate the plates at 37°C for 1 hour, and then wash five times with 0.05% Tween 20 in PBS.

vii) Add hydrogen peroxide to the substrate solution (0.04% orthophenylenediamine in phosphate/citrate buffer, pH 5.0) at the rate of 10 µl/25 ml, and add 100 µl of substrate to each well.

viii) Incubate at room temperature for around 10 minutes; the time necessary for the colour to develop will depend on both the temperature of the substrate when added to the wells, and the room temperature.

ix) Stop the reaction by adding 100 µl of 3 N sulphuric acid to each well.

x) *Reading the results:* Positive sera have a clear yellow colour and can be read by eye, but to ensure that all positive sera are identified, it is necessary to read the absorbance in each well spectrophotometrically, at 492 nm, in an ELISA reader. Any serum is considered to be positive if it has an absorbance value of more than twice the mean absorbance value of the control negative sera on that plate.

b) Indirect fluorescent antibody test

This test (10) should be used as a confirmatory test for sera from areas that are free from ASF and are positive in the ELISA, and for sera from endemic areas that give an inconclusive result in the ELISA.

- **Test procedure**

i) Prepare a suspension of ASFV-infected pig kidney or monkey cells at a concentration of 5×10^5 cells/ml, spread small drops on glass slides, air dry and fix with acetone at room temperature for 10 minutes. Note that slides can be stored at –20°C until ready for use.

ii) Heat inactivate test sera at 56°C for 30 minutes.

iii) Add appropriate dilutions of test sera and positive and negative control sera in buffered saline to slides of both infected and uninfected control cells, and incubate for 1 hour at 37°C in a humid chamber.

iv) Wash the slides with PBS and then distilled water.

v) Add predetermined or recommended dilutions of anti-pig immunoglobulin-FITC or protein A-FITC conjugate to all slides, and incubate for 1 hour at 37°C in a humid chamber.

vi) Wash the slides with PBS and then distilled water, mount in PBS/glycerol, and examine under an ultraviolet light microscope with suitable barrier and exciter filters.

vii) *Reading the results:* The control positive serum on infected cells must be positive and all other controls must be negative before the test can be read. Sera are positive if infected cultures show specific fluorescence.

c) Immunoblotting test

This test should be used as an alternative to the IFA test to confirm equivocal results with individual sera.

- **Preparation of antigen strips**

i) Prepare cytoplasmic soluble virus proteins as described for the preparation of ELISA antigen in Section A.2.a.

ii) Electrophorese through 17% acryl-amide/N,N'-diallyltartardiamide (DATD) gels with appropriate molecular weight standards.

iii) Transfer the proteins onto a 14×14 cm^2 nitrocellulose membrane by electrophoresis at a constant current of 5 mA/cm in transfer buffer (20% methanol in 196 mM glycine, 25 mM Tris-HCl, pH 8.3).

iv) Dry the membrane and label the side on to which the proteins were electrophoresed.

v) Cut one strip from the edge of the filter and carry out the immunoblotting procedure described below. Identify the region containing proteins of 23–35 kDa by comparison with the molecular weight standards run in parallel, and cut this region into 0.5 cm wide strips. Label each strip on the side on to which the proteins were electrophoresed.

These strips (approximately 4 cm long) constitute the antigen strips used for immunoblotting and contain proteins with which antibodies in both acute and convalescent pig sera will react. These antibodies persist for life in some pigs.

- **Preparation of chloranaphthol substrate solution**

This solution must be prepared immediately before use.

i) Dissolve 6 mg of 4-chloro-1-naphthol in 2 ml of methanol and add this solution slowly to 10 ml of PBS while it is being stirred.

ii) Remove the white precipitate that is formed by filtation through Whatman No.1 filter paper (optional).

iii) Add 4 µl of 30% hydrogen peroxide.

- **Test procedure**

The antigen strips must be kept with the labelled side uppermost during the immunoreaction procedure.

i) Incubate the antigen strips in blocking buffer (2% nonfat dried milk in PBS) at 37°C for 30 minutes with continuous agitation.

ii) Prepare 1/40 dilutions of test sera and positive and negative control sera in blocking buffer.

iii) Incubate the antigen strips in the appropriate serum at 37°C for 45 minutes with continuous agitation. Incubate one antigen strip in positive control serum and one in negative control serum. These two strips are controls. Wash four times in blocking buffer; the final wash should be for 5 minutes with continuous agitation.

iv) Add protein-A/horseradish-peroxidase conjugate at the recommended or pretitrated dilution in blocking buffer to all antigen strips. Incubate at 37°C for 45 minutes with continuous agitation. Wash four times in blocking buffer; the final wash should be for 5 minutes with continuous agitation.

v) Prepare the substrate solution, add to the antigen strips, and incubate at room temperature for 5–15 minutes with continuous agitation.

vi) Stop the reaction with distilled water when the protein bands are suitably dark.

vii) *Reading the results:* Positive sera react with more than one virus protein in the antigen strip; they must give a similar protein pattern and have the same intensity of colour as the antigen strips stained with positive control serum.

d) Counter immunoelectrophoresis (immunoelectro-osmophoresis) test

This test (6) can be carried out rapidly and specific antibody can be detected in some sera 30 minutes after the test is set up. It requires the use of electrophoresis equipment (electrophoresis chamber, slide frames, gel cutter) and a 500-volt constant-current power supply. Due to its low sensitivity, this test is recommended for screening groups of pigs, but not individual animals.

- **Test procedure**

i) Place the required number of 2.5 × 10 cm glass slides in the slide frame on a level table and cover with the recommended volume of 0.6% agarose in veronal/acetate buffer, pH 8.6 (ionic strength 0.025) containing 0.1% sodium azide, and allow to set.

ii) Cut four pairs of wells, 3 mm in diameter, 10 mm apart in the gel on each slide as shown below.

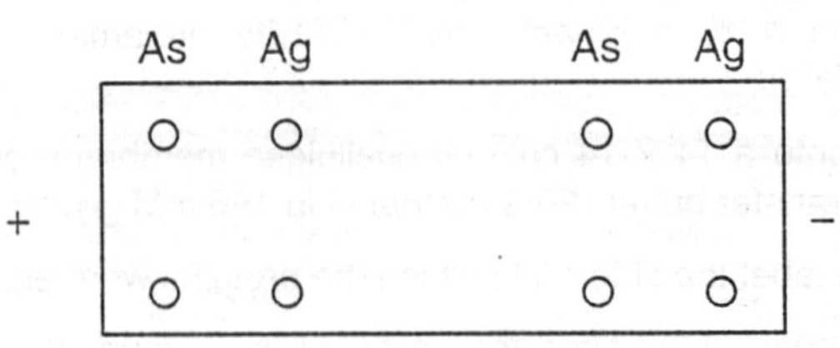

As = antiserum; Ag = antigen; + = positive electrode; – = negative electrode)

iii) Fill the wells with the appropriate reagents, including control positive and negative antigens and antisera, using capillary (haematocrit) tubes.

iv) Place the frames in the electrophoresis chamber and run for 30 minutes with a constant voltage of 19 volts/cm.

v) After electrophoresis, examine the slides over an indirect light source for specific lines of precipitation.

vi) Wash the slides in 2% NaCl solution overnight and for 2 hours in several changes of distilled water before drying.

vii) Stain dried slides with 0.075% amido black in equal volumes of methanol, 12% acetic acid and 1.6% sodium acetate, containing 0.007% glycerol, for 5–10 minutes and destain with three 10-minute washes in an aqueous solution of 45% methanol and 10% glacial acetic acid.

viii) *Reading the results:* Lines of precipitation observed between the wells containing antigen and antiserum on the stained slides should be similar to that of the positive control to be considered positive.

B. REQUIREMENTS FOR VACCINES AND DIAGNOSTIC BIOLOGICALS

At present there is no vaccine for ASF.

REFERENCES

1. ARIAS M. & SANCHEZ VIZCAINO J.M. (1992). Manual de diagnóstico serológico de la peste porcina africana. (Manual of diagnostic serology for African swine fever.) Ministry of Agriculture, CISA-INIA, Valdeolmos-28130 Madrid, Spain, 1–44.

2. BOOL P.H., ORDAS A. & SANCHEZ BOTIJA C. (1969). El diagnostico de la peste porcina africana por inmunofluorescencia. (The diagnosis of African swine fever by immunofluorescence). *Bull. OIE*, **72**, 819–839.

3. ESCRIBANO J.M., PASTOR M.J., ARIAS M. & SANCHEZ VIZCAINO J.M. (1990). Confirmación de sueros positivos a ELISA-peste porcina africana, mediante la técnica de 'Immunoblotting'. Utilización de las proteínas inducidas por el virus cone pesosmoleculares comprendidos entre 23 y 35 kilodaltons, en el desarrollo de un 'kit' de diagnóstico. (Confirmation of sera positive by ASF ELISA with the immunoblotting technique. Use of virus-induced proteins of 23–25 kDa in the development of a diagnostic kit.) *Med. Vet.*, **7**, 135–141.

4. ESCRIBANO J.M., PASTOR M.J. & SANCHEZ VIZCAINO J.M. (1989). Antibodies to bovine serum albumin in swine sera: implications for false positive reactions in the serodiagnosis of African swine fever. *Am. J. Vet. Res.*, **50**, 1118–1122.

5. MALMQUIST W.A. & HAY D. (1960). Haemadsorption and cytopathic effect produced by African swine fever virus in swine bone marrow and buffy coat cultures. *Am. J. Vet. Res.*, **21**, 104–108.

6. PAN I.C., DE BOER C.J. & HESS W.R. (1972). African swine fever: application of immuno-electro-osmophoresis for the detection of antibody. *Can. J. Comp. Med.*, **36**, 309–316.

7. PAN I.C., TRAUTMAN R., HESS W.R., DE BOER C.J., TESSLER J., ORDAS A., SANCHEZ BOTIJA C., OVEJERO J. & SANCHEZ M.C. (1974). African swine fever: comparison of four serotests on porcine serums in Spain. *Am. J. Vet. Res.*, **35**, 787–790.

8. PASTOR M.J., ARIAS M. & ESCRIBANO J.M. (1990). Comparison of two antigens for use in an enzyme-linked immunosorbent assay to detect African swine fever antibody. *Am. J. Vet. Res.*, **51**, 1540–1543.

9. PASTOR M.J., LAVIADA M.D., SANCHEZ VIZCAINO J.M. & ESCRIBANO J.M. (1989). Detection of African swine fever virus antibodies by immunoblotting assay. *Can. J. Vet. Res.*, **53**, 105–107.

10. SANCHEZ BOTIJA C., ORDAS A. & GONZALES J.G. (1970). La immunofluorescencia indirecta aplicada a la investigación de anticuerpos de la peste porcina africana. Su valor para el diagnóstico. (Indirect immunofluorescence for the investigation of African swine fever antibodies. Its value for diagnosis). *Rev. Patron. Biol. Anim.*, **14**, 159–180.

11. SANCHEZ VIZCAINO J.M. (1987). African swine fever diagnosis. *In:* African Swine Fever, Becker Y., ed. Martinus Nijhoff, Boston, USA, 63–71.

12. SANCHEZ VIZCAINO J.M., CROWTHER J.R. & WARDLEY R.C. (1983). A collaborative study on the use of the ELISA in the diagnosis of African swine fever. *In:* African Swine Fever. (CEC/FAO Research Seminar, Sardinia, Sept. 1981). Wilkinson P.J., ed. Commission of the European Communities Publication EUR 8466 EN, 297–325.

13. Vinuela E. (1985). African swine fever. *Curr. Top. Microbiol. Immunol.*, **116**, 151–170.

14. Wardley R.C., Abu Elzein E.M.E., Crowther J.R. & Wilkinson P.J. (1979). A solid-phase enzyme-linked immunosorbent assay for the detection of African swine fever antigen and antibody. *J. Hyg.*, **83**, 363–369.

*
* *

CHAPTER 2.1.13.

CLASSICAL SWINE FEVER (hog cholera)

SUMMARY

Classical swine fever (CSF), also known as hog cholera, is a contagious viral disease of pigs. The causative virus is a member of the genus Pestivirus of the family Flaviviridae, and is closely related to the viruses of bovine viral diarrhoea and border disease. There is only one serotype of CSF virus (CSFV).

The disease may run an acute, subacute, chronic or inapparent course, depending on a variety of viral and host factors of which the age of the animals, the virulence of the virus and the time of infection (pre- or post-natal) are of greatest importance. Adult pigs usually display less severe signs of disease than young animals and stand a better chance of survival. In pregnant sows, the virus may cross the placental barrier and reach the fetuses. In-utero *infection with strains of the virus of moderate or low virulence can result in what is referred to as the 'carrier sow' syndrome followed by prenatal or early post-natal death, the birth of diseased piglets or an apparently 'healthy' but infected litter. An outbreak of CSF has serious consequences for trade in pigs and pig products.*

The highly variable clinical picture of CSF often precludes a diagnosis on clinical and pathological grounds alone. Laboratory methods are therefore essential for an unambiguous diagnosis. Detection of virus in whole blood and of antibodies in serum are the methods of choice for diagnosing CSF in live pigs, whereas detection of virus or antigen in organ samples is most suitable when the pig is dead.

Identification of the agent: *The direct fluorescent antibody test (FAT) on cryostat sections of organs from affected pigs is used for the detection of CSF antigen. A panel of monoclonal antibodies (MAbs) is used to determine whether the fluorescence is due to CSF or non-CSF pestivirus antigens. In negative FAT cases, the isolation of CSFV in the PK-15 cell line, or other suitable cell lines, should be attempted. The cultures are examined for virus growth by direct immunofluorescence or direct peroxidase staining; positive results are further characterised by the use of MAbs.*

Serological tests: *Detection of virus-specific antibodies is particularly useful in herds suspected of being infected at least 30 days previously with CSFV. Serological methods are also valuable for monitoring and for prevalence studies, and are essential if a country wishes to be internationally recognised as being free from the disease in the absence of vaccination.*

As antibodies against ruminant pestivirus are regularly observed in breeding pigs, screening tests have to be followed by confirmatory tests. Only tests that differentiate between bovine viral diarrhoea, border disease and CSF antibodies are relevant. For this purpose, the neutralising peroxidase-linked assay (NPLA), the fluorescent antibody virus neutralisation test and the enzyme-linked immunosorbent assay (ELISA) are very suitable. All three tests are specific and sensitive. The NPLA and ELISA can be read macroscopically and can be automated.

Requirements for vaccines and diagnostic biologicals: *Vaccines against CSF are based on live virus that has been attenuated by passage through cell cultures or through a suitable host species that is not of the family Suidae. The production of these modified live virus (MLV) vaccines is based on a seed-lot system that has been validated with respect to virus identity, sterility, purity, safety, nontransmissibility, stability and immunogenicity.*

Effective inactivated, conventional whole virus vaccines are not available. In recent years 'marker vaccines' have been developed, which in contrast to MLV vaccines induce antibodies that can be distinguished from antibodies induced by field virus using an accompanying diagnostic test. The presently registered 'marker vaccines' are based on the major envelope glycoprotein (E2-subunit) of CSFV, and are produced in insect cells using recombinant DNA technology.

A. DIAGNOSTIC TECHNIQUES

The viruses that cause classical swine fever (CSF), bovine viral diarrhoea (BVD) and border disease (BD) are members of the family Flaviviridae, genus Pestivirus, and are closely related, both antigenically and structurally. The term BVD is used generically in this chapter to include all ruminant pestiviruses.

Clinical signs and lesions seen post-mortem in pigs affected with CSF are highly variable due to both viral and host factors. Furthermore, congenital infections with BVD virus (BVDV) strains in pigs can give rise to a clinical disease that is indistinguishable from CSF (14–16).

Spread of disease in all age groups, accompanied by pyrexia, huddling, inappetance, dullness, weakness, conjunctivitis, constipation followed by diarrhoea, and an unsteady gait are the prevailing signs. Several days after the onset of clinical signs, the ears, abdomen and inner thighs may show a purple discoloration. Animals with acute disease die within 1–2 weeks. Sudden death in the absence of clinical illness is not symptomatic of CSF.

Under certain circumstances related to the animals' age and condition, as well as to the virus strain involved, subacute or chronic clinical illness may develop, which can be protracted for 2–4 weeks or even months. Chronic illness leads to a stunting of growth, anorexia, intermittent pyrexia and diarrhoea. Congenital persistent infections may go undetected for months and may be confined to only a few piglets in the herd. The clinical signs are nonspecific: wasting in the absence of pyrexia. Chronic, persistent infections always lead to the death of the animal. Herd mortality rates may be slightly above the expected level. CSF affects the immune system, a main characteristic being generalised leukopenia, which can often be detected before the onset of fever. Immunosuppression may lead to concurrent infections.

In acute cases, gross pathological lesions are often inconspicuous or absent. In typical cases, the lymph nodes are marbled red, and haemorrhages occur on the epicardium, and in the kidneys, urinary bladder, the skin and subcutis. In subacute and chronic cases, necrotic or 'button' ulcers may be observed in the mucosae of the gastrointestinal tract, epiglottis and larynx, in addition to the above lesions.

Histopathological findings are not pathognomonic. Lesions may include parenchymatous degeneration of lymphatic tissue, cellular proliferation of vascular interstitial tissue, and a nonsuppurative meningo-encephalomyelitis, with or without vascular cuffing.

The variability of the clinical signs and post-mortem lesions do not provide firm evidence for unequivocal diagnosis. Other septicaemic diseases, such as African swine fever, salmonellosis, pasteurellosis, actinobacillosis and *Haemophillus suis* infections may be confused with acute CSF. In fact, these bacteria often cause concurrent infections, and isolating these pathogens may obscure the real cause of disease, the CSF virus (CSFV).

A tentative diagnosis based on clinical signs and post-mortem lesions must therefore be confirmed by laboratory investigations. This is all the more necessary in view of the serious consequences of an outbreak of CSF for trade in pigs and pig products.

Laboratory methods for diagnosis of CSF are aimed at detection of the virus or viral antigens, or detection of specific antibodies. For a correct interpretation of the test results the inspecting veterinarian should pay particular attention to the simultaneous and clustered occurrence of two or more of the prevailing signs of disease listed above. Random sampling is unsuitable for CSF diagnosis. As pyrexia is one of the first signs of CSF and is accompanied by viraemia (3), virus detection in whole heparinised blood or tissues collected from a few febrile animals is the method of choice for detecting infected herds at an early stage. Additionally, whole blood samples for virus detection can be collected from a larger group of pigs.

Antibodies develop in the third week of illness and persist in the surviving animal for life. Samples for antibody detection are collected in ordinary (nonheparinised) tubes from convalescent pigs and from contact herds when ≥30 days have elapsed since the suspected contact with a confirmed outbreak took place.

1. Identification of the agent

a) Immunological methods

- **Fluorescent antibody test**

The fluorescent antibody test (FAT) is a rapid test that can be used to detect CSFV antigen in cryostat sections of tonsils, spleen, kidney, or distal portions of the ileum. Tissues should be collected from several animals and transported without preservatives under cool conditions, but not frozen. Cryostat sections are stained directly with anti-CSF immunoglobulin conjugated to fluorescein isothiocyanate (FITC) or indirectly using a secondary FITC conjugate and examined by fluorescence microscopy. Tonsillar tissue is the most suitable, as this is the first to become affected by the virus irrespective of the route of infection (10). In subacute and chronic cases, the ileum is frequently positive and occasionally may be the only tissue to display fluorescence. A negative FAT result does not completely rule out CSF infection. When suspicion of CSF continues, further samples should be obtained or attempts made at virus isolation in cell culture (e.g. PK-15) or another cell line of pig origin that is as sensitive and known to be free from pestivirus contamination.

- **Test procedure**

Include positive and negative control sections in each series of organ samples to be examined.

i) Cut out a piece of tonsil, spleen, kidney and ileum of approximately 1 × 1 × 0.5 cm, and mount it with a cryo-embedding compound or distilled water on a cryostat table.

ii) Freeze the piece of organ on to the cryostat table.

iii) Cut sections not more than 4 µm thick and mount these on to 10 × 32 mm grease-free cover-slips with one corner cut-off. All sections are mounted with this corner in the same position (e.g. top right).

iv) Fix the mounted sections for 10 minutes at room temperature in acetone (analytical grade) or air-dry for 20 minutes at 37°C.

v) Immerse the sections briefly in phosphate buffered saline (PBS), remove excess fluid with tissue paper and place them (cut off corner top right) on a frame in an incubation chamber humidified with a small volume of water placed in the bottom of the chamber.

vi) Dispense the anti-CSF immunoglobulin at working dilution on to the entire section and incubate in the closed chamber for 30 minutes at 37°C. If a secondary FITC conjugate is required, wash the section five times for 2 minutes each in PBS at room temperature, then add the FITC conjugate at working dilution and incubate as previously described.

vii) Wash the sections five times for 2 minutes each in PBS at room temperature.

viii) Remove the remaining PBS by touching the cover-slip against tissue paper and mount the cover-slip (with the section between cover-slip and slide) with mounting buffer on to a microscope slide.

ix) Remove excess mounting fluid with tissue paper and examine the sections for fluorescence using a UV microscope. A CSF-positive section shows brilliant green fluorescing cells. In the tonsils, fluorescence in the epithelial lining of the crypts is particularly evident. In kidney sections, fluorescence is most abundant in the proximal and distal tubules of the renal cortex and the collecting ducts in the medulla. In the ileum, fluorescence is most prominent in the epithelial cells of the Lieberkühn glands, whereas in the spleen reactivity is more diffuse, with concentrations of lymphoid cells in the periarterial lymphoid sheath (PALS).

The FAT involves the use of an anti-CSF immunoglobulin prepared from a polyclonal antibody to CSFV that will not distinguish between the antigens of different pestiviruses. Conjugates used for the FAT on cryostat sections or inoculated cell cultures should be prepared from anti-CSFV gamma-globulins raised in specific pathogen free pigs. The working dilution of the conjugates (at least 1/30) should combine a maximum brilliance with a minimum of background.

Strains of modified live virus (MLV) vaccine multiply mainly in the regional lymph nodes and in the crypt epithelium of the tonsils. Pigs vaccinated with MLV strains may yield a positive FAT for 2 weeks after vaccination (9, 11). Rabbit inoculation is used to differentiate between lapinised and field strains of CSFV. In contrast to field strains, lapinised strains given intravenously cause a febrile reaction and induce an immune response in rabbits.

Pigs infected with BVDV can give false-positive FAT reactions. Congenital infections with BVDV can cause clinical signs and pathological lesions indistinguishable from those in chronic CSF (14–16). Infections by CSFV or BVDV can be differentiated by testing sera from the dam and litter mates, or from other contacts of an FAT-positive piglet, for neutralising antibodies to either virus. Another method of differentiating these viruses is by the inoculation of seronegative piglets with a suspension of suspect material, followed 5 weeks later by virus neutralisation (VN) tests on their sera for the respective antibodies. However, VN tests may take several days, and animal inoculation methods take several weeks.

- **Immunoperoxidase procedure for differentiation of pestiviruses by monoclonal antibodies**

The use of a panel of three horseradish peroxidase (HRPO) or FITC-conjugated monoclonal antibodies (MAbs) specifically detecting all field strains of CSFV, vaccine strains of CSFV and BVDV/BDV, respectively, would allow an unambiguous differentiation between field and vaccine strains of CSFV on the one hand, and between CSFV and other pestiviruses on the other (6, 17, 19). A prerequisite is that the MAb against CSFV recognises all field strains and that the anti-vaccine MAb recognises all vaccine strains used in the country. *No single MAb against BVDV recognises all BVDV/BDV strains* (6). The use of an MAb to differentiate a CSF vaccine strain can be omitted in nonvaccination areas. A polyclonal anti-CSF immunoglobulin conjugated to HRPO serves as a positive control.

- **Test procedure**

i) Cut eight or more cryostat sections (4 µm) of the FAT-positive tonsil, or another positive organ if the tonsil is not available.

ii) Fix the sections on to flying cover-slips for 10 minutes in acetone (analytical grade) and allow to air dry.

iii) Prepare working dilutions of the respective MAb-peroxidase conjugates in PBS + 0.01% Tween 80 + 5% horse serum, pH 7.6. (FITC–MAb can also be used, as well as unconjugated MAb provided that a secondary conjugate is used.)

iv) After rinsing with PBS, overlay two sections with the working dilution of the respective monoclonal conjugates, and two sections with the working dilution of the polyclonal conjugate (controls).

v) Incubate for 1 hour at 37°C in a humid chamber.

vi) Wash the sections six times for 10 seconds each in PBS.

vii) Stain the sections with freshly prepared chromogen–substrate solution* for 5–15 minutes at room temperature.

viii) Rinse the sections in 0.05 M sodium acetate, pH 5.0, in distilled water and mount them on microscope slides.

ix) Examine sections with a light microscope. Dark red staining of the cytoplasm of the epithelial cells lining the tonsillar crypts indicates recognition of the virus isolate by the respective conjugate, and is considered to be positive.

x) Interpretation of the test:

Polyclonal antibody	Monoclonal antibody specific for			Interpretation
	CSF strain	CSF vaccine strain	BVD/BD strain	
+	+	–	–	CSF field strain
+	+	+	–	CSF vaccine strain
+	–	–	+	BVD/BD strain
+	–	–	–	Other non-CSF pestivirus

- **Antigen-capture assay**

For early diagnosis of CSF in live pigs, antigen-capture enzyme-linked immunosorbent assays (ELISAs) have been developed for screening herds suspected to have been infected recently. The ELISAs are of the

* **Chromogen–substrate solution**

A. Stock solution of chromogen: 0.4% 3-amino-9-ethyl carbazole; N,N-dimethyl-formamide (1 ml). Caution **TOXIC compound.**

B. 0.05 M sodium acetate, pH 5.0; 19 ml (sterile filtered through a membrane).

C. Stock solution of substrate (30% hydrogen peroxide).

Keep stock solutions A and C at 4°C in the dark and solution B at room temperature. Stock solution A can be kept at 4°C for at least 6 months and solution C for 1 year. Immediately before use, dilute 1 ml of solution A in 19 ml of solution B. Then add 10 µl of stock solution C. Mix well and stain the sections.

double-antibody sandwich type, using monoclonal and/or polyclonal antibodies against a variety of viral proteins in either serum, the blood leukocyte fraction or anticoagulated whole blood (4). The technique is relatively simple to perform, does not require tissue culture facilities, is suitable for automation and provides results within 36 hours. The disadvantage of being less sensitive than virus isolation, especially in adult pigs and mild or subclinical cases, may be compensated by testing all pigs of the suspect herd showing pyrexia. However, the lowered specificity of these tests should also be taken into consideration.

b) Isolation of virus

Isolation of virus in cell cultures is a more sensitive but slower method for diagnosis of CSF than immunofluorescence on frozen sections. Isolation is best performed in rapidly dividing PK-15 cells seeded on to cover-slips simultaneously with a 2% suspension of the tonsil in growth medium. Other pig cell lines may be used, but should be demonstrably at least as sensitive as PK-15 cells for isolation of CSFV. The cultures are examined for fluorescent foci by FAT after 24–72 hours.

The tonsil is the organ of choice for virus isolation from pigs that died or were killed for diagnostic purposes. If the tonsil is not available, the spleen, kidney or lymph nodes can be used.

A detailed procedure for virus isolation is as follows:

i) Prepare a 100-fold strength glutamine–antibiotic stock solution: dissolve glutamine (2.92 g) in 50 ml distilled water (solution A) and sterilise by filtration. Dissolve each of the following antibiotics in 5–10 ml sterile distilled water: penicillin (10^6 Internatinal Units [IU]); streptomycin (1 g); mycostatin (5×10^5 U); polymixin B (15×10^4 U); and kanamycin (1 g). Pool these solutions (solution B). Mix aseptically solutions A and B, make up to 100 ml with sterile distilled water, and store in aliquots at –20°C. For use, thaw one bottle of stock solution and add 1–10 ml of tissue suspension or 0.2–10 ml of cell suspension, respectively.

ii) Cut 1–2 g of tonsillar tissue into small pieces and, using a mortar and pestle, grind in a small amount of cell culture medium with sterile sand into a homogeneous paste. Alternatively, use an appropriate crushing machine at 4°C.

iii) Make a 20% (w/v) suspension by adding Hanks' balanced salts solution (BSS) or Hanks' minimum essential medium (MEM); 1 ml of the glutamine–antibiotic stock is added for each 10 ml of suspension. This mixture is held at room temperature for 1 hour.

iv) Centrifuge at 1000 ***g*** for 15 minutes.

v) A PK-15 monolayer is trypsinised, the cell suspension is centrifuged at 160 ***g*** for 10 minutes, and resuspended to contain 2×10^6 cells/ml in growth medium (Eagle's MEM with Earle's salts; 5% fetal bovine serum free from antibodies to BVD; and 0.2 ml of the glutamine–antibiotic stock solution per 10 ml cell suspension).

vi) Mix nine parts of cell suspension (from step v) and one part of supernatant fluid (from step iv) and inoculate into 6–8 Leighton tubes with cover-slips or other appropriate cell culture flasks. Three tubes are inoculated with cell suspension alone as controls. After completion of the sample inoculations, three tubes are inoculated with CSFV as positive controls. Careful precautions must be taken to avoid cross-contamination with this known positive virus suspension.

vii) At 1, 2 and 3 days after inoculation, two cultures together with a control culture are washed twice for 5 minutes each in Hanks' BSS or Hanks' MEM, fixed with cold acetone (analytical grade) for 10 minutes, and stained with a direct anti-CSFV conjugate at its appropriate working dilution or indirectly, as described in Section 1.a.

    If the 2% tonsil suspension proves to be toxic for the cells, then the test should be repeated using a higher dilution or another organ.

viii) After washing in PBS three times for 5 minutes each, the cover-slip cultures are mounted in 90% carbonate–bicarbonate buffered glycerol, pH>8.0, and examined for fluorescent foci.

Instead of Leighton tubes, flat-bottomed microtitre plates or M24-plates can be used for virus isolation. Plates are fixed and stained as described later for the neutralising peroxidase-linked assay (NPLA).

Whole blood (heparin or ethylene diamine tetra-acetic acid treated) from clinically diseased pigs is a suitable sample for early CSF diagnosis. The leukocyte fraction or other components may be used, but for reasons of sensitivity and simplicity whole blood is preferred (5). The procedure is as follows:

i) Freeze a sample of whole blood at –20°C and thaw in a waterbath at 37°C.

ii) Inoculate 300 µl haemolysed blood on to a PK-15-monolayer grown to approximately 75% confluence* in an M24-plate, and allow adsorption for 1 hour at 37°C.

ii) Remove inoculum, wash the monolayer once with Hanks' BSS or Hanks' MEM, and add growth medium.

iv) After a further incubation period of 3–4 days, the plates are washed, fixed and stained, as described later for the NPLA, using in each step a volume of 300 µl to compensate for the larger cell surface.

- **Reverse-transcription polymerase chain reaction**

Methods for reverse-transcription polymerase chain reaction (RT-PCR) are under development. A promising alternative to the antigen-capture ELISA and the virus isolation method is a single tube reverse-transcription nested polymerase chain reaction (RT-nPCR) (8). This method, which is under development, is rapid and more sensitive than antigen-capture ELISAs or virus isolation or the RT-PCR. It has the additional advantage of reducing the risk of carry-over contamination because tubes are not opened between the successive RT, first PCR and nested PCR reaction steps. No internationally standardised method is yet available. Examples of a suitable protocol may be obtained from the literature or from the OIE Reference Laboratories for CSF (see Table given in Part 4 of this *Manual*).

The molecular epidemiology of CSF is based on the comparison of genetic differences between virus isolates. RT-PCR amplification of CSFV RNA followed by nucleotide sequencing is the simplest way of obtaining the sequence data to make these comparisons. A number of different regions of the CSFV genome may be targeted for molecular epidemiological studies. Two regions have been extensively studied and provide large sets of sequence data with which new isolates can be compared. One of these regions lies within the 5'-noncoding region (5'NCR) of the genome (150 nucleotides) and the other lies within the E2 major glycoprotein gene (190 nucleotides). In brief, the method used is to extract virus RNA from infected PK-15 cell cultures, perform RT-PCR to amplify one or both targets within the 5'NCR or the E2 gene, and then determine the nucleotide sequence of the products and compare with stored sequence information held in the databases. A database of these sequences is available from the OIE Reference Laboratory for CSF (Hanover, Germany). CSFV isolates from primary outbreaks should be sent to the OIE Reference Laboratory in Germany for investigation of molecular epidemiology. An unlimited import permit is available there.

2. Serological tests

Detection of virus-specific antibodies is particularly useful on premises suspected of having infections with CSF strains of low virulence. Due to the immunosuppressive effect of CSFV, antibodies cannot be detected with certainty until 30 days post-infection. Serological investigations aimed at detecting residual foci of infection, especially in breeding herds, may also be useful in a terminal phase of CSF eradication.

As the incidence of BVD infection may be high in breeding stock, only tests that will discriminate between CSF and BVD antibodies are useful. For this purpose, VN and the ELISA using MAbs satisfy the requirements for specificity and sensitivity.

Neutralisation tests are performed in cell cultures using a constant-virus/varying-serum method. As CSFV is noncytopathic, any non-neutralised virus must be detected, after multiplication, by an indicator system. The fluorescent antibody virus neutralisation (FAVN) test (7) and the NPLA (12) are the most commonly used techniques. Both tests can be carried out in microtitre plates. The peroxidase system has the advantage that the results can be read by the naked eye.

a) Fluorescent antibody virus neutralisation test (a prescribed test for international trade)

i) Seed a suspension of PK-15 cells at a concentration of 2×10^5 cells/ml into 5 cm Petri dishes with cover-slips spread over the bottom, or into Leighton tubes with a cover-slip or into flat-bottomed microtitre plates.

ii) Incubate the cultures for 1–2 days at 37°C in a CO_2 cabinet until they reach 70–80% confluency. An ordinary incubator may be used for stoppered Leighton tubes.

iii) Inactivate the sera for 30 minutes at 56°C. For international trade purposes, it is best to test with an initial serum dilution of 1/5 (1/10 final dilution).

---

* Simultaneous inoculation, though slightly more sensitive, is less suitable as the anticoagulant may interfere with the adhesion of cells on to the surface.

iv) Incubate equal volumes of diluted serum and virus suspension containing 200 $TCID_{50}$ (50% tissue culture infective dose) per 0.1 ml for 1–2 hours at 37°C.

v) Remove the cover-slips from Petri dishes or Leighton tubes, wash briefly in serum-free medium, overlay the cell sheet with the serum/virus mixture (from step iii) and incubate for 1 hour at 37°C in a humid atmosphere.

vi) Place the cover-slip in a clean Leighton tube and incubate the cultures in maintenance medium for 2 more days.

vii) Remove the cover-slips from the Leighton tubes, wash the monolayers twice for 5 minutes each in PBS, pH 7.2, fix in pure acetone for 10 minutes and stain with the working dilution of the conjugate for 30 minutes at 37°C before washing.

viii) Mount the cover-slips on grease-free microscope slides with 90% carbonate–bicarbonate buffered glycerol, pH>8.0, and examine for fluorescence.

When the FAVN test is performed in microtitre plates, the procedure for the NPLA (see below) can be followed up to step viii. The plates are then stained with the working dilution of the conjugate for 30 minutes at 37°C and examined for fluorescence.

b) Neutralising peroxidase-linked assay (a prescribed test for international trade)

The NPLA is carried out in flat-bottomed microtitre plates. Sera are first inactivated for 30 minutes at 56°C. For international trade purposes, it is best to test with an initial serum dilution of 1/5 (1/10 final dilution). For surveillance schemes within a country, a screening dilution of 1/10 may suffice. Appropriate controls to ensure specificity and sensitivity of reactions are incorporated into each test.

- **Test procedure**

i) Dispense dilutions of serum in growth medium (Eagle's MEM, 5% fetal bovine serum and antibiotics) in 50 µl volumes into duplicate wells of a microtitre plate. The fetal bovine serum must be free from both BVDV and antibodies to it. A third well may be included for each sample. This well contains serum and not virus and is used as a serum control (for cytotoxicity and/or nonspecific staining).

ii) Add 50 µl of virus suspension to the wells, diluted in growth medium to contain approximately 200 $TCID_{50}$/50 µl, and mix the contents on a microplate shaker for 20 seconds.

iii) Incubate the plates in a CO_2 incubator for 1 hour at 37°C.

iv) Add to all wells 50 µl of growth medium containing 2×10^5 cells/ml.

v) Allow the cells to grow in 5% CO_2 to become confluent, usually within 4 days.

vi) Discard the growth medium and rinse the plates once in 0.15 M NaCl.

vii) Drain the plates by blotting on a towel.

viii) The cell monolayers may be fixed in one of several ways:

- The plates are incubated for 45 minutes at 37°C, and then for at least a further 45 minutes at –20°C. The plates are removed from the freezer, the wells are filled with 100 µl 4% paraformaldehyde in PBS and reincubated for 5–10 minutes at room temperature. The paraformaldehyde is discarded and the plates are rinsed with 0.15 M NaCl; or
- The plates are incubated at 70–80°C for 1–2 hours; or
- The plates are fixed in 20% acetone in PBS for 10 minutes followed by thorough drying at 25–30°C for 4 hours. (This can be done quickly with the aid of a hair dryer – after 3–5 minutes complete dryness is obtained as observed by the whitish colour of the cell monolayer.)

ix) Add to each well 50 µl of a hyperimmune porcine CSF antiserum, diluted in 0.5 M NaCl containing 1% Tween 80 + 0.1% sodium azide, pH 7.6. Incubate at 37°C for 15 minutes. The working dilution of the antiserum should be determined by prior titration: i.e. a serum with an NPLA titre of 1/30,000 could be used at 1/100.

x) Wash the plates five times in 0.15 M NaCl containing 1% Tween 80, pH 7.6.

xi) Add to each well 50 µl of an anti-porcine IgG-HRPO conjugate, diluted to its working concentration in 0.5 M NaCl with 1% Tween 80, pH 7.6, and then incubate for 10 minutes at 37°C.

xii) Wash the plates five times in 0.15 M NaCl containing 1% Tween 80, pH 7.6.

xiii) Add 50 µl of chromogen–substrate solution to each well and stain for 15–30 minutes at room temperature. This solution is described in Section A.1.a. 'Immunoperoxidase procedure for differentiation of pestiviruses by monoclonal antibodies'.

xiv) The test is read visually. Infected cell sheets are completely or partially stained reddish brown. In doubtful cases, the monolayer should be examined by low power microscopy. The cytoplasm of infected cells is stained dark red.

Occasionally, sera from pigs infected with BVDV react in the FAVN or NPLA at low dilution as if they were infected with CSFV. The extent of cross-reactivity depends on the strain of BVDV involved and the interval between infection and time of sampling (18). The usually high antibody levels reached after exposure to CSF infection, including strains of low virulence, allow the use of comparatively high initial dilutions in NPLA tests for CSF antibody, thus avoiding most, but not all, cross-reactions (12, 13). In case of continued doubt, comparative tests using a strain of CSFV, a strain of BVDV and a strain of BDV, that are representative for the country or region, have proved useful. Comparative neutralisation tests are end-point titrations in which the same series of twofold dilutions of the suspected serum sample is tested in duplicate against 200 $TCID_{50}$ of each selected virus strain. The comparative tests are performed according to the protocols described for the FAVN or NPLA. Neutralisation titres are expressed as the reciprocal of the highest serum dilution that prevents virus growth in 50% of two replicate wells. A four-fold difference or more between end-points of two titrations should be considered decisive for an infection by the virus species yielding the highest titre.

c) Enzyme-linked immunosorbent assay (a prescribed test for international trade)

Competitive, blocking and indirect techniques may be used on any suitable support. The tests used should minimise cross-reactions with BVDV and other pestiviruses. However, the test system must ensure identification of all CSF infections, and at all stages of the immune response to infection.

Antigen: The antigen should be derived from or correspond to viral proteins of one of the recommended CSFV strains. Cells used to prepare antigen must be free from any other pestivirus infection.

Antisera: Polyclonal antisera for competitive or blocking assays should be raised in pigs or rabbits by infection with one of the recommended CSFV strains or with the lapinised C strain. MAbs should be directed against or correspond to an immunodominant viral protein of CSFV. Indirect assays should use an anti-porcine immunoglobulin reagent that detects both IgG and IgM.

The sensitivity of the ELISA should be high enough to score positive any serum that reacts in the neutralisation test. The ELISA may only be used with serum or plasma samples derived from individual pigs. If the ELISA procedure used is not CSF-specific, then positive samples should be further examined by differential tests to distinguish between CSF and other pestiviruses.

An example of a specific ELISA is the complex-trapping-blocking ELISA (1), which is designed to screen a large number of pig sera for antibodies against CSFV. Its major components are two MAbs, each of which recognises a different epitope on the envelope protein E2 (gp55) of the CSFV. The E2 antigen is produced in insect cells that are infected with baculovirus containing the E2 gene of CSFV.

The complex trapping blocking ELISA is a one-step method and is suitable for use in automated ELISA systems e.g. robots. The sera are tested undiluted. The test is fast and easy to perform, and detects antibodies against low virulence strains of CSFV at an early stage after infection. As the MAbs are specific for CSFV, the complex trapping blocking ELISA will only rarely detect antibodies against BVDV, although BD antibodies can be more problematic. Positive sera are retested for confirmation by the NPLA.

More information on the commercial kits can be obtained from the OIE Reference Laboratories.

B. REQUIREMENTS FOR VACCINES AND DIAGNOSTIC BIOLOGICALS

Effective inactivated whole virus vaccines against CSF are not available.

B1. Modified live virus vaccines

MLV vaccines are produced from CSFV strains that have been attenuated by passage either in cell cultures or in a suitable host species not belonging to the family Suidae. Production is carried out in cell cultures, or in non-Suidae animals, based on a seed-lot system. This must be validated with respect to identity, sterility, purity, safety, nontransmissibility, stability and immunogenicity.

To produce a seed lot and a final vaccine of high quality, the optimal conditions for virus yield must be determined. For vaccines produced in cell cultures, growth curve experiments must be done to study the effect of composition of the medium, regulation of pH and atmospheric CO_2 content, starting concentration of seeded cells, ratio between cell sheet surface and medium volume, phase of the cell growth at the time of viral infection, stationary or rolling conditions during viral replication, etc. For vaccines produced in animals, their age, breed, weight, the size of inoculum (number of animal ID_{50} [50% infectious dose]), pathogenesis of the infection, and the clinical signs are factors that must be investigated to determine the peak of virus growth and the tissues to be harvested.

Regardless of the production method, the substrate should be harvested under aseptic conditions and be subjected to a freeze–thaw cycle to release cell-associated virus. Coarse cell or tissue elements are removed by filtration or low speed centrifugation. A stabiliser is added, such as lactose at a final concentration of 5%. The vaccine is homogenised before lyophilisation to ensure a uniform batch.

The vaccine virus in the final product should not differ by more than five passages from the material used for validating the seed lot. The commercial vaccine should be produced in batches in lyophilised form as a homogeneous product.

1. Seed management

a) Characteristics of the seed

To validate a seed lot for an MLV CSF vaccine, samples of the seed lot must first pass pilot experiments. Except for tests to confirm identity, sterility, purity and stability of attenuation, pilot experiments may also be performed with representative samples of the final commercial product. These samples must originate from the same seed lot as tested above.

Except where otherwise specified, all pigs used in pilot tests are 6–8 weeks of age, healthy, free from antibodies against CSFV and BVDV, of the same breed and origin, grouped at random if necessary, and kept under the same conditions. Pregnant sows must be of equal parity.

The seed virus must be sterile and induce specific neutralising antibodies against a virulent strain of CSFV in pigs.

b) Method of culture

Production is performed in cell cultures or in a suitable host of a species not of the family Suidae.

c) Validation as a vaccine

i) *Purity*

Vaccine must be virologically pure.

Each of three seronegative pigs is inoculated intramuscularly with an amount of seed-lot virus equivalent to tenfold the amount of virus contained in one dose of vaccine. This is repeated 3 weeks later using the same dose and route of administration. Serum samples are collected 2 weeks after the last inoculation, and tested by the most sensitive method for freedom from antibodies to the viruses of African swine fever, Aujeszky's disease, BVD, foot and mouth disease (all types), transmissible gastroenteritis, swine vesicular disease, porcine reproductive and respiratory disease, and porcine influenza (types H1N1 and H3N2); and for porcine adenoviruses, porcine enteroviruses (types 1 and 2), porcine parvovirus and circovirus.

ii) *Safety*

For tests of safety, each of ten seronegative pigs is inoculated intramuscularly with ten vaccine doses. Ten other pigs serve as controls. All pigs are observed for 3 weeks thereafter. Body temperatures are recorded and blood samples are collected daily, with an anticoagulant, for the first week. Body weights are recorded at inoculation and 2 weeks later. No animal should die or show signs of illness caused by the vaccine (seed-lot) virus. A daily group average body temperature should not reach 40.5°C or more throughout the trial period. The average weight gain should not fall significantly (p <0.05) below that of the controls. Leukopenia (white blood cell [WBC] count $<7 \times 10^6$ cells/ml) may be disregarded if it is only in one pig for 1 day.

Each of ten pigs is immunosuppressed by daily injections, each of 2 mg prednisolone/kg body weight, for 5 consecutive days. On day 3, each animal is inoculated with the equivalent of one dose of vaccine, and kept under observation for 3 weeks thereafter. No animal should die or become ill due to the vaccine virus.

Each of ten sows, 25–35 days pregnant, is inoculated intramuscularly with the equivalent of one dose of vaccine. A further ten animals of the same parity and gestation serve as controls. The vaccination should not interfere with normal gestation to term, and the number of live piglets born from the test group should not be significantly fewer ($p < 0.05$) than that for the control pigs.

For field trials, a minimum of 200 pigs is used, farrowed and reared by at least 20 dams, and seronegative for CSF and BVD. The litters are equally distributed over at least two farms. Half of the piglets in each litter are inoculated intramuscularly at 7–14 days of age with the equivalent of one dose of vaccine. The uninoculated littermates are controls. All piglets are weighed at inoculation and 2 weeks later, and are kept under observation for 3 weeks. A mortality rate that exceeds 5% due to causes other than vaccination invalidates the trial. No animal should die or show signs of disease due to the vaccine virus. The average weight gain of the inoculated pigs in the litters should not be more than 20% below that of the controls during the 2 weeks post-inoculation.

iii) *Nontransmissibility*

To confirm nontransmissibility, 24 seronegative pigs are divided into four groups of equal size. Five pigs in each group are inoculated intramuscularly with the equivalent of one dose of vaccine. The remaining pigs represent in-contact controls. All pigs are challenged 6 weeks later with at least 10^5 PID_{50} (50% pig infectious dose) of a virulent strain of CSFV. All in-contact animals should be serologically negative at the time of challenge, and then die within 3 weeks. All vaccinated pigs should remain healthy and survive.

iv) *Stability of attenuation*

To confirm stability of virus attenuation, two pigs are each inoculated intramuscularly with an amount of seed-lot virus equivalent to 100 doses of vaccine, and then killed 6–7 days later. The tonsils of both pigs are pooled and made into a 10% suspension in PBS, pH 7.2. This is used to inoculate two further pigs intramuscularly with 2 ml, and these are then killed 6–7 days later. This protocol is repeated five times. During these passages, the tonsillar tissue may be stored at 4°C, if storage is to be under 24 hours, or at –70°C for longer periods. At the same time, the presence of CSF antigen is confirmed at each passage by the direct FAT in cryostat sections of the tonsils, or by virus isolation in a suitable substrate. If CSFV or antigen cannot be demonstrated after a certain passage, a second series of passages is performed to show infection, commencing with the last two pigs of the previous series.

Five pigs are inoculated intramuscularly with the sixth pig passage of the seed-lot virus, equivalent to one vaccine dose or, if this passage has not been reached, the highest passage of the two series where virus or viral antigen was detected. Five further pigs are similarly inoculated with one dose of the seed-lot virus, equivalent to one vaccine dose. All pigs are weighed at the time of inoculation and again 2 weeks later. Blood is collected daily into anticoagulant during the first week, and all pigs are kept under observation for 3 weeks. No animal should die or become ill from the vaccine virus. The average weight gain of the two groups during the first 2 weeks should not differ significantly ($p < 0.05$). Leukopenia (WBC count of $<7 \times 10^6$/ml) is permitted, at the most, in one pig of either group for 1 day.

v) *Immunogenicity*

To demonstrate adequate immunogenicity, ten pigs are each inoculated with an amount of virus equivalent to one dose of vaccine, and two other pigs are housed separately as uninoculated controls. All pigs are challenged 7 days later with 10^5 PID_{50} of a virulent strain of CSFV. Only the controls should die.

In a test for duration of immunity, ten pigs are each inoculated with one dose, and two others are maintained separately as controls. Six months later, the sera of the inoculated pigs are tested for CSF antibodies; at least eight pigs should be positive. All pigs are then challenged with at least 10^5 PID_{50} of a virulent strain of CSFV, and observed for 3 weeks. Only the controls should die.

To test protection of the development of the carrier sow syndrome, 20 pregnant sows at the same stage of gestation are randomly divided into two groups. The sows of one group are vaccinated once or twice with an amount of virus equivalent to one dose of vaccine, and intranasally challenged 4 weeks after the last vaccination with a field strain of low virulence, together with the unvaccinated control sows. All sows are killed 4 weeks after challenge and the fetuses are examined for the presence of CSFV or viral antigen. Vaccination should significantly reduce transplacental transmission of the virus.

Under the storage conditions prescribed by the manufacturer for the final product, a volume of virus equivalent to one dose of vaccine must maintain its immunogenicity at least until the end of the stated shelf life.

2. Method of manufacture

Each batch of MLV CSF vaccine must be derived from the same seed lot that has been used for the pilot tests. Also, each batch must be prepared according to the production protocol and under the conditions laid down for the registration of the final product. The properties of each batch and those of the seed lot must be verified as uniform.

3. In-process control

The protocol for production will depend on the vaccine strain, the production system (animals or cell cultures), and available facilities. The norms for cell culture vaccines may vary according to the production system, namely, primary cultures, cell lines, monolayers or suspension cultures.

4. Batch control

All pigs used in batch control tests must be 6–8 weeks of age and free from antibodies to CSFV and BVDV. They must be uniform in origin, breed, husbandry, and randomly distributed into any groups where necessary.

a) Identity

The vaccine must induce specific neutralising antibodies against a virulent strain of CSFV.

b) Sterility

Tests for sterility and freedom from contamination of biological material may be found in Chapter I.4.

c) Safety

Each of three pigs is inoculated intramuscularly with ten doses of the reconstituted vaccine as a single injection. The pigs are observed for 3 weeks thereafter and body temperatures are taken daily for the first week. No pig should die or show signs of disease attributable to the vaccine, the average daily body temperature must at no time reach 40.5°C or more, and the pigs should grow normally.

d) Purity

The batch must be virologically pure. To test for this, three pigs are each inoculated intramuscularly with ten vaccine doses. Serum samples are collected at the time of inoculation and again 5 weeks later. These are tested for antibodies to BVD (neutralisation for 1 hour at 37°C) and porcine parvovirus (haemagglutination inhibition using four haemagglutinating units). All three pigs must remain disease free. Tests for virological purity need not be carried out when using vaccines produced in rabbits.

e) Potency

Potency is expressed as the number of 50% protective doses (PD_{50}) contained in one vaccine dose. One vaccine dose is at least 100 PD_{50}.

Two groups of five 6–8-week-old piglets are inoculated intramuscularly with a 1/40 and a 1/160 dilution of the reconstituted vaccine, respectively, using buffered salt solution, pH 7.2. The vaccinated pigs together with two controls are challenged intramuscularly with 10^5 PID_{50} of a virulent strain of CSFV 2 weeks later. The pigs are observed for 2 weeks thereafter, during which time the controls should die. From the pigs that survive without showing any signs of CSF, the number of PD_{50} contained in the vaccine is calculated using the usual statistical methods.

This potency test may be replaced by an infectivity assay, provided that the manufacturer can show that there is a distinct and reproducible relationship between the virus content of the vaccine and the protection it will confer on pigs against challenge.

f) Stability

The period of validity of a batch of lyophilised CSF vaccine should not be under 1 year.

B2. Marker vaccines

Despite the existence of safe and effective MLV vaccines against CSF, their use has been discouraged in the European Union (EU) and some other CSF-free or near free countries, because antibodies provoked by such vaccines cannot be distinguished from antibodies induced by the wild-type virus. A 'marker vaccine' does not have this disadvantage: it can elicit a protective immune response that can be distinguished from the immune response induced by field virus. A prerequisite for the distinction between vaccinated and naturally infected animals is the availability of a companion serological test that is highly discriminatory, for tracing residual infections.

The minimum demands for CSF marker vaccines and the companion discriminatory tests have been formulated as follows (2):

a) Vaccine

The vaccine should provide protection against any natural-contact challenge. The efficacy of vaccination should be shown experimentally by studies in which transmission of wild-type virus in vaccinated groups of pigs is studied. The protective effect of vaccination should be achieved within the shortest possible period. A fast and reliable protection should preferably be obtained after one single application. Furthermore, it should be ensured that infection of vaccinated pregnant sows does not lead to transplacental infection and the birth of litters congenitally infected with CSFV. Duration of immunity should be at least 6 months.

b) Companion discriminatory test

The companion discriminatory serological test should be very sensitive because vaccination will reduce the prevalence of the disease. It should be used as a herd test. If a high sensitivity reduces the specificity of the test, already compromised by the presence of antibodies to other pestiviruses, good and fast confirmatory assays should be available to discriminate positive from false-positive results.

So far, two marker vaccines for CSF have been registered in the EU. Both vaccines are based on the E2 glycoprotein of CSFV as immunogen. The E2 subunit is produced by insect cells that are infected by genetically modified baculovirus, which contains the E2 gene of CSFV. The vaccines, therefore, do not contain any CSFV, while the baculo (vector) virus is chemically inactivated. The final preparations are adjuvanted with mineral oils to form a double (water/oil/water), or a single (water in oil) emulsion.

REFERENCES

1. COLIJN E.O., BLOEMRAAD M. & WENSVOORT G. (1997). An improved ELISA for the detection of serum antibodies directed against classical swine fever virus. *Vet. Microbiol.*, **59**, 15–25.

2. COMMISSION OF THE EUROPEAN COMMUNITIES (1997). The Use of Marker Vaccines in the Control of Infectious Diseases in Particular, Classical Swine Fever. Report Sci. Vet. Comm. Commission of the European Communities, DGVI, BII2, doc VI/8119, 1–13.

3. DEPNER K., GRUBER A. & LIESS B. (1994). Experimental infection of weaner pigs with a field isolate of HC/CSF virus derived from a recent outbreak in Lower Saxony. I: Clinical, virological and serological findings. *Wien. Tierarztl. Monatsschr.*, **81**, 370–373.

4. DEPNER K., PATON D.J., CRUCIERE C., DE MIA G.M., MULLER A., KOENEN F., STARK R. & LIESS B. (1995). Evaluation of the enzyme-linked immunosorbent assay for the rapid screening and detection of classical swine fever virus antigens in the blood of pigs. *Rev. sci. tech. Off. int. Epiz.*, **14**, 677–689.

5. DE SMIT A.J., TERPSTRA C. & WENSVOORT G. (1994). Comparison of Viral Isolation Methods from Whole Blood or Blood Components for Early Diagnosis of CSF. Rep. Meeting Nat. Swine Fever Lab. Brussels 24–25 November. Commission of the European Communities, DGVI/5848/95, 21–22.

6. EDWARDS S., MOENNIG V. & WENSVOORT G. (1991). The development of an international reference panel of monoclonal antibodies for the differentiation of hog cholera virus from other pestiviruses. *Vet. Microbiol.*, **29**, 101–108.

7. LIESS B. & PRAGER D. (1976). Detection of neutralising antibodies (NIF) test: use of new technical equipment for laboratory swine fever diagnosis. *In:* CEC Seminar on Diagnosis and Epizootiology of Classical Swine Fever. EUR 5486, 187–197.

8. McGoldrick A., Lowings J.P., Ibata G., Sands J.J., Belak S. & Paton D.J. (1998). A novel approach to the detection of classical swine fever virus by TR-PCR with a fluorogenic probe (Taq Man). *J. Virol. Methods,* **72**, 125–135.

9. Ogawa N., Nakagawa H., Yamamoto H., Sawada M., Hanaki T. & Sazawa H. (1973). Viral detection in pigs inoculated with the GPE-strain of hog cholera attenuated virus. *Ann. Rep. Nat. Vet. Assay Lab.* (Japan), **10**, 15–19.

10. Ressang A.A. (1973). Studies on the pathogenesis of hog cholera. *Zentralbl. Veterinarmed. [B],* **20**, 256–271.

11. Terpstra C. (1978). Detection of C-strain virus in pigs following vaccination against swine fever. *Tijdschr. Diergeneeskd,* **103**, 678–684.

12. Terpstra C., Bloemraad M. & Gielkens A.J.L. (1984). The neutralising peroxidase-linked assay for detection of antibody against swine fever virus. *Vet. Microbiol.*, **9**, 113–120.

13. Terpstra C. & Wensvoort G. (1988). The protective value of vaccine-induced neutralising antibody titres in swine fever. *Vet. Microbiol.*, **16**, 123–128.

14. Terpstra C. & Wensvoort G. (1988). Natural infections of pigs with bovine viral diarrhoea virus associated with signs resembling swine fever. *Res. Vet. Sci.*, **45**, 137–142.

15. Vannier P. & Carnero R. (1985). Effets pour le porc d'un virus propagé par un vaccin contre la maladie d'Aujeszky. *Point Vet.*, **17**, 325–331.

16. Wensvoort G. & Terpstra C. (1988). Bovine viral diarrhoea infections in piglets born from sows vaccinated against swine fever with contaminated vaccine. *Res. Vet. Sci.*, **45**, 143–148.

17. Wensvoort G., Terpstra C., Boonstra J., Bloemraad M. & Van Zaane D. (1986). Production of monoclonal antibodies against swine fever virus and their use in laboratory diagnosis. *Vet. Microbiol.*, **12**, 101–108.

18. Wensvoort G., Terpstra C., De Kluyver E.P (1989). Characterization of porcine and some ruminant pestiviruses by cross-neutralisation. *Vet. Microbiol.*, **20**, 291–306.

19. Wensvoort G., Terpstra C., De Kluyver E.P., Kraghten C. & Warnaar J.C. (1989). Antigenic differentiation of pestivirus strains with monoclonal antibodies against hog cholera virus. *Vet. Microbiol.*, **21**, 9–20.

*

* *

CHAPTER 2.1.14.

HIGHLY PATHOGENIC AVIAN INFLUENZA

SUMMARY

Highly pathogenic avian influenza (HPAI), also known as fowl plague, is caused by specified influenza A viruses, which are members of the family Orthomyxoviridae. There are three influenza types – A, B and C; only influenza A viruses are known to infect birds. Diagnosis is by isolation and characterisation of the virus. This is because infections in birds can give rise to a wide variety of clinical signs that may vary according to the host, strain of virus, the host's immune status, presence of any secondary exacerbating organisms and environmental conditions.

Identification of the agent: *Suspensions in antibiotic solution of tracheal and cloacal swabs (or faeces) taken from live birds, or of faeces and pooled samples of organs from dead birds, are inoculated into the allantoic cavity of 9–11-day-old embryonated fowl eggs. The eggs are incubated at 35–37°C for 4–7 days. The allantoic fluid of any eggs containing dead or dying embryos as they arise, and all eggs at the end of the incubation period, are tested for the presence of haemagglutinating activity. The presence of influenza A virus can be confirmed by an immunodiffusion test between concentrated virus and an antiserum to the nucleocapsid or matrix antigens, both of which are common to all influenza A viruses.*

For subtyping the virus, the laboratory must have monospecific antisera prepared against the isolated antigens of each of the 15 haemagglutinin (H1–H15) and 9 neuraminidase (N1–N9) subtypes of influenza A viruses that can be used in immunodiffusion tests. Alternatively, the newly isolated virus may be examined by haemagglutination and neuraminidase inhibition tests against a battery of polyclonal antisera to a wide range of strains covering all the subtypes.

As the terms HPAI and 'fowl plague' refer to infection with virulent strains of influenza A virus, it is necessary to assess the virulence of an isolate for domestic poultry. Whereas all virulent strains isolated to date have been either of the H5 or H7 subtype, most H5 or H7 isolates have been of low virulence. The methods used for the determination of strain virulence for birds have evolved over recent years with a greater understanding of the molecular basis of pathogenicity, but still primarily involve the inoculation of a minimum of eight susceptible 4–8-week-old chickens with infectious virus; strains are considered to be highly pathogenic if they cause more than 75% mortality within 10 days.

Serological tests: *As all influenza A viruses have antigenically similar nucleocapsid and antigenically similar matrix antigens, agar gel immunodiffusion tests are used to detect antibodies to these antigens. Concentrated virus preparations containing either or both type of antigens are used in such tests. Not all birds develop demonstrable precipitating antibodies. Haemagglutination inhibition tests have also been employed in routine diagnostic serology, but it is possible that this technique may miss some particular infections because the haemagglutinin is subtype specific. Enzyme-linked immunosorbent assays have been used to detect antibodies to influenza A type specific antigens.*

Requirements for vaccines and diagnostic biologicals: *In most countries, vaccines specifically designed to contain or prevent HPAI are banned or discouraged by government agencies because they may interfere with stamping-out control policies. During the 1990s the prophylactic use of inactivated oil-emulsion vaccines was employed in Mexico and Pakistan to control widespread outbreaks of HPAI, and a recombinant fowlpox virus vaccine expressing the homologous HA gene was also tested in field trials in Mexico.*

A. DIAGNOSTIC TECHNIQUES

Highly pathogenic avian influenza (HPAI), which is also known as fowl plague, is caused by infection with influenza A viruses of the family Orthomyxoviridae. Influenza A viruses are the only orthomyxoviruses known to affect birds. Many species of birds have been shown to be susceptible to infection with influenza A viruses and aquatic birds form a major reservoir of these viruses, but the overwhelming majority of isolates have been of low pathogenicity for chickens and turkeys, the main birds of economic importance to be affected. Influenza A viruses have antigenically related nucleocapsid and antigenically related matrix proteins, but are classified into subtypes on the basis of their haemagglutinin (H) and neuraminidase (N) antigens (29). At present, 15 H subtypes (H1–H15) and 9 neuraminidase subtypes (N1–N9) are recognised. To date, the highly virulent influenza A viruses that produce acute clinical disease in chickens and turkeys have been associated only with the H5 and H7 subtypes (with the exception of two H10 subtypes that would also have fulfilled the OIE and European Union [EU] definitions), although the reasons for this are not clear. Many viruses of H5 and H7 subtype isolated from birds have been of low virulence for poultry (1).

Depending on the age and type of bird and on environmental factors, the highly pathogenic disease may vary from one of sudden death with little or no overt signs to a more characteristic disease with respiratory signs, excessive lacrimation, sinusitis, oedema of the head, cyanosis of the unfeathered skin and diarrhoea. However, none of these signs can be considered pathognomonic. Diagnosis of the disease, therefore, depends on the isolation of the virus and a demonstration of its virulence for an appropriate host. Testing sera from suspect birds using immunological methods may supplement diagnosis, but these methods are not suitable for a detailed identification. Diagnosis for official control purposes is established on the basis of agreed official criteria for pathogenicity, according to *in-vivo* tests or to molecular determinants (i.e. the presence of multiple amino acids at the cleavage site of the haemagglutinin). These definitions evolve as scientific knowledge of the disease increases.

1. Identification of the agent

Samples taken from dead birds should include intestinal contents (faeces) or cloacal swabs and oro-nasal swabs. Samples from trachea, lungs, air sacs, intestine, spleen, kidney, brain, liver and heart may also be collected and processed either separately or as a pool.

Samples from live birds should include both tracheal and cloacal swabs, although swabs of the latter site are the most likely to yield virus. As small delicate birds may be harmed by swabbing, the collection of fresh faeces may serve as an adequate alternative.

The samples should be placed in isotonic phosphate buffered saline (PBS), pH 7.0–7.4, containing antibiotics. The antibiotics can be varied according to local conditions, but could be, for example, penicillin (2000 units/ml), streptomycin (2 mg/ml), gentamicin (50 µg/ml) and mycostatin (1000 units/ml) for tissues and tracheal swabs, but at five-fold higher concentrations for faeces and cloacal swabs. It is important to readjust the pH of the solution to pH 7.0–7.4 following the addition of the antibiotics. Faeces and finely minced tissues should be prepared as 10–20% (w/v) suspensions in the antibiotic solution. Suspensions should be processed as soon as possible after incubation for 1–2 hours at room temperature. Where this is not possible, they may be stored for several days at 4°C.

The preferred method of growing avian influenza A viruses is by the inoculation of embryonated specific pathogen free (SPF) fowl eggs, or at least specific antibody negative (SAN) eggs. The supernatant fluids of faeces or tissue suspensions obtained through clarification by centrifugation at 1000 ***g*** are inoculated into the allantoic sac of at least five embryonated SPF fowl eggs of 9–11 days' incubation. The eggs are incubated at 35–37°C for 4–7 days. Eggs containing dead or dying embryos as they arise, and all eggs remaining at the end of the incubation period, should first be chilled to 4°C and the allantoic fluids should then be tested for haemagglutination (HA) activity (see Section A.3.b.). Detection of HA activity indicates a high probability of the presence of an influenza A virus or of an avian paramyxovirus. Fluids that give a negative reaction should be passaged into at least one further batch of eggs.

The presence of influenza A virus can be confirmed in agar gel immunodiffusion (AGID) tests by demonstrating the presence of the nucleocapsid or matrix antigens, both of which are common to all influenza A viruses (see Section A.3.a.). The antigens may be prepared by concentrating the virus from infective allantoic fluid or extracting the infected chorioallantoic membranes; these are tested against known positive antisera. Virus may be concentrated from infective allantoic fluid by ultracentrifugation, or by precipitation under acid conditions. The latter method consists of the addition of 1.0 M HCl to infective allantoic fluid until it is approximately pH 4.0. The mixture is placed in an ice bath for 1 hour and then clarified by centrifugation at 1000 ***g*** at 4°C. The supernatant fluid is discarded. The virus concentrates are resuspended in glycine-sarcosyl buffer: this consists of 1% (w/v) sodium lauroyl sarcosinate buffered to pH 9.0 with 0.5 M glycine. These concentrates contain both nucleocapsid and matrix polypeptides.

Preparations of nucleocapsid-rich antigen can also be obtained from chorioallantoic membranes for use in the AGID test (5). This latter method involves removal of the chorioallantoic membranes from infected eggs that have allantoic fluids with HA activity. The membranes are then homogenised or ground to a paste. This is subjected to three freeze–thaw cycles, followed by centrifugation at 1000 ***g*** for 10 minutes. The pellet is discarded and the supernatant is used as an antigen following treatment with 0.1% formalin.

Use of the AGID test to demonstrate nucleocapsid or matrix antigens is a satisfactory way to indicate the presence of avian influenza virus in amnioallantoic fluid, but various enzyme-linked immunosorbent assays (ELISAs) are now also available. There is a sensitive and specific ELISA that demonstrates nucleoprotein of Type A influenza virus using a monoclonal antibody against Type A influenza nucleoprotein (19, 20, 22). This is available as a commercial kit.

Any HA activity of sterile fluids harvested from the inoculated eggs is most likely to be due to an influenza A virus or to an avian paramyxovirus (a few strains of avian reovirus will do this, or nonsterile fluid could contain HA of bacterial origin). There are currently nine recognised serotypes of avian paramyxoviruses. Most laboratories will have antiserum specific for Newcastle disease virus (avian paramyxovirus type 1), and in view of its widespread occurrence and almost universal use as a live vaccine in poultry, it is best to evaluate its presence by haemagglutination inhibition (HI) tests (see Chapter 2.1.15.).

Alternatively, the presence of influenza virus can be confirmed by the use of reverse-transcription polymerase chain reaction (RT-PCR) using nucleoprotein-specific conserved primers (2). Also, the presence of subtype H5 or H7 influenza virus can be confirmed by using H5- or H7-specific primers (9, 18, 28). Standardised procedures for these methods have yet to be established and agreed internationally.

The method recommended for definitive antigenic subtyping of influenza A viruses by the World Health Organization (WHO) Expert Committee (29) involves the use of highly specific antisera, prepared in an animal giving minimum nonspecific reactions (e.g. goat), directed against the H and N subtypes (17). An alternative technique is the use of polyclonal antisera raised against a battery of intact influenza viruses. Subtype identification by this technique is beyond the scope of most diagnostic laboratories not specialising in influenza viruses. Assistance is available from the OIE Reference Laboratories (see Table given in Part 4 of this *Manual*).

2. Assessment of pathogenicity

The term highly pathogenic avian influenza implies the involvement of virulent strains of virus. It is used to describe a disease of chickens with clinical signs such as excessive lacrimation, respiratory distress, sinusitis, oedema of the head and face, cyanosis of the unfeathered skin, and diarrhoea. Sudden death may be the only sign. These signs may vary enormously depending on the host, age of the bird, presence of other organisms and environmental conditions. In addition, viruses that normally cause only a mild or no clinical disease may mimic highly pathogenic avian influenza if exacerbating conditions exist.

At the First International Symposium on Avian Influenza held in 1981 (3), it was resolved to abandon the term 'fowl plague' and to define highly pathogenic strains on the basis of their ability to produce not less than 75% mortality within 8 days in at least eight susceptible 4–8-week-old chickens inoculated by the intramuscular, intravenous or caudal air sac route. However, this definition proved unsatisfactory when applied to the viruses responsible for the widespread outbreaks in chickens occurring in 1983 in Pennsylvania and the surrounding states of the United States of America (USA). The problem was mainly caused by the presence of a virus of demonstrable low pathogenicity in laboratory tests, but which was shown to be fully pathogenic following a single point mutation. Further consideration of a definition to include such 'potentially pathogenic' viruses was undertaken by several international groups.

The eventual recommendations made were based on the finding that while there have been numerous isolations of strains of H5 and H7 subtypes of low pathogenicity, all the highly pathogenic influenza strains isolated to date have possessed either the H5 or H7 haemagglutinin. Further information concerning the pathogenicity or potential pathogenicity of H5 and H7 subtypes may be obtained by sequencing the genome, as pathogenicity is associated with the presence of multiple basic amino acids at the cleavage site of the haemagglutinin. For example, all H7 subtype viruses of low virulence have had the amino acid motif at the HA0 cleavage site of either -PEIPKGR*GLF- or -PENPKGR*GLF-, whereas examples of amino acids motifs for HPAI H7 viruses are: -PEIPKKKKR*GLF-, PETPKRKRKR*GLF-, -PEIPKKREKR*GLF-, -PETPKRRRR*GLF-. Amino acid sequencing of the cleavage sites of H5 and H7 subtype influenza isolates of low virulence for birds should identify viruses that have the capacity, following simple mutation, to become highly pathogenic for poultry.

The OIE subsequently adopted the following criteria for classifying an avian influenza virus as highly pathogenic:

a) Any influenza virus that is lethal for six, seven or eight of eight 4–8-week-old susceptible chickens within 10 days following intravenous inoculation with 0.2 ml of a 1/10 dilution of a bacteria-free, infective allantoic fluid.

b) The following additional test is required if the isolate kills from one to five chickens but is not of the H5 or H7 subtype: growth of the virus in cell culture[1] with cytopathic effect or plaque formation in the absence of trypsin. If no growth is observed, the isolate is not considered to be a HPAI isolate.

c) For all H5 and H7 viruses of low pathogenicity and for other influenza viruses, if growth is observed in cell culture without trypsin, the amino acid sequence of the connecting peptide of the haemagglutinin must be determined. If the sequence is similar to that observed for other HPAI isolates, the isolate being tested will be considered to be highly pathogenic.

In the EU, a similar definition was adopted in Directive 92/40/EEC (7), although in this case the intravenous pathogenicity index (IVPI) test was used as a method of assessing virulence. For the purposes of confirming disease and implementing the control measures in the Directive, the following definition applies:

'an infection of poultry caused by an influenza A virus that has an intravenous pathogenicity index in 6-week-old chickens >1.2 or any infection with influenza A viruses of H5 or H7 subtype for which nucleotide sequencing has demonstrated the presence of multiple basic amino acids at the cleavage site of the haemagglutinin.'

The IVPI test is carried out as follows.

i) Fresh infective allantoic fluid with a HA titre >1/16 ($>2^4$ or $>\log_2 4$ when expressed as the reciprocal) is diluted 1/10 in sterile isotonic saline.

ii) 0.1 ml of the diluted virus is injected intravenously into each of ten 6-week-old SPF chickens.

iii) Birds are examined at 24-hour intervals for 10 days. At each observation, each bird is scored 0 if normal, 1 if sick, 2 if severely sick, 3 if dead. (The judgement of sick and severely sick birds is a subjective clinical assessment. Normally, 'sick' birds would show one of the following signs and 'severely sick' more than one of the following signs: respiratory involvement, depression, diarrhoea, cyanosis of the exposed skin or wattles, oedema of the face and/or head, nervous signs. Dead individuals must be scored as 3 at each of the remaining daily observations after death.)

iv) The intravenous pathogenicity index (IVPI) is the mean score per bird per observation over the 10-day period. An index of 3.00 means that all birds died within 24 hours, an index of 0.00 means that no bird showed any clinical sign during the 10-day observation period.

A variety of strategies and techniques have been used successfully to sequence the nucleotides at that portion of the HA gene coding for the cleavage site region of the haemagglutinin of H5 and H7 subtypes of avian influenza, enabling the amino acids there to be deduced. The most commonly used method has been RT-PCR using oligonucleotide primers complementing areas of the gene either side of the cleavage site coding region, followed by cycle sequencing (27). Various stages in the procedure can be facilitated using commercially available kits and automatic sequencers.

Although all the truly HPAI viruses isolated to date have been of H5 or H7 subtypes, at least two isolates, both of H10 subtype (H10 N4 and H10 N5), have been reported that would have fulfilled both the OIE and EU definitions for HPAI viruses (25) as they killed 7/10 and 8/10 chickens with IVPI values >1.2 when the birds were inoculated intravenously. However, they produced no deaths or disease signs when inoculated intranasally and these viruses did not have multiple basic amino acids at their haemagglutinin cleavage sites.

3. Serological tests

a) Agar gel immunodiffusion

All influenza A viruses have antigenically similar nucleocapsid and antigenically similar matrix antigens. This fact enables the presence or absence of antibodies to any influenza A virus to be detected by AGID tests. Concentrated virus preparations, as described above, contain both matrix and nucleocapsid antigens; the matrix antigen diffuses more rapidly than the nucleocapsid antigen. AGID tests have been widely and routinely used to detect specific antibodies in chicken and turkey flocks as an indication of infection. These have generally employed nucleocapsid-enriched preparations made from the chorioallantoic membranes of embryonated fowl eggs (5) that have been infected at 10 days of age, homogenised, freeze–thawed three times, and centrifuged at 1000 ***g***. The supernatant fluids are inactivated by the addition of 0.1% formalin or 1% betapropiolactone, recentrifuged and used as antigen. Not all avian species may produce precipitating antibodies following infection with influenza viruses.

1 For example primary cells such as chick embryo cells or cell lines such as MDCK cells, although most cell cultures support the growth of HPAI influenza viruses or those of low pathogenicity in the presence of trypsin.

Tests are usually carried out using gels of 1% (w/v) agarose or purified agar and 8% (w/v) NaCl in 0.1 M phosphate buffer, pH 7.2, poured to a thickness of 2–3 mm in Petri dishes or on microscope slides. Using a template and cutter, wells of approximately 5 mm in diameter, and 2–5 mm apart, are cut in the agar. A pattern of wells must place each suspect serum adjacent to a known positive serum and antigen. This will make a continuous line of identity between the known positive, the suspect serum and the nucleocapsid antigen. Approximately 50 µl of each reagent should be added to each well.

Precipitin lines can be detected after approximately 24–48 hours, but this may be dependent on the concentrations of the antibody and the antigen. These lines are best observed against a dark background that is illuminated from behind. A specific, positive result is recorded when the precipitin line between the known positive control wells is continuous with the line between the antigen and the test well. Crossed lines are interpreted to be due to the test serum lacking identity with the antibodies in the positive control well.

b) Haemagglutination and haemagglutination inhibition tests

Variations of the procedures for HA and HI tests are practised in different laboratories. The following recommended examples apply in the use of V-bottomed microwell plastic plates in which the final volume for both types of test is 0.075 ml. The reagents required for these tests are: isotonic PBS (0.1 M), pH 7.0–7.2; and red blood cells (RBCs) taken from a minimum of three SPF chickens (if SPF chickens are not available blood may be taken from birds that are regularly monitored and shown to be free from antibodies to avian influenza) and pooled in an equal volume of Alsever's solution. Cells should be washed three times in PBS before use as a 1% (packed cell v/v) suspension. Positive and negative control antigens and antisera should be run with each test, as appropriate.

- **Haemagglutination test**

i) Dispense 0.025 ml PBS into each well of a plastic V-bottomed microtitre plate.

ii) Place 0.025 ml virus suspension (i.e. infective allantoic fluid) in the first well. For accurate determination of the HA content, this should be done from a close range of an initial series of dilutions, i.e. 1/3,1/4, 1/5, 1/6, etc.

iii) Make twofold dilutions of 0.025 ml volumes of the virus suspension across the plate.

iv) Dispense a further 0.025 ml PBS to each well.

v) Dispense 0.025 ml of 1% (v/v) chicken RBCs to each well.

vi) Mix by tapping the plate gently and then allow the RBCs to settle for about 40 minutes at room temperature, i.e. about 20°C, or for 60 minutes at 4°C if ambient temperatures are high, by which time control RBCs should be settled to a distinct button.

vii) HA is determined by tilting the plate and observing the presence or absence of tear-shaped streaming of the RBCs. The titration should be read to the highest dilution giving complete HA (no streaming); this represents 1 HA unit (HAU) and can be calculated accurately from the initial range of dilutions.

- **Haemagglutination inhibition test**

i) Dispense 0.025 ml PBS into each well of a plastic V-bottomed microtitre plate.

ii) Place 0.025 ml of serum into the first well of the plate.

iii) Make twofold dilutions of 0.025 ml volumes of the serum across the plate.

iv) Add 4 HAU of virus/antigen in 0.025 ml to each well and leave for a minimum of 30 minutes at room temperature (i.e. about 20°C) or 60 minutes at 4°C.

v) Add 0.025 ml of 1% (v/v) chicken RBCs to each well and after gentle mixing, allow the RBCs to settle for about 40 minutes at room temperature, i.e. about 20°C, or for 60 minutes at 4°C if ambient temperatures are high, by which time control RBCs should be settled to a distinct button.

vi) The HI titre is the highest dilution of serum causing complete inhibition of 4 HAU of antigen. The agglutination is assessed by tilting the plates. Only those wells in which the RBCs stream at the same rate as the control wells (containing 0.025 ml RBCs and 0.05 ml PBS only) should be considered to show inhibition.

vii) The validity of results should be assessed against a negative control serum, which should not give a titre >1/4 (>2^2 or >$\log_2$ when expressed as the reciprocal), and a positive control serum for which the titre should be within one dilution of the known titre.

HI titres may be regarded as being positive if there is inhibition at a serum dilution of 1/16 (2^4 or $\log_2$ 4 when expressed as the reciprocal) or more against 4 HAU of antigen. Some laboratories prefer to use 8 HAU in

HI tests. While this is permissible, it affects the interpretation of results so that a positive titre is 1/8 (2^3 or $\log_2 3$) or more.

Chicken sera rarely give nonspecific positive reactions in this test and any pretreatment of the sera is unnecessary. Sera from species other than chickens may sometimes cause agglutination of chicken RBCs, so this property should first be determined and then removed by adsorption of the serum with chicken RBCs. This is done by adding 0.025 ml of packed chicken RBCs to each 0.5 ml of antisera, shaking gently and leaving for at least 30 minutes; the RBCs are then pelleted by centrifugation at 800 ***g*** for 2–5 minutes and the adsorbed sera are decanted. Alternatively, RBCs of the avian species under investigation could be used.

B. REQUIREMENTS FOR VACCINES AND DIAGNOSTIC BIOLOGICALS

In some countries, vaccines designed to contain or prevent HPAI are specifically banned or discouraged by government agencies because they may interfere with stamping-out control policies. However, most HPAI control regulations reserve the right to use vaccines in emergencies, and this has been done in Mexico and Pakistan.

Since the 1970s in the USA there has been widespread use of inactivated vaccines produced under special licence on a commercial basis (12, 14, 16). These vaccines have been used primarily in turkeys against viruses that are not highly pathogenic but which may cause serious problems, especially in exacerbating circumstances. Significant quantities of vaccine have been used (12, 14).

The existence of a large number of virus subtypes, together with the known variation of different strains within a subtype, pose serious problems when selecting strains to produce influenza vaccines. In addition, some isolates do not grow to a sufficiently high titre to produce adequately potent vaccines without costly prior concentration. The vaccines produced have either been autogenous, i.e. prepared from isolates specifically involved in an epizootic, or have been prepared from viruses possessing the same haemagglutinin subtype that yield high concentrations of antigen. In the USA, some standardisation of the latter has been carried out in that the National Veterinary Services Laboratories have propagated and hold influenza viruses of each subtype for use as seed virus in the preparation of inactivated vaccines (4). These vaccines and those for use in Italy (8) against viruses of low pathogenicity, and against HPAI in Mexico (10) and Pakistan (15), have been prepared from infective allantoic fluid inactivated by beta-propiolactone or formalin and emulsified with mineral oil.

The information below is based primarily on the experiences in the USA and the guidance and policy for licensing avian influenza vaccines in that country (23). The basic principles for producing vaccines, particularly inactivated vaccines, are common to several viruses e.g. Newcastle disease (Chapter 2.1.15.).

Live conventional influenza vaccines against any subtype are not recommended.

1. Seed management

a) Characteristics of the seed

For any subtype only well characterised influenza A virus of proven low pathogenicity, preferably obtained from an international or national repository, should be used to establish a master seed for inactivated vaccines.

b) Method of culture

A master seed is established, and from this a working seed. If the strain has been cloned, the establishment of a master culture may only involve producing a large volume of infective allantoic fluid (minimum 100 ml), which can be stored as lyophilised aliquots (0.5 ml).

c) Validation as a vaccine

The master seed should be checked after preparation for sterility, safety, potency and absence of specified extraneous agents.

2. Method of manufacture

For vaccine production, a working seed, from which batches of vaccine are produced, is first established by expansion of an aliquot of master seed to a sufficient volume to allow vaccine production for 12–18 months. It is best to store the working seed in liquid form at below –60°C as lyophilised virus does not always multiply to high titre on subsequent first passage.

The inactivated influenza vaccines prepared from conventional virus are produced in embryonated fowl eggs. The method of production is basically that of propagating the virus aseptically; all procedures are performed under sterile conditions.

It is usual to dilute the working seed in sterile PBS, pH 7.2, so that about 10^3–10^4 EID_{50}/0.1 ml are inoculated into the allantoic cavity of 9- or 10-day-old embryonated SPF fowl eggs. These are then incubated at 37°C. Eggs containing embryos that die within 24 hours should be discarded. The incubation time will depend on the virus strain being used and will be predetermined to ensure maximum yield with the minimum number of embryo deaths.

The infected eggs should be chilled at 4°C before being harvested. The tops of the eggs are removed and the allantoic fluids aspirated after depression of the embryo. The inclusion of any yolk material and albumin should be avoided. All fluids should be stored immediately at 4°C and tested for bacterial contamination before large pools are made for inactivation.

In the manufacture of inactivated vaccines, the harvested allantoic fluid is treated with either formaldehyde (a typical final concentration is 1/1000) or beta-propiolactone (a typical final concentration is 1/2000–1/4000). The time required must be sufficient to ensure freedom from live virus. Most inactivated vaccines are not concentrated; the inactivated allantoic fluid is usually emulsified with mineral or vegetable oil. The exact formulations are generally commercial secrets.

3. In-process control

For inactivated vaccines, the efficacy of the process of inactivation should be tested in embryonated eggs, taking 25 aliquots of 0.2 ml from each batch and passaging each aliquot three times through SPF embryos.

4. Batch control

Most countries have published specifications for the control of production and testing of vaccines, which include the definition of the obligatory tests on vaccines during and after manufacture.

a) Sterility

Tests for sterility and freedom from contamination of biological materials may be found in Chapter I.4.

b) Safety

For inactivated vaccines, a double dose is administered by the recommended route to ten 3-week-old birds, and these are observed for 2 weeks for absence of clinical signs of disease or local lesions.

c) Potency

Conventional potency testing involving the use of three diluted doses and challenge with virulent virus (e.g. chapter 2.1.15.) may be used for vaccines prepared to give protection against HPAI or H5 and H7 subtypes generally. For inactivated vaccines to other subtypes where virulent viruses are not available, potency tests may rely on measurement of immune response or challenge and assessment of morbidity. Assessment of haemagglutinin antigen content (26) could allow *in-vitro* extrapolation to potency for subsequent vaccine batches.

d) Stability

When stored under the recommended conditions, the final vaccine product should maintain its potency for at least 1 year. Inactivated vaccines must not be frozen.

e) Preservatives

A preservative may be used for vaccine in multidose containers.

f) Precautions (hazards)

Care must be taken to avoid self-injection with oil emulsion vaccines.

5. Tests on the final product

a) Safety

See Section B.4.b. above

b) Potency

See Section B.4.c. above.

6. Novel vaccines

Recombinant fowl pox virus vaccines containing H5 HA have been prepared, evaluated (6, 21) and used in field trials in Mexico (11).

A baculovirus-expression system has been used to produce recombinant H5 and H7 antigens for incorporation into vaccines (24).

DNA encoding H5 haemagglutinin has been evaluated as a potential vaccine in poultry (13).

REFERENCES

1. ALEXANDER D.J. (1993). Orthomyxovirus infections. *In:* Viral Infections of Vertebrates, Volume 3: Viral Infections of Birds, McFerran J.B. & McNulty M.S., eds. Horzinek M.C., Series editor. Elsevier, Amsterdam, The Netherlands, 287–316.

2. ALTMULLER A., KUNERL M., MULLER K., HINSHAW V.S., FITCH W.M. & SCHOLTISSEK C. (1991). Genetic relatedness of the nucleoprotein (NP) of recent swine, turkey and human influenza A virus (H1N1) isolates. *Virus Res.*, **22**, 79–87.

3. BANKOWSKI R.A. (1982). Proceedings of the First International Symposium on Avian Influenza, 1981. Carter Comp., Richmond, USA.

4. BANKOWSKI RA. (1985). Report of the Committee on Transmissible Diseases of Poultry and Other Avian Species. Proceedings of the 88th Annual Meeting of the U.S. Animal Health Association, 474–483.

5. BEARD C.W. (1970). Demonstration of type-specific influenza antibody in mammalian and avian sera by immunodiffusion. *Bull. WHO*, **42**, 779–785.

6. BEARD C.W., SCHNITZLEIN W.M. & TRIPATHY D.N. (1991). Protection of chickens against highly pathogenic avian influenza virus (H5N2) by recombinant fowlpox viruses. *Avian Dis.*, **35**, 356–359.

7. COUNCIL OF THE EUROPEAN COMMUNITIES (1992). Council Directive 92/40/EEC of 19th May 1992 introducing Community measures for the control of avian influenza. *Off. J. European Communities*, **L167**, 1–15.

8. DAPRILE P.N. (1986). Current situation of avian influenza in Italy and approaches to its control. *In:* Acute Virus Infections of Poultry, McFerran J.B. & McNulty M.S., eds. Martinus Nijhoff, Dordrecht, The Netherlands, 29–35.

9. GARCIA A., CRAWFORD J.M., LATIMER J.W., RIVERA-CRUZ E. & PERDUE M.L. (1996). Heterogeneity in the haemagglutinin gene and emergence of the highly pathogenic phenotype among recent H5N2 avian influenza viruses from Mexico. *J. Gen. Virol.*, **77**, 1493–1504.

10. GARCIA A., JOHNSON H., KUMAR SRIVASTAVA D., JAYAWARDENE D.A., WEHR D.R. & WEBSTER R.G. (1998). Efficacy of inactivated H5N2 influenza vaccines against lethal A/chicken/Queretaro/19/95 infection. *Avian Dis.*, **42**, 248–256.

11. GARCIA-GARCIA J., RODRIGUEZ V.H. & HERNANDEZ M.A. (1998). Experimental studies in field trials with recombinant fowlpox vaccine in broilers in Mexico. Proceedings of the Fourth International Symposium on Avian Influenza, Athens, Georgia. Swayne D.E. & Slemons R.D., eds. U.S. Animal Health Association, 245–252.

12. HALVORSON D.A. (1998). Strengths and weaknesses of vaccines as a control tool. Proceedings of the Fourth International Symposium on Avian Influenza, Athens, Georgia. Swayne D.E. & Slemons R.D., eds. U.S. Animal Health Association, 223–227.

13. KODIHALLI S. & WEBSTER R.G. (1998). DNA vaccines for avian influenza – a model for future poultry vaccines? Proceedings of the Fourth International Symposium on Avian Influenza, Athens, Georgia. Swayne D.E. & Slemons R.D., eds. U.S. Animal Health Association, 263–280.

14. MCCAPES R.H. & BANKOWSKI R.A. (1985). Use of avian influenza vaccines in California turkey breeders – medical rationale. Proceedings of the Second International Symposium on Avian Influenza, Athens, Georgia. U.S. Animal Health Association, 271–278.

15. NAEEM K. (1998). The avian influenza H7N3 outbreak in South Central Asia. Proceedings of the Fourth International Symposium on Avian Influenza, Athens, Georgia. Swayne D.E. & Slemons R.D., eds. U.S. Animal Health Association, 31–35.

16. PRICE R.J. (1982). Commercial avian influenza vaccines. *In:* Proceedings of the First Avian Influenza Symposium, 1981. Carter Comp., Richmond USA, 178–179.

17. SCHILD G.C., NEWMAN R.W., WEBSTER R.G., MAJOR D. & HINSHAW V.S. (1980). Antigenic analysis of influenza A virus surface antigens: considerations for the nomenclature of influenza virus. *Arch. Virol.*, **83,** 171–1 84.

18. SENNE D.A., PANIGRAHY B., KAWAOKA Y., PEARSON J.E., SUSS J., LIPKIND M., KIDA H. & WEBSTER R.G. (1996). Survey of the haemagglutinin (HA) cleavage site sequence of H5 and H7 avian influenza viruses: amino acid sequence at the cleavage site as a marker of pathogenicity potential. *Avian Dis.*, **40**, 425–437.

19. SHAFER A.L., KATZ J.B. & EERNISSE K.A. (1998). Development and validation of a competitive enzyme-linked immunosorbent assay for detection of Type A influenza antibodies in avian sera. *Avian Dis.*, **42**, 28–34.

20. SLEMONS R.D. & BRUGH M. (1998). Rapid antigen detection as an aid in early diagnosis and control of avian influenza. *In:* Proceedings of the Fourth International Symposium on Avian Influenza, Athens, Georgia. Swayne D.E. & Slemons R.D., eds. U.S. Animal Health Association, Richmond, Virginia, USA, 313–317.

21. SWAYNE D.E. & MICKLE T.R. (1997). Protection of chickens against highly pathogenic Mexican-origin H5N2 avian influenza virus by a recombinant fowlpox vaccine. Proceedings the 100th Annual Meeting of the U.S. Animal Health Association, Little Rock, USA, 1996, 557–563.

22. SWAYNE D.E., SENNE D.A. & BEARD C.W. (1998). Influenza. *In:* Isolation and Identification of Avian Pathogens, Fourth Edition, Swayne D.E., Glisson J.R., Jackwood M.W., Pearson J.E. & Reed W.M., eds. American Association of Avian Pathologists, Kennett Square, Pennsylvania, USA, 150–155.

23. UNITED STATES DEPARTMENT OF AGRICULTURE (USDA) (1995). Memorandum No. 800.85. Avian influenza vaccines. USDA, Veterinary Biologics, Animal and Plant Health Inspection Services.

24. WILKINSON B.E. (1998). Recombinant hemagglutinin subunit vaccine produced in a baculovirus expression vector system. Proceedings of the Fourth International Symposium on Avian Influenza, Athens, Georgia. Swayne D.E. & Slemons R.D., eds. U.S. Animal Health Association, 253–262.

25. WOOD G.W., BANKS J., STRONG I., PARSONS G. & ALEXANDER D.J. (1996). An avian influenza virus of H10 subtype that is highly pathogenic for chickens but lacks multiple basic amino acids at the haemagglutinin cleavage site. *Avian Pathol.*, **25,** 799–806.

26. WOOD J.M., KAWAOKA Y., NEWBERRY L.A., BORDWELL E. & WEBSTER R.G. (1985). Standardisation of inactivated H5N2 influenza vaccine and efficacy against lethal A/chicken/Pennsylvania/1370/83 infection. *Avian Dis.,* **29,** 867–872.

27. WOOD G.W., MCCAULEY J.W., BASHIRUDDIN J.B. & ALEXANDER D.J. (1993). Deduced amino acid sequences at the haemagglutinin cleavage site of avian influenza A viruses of H5 and H7 subtypes. *Arch. Virol.,* **130,** 209–217.

28. WOOD G.W., PARSONS G. & ALEXANDER D.J. (1995). Replication of influenza A viruses of high and low pathogenicity for chickens at different sites in chickens and ducks following intranasal inoculation. *Avian Pathol.*, **24**, 545–551.

29. WORLD HEALTH ORGANIZATION EXPERT COMMITTEE (1980). A revision of the system of nomenclature for influenza viruses: a WHO Memorandum. *Bull. WHO,* **58**, 585–591.

CHAPTER 2.1.15.

NEWCASTLE DISEASE

SUMMARY

Newcastle disease (ND) is caused by specified viruses of the avian paramyxovirus type I (APMV-I) serotype of the genus Rubulavirus *belonging to the family Paramyxoviridae. There are nine serotypes of avian paramyxoviruses designated APMV-I to APMV-9.*

Strains of ND virus vary widely in the severity of the disease they may produce in birds. The less pathogenic strains may induce severe disease when exacerbated by the presence of other organisms or by adverse environmental conditions. The preferred method of diagnosis is virus isolation and subsequent characterisation.

***Identification of the agent:** Suspensions in an antibiotic solution prepared from tracheal and cloacal swabs (or faeces) obtained from live birds, or of faeces and pooled organ samples taken from dead birds, are inoculated into the allantoic cavity of 9–11-day-old embryonating fowl eggs. The eggs are incubated at 37°C for 4–7 days. The allantoic fluids of any egg containing dead or dying embryos as they arise, and all eggs at the end of the incubation period, are tested for haemagglutinating activity.*

Any haemagglutinating agents should be tested for specific inhibition with a monospecific antiserum to ND virus. ND virus (APMV-1) may show some antigenic cross-relationship with some of the other avian paramyxovirus serotypes, particularly APMV-3 and APMV-7.

The pathogenicity of any newly isolated virus can be assessed by determining the mean death time in eggs, the intracerebral pathogenicity index in 1-day-old chicks or by the intravenous pathogenicity index in 6-week-old chickens. In some countries, variations of these standard techniques are used. The pathogenicity of isolates can also be evaluated using molecular biological techniques, i.e. reverse-transcription polymerase chain reaction and sequencing.

***Serological tests:** The haemagglutination inhibition test is used most widely in ND virus serology, its usefulness in diagnosis depends on the vaccinal immune status of the birds to be tested and on prevailing disease conditions.*

***Requirements for vaccines and diagnostic biologicals:** Live viruses of low virulence (lentogenic) or of moderate virulence (mesogenic) are used for the vaccination of poultry depending on the disease situation. Inactivated vaccines are also used.*

Live vaccines may be administered to poultry by various routes. They are usually produced by harvesting the infective allantoic/amniotic fluids from inoculated embryonating fowl eggs; some are prepared from infective cell cultures. The final product should be derived from the expansion of master and working seeds.

Inactivated vaccines are given intramuscularly or subcutaneously. They are usually produced by the addition of formaldehyde to infective virus preparations, or by treatment with beta-propiolactone. Most inactivated vaccines are prepared for use by emulsification with a mineral or vegetable oil.

A. DIAGNOSTIC TECHNIQUES

Newcastle disease (ND) is caused by ND virus, which is a member of the genus *Rubulavirus* of the family Paramyxoviridae. The paramyxoviruses isolated from avian species have been classified by serological testing into nine serotypes designated APMV-1 to APMV-9; ND virus has been designated APMV-1 (1).

Since its recognition in 1926, ND is regarded as being endemic in many countries. Prophylactic vaccination is practised in all but a few of the countries that produce poultry on a commercial scale.

One of the most characteristic properties of different strains of ND virus has been their great variation in pathogenicity for chickens. Strains of ND virus have been grouped into five pathotypes on the basis of the clinical signs seen in infected chickens (8). These are:

1. Viscerotropic velogenic – a highly pathogenic form in which haemorrhagic intestinal lesions are frequently seen;

2. Neurotropic velogenic – a form that presents with high mortality, usually following respiratory and nervous signs;

3. Mesogenic – a form that presents with respiratory signs, occasional nervous signs, but low mortality;

4. Lentogenic or respiratory – a form that presents with mild or subclinical respiratory infection;

5. Asymptomatic enteric – a form that usually consists of a subclinical enteric infection.

Pathotype groupings are rarely clear-cut (2) and even in infections of specific pathogen free (SPF) birds, considerable overlapping may be seen. In addition, exacerbation of the clinical signs induced by the milder strains may occur in superimposed infections by other organisms or when adverse environmental conditions are present.

As signs of clinical disease in chickens vary widely and diagnosis may be complicated further by the different responses to infection by different hosts, clinical signs alone do not present a reliable basis for diagnosis of ND. However, the characteristic signs and lesions associated with the virulent pathotypes will give rise to strong suspicions of the disease.

1. Identification of the agent

a) Samples for virus isolation

When investigations of ND are the result of severe disease and high mortality in poultry flocks, it is usual to attempt virus isolation from recently dead birds or moribund birds that have been killed humanely. Samples from dead birds should consist of oro-nasal swabs, as well as samples collected from lung, kidneys, intestine (including contents), spleen, brain, liver and heart tissues. These may be collected separately or as a pool, although intestinal samples are usually processed separately from other samples.

Samples from live birds should include both tracheal and cloacal swabs, the latter should be visibly coated with faecal material. Small delicate birds may be harmed by swabbing, but the collection of fresh faeces may serve as an adequate alternative.

Where opportunities for obtaining samples are limited, it is important that cloacal swabs (or faeces) and tracheal swabs (or tracheal tissue) be examined as well as organs or tissues that are grossly affected or associated with the clinical disease. Samples should be taken in the early stages of the disease.

The samples should be placed in isotonic phosphate buffered saline (PBS), pH 7.0–7.4, containing antibiotics. The antibiotics can be varied according to local conditions, but could be, for example: penicillin (2000 units/ml); streptomycin (2 mg/ml); gentamycin (50 µg/ml); and mycostatin (1000 units/ml) for tissues and tracheal swabs, but at five-fold higher concentrations for faeces and cloacal swabs. It is important to readjust the solution to pH 7.0–7.4 following the addition of the antibiotics. Faeces and finely minced tissues should be prepared as 10–20% (w/v) suspensions in the antibiotic solution. Suspensions should be processed as soon as possible after leaving them for 1–2 hours at room temperature. When immediate processing is impracticable, samples may be stored at 4°C for up to 4 days.

b) Virus culture

The supernatant fluids of faeces or tissue suspensions obtained through clarification by centrifugation at 1000 ***g*** for about 10 minutes at a temperature not exceeding 25°C are inoculated in 0.2 ml volumes into the allantoic cavity of each of at least five embryonated SPF fowl eggs of 9–11 days' incubation. After inoculation, these are incubated at 35–37°C for 4–7 days. Eggs containing dead or dying embryos as they arise, and all eggs remaining at the end of the incubation period, should first be chilled to 4°C and the allantoic fluids tested for haemagglutination (HA) activity. Fluids that give a negative reaction should be passaged into at least one further batch of eggs.

c) **Virus identification**

HA activity detected in bacteriologically sterile fluids harvested from inoculated eggs may be due to the presence of any of the 15 haemagglutinin subtypes of influenza A viruses or of the eight other paramyxovirus serotypes. (Nonsterile fluid could contain bacterial HA.) ND virus can be confirmed by the use of specific antiserum in a haemagglutination inhibition (HI) test. Usually chicken antiserum that has been prepared against one of the strains of ND virus is used.

Cross-reactions in HI tests between ND virus and APMV-3 serotype virus may cause some problems (1) that can be resolved by the use of suitable antigen and antiserum controls.

d) **Pathogenicity indices**

The extreme variation in virulence of different ND virus isolates and the widespread use of live vaccines means that the identification of an isolate as ND virus from birds showing clinical signs does not confirm a diagnosis of ND, so that an assessment of the virulence of the isolate is also required (see Section 1.f. below 'Definition of Newcastle disease'). Several potential *in-vitro* tests for establishing virulence usually related to the molecular basis for pathogenicity (Section 1.e. below) are being investigated by various groups around the world. At present, a definitive assessment of virus virulence is usually based on one or more of the following *in-vivo* tests, although the current OIE definition (Section A.1.f. below) allows molecular assessment of virulence:

- **Mean death time in eggs**

i) Fresh infective allantoic fluid is diluted in sterile saline to give a tenfold dilution series between 10^{-6} and 10^{-9}.

ii) For each dilution, 0.1 ml is inoculated into the allantoic cavity of each of five 9–10-day-old embryonated SPF fowl eggs, which are then incubated at 37°C.

iii) The remaining virus dilutions are retained at 4°C and another five eggs are inoculated with 0.1 ml of each dilution 8 hours later and left at 37°C.

iv) Each egg is examined twice daily for 7 days and the times of any embryo deaths are recorded.

v) The minimum lethal dose is the highest virus dilution that causes all the embryos inoculated with that dilution to die.

vi) The mean death time (MDT) is the mean time in hours for the minimum lethal dose to kill all the inoculated embryos.

vii) The MDT has been used to classify ND virus strains into velogenic (taking under 60 hours to kill); mesogenic (taking between 60 and 90 hours to kill); and lentogenic (taking more than 90 hours to kill).

- **Intracerebral pathogenicity index**

i) Fresh infective allantoic fluid with a HA titre $>2^4$ (>1/16) is diluted 1/10 in sterile isotonic saline with no additives, such as antibiotics.

ii) 0.05 ml of the diluted virus is injected intracerebrally into each of ten chicks hatched from eggs from an SPF flock. These chicks must be over 24-hours and under 40-hours old at the time of inoculation.

iii) The birds are examined every 24 hours for 8 days.

iv) At each observation, the birds are scored: 0 if normal, 1 if sick, and 2 if dead. (Dead individuals must be scored as 2 at each of the remaining daily observations after death.)

v) The intracerebral pathogenicity index (ICPI) is the mean score per bird per observation over the 8 day period.

The most virulent viruses will give indices that approach the maximum score of 2.0, whereas lentogenic strains will give values close to 0.0.

- **Intravenous pathogenicity index**

i) Freshly collected infective allantoic fluid (which should be no older than 24–48 hours and should have tested negative for bacterial contamination) with a HA titre of $>2^4$ (>1/16) is diluted 1/10 in sterile isotonic saline.

ii) 0.1 ml of the diluted virus is injected intravenously into each of ten 6-week-old SPF chickens.

iii) Birds are examined at 24-hour intervals for 10 days and scored at each observation: 0 if normal, 1 if sick, 2 if paralysed or showing other nervous signs, and 3 if dead. (Dead individuals must be scored as 3 at each of the remaining daily observations after death.)

iv) The intravenous pathogenicity index (IVPI) is the mean score per bird per observation over the 10-day period.

Lentogenic strains and some mesogenic strains will have IVPI values of 0, whereas the indices for virulent strains will approach 3.0.

Some variations have been recommended in these tests. Swabbing of the cloaca and conjunctiva of 8-week-old chickens with undiluted allantoic fluid has been substituted for the IVPI test (16). The intention is to distinguish between viscerotropic velogenic and other velogenic viruses.

- **Interpretation of pathogenicity indices**

Interpretation of the pathogenicity indices obtained with a view to imposing trade or movement restrictions, or other policies, is not straightforward. The objective is to control strains significantly more virulent than lentogenic strains, such as Hitchner-B_1 or La Sota. As viruses capable of producing quite severe disease may have IVPI values of 0, the ICPI test is used most often for such assessments. However, as different strains show a range of values from 0.00 to 2.00 in this test, it is clear that any value used for definition must be governed by practicable considerations.

e) Molecular basis for pathogenicity

During replication, ND virus particles are produced with a precursor glycoprotein, F0, which has to be cleaved to F1 and F2 for the virus particles to be infectious. This post-translation cleavage is mediated by host-cell proteases. Trypsin is capable of cleaving F0 for all ND virus strains.

It would appear that the F0 molecules of viruses virulent for chickens can be cleaved by a host protease or proteases found in a wide range of cells and tissues thus spreading throughout the host, damaging vital organs, but F0 molecules in viruses of low virulence are restricted in their sensitivity to host proteases resulting in restriction of these viruses to growth only in certain host-cell types.

Most ND viruses that are pathogenic for chickens have the sequence ^{112}R/K-R-Q-K/R-R^{116} at the C-terminus of the F2 protein and F (phenylalanine) at residue 117, the N-terminus of the F1 protein, whereas the viruses of low virulence have sequences in the same region of ^{112}G/E-K/R-Q-G/E-R^{116} and L (leucine) at residue 117. Some of the pigeon variant viruses (PPMV-1) examined have the sequence ^{112}G-R-Q-K-R-F^{117}, but give high ICPI values. Thus there appears to be the requirement of at least one pair of basic amino acids at residues 116 and 115 plus a phenylalanine at residue 117 and a basic amino acid (R) at 113 if the virus is to show virulence for chickens.

Several studies have been done using molecular techniques to determine the F0 cleavage site sequence by reverse-transcription polymerase chain reaction (RT-PCR), either on the isolated virus or on tissues and faeces from infected birds, with a view to establishing a routine *in-vitro* test for virulence (17, 18, 22). Determination of the F0 cleavage sequence gives a clear indication of the virulence of the virus, but, for a variety of reasons relating to the sensitivity of detection and the variations seen around the cleavage site for different viruses, the method is not yet in general use. None of the molecular techniques for assessing virulence offers a clear advantage in terms of speed, reproducibility and ability to detect all known viruses compared with virus isolation and *in-vivo* assessment. Thus, to date they have not fully replaced the conventional methods. However, it seems highly likely that with the continued rapid advancement of such techniques and the desire to avoid the use of animals for such tests that in the future molecular-based techniques will be sufficiently developed to be used for the assessment of virulence on a routine basis.

f) Definition of Newcastle disease

It seems likely that the vast majority of birds are susceptible to infection with ND viruses of both high and low virulence for chickens, although the clinical signs seen in birds infected with ND virus vary widely and are dependent on factors such as: the virus, host species, age of host, infection with other organisms, environmental stress and immune status. In some circumstances infection with the extremely virulent viruses may result in sudden high mortality with comparatively few clinical signs. Thus the clinical signs are variable and influenced by other factors so that none can be regarded as pathognomonic.

Even for susceptible hosts, such as chickens, ND viruses show a considerable range of virulence. Generally, variation consists of clusters around the two extremes in tests used to assess virulence, but, for a variety of reasons, some viruses may show intermediate virulence.

The enormous variation in virulence and clinical signs means it is necessary to define carefully what constitutes ND for the purposes of trade, control measures and policies. The definition of ND currently in use in all member states of the European Union is defined in Directive 92/66/EEC (12).

The OIE definition for reporting an outbreak of ND is:

'Newcastle disease is defined as an infection of birds caused by a virus of avian paramyxovirus serotype 1 (APMV-1) that meets one of the following criteria for virulence:

a) *The virus has an intracerebral pathogenicity index (ICPI) in day-old chicks* (Gallus gallus) *of 0.7 or greater.*

or

b) *Multiple basic amino acids have been demonstrated in the virus (either directly or by deduction) at the C-terminus of the F2 protein and phenylalanine at residue 117, which is the N-terminus of the F1 protein. The term 'multiple basic amino acids' refers to at least three arginine or lysine residues between residues 113 and 116. Failure to demonstrate the characteristic pattern of amino acid residues as described above would require characterisation of the isolated virus by an ICPI test.'*

In this definition, amino acid residues are numbered from the N-terminus of the amino acid sequence deduced from the nucleotide sequence of the F0 gene, 113–116 corresponds to residues –4 to –1 from the cleavage site.'

g) Monoclonal antibodies

Mouse monoclonal antibodies (MAbs) directed against strains of ND virus have been used in HI tests to allow rapid identification of ND virus without the possible cross-reactions with other APMV serotypes that may occur with polyclonal sera. MAbs have been produced that give reactions in HI tests that are specific for particular strains or variant ND virus isolates (1, 5).

Panels of MAbs have been used to establish antigenic profiles of ND virus isolates based on whether or not they react with the viruses. This has proven to be a valuable method for grouping and differentiating isolates of ND virus, and has been particularly valuable in understanding the epidemiology of outbreaks (5).

h) Phylogenetic studies

Development of improved techniques for nucleotide sequencing, the availability of sequence data of more ND viruses in computer databases and the demonstration that even relatively short sequence lengths could give meaningful results in phylogenetic analyses have led to a considerable increase is such studies in recent years. Considerable genetic diversity has been detected, but viruses sharing temporal, geographical, antigenic or epidemiological parameters tend to fall into specific lineages or clades and this has proven valuable in assessing both the global epidemiology and local spread of ND (4, 11, 20, 24, 26).

Although in the past phylogenetic studies have been impracticable as a routine tool, the greater availability and increased speed for the production of results of sophisticated, commercially available kits for RT-PCR and automatic sequencers now means such studies are within the capabilities of many more diagnostic laboratories and can give meaningful results that are contemporaneous rather that retrospective.

2. Serological tests

ND virus may be employed as an antigen in a wide variety of serological tests, enabling neutralisation or enzyme-linked immunosorbent assays (ELISA) to be used for diagnosis. At present, the HI test is most widely used. Chicken sera rarely give nonspecific positive reactions in this test and any pretreatment of the sera is unnecessary. Sera from species other than chickens may sometimes cause agglutination of chicken red blood cells (RBCs), so this property should first be determined and then removed by adsorption of the serum with chicken RBCs. This is done by adding 0.025 ml of packed chicken RBCs to each 0.5 ml of antisera, shaking gently and leaving for at least 30 minutes; the RBCs are then pelleted by centrifugation at 800 ***g*** for 2–5 minutes and the adsorbed sera are decanted.

Variations of the procedures for HA and HI tests are practised in different laboratories. The following recommended examples apply in the use of V-bottomed microwell plastic plates in which the final volume for both types of test is 0.075 ml. The reagents required for these tests are isotonic PBS (0.1 M), pH 7.0–7.2, and RBC taken from a minimum of three SPF chickens and pooled into an equal volume of Alsever's solution. (If SPF chickens are not available, blood may be taken from unvaccinated birds monitored regularly and shown to be free from antibodies to ND virus.) Cells should be washed three times in PBS before use as a 1% (packed cell v/v) suspension. Positive and negative control antigens and antisera should be run with each test, as appropriate.

a) Haemagglutination and haemagglutination inhibition tests

- **Haemagglutination test**

i) 0.025 ml of PBS is dispensed into each well of a plastic V-bottomed microtitre plate.

ii) 0.025 ml of the virus suspension (i.e. infective allantoic fluid) is placed in the first well. For accurate determination of the HA content, this should be done from a close range of an initial series of dilutions, i.e. 1/3, 1/5, 1/7, etc.

iii) Twofold dilutions of 0.025 ml volumes of the virus suspension are made across the plate.

iv) A further 0.025 ml of PBS is dispensed to each well.

v) 0.025 ml of 1% (v/v) chicken RBCs is dispensed to each well.

vi) The solution is mixed by tapping the plate gently. The RBCs are allowed to settle for about 40 minutes at room temperature, i.e. about 20°C, or for 60 minutes at 4°C if ambient temperatures are high, when control RBCs should be settled to a distinct button.

vii) HA is determined by tilting the plate and observing the presence or absence of tear-shaped streaming of the RBCs. The titration should be read to the highest dilution giving complete HA (no streaming); this represents 1 HA unit (HAU) and can be calculated accurately from the initial range of dilutions.

- **Haemagglutination inhibition test**

i) 0.025 ml of PBS is dispensed into each well of a plastic V-bottomed microtitre plate.

ii) 0.025 ml of serum is placed into the first well of the plate.

iii) Twofold dilutions of 0.025 ml volumes of the serum are made across the plate.

iv) 4 HAU virus/antigen in 0.025 ml is added to each well and the plate is left for a minimum of 30 minutes at room temperature, i.e. about 20°C, or 60 minutes at 4°C.

v) 0.025 ml of 1% (v/v) chicken RBCs is added to each well and, after gentle mixing, the RBCs are allowed to settle for about 40 minutes at room temperature, i.e. about 20°C, or for about 60 minutes at 4°C if ambient temperatures are high, when control RBCs should be settled to a distinct button.

vi) The HI titre is the highest dilution of serum causing complete inhibition of 4 HAU of antigen. The agglutination is assessed by tilting the plates. Only those wells in which the RBCs stream at the same rate as the control wells (containing 0.025 ml RBCs and 0.05 ml PBS only) should be considered to show inhibition.

vii) The validity of results should be assessed against a negative control serum, which should not give a titre >1/4 ($>2^2$ or $>\log_2 2$ when expressed as the reciprocal), and a positive control serum for which the titre should be within one dilution of the known titre.

The value of serology in diagnosis is clearly related to the expected immune status of the affected birds. HI titres may be regarded as being positive if there is inhibition at a serum dilution of 1/16 (2^4 or $\log_2 4$ when expressed as the reciprocal) or more against 4 HAU of antigen. Some laboratories prefer to use 8 HAU in HI tests. While this is permissible, it affects the interpretation of results so that a positive titre is 1/8 (2^3 or $\log_2 3$) or more. Back titration of antigen should be included in all tests to verify the number of HAU used.

HI titres may be used to assess the immune status of a flock. In vaccinated flocks that are being monitored serologically, it may be possible to identify anamnestic responses as the result of a challenge infection with field virus (7), but great care should be exercised as variations may occur from other causes. For example, it has been demonstrated that APMV-3 virus infections of ND-virus-vaccinated turkeys will result in substantially increased titres to ND virus (3).

There are a variety of commercial ELISA kits available and these are based on several different strategies for the detection of ND virus antibodies, including indirect, sandwich and blocking or competitive ELISAs using MAbs. At least one kit uses a subunit antigen. Usually such tests have been evaluated and validated by the manufacturer, and it is therefore important that the instructions specified for their use be followed carefully.

B. REQUIREMENTS FOR VACCINES AND DIAGNOSTIC BIOLOGICALS

A detailed account of all aspects of ND virus vaccines, including their production and use, has been published (7) and should be referred to for details of the procedures outlined here,

In this section, conventional live and inactivated vaccines will be considered, as these are still used universally. However, it should be remembered that there has been much recent work on the application of molecular biology techniques to the production of new vaccines, and success has been reported in obtaining protective immunity with recombinant fowlpox virus, vaccinia virus, pigeonpox virus, turkey herpesvirus and avian cells in which the HN gene, the F gene, or both, of ND virus are expressed. Several of these recombinant viruses have been licensed for use in certain countries.

ND virus strains used in commercial live virus vaccines fall into two groups: lentogenic vaccines, such as Hitchner-B_1, La Sota, V4, NDW and F, and mesogenic vaccines, such as Roakin, Mukteswar and Komarov. Strains from both these groups have been subjected to selection and cloning to fulfil different criteria in their production and application. The mesogenic vaccine viruses all have two pairs of basic amino acids at the F0 cleavage site and ICPI values of around 1.4. This means that infections of birds with these viruses would fall within the proposed definition of ND (Section A.1.f.); as these vaccines are primarily used in countries where ND is endemic this may not necessarily preclude their use.

Most live virus vaccines are grown in the allantoic cavity of embryonated fowl eggs but some, notably some mesogenic strains, have been adapted to a variety of tissue culture systems.

Live virus vaccines may be administered to birds by incorporation in the drinking water, delivered as a coarse spray, or by intranasal or conjunctival instillation. Some mesogenic strains are given by wing-web intradermal inoculation. Vaccines have been constructed to give optimum results through application by specific routes. In general, the more immunogenic live vaccines are more virulent, and are therefore more likely to cause adverse side-effects. For example, vaccination with the La Sota strain will cause considerably greater problems in young susceptible birds than the Hitchner-B_1 strain, although La Sota induces a stronger immune response.

Inactivated vaccines are considerably more expensive than live vaccines, and their use entails handling and injecting individual birds. They are prepared from allantoic fluid that has had its infectivity inactivated by the addition of formaldehyde or beta-propiolactone. This is incorporated into an emulsion with mineral oil, and is administered intramuscularly or subcutaneously. Individual birds thus receive a standard dose. There is no subsequent spread of virus or adverse respiratory reactions. Both virulent and avirulent strains are used as seed virus although, from the aspect of safety control, the use of the latter appears more suitable. As no virus multiplication takes place after administration, a much larger amount of antigen is required for immunisation than for live virus vaccination. A high yield of virus to produce a potent vaccine is important, and the Ulster 2C strain is very suitable for this purpose.

The duration of immunity depends on the vaccination programme chosen. One of the most important considerations affecting vaccination programmes is the level of maternal immunity in young chickens, which may vary considerably from farm to farm, batch to batch, and among individual chickens. For this reason, one of several strategies is employed. Either the birds are not vaccinated until 2–4 weeks of age when most of them will be susceptible, or 1-day-old birds are vaccinated by conjunctival instillation or by the application of a coarse spray. This will establish active infection in some birds that will persist until maternal immunity has waned. Revaccination is then carried out 3–4 weeks later. It has been demonstrated that inactivated vaccines may also be usefully employed to vaccinate 1-day-old chicks that have a degree of maternal immunity (10), and the best results of all were obtained when 1-day-old maternally immune chicks were given a combination of live and inactivated vaccines, compared with live or inactivated vaccines given alone (9). Vaccination of fully susceptible 1-day-old birds, even with the most mild of live vaccines, may result in respiratory disease, especially if common pathogenic bacteria are present in significant numbers.

Vaccination after 3 weeks of age is normally practised in breeding hens and hens laying table eggs only, and should be done at sufficiently frequent intervals to maintain an adequate immunity. Vaccination programmes often employ slightly more pathogenic live virus vaccines to boost immunity than those used initially or when oil emulsion inactivated vaccines have been used.

When devising a vaccination programme, consideration should be given to the type of vaccine used, the immune and disease status of the birds to be vaccinated, and the level of protection required in relation to any possibility of infection with field virus under local conditions (7). Two examples of vaccination programmes that may be used in different disease circumstances are listed here. For the first example, when the disease is mild and sporadic, it is suggested that the following order of vaccination be adopted: live Hitchner-B_1 by conjunctival or spray administration at 1 day of age; live Hitchner-B_1 or La Sota at 18–21 days of age in the drinking water; live La Sota in the drinking water at 10 weeks of age, and an inactivated oil emulsion vaccine at point of lay. For the second example, when the disease is severe and more widespread, the same protocol as above is adopted up to

21 days of age, and this is followed by revaccination at 35–42 days of age with live La Sota in the drinking water or as an aerosol; this revaccination is repeated at 10 weeks of age with an inactivated vaccine (or a mesogenic live vaccine) and again repeated at point of lay (7).

1. Seed management

a) Characteristics of the seed

The first principle to consider when selecting a strain for a live ND virus vaccine is whether it is to be used as a primary or a secondary vaccine, the main consideration being its pathogenicity. The methods of application and frequency of use are valid considerations. The use of MAbs has demonstrated considerable variation in the antigenicity of different strains (5). This may indicate a need to tailor vaccines more carefully to relate antigenically to any prevalent field virus.

A live vaccine based on ND virus strain V4, selected for heat stability, has been introduced to combat the specific problems associated with village chicken rearing in developing countries. The intention is that this vaccine could be coated on food fed to scavenging chickens. To date, trials in different countries have produced mixed results; it may well be that local factors are extremely important in affecting the success of this strategy (25).

Use of live vaccines may be restricted by legislation. For example, Commission Decision 93/152/EEC (13) restricts the use of vaccines in member states of the European Union from 1 January 1995 to those for which the master seed has been tested and shown to have an ICPI of <0.4 if no fewer than 10^7 mean egg infectious doses (EID_{50}) are administered to each bird, or <0.5 if no fewer than 10^8 EID_{50} are administered to each bird.

The most important consideration in selecting a seed for the preparation of inactivated vaccine is the amount of antigen produced when grown in embryonated eggs; it is rarely cost-effective to concentrate virus. Both virulent and lentogenic strains have been used as inactivated vaccines, but the former offer an unnecessary risk because the manipulation of large quantities of virulent virus is involved, as well as the dangers of inadequate inactivation and possible subsequent contamination. This risk is reflected in Commission Decision 93/152/EEC (13), which restricts the use of viruses used for inactivated vaccine in member states of the European Union from 1 January 1995 to those for which the master seed has been tested and shown to have an ICPI of <0.7 if no fewer than 10^8 EID_{50} are administered to each bird. Some lentogenic strains grow to very high titres in eggs. Exceptionally high titres can be obtained by the Ulster 2C strain, which has been recommended as a seed for inactivated vaccine (15). However, successful commercial inactivated vaccines are produced when the Hitchner B_1, La Sota or F strains are used as seeds.

b) Method of culture

A master seed is established, and from this a working seed. If the strain has been cloned by limiting dilution or plaque selection, the establishment of a master culture may only involve producing a large volume of infective allantoic fluid (minimum 100 ml), which can be stored as lyophilised aliquots (0.5 ml).

c) Validation as a vaccine

Seed viruses of unknown pedigree should be passaged through SPF eggs and cloned before producing the master seed. Some passage through SPF chickens may also be desirable (7). In either case, the master seed should be checked after preparation for sterility, safety, potency and extraneous agents.

2. Method of manufacture

For vaccine production, a working seed, from which batches of vaccine are produced, is first established by expansion of an aliquot of master seed to a sufficient volume to allow vaccine production for 12–18 months. It is best to store the working seed in liquid form at –60°C or lower as lyophilised virus does not always multiply to high titre on subsequent first passage (7).

Most ND vaccines are produced in embryonated fowl eggs, and live virus vaccines should be produced in SPF eggs. The method of production is large-scale aseptic propagation of the virus; all procedures are performed under sterile conditions.

It is usual to dilute the working seed in sterile PBS, pH 7.2, so that about 10^3–10^4 EID_{50}/0.1 ml is inoculated into the allantoic cavity of 9- or 10-day-old embryonated SPF fowl eggs. These are then incubated at 37°C. Eggs containing embryos that die within 24 hours should be discarded. The incubation time will depend on the virus strain being used and will be predetermined to ensure maximum yield with the minimum number of embryo deaths.

The infected eggs should be chilled at 4°C before being harvested. The tops of the eggs are removed and the allantoic fluids aspirated after depression of the embryo. The inclusion of any yolk material and albumin should be avoided. All fluids should be stored immediately at 4°C and tested for bacterial contamination before large pools are made for lyophilisation or inactivation. Live vaccines are usually lyophilised. The methodology depends on the machinery used and the expertise of the manufacturers, but this is a very important step as inadequate lyophilisation results in both loss of titre and a reduced shelf life.

In the manufacture of inactivated vaccines, the harvested allantoic fluid is treated with either formaldehyde (a typical final concentration is 1/1000) or beta-propiolactone (a typical final concentration is 1/2000–1/4000). The time required must be sufficient to ensure freedom from live virus. Most inactivated vaccines are not concentrated; the inactivated allantoic fluid is usually emulsified with mineral or vegetable oil. The exact formulations are generally commercial secrets.

Generally oil-based inactivated vaccines are prepared as primary emulsions of water-in-oil. The oil phase usually consists of nine volumes of highly refined mineral oil, such as Marcol 52, Drakeol 6VR and BayolF, plus one volume of emulsifying agent, such as Arlacel A, Montanide 80 and Montanide 888 (23). The aqueous phase is the inactivated virus to which a non-ionic emulsifier such as Tween 80 has been added. The oil phase to aqueous phase ratio is usually 1:1 to 1:4. Manufacturers strive to reach a balance between adjuvant effect, viscosity and stability. Too high viscosity and the vaccine is difficult to inject; too low viscosity and the vaccine is unstable.

3. In-process control

Each batch of live virus vaccine should be tested for viability and potency. For those produced in eggs, the most important process control is testing for bacterial and fungal contamination. This is necessary because of the occasional occurrence of putrefying eggs, which may remain undetected at the time of harvest.

For inactivated vaccines, the efficacy of the process of inactivation should be tested in embryonated eggs, taking 25 aliquots (0.2 ml) from each batch and passaging each three times through SPF embryos (7).

4. Batch control

Most countries have published specifications for the control of production and testing of ND virus vaccines (e.g. ref. 21), which include the definition of the obligatory tests on vaccines during and after manufacture.

It is necessary to test the infectivity of live virus vaccines to enable adequate levels of virus to be administered. This is usually titrated in embryonated fowl eggs to give the EID_{50}. This involves making tenfold dilutions of virus; 0.1 ml of each dilution is inoculated into between five and seven 9–10-day-old embryonated fowl eggs. After 5–7 days incubation at 37°C, the eggs are chilled and tested for the presence of haemagglutinin activity, which is an indication of the presence of live virus. The EID_{50} end-point is calculated using a standard formula such as Spearman–Kärber (6).

a) Sterility

Tests for sterility and freedom from contamination of biological materials may be found in Chapter I.4.

b) Safety

The use of chickens for the testing of vaccines involves the inoculation of ten or more birds of stated age that originate from an SPF flock. Ten doses of live vaccine are administered supraconjunctivally to each bird and the birds are then observed for 21 days. No chicken should show serious clinical signs and none should die from causes attributable to the vaccine (14).

For inactivated vaccines, a double dose is administered by the recommended route to ten 3-week-old birds, and these are observed for 2 weeks for absence of clinical signs of disease or local lesions.

c) Potency

Various methods for the testing of ND virus vaccines for potency have been proposed. The importance of using a suitable challenge strain for assessment has been stressed (7). A suitable strain is the Herts 33 strain. For live vaccines, the method recommended (14) involves the vaccination of 20 SPF or other fully susceptible birds at the minimum recommended age by the suggested route using the minimum recommended dose. After 14–21 days, each vaccinated bird and ten control birds are challenged intramuscularly with 10^5 LD_{50} (50% lethal dose) of ND challenge virus The vaccine passes the test if at the end of 10 days, 90% of the vaccinated chickens survive with no signs of disease, but all controls die within 6 days.

For inactivated vaccines, 21–28-day-old SPF or susceptible chickens are used. Three groups of 20 birds are injected intramuscularly with volumes of vaccine equivalent to 1/25, 1/50 and 1/100 of a dose. A group of ten chickens is kept as controls. All the birds are challenged by intramuscular injection of 10^6 LD_{50} of ND challenge virus, 17–21 days later. Chickens are observed for 21 days. The PD_{50} (50% protective dose) is calculated by standard statistical methods. The test is only valid if challenged control birds all die within 6 days. The vaccine complies with the test if the PD_{50} is not less than 50 per dose and if the lower confidence limit is not less than 35 PD_{50} per dose. Some control authorities accept a test at 1/50 only, for animal welfare reasons.

It is not necessary to repeat the potency test on each batch if it has been shown that a representative batch of the final product from the master seed has passed the test.

d) Duration of immunity

The level of immunity reached with any single dose or regimen of ND vaccination will vary enormously with both vaccine and host species. The level of immunity required in a given host (i.e. to protect against death, disease, meat or egg production losses) is extremely complex and difficult to evaluate. Generally some assessment of the longevity of serum antibodies should be made and vaccine regimens adopted to maintain these above an acceptable level (7).

e) Stability

When stored under the recommended conditions the final vaccine product should maintain its potency for at least 1 year. Accelerated stability tests such as reduction of infectivity following incubation at 37°C for 7 days (19) may be used as a guide to the storage capabilities of a batch of live vaccine. Oil emulsion vaccines should also be subjected to accelerated ageing by storing at 37°C, for a minimum of 1 month, without separation of the aqueous and oil phases. Live virus vaccines must be used immediately after reconstitution. Inactivated vaccines must not be frozen.

f) Preservatives

For live vaccines preservatives must not be included in the freeze-dried product, but antimicrobial preservatives may be incorporated in the diluent used to reconstitute the vaccine.

g) Precautions (hazards)

Live ND virus vaccines may represent a hazard to humans. ND viruses, both virulent and of low virulence for chickens have been reported to have infected humans, usually causing acute conjunctivitis following direct introduction to the eye. Infections are usually transient and the cornea is not involved.

Mineral oil emulsion vaccines represent a serious hazard. Accidental injection of humans should be treated promptly by incision and washing of the site.

5. Tests on the final product

a) Safety

See Section B.4.b. above

b) Potency

See Section B.4.c. above.

REFERENCES

1. ALEXANDER D.J. (1997). Newcastle disease and other avian Paramyxoviridae infections. *In:* Diseases of Poultry, Tenth Edition, Calnek B.W., Barnes H.J., Beard C.W., McDougald L.R. & Saif Y.M., eds. 541–570.

2. ALEXANDER D.J. & ALLAN W.H. (1974). Newcastle disease virus pathotypes. *Avian Pathol.*, **3**, 269–278.

3. ALEXANDER D.J., PATTISON M. & MACPHERSON I. (1983). Avian paramyxovirus of PMV-3 serotype in British turkeys. *Avian Pathol.,* **12,** 469–482.

4. ALEXANDER D.J., BANKS J., COLLINS M.S., MANVELL R.J., FROST K.M., SPEIDEL E.C. & ALDOUS E.W. (1999). Antigenic and genetic characterisation of Newcastle disease viruses isolated from outbreaks in domestic fowl and turkeys in Great Britain during 1997. *Vet. Rec.,* **145**, 417–421.

5. ALEXANDER D.J., MANVELL R.J., LOWINGS J.P., FROST K.M., COLLINS M.S., RUSSELL P.H. & SMITH J.E. (1997). Antigenic diversity and similarities detected in avian paramyxovirus type 1 (Newcastle disease virus) isolates using monoclonal antibodies. *Avian Pathol.,* **26**, 399–418.

6. ALLAN W.H. & HEBERT C.N. (1968). The precision of virus endpoint determinations. *Arch. Gesamte Virusforsch.,* **25**, 330–336.

7. ALLAN W.H., LANCASTER J.E. & TOTH B. (1978). Newcastle Disease Vaccines. Food and Agriculture Organization of the United Nations, Rome, Italy.

8. BEARD C.W. & HANSON R.P (1981). Newcastle disease. *In:* Diseases of Poultry, Eighth Edition, Hofstad M.S., Barnes H.J., Calnek B.W., Reid W.M. & Yoder H.W., eds. Iowa State University Press, Ames, Iowa, USA, 452–470.

9. BENNEJEAN G., GUITTET M., PICAULT J.P., BOUQUET J.F., DEVAUX B., GAUDRY D. & MOREAU Y. (1978). Vaccination of day-old chicks against Newcastle disease using inactivated oil adjuvant vaccine and/or live vaccine. *Avian Pathol.,* **7**, 15–27.

10. BOX P.G., FURMINGER G.S., ROBERTSON W.W. & WARDEN D. (1976). The effect of Mareks disease vaccination on the immunisation of day-old chicks against Newcastle disease using B1 and oil emulsion vaccine. *Avian Pathol.*, **5**, 299–306.

11. COLLINS M.S., FRANKLIN S., STRONG I, MEULEMANS G. & ALEXANDER D.J. (1998). Antigenic and phylogenetic studies on a variant Newcastle disease virus using anti-fusion protein monoclonal antibodies and partial sequencing of the fusion protein gene. *Avian Pathol.,* **27**, 90–96.

12. COMMISSION OF THE EUROPEAN COMMUNITIES (1992). Council directive 92/66/EEC of 14 July 1992 introducing Community measures for the control of Newcastle disease. *Off. J. European Communities*, **L260,** 1–20.

13. COMMISSION OF THE EUROPEAN COMMUNITIES (1993). Commission Decision of 8 February 1993 laying down the criteria for vaccines to be used against Newcastle disease in the context of routine vaccination programmes. *Off. J. European Communities*, **L59**, 35

14. COUNCIL OF EUROPE (1997). European Pharmacopoeia, Third Edition. Editions of the Council of Europe, Strasbourg, France.

15. GOUGH R.E., ALLAN W.H. & NEDELCIU D. (1977). Immune response to monovalent and bivalent Newcastle disease and infectious bronchitis inactivated vaccines. *Avian Pathol.,* **6**, 131–142.

16. HANSON R.P. (1980). Newcastle disease. *In:* Isolation and Identification of Avian Pathogens, Hitchner SB., Purchase HG. & Williams J.E., eds. AAAP, College Station, Texas, USA, 63–66.

17. JESTIN V., CHERBONNEL M. & ARNAULD C. (1994). Direct identification and characterisation of APMV-1 from suspicious organs by nested PCR and automated sequencing, Alexander D.J., ed. Proceedings of the Joint First Annual Meetings of the National Newcastle Disease and Avian Influenza Laboratories of the European Communities, Brussels, Belgium, 1993, 89–97.

18. KANT A., KOCH G., VAN ROOZELAAR D.J., BALK F. & TER HUURNE A. (1997). Differentiation of virulent and non-virulent strains of Newcastle disease virus within 24 hours by polymerase chain reaction. *Avian Pathol.,* **26**, 837–6849.

19. LENSING. H.H. (1974). Newcastle disease – live vaccine testing. *Dev. Biol. Stand.,* **25**, 189–1 94.

20. LOMNICIZI B., WEHMANN E., HERCZEG J., BALLAGI-PORDANY A., KALETA E.F., WERNER O., MEULEMANS G., JORGENSEN P.H., MANTE A.P., GIELKENS A.L.J., CAPUA I. & DAMOSER J. (1998). Newcastle disease outbreaks in recent years in Western Europe were caused by an old (VI) and a novel genotype (VII). *Arch. Virol.,* **143**, 49–64.

21. MINISTRY OF AGRICULTURE, FISHERIES AND FOOD (1993). Specifications for the Production and Control of Avian Live Virus Vaccines. Her Majesty's Stationery Office, London, UK.

22. OBERDORFER A. & WERNER O. (1998). Newcastle disease virus: detection and characterization by PCR of recent German isolates differing in pathogenicity. *Avian Pathol.*, **27**, 237–243.

23. PALYA V. & RWEYEMAMU M.M. (1992). Live versus inactivated Newcastle disease vaccines. Proceedings of the FAO Symposium Newcastle Disease Vaccines for Rural Africa, Debre Zeit, Ethiopia, April 1991, 107–119.

24. SEAL B., KING D.J. & BENNETT J.D. (1995). Characterisation of Newcastle disease virus isolates by reverse transcription PCR coupled to direct nucleotide sequencing and development of sequence database for pathotype prediction and molecular epidemiological analysis. *J. Clin. Microbiol.*, **33**, 2624–2630.

25. SPRADBROW P.B., ed. (1992). Newcastle Disease in Village Chickens. Proceedings No. 39, Australian Centre for International Agricultural Research, Canberra, Australia, 189 pp.

26. TAKAKUWA H., ITO T., TAKADA A., OKAZAKI K. & KIDA H. (1998). Potentially virulent Newcastle disease viruses are maintained in migratory waterfowl populations. *Jpn J. Vet. Res.*, **45**, 207–215.

*
* *

SECTION 2.2.

MULTIPLE SPECIES DISEASES IN LIST B

CHAPTER 2.2.1.

ANTHRAX

SUMMARY

Anthrax is primarily a disease of herbivorous animals, although all mammals including humans, and at least some avian species can contract it. Mortality can be very high, especially in herbivores. The aetiological agent is the spore-forming, Gram-positive rod-shaped Bacillus anthracis. *The disease has world-wide distribution and is a zoonosis. Anthrax is not only of importance to the livestock industry, certain populations of wildlife and humans, especially those who are occupationally exposed, it also supplies numerous models of historical as well as present-day significance to the current understanding of bacteriology, molecular biology, toxinology, immunology, and the pathogenesis and epidemiology of infectious diseases.*

The disease is mediated by exotoxins. Peracute, acute, subacute and, rarely, chronic forms of the disease are reported. Ante-mortem clinical signs may be virtually absent in peracute and acute forms of the disease. Subacute disease may be accompanied by progressive fever, depression, inappetence, weakness, prostration and death. Chronic disease may show localised swelling, fever and enlarged lymph glands; death may occur if the airway becomes obstructed. Post-mortem examination of recently dead animals (which must be performed with great care to avoid infection of the operator or contamination of the environment) may show any number of lesions, none of which is pathognomonic or entirely consistent. Lesions most commonly seen are those of a generalised septicaemia often accompanied by an enlarged spleen having a 'blackberry jam' consistency and poorly clotted blood. Haemhorrage from the nose, mouth and/or anus at death is a common sign.

Identification of the agent: *Visualisation of the capsulated bacilli, usually in large numbers, in a blood smear stained with polychrome methylene blue (M'Fadyean reaction) is fully diagnostic.* Bacillus anthracis *is readily isolated in relatively high numbers from blood or tissues of a recently dead animal that died of anthrax, and in pure culture, on any nutrient agar incubated aerobically at 37°C. Its characteristic appearance on blood agar makes this the medium of choice. As the carcass decomposes, especially in a warm climate, the putrefactive bacteria out compete and eventually eliminate the infective organism within the carcass. Confirmation of anthrax in these cases may depend on isolation from soil contaminated by the terminal discharges.*

Colony morphology of B. anthracis *is quite characteristic after overnight incubation on blood agar. The colony is relatively large, measuring approximately 0.3–0.5 cm in diameter. It is white to grey-white, nonhaemolytic with a rough, ground-glass appearance and has a very tacky, butyrous consistency. Prominent wisps of growth trailing back toward the parent colony, all in the same direction, are sometimes seen. This characteristic has been described as a 'medusa head' appearance.*

The vegetative cells of B. anthracis *are large, measuring 3–5 µm in length and approximately 1 µm in width. Ellipsoidal central spores, which do not swell the sporangium, are formed at the end of the exponential cell growth phase. The cells stain strongly Gram positive, and long chains are often seen* in vitro, *while paired or short chains are seen* in vivo. *The bacilli in infected tissue are encapsulated, but this characteristic is lost when the bacterium is grown aerobically* in vitro. *The* *capsule can be induced by incubating in defibrinated horse blood for at least 5 hours, or by culturing the isolate on nutrient agar containing 0.7% sodium bicarbonate with incubation at 37°C in the presence of CO_2.*

Additional useful laboratory confirmatory tests are the absence of motility, susceptibility to the specific diagnostic ('gamma') bacteriophage and sensitivity to penicillin. Primers are now available that can be used to show the presence of the toxin and capsule genes by polymerase chain reaction as confirmation of virulence, replacing animal inoculation. A thermoprecipitin test described by Ascoli in 1911 is still used in some countries to supply retrospective evidence of anthrax in decomposed carcasses or animal products.

***Serological tests:** Antibody detection in serum from infected animals is rarely used for diagnostic purposes and is essentially a research tool. The predominant procedure today is the enzyme-linked immunosorbent assay (ELISA).*

***Requirements for vaccines and diagnostic biologicals:** The most widely used anthrax vaccine for immunising livestock is a suspension of live spores prepared from the noncapsulated Sterne strain of* B. anthracis. *An equivalent strain is used in Russia (strain 55). The older Pasteur vaccine is still used in Italy. A list of producers is given in the World Health Organization anthrax guidelines (14).*

There are no standardised requirements for diagnostic biologicals. Diagnostic 'gamma' phage may be obtained from, for example the United States Centre for Disease Control (CDC[1]) or various central veterinary or anthrax reference laboratories.

A. DIAGNOSTIC TECHNIQUES

Anthrax is primarily a disease of herbivorous animals, although all mammals including humans, and at least some avian species can contract it. Mortality can be very high, especially in herbivores. The aetiological agent is the spore-forming, Gram-positive rod-shaped *Bacillus anthracis,* the only obligate pathogen within the genus *Bacillus.* Most of the other species of *Bacillus* are common ubiquitous environmental saprophytes, although a number, notably *B. cereus, B. licheniformis* and *B. subtilis,* are occasionally associated with food poisoning in humans and with other clinical manifestations in both humans and animals.

Animal anthrax occurs in at least three different forms: peracute or apoplectic form, acute form, and subacute to chronic form. Ruminants are most likely to manifest the peracute and acute forms, horses the acute form, and dogs, cats, and pigs a subacute to chronic or localised condition. In the peracute disease, signs preceding death often go unobserved. The clinical history usually describes the animal to be in good health a few hours before death. If the animal is observed shortly before death, fever up to 42°C (107°F), muscle tremors, dyspnoea, and mucosal congestion are the most common signs. Shortly afterwards, the animal will often have terminal convulsions, collapse and then die. Following death, unclotted blood may exude from the anus, vulva, nostrils, and/or mouth. Incomplete rigor mortis is also common.

The acute form may occur in cattle and clinical signs, such as depression, anorexia, fever, rapid respiration, increased heart rate, congested mucous membranes, or oedematous swellings, may be observed up to 48 hours before death. The acute form is usually seen in horses and varies with the site of exposure. Enteritis and colic are accompanied by high fever and depression. Death usually occurs within 48–96 hours. Spores introduced subcutaneously, for example by biting insects, result in a hot, oedematous swelling at the site that spreads to the throat, thorax, abdomen, prepuce or mammary gland. Dyspnoea due to throat swelling with resulting compression of the trachea may also be apparent. The course of the disease is usually 1–3 days, with some animals surviving for 1 week or more.

The subacute to chronic form of anthrax occurs in domestic and wild pigs, dogs and cats. The infectious bacteria are usually ingested when the host feeds on a contaminated source. The organism tends to localise in the regional lymph nodes of the pharyngeal area, where severe swelling may occur, resulting in death by occlusion of the airway. In cases where this does not occur, a fatal bacteraemia may develop, although recovery after a few days of illness is not uncommon. An intestinal form with severe acute gastroenteritis is also seen in carnivores and omnivores.

1 The Division of Bacterial and Mycotic Diseases, Centers for Disease Control (CDC), 1600 Clifton Road, Atlanta, Georgia 30333, United States of America (USA).

Suspicion of anthrax will depend on signs, such as sudden death with haemorrhaging from the orifices and incomplete rigor mortis, or on the history of the site, herd, etc. If anthrax is suspected, a thin smear is made on a microscope slide from a small drop of blood. This may be obtained by making a small cut in an ear vein or with a syringe from any available vein (care must be taken to avoid contaminating the environment or the operator). The blood smear is air-dried, fixed by immersion in 95–100% alcohol for 1 minute and stained with polychrome methylene blue (further details below). The presence of the capsulated 'box-car' bacilli in pairs or short chains, usually in large numbers, is definitive for anthrax. Smears made from swabs of the blood emerging from any of the orifices will also reveal the capsulated bacilli, but may be contaminated with other organisms or artefacts. Samples of the blood can also be taken for culture.

It is best **not** to perform a necropsy in order to prevent environmental contamination. In opening up the carcass, vegetative *B. anthracis* are exposed to the air allowing them to sporulate and contaminate the premises wherever blood or other body fluids have been spilled. In some countries post-mortem is forbidden. Post-mortem findings are well documented, however. There are no consistent pathognomonic lesions and considerable similarities are seen to other infectious and toxic causes of acute death. Poorly clotted dark blood, enlarged pulpy spleen with a 'blackberry jam' consistency, and multiple petechial haemorrhages characteristic of a septicaemia are usual. In horses, post-mortem findings may be similar to those of ruminants, but sometimes may just consist of oedematous lesions confined to the throat and neck with no involvement of internal organs. In omnivores (pigs) and carnivores, findings of septicaemia as described for ruminants may occur, but more often there is extensive oedema and inflammation in the pharyngeal area. If the focus of infection is in the gastrointestinal tract, severe inflammation, sometimes with haemorrhage and necrosis, may be seen in the stomach, intestines, and mesenteric lymph nodes, accompanied by peritonitis and excessive peritoneal fluid.

Natural decomposition of a carcass destroys most of the vegetative organisms through the action of putrefactive bacteria. This can occur within a day or two in hot climates. The capsulated bacilli may not be readily seen in smears of blood samples taken after this has occurred, though the blood may remain culture positive for a day or so more. Some sporulation may have occurred in fluids exuded through natural body openings, and, particularly if a carcass has been opened by scavengers, many spores may be dispersed into the environment. Swabs of congealed fluids or samples of soil contaminated by the fluids are likely to yield *B. anthracis* on culture. Culture of soil samples may be the best way to confirm that death was due to anthrax in well putrefied carcasses.

- **Disposal after sample collection**

Proper disposal of an infected carcass by incineration (although labour intensive and fuel consumptive) is the most desirable method and is often required by law. The contaminated soil, bedding, etc. should be incinerated together with the carcass and, ideally, the site should also be chemically disinfected for extra certainty. In some countries, it is considered that the best approach is to take the carcass for rendering. Contaminated soil, bedding, etc. would still need to be incinerated. Where incineration or rendering are not feasible, deep burial and covering with quicklime is the alternative, although periodic recovery of anthrax spores from some old carcass burial sites have shown that this is the least satisfactory alternative.

- **Risk factors for handlers of anthrax carcasses**

More than 95% of human anthrax cases take the cutaneous form and result from handling carcasses or hides, hair, meat or bones from such carcasses. *Bacillus anthracis* is not invasive and requires a lesion to infect. Protection for veterinarians and other animal handlers involves wearing gloves and other protective clothing when handling specimens from suspected anthrax carcasses and never rubbing the face or eyes. The risk of pulmonary anthrax from airborne spores is negligible for these types of occupations; the potential for inhalation of infectious doses is near zero. The risk of gastrointestinal anthrax only arises if the individuals go on to eat the meat or other food that has been cross-contaminated.

The risk of inhaling infectious doses becomes significant in occupations involving the processing of animal by-products for manufacturing goods (industrial anthrax). These include the tanning, woollen, carpet, bone processing, and other such industries, where the potential for aerosolisation of substantial numbers of spores within particles of less than 10 µm increases the risk of inhalation exposure to infectious doses. Laboratory workers should use good laboratory practice when working with specimens from suspected anthrax cases and when culturing *B. anthracis*. Use of a safety cabinet is desirable for diagnostic procedures, becoming mandatory if the need for manipulation of broth cultures or spore suspensions arises. As soon as they are finished with, tissues and cultures should be binned or bagged for autoclaving, followed by incineration. There is little need nowadays to use laboratory animals for diagnostic purposes, but if they are used, the bedding and cages should be autoclaved after use and the bedding incinerated afterwards. Care should be taken not to create dusty aerosols when handling the bedding.

1. Identification of the agent

Demonstration of encapsulated *B. anthracis* in smears of blood or tissues from fresh anthrax-infected carcasses and growth of the organism on blood agar plates is relatively uncomplicated and within the capability of most bacteriology laboratories. Difficulty may be encountered in the case of pigs and carnivores in which the terminal bacteraemia is frequently not marked, or in animals that received antibiotics before death.

Recovery of *B. anthracis* from old decomposed carcasses, processed specimens (bone meal, hides), or environmental samples (contaminated soil) is also often difficult, requiring demanding and labour-intensive procedures.

a) Fresh specimens

- **Capsule visualisation**

As described above, virulent encapsulated *B. anthracis* present in tissues and blood and other body fluids from animals that have died from anthrax should be looked for in smears of these specimens that have been dried, fixed and stained with polychrome methylene blue (M'Fadyean's reaction). The capsule stains pink whereas the bacillus cells stain dark blue. The cells are found in pairs or short chains and are often square-ended (the chains are sometimes likened to a set of railway carriages – so-called 'box-car' appearance). The Gram and regular Giemsa stains do not reveal the capsule. The capsule is not present on *B. anthracis* grown aerobically on nutrient agar or in nutrient broths, but can be seen when the virulent bacterium is cultured for a few hours in a few millilitres of blood (defribrinated horse blood seems to work best). Alternatively, the capsule is produced when the virulent *B. anthracis* is cultured on nutrient agar containing 0.7% sodium bicarbonate and incubated in the presence of CO_2 (20% is optimal, but a candle jar works well). The agar is prepared by reconstituting enough nutrient agar base powder for 100 ml of agar in 90 ml of water. Autoclave and cool to 50°C in a water bath. Add 10 ml of a filter-sterilised (0.22–0.45 µm filter) 7% solution of sodium bicarbonate. Mix and pour into Petri dishes. The encapsulated *B. anthracis* will form mucoid colonies and the capsule can be visualised by making thin smears on microscope slides, fixing and staining with polychrome methylene blue as before.

- **Polychrome methylene blue (M'Fadyean's stain)**

Polychrome methylene blue is prepared as follows: 0.3 g of methylene blue is dissolved in 30 ml of 95% ethanol; 100 ml of 0.01% potassium hydroxide (KOH) is mixed with the methylene blue solution. Ideally, this should be allowed to stand exposed to the air, with occasional shaking, for at least 1 year to oxidise and mature. Addition of K_2CO_3 (to a final concentration of 1%) hastens the 'ripening' of the stain, but before it is regarded as diagnostically reliable, its efficacy should be established by testing it in parallel with an earlier, functional batch of stain on *bona fide* samples. It has now been found that stains that give positive reactions with cultures of *B. anthracis* cultured artificially in horse blood sometimes do not give positive results in the field. Well quality-controlled polychrome methylene blue (M'Fadyean) stain is becoming increasingly hard to obtain; in some parts of the world, this is already leading to missed diagnosis.

In making smears for staining, only small drops of blood or tissue fluid are needed and a thin, small smear is best. After fixing and drying, a small (approximately 20 µl) drop of stain is placed on the smear and spread over it with an inoculating loop. After 1 minute the stain is washed with water into a hypochlorite solution (10,000 ppm available chlorine). The slide is blotted, air-dried and observed initially using the ×10 objective lens under which the short chains appear like short hairs; once found, these can be observed under oil immersion (×1000) for the presence of the pink capsule surrounding the blue/black-staining bacilli. To avoid laboratory contamination, the slide and blotting paper should be autoclaved or left for some hours in hypochlorite disinfectant.

- **Culture and identification of *Bacillus anthracis***

Bacillus anthracis grows readily on most types of nutrient agar, however, 5–7% horse or sheep blood agar is the diagnostic medium of choice. Blood is the primary clinical material to examine. Swabs of blood, other body fluids or swabs taken from incisions in tissues or organs can be spread over blood agar plates. After overnight incubation at 37°C, *B. anthracis* colonies are white or grey-white, 0.3–0.5 mm in diameter, nonhaemolytic, with a ground-glass moist surface, and very tacky when teased with an inoculating loop. Tailing and prominent wisps of growth trailing back toward the parent colony, all in the same direction, are sometimes seen. This characteristic has been described as a 'medusa head' appearance. Confirmation of identity as *B. anthracis* can be accomplished by testing for diagnostic 'gamma' phage and penicillin susceptibility and capsule induction. Absence of motility is an additional test that can be done.

The susceptibility of *B. anthracis* to the gamma bacteriophage was first described by Brown & Cherry in 1955 (3). The phage is available from CDC (see footnote 1), various national central veterinary laboratories and other anthrax reference laboratories. The procedure for the test is simply to streak a blood or nutrient agar plate, or portion of a plate (several tests can be done on one plate) with the suspect organism and place a 10–15 µl drop of the phage suspension to one side of the streaked area. A 10-unit penicillin disk can be placed to the other side. Allow the drop of phage suspension to soak in and incubate the plate at 37°C. A control culture should be included; the vaccine strain can be used for this. After several hours' incubation, if the culture is *B. anthracis*, the area under the phage will be devoid of bacterial growth, due to lysis of the *B. anthracis*, and a clear zone will be seen around the penicillin disk. *(Note: phage-resistant* B. anthracis *isolates are encountered very occasionally; similarly, there are a few reports in the literature of penicillin-resistant strains.)*

Induction of the capsule is described above.

- **Confirmation of virulence with the polymerase chain reaction**

Full confirmation of virulence can be carried out using the polymerase chain reaction (PCR). The following instructions are taken from ref. 14. Template DNA for PCR can be prepared from a fresh colony of *B. anthracis* on nutrient agar by resuspension of a loopful of growth in 25 µl sterile deionised (or distilled) water and heating to 95°C for 10 minutes. Following cooling to approximately 4°C, and brief centrifugation, the supernatant can be used for the PCR reaction.

Suitable primers (2, 6) for confirming the presence of the pX01 and pX02 plasmids are given in the table below.

Target	Primer ID	Sequence 5'–3'	Product size	Concentration
Protective antigen (PA)	PA 5 3048–3029	TCC-TAA-CAC-TAA-CGA-AGT-CG	596 bp	1 mM
	PA 8 2452–2471	GAG-GTA-GAA-GGA-TAT-ACG-GT		
Capsule	1234 1411–1430	CTG-AGC-CAT-TAA-TCG-ATA-TG	846 bp	0.2 mM
	1301 2257–2238	TCC-CAC-TTA-CGT-AAT-CTG-AG		

PCR can be carried out in 50 µl volumes using the above primers, 200 µM each of dATP, dCTP, dTTP and dGTP, 1.5 mM $MgCl_2$ and 2.5 units of amplitaq polymerase, all in NH_4 buffer, followed by the addition of 5 µl of template DNA.

Alternatively, 'Ready-To-Go™' beads are available from Pharmacia Biotech[2]. These are premixed, predispensed, dried beads, stable at room temperature, containing all the necessary reagents, except primer and template, for performing 25 µl PCR reactions. The template can be added in a 2.5 µl volume.

The following PCR cycle can be used: 1 × 95°C for 5 minutes; 30 × 95°C for 0.5 minute followed by 55°C for 0.5 minute followed by 72°C for 0.5 minute; 1 × 72°C for 5 minutes; cool to 4°C.

It should be noted that, in use for some years now in an anthrax reference facility, the primers given in the table above have proved themselves well for the purpose specified, namely to confirm the presence or absence of pXO1 and/or pXO2 in pure cultures of isolates from animal (including human) or environmental specimens or samples. They are unsuitable, however, for direct detection of *B. anthracis* in such specimens or samples. A choice of alternatives can be found in ref. 7. For the rare possibility that an isolate may lack both pXO1 and pXO2, a chromosomal marker should also be run; primers for these are also supplied in ref. 7

b) Agent identification from old, decomposed specimens, processed materials, and environmental samples, including soil

These specimens more often than not have saprophytic contaminants that outgrow and obscure *B. anthracis* on nonselective agars. The following procedure is suggested:

i) The sample is blended in two volumes of sterile distilled or deionised water and placed in a water bath at 62.5 ± 0.5°C for 15 minutes.

ii) Tenfold dilutions to 10^{-2} or 10^{-3} are then prepared. From each dilution, 10–100 µl are plated on to blood agar (optional) and 250–300 µl on to PLET agar (polymyxin, lysozyme, EDTA [ethylene diamine tetra-acetic acid], thallous acetate) (8, 14). All plates are incubated at 37°C.

2 Uppsala, Sweden, product number 27-9555-01.

iii) Blood agar plates, if included, are examined for typical colonies as previously described after overnight incubation, and the PLET plates are examined after 40–48 hours. Confirmation of the identity of suspect colonies as *B. anthracis* is done as described above. *(It is rare, following this scheme, to find* B. anthracis *on blood agar plates and not on the PLET and the costs of inclusion of the blood plates may not be considered to be justified by the relatively poor returns they supply.)*

PLET medium (8, 14) is prepared by using heart-infusion agar base (DIFCO) made up to the manufacturer's instructions with the addition of 0.25–0.3 g/litre EDTA and 0.04 g/litre thallous acetate. *(NOTE: thallous acetate is poisonous and should be handled with care.)* The mixture is autoclaved and uniformly cooled to 50°C before adding the polymyxin at 30,000 units/litre and lysozyme at 300,000 units/litre. After mixing thoroughly, the agar is dispensed into Petri dishes.

Reports of procedures for direct detection of *B. anthracis* in soils and other environmental specimens using the PCR are emerging. None of these has become routinely applicable at the present time and sensitivity levels remain at least 100-fold less than the conventional PLET-based procedure given above.

Animal inoculation may be considered for recovery of *B. anthracis* if all other methods fail. Examples of when this might occur are specimens from animals that received antibiotic therapy before death or environmental samples containing sporostatic chemicals. Due to the increasing concern to eliminate the use of animals for biological testing, this approach should be used as a last resort and only if justified. Adult mice or guinea-pigs are the animals of choice. If the samples involved are soils, the animals should be pretreated, the day before testing, with both tetanus and gas gangrene antiserum. The samples are prepared as described for culturing (Section A.1.b. above), including heat-shocking at 62.5°C for 15 minutes. Mice are injected subcutaneously with 0.05–0.1 ml; guinea-pigs are inoculated intramuscularly with up to 0.4 ml (0.2 ml in each thigh muscle). Any *B. anthracis* present will result in death in 48–72 hours and the organism can be cultured from the blood as described above.

c) Immunological detection and diagnosis

It needs to be borne in mind that *B. anthracis* is antigenically very closely related to *B. cereus,* which is an almost ubiquitous component of the environmental microflora. The only unshared antigens that lend themselves to differentiating these two species by immunological approaches are the anthrax toxin antigens, produced during the exponential phase of growth, and the capsule of *B. anthracis.* This places considerable constraints on the extent to which immunological methods can be used in routine detection methodology.

- **Ascoli test (1)**

In 1911, Ascoli (1) published a procedure for the detection of thermostable anthrax antigen in animal tissue being used for by-products. This uses antiserum raised in rabbits to produce a precipitin reaction. The test lacks high specificity, in that the thermostable antigens of *B. anthracis* are shared by other *Bacillus* spp., and is dependent on the probability that only *B. anthracis* would proliferate throughout the animal and deposit sufficient antigen to give a positive reaction. Nowadays, it appears to be used in Eastern Europe only.

To perform the Ascoli test, put approximately 2 g of sample in 5 ml of saline containing 1/100 final concentration of acetic acid and boil for 5 minutes. The resultant solution is cooled and filtered through filter paper. A few drops of rabbit antiserum (see preparation below) are placed in a small test tube. The filtrate from the previous step is gently layered over the top of the antiserum. A positive test is the formation of a visible precipitin band in under 15 minutes. Positive and negative control specimen suspensions should be included.

Antiserum is prepared in rabbits by the subcutaneous inoculation of Sterne strain anthrax vaccine on days 1 and 14. On days 28 and 35, the rabbits receive 0.5 ml of a mixture of several strains of virulent *B. anthracis* not exceeding 10^5 colony-forming units (cfu)/ml suspended in saline. Alternatively, the live virulent bacteria can be inactivated by prolonged suspension in 0.2% formalised saline, but the antigen mass needs to be increased to 10^8–10^9 cfu/ml. The suspension should be checked for inactivation of the *B. anthracis* before animal inoculation by culture of 0.1 ml into 100 ml of nutrient broth containing 0.1% histidine and, after incubation at 37°C for 7 days, subculture on to blood or nutrient agar. The dose regimen for the formalised suspension after initial vaccination on days 1 and 14 is increasing doses of 0.1, 0.5, 1, and 2 ml given intravenously at intervals of 4–5 days. Following either procedure, a test bleed at 10 days after the last injection should determine whether additional 2 ml doses should be administered to boost the precipitin titre.

- **Immunofluorescence**

While some success has been achieved with immunofluorescence for capsule observation in the research situation (4), it does not lend itself to routine diagnosis.

2. Serological tests

Historically, there has been little need for serological support for the diagnosis of anthrax in animals. Either the animal had anthrax, recognised from the recent history of the herd or site, and was treated accordingly, or it died. Most of the interest in developing serological testing has been for research on humoral responses in humans, and to a lesser extent in animals, for evaluating vaccines and for epidemiological studies involving naturally acquired seroconversion in humans, livestock and wild mammals.

Currently accepted as the best serological procedure is the enzyme-linked immunosorbent assay (ELISA) in microtitre plates coated with the protective antigen (PA) component of the anthrax toxin at 3–5 µg/ml in high pH (9.5) carbonate-coating buffer. The toxin antigens appear to be truly specific for *B. anthracis*, although there is at present no commercial source of these. This means that anthrax serology is currently confined to a few specialist laboratories. Various versions of the ELISA exist and can be found in standard laboratory manuals; any version will do for anthrax serology, although certain sera appear to be more 'sticky' than others. A useful tip is to use reconstituted dried milk as the blocking agent and to raise its concentration until control negative sera are giving reliable negative results. For bovine sera, this may be a 10% suspension or higher.

Examples of the successful field application of anthrax serology are given elsewhere (5, 11, 15).

3. Hypersensitivity test (Anthraxin™)

In Central and Eastern Europe, a skin test using Anthraxin™[3], first licensed in the former USSR in 1962, has become widely used for retrospective diagnosis of human and animal anthrax and for vaccine evaluation (12). This is a commercially produced heat-stable protein/polysaccharide/nucleic acid complex, derived from oedematous fluid of animals injected with the vaccine STI or the Zenkowsky strains of *B. anthracis*. The test involves intradermal injection of 0.1 ml of Anthraxin and inspection after 24 hours for erythema and induration at the site lasting for 48 hours after the injection. This delayed-type hypersensitivity is seen as reflecting anthrax cell-mediated immunity and was the test reportedly capable of diagnosing anthrax retrospectively some 31 years after primary infection in up to 72% of cases. It was used with success in a retrospective investigation of a series of cases occurring in a spinning mill in Switzerland where synthetic fibres were combined with goat hair from Pakistan (10). The diagnostic reliability of Anthraxin, like Ascoli test antigen, depends on the nature of anthrax rather than on the specificity of the antigens involved.

B1. REQUIREMENTS FOR VACCINES AND DIAGNOSTIC BIOLOGICALS: VACCINES

The most widely used vaccine for prevention of anthrax in animals was developed by Sterne in 1937 (13). He derived a rough variant of virulent *B. anthracis* from culture on serum agar in an elevated CO_2 atmosphere. This variant, named 34F2, was incapable of forming a capsule and was subsequently found to have lost the pX02 plasmid, which codes for capsule formation. It has become the most widely used strain world-wide for animal anthrax vaccine production. In Central and Eastern Europe, an equivalent pX02$^-$ derivative, Strain 55, is the active ingredient of the current livestock vaccine. A list of manufacturers of anthrax vaccine for use in animals is given in Appendix V of ref. 14.

The following information concerning preparation of the anthrax vaccine for use in animals is based on refs 9 and 16. Generalised procedures are given; national regulatory authorities should be consulted in relation to Standard Operating Procedures that may pertain locally.

1. Seed management

a) Characteristics of the seed

Anthrax vaccine production is based on the seed-lot system. A seed lot is a quantity of spores of uniform composition processed at one time and maintained for the purpose of vaccine preparation. Each seed lot is no more than three passages from the parent culture and must produce a vaccine that is efficacious and safe for use in animals. It is recommended that a large seed lot be prepared from the parent strain and preserved by lyophilisation for future production lots. The parent culture can be purchased[4]. The seed lot is acceptable for anthrax vaccine if a vaccine prepared from the seed lot or a suspension harvested from a culture derived from a seed lot meets the requirements for control of final bulk with respect to freedom from bacterial contamination, safety and efficacy (immunogenicity).

3 V.O. Medexport, 113461 Moscow, Russia.

4 National Institute for Biological Standards and Control, Blanche Lane, South Mimms, Potters Bar, Hertfordshire EN6 3QG, United Kingdom.

b) **Preparation of master seed**

Seed lots are cultured on solid media formulated to promote sporulation of the organism (see Section B1.2. below). The solid medium formula given in ref. 9 is: 50 g tryptic digest of casein; 10 g yeast extract; 0.1 g $CaCl_2.6H_2O$; 0.01 g $FeSO_4.7H_2O$; 0.05 g $MgSO_4.7H_2O$; 0.03 g $MnSO_4.4H_2O$; 5.0 g K_2HPO_4; 1.0 g KH_2PO_4; 22 g agar; 1000 ml deionised or distilled water. The ingredients are dissolved in the water with the appropriate amount of heating; the solution is adjusted to pH 7.4, distributed into Roux bottles (120 ml per bottle) or other appropriate container, sterilised by autoclaving and cooled in the horizontal position. After the agar has solidified, excess liquid should be removed aseptically and the bottles left in an incubator (37°C) for at least 2 days to dry and to check the sterility.

Volumes of 2 ml of vaccine seed from a reference laboratory should be spread across the agar in Roux bottles, which should be incubated at 37°C until at least 80% sporulation is apparent by microscopic examination of aseptically extracted loopfuls (at least 72 hours). The growth is harvested with 10 ml per bottle of sterile deionised or distilled water and checked for purity. After washing three times in sterile deionised or distilled water with final suspension, also in sterile deionised or distilled water, sterilised lyophilisation stabiliser is added and the suspension is dispensed into lyophilisation vials and freeze-dried.

c) **Preparation and testing of working seed**

Reconstitute a vial of seed stock and inoculate several slants (approximately 10 ml) of sporulation (casein digest) agar. Incubate at 37°C for 72 hours and store in a refrigerator. Test the slants for purity by culture on to nutrient agar plates and in nutrient broth (0.1 ml in 100 ml of nutrient broth). The latter should be subcultured on to nutrient agar after incubation at 37°C for 7 days and should be a pure culture of *B. anthracis.* A sample of the broth culture should also be checked for lack of motility.

Volumes of seed needed for a production run should be calculated on the basis of harvesting the spores from each slant with 10 ml of sterile deionised or distilled water and using this to inoculate five Roux bottles.

d) **Safety of seed-lot**

Not less than 5×10^9 culturable spores should be injected subcutaneously into each of three healthy, 1–2-year-old, unvaccinated sheep, which must survive an observation period of at least 10 days.

e) **Immunogenicity of seed-lot**

At least 10 healthy guinea-pigs, 300–500 g in weight should be inoculated with 5×10^6 viable spores and observed for 21 days. At least 80% of the animals should survive. The immunised animals, together with three unimmunised controls, should then be challenged with 10 median lethal doses (LD_{50}) of the strain 17 JB of *B. anthracis.* During a 10-day observation period, none of the immunised animals should succumb to the challenge while all the controls should die from anthrax. The test should be repeated if one of the immunised animals dies.

2. Method of production

a) **Preparation of vaccine concentrate**

Roux bottles with casein digest agar are prepared as for the master seed in Section B1.1.b. above. One Roux bottle can be expected to yield about 2000 doses of vaccine. Each Roux bottle is inoculated with 2 ml of working seed suspension and incubated at 37°C with porous plugs for several days until small loopfuls of culture from randomly selected bottles show at least 90% of the organisms to be in sporulated forms when examined in wet mounts by phase contrast (phase bright spores) or following staining for spores. The growth from each bottle is then harvested with 20 ml of physiological saline. Tests for contaminants should be carried out by subculture to nutrient agar plates and inoculation of 100 ml nutrient broth with 0.1 ml of harvested spores followed by subculture to nutrient agar after 7 days at 37°C and by tests for motility. Acceptable harvests (i.e. those showing no evidence of contaminants) are pooled.

b) **Glycerination**

Twice the volume of sterile, pure, neutral glycerol should be added to the bulk pool. Saponin (0.1% final concentration) may also be added at this point if it is to be included as an adjuvant. Mix thoroughly (the inclusion of sterilised glass beads may be helpful). Carry out a purity test as before and hold for 3 weeks at ambient temperature to allow lysis of any vegetative bacteria, determine the viable spore count and store under refrigeration thereafter.

c) **Determining titre and dilution for use**

The number of culturable spores in the product is then calculated by spreading ten-fold dilutions on nutrient agar plates. The suspension is diluted so that the final bulk contains the number of culturable spores desired. The diluent should contain the same proportions of saline, glycerol and (if being included) saponin as present in the vaccine concentrate. The vaccine should contain not less than 10 million viable spores per dose for cattle, buffaloes and horses, and not less than 5 million spores per dose for sheep, goats and pigs.

d) **Safety**

Safety testing is performed on two healthy sheep or goats and consists of inoculating subcutaneously twice the recommended vaccination dose. The animals are observed for 10 days. The final bulk passes the test if no systemic reactions develop and if not more than a transient oedema is observed at the injection site. If the test is carried out in sheep only, a progressive oedema indicates that the vaccine may be unsuitable for goats.

e) **Filling the containers**

Distribution of aliquots of vaccine into single and multidose containers is performed as outlined in World Health Organization Technical Report No. 363 series entitled *General Requirements for Manufacturing Establishments and Control Laboratories* (Requirements for Biological Substances No. 1), 1965, 16–17. Basically, the final bulk is distributed to containers in an aseptic manner in an area not used for production, and any contamination or alteration of the product must be avoided. The vaccine may be lyophilised after distribution into appropriate dosage containers. Containers are sealed as soon as possible with a material that is not detrimental to the product and that is capable of maintaining a hermetic seal for the life of the vaccine.

3. In-process control

Purity tests consist of microscopic examination of stained smears with culture and motility tests as described in Section B1.2.a.

4. Batch control and tests on the final product

a) **Sterility**

The vaccine is a live culture of *B. anthracis* spores; sterility does not apply, but the batches must be tested for freedom from contamination (see Chapter I.4.).

b) **Efficacy**

Efficacy or immunogenicity is tested on the final bulk as follows: at least ten healthy 300–500 g guinea-pigs are inoculated with a sheep dose of the vaccine. The guinea-pigs are observed for 21 days, and at least 80% of the animals must survive the observation period. Surviving immunised guinea-pigs and three nonvaccinated controls are challenged with an appropriate dose of virulent *B. anthracis*. A recommended challenge is 200 LD_{50} of the Pasteur II strain (17JB), which is available from the same source as the Sterne 34F2 vaccine strain. If, by 10 days after challenge, all vaccinated guinea-pigs survive and control animals die, the final bulk is deemed to be satisfactory. If any vaccinated animals die during the post-challenge observation period from a cause other than anthrax, and death is not associated with the vaccine, the test may be repeated.

c) **Dose**

The recommended dose for cattle and horses is a minimum of 10×10^6 culturable spores; for sheep, goats and pigs, it is $1–5 \times 10^6$ culturable spores. The vaccine should contain these spores in an appropriate volume, e.g. 1×10^7/ml.

d) **Duration of immunity**

Most experts agree that immunity is good for at least 1 year and it is recommended that an annual booster be given. Horses may be slow to develop immunity following initial vaccination; some manufacturers therefore recommend a two-dose initial vaccination, administered 1 month apart, followed by a single annual booster.

e) Stability

As there is no generally acceptable test for stability of anthrax vaccines, it is recommended that, in each filling lot, the number of culturable spores be determined before and after holding at an appropriate temperature for an appropriate period. There should be no evidence of a fall in the number of culturable spores.

f) Preservatives and storage

Bacillus anthracis spores are stable in unlyophilised or lyophilised vaccine and preservatives are not required. Storage under refrigeration is recommended (4°C).

g) Precautions (hazards)

The vaccine has been shown to cause disease in some goats and llamas; this may be related to the saponin adjuvant. The vaccine is not recommended for use in pregnant animals, nor in animals destined for slaughter within 2–3 weeks of vaccination. Local regulations may specify other time periods in some countries or regions, but there is no scientific reason for regarding meat from clinically healthy animals as unfit for human handling or consumption after a holding period of 2 weeks following vaccination. Concurrent administration of antibiotics to vaccinated animals is contraindicated as the antibiotic will interfere with the vaccine. Antibiotics should not be given for several days before and after vaccination. Left over vaccine, empty vials, and equipment used for vaccinating are contaminated with the live spores and should be autoclaved, disinfected, or incinerated. Accidental human inoculation is treated by expressing as much of the inoculum as possible from the injection site and washing the wound thoroughly with soap and water. Medical attention should be sought if infection develops.

5. Tests on the final product

a) Safety

Every batch of vaccine will be tested for safety as described in Section B1.2.d.

b) Potency

Every batch of vaccine will be tested for potency, as described in Section B1.4.b.

B2. REQUIREMENTS FOR VACCINES AND DIAGNOSTIC BIOLOGICALS: DIAGNOSTIC BIOLOGICALS

- **Propagation of the diagnostic 'gamma' bacteriophage**
  - **The bacteriophage can be propagated and concentrated by the following protocol (taken from ref. 14):**

Stage one

i) Spread a blood agar plate of the Sterne vaccine strain of *B. anthracis*. Incubate at 37°C overnight.

ii) Inoculate approximately 10 ml of nutrient broth with growth from the blood agar plate and incubate at 37°C for about 4 hours (until just cloudy), then refrigerate.

iii) Spread 100 µl of the culture from step ii on three predried blood agar plates and incubate at 37°C for 30–60 minutes.

iv) Spread 100 µl of the phage suspension to be amplified over the same plates. Incubate at 37°C overnight.

v) Harvest the phage-lysed growth on the blood agar plate in 5 ml of nutrient broth followed by a second 'wash' of 5 ml nutrient broth. Incubate at 37°C overnight.

vi) Filter (0.45 µm) and count by dropping 20 µl drops (3 drops per dilution) of tenfold dilutions of the filtrate in saline on to lawns of the *B. anthracis* culture prepared as in step iii.

Stage two

This is essentially the same procedure as Stage one, only using the filtrate from step vi to harvest the phage from the plates, i.e.:

vii) Prepare three Sterne strain lawns on blood agar, as in step iii. Incubate at 37°C 30–60 minutes.

viii) Spread 100 µl phage from step vi. Incubate at 37°C overnight.

ix) To 9 ml of filtrate from step vi, add 1 ml of 10 × concentrated nutrient broth.

x) Harvest the phage from step viii with 5 ml of the solution from step ix, followed by a second 5 ml wash with the rest of the solution from step ix.

xi) Add 10 ml of 1 × nutrient broth.

xii) Incubate at 37°C overnight, centrifuge with appropriate precautions, filter and count.

Stage three

xiii) Inoculate 100 ml of brain–heart infusion broth with approximately 2.5 ml of the culture from step ii. Incubate on a rotary shaker at 37°C until just turbid.

xiv) Add the 20 ml of filtrate from step xii and continue incubation overnight.

xv) Centrifuge (with appropriate precautions) and filter.

xvi) The resultant filtrate is checked for freedom from contamination and titrated in tenfold dilutions on lawns of the vaccine strain as in step vi to determine the concentration of the phage. This should be of the order of 10^8–10^9 plaque forming units per ml. This must be kept refrigerated at a temperature of between 2°C and 8°C, not frozen.

REFERENCES

1. ASCOLI A. (1911). Die Präzipitindiagnose bei Milzbrand. *Centralbl. Bakt. Parasit. Infeckt.*, **58**, 63–70.

2. BEYER W., GLOCKNER P., OTTO J. & BOHM R. (1996). A nested PCR and DNA-amplification-fingerprinting method for detection and identification of *Bacillus anthracis* in soil samples from former tanneries. *Salisbury Med. Bull.,* No. 87, Special Suppl., 47–49.

3. BROWN E.R. & CHERRY W.B. (1955). Specific identification of *Bacillus anthracis* by means of a variant bacteriophage. *J. Infect. Dis.*, **96**, 34–39.

4. EZZELL J.W. & ABSHIRE T.G. (1996). Encapsulation of *Bacillus anthracis* spores and spore identification. *Salisbury Med. Bull.,* No 87, Special Suppl., 42.

5. HARRISON L.H., EZZELL J.W., ABSHIRE T.G., KIDD S. & KAUFMANN A.F. (1989). Evaluation of serologic tests for diagnosis of anthrax after an outbreak of cutaneous anthrax in Paraguay. *J. Infect. Dis.*, **160**, 706–710.

6. HUTSON R.A., DUGGLEBY C.J., LOWE J.R., MANCHEE R.J. & TURNBULL P.C.B. (1993). The development and assessment of DNA and oligonucleotide probes for the specific detection of *Bacillus anthracis*. *J. Appl. Bacteriol.,* **75**, 463–472

7. JACKSON P.J., HUGH-JONES M.E., ADAIR D.M., GREEN G., HILL K.K., KUSKE C.R., GRINBERG L.M., ABRAMOVA, F.A. & KEIM P. (1998). PCR analysis of tissue samples from the 1979 Sverdlovsk anthrax victims: The presence of multiple *Bacillus anthracis* strains in different victims. *Proc. Natl Acad. Sci. USA*, **95**, 1224–1229.

8. KNISELY R.F. (1966). Selective medium for *Bacillus anthracis*. *J. Bacteriol.*, **92**, 784–786.

9. MISRA R.P. (1991). Manual for the Production of Anthrax and Blackleg Vaccines. Food and Agriculture Organisation of the United Nations (FAO) Animal Production and Health Paper 87, FAO, Rome, Italy.

10. PFISTERER R.M. (1990). Retrospective verification of the diagnosis of anthrax by means of the intracutaneous skin test with the Russian allergen 'Anthraxin' in a recent epidemic in Switzerland. *Salisbury Med. Bull.,* No. 68, Special Suppl., 80.

11. REDMOND C., HALL G.A., TURNBULL P.C.B. & GILLGAN J.S. (1996). Experimentally assessed public health risks associated with pigs from farms experiencing anthrax. *Vet. Rec.*, **141**, 244–247.

12. SHLYAKHOVE E., RUBINSTEIN E. & NOVIKOV I. (1997). Anthrax post-vaccinal cell-mediated immunity in humans: kinetics pattern. *Vaccine*, **15**, 631–636.

13. STERNE M. (1937). The effect of different carbon dioxide concentrations on the growth of virulent anthrax strains. *Onderstepoort J. Vet. Sci. Anim. Ind.*, **9**, 49–67.

14. TURNBULL P.C.B., BOEHM R., COSIVI O., DOGANAY M., HUGH-JONES M.E., LALITHA M.K. & DE VOS V. (1998). Guidelines for the Surveillance and Control of Anthrax in Humans and Animals. WHO/EMC/ZDI/98.6. World Health Organization, Geneva, Switzerland.

15. TURNBULL P.C.B., DOGANAY M., LINDEQUE P.M., AYGEN B. & MCLAUGHLIN J. (1992). Serology and anthrax in humans, livestock and Etosha National Park wildlife. *Epidemiol. Infect.*, **108**, 299–313.

16. WORLD HEALTH ORGANIZATION EXPERT COMMITTEE ON BIOLOGICAL STANDARDIZATION (1967). Requirements for Anthrax Spore Vaccine (Live – for Veterinary Use) (Requirements for Bioiogical Substances No. 13). World Health Organization (WHO) Technical Report Series No. 361. WHO, Geneva, Switzerland.

FURTHER READING

A. LOGAN N.A. & TURNBULL P.C.B. (1998). *Bacillus* and recently derived genera. *In:* Manual of Clinical Microbiology, Seventh Edition, Murray P.R., Baron E.J., Pfaller M.A., Tenover F.C. & Yolken R.H., eds. American Society for Microbiology, Washington DC, USA, 357–369.

B. QUINN C.P. & TURNBULL P.C.B. (1998). Anthrax. *In:* Topley & Wilson's Microbiology and Microbial Infections, Vol. 3, Ninth Edition, Collier L., Balows A. & Sussman M., eds. Arnold, London, UK, 799–818.

C. TURNBULL P.C.B., (ED.) (1996). Proceedings of the International Workshop on Anthrax. *Salisbury Med. Bull.*, Special Supple. No. 87, 139 pages.

D. TURNBULL P.C.B. (1998). Anthrax. *In:* Zoonoses. Biology, Clinical Practice, and Public Health Control. Palmer S.R., Soulsby E.J.L. & Simpson D.I.H., eds. Oxford University Press, Oxford, UK, 3–16.

E. WHITFORD H.W. & HUGH-JONES M.E. (1994). Anthrax. *In:* Handbook Series in Zoonoses, Second Edition, Beran G.W., editor-in-chief. CRC Press, Boca Raton, Florida, USA, 61–82.

*
* *

CHAPTER 2.2.2.

AUJESZKY'S DISEASE

SUMMARY

Aujeszky's disease, also known as pseudorabies, is caused by an alphaherpesvirus that infects the central nervous system and other organs, such as the respiratory tract, in virtually all mammals except humans and the tailless apes. It is associated primarily with pigs, the natural host, which remain latently infected following clinical recovery. The disease is controlled by containment of infected herds and by the use of vaccines and removal of latently infected animals.

A diagnosis of Aujeszky's disease is established by detecting the agent (virus isolation, polymerase chain reaction [PCR]), as well as by detecting a serological response in the live animal.

***Identification of the agent:** Isolation of Aujeszky's disease virus can be made by inoculating a tissue homogenate, for example of brain and tonsil or material collected from the nose/throat, into a susceptible cell line such as porcine kidney (PK-15) or SK6, or primary or secondary kidney cells. The specificity of the cytopathic effect is verified by immunofluorescence, immunoperoxidase or neutralisation with specific antiserum. The virus can also be identified using PCR, but this technique is still quite new.*

***Serological tests:** Aujeszky's disease antibodies are demonstrated by virus neutralisation, latex agglutination or enzyme-linked immunosorbent assay (ELISA). A number of ELISA kits are commercially available world-wide. An OIE international standard serum defines the lower limit of sensitivity for routine testing by laboratories that undertake the serological diagnosis of Aujeszky's disease.*

Since about 1990, it has become possible to distinguish between antibodies resulting from natural infection and those from vaccination by use of gene-deleted vaccines.

***Requirements for vaccines and diagnostic biologicals:** The spread of Aujeszky's disease may be diminished by the use of vaccines containing either modified live virus or inactivated virus antigens. More recently, these conventional vaccines have been supplemented by rDNA-derived gene-deleted or naturally deleted live pseudorabies virus vaccines. The virus used in these new vaccines, sometimes referred to as marker vaccines, lacks a specific glycoprotein (gG, gE, or gC).*

A. DIAGNOSTIC TECHNIQUES

Aujeszky's disease, also known as pseudorabies, is caused by an alphaherpesvirus, a member of the family Herpesviridae. The pseudorabies virus (PRV) principally affects pigs, herbivores and carnivores, but can infect all mammalian species other than humans and most species of primates.

Whereas isolation of PRV will assist in a provisional diagnosis in the case of lethal forms of Aujeszky's disease or clinical disease in pigs, other techniques and serological tests are required for diagnosis of latent infections. Many affected animals, however, except pigs, do not live long enough to produce any marked serological response.

1. Identification of the agent

a) Virus isolation

The diagnosis of Aujeszky's disease can be confirmed by isolating PRV from the oro-pharyngeal fluid, nasal fluid (swabs) or tonsil biopsies of living pigs, or from samples from dead pigs or following the presentation of clinical signs such as encephalitis in herbivores or carnivores. For post-mortem isolation of PRV, samples of brain and tonsil are the preferred specimens. In cattle, infection is usually characterised by a pruritus, in which case a sample of the corresponding section of the spinal cord may be required in order to isolate the virus. In latently infected pigs, the trigeminal ganglion is the most consistent site for virus isolation, although latent virus is usually difficult to culture.

The samples are homogenised in normal saline or cell culture medium and the resulting suspension is clarified by low speed centrifugation at 900 ***g*** for 10 minutes. The supernatant fluid is used to inoculate any sensitive cell culture system. Numerous types of cell line or primary cell cultures are sensitive to PRV, but a porcine kidney cell line (PK-15) is generally employed. The overlay medium for the cultures should contain antibiotics (such as: 200 IU/ml penicillin; 100 µg/ml streptomycin; 100 µg/ml polymyxin; and 3 µg/ml fungizone).

PRV induces a cytopathic effect (CPE) that usually appears within 24–72 hours, but cell cultures may be incubated for 5–6 days. The monolayer develops accumulations of birefringent cells, followed by complete detachment of the cell sheet. Syncytia also develop, the appearance and size of which are variable. In the absence of any obvious CPE, it is advisable to make one blind passage into further cultures. Additional evidence may be obtained by staining infected cover-slip cultures with haematoxylin and eosin to demonstrate the characteristic herpesviral acidophilic intranuclear inclusions with margination of the chromatin. The virus identity should be confirmed by immunofluorescence, immunoperoxidase, or neutralisation using specific antiserum.

The isolation of PRV makes it possible to confirm Aujeszky's disease, but failure to isolate does not guarantee freedom from infection.

b) Identification of virus by the polymerase chain reaction

The polymerase chain reaction (PCR) can be used to identify PRV genomes in secretions or organ samples. As this technique is still quite new, it is not yet possible to specify a standard procedure. Only some general information can be given.

PCR is based on the selective amplification of a specific part of the genome using two primers located at each end of the selected sequence. In a first step, the complete DNA may be isolated using standard procedures (e.g. proteinase K digestion and phenol–chloroform extraction). Using cycles of DNA denaturation to give single-stranded DNA templates, hybridisation of the primers, and synthesis of complementary sequences using a thermostable DNA polymerase, the target sequence can be amplified up to 10^6-fold. The primers must be designed to amplify a sequence conserved among PRV strains, for example parts of the gB or gD genes, which code for essential glycoproteins, have been used.

The amplified product may be identified from its molecular weight as determined by migration in agarose gel, with further confirmation where possible by Southern hybridisation using a complementary probe. More recent techniques involve liquid hybridisation using enzyme-labelled probes, which give a colour reaction after incubation with the appropriate substrate. An improvement of the technique is known as 'nested PCR' and uses two sets of primers, one of which is located within the sequence amplified by the first set of primers. By using appropriate hybridisation temperatures in a two-step reaction, both the sensitivity and specificity of the PCR can be improved.

In all cases, the main advantage of PCR when compared with conventional virus isolation techniques is its rapidity, as preliminary identification can be completed within one day with confirmation of the PCR product on the second day. With the most modern equipment the whole process can be completed in one day. However, because of the nature of the test, many precautions need to be taken to avoid contamination of samples with extraneous DNA from previous tests or from general environmental contamination in the laboratory (see chapter I.4.). This may limit the value of the test for many laboratories, and therefore this technique cannot be fully recommended for routine diagnosis, although methods are available for preventing DNA carry-over contamination (e.g. dUTP-UNG system [d-uracil triphosphate/uracil-N-glycosylase]). Many diagnostic laboratories would restrict the use of PCR to the detection of latent infection.

2. Serological tests

Any serological technique used should be sufficiently sensitive to give a positive result with the OIE International Standard Reference Serum. This serum is obtainable from the OIE Reference Laboratory for Aujeszky's Disease in France (see Table given in Part 4 of this *Manual*) and should be reconstituted before use according to the data sheet instructions. For international trade purposes, the test should be sensitive enough to detect the standard serum diluted 1/2.

Virus neutralisation (VN) has been recognised as the reference method for serology (4, 27), but for general diagnostic purposes it has been widely replaced by the enzyme-linked immunosorbent assay (ELISA) because of its suitability for large-scale testing (2, 11, 15, 17).

A latex agglutination test has also been developed and can be used for screening for antibodies. Kits for the test are commercially available.

a) Virus neutralisation (a prescribed test for international trade)

VN in cell culture can be performed in several ways, which vary according to the length of incubation of the virus/serum mixtures (e.g. 1 hour at 37°C or 24 hours at 4°C), and the presence or absence of complement. Most laboratories use a reaction period of 1 hour at 37°C in the absence of complement, because this is easy and rapid. However, the sensitivity can be improved by increasing the incubation period to 24 hours at 4°C, which facilitates the detection of antibody levels 10–15 times lower than in the 1-hour method. For international trade purposes, the test method should be validated as being sensitive enough to detect the OIE Standard Reference Serum diluted 1/2.

VN cannot be used to differentiate antibodies of vaccinal origin from those caused by natural infection. It is one of the two tests available to comply with the requirement in the OIE *International Animal Health Code* chapter when it refers to 'a diagnostic test to the whole virus'.

Cells: Cells susceptible to infection with PRV are used; they may be cell lines (e.g. PK-15, SK6), or primary or secondary cell cultures.

Cell culture medium: The medium depends on the type of cells. For example, the medium for PK-15 cells is Eagle's minimal essential medium (MEM) + 10% fetal bovine serum and antibiotics (100 IU/ml penicillin and 100 µg/ml streptomycin, or alternatively, 50 µg/ml gentamycin).

Maintenance of the cells: The cells are cultured in cell culture vessels of, for example, 75 cm^2. They are trypsinised once or twice per week. For weekly trypsinisation, the cells are cultured in 50 ml of medium, with a multiplication rate of 5. For two trypsinisations a week, the cells are cultured in 30 ml of medium, with a multiplication rate of 3.

For trypsinisation, the growth medium is removed once the cell sheet is complete. The cell sheet is washed with about 5 ml of recently thawed trypsin/ethylene diamine tetra-acetic acid (EDTA) (0.25%). The washing fluid is discarded and the preparation is washed again, retaining only a few drops of trypsin. The container is placed in an incubator at 37°C for 5–10 minutes until the cells have become detached. Once the sheet is detached and the cells are well separated, they are suspended in 90 ml of growth medium, and this suspension is distributed into three 75 cm^2 cell culture bottles.

Virus: A suitable strain of PRV, such as the Kojnok strain, or NIA-3 strain, is stored at a temperature of –70°C or below, or in freeze-dried form at 4°C.

Preparation of stock virus suspension: The culture fluid is removed from a cell culture bottle containing a complete cell sheet. About 1 ml of stock virus suspension of known titre (about 10^7 $TCID_{50}$/ml [50% tissue culture infective dose]) is added, and the bottle is incubated at 37°C for 1 hour. Then, 30 ml of culture medium is added and the bottle is again incubated at 37°C. The bottle is examined frequently until there is about 75% cell destruction (after about 36–48 hours). It is then frozen at a temperature of –20°C or lower in order to disrupt the cells.

The bottle is then thawed and shaken vigorously. Medium is collected and centrifuged at 1500 ***g*** for 15 minutes. The supernatant fluid is divided into portions (of about 0.5 ml) in small tubes that are labelled (date and virus reference) before being stored at a temperature of –70°C or lower until required.

Titration of the stock virus suspension: Titration of the stock suspension is performed by the method of Reed & Muench or that of Kärber, and the titre is expressed per 50 µl and per ml.

The VN test requires an internal quality control serum with a known titre of neutralising antibody to PRV (it must be calibrated against an international standard serum or a secondary standard prepared from that serum), and a negative control serum (from a specific antibody free pig, e.g. from an official Aujeszky's disease free herd). The test sera themselves should be of good quality. Serum should be separated from the coagulum without delay, thereby preventing toxicity.

There are qualitative and quantitative procedures for VN, both of which are described below.

- **Qualitative technique**

i) Complement in the serum samples is destroyed by heating in a water bath at 56°C for 30 minutes.

ii) Each undiluted serum is placed in three wells, at 50 µl per well, of a 96-well cell-culture grade microtitre plate.

iii) 50 µl of virus suspension containing 100 $TCID_{50}$/50 µl (or 2×10^3 $TCID_{50}$/ml), obtained by diluting stock virus suspension of known titre with MEM, is added to each well.

iv) The plate is shaken and placed in an incubator for 1 hour at 37°C (CO_2 optional).

v) 150 µl of cell suspension containing about 150,000 cells/ml is added to each well.

vi) The plate is covered (for incubation in CO_2), or a plastic sheet is sealed carefully around the edges of the plate (for incubation in air). The plate is shaken lightly to obtain an even distribution of cells at the bottom of the wells, and placed in the incubator at 37°C (CO_2 optional).

vii) *Controls:* Each set of plates must include the following controls:

Virus control: This is to verify the amount of virus actually used for the test. The virus dose used for serum neutralisation (target titre 100 $TCID_{50}$/50 µl) is diluted with MEM at 1/10, 1/100 and 1/1000. Of each dilution, 50 µl is placed in at least five wells, to which 50 µl of medium is added before the wells are incubated for 1 hour at 37°C. The cell suspension is added in the same way as for the sera under test.

Cell control: 150 µl cell suspension and 100 µl MEM are placed in each of at least two wells.

Positive serum control: A serum of known PRV neutralising antibody titre is used. Five dilutions are prepared in the same way as for the sera under test: a dilution corresponding to the serum titre, two-fold and four-fold dilutions, and 1/2 and 1/4 dilutions (equivalent to T, T/2, T/4, 2T and 4T, where T is the serum titre, i.e. undiluted serum for the qualitative test).

Serum control: This is to verify the absence of a toxic effect of the sera on the cells. Wells containing 50 µl of each serum are incubated for 1 hour at 37°C in the presence of 50 µl of medium. Then, 150 µl of cell suspension is added in the same way as for the sera under test.

Negative serum control: This is done in the same way as for sera under test.

viii) *Reading the results:* An inverted-image microscope (×100) is used to examine the wells for toxic effects and CPEs after 48 and 72 hours. The controls must give the following results if the tests are to be considered valid:

Virus control: The titre of the viral suspension should be between 30 and 300 $TCID_{50}$/50 µl.

Cell control: The cell sheet must be intact.

Positive serum control: The titre obtained must be equal to the predicted titre, within one dilution.

Serum control: Examination for a CPE should take into account a possible toxic effect on cells.

Negative serum control: A CPE should be present.

ix) For the sera under test, the following results may be seen: presence of a CPE in three wells = negative result; absence of a CPE in three wells on day 3 = positive result; presence of a CPE in one well but not in the others = doubtful result, test must be repeated; small plaques indicating a CPE on day 3 = doubtful result, test must be repeated; toxicity in serum control and test wells = unreadable result, test must be repeated (NB replacement of medium with fresh medium after 16 hours' incubation will reduce the toxicity without affecting the titre of specific antibody).

x) *Interpretation of the results:* This test is capable of detecting the presence or absence of neutralising antibody to PRV. It is incapable of distinguishing vaccinated animals from infected animals.

The technique described (VN for 1 hour at 37°C) can give false-negative and false-positive results. The sensitivity can be increased (leading to fewer false negatives) by adopting a method based on neutralisation involving 24 hours of contact between virus and serum at 4°C, before the addition of cells.

A qualitative technique such as this one, which employs undiluted serum (1/2 final dilution), can give a false-positive result in certain cases due to nonspecific neutralisation of the virus. This problem can be addressed by carrying out a confirmatory test using the quantitative technique (see below).

- **Quantitative technique**

This is similar to the qualitative procedure, but each serum is used both undiluted and in a series of dilutions. Depending on the desired precision, the purpose of testing and the expected titre, one or more wells are used for each dilution of serum, and a greater or smaller range of dilutions. Ideally, the procedure may be described for a range of dilutions reaching an initial maximum of 1/256, with three wells for each dilution.

i) Complement in the serum samples is destroyed by heating in a water bath at 56°C for 30 minutes.

ii) 50 µl of MEM is added to wells A3 to A6 of a 96-well cell-culture grade microtitre plate.

iii) 50 µl of undiluted serum is added to wells A1 to A3, and continued for wells in rows B, C, etc., with other serum samples.

iv) Using a multichannel pipette, the contents of wells in row 3 are mixed, then 50 µl is transferred to row 4, and so on to row 6, using the same nozzles. The 50 µl portions remaining after row 6 are discarded.

v) 50 µl of MEM is added to row 1 instead of virus: this is a control row of sera. Viral suspension is deposited in the wells of the other rows. Subsequent manipulations are the same as described for the qualitative technique.

vi) *Reading the results:* The neutralising titre of a serum is expressed by the denominator of the highest initial dilution that brings about complete neutralisation of the CPE of the virus in 50% of the wells. Neutralisation at any dilution (even undiluted, equivalent to a final dilution of 1/2) is considered to be positive. If the serum shows neutralisation only when undiluted (with growth of virus and CPE at the 1/2 and subsequent dilutions), it would be advisable to apply alternative tests (ELISA or latex agglutination) to provide confirmation of the result, or to request another sampling of the animal, at least 8 days after the first.

b) Enzyme-linked immunosorbent assay (a prescribed test for international trade)

The sensitivity of the ELISA is generally superior to that of the VN test using 1-hour neutralisation without complement. Some weak positive sera are more readily detected by VN tests using 24-hour neutralisation, while others are more readily detectable by ELISA.

ELISA kits, which are available commercially, use indirect or competitive techniques for measuring antibody levels. They differ in their mode of preparation of antigen, conjugate, or substrate, in the period of incubation and in the interpretation of the results. Their general advantage is that they enable the rapid processing of large numbers of samples. This can also be automated and the results analysed by computer. Some of these kits make it possible to differentiate between vaccinated and naturally infected animals when used with a 'matching' vaccine (6, 20, 21). Alternatively, noncommercial ELISA protocols may be adopted (2, 17) provided they are shown to detect the OIE International Standard Reference Serum as positive at a dilution of 1/2 (the minimum sensitivity for international trade purposes). It is recommended to use a kit or in-house assay that has been validated to this standard by external quality control tests by an independent laboratory. A suitable test protocol for whole virus antibodies is presented below (17).

- **Preparation of antigen**

i) A cell line sensitive to PRV is used, such as PK-15 or fetal pig testis. It must be free from extraneous viruses, such as bovine viral diarrhoea virus. The cells should be split and seeded into fresh 75 cm^2 flasks the day before inoculation. A suitable medium such as MEM, without serum, is used to overlay the cultures.

ii) Virus inoculated, and control uninoculated flasks are processed in parallel throughout. A suitable well characterised strain of PRV is used, e.g. Kojnock strain. When a confluent cell monolayer has developed (approximately 24 hours after seeding), it is inoculated with 10^8 $TCID_{50}$ PRV in 5 ml medium; and 5 ml medium (without virus) is placed in control flasks. The cultures are left for adsorption for 30 minutes at 37°C, and then overlaid with 20 ml medium.

iii) When CPE is just beginning, the supernatant medium is discarded and 4 ml KCl (4 mM solution) and glass beads are added. The flasks are shaken gently to detach cells.

iv) Cells are washed by centrifuging three times at 770 ***g*** in 4 mM KCl. The pellet is resuspended in 4 mM KCl with 0.2% Triton X-100 (1 ml per flask) by applying 60 strokes with a glass homogeniser

v) The cell homogenate is layered on to 0.25 mM sucrose in 4 mM KCl and centrifuged for 10 minutes at 770 ***g***.

vi) The pellet is resuspended in antigen-diluting buffer, pH 9.6 (0.1 M Tris, 2 mM EDTA, 0.15 mM NaCl) at 1/50 the volume of the original culture medium. It may then be stored in small aliquots at –70°C. Antigen is stable in this form for 2 years.

- **Coating microtitre plates**

i) Virus antigen and control (no virus) antigen are diluted in diluting buffer, pH 9.6 (see above) to a dilution predetermined in chequerboard titrations.

ii) 200 µl of antigen is dispensed into each well of 96-well ELISA-grade plates, coating alternate rows with PRV positive and control antigen. Incubation is for 18 hours at 4°C.

iii) The plates are washed three times with washing solution (Tween 20, 0.5 ml/litre).

iv) Coated plates are stored at –20°C or –70°C. They are stable for several months.

- **Test procedure**

i) Test serum samples are diluted 1/30 in PBS/Tween buffer, pH 7.2 (137 mM NaCl, 9.5 mM phosphate buffer, 0.5 ml/litre Tween 20).

ii) Diluted samples are added to virus and control antigen coated wells, and incubated at 37°C for 30 minutes.

iii) The plates are washed three times with washing solution (0.5 ml/litre Tween 20).

iv) Protein A/peroxidase conjugate is added to all wells at a predetermined dilution in PBS/Tween buffer, pH 7.2 (see above), with added bovine serum albumen fraction V (10 g/litre), and the plates are incubated at 37°C for 30 minutes.

v) The plates are washed three times with washing solution (0.5 ml/litre Tween 20).

vi) A suitable chromogen/substrate mixture, such as tetra methyl benzidine (TMB)/hydrogen peroxide, is added to each plate.

vii) The reaction is stopped with 2 M sulphuric acid. The absorbance is read at 492 nm.

The test must be fully validated using known positive and negative sera, and calibrated against the OIE International Standard Reference Serum. All tests must include positive and negative internal controls, including a weak positive that, when diluted at the appropriate dilution for the test, has equivalent activity to a 1/2 dilution of the OIE International Standard Reference Serum. For further details see reference 17 and Chapter I.3. Principles of validation of diagnostic assays for infectious diseases. Commercial ELISA kits also have to be validated in the setting in which they are going to be used.

As well as testing sera, the ELISA can be adapted to test filter paper disks that have been moistened with a small quantity of blood obtained by puncturing a superficial vein. This technique makes it convenient to collect blood samples from large numbers of pigs (3, 18). The disks are air-dried before shipment to the laboratory.

Requirements for the detection of gE antibodies by ELISA in pigs that are to be introduced into zones free from Aujeszky's disease have been defined by several control authorities for slaughter. The OIE *International Animal Health Code* specifies[1] circumstances in which gE-specific tests may be used. The gE ELISAs can also be adapted to test blood on filter paper disks.

B. REQUIREMENTS FOR VACCINES AND DIAGNOSTIC BIOLOGICALS

Aujeszky's disease may be controlled by the use of vaccines containing either modified live or inactivated virus antigens. More recently, these conventional vaccines have been supplemented by recombinant DNA-derived gene-deleted or naturally deleted live PRV vaccines. These new vaccines, sometimes referred to as marker vaccines, are made with a virus that lacks a specific glycoprotein (most commonly gE-, although gG- or gC-deleted vaccines have also been described). At least one commercially available vaccine has dual deletions. These gene-deleted marker vaccines have the advantage over conventional whole virus vaccines that it is possible to distinguish noninfected vaccinated animals from those with field infection. This is done by testing for the antibodies directed against the protein coded for by the deleted gene, which will be absent in noninfected marker-vaccinated pigs but present in field-infected pigs. Therefore, in countries with infected pigs, where the eradication of Aujeszky's disease is planned, these marker vaccines are the vaccines of choice. Standards applicable to the manufacture of live and inactivated virus vaccines are described. For marker vaccines, the tests should include demonstrable absence of a serological response in vaccinated pigs to the protein coded for by the deleted gene, and in addition a demonstrable response to the same protein in vaccinated pigs that become infected by field virus.

1. Seed management

a) Characteristics of the seed

Vaccines are made using a seed-lot system in which a master seed virus (MSV) is prepared from a suitable strain of Aujeszky's disease virus. A number of strains are used for vaccine manufacture. The antigen in an

1 Subject to approval of a revised chapter in the *International Animal Health Code* by the OIE International Committee.

inactivated vaccine can be one of a number of wild-type strains, or the naturally deleted Bucharest virus, or rDNA-derived gene-deleted virus. Modified live conventional vaccines and rDNA-engineered vaccines use numerous strains, such as Bartha (8–10, 14, 16, 22, 26), or are derived from Aujeszky's original isolate or from other field isolates, such as the NIA-3 strain.

It is recommended that for differentiating between infected and vaccinated animals, deleted strains should be used.

A virus identity test (using either a fluorescent antibody test, neutralisation test, [constant serum/decreasing virus method], or any other suitable identity test) must be conducted on the MSV.

The MSV must be shown to be free from mycoplasma, bacteria, fungi, cytopathogenic or haemadsorbing viruses, porcine parvovirus, cytopathic and noncytopathic ovine and bovine pestiviruses and other extraneous agents, such as circovirus, as determined by culturing and by fluorescent antibody procedures or others, such as PCR.

b) Method of culture

Most of the cell lines used to propagate PRV are continuous lines, such as the PK-15 line. A master cell stock (MCS) is established at a specified passage level. The MCS and the highest passage level (MCS × n) intended for use in the preparation of a biological product is specified in an Outline of Production. Both MCS and MCS × n are monitored by a variety of procedures to characterise the cell line and to ensure freedom from adventitious agents. Porcine cells are tested for porcine cytomegalovirus, bovine viral diarrhoea/ classical swine fever virus, the rabies viruses, African swine fever, porcine influenza, porcine respiratory and reproductive syndrome, and vesicular stomatitis. This list may be modified if the country of origin of the cells is free from a certain infection.

The MCS must be monitored for species of origin. A minimum of 50 mitotic cells should be examined at both the MCS and MCS × n passage levels. The modal number in the MCS × n must not exceed 15% of the modal number of the MCS. Any marker chromosomes in the MCS must also be present in the highest cell passage.

If there is evidence that the cell line may induce malignancies in the species for which the product is intended, the cell line is tested for tumorgenicity and oncogenicity.

c) Validation as a vaccine

i) *Purity*

The MSV must be shown to be free from mycoplasma, bacteria, fungi, cytopathogenic or haemadsorbing viruses, porcine parvovirus, cytopathic and noncytopathic ovine and bovine pestiviruses and other extraneous agents, such as circovirus, as determined by culturing and by fluorescent antibody procedures or others, such as PCR.

ii) *Stability tests*

Tests have to be carried out to verify the shelf life proposed by the manufacturer. These tests must always be real-time studies; they must be carried out on a sufficient number of batches (at least three) produced according to the described production process and on products stored in the final container, and normally include biological and physicochemical stability tests. The manufacturer has to provide the results of analyses that support the proposed shelf life under all proposed storage conditions. Usually, the proposed shelf life corresponds to the period for which the product is considered to be stable minus 3 months.

iii) *Safety tests*

Local and general reactions must be examined. When a live vaccine is used, it is necessary to differentiate the exact safety properties of the vaccinal strain from those of the finished product if this includes an adjuvant.

In general, safety is tested initially under experimental conditions. When the results of these preliminary tests are known, it is necessary to increase the number of animals vaccinated in order to evaluate the safety of the vaccine under practical conditions.

- **Laboratory testing**

All tests must be carried out on pigs that do not have antibodies against Aujeszky's disease virus or against a fraction of the virus.

a. General effects

1. Live vaccines

Intranasal tests and vaccination of 3–5-day-old piglets are very useful for ascertaining the degree of safety of a strain. At least five piglets should be used.

It is also essential to assess the properties of a vaccine, especially live ones, in the target animals under normal conditions of use, e.g. fattening pigs, which are generally vaccinated when they are between 9 and 12 weeks old, and for pregnant sows when this use of the vaccine is claimed by the manufacturer and is authorised. No clinical signs, including significant thermal reactions, should be observed after vaccination. These assays have to be performed on at least ten vaccinated pigs, with unvaccinated pigs as controls.

Reversion to virulence following serial passage must be examined. Primary vaccination is done by the intranasal route. Series of at least five passages in piglets are made. If necessary, the organism is propagated *in vitro* between two *in-vivo* passages. No fewer than two fully susceptible animals must be used for each passage.

The object of these assays is to test the genetic stability of live vaccine strains. The tests appear to be less necessary when a genetically modified live strain is concerned, especially if it is processed by gene deletion.

It is recommended to test for possible excretion of the vaccine strain. For this purpose, no fewer than 14 piglets, 3–4 weeks old each receive one dose of vaccine by the recommended route and at the recommended site. Four unvaccinated piglets are kept as contact controls. Suitably sensitive tests for the virus are carried out individually on the nasal and oral secretions as follows: nasal and oral swabs are collected daily from 1 day before vaccination to 10 days after vaccination. Vaccine strains that are isolated from the nasal/oral secretion collected from pigs in which the vaccine was administered by the parenteral route are not recommended.

The ability of the PRV vaccine strain to spread from a vaccinated pig to unvaccinated ones (diffusibility) must be tested by using the recommended route of administration that presents the greatest risk of spreading. A repetition of the assays (four times) is necessary as this phenomenon is difficult to detect. Four piglets should be used each time for vaccination and placed in contact, 1 day later, with two unvaccinated piglets. It may also be necessary to examine the diffusibility of the strain to nontarget species that may be susceptible to the vaccinal strain.

Finally, most of the live attenuated vaccine strains are tested with regard to their general effects by administering to 5–10-day-old piglets ten times the field dose. This administration of an overdose makes it possible to detect reactions not produced under normal conditions of use. Such reactions may be produced inadvertently when large numbers of animals are vaccinated.

2. Inactivated vaccines

It is essential to test inactivated vaccines in the target animals under normal conditions of use for fattening pigs and for sows when this use is claimed by the manufacturer and authorised (25). As described previously, it is fundamental to use objective and quantifiable criteria to detect and to measure adverse reactions, such as temperature changes, weight performance, litter size, reproductive performance, etc., on vaccinated and control groups. The tests must be performed by administering the vaccine in the recommended dose and at each recommended route of administration to the pigs for which it is intended.

Pigs or sows are usually kept under observation and submitted to examinations until any reaction has disappeared. The period of observation must not be fewer than 14 days from the day of administration. This period has to be extended when, for example, the vaccine is used in pregnant sows and it is necessary to assess the possible effects of the vaccine on reproductive performance. In this case, the period of observation lasts the full duration of the pregnancy.

Control authorities generally request vaccination with a double dose so that adverse reactions, which may be at the limit of detection when a single dose is administered, are more likely to be detected.

b. Local reactions

Local reactions are often associated with the use of inactivated vaccines, as these side-effects can be induced by adjuvants, particularly oil adjuvants (23). However, some Aujeszky's disease live vaccines are mixed with different adjuvants, which modify what has been observed in the past.

Local reactions are mainly inflammatory and can be more or less complicated (necrotic or suppurative), depending on the nature of the adjuvants used and the aseptic conditions of the vaccination. Oil adjuvants can induce a variety of effects including muscular degeneration, granuloma, fibrosis and abscessation. In addition to the nature of the oil used (the intensity of the reaction is reduced when metabolisable oils are used in the vaccine), the type of emulsion used (water/oil,

oil/water, water/oil/water) induces these reactions to a greater or lesser extent. In consequence, it is necessary to observe the site of injection not only from the outside, but also by dissection after slaughter, especially for final product pigs.

- **Field testing**

All tests must be carried out on pigs that do not have antibodies against Aujeszky's disease virus or against a fraction of the virus, except that some tests may be done using maternally immune animals.

Field trials are necessary to assess the safety of an Aujeszky's disease vaccine in a large number of pigs or sows. In Europe (7), tests must be carried out in each category of animals for which the vaccine is intended (sows, fattening pigs). At least three groups of no fewer than 20 animals each are used with corresponding groups of no fewer than 10 controls. The rectal temperature of each animal is measured at the time of vaccination, and 24 and 48 hours later. At slaughter, the injection site must be examined for local reactions. If the vaccine is intended to be used in sows, reproductive performances have to be recorded. Field trials are supplemented by laboratory studies of efficacy correlated to vaccine potency.

iv) *Efficacy tests*

- **Laboratory trials**

All tests must be carried out on pigs that do not have antibodies against Aujeszky's disease virus or against a fraction of the virus, except that some tests may be done using maternally immune animals.

a. Assessment of passive immunity

To test the efficacy of vaccines, it is important to mimic the natural infection conditions (1). PRV infection gives rise to important losses of young piglets from nonimmune sows. Thus, when vaccinating sows, the main goal is to protect the young piglets through passive immunity conferred by the colostrum ingested immediately after birth, with the secondary objective of preventing abortion.

To measure this passive immunity and the protection induced by vaccinating the sows, experimental models have been established. The sows are vaccinated according to the vaccinal protocol during pregnancy. When the piglets are, for example, 6–10 days old they are given an intranasal challenge exposure with a virulent PRV strain. It is preferable to use a strain titrated in median lethal doses (LD_{50}). Pigs should be inoculated by the nasal route, 10^2 pig LD_{50} per pig in 1 ml. The efficacy of the vaccine is assessed by comparing clinical signs, but also and more importantly, mortality in piglets from unvaccinated dams with that observed in piglets from vaccinated sows.

Piglets from vaccinated sows can be found to have 80% protection against mortality compared with those from the control sows. In order for the results to be significant, it is recommended that eight vaccinated sows and four control sows be used (subject to satisfactory numbers of piglets from each sow).

b. Assessment of active immunity

1. Clinical protection

Several criteria can be considered when measuring active immunity induced by vaccinating pigs. Generally, pigs are vaccinated at the beginning of the growing period, i.e. when they are between 9 and 12 weeks old. Laboratory trials are performed by challenging pigs at the end of the finishing period, when they weigh between 80 and 90 kg.

In general, at least three criteria, such as rectal temperatures, weight losses and clinical signs, along with mortality, are used to measure the clinical protection of pigs after vaccination and challenge (5). The antibody titres have little predictive value for the efficacy of the vaccines. Weight loss compared between the vaccinated and control groups is certainly the most reproducible and reliable parameter when the challenge conditions are well standardised. The measure of the difference in weight gain or loss between the two groups of pigs and, in the interval of time between challenge (day 0 and day 7), has a very good predictive value for the efficacy of the vaccines (13). Significant results can be obtained when weight performances are compared between one group of at least eight vaccinated pigs and another group of eight unvaccinated control pigs

For challenge, it is usually preferable to use a high titre of a virulent strain, as this makes it possible to obtain a more marked difference between vaccinated and control pigs. On the basis of previous work, a challenge dose with at least 10^6 $TCID_{50}$/ml virulent strain having undergone not more that three passages on primary cells can be sufficient, but a higher titre ($10^{7.5}$ $TCID_{50}$/ml) is recommended. The oro-nasal route should be used to challenge the pigs by introducing the virulent strain in an appropriately high volume (≥4 ml).

This method of evaluating the efficacy of PRV vaccines is now well tested and has made it possible to establish an objective index for determining the efficacy of a vaccine. This index, which compares the relative weight losses between vaccinated and control pigs, can also be used for potency testing batches before release and for batch efficacy testing. However, the value of the cut-off index will be different as the conditions of the assay will not be identical. The influence of passively acquired, maternally derived antibodies on the efficacy of a vaccine must be evaluated adequately.

2. Virulent virus excretion

Additionally, it is desirable that vaccines should prevent or at least limit viral excretion from infected pigs (12, 19, 24). When a control programme against Aujeszky's disease is based on large-scale vaccination, it is essential to choose the vaccines or the vaccinal scheme that best limits the replication of virulent virus in infected pigs. Several assays have been performed to compare vaccines on that basis.

Generally, the pigs are vaccinated and challenged at different periods. It is better, but more time-consuming, to infect pigs at the end of the finishing period. To measure the virus excretion, nasal swabs (taken at 10 cm depth in the nostrils) are taken daily from each pig from the day before challenge to at least 12 days after challenge. The swabs can be weighed before the sampling and immediately after to calculate the exact weight of collected mucus. Medium is then added to each tube containing a swab. The virus is titrated from the frozen and thawed medium.

Different arbitrary indexes can be used to express the quantity of virulent virus excreted by pigs, taking into consideration the duration and the level of viral excretion, and the number of pigs excreting virulent virus.

3. Duration of immunity

It is recommended that any claims regarding the onset and duration of immunity should be supported by data from trials. Assessment of duration of immunity can be based on challenge trials or, as far as it is possible, on immunological and serological tests.

- **Field trials**

  In general terms, it is extremely difficult to assess vaccine efficacy in animal populations. In order to do this, it would be necessary to vaccinate the animals in the absence of the pathogen that the vaccine protects against, then to await the moment of infection and to compare the effects of infection in vaccinated animals (or the offspring of vaccinated dams) with the effects in the unvaccinated animals of the same age, in the same building and in the same batch as the vaccinated animals (or those protected passively). As all these conditions are difficult to achieve in the field, field trials are certainly more appropriate to safety testing than to efficacy testing.

2. Method of manufacture

Only MSV that has been established as pure, safe and immunogenic may be used as seed for a vaccine product. Cells from the MCS are propagated in a variety of growth media. All batches of vaccine must be from the first to the twentieth passage of MCS.

3. In-process control

It is necessary to carry out tests at each critical step of the manufacturing process. The control tests are also carried out on intermediate products with a view to verifying the consistency of the production process and the final product.

4. Batch control

It is essential to differentiate the tests that are carried out on a routine basis to release batches of final product from those that are performed to define the biological properties of a vaccine. The trials carried out for batch release are not the same as the ones carried out once only to determine the safety and efficacy of a vaccine. The batch release controls are always short-term trials, as inexpensive as possible, and not always carried out in pigs. Their purpose is mainly to attest to the reproducibility of the quality of the finished product, which has to conform with the quality initially defined in the application for marketing authorisation.

a) Sterility and purity tests

Tests must be carried out for sterility and freedom from contamination (see Chapter I.4.)

Each batch of PRV vaccines must be tested for freedom from extraneous viruses. Using a minimum amount of a monospecific antiserum, the live vaccinal strain is neutralised and inoculated into cell cultures known to be sensitive to viruses pathogenic for pigs. No CPE and no haemadsorbing agents should be detected. The vaccines have to be free from pestiviruses.

b) Inactivation

For inactivated vaccines, inactivation must be checked using two passages in the same type of cell culture as used in the production of the vaccine. Tests can be carried out by vaccinating susceptible animals such as rabbits.

c) Identity

Where necessary, a specific test for virus identification should be carried out.

d) Safety

Safety of live vaccines is tested by administering ten doses of the reconstituted vaccine by the route stated on the leaflet to each of at least two piglets of the minimum age recommended for vaccination that are free from PRV antibodies. Two piglets of the same origin and age are kept as controls. No abnormal local or systemic reaction should occur. The weight curve of the vaccinated piglets must not differ significantly from that of the controls.

For inactivated vaccines, safety is tested by injecting two doses into piglets under the same conditions as described previously.

e) Potency

The potency of the vaccine must be demonstrated using a suitable method, the results of which have to be correlated with the efficacy tests described previously.

In this kind of test, the most difficult point is to determine an acceptability threshold for using or rejecting the batch according to the results that are obtained.

Virus content tests should be carried out using each of at least three containers. The virus titre of the vaccine must be determined and must normally not be higher than 1/10 of the dose at which the vaccine has been shown to be safe, and not lower than the minimum release titre.

f) Preservatives

If no preservative is included in the final product, the manufacturer must demonstrate that the product remains acceptable for its recommended period of use after opening the vial.

The efficacy of preservatives in multidose containers must be demonstrated. The concentration of the preservative in the final filled vaccine and its persistence throughout shelf life must be checked.

g) Precautions (hazards)

All information about possible adverse reactions induced by the vaccine must be indicated. Any putative risk for human health if the user is accidentally given a small quantity of the product has to be indicated. The manufacturer should indicate all the conditions of use of the vaccine: mixing, reconstitution, storage, asepsis, length of needle, route of administration, health status of the vaccinated animals, etc.

5. Tests on the final product

a) Safety

Every batch of vaccine must be tested for safety, as described in Section B.4.d.

b) Potency

Every batch of vaccine must be tested for potency, as described in Section B.4.e.

REFERENCES

1. ANDRIES K., PENSAERT M. B. & VANDEPUTTE J. (1978). Effect of experimental infection with pseudorabies (Aujeszky's disease) virus on pigs with maternal immunity from vaccinated sows. *Am. J. Vet. Res.*, **39**, 1282–1285.

2. BANKS M. (1983). Rapid ELISA for Aujeszky's disease eradication. *Vet. Rec.*, **113**, 94–95.

3. BANKS M. (1985). Detection of antibodies to Aujeszky's disease virus in whole blood by ELISA-disc. *J. Virol. Methods*, **12**, 41–45.

4. BITSCH V. & EKILDSEN M. (1982). Complement-dependent neutralization of Aujeszky's disease virus by antibody. *In:* Current Topics in Veterinary Medicine and Animal Science 17. Aujeszky's Disease, Wittmann G. & Hall S.A., eds. Martinus Nijhoff, The Hague, The Netherlands, 41.

5. DE LEEUW P.W. & VAN OIRSCHOT J.T. (1985). Vaccines against Aujeszky's disease: evaluation of their efficacy under standardized laboratory conditions. *Vet. Q.*, **7**, 780–786.

6. ELOIT M., FARGEAUD D., VANNIER P. & TOMA B. (1989). Development of an ELISA to differentiate between animals either vaccinated with or infected by Aujeszky's disease virus. *Vet. Rec.*, **124**, 91–94.

7. EUROPEAN PHARMACOPOEIA, THIRD EDITION (1997). Monograph 0744: Vaccinum morbi Aujeszky ad suem inactivatum (inactivated Aujeszky's disease vaccine for pigs). Monograph 0745: Vaccinum morbi Aujeszky ad suem vivum cryodesiccatum ad usum parenterale (Freeze-dried Aujeszky disease live vaccine for pigs for parenteral administration). Council of Europe, Strasbourg, France.

8. KIT S. (1988). Safety and efficacy of genetically engineered Aujeszky's disease vaccines. *In:* Vaccination and Control of Aujeszky's Disease, Van Oirschot J.T., ed. Kluwer Academic Publishers, The Netherlands, 45–55.

9. MARCHIOLI C.C., YANCEY R.J., WARDLEY R.C., THOMSEN D.R. & POST L.E. (1987). A vaccine strain of pseudorabies virus with deletions in the thymidine kinase and glycoprotein genes. *Am. J. Vet. Res.*, **48**, 1577–1583.

10. MCFERRAN J.B. & DOW C. (1975). Studies on immunisation of pigs with the Bartha strain of Aujeszky's disease virus. *Res. Vet. Sci.*, **19**, 17–22.

11. MOENNING V., WOLDESENBERT P., FEY H.R., LIESS B., DOPOTKA H.D. & BEHRENS F. (1982). Comparative evaluation of ELISA and neutralization test for the diagnosis of Aujeszky's disease. *In:* Current Topics in Veterinary Medicine and Animal Science 17. Aujeszky's Disease, Wittmann G. & Hall S.A., eds. Martinus Nijhoff, The Hague, The Netherlands, 51.

12. PENSAERT M.B., DE SMET K. & DE WAELE K. (1990). Extent and duration of virulent virus excretion upon challenge of pigs vaccinated with different glycoprotein-deleted Aujeszky's disease vaccines. *Vet. Microbiol.*, **22**, 107–117.

13. STELLMANN C., VANNIER P., CHAPPUIS G., BRUN A., DAUVERGNE M., FARGEAUD D., BUGAUD M. & COLSON X. (1989). The potency testing of pseudorabies vaccines in pigs. A proposal for a quantitative criterion and a minimum requirement. *J. Biol. Stand.*, **17**, 17–27.

14. TOMA B. (1979). Obtention et caracterisation d'une souche thermosensible de virus de la maladie d'Aujeszky (souche ALFORT 26). *Rec. Med. Vet.*, **155**, 131–137.

15. TOMA B. (1982). Serological diagnosis of Aujeszky's disease using enzyme-linked immunosorbent assay (ELISA). *In:* Current Topics in Veterinary Medicine and Animal Science 17. Aujesky's Disease, Wittmann G. & Hall S.A., eds. Martinus Nijhoff, The Hague, The Netherlands, 65.

16. TOMA B., BRUN, A., CHAPPUIS G. & TERRE J. (1979). Propriétés biologiques d'une souche thermosensible (ALFORT 26) de virus de la maladie d'Aujeszky. *Rec. Med. Vet.*, **155**, 245–252.

17. TOMA B. & ELOIT M. (1986). Pseudorabies virus antibodies (Aujeszky's disease). *In:* Methods of Enzymatic Analysis X, Antigens and Antibodies 1, Bergmeyer V.C.H., ed. D-6940 Weinheim, Germany.

18. TOMA B., ELOIT M. & TILMANT P. (1986). Sérodiagnostic de la maladie d'Aujeszky: utilisation de prélèvements de sang sur papier filtre. *Rec. Med. Vet.*, **162**, 1111–1117.

19. VAN OIRSCHOT J.T. & GIELKENS A.L.J. (1984). Intranasal vaccination of pigs against pseudorabies: absence of vaccinal virus latency and failure to prevent latency of virulent virus. *Am. J. Vet. Res.*, **45**, 2099–2103.

20. VAN OIRSCHOT J.T. & OEI H.L. (1989). Comparison of two ELISAs for detecting antibodies to glycoprotein I of Aujeszky's disease virus. *Vet. Rec.*, **125**, 63–64.

21. VAN OIRSCHOT J.T., RZIHA M.J., MOONEN, P.J.L.M., POL J.M. & VAN ZAANE D. (1986). Differentiation of serum antibodies from pigs vaccinated or infected with Aujeszky's disease virus by a competitive immunoassay. *J. Gen. Virol.*, **67**, 1179–1182.

22. VAN OIRSCHOT J.T., TERPSTRA C., MOORMANN R.J.M., BERNS A.J.M. & GIELKENS A.L.J. (1990). Safety of an Aujeszky's disease vaccine based on deletion mutant strain 783 which does not express thymidine kinase and glycoprotein I. *Vet. Rec.*, **127**, 443–446.

23. VANNIER P. (1986). Immunisation de porcs charcutiers contre la maladie d'Aujeszky avec deux vaccins à adjuvants huileux. Etude des réactions locales. *Rec. Med. Vet.*, **162**, 37–44.

24. VANNIER P., HUTET E., BOURGUEIL E. & CARIOLET R. (1991). Level of virulent virus excreted by infected pigs previously vaccinated with different glycoprotein deleted Aujeszky's disease vaccines. *Vet. Microbiol.*, **29**, 213–223.

25. VANNIER P., TILLON J.P., TOMA B., DELAGNEAU J.F., LOQUERIE R. & PRUNET P. (1976). Protection conférée au porc par un nouveau vaccin huileux à virus inactivé contre la maladie d'Aujeszky. Conséquences pratiques. *J. Rech. Porc Fr.*, 281–290.

26. VISSER N. & LUTTICKEN D. (1988). Experiences with a gI-/TK-modified live pseudorabies virus vaccine: strain Begonia. *In:* Vaccination and Control of Aujeszky's Disease, Van Oirschot J.T., ed. Kluwer Academic Publishers, The Netherlands, 37–44.

27. WITTMANN G. & LEITZKE I.I. (1985). Die Beeinflussung des Aujeszkyvirus-neutralizationstests durch verschiedene Testbedingungen. *Dtsch. Tierarztl. Wochenschr.*, **92**, 262–266.

*

* *

CHAPTER 2.2.3.

ECHINOCOCCOSIS/HYDATIDOSIS

SUMMARY

Diagnosis of echinococcosis in dogs or other susceptible carnivores depends on the demonstration of adult cestodes of the Echinococcus *genus in their faeces or small intestine. In intermediate hosts, this depends on detection of the larval cyst form that can infect almost any organ, particularly the liver and lungs.*

Identification of the agent: *At present, four species of the genus* Echinococcus *are regarded as taxonomically valid. These are* E. granulosus, E. multilocularis, E. oligarthrus *and* E. vogeli. *The latter two species are rare infections. These four species are morphologically distinct in both adult and larval stages. Also, a number of inter- and intraspecific variants have been described especially for* E. granulosus, *but can only be differentiated reliably on the basis of DNA analysis.*

Larval forms of Echinococcus *can usually be visually detected in organs. Special care has to be taken for a specific diagnosis of echinococcosis in instances where* Taenia hydatigena *in sheep is also a problem. Histological examination may confirm the diagnosis after formalin-fixed material is processed by conventional staining methods. The presence of a periodic-acid-Schiff positive, acellular laminated layer with or without an internal cellular, nucleated germinal membrane can be regarded as a specific characteristic of metacestodes of* Echinococcus.

The small intestine is required at necropsy for the collection of adult Echinococcus *spp. in wildlife or in domestic dogs. The technique of carrying out surveys with the use of arecoline has been generally adopted for determining the prevalence of* Echinococcus *spp. in dogs. Handling infected material presents a risk to the operator of contracting a potentially fatal disease. Significant progress is being made in the development of immunological tests for adult infections by use of coproantigen detection.*

Progress has been made in the detection of E. multilocularis *in definitive hosts using polymerase chain reaction/DNA methods, but not yet in the detection of* E. granulosus.

Serological tests: *Oncosphere, cyst fluid and protoscolex antibodies can be detected in the serum of infected dogs and sheep, but this has not yet reached a practical stage as it does not distinguish between current and previous infections. Cross-reactivity between* Echinococcus *and* Taenia *species also may occur.*

Requirements for vaccines and diagnostic biologicals: *Excellent progress is being made in the development of a vaccine for the larval, but not the adult stage of* E. granulosus.

A. DIAGNOSTIC TECHNIQUES

At present, four species of the genus *Echinococcus* are accepted taxonomically, namely *E. granulosus, E. multilocularis, E. oligarthrus,* and *E. vogeli.* The latter two species are confined to Central and South America. These are morphologically distinct both in their adult and larval stages. A number of interspecific and intraspecific variants have been described. Only the four species described above are accepted taxonomically although genotypes of *E. granulosus* are now considered. Further studies are needed to define the full range of genetic diversity (11, 13, 14, 17).

- ***Echinococcus granulosus***

The parasite is transmitted between the domestic dog and a number of domestic ungulate species. The dog/sheep cycle is most important. Sylvatic definitive and intermediate hosts may also occur, e.g. wolf/cervid.

The adult varies between 2 and 7 mm in length and usually possesses from three to four segments, rarely up to six. The penultimate segment is mature, and the genital pore normally opens posterior to the middle in both mature and gravid segments. The last (gravid) segment is usually more than half the length of the entire worm. There are rostellar hooks on the protoscolex in two rows. The size of the hooks varies between 22 and 45 µm in the first row, and between 18 and 38 µm in the second row. The gravid uterus has well-developed sacculations.

The larval stage is a fluid-filled bladder or hydatid cyst that is unilocular, although communicating chambers also occur. Growth is expansive, and endogenous daughter cysts may be produced. Individual bladders may reach up to 30 cm in diameter and occur most frequently in liver and lungs, but may develop in other internal organs. It is referred to as cystic echinococcosis.

The strain specificities of *E. granulosus* in domestic cycles include, dog/sheep in the Mediterranean region, South America (Argentina, Brazil, Chile, Peru and Uruguay), Africa (Ethiopia, Kenya and Sudan), the Middle East and Levant regions, Russia, Central Asia (Kazakhstan, Kyrgyzstan and Uzbekistan), Mongolia, the People's Republic of China and Oceania; dog/horse in Belgium, Ireland, Italy, Switzerland and the United Kingdom; dog/cattle in Belgium, Germany, South Africa and Switzerland; dog/swine in Poland; and dog/reindeer in subarctic regions of Norway, Sweden and Alaska. The status of dog/camel strains requires further elucidation.

- ***Echinococcus multilocularis***

The parasite is transmitted between wild definitive hosts (e.g. *Vulpes vulpes, Alopex lagopus, Canis latrans*) and small arvicolid rodents (voles and lemmings). Domestic dogs and cats are susceptible, although cats less so than dogs. The adult varies between 1.2 and 3.7 mm in length and usually possesses from four to five segments. The penultimate segment is characteristically mature, and the genital pore is anterior to the midline in both mature and gravid segments. The gravid uterus is sac-like. On the rostellum, there are hooks that vary in size between 27.6 and 34.3 µm (large) and between 22.7 and 31.0 µm (small).

The metacestode is a multivesicular structure consisting of conglomerates of small vesicles, usually not exceeding a few millimetres in diameter. Unlike *E. granulosus*, the larval mass often contains a semisolid rather than a fluid matrix. It proliferates by exogenous budding, and this results in infiltration of tissues. It is commonly referred to as alveolar echinococcosis. Evidence for strains or genotypes of *E. multilocularis* is much less defined than for *E. granulosus.*

- ***Echinococcus oligarthrus***

The parasite typically uses wild felids as definitive hosts (e.g. *Felis concolor, F. jaguarundi*) and large rodents (e.g. *Dasyprocta* sp., *Cuniculus paca*) as intermediate hosts. The adult varies between 1.9 and 2.9 mm in length, and normally possesses three segments, the penultimate of which is mature. The genital pore is anterior to the middle in mature segments and approximately at the middle in gravid segments. The gravid uterus is sac-like.

The metacestode is polycystic and fluid-filled with a tendency to become septate and multichambered. The rostellar hooks of the protoscolex vary in length between 25.9 and 27.9 µm. The single cyst may reach a diameter of approximately 5 cm. Preferred sites are internal organs and muscles. To date, only three reports of human disease are on record. The parasite appears not to mature in dogs.

- ***Echinococcus vogeli***

The parasite typically uses the bush dog *(Speothus venaticus)* as a wild definitive host, but the domestic dog is susceptible, as are large rodents (e.g. *Cuniculus paca*) as intermediate hosts. The adult varies between 3.9 and 5.6 mm in length, and usually has three segments, the penultimate of which is mature. The genital pore is situated posterior to the middle in both the mature and gravid segments. The gravid uterus has no lateral sacculations and is characterised by being relatively long and tubular in form, compared with the other segments, which are sac-like.

The metacestode is similar to that of *E. oligarthrus*. It has been reported that the two species can be distinguished by comparing differences in the dimensions and proportions of the rostellar hooks on the protoscolex. The hooks of *E. oligarthrus* vary in length between 25.9 and 37.9 µm (average 33.4 µm) and between 22.6 and 29.5 µm (average 25.45 µm) for large and small hooks, respectively. Those of *E. vogeli* vary between 19.1 and 43.9 µm (average 41.64 µm) and between 30.4 and 36.5 µm (average 33.6 µm) for the large and small hooks, respectively. Also the hook-guard for *E. oligarthrus* divides the hook 50:50, compared with 30:70 for *E. vogeli.*

E. vogeli is a zoonosis with >40 human cases on record; most infections probably occur from a domestic dog. It appears not to mature in cats. It is commonly referred to as polycystic echinococcosis.

1. Identification of the agent

In the intermediate host, diagnosis depends on the detection of the larval cyst form, which can occur in almost any organ, but particularly in the liver and lungs. The diagnosis of echinococcosis in dogs or other carnivores requires the demonstration of the cestodes of *Echinococcus* spp. in their faeces or the small intestine.

a) Diagnosis of larval echinococcosis

- **Necropsy**

Whereas diagnosis of *E. granulosus* in domestic animals may take place in licensed slaughter houses, that for *Echinococcus* sp. in wildlife must be done by field surveys. Specimens should be preserved by removal of tissue and fixation in 4–10% formol saline or kept cool and deep-frozen for subsequent examination.

Larvae can be observed in many organs, but in large animals, such as sheep and cattle, palpation or incision should be done. Pigs, sheep and goats may be infected with *Taenia hydatigena*, and it is sometimes difficult to differentiate between these two parasites when they occur in the liver. *Ascaris suum* has also been implicated as a cause of 'white spot' in sheep livers. In wild animals, such as ruminants and rodents, several other larval cestodes should be considered for differential diagnosis.

Formalin-fixed material can be stained by conventional histological techniques. The presence of a periodic-acid-Schiff (PAS) positive acellular laminated layer with or without an internal cellular, nucleated germinal membrane can be regarded as a specific characteristic of the metacestodes of *Echinococcus*. The presence of protoscoleces within brood-capsules or in hydatid sand is also diagnostic for the genus. Genotyping of *E. granulosus* is usually done on DNA derived from protoscoleces preserved in 90% ethanol.

b) Diagnosis of adult parasites in carnivores

- **Necropsy**

Necropsy is invariably employed in studies of echinococcosis in wildlife and is useful if domestic dogs are humanely culled. It should be emphasised that it is necessary to isolate and identify the adult *Echinococcus*, because under normal conditions of faecal examination, the eggs of *Echinococcus* cannot be differentiated from those of *Taenia* spp.

The small intestine is removed as soon as possible after death, and tied at both ends. If the material is not frozen or formalin fixed (4–10%), it should be examined quickly, as the parasite can be digested within 24 hours. Formalin does not kill eggs. The fresh intestine is divided into several sections and immersed in saline at 37°C for examination. Worms adhering to the intestinal wall may be observed and counted by means of a hand lens (for *E. granulosus* and *E. vogeli*). For accurate counts, the unfixed intestine is best divided into four or six sections, opened up and immersed in saline at 37°C for 30 minutes to release the parasites. The contents are washed into another container for detailed examination, and the intestinal wall is scraped with a spatula. All material is boiled and washed by sieving to eliminate most of the particulate material. The washed intestinal contents and scrapings are placed on a black tray, and the worms are counted with the aid of a hand lens or stereoscopic microscope. *Echinococcus granulosus* is usually found in the first third of the small intestine of dogs.

- **Mucosal scrapings**

For necropsy of foxes (or dogs) for *E. multilocularis* carcasses or intestines should be deep frozen at –70°C to –80°C for 3–7 days before necropsy. Eggs of *E. multilocularis* are resistant to freezing down to –50°C. Deep mucosal scrapings should be made using microscope slides and adherent material transferred to a square plastic Petri dish. Scrapings are squashed between slides and examined under a stereoscopic light microscope (×120). Five mucosal scrapings from proximal, middle and posterior thirds of the small intestine (total 15) are recommended. *Echinococcus multilocularis* is usually found in the second half of the small intestine.

- **Preserving specimens**

Intact worms are fragile and for morphological studies are best handled in normal saline with a Pasteur pipette. They are washed free of other material and left for approximately 30 minutes for all movement to cease. After removal of the fluid, cold 5–10% formalin (5°C) or FAA fixative (95% ethanol [80 ml], 37–40% formaldehyde [10 ml], and glacial acetic acid [5 ml]) is added and the worms are left for a further 12 hours. For staining, the worms are washed in water for 15 minutes and transferred to Mayer's paracarmine (carminic acid [1.0 g], aluminium chloride [0.5 g], calcium chloride [4.0 g], and 70% ethanol [100 ml]) for 12–24 hours. Excess stain is removed by immersion in 0.5–1.0% hydrochloric acid solution for a few seconds. Dehydration is accomplished by serial passage in ascending concentrations of alcohol (35, 50, 70, 85, 95, 100%) for at least 15 minutes in each, with two changes in 100%. The alcohol is removed by xylol (10 minutes) and cleared with methyl salicylate or creosote. Prior to mounting in any suitable medium such as balsam, picolyte, etc., the specimens should be returned to the xylol for few minutes.

Investigators carrying out these procedures are exposed to risk of infection and severe disease, which must be minimised by appropriate procedures. Infective material can be decontaminated by freezing at –80°C (core temperature) for 48 hours, or –70°C for 4 days. Face masks, disposable gloves and an apron must be worn. Chemical disinfection is not reliable, although sodium hypochlorite may destroy a proportion of eggs (3). Contaminated material must be destroyed by heat. The decontamination of laboratories can be achieved at reduced humidity (40%) combined with increased room temperature (30°C) for at least 48 hours.

Recently, some methods have been developed with the aim of simplifying and improving epidemiological investigations in final host populations and of allowing diagnosis in living animals. These methods include the detection of coproantigens and polymerase chain reaction (PCR) DNA detection (see below).

c) Arecoline surveys and surveillance

Arecoline is used to perform surveys of tapeworm infections in dog populations. Its use as a control agent has now been superseded by praziquantel. Arecoline is a parasympathomimetic agent. Its action results in sweating, and stimulation of salivary, lachrymal, gastric, pancreatic, and intestinal glands. It increases intestinal tonus and the mobility of smooth muscle, and this effect is responsible for purgation. The liver is the principal site of detoxification. Arecoline also has a direct action on the worm itself, by causing paralysis, but not death, and thereby making it relax its hold on the intestinal wall. Thus, it must be administered by the oral route. The accompanying purgation carries the worms out with the faeces. It is particularly suitable for baseline surveys of *E. granulosus,* however, 15–25% of dogs may not purge. The accepted dose rates for tablets each containing 25 mg arecoline hydrobromide are: 1 tablet per 14 kg body weight (minimum); 1 tablet per 7 kg body weight (maximum); 1 tablet per 10 kg body weight (optimum). Pregnant bitches and animals with cardiac abnormalities should not be treated with arecoline. As some dogs resist purgation, the additional use of arecoline hydrobromide as an enema has been recommended, but the worms may not be paralysed by this procedure and it may thus lead to false-negative interpretations. Such dogs should be dosed again after a rest of 3–4 days.

Dogs that are purged successfully may produce at least two motions; the first will be formed faeces and can be ignored, but the mucus that follows may be productive. This can be divided into several samples and each examined separately, but this method is not recommended as the worms will be difficult to detect. Preferably, the mucus sample (about 4 ml) is diluted with 100 ml of tap water, covered with a thin layer of 1 ml of kerosene (paraffin) and boiled for 5 minutes. The kerosene prevents foaming and reduces the smell.

Investigators carrying out these procedures are exposed to risk of infection and severe disease. Personnel should wear whole body coveralls, boots, disposable gloves and face mask. Coveralls should be boil washed after use, and boots disinfected in 10% sodium hypochlorite solution. The purge should be boiled as soon as possible after collection. Dogs may continue to pass eggs, proglottides and worms after first purge, therefore, they should remain tethered for 2 hours after purgation and given access to drinking water. After arecoline testing, the area of ground used to tether dogs should be sprayed with kerosene and flamed.

d) Coproantigen tests

An alternative to arecoline testing, based on a faecal antigen-detection antibody sandwich enzyme-linked immunosorbent assay (ELISA), has been developed recently and has shown particular promise as coproantigens can be detected shortly after infection (10–14 days) and the level declines rapidly following expulsion of the worms. The sensitivity and specificity of the test has been estimated at 70% and 98%, respectively (1, 3, 7, 8).

Both qualitative and quantitative results can be obtained from arecoline testing, which is most useful for base-line epidemiological studies on the comparative rates of infection with Taeniidae in dogs. Further studies may show that the coproantigen test may be more cost-effective than arecoline testing during routine surveillance of *E. granulosus* in the dog population. The practical role to be played by this technology in the surveillance of *E. multilocularis* in foxes in comparison with necropsy has yet to be determined (6).

Specific coproantigen ELISAs[1] have now been developed and have sufficient specificity and sensitivity to consider replacement of arecoline testing for *Echinococcus* detection in dogs and other definitive hosts (3). Specificity of detection of genus-specific *Echinococcus* coproantigens is around 98%, and overall sensitivity approximately 70%; however, when mean worm burdens are >50–100, sensitivity approaches 100% (1, 3, 4, 8). Dogs, dingoes, foxes and wolves have been screened successfully by coproantigen ELISAs and, importantly, *E. multilocularis* worm infections are also detectable in red foxes and domestic dogs (8, 15). When the capture ELISA uses either anti-ES or anti-somatic proglottis antibodies to *E. granulosus*, the sensitivity for *E. multilocularis* infection may be reduced, though genus specificity remains intact. Polyclonal- or monoclonal-antibody-based coproantigen ELISAs, developed for *E. multilocularis* rather than primarily for *E. granulosus* infection, exhibited higher sensitivity and specificity, even against *E. granulosus* infections (~80%) (6, 15). However, for low worm burdens (<50) sensitivity of *E. multilocularis* coproantigen ELISA is below that of the mucosal smear method at necropsy (6).

The exact nature of *Echinococcus* antigens released in faeces for coproantigen detection have not been characterised. However, their stability in 5% formal saline after boiling and susceptibility to periodate treatment suggest involvement of carbohydrate antigen(s) (3).

Coproantigens can be detected prior to release of eggs by *Echinococcus* worms, and therefore are not related to egg antigen(s) (8, 15). This has the advantage of detection of prepatent infections. Furthermore, coproantigen levels return to the preinfection baseline within 5 days of anthelminthic treatment of infected dogs (8).

For detection of *E. multilocularis* infection of foxes, necropsy is time-consuming. Coproantigen testing by ELISA offers a specific practical alternative. Fox faecal samples should be taken at post-mortem from the rectum rather than from the intestinal tract. *Echinococcus* coproantigens are also stable in fox or dog faeces left at 20°C for 1 week.

- **Coproantigen test procedure *(Echinococcus granulosus)* (1, 4)**

i) The faecal sample is mixed with an equal volume of phosphate buffered saline (PBS), pH 7.2, containing 0.3% Tween 20 (PBST), in a capped 5 ml disposable tube. This is shaken vigorously and centrifuged at 2000 *g* for 20 minutes at room temperature. Faecal supernatants can be tested immediately or stored at –20°C or lower. Supernatants that appear very dark or viscous are still acceptable for use.

ii) A 96-well ELISA microtitre plate (Immulon #4, Dynex Technologies) is coated with optimal concentration (typically 5 µg per ml) of a protein A purified IgG fraction of rabbit anti-*E. granulosus* proglottis extract (1) in 0.05 M bicarbonate/carbonate buffer, pH 9.6 (100 µl per well). The plate is covered and incubated overnight at 4°C.

iii) The wells are rinsed three times in PBST with 1 minute between washes; 100 µl of the same buffer is added to each well, and the plate is incubated for 1 hour at room temperature.

iv) The PBST is discarded and 50 µl per well of faecal sample supernatants is added (in duplicate wells) to 50 µl of neat fetal calf serum. The plate is incubated at room temperature for 1 hour with clingfilm seal covering the plate.

v) The wells are rinsed as in step iii, but the contents are discarded into a 10% bleach (hypochlorite) solution.

vi) An optimal dilution of an IgG rabbit anti-*E.-granulosus* proglottis extract peroxidase conjugate (1) in PBST is prepared and 100 µl per well is added to all wells. The plate is incubated for 1 hour at room temperature.

vii) The wells are rinsed as in step iii.

viii) Next, 100 µl per well of tetramethyl benzidene substrate (TMB, KPL Labs) is added and the plate is left in the dark for 20 minutes at room temperature.

ix) The enzyme-substrate reaction is stopped by adding 100 µl of 1 M phosphoric acid (H_3PO_4) to each well. The colour turns from blue to yellow if positive. Absorbance of wells is read at 450 nm.

x) Laboratories should establish their own end-point criteria using standard positive and negative samples. Standards can also be obtained from the OIE Reference Laboratories (see Table given in Part 4 of this *Manual*). Usually, the positive to negative threshold is taken as 3 standard deviations above the mean absorbance value of control negatives, or against a reference standard control positive using absorbance units equivalence.

---

1 *Echinococcus* coproantigen ELISA is available commercially as a kit from: Genzyme Virotech GmbH, Lowenplatz 5, 65428 Russelsheim, Germany; and Dr Brommeli AG, Liebefeld-Berne, Switzerland.

e) DNA recognition methods

Definitive hosts: Differential diagnosis of *E. granulosus* and *E. multilocularis* infections in definitive hosts may be achieved by specific detection of PCR-amplified DNA from *E. multilocularis* eggs present in faeces (2, 12). Primers from the Ulsn RNA gene of *E. multilocularis* are species specific, exhibiting 100% specificity following zinc chloride flotation purification of eggs from faeces, and gave a sensitivity of 94% for *E. multilocularis* infection in red foxes (12). In practice, it is recommended to screen definitive hosts (e.g. foxes) using the coproantigen test and confirm with the PCR DNA test. In Europe, transmission of *E. multilocularis* generally occurs in regions where *E. granulosus* is not endemic or appears very infrequently. In other regions including parts of the Near East (Turkey and Iran), Central Asia, Russia and the People's Republic of China, these two species may occur together (5). Further evaluation of *E. multilocularis* infection is required to investigate intermittent shedding and duration of shedding of parasite DNA. There is currently no PCR DNA test for *E. granulosus.*

Intermediate hosts: DNA hybridisation methods are not currently used for the detection of *E. granulosus* in livestock intermediate hosts. These methods are, however, important in identification of isolates or strains of *E. granulosus* for epidemiological purposes (13).

For small lesions of *E. multilocularis* in wild or aberrant domestic intermediate hosts, DNA hybridisation techniques may be useful (10).

2. Serological tests

a) Intermediate hosts

Immunological tests, useful in humans, are less sensitive and specific in livestock and at present cannot replace necropsy (3, 10).

b) Definitive hosts

An extensive programme has been initiated to develop immunodiagnostic tests for use against canine echinococcosis. Following ingestion of a cyst, dogs will be exposed at the intestinal level to various antigens during the establishment of the parasite and its development and oogenesis. Oncosphere and protoscolex antibodies can be readily detected in the serum of infected dogs. This has not reached a practical stage as it does not differentiate between current and previous infections.

B. REQUIREMENTS FOR VACCINES AND DIAGNOSTIC BIOLOGICALS

1. Intermediate hosts

A vaccine, based on a single polypeptide antigen derived from oncospheres and produced in *Escherichia coli* using recombinant DNA technology has been successfully developed for use against *T. ovis* in sheep. This technology has now been successfully applied to *E. granulosus* (9).

Phase I trials using the recombinant oncosphere antigen vaccine EG95 gave 96–98% protection against experimental challenge of sheep with *E. granulosus.* Protection may last up to 12 months and can be transferred to lambs via colostrum. Phase II trials with natural challenge of vaccinated lambs resulted in similar levels of protection. EG95 vaccine for *E. granulosus* can now be mass produced and has the potential to significantly reduce the time for the attack phase of hydatid control programmes. The vaccine for ovine hydatidosis would be used in parallel with dog-dosing measures and health education programmes.

2. Definitive hosts

While considerable research has been undertaken with crude antigens to protect dogs from echinococcosis, no real success has been demonstrated so far. Basic research on canine mucosal immunology and *Echinococcus* infection is required for progress.

REFERENCES

1. ALLAN J.C., CRAIG P.S., GARCIA NOVAL J., MENCOS F., LIU D., WANG Y., WEN H., ZHOU P., STRINGER R., ROGAN M.T. & ZEYHLE E. (1992). Coproantigen detection for the immunodiagnosis of echinococcosis and taeniasis in dogs and humans. *Parasitology*, **104**, 79–85.

2. BRETAGNE S., GUILLOUN J.P., MORAND M. & HOUIN R. (1993). Detection of *Echinococcus multilocularis* DNA in fox faeces using DNA hybridization. *Parasitology,* **106**, 193–199.

3. CRAIG P.S. (1997). Immunodiagnosis of *Echinococcus granulosus* and a comparison of techniques for diagnosis of canine echinococcosis. *In:* Compendium on Cystic Echinococcosis in Africa and in Middle Eastern Countries with Special Reference to Morocco, Andersen F.L., Ouhelli H. & Kachani M., eds. Brigham Young University Print Services, Provo, Utah, USA.

4. CRAIG P.S., GASSER R.B., PARADA L., CABRERA P., PARIETTI S., BORGUES C., ACUTTIS A., AGULLA J., SNOWDEN R. & PAOLILLO E. (1995). Diagnosis of canine echinococcosis: comparison of coproantigen and serum antibody tests with arecoline purgation in Uruguay. *Vet. Parasitol.*, **56**, 293–301.

5. CRAIG P.S., ROGAN M.T. & ALLAN J.C. (1996). Detection, screening and community epidemiology of taeniid cestode zoonoses: cystic echinococcosis, alveolar echinococcosis and neurocysticercosis. *Adv. Parasitol.* **38**, 169–250.

6. DEPLAZES P., ALTHER P., TANNER I., THOMPSON R.C.A & ECKERT J. (1999). *Echinococcus multilocularis* coproantigen detection by enzyme-linked immunosorbent assay in fox, dog and cat populations. *J. Parasitol.*, **85**, 115–121.

7. DEPLAZES P. & ECKERT J. (1996). Diagnosis of *Echinococcus multilocularis* infection in final hosts. *Appl. Parasitol.*, **37**, 245–252.

8. DEPLAZES P., GOTTSTEIN B., ECKERT J., JENKINS D.J., WALD D. & JIMENEZ-PALACIOS S. (1992). Detection of *Echinococcus* coproantigens by enzyme-linked immunosorbent assay in dogs, dingoes and foxes. *Parasitol. Res.*, **78**, 303–308.

9. LIGHTOWLERS M.W, LAWRENCE S.B., GAUCI C.G., YOUNG J., RALSTON M.J., MAAS D. & HEATH D.D. (1996). Vaccination against hydatidosis using a defined recombinant antigen. *Int. J. Parasitol.*, **18**, 457–462.

10. LIGHTOWLERS M.W. & GOTTSTEIN B. (1995). Echinococcosis/hydatidosis: Antigens, immunological and molecular diagnosis. *In: Echinococcus* and Hydatid Disease, Thompson R.C.A. & Lymbery A.J., eds. CAB International, Wallingford, UK, 355–410.

11. LYMBERY A.J. (1995). Genetic diversity, genetic differentiation and speciation, in the genus *Echinococcus* Rudolphi 1801. *In: Echinococcus* and Hydatid Disease, Thompson R.C.A. & Lymbery A.J., eds. CAB International, Wallingford, UK, 51–87.

12. MATHIS A., DEPLAZES P. & ECKERT J. (1996). An improved test system for PCR-based specific detection of *Echinococcus multilocularis* eggs. *J. Helminthol.*, **70**, 219–222.

13. MCMANUS D.P. & BRYANT C. (1995). Biochemistry, Physiology and Molecular Biology of *Echinococcus. In: Echinococcus* and Hydatid Disease, Thompson R.C.A. & Lymbery A.J., eds. CAB International, Wallingford, UK, 135–182.

14. RAUSCH R.L. (1995). Life cycle patterns and geographical distribution of *Echinococcus* species. *In: Echinococcus* and Hydatid Disease, Thompson R.C.A. & Lymbery A.J., eds. CAB International, Wallingford, UK, 89–134.

15. SAKASHITA M., SAKAI H., KOHNO H., OOI H., OKU Y., YAGI K., ITO M. & KAMIYA M. (1995). Detection of *Echinococcus multilocularis* coproantigens in experimentally infected dogs using murine monoclonal antibody against adult worms. *Jpn J. Parasitol.*, **44**, 413–420.

16. SCHANTZ P.M. (1993). Surveillance and surveys for cystic echinococcosis. *In:* Compendium on Cystic Echinococcosis with Special Reference to the Xinjiang Uygur Autonomous Region, The People's Republic of China, Andersen F., ed. Brigham Young University, Provo, Utah, USA, 74–84.

17. THOMPSON R.C.A. (1995). Biology and systematics of *Echinococcus. In: Echinococcus* and Hydatid Disease, Thompson R.C.A. & Lymbery A.J., eds. CAB International, Wallingford, UK, 1–50.

*
* *

CHAPTER 2.2.4.

LEPTOSPIROSIS

SUMMARY

Leptospirosis is a contagious disease of animals and humans caused by infection with the spirochete Leptospira. *Laboratory diagnostic procedures for leptospirosis fall into two groups. The first group consists of tests for the demonstration of leptospires or their genetic material in animal tissues or body fluids. The second contains the tests for antibody detection. The selection of tests to be carried out depends on the purpose for which a diagnosis is to be made and the resources available.*

Identification of the agent: *The isolation or demonstration of leptospires in:*

a) the internal organs (such as liver, lung, brain, and kidney) and body fluids (blood, milk, cerebrospinal, thoracic, and peritoneal fluids) of clinically affected animals gives a definitive diagnosis of acute clinical disease or, in the case of a fetus, chronic infection of its mother.

b) the kidney, urine, or genital tract of animals without clinical signs is diagnostic only of a chronic carrier state.

Isolation of leptospires from clinical material and identification of isolates are time-consuming and are tasks for specialised reference laboratories. Isolation followed by typing from renal carriers is very useful in epidemiological studies to determine which serovars are present within a particular group of animals, an animal species, or a geographical location.

The demonstration of leptospires by immunochemical tests (immunofluorescence and immunohistochemistry) is more suited to most laboratory situations. However, the efficacy of these tests is dependant on the number of organisms present within the tissue, and the tests lack the sensitivity of culture. Unless specially prepared reagents are used, immunochemical tests provide no useful information as to the infecting serovar. Reagents for immunofluorescence are best prepared with high IgG titre anti-leptospire sera, which are not available commercially. Rabbit leptospiral typing serum can be used for immunohistochemistry and is available from leptospiral reference laboratories.

Genetic material of leptospires can be demonstrated in tissues or body fluids using a variety of assays based on the polymerase chain reaction (PCR). PCR assays are sensitive but false-positive results can be a problem. In addition, sample processing for PCR is critical and must be adjusted to the tissue, fluid, and species being tested.

Serological tests: *Serological testing is the most widely used means for diagnosis of leptospirosis, and the microscopic agglutination test (MAT) is the standard serological test. Minimum antigen requirements include representative strains of all the serogroups known to exist in the particular country plus those known to be maintained elsewhere by the host species under test.*

The MAT is used primarily as a herd test. To obtain useful information, at least ten animals or 10% of the herd, whichever is greater, should be tested. As an individual animal test, the MAT is very useful for diagnosing acute infection: a four-fold rise in antibody titres in paired acute and convalescent serum samples is diagnostic.

The MAT has limitations in the diagnosis of chronic infection in individual animals: both in the diagnosis of abortion and identification of renal or genital carriers (of particular interest to those involved in the import/export of live animals). Infected animals may have MAT titres below the widely accepted minimum significant titre of 1/100 (final dilution).

Enzyme-linked immunosorbent assays can also be useful for detection of antibodies against leptospires. Numerous assays have been developed and are primarily used for the detection of recent infections and the screening of experimental animals for use in challenge studies.

Requirements for vaccines and diagnostic biologicals: *Vaccines for veterinary use are suspensions of one or more serovars of* Leptospira *spp. inactivated in such a manner that immunogenic activity is retained. While a range of experimental vaccines based on cellular extracts have been tested, commercial vaccines are, with few exceptions, whole cell products. The leptospires are grown in suitable culture media, which often contain serum or serum proteins. If used, serum or serum proteins should be removed from the final products. Vaccines may contain suitable adjuvants.*

A. DIAGNOSTIC TECHNIQUES

Leptospirosis is a contagious disease of animals and humans caused by infection with the spirochete *Leptospira*. All the pathogenic leptospires were formerly classified as members of the species *Leptospira interrogans*; the genus has recently been reorganised and pathogenic leptospires are now identified in several species of *Leptospira* (9, 55, 77). There are more than 200 distinct leptospiral serovars recognised and these are arranged in 23 serogroups (42). A recently published textbook (28) reviews *Leptospira* and leptospirosis.

The use, interpretation, and value of laboratory diagnostic procedures for leptospirosis varies with the clinical history of the animal or herd, the duration of infection, and the infecting serovar. Acute leptospirosis should be suspected in the following cases: sudden onset of agalactia (in adult milking cattle and sheep); icterus and haemoglobinuria, especially in young animals; meningitis; and nephritis and hepatitis in dogs. Chronic leptospirosis should be considered in the following cases: abortion, stillbirth, birth of weak offspring (may be premature); infertility; and cases of periodic ophthalmia in horses. Two major chronic microbiological sequelae of leptospiral infection present particular diagnostic problems: the localisation and persistence of leptospires in the kidney and in the male and female genital tract. Chronically infected animals may remain carriers for life and serve as reservoirs of the infection for other animals and humans.

1. Identification of the agent

The demonstration of leptospires in blood and milk of animals showing clinical signs suggestive of acute leptospirosis is considered to be diagnostic. However, isolation from blood is not often successful because bacteraemia is transient and not always accompanied by clinical signs. The demonstration of generalised leptospiral infection in a range of organs taken at necropsy is also considered to be diagnostic. However, the demonstration of leptospires in the genital tract, kidneys, or urine merely indicates that the animal was a carrier.

Failure to demonstrate leptospires in the urine of an animal does not eliminate the possibility that the animal is a chronic renal carrier; it merely indicates that the animal was not excreting detectable numbers of leptospires at the time of testing. Collection of urine following treatment of the animal with a diuretic will enhance the chances of detecting the organism (50).

The demonstration of leptospires in body fluids or internal organs (usually kidney, liver, lung, brain, or adrenal gland) of aborted or stillborn fetuses is considered to be diagnostic of chronic leptospirosis of the mother, and is evidence of active infection of the fetus.

The isolation of leptospires is the most sensitive method of demonstrating their presence, provided that antibiotic residues are absent, that tissue autolysis is not advanced, that tissues are processed for culture rapidly after collection, and – in the case of urine – at a suitable pH. If tissues or fluids cannot be transported promptly to the laboratory for leptospiral culture, the sample should be kept at 4°C to prevent overgrowth of other bacteria and autolysis of tissue samples. Liquid culture medium or 1% bovine serum albumin (BSA) solution containing 5-fluorouracil at 100–200 µg/ml should be used as transport media for the submission of samples.

Culture should be carried out in a semisolid (0.1–0.2% agar) medium containing BSA and either Tween 80 (e.g. Tween 80/BSA medium or EMJH) (39) or containing BSA and a combination of Tween 80 and Tween 40 (23). Contamination may be controlled by the addition of a variety of selective agents, e.g. 5-fluorouracil (40), nalidixic acid (41), fosfomycin (51), and a mixture of rifamycin, polymyxin, neomycin, 5-fluorouracil, bacitracin, and actidione (1). However, use of selective agents, especially those used by Adler *et al.* (1), may reduce the chances of isolation when there are only small numbers of viable leptospires, and many strains of leptospires will not grow in selective media containing multiple antibiotics. Addition of 0.5–1% rabbit serum to semisolid culture medium enhances the chances of isolating some fastidious leptospiral serovars.

Cultures should be incubated at 29±1°C for at least 16 weeks, and preferably for 26 weeks (23). The time required for detection of a positive culture varies with the leptospiral serovar and the numbers of organisms present in the sample. Cultures should be examined by dark-field microscopy every 1–2 weeks. It is important to use a 100 watt light source and a good quality microscope.

Leptospires may also be demonstrated by a variety of immunochemical staining techniques, e.g. immunofluorescence (24), and various immunohistochemical techniques (3, 26, 59, 61, 78). These are useful in diagnosing infection in pathological material that is unsuitable for culture or where a rapid diagnosis is required. As the success of these techniques is dependant on the number of organisms present, they are less suitable for diagnosing the chronic carrier state, where the numbers of organisms may be very low or very localised. Leptospires do not stain satisfactorily with aniline dyes, and silver staining techniques lack sensitivity and specificity, although they are a useful adjunct for histopathological diagnosis (4).

Initial reports suggested that DNA probes (7, 48, 65) and time-resolved immunofluorescent assays (72) would prove to be very useful techniques for the detection of leptospires. Further evaluation on field material has reduced the use of DNA probes, but polymerase chain reaction (PCR)-based assays are now used in some diagnostic and most reference laboratories. A variety of primer sets for the conduct of PCR assays have been described (29, 31, 36, 47, 71, 76) with some primers specific for the genus *Leptospira* and others that are serovar specific. PCR assays can be quite sensitive, but lack of specificity (i.e. false-positive results) can be a problem. Quality control of PCR assays used for diagnosis of leptospirosis requires careful attention to laboratory design and workflow to prevent contamination of reagents, and use of appropriate control samples (22, 45). In addition, sample processing for PCR is critical and must be suited to the tissue, fluid, and species being tested. A newly described procedure for the preparation of urine samples for PCR using magnetic beads coated with anti-leptospire antibody shows promise in enhancing the detection of pathogenic leptospires in urine (62).

The identification of leptospiral isolates is a task for specialised reference laboratories. For complete identification, a combination of procedures must be used to determine: 1) if the isolate is a pathogen or a saprophyte; 2) the species of *Leptospira* to which the isolate belongs; and 3) the serogroup and serovar of the isolate. A pure leptospiral culture is identified as belonging to a pathogenic or saprophytic species by a variety of tests: the ability to infect animals; the relative resistance to 8-azaguanine; lipase activity; salt and temperature tolerance (38, 39); PCR-assay-based amplification of 23S rDNA (75); and G+C content of DNA (38).

New leptospiral species have been identified based on DNA–DNA hybridisation analysis (9, 55, 77). In most cases, the type strain for each serovar was used in these analyses; for a few serovars, clinical isolates have also been tested to determine the new genospecies designations. Different isolates belonging to a single serovar usually belong to the same species, but this is not always the case. Species identification of field isolates is still cumbersome but can be done by sequence analysis of the 16S rDNA or by genetic analysis of the 16S or 23S ribosomal RNA genes (12, 43, 52, 54, 73, 74).

Strains belonging to *Leptospira* can be differentiated to the serogroup level by cross-agglutination reactions (21). Further differentiation to the serovar level is traditionally done by cross-agglutination absorption, although for most isolates this is now being done using less time-consuming methods: factor analysis (21), monoclonal antibodies (MAbs) (63, 64), restriction endonuclease analysis (35, 44, 66, 67), and various PCR strategies (12, 16, 20, 30, 53, 54, 56, 58, 79, 80). However, these may not give exactly the same results as the cross-agglutination absorption test.

2. Serological tests

Serological testing is the laboratory procedure most frequently used to confirm the clinical diagnosis, to determine herd prevalence, and to conduct epidemiological studies. Leptospiral antibodies appear within a few days of onset of illness and persist for weeks or months and, in some cases, years. Unfortunately, antibody titres frequently fall to undetectable levels while animals remain chronically infected. To overcome this problem, sensitive methods are needed to detect the organism in the urine or genital tract of chronic carriers.

A wide variety of serological tests, which show varying degrees of serogroup and serovar specificity, have been described. Two tests have a role in veterinary diagnosis: the microscopic agglutination test (MAT) and the enzyme-linked immunosorbent assay (ELISA).

a) Microscopic agglutination test

The MAT, using live antigens, is the most widely used serological test. It is the reference test against which all other serological tests are evaluated and is the test used for import/export testing. For optimum sensitivity, it should employ serovars of all the serogroups known to exist in the country in which the animals are found and, preferably, strains representing all the known serogroups. The presence of a serogroup is usually indicated by frequent reaction in serological screening or isolation of a serovar from clinically affected animals. The sensitivity of the test can be improved by using local isolates rather than reference strains, but reference strains assist in the interpretation of results between laboratories. The specificity of the MAT is good; antibodies against other bacteria usually do not cross-react with *Leptospira* to a significant extent. However, there is significant serological cross-reactivity between serovars of *Leptospira* and an animal infected with one serovar is likely to have antibodies against the infecting serovar that cross-react with other serovars (usually at a lower level) in the MAT. The two methods for carrying out the test have been described in detail (34, 49).

The strains selected should be grown in Tween 80 BSA medium at 29±1°C and the culture should be at least 4 days old, but no more than 8 days. The transmittance of the antigen should be 60–70% using a spectrophotometer with a 400 nm filter. The number of antigens to be used is determined and a screening test may be performed with a 1/50 serum dilution. A volume of each antigen, equal to the diluted serum volume, is added to each well, making the final serum dilution 1/100 in the screening test. The microtitration plates are incubated at 29±1°C for 2 hours. The plates are examined by dark-field microscopy. The degree of reaction is interpreted by estimating the percentage of leptospires that are agglutinated. If 100% of the leptospires are agglutinated, the reaction is 4+; 3+ = approximately 75% agglutination; 2+ = 50%; and 1+ = less than 50%. If a screening test is performed, any serum that has a 2+ reaction at a 1/100 dilution is titrated to an end-point using doubling dilutions of serum, starting at a final dilution of 1/100 through to 1/12,800 or higher. The end-point titre is the highest dilution with a 2+ or greater reaction.

Identity of antigens is a crucial factor in conducting the MAT. Antigens should be evaluated for identity, using hyperimmune rabbit sera or MAbs, at least twice a year. Hyperimmune rabbit serum for this purpose can be prepared using a protocol such as that given by the Subcommittee on the Taxonomy of *Leptospira* (37). Briefly, healthy rabbits weighing 2–4 kg that lack detectable anti-leptospire antibodies are selected. Each rabbit is given an intravenous injection in a marginal vein of the ear with a well-growing live or formalin-treated cloned culture with a density of approximately 2×10^8 leptospires/ml. The culture should be grown in Tween 80 BSA medium or another appropriate medium. Five injections of 1, 2, 4, 6, and 6 ml are given at 7-day intervals. One week following the final injection, the homologous antibody titre is determined by MAT. If the titre is ≥1/12,800, the rabbit is anaesthetised and bled by cardiac puncture 7 days later (i.e. 14 days after the final injection). If the titre is <1/12,800, a further injection of 6 ml of culture can be given; 7 days after this injection the homologous titre is again determined. Unless the titre is ≥1/12,800 the procedure should be repeated with another rabbit. Two rabbits are used to prepare each antiserum. If the titres are satisfactory in both rabbits, the sera may be pooled. To preserve potency, it is preferable to freeze-dry the antiserum in 2 ml volumes and store it at 4°C. Alternatively, the serum can be stored in 2 ml volumes at –20°C.

Purity of antigens used in the MAT should be checked regularly by culture on blood agar and in thioglycolate broth. Stock cultures of antigens may be stored at –70°C or in liquid nitrogen. There may be a low survival rate of leptospires after lyophilisation. Repeated passage of antigens in liquid medium results in a loss of antigenicity. In this case, a new liquid culture should be derived from the stock culture.

In some situations, formalinised or lyophilised cultures may be used in the MAT. The main advantages of the use of nonliving organisms are that the antigens can be standardised and the expense, difficulty, and risk of maintaining live cultures of *Leptospira* can be avoided. Titres determined using live antigens and killed antigens may not be directly comparable and many diagnosticians feel that maximum sensitivity of the MAT is obtained using live antigens.

As an individual animal test, the MAT is very useful in diagnosing acute infection; the demonstration of a four-fold change in antibody titres in paired acute and convalescent serum samples is diagnostic. The test has limitations in diagnosis of chronic infection in individual animals, both in the diagnosis of abortion (25) and in the identification of renal or genital carriers (23). This is particularly true with the host-adapted leptospiral infections, e.g. serovar *hardjo* infection in cattle: when a titre of 1/100 or greater is taken as significant, the sensitivity of the test is only 41%, and even when the minimum significant titre is reduced to 1/10, the sensitivity of the test is only 67% (23). The demonstration of antibodies in fetal blood is diagnostic.

As leptospirosis is a herd problem, the MAT has much greater use as a herd test. To obtain useful information, Cole *et al.* (15) have suggested that samples be taken from at least 10 animals, or 10% of the herd, whichever is the greater. In a study of *hardjo* infection in cattle, Hathaway *et al.* (34) found that a ten-cow sample usually indicated the presence or absence of infection in a herd. Increasing the sample size markedly improved epidemiological information, investigations of clinical disease, and public health tracebacks.

In making a serological diagnosis of leptospirosis, account must be taken of the infecting serovar and of the clinical condition involved. In the case of *pomona*-induced abortion in cattle, a high titre is commonly found at the time of abortion because the clinical incident occurs during the acute phase of infection. Abortion in cattle due to *hardjo* is a chronic event; in this case, the serological response at the time of abortion is more variable, with some animals seronegative and others showing high titres. Cattle may experience a drop in milk production during the acute phase of *hardjo* infection and this clinical sign is associated with high titres. Vaccination history must also be considered in the interpretation of MAT results as widespread vaccination contributes significantly to the number of seropositive animals.

b) Enzyme-linked immunosorbent assays

ELISAs for detection of anti-leptospiral antibodies have been developed using a number of different antigen preparations, assay protocols and assay platforms, including plate tests and dipstick tests. In general, ELISAs are quite sensitive, but lack the serovar specificity of the MAT. An ELISA that measures canine IgG and IgM against various leptospiral serovars has been developed and evaluated in Europe (32, 33). Anti-leptospiral IgM is detectable in this assay as early as 1 week after infection, before agglutinating antibodies are present. IgG antibodies are detectable in infected dogs beginning 2 weeks after infection and persist for long periods of time. Therefore, dogs with acute leptospirosis have high IgM titres and relatively low IgG titres; dogs that are vaccinated or have had previous leptospiral infections have high IgG titres but low IgM titres. Similar assays to detect anti-leptospiral bovine, porcine, and ovine antibodies have also been developed (2, 14, 19, 46, 68). The major identified role of ELISA in livestock species is the use of an IgM ELISA for identification of recent infections (19). A total-Ig ELISA is useful in identification of fully susceptible animals suitable for experimental challenge work (27). ELISAs have also been developed for use in milk from individual cows or in bulk tank milk for the detection of serovar *hardjo* antibodies. These tests have been helpful in identifying *hardjo*-infected herds.

B. REQUIREMENTS FOR VACCINES AND DIAGNOSTIC BIOLOGICALS

Leptospiral vaccines for veterinary use are suspensions of one or more strains of pathogenic *Leptospira* inactivated in such a manner that immunogenic activity is retained. While experimental vaccines based on cellular extracts have been tested (6), commercial vaccines are, with few exceptions, whole cell products. The leptospires are grown in suitable culture media that may contain serum or serum proteins. If used, serum or serum proteins should be removed from the final product. Vaccines may contain suitable adjuvants.

1. Seed management

a) Characteristics of the seed

Proper selection of vaccine production strains is of utmost importance. Immunity induced by vaccination is largely serovar-specific (13). A vaccine should be formulated for use in a particular animal species in a particular geographical region. It should contain only those serovars – and preferably those genotypes – that cause problems in the animal species, or that are transmitted by the animal species to other species in the geographical location. Strains selected for use as master seed culture should be cloned on solid medium to ensure the absence of saprophytic leptospire contaminants and uniformity of the culture.

Suitable strains should be further selected by their ability to grow to high yields under batch culture conditions.

b) Methods of culture

Each component strain to be included in the final vaccine should be grown separately in liquid medium; preferably in a protein-free (5, 60) or low-protein medium (5).

The volume of each master seed culture should be amplified by growth for 2–10 days at 29±1°C in a series of subcultures until a volume sufficient for use as a production seed culture is achieved. Cultures should be aerated and agitated as required.

Each subculture of the master seed culture should be checked for purity and for satisfactory growth. Purity can be checked by inoculating a loopful of culture into blood agar plates or into thioglycolate broth for incubation at 37°C for 2–5 days, and by examining a Gram-stained smear of culture sediment. Growth can be checked by dark-field microscopy. Each production seed culture should also be checked against its' homologous rabbit antiserum (21) to ensure purity and homology. MAbs may also be used for this purpose.

c) Validation as a vaccine

There is a large volume of literature describing the efficacy of leptospiral vaccines. In most cases, vaccines provide excellent protection against disease produced by homologous challenge under field conditions.

Vaccines are less efficacious at preventing infection in animals and a percentage of vaccinated animals will become infected with the relevant serovar and may shed the organism in their urine despite a lack of clinical signs of disease.

Efficacy trials and vaccine validation must be conducted in the target species for the vaccine. The vaccine should be administered as recommended on the label and immunity should be tested by challenge with virulent field strains of each serovar by natural routes of infection, i.e. by conjunctival and/or vaginal challenge. In the past, validation studies were conducted with challenge of immunity by intravenous or intramuscular injections of leptospires. Vaccines validated in this way have not always been shown to be protective against field challenge, which occurs by exposure of mucous membranes of the eye, mouth, and genital tract to leptospires. Most notably, commercial leptospiral vaccines containing serovar *hardjo* have not always protected cattle from conjunctival or field challenge with serovar *hardjo* (8).

2. Method of manufacture

Manufacture is carried out by batch culture in appropriately sized fermentor vessels. These should be equipped with ports for the sterile addition of seed culture, air, and additional medium. They should also have sampling ports so that the purity and growth of the production culture can be monitored.

Ideally, low-protein or protein-free media are used for production. However, some strains require the presence of animal protein to achieve suitable yields; this is usually supplied as bovine serum albumin. All media components that are not degraded by heat should be heat sterilised. This reduces the risk of contamination by water-borne saprophytic leptospires that are not removed by filter sterilisation.

After addition of the seed culture, the growth of the production culture is monitored at frequent intervals for the start of log-phase growth. Once this is observed, the vessel is then agitated and aerated. The final yield can often be improved by the addition of more Tween 80 to the culture when log-growth is first observed to be slowing down. Adequate growth may require up to 10 days of incubation at 29±1°C.

Inactivation is usually by the addition of formalin, but phenol, merthiolate, and heat inactivation have also been used.

After the appropriate inactivation period, the culture may be concentrated and extraneous protein material may be removed by ultrafiltration. Suitable volumes of the various strains to be included in the final vaccine can then be blended, and adjuvant and preservative added, if appropriate.

3. In-process control

During production, daily or twice daily subsamples should be taken and monitored for growth of leptospires and absence of contaminants. Growth is monitored either by counting leptospires in a counting chamber under dark-field microscopy or by a nephelometer. The absence of contamination can be monitored by the microscopic examination of Gram-stained preparations of centrifuged culture.

Immediately prior to inactivation, a sample should be taken for checking against its' homologous antiserum (or MAbs) in a MAT. The inactivated culture must be checked for freedom from viable leptospires. This is done by inoculating aliquots of inactivated culture into an appropriate growth medium, such as the medium of Johnson & Harris (39), incubating at 29±1°C for at least 4 weeks, and examining weekly by dark-field microscopy for the presence of viable leptospires.

After blending, the levels of free inactivating agents, minerals present in adjuvants (such as aluminum), and preservative (such as thiomersal) must be within prescribed limits.

4. Batch control

a) Sterility

Selected samples of the completed vaccine should be tested for the absence of viable bacteria and fungi (11, 17, 18, 69). Tests for sterility and freedom from contamination of biological materials may be found in Chapter I.4.

b) Safety

Samples of completed product should be tested for safety. Methods for this have been described elsewhere (10, 17, 70). A suitable test is to take two healthy animals of one of the species for which the vaccine is intended. The animals must be susceptible to the serovars used in the vaccine and their sera must be free from agglutinating antibodies to those serovars. Each animal is given an injection of the vaccine by the recommended route with twice the recommended dose, as stated on the label. The animals are observed for 14 days and should show no adverse effects attributable to the vaccine.

c) **Potency**

Samples of completed vaccine should be tested for potency in hamsters or guinea-pigs. Potency is usually measured by the vaccine's ability to prevent the death of the animal when challenged with between 10 and 10,000 LD_{50} (50% lethal dose). With some serovars that are not hamster or guinea-pig lethal, such as serovar *hardjo*, potency is measured against prevention of renal infection when the animals are challenged with between 10 and 10,000 ID_{50} (50% infectious dose) or by induction of a suitable antibody titre in rabbits.

An example protocol is to inject 1/40 dog dose of the vaccine into each of ten healthy hamsters no more than 3 months old and drawn from the same stock. After 15–30 days, each vaccinated hamster, and each of ten unvaccinated hamsters of the same age, are injected intraperitoneally with a suitable quantity of a virulent culture of leptospires of the serovar used to make the vaccine (or a suspension of liver or kidney tissue collected from an experimentally infected animal). In the case of bivalent vaccines, each serovar is tested separately. For the vaccine to pass the test, at least 8/10 of the unvaccinated animals must die with typical signs of leptospirosis within 14 days and at least 8/10 of the vaccinated animals should remain in good health for 14 days after the death of the controls. Other protocols apply to cattle and pig vaccines, which contain as many as five or six components.

In-vitro potency tests for leptospiral vaccines are being developed based on quantifying the protective antigen in the vaccine using MAbs in a capture ELISA (57). These assays are being standardised using reference vaccines and correlation with existing hamster or antibody-based potency assays and target–host efficacy data.

d) **Duration of immunity**

Duration of immunity should be checked in the animal species for which the vaccine is intended using natural routes of challenge (8). Vaccinal immunity should persist for at least 6 months.

e) **Stability**

When stored under the prescribed conditions, the vaccines may be expected to retain their potency for 1 2 years. Stability should be assessed by determining potency after storage at 4°C, room temperature, and 37°C.

5. Tests on the final product

a) **Safety**

See Section B.4.b.

b) **Potency**

See Section B.4.c

REFERENCES

1. ADLER B., FAINE S., CHRISTOPHER W.L. & CHAPPEL R.J. (1986). Development of an improved selective medium for isolation of leptospires from clinical material. *Vet. Microbiol.*, **12**, 377–381.

2. ADLER B., FAINE S. & GORDON L.M. (1981). The enzyme-linked immunosorbent assay as a serological test for detecting antibodies against *Leptospira interrogans* serovar *hardjo* in sheep. *Aust. Vet. J.*, **57**, 414–417.

3. BARNETT J.K., BARNETT D., BOLIN C.A., SUMMERS T.A., WAGAR E., CHEVILLE N.F., HARTSKEERL R. & HAAKE D. (1999). Expression and distribution of leptospiral outer membrane components during renal infection of hamsters. *Infect. Immun.*, **67**, 853–861.

4. BASKERVILLE A. (1986). Histopathological aspects of diagnosis of leptospirosis. *Curr. Top. Vet. Med. Anim. Sci.*, **36**, 33–43.

5. BEY R.F. & JOHNSON R.C. (1978). Protein-free and low-protein media for the cultivation of *Leptospira. Infect. Immun.*, **19**, 562–569.

6. BEY R.F. & JOHNSON R.C. (1986). Current status of leptospiral vaccines. *Prog. Vet. Microbiol. Immunol.*, **2**, 175–197.

7. BOLIN C.A., ZUERNER R.L. & TRUEBA G. (1989). Comparison of three techniques to detect *Leptospira interrogans* serovar *hardjo* type *hardjo*-bovis in bovine urine. *Am. J. Vet. Res.*, **50**, 1001–1003.

8. BOLIN C.A., ZUERNER R.L. & TRUEBA G. (1989). Effect of vaccination with a pentavalent leptospiral vaccine containing *Leptospira interrogans* serovar *hardjo* type *hardjo*-bovis on type *hardjo*-bovis infection of cattle. *Am. J. Vet. Res.*, **50**, 2004–2008.

9. BRENNER J., KAUFMANN A.F., SULZER K.R., STEIGERWALT A.G., ROGERS F.C. & WEYANT R.S. (1999). Further determination of DNA relatedness between serogroups and serovars in the family Leptospiraceae with a proposal for *Leptospira alexanderi* sp. nov. and four new *Leptospira genomospecies. Int. J. Syst. Bact.*, **49**, 839–858.

10. BRITISH PHARMACOPOEIA (VETERINARY) (1985). Leptospira veterinary vaccines. 117.

11. BRITISH PHARMACOPOEIA (VETERINARY) (1985). Test for sterility of veterinary immunological products. Appendix xviA, (vet). 2, A127–A128.

12. BROWN P.D. & LEVETT P.N. (1997). Differentiation of *Leptospira* species and serovars by PCR-restriction endonuclease analysis, arbitrarily primed PCR and low-stringency PCR. *J. Med. Microbiol.*, **46**, 173–181.

13. CHEN T.Z. (1986). Development and present status of leptospiral vaccine and technology of production of the vaccine in China. *Ann. Immunol. Hung.*, **26**, 125–151.

14. CHO H.J., GALE S.P., MASRI S.A. & MALKIN K.L. (1989). Diagnostic specificity, sensitivity and cross-reactivity of an enzyme-linked immunosorbent assay for the detection of antibody against *Leptospira interrogans* serovars *pomona, sejroe* and *hardjo* in cattle. *Can. J. Vet. Res.*, **53**, 285–289.

15. COLE J.R., ELLINGHAUSEN H.C. & RUBIN H.L. (1980). Laboratory diagnosis of leptospirosis of domestic animals. *Proc. U.S. Anim. Health Assoc.*, **83**, 189–199.

16. CORNEY B.G., COLLEY J., DJORDJEVIC S.P., WHITTINGTON R. & GRAHAM G.C. (1993). Rapid identification of some *Leptospira* isolates from cattle by random amplified polymorphic DNA fingerprinting. *J. Clin. Microbiol.*, **31**, 2927–2932.

17. COUNCIL OF EUROPE (1997). Monograph 62: vaccines for veterinary use. *In:* European Pharmacopoeia, Third Edition. Editions of the Council of Europe, Strasbourg, France, 1823–1827.

18. COUNCIL OF EUROPE (1997). Chapter 2. *In:* European Pharmacopoeia, Third Edition. Editions of the Council of Europe, Strasbourg, France, 11–153.

19. COUSINS D.V., ROBERTSON G.M. & HUSTAS L. (1985). The use of the enzyme-linked immunosorbent assay (ELISA) to detect the IgM and IgG antibody response to *Leptospira interrogans* serovars *hardjo, pomona* and *tarassovi* in cattle. *Vet. Microbiol.*, **10**, 439–450.

20. DE CABALLERO O.L., DIAS NETO E., KOURY M.C., ROMANHA A.J. & SIMPSON A.J. (1994). Low-stringency PCR with diagnostically useful primers for identification of *Leptospira* serovars. *J. Clin. Microbiol.*, **32**, 1369–1372.

21. DIKKEN H. & KMETY E. (1978). Serological typing methods of leptospires. *Methods Microbiol.*, **11**, 259–307.

22. DRAGON E.A., SPADORO J.P. & MADEJ R. (1993). Quality control of polymerase chain reaction. *In:* Diagnostic Molecular Microbiology. Principals and Applications, Persing D.H., Smith T.F., Tenover F.C. & White T.J., eds. American Society for Microbiology, Washington D.C., USA, 160–168.

23. ELLIS W.A. (1986). The diagnosis of leptospirosis in farm animals. *In:* The Present State of Leptospirosis Diagnosis and Control, Ellis W.A. & Little T.W.A., eds. Martinus Nijhoff, Dordrecht, The Netherlands, 13–31.

24. ELLIS W.A., O'BRIEN J.J., NEILL S.D., FERGUSON H.W. & HANNA J. (1982). Bovine leptospirosis: microbiological and serological findings in aborted cows. *Vet. Rec.*, **110**, 147–150.

25. ELLIS W.A., O'BRIEN J.J., NEILL S.D. & HANNA J. (1982). Bovine leptospirosis: Serological findings in aborting cows. *Vet. Rec.*, **110**, 178–180.

26. ELLIS T.M., ROBERTSON G.M., HUSTAS L. & KIRBY M. (1983). Detection of leptospires in tissue using an immunoperoxidase staining procedure. *Aust. Vet. J.*, **60**, 364–367.

27. ELLIS W.A. & ZYGRAICH N. (1986). Experimental studies with a *Leptospira interrogans* serovar *hardjo* vaccine. Proceedings of the XIVth World Congress on Diseases of Cattle, Dublin, Eire, 971–974.

28. FAINE S. (1994). *Leptospira* and leptospirosis. CRC Press, Boca Raton, Florida, USA.

29. GERRITSEN M.J., OLYHOEK T., SMITS M.A. & BOKHOUT B.A. (1991). Sample preparation method for polymerase chain reaction-based semiquantitative detection of *Leptospira interrogans* serovar *hardjo* subtype *hardjo*-bovis in bovine urine. *J. Clin. Microbiol.*, **29**, 2805–2808.

30. GERRITSEN M.A., SMITS M.A. & OLYHOEK T. (1995). Random amplified polymorphic DNA fingerprinting for rapid identification of leptospiras of serogroup Sejroe. *J. Med. Microbiol.*, **42**, 336–339.

31. GRAVEKAMP C., VAN DE KAMP H., FRANZEN M., CARRINGTON D., SCHOONE G.J., VAN EYS G.J.J.M., EVERARD C.O.R., HARTSKEERL R.A. & TERPSTRA W.J. (1993). Detection of seven species of pathogenic leptospires by PCR using two sets of primers. *J. Gen. Microbiol.*, **139**, 1691–1700.

32. HARTMAN E.G., VAN DEN INGH T.S.G.A.M. & ROTHUIZEN J. (1986). Clinical, pathological and serological features of spontaneous canine leptospirosis. An evaluation of the IgM- and IgG-specific ELISA. *Vet. Immunol. Immunopathol.*, **13**, 261–271.

33. HARTMAN E.G., VAN HOUTEN M., FRIK J.F. & VAN DER DONK J.A. (1984). Humoral immune response of dogs after vaccination against leptospirosis measured by an IgM- and IgG-specific ELISA. *Vet. Immunol. Immunopathol.*, **7**, 245–254.

34. HATHAWAY S.C., LITTLE T.W.A. & PRITCHARD D.G. (1986). Problems associated with the diagnosis of *Leptospira interrogans* serovar *hardjo* infection in bovine populations. *Vet. Rec.*, **119**, 84–86.

35. HERRMANN J.L., BELLENGER E., PEROLAT P., BARANTON G. & SAINT GIRONS I. (1992). Pulsed-field gel electrophoresis of *notI* digests of leptospiral DNA – A new rapid method of serovar identification. *J. Clin. Microbiol.*, **30**, 1696–1702.

36. HOOKEY J.V. (1992). Detection of Leptospiraceae by amplification of 16S ribosomal DNA. *FEMS Microbiol. Lett.*, **90**, 267–274.

37. INTERNATIONAL COMMITTEE ON SYSTEMATIC BACTERIOLOGY (1984). Subcommittee on the taxonomy of *Leptospira*. *Int. J. Syst. Bacteriol.*, **34**, 258–259.

38. JOHNSON R.C. & FAINE S. (1984). Leptospiraceae. *In:* Bergey's Manual of Systematic Bacteriology, Vol. 1. Williams & Wilkins, Baltimore, USA, 62–67.

39. JOHNSON R.C. & HARRIS V.G. (1967). Differentiation of pathogenic and saprophytic leptospires. I. Growth at low temperatures. *J. Bacteriol.*, **94**, 27–31.

40. JOHNSON R.C. & ROGERS P. (1964). 5-Fluorouracil as a selective agent for growth of Leptospirae. *J. Bacteriol.*, **87**, 422–426.

41. JOHNSON R.C. & SEITER C.W. (1977). The *Leptospira* and their cultivation – a monograph. Reheis Chemical (a division of Armour Pharmaceutical), Phoenix, Arizona, USA.

42. KMETY E. & DIKKEN H. (1993). Classification of the Species *Leptospira interogans* and History of its Serovars. University Press, Groningen, The Netherlands.

43. LETOCART M., BARANTON G. & PEROLAT P. (1997). Rapid identification of pathogenic *Leptospira* species *(Leptospira interrogans, L. borgpetersenii,* and *L. kirschneri)* with species-specific DNA probes produced by arbitrarily primed PCR. *J. Clin. Microbiol.*, **35**, 248–253.

44. Marshall R.B., Wilton B.E. & Robinson A.J. (1981). Identification of *Leptospira* serovars by restriction-endonuclease analysis. *J. Med. Microbiol.*, **14**, 163–166.

45. McCreedy B.J. & Callaway T.H. (1993). Laboratory design and work flow. *In:* Diagnostic Molecular Microbiology. Principals and Applications, Persing D.H., Smith T.F., Tenover F.C. & White T.J., eds. American Society for Microbiology, Washington D.C., USA, 149–159.

46. Mendoza L. & Prescott J.F. (1992). Serodiagnosis of leptospirosis in pigs using an axial filament enzyme-linked immunosorbent assay. *Vet. Microbiol.*, **31**, 55–70.

47. Merien F., Amouriaux P., Perolat P., Baranton G. & Saint Giron I. (1992). Polymerase chain reaction for detection of *Leptospira* spp. in clinical samples. *J. Clin. Microbiol.*, **30**, 2219–2224.

48. Millar B.D., Chappel R.J. & Adler B. (1987). Detection of leptospires in biological fluids using DNA hybridisation. *Vet. Microbiol.*, **15**, 71–78.

49. National Veterinary Services Laboratories (1987). Microtiter technique for detection of *Leptospira* antibodies. *Proc. U.S. Anim. Health Assoc.*, **91**, 65–73.

50. Nervig R.M. & Garrett L.A. (1979). Use of furosemide to obtain bovine urine samples for leptospiral isolation. *Am. J. Vet. Res.*, **40**, 1197–1200.

51. Oie S., Koshiro A., Konishi H. & Yoshsii Z. (1986). *In vitro* evaluation of combined usage of fosfomycin and 5-fluorouracil for selective isolation of *Leptospira* species. *J. Clin. Microbiol.*, **23**, 1084–1087.

52. Perolat P., Lecuyer I., Postic D. & Baranton G. (1993). Diversity of ribosomal DNA fingerprints of *Leptospira* serovars provides a database for subtyping and species assignation. *Res. Microbiol.*, **144**, 5–15.

53. Perolat P., Merien F., Ellis W.A. & Baranton G. (1994). Characterization of *Leptospira* isolates from serovar *hardjo* by ribotyping, arbitrarily primed PCR, and mapped restriction site polymorphisms. *J. Clin. Microbiol.*, **32**, 1949–1957.

54. Ralph D., McClelland M., Welsh J., Barabton G. & Perolat P. (1993). *Leptospira* species categorized by arbitrarily primed polymerase chain reaction (PCR) and by mapped restriction polymorphisms in PCR-amplified rRNA genes. *J. Bacteriol.*, **175**, 973–981.

55. Ramadass P., Jarvis B.D.W., Corner R.J., Penny D. & Marshall R.B. (1992). Genetic characterization of pathogenic *Leptospira* spp. by DNA hybridization. *Int. J. Syst. Bacteriol.*, **42**, 215–219.

56. Ramadass P., Meerarani S., Venkatesha M.D., Senthilkumar A. & Nachimuthu K. (1997). Characterization of leptospiral serovars by randomly amplified polymorphic DNA fingerprinting. *Int. J. Syst. Bacteriol.*, **47**, 575–576.

57. Ruby K.W., Cardella M.A. & Knudtson W.U. (1992). Assay for measuring relative potency of leptospiral bacterins containing serovar *pomona*. *Biologicals*, **20**, 259–266.

58. Savio M.L., Rossi C., Fusi P., Tagliabue S. & Pacciarini M.L. (1994). Detection and identification of *Leptospira interrogans* serovars by PCR coupled with restriction endonuclease analysis of amplified DNA. *J. Clin. Microbiol.*, **32**, 935–941.

59. Scanziani E. (1991). Comparison between specific immunoperoxidase staining and bacteriological culture in the diagnosis of renal leptospirosis of pigs. *Res. Vet. Sci.*, **50**, 229–232.

60. Shenberg E. (1967). Growth of pathogenic *Leptospira* in chemically defined media. *J. Bacteriol.*, **93**, 1598–1606.

61. Skilbeck N.W. & Chappel R.J. (1987). Immunogold silver staining for visualization of leptospires in histologic sections. *J. Clin. Microbiol.*, **25**, 85–86.

62. Taylor M.J., Ellis W.A., Montgomery J.J., Yan K.T., McDowell S.W. & Mackie D. (1997). Magnetic immunocapture PCR (MIPA): detection of *Leptospira borgpetersenii* serovar *hardjo*. *Vet. Microbiol.*, **56**, 135–145.

63. TERPSTRA W.J., KORVER H., SCHOONE G.J., VAN LEEUWEN J., SCHONEMANN C.E., DE JONGE-AGLIBUT S. & KOLK A.H.J. (1987). Comparative classification of *Leptospira* serovars of the pomona group by monoclonal antibodies and restriction-endonuclease analysis. *Zentralbl. Bakteriol. Mikrobiol. Hyg.* [A], **266**, 412–421.

64. TERPSTRA W.J., KORVER H., VAN LEEUWEN J., KLATSER P.R. & KOLK A.H.J. (1985). The classification of Sejroe group serovars of *Leptospira interrogans* with monoclonal antibodies. *Zentralbl. Bakteriol. Mikrobiol. Hyg.* [A], **259**, 498–506.

65. TERPSTRA W.J., SCHOONE G.J., LIGHTART G.S. & TER SCHEGGET J. (1987). Detection of *Leptospira interrogans* in clinical specimens by *in situ* hybridization using biotin-labeled DNA probes. *J. Gen. Microbiol.*, **133**, 911–914.

66. THIERMANN A.B., HANDSAKER A.L., FOLEY J.W., WHITE F.H. & KINGSCOTE B.F. (1986). Reclassification of North American leptospiral isolates belonging to serogroups Mini and Sejroe by restriction endonuclease analysis. *Am. J. Vet. Res.*, **47**, 61–66.

67. THIERMANN A.B., HANDSAKER A.L., MOSELEY S.L. & KINGSCOTE B. (1985). New method for classification of leptospiral isolates belonging to serogroup Pomona by restriction endonuclease analysis: serovar *kennewicki*. *J. Clin. Microbiol.*, **21**, 585–587.

68. TRUEBA G.A., BOLIN C.A. & THOEN C.O. (1990). Evaluation of an enzyme immunoassay for diagnosis of bovine leptospirosis caused by *Leptospira interrogans* serovar *hardjo* type *hardjo*-bovis. *J. Vet. Diagn. Invest.*, **2**, 323–329.

69. UNITED STATES DEPARTMENT OF AGRICULTURE STANDARD REQUIREMENTS §113.26.

70. UNITED STATES DEPARTMENT OF AGRICULTURE STANDARD REQUIREMENTS §113.38.

71. VAN EYS G.J.J.M., GRAVEKAMP C., GERRITSEN M.J., QUINT W., CORNELISSEN M.T., TER SCHEGGET J. & TERPSTRA W.J. (1989). Detection of leptospires in urine by polymerase chain reaction. *J. Clin. Microbiol.*, **27**, 2258–2262.

72. WAITKINS S.A. & HOOKEY J.V. (1988). The detection and enumeration of *Leptospira interrogans* serovar *hardjo* by time-resolved fluoroimmunoassay. *Serodiagn. Immunother. Infect. Dis.*, **2**, 142–150.

73. WOO T.H., PATEL B.K., SMYTHE L.D., SYMONDS M.L., NORRIS M. & DOHNT M.F. (1997). Comparison of two PCR methods for rapid identification of *Leptospira* genospecies *interrogans*. *FEMS Microbiol. Lett.*, **155**, 169–177.

74. WOO T.H., PATEL B.K., SMYTHE L.D., SYMONDS M.L., NORRIS M. & DOHNY M.F. (1997). Identification of pathogenic *Leptospira* genospecies by continuous monitoring of fluorogenic hybridization probes during rapid-cycle PCR. *J. Clin. Microbiol.*, **35**, 3140–3146.

75. WOO T.H.S., SMYTHE L.D., SYMONDS M.L., NORRIS M.A., DOHNT M.F. & PATEL B.K.C. (1997). Rapid distinction between *Leptospira interrogans* and *Leptospira biflexa* by PCR amplification of 23S ribosomal DNA. *FEMS Microbiol. Lett.*, **150**, 9–18.

76. WOODWARD M.J., SULLIVAN G.J., PALMER N.M.A., WOOLLEY J.C. & REDSTONE J.S. (1991). Development of a PCR test specific for *Leptospira hardjo* genotype bovis. *Vet. Rec.*, **128**, 282–283.

77. YASUDA P.H., STEIGERWALT A.G., SULZER K.R., KAUFMANN A.F., ROGERS F. & BRENNER D.J. (1987). Deoxyribonucleic acid relatedness between serogroups and serovars in the family Leptospiraceae with proposals for seven new *Leptospira* species. *Int. J. Syst. Bacteriol.*, **37**, 407–415.

78. ZAKI S.R., SHIEH W.J., EPIDEMIC WORKING GROUP NADC, EPIDEMIC WORKING GROUP MINISTRY OF HEALTH, EPIDEMIC WORKING GROUP PAHO & EPIDEMIC WORKING GROUP CDC (1996). Leptospirosis associated with an outbreak of acute febrile illness and pulmonary hemorrhage, Nicaragua, 1995. *Lancet*, **347**, 535.

79. ZUERNER R.L., ALT D.P. & BOLIN C.A. (1995). IS1533-based PCR assay for identification of *Leptospira interrogans* sensu lato serovars. *J. Clin. Microbiol.*, **33**, 3284–3289.

80. ZUERNER R.L. & BOLIN C.A. (1997). Differentiation of *Leptospira interrogans* isolates by IS1500 hybridization and PCR assays. *J. Clin. Microbiol.*, **35**, 2612–2617.

CHAPTER 2.2.5.

RABIES

SUMMARY

Rabies is a major zoonosis for which diagnostic techniques have been standardised internationally. As there is no gross pathognomonic lesion for rabies, diagnosis can only be made in the laboratory. Laboratory techniques are preferably conducted on central nervous system (CNS) tissue removed from the cranium. The hippocampus (Ammon's horn), cerebellum and the medulla oblongata are the tissues of choice.

Identification of the agent: *This is preferably done using the fluorescent antibody test (FAT). A drop of purified immunoglobulin previously conjugated with fluorescein isothiocyanate is added to a fixed brain tissue smear, preferably made from several parts of the brain including the hippocampus, cerebellum and medulla oblongata. For a large number of samples, as in an epidemiological survey, the immunoenzyme technique can provide rapid results (the rapid rabies enzyme immunodiagnosis [RREID]). Both the FAT and RREID provide a reliable diagnosis in 98–100% of cases.*

To demonstrate infected neuronal cells, histological tests can be used. These procedures will reveal aggregates of viral material (the Negri bodies) in the cytoplasm of neurones. Nevertheless, the sensitivity of histological techniques is not high, specially where there is some autolysis of the specimen. Even in fresh specimens, up to 40% false-negative results may be observed.

As a single negative test on fresh material does not rule out the possibility of infection, inoculation tests should be carried out simultaneously. Newborn mice or 3–4-week-old mice are inoculated intracerebrally with a suspension of hippocampal tissue, or pool of several CNS tissues, and then kept under observation for 28 days. For any mouse that dies between 5 and 28 days, the cause of death should be confirmed by FAT. Alternatively, a monolayer culture of susceptible cells is inoculated with the same material as used for mice. FAT carried out after appropriate incubation will demonstrate the presence or absence of viral antigen. Wherever possible, virus isolation in cell culture should replace mouse inoculation tests.

The identification of the agent can be supplemented in specialised laboratories by identifying any variant virus strains through the use of monoclonal antibodies, specific nucleic acid probes, or the polymerase chain reaction followed by DNA sequencing of genomic areas. Such techniques can distinguish between field and vaccine strains, and possibly identify the geographical origin of the field strains.

Serological tests: *Virus neutralisation (VN) assays in cell cultures are the prescribed tests for international trade. Alternatively, use may be made of a test that is known to correlate with these, notably an enzyme-linked immunosorbent assay using antibody to the G protein or the neutralisation test in mice. Results are expressed in International Units or equivalent units relative to an international standard antiserum.*

Requirements for vaccines and diagnostic biologicals: *Rabies vaccines for use in animals contain either live virus attenuated for the target species (such as Flury low egg passage, Flury high egg passage, Street-Alabama-Dufferin or Kelev), or virus inactivated by chemical or physical means, or are recombinant vaccines. The virus is cultivated in the CNS tissue of newborn animals, in embryonated eggs, or in cell cultures.*

Rabies vaccines are usually lyophilised, but inactivated virus vaccines, preferably with an adjuvant, may be stored in fluid form.

Before newly developed vaccines can be licensed, the duration of immunity resulting from their use should be determined in vaccinated animals of the target species. All vaccines should remain stable for at least 1 year.

For live virus vaccines, the minimum virus content that will elicit an adequate immune response must be established.

The potency of inactivated virus vaccines is established by mouse vaccination followed by intracerebral challenge using tests formulated by the National Institutes of Health in the United States of America or the European Pharmacopoeia elsewhere. The final products of both types of vaccine are subjected to tests for innocuity and absence of toxicity.

For live vaccines that are prepared for oral vaccination of wild (or domestic) animals, innocuity and efficacy in target animals and safety in nontarget species must be demonstrated.

A. DIAGNOSTIC TECHNIQUES

Rabies is caused by a neurotropic virus of the genus Lyssavirus of the family Rhabdoviridae, and is transmissible to all mammals. As it is transmissible to humans by inoculation or inhalation of infectious virus, all suspected infected material must be handled under the appropriate safety conditions specified by the World Health Organisation (WHO) (38).

Seven distinct genetic lineages can be distinguished within the genus Lyssavirus by cross-protection tests and molecular biological analysis (5, 13, 21), namely the classical rabies virus itself (RV, genotype 1, serotype 1), Lagos bat virus (LBV, genotype 2, serotype 2), Mokola virus (MV, genotype 3, serotype 3), and Duvenhage virus (DV, genotype 4, serotype 4). The European bat viruses (EBV), subdivided into two biotypes (EBV1, genotype 5 and EBV2, genotype 6) and the Australian bat virus (ABV, genotype 7), recently isolated in Australia (24), are also members of the Lyssavirus genus, but are not yet classified into serotypes. Viruses of serotypes 2–4, EBV and ABV are known as rabies-related viruses. The use of monoclonal antibodies (MAbs) directed against viral nucleocapsid or glycoprotein antigens, and the sequencing of defined genomic areas has made possible the definition of numerous subtypes within each serotype. Lyssaviruses cause a clinical disease indistinguishable from classical rabies. Conserved antigenic sites on the nucleocapsid proteins permit recognition of all lyssaviruses with modern commercial preparations of anti-rabies antibody conjugates used for diagnostic tests on brain tissue. For RV, DV, EBV and ABV, conserved antigenic sites on the surface glycoproteins allow cross-neutralisation and cross-protective immunity to be elicited by rabies vaccination. Little or no cross-protection against infection with MV or LBV is elicited by rabies vaccination and most anti-rabies virus antisera do not neutralise these latter lyssaviruses.

Humans working with suspect material must be vaccinated against lyssaviruses or other pathogens that may be present in diagnostic samples. The laboratory must comply with national biocontainment and biosafety regulations to protect staff from contact with pathogens.

WHO recommends the preventive immunisation of the exposed staff. The immunisation protocol includes three injections at day 0, 7, and 28. The serological evaluation of immunisation is made 1–3 weeks after the last injection, and checked every 6 months in the case of laboratory workers or every 2 years for other diagnosticians, in order to practice booster vaccination when the titre is below 0.5 International Units (IU) per ml.

As no clinical sign or gross post-mortem lesion can be considered to be pathognomonic, the diagnosis of rabies has to rely on laboratory testing. Serological evidence of infection is rarely obtained because of late seroconversion and the high mortality rate of host species, although such evidence may be used in some epidemiological surveys.

1. Identification of the agent

Clinical observation may only lead to a suspicion of rabies because signs of the disease are not characteristic and may vary greatly from one animal to another (37). The only way to perform a reliable diagnosis of rabies is to identify the virus or some of its specific components using laboratory tests.

Specimens for rabies diagnosis must be sent to the laboratory rapidly under cold conditions, because rabies virus is rapidly inactivated. Shipment conditions must be considered to be part of the 'rabies diagnosis chain'.

Several laboratory techniques may be used, and have been detailed and standardised in the fourth edition of the WHO's *Laboratory Techniques in Rabies* (38). The methods vary in their efficiency, specificity and reliability. They are classically applied to brain tissue, but they can also be applied, though less effectively, to other organs (e.g. salivary glands). In the brain, rabies virus is particularly abundant in the Hippocampus (Ammon's horn), cerebellum and the medulla oblongata. To reach these parts of the brain, it is necessary to remove the entire organ after having opened the skull in a necropsy room. Under some conditions (e.g. in the field or when sampling for large epidemiological studies), a simplified method of sampling through the occipital foramen (11), or through the orbital cavity (26), can be used.

a) Shipment of samples

During the shipment of suspect material for diagnosis (animal heads or brain samples), no risk of human contamination should arise: brains must be placed in a leak-proof rigid container, (animal heads will be wrapped in absorbent material), and sealed in a plastic bag within insulated boxes containing refrigerant. Transport regulations for dangerous materials must be observed.

When these conditions cannot be fulfilled, different preservation techniques may be used. The choice of the preservative is closely linked to the tests to be used for diagnosis:

- Formalin inactivates the virus, thus the isolation tests cannot be used and diagnosis depends on using a modified direct fluorescent antibody test (FAT), immunohistochemistry or histology (35, 38);
- Infectivity may be maintained at room temperature for a prolonged period of time if small pieces of brain are kept in a mixture of 50% glycerol in phosphate buffered saline (PBS). As the virus is not inactivated, all laboratory tests can be used. Note that if glycerol is used, several washes in PBS will be required and that intensity of fluorescence may be reduced if acetone is used as the fixative.

b) Collection of samples

Usually the brain is collected following the opening of the skull in a necropsy room, and different samples are taken for diagnosis. This step may be hazardous if laboratory technicians are not fully trained, or under field conditions. In such cases, there are two possible methods of collecting some brain samples without opening the skull:

- **Occipital foramen route for brain sampling**

A 5 mm drinking straw (11) or a 2 ml disposable plastic pipette (15) is introduced into the occipital foramen in the direction of an eye. Samples can be collected from the rachidian bulb, the base of the cerebellum, hippocampus, cortex, and medulla oblongata.

- **Retro-orbital route for brain sampling**

In this technique (26), a trocar is used to make a hole in the posterior wall of the eye socket, and a plastic pipette is then introduced through this hole. The sampled parts of the brain are the same as in the former technique, but they are taken in the opposite direction.

c) Routine laboratory tests

Laboratory diagnosis can be performed by using three kinds of procedure.

- **Histological identification of characteristic cell lesions**

Negri bodies correspond to aggregation of viral proteins, but the classical staining techniques detect only an affinity of these structures for acidophilic stains. Immunohistochemical tests are the only histological test specific to rabies.

A direct unfixed tissue smear may be stained by the Seller method, diagnosis is then obtained in under 1 hour. Generally, histological tests, such as Mann's test, are performed on fixed material after a paraffin-embedding step, and the result of the test is obtained within 3 days. Whichever staining method is used, the evidence of infection is provided by intracytoplasmic acidophilic bodies. These histological methods are tending to be abandoned, especially the Seller method, because they are sensitive to sample decomposition. If the specimen is well conserved, they may detect a high percentage of positive cases after up to 20 days in formalin. If the specimen is putrefied or even in fresh specimens, histology may yield 15–40% false-negative results. These techniques have advantages in that the laboratory equipment needed to perform them is inexpensive and any need to keep specimens cold after fixation is avoided – which is important under tropical conditions.

- **Immunochemical identification of rabies virus antigen**

i) *Fluorescent antibody test*

The most widely used test for rabies diagnosis is the FAT, which is recommended by both WHO and OIE. This test may be used directly on a smear, and can also be used to confirm the presence of rabies antigen in cell culture or in brain tissue of mice that have been inoculated for diagnosis. The FAT gives reliable results on fresh specimens within a few hours in 95–99% of cases. The sensitivity of the FAT depends on the specimen (the animal species involved and the degree of autolysis) (1, 9), on the type of lyssavirus and on the proficiency of the diagnostic staff. Sensitivity may be lower in samples from vaccinated animals. For direct rabies diagnosis, smears prepared from hippocampus, cerebellum or medulla oblongata are fixed in high-grade cold acetone and then stained with a drop of specific conjugate. Anti-rabies fluorescent conjugates may be prepared in the laboratory. Those available commercially are either polyclonal conjugates specific to the entire virus or specific to the rabies nucleoprotein, or they may be prepared from a mix of different MAbs. In the FAT, the specific aggregates of nucleocapsid are identified by their fluorescence.

The FAT may be applied to glycerol-preserved specimens after a washing step. If the specimen has been preserved in a formalin solution, the FAT may be used only after the specimen has been treated with an enzyme (6, 7, 33, 35).

ii) *Immunochemical tests*

The antibody may be conjugated to an enzyme such as peroxidase instead of fluorescein isothiocyanate (FITC). This conjugate may be used for direct diagnosis with the same sensitivity as FAT (22), but attention must be paid to the risk of nonspecific false-positive results. This risk is considerably reduced by the thorough training of the technicians. It must also be emphasised that this technique needs one incubation step more than FAT when it is done on fresh acetone-fixed smears.

Peroxidase conjugate may be used on sections of formalin-fixed tissue for immunohistochemical tests.

An enzyme-linked immunosorbent assay (ELISA) that detects rabies antigen is one variation of the immunochemical test. This rapid rabies enzyme immunodiagnosis test (RREID) is available commercially (29): a plastic microplate coated with antibodies specific to rabies nucleoprotein is incubated with the clarified supernatant of the homogenised tissue to be tested. Any bound antigen is revealed by anti-rabies nucleocaspid antibodies conjugated to peroxide. It is possible to read this test by eye, but preferable to use a spectrophometer, in which case it may be automated, which is useful for large-scale epidemiological surveys. The correlation between the FAT and the RREID ranges between 96% and 99% (8, 14). The 'routine' version of this test is not sensitive to rabies-related viruses. In such cases, the RREID-Lyssa (27) is recommended.

- **Detection of the replication of uninactivated rabies virus after inoculation**

These tests detect the infectivity of a tissue suspension for tissue culture or an animal. They should be used if the FAT gives an uncertain result or where the FAT is negative in the case of known human exposure.

i) *Mouse inoculation test*

Five-to-ten mice, 3–4 weeks old (12–14 g), or a litter of 2-day-old newborn mice, are inoculated intracerebrally. It is an advantage, though not strictly essential, to use specific pathogen free (SPF) mice. The inoculum is the clarified supernatant of a 20% (w/v) homogenate of brain material (cortex, Ammon's horn, cerebellum, medulla oblongata) in an isotonic buffered solution containing antibiotics. The young adult mice are observed for 28 days, and every dead mouse is examined for rabies using the FAT. For street fox rabies strains, deaths due to rabies generally begin 9 days post-inoculation. For faster results in newborn mice, it is possible to check one baby mouse by FAT on days 5, 7, 9 and 11 post-inoculation.

This *in-vivo* test is quite expensive, particularly if SPF mice are used, and should be avoided where possible. It does not give rapid results (compared with *in-vitro* inoculation tests), but when the test is positive, a large amount of virus can be isolated from a single mouse brain for strain identification purposes.

ii) *Cell culture test*

A neuroblastoma cell line, identified as CCL-131 in the American Type Culture Collection (ATCC)[1], is used for routine diagnosis of rabies. The cells are grown in Dulbecco's modified Eagle's medium (DMEM) with 5% fetal calf serum (FCS), incubated at 36°C with 5% CO_2. Its sensitivity has been compared with that of baby hamster kidney (BHK-21) cells (30). This cell line is sensitive to street isolates without any adaptation step, but should be checked for susceptibility to locally predominant virus variants before use. Replication of rabies virus in the cells is revealed by the FAT. The result of the test is obtained after at least 18 hours (one replication cycle of virus in the cells); generally incubation continues for 48 hours (10) or in some laboratories up to 4 days.

This test is as sensitive as the mouse inoculation test. Once a cell culture unit exists in the laboratory, this test should replace the mouse inoculation test as it avoids the use of live animals, is less expensive and gives a more rapid result.

1 American Type Culture Collection (ATCC), 10801 University Boulevard, Manassas, Virginia 20110-2209, United States of America (USA).

It is often advisable to carry out more than one type of test on each sample, at least where there has been human contact.

d) Other identification tests

The tests above may be complemented in specialised laboratories (such as OIE or WHO Reference Laboratories) using MAbs, nucleic acid probes, or the polymerase chain reaction (PCR), followed by DNA sequencing of genomic areas for typing the virus (15). This enables a distinction to be made between vaccine virus and a field strain of virus, and possibly the geographical origin of the latter.

2. Serological tests

Serological tests are rarely used in epidemiological surveys, due to late seroconversion and the low percentage of animals surviving the disease and therefore having post-infection antibodies. Oral immunisation of rabies reservoirs is becoming the method of choice for rabies control. For follow-up investigations in oral vaccination campaigns, virus neutralisation (VN) tests using antibody to rabies G protein in cell culture are preferred. However, with poor quality sera obtained in the field, these VN tests on cells are too sensitive to cytotoxicity and could possibly lead to false-positive responses. For such samples, the use of an indirect ELISA with rabies glycoprotein-coated plates has been shown to be as sensitive and specific as the VN test on cells (19).

a) Virus neutralisation test in cell culture: fluorescent antibody virus neutralisation test (a prescribed test for international trade)

The principle of the fluorescent antibody virus neutralisation (FAVN) test (18) is the neutralisation *in vitro* of a constant amount of rabies virus ('challenge virus standard' [CVS] strain adapted to cell culture) before inoculating cells susceptible to rabies virus: BHK-21 C13 or MNA cells.

The serum titre is the dilution at which 100% of the virus is neutralised in 50% of the wells. This titre is expressed in IU/ml by comparing it with the neutralising dilution of a standard serum under the same experimental conditions (OIE serum of dog origin or WHO standard for rabies immunoglobulin [human] No. 2, or both).

This microtitration method uses 96-well microplates, and is an adaptation of the technique of Smith *et al.* (31), modified by Zalan *et al.* (39) and by Perrin *et al.* (28). A recent publication (16) has shown that the FAVN and the rapid fluorescent focus inhibition test (RFFIT) give equivalent results.

- **Essential equipment**

  Humidified incubator at 37°C with 5% CO_2; dry incubator at 37°C; biocontainment cabinet; fluorescence microscope suitable for FITC fluorescence equipped with ×10 eye-piece and ×10 objective. The global magnification of the microscope ranges between 100 and 125 due to the extra magnification of some epi-fluorescence systems.

- **Reagents and biologicals**

  PBS buffer, pH 7.2, without Ca^{2+} and Mg^{2+}, stored at 4°C;

  Trypsin ethylene diamine tetra-acetic acid (EDTA);

  High-grade acetone 80% (diluted with deionised water), stored at 4°C;

  Dulbecco's modified Eagle's medium (DMEM) + 10% decomplemented FCS;

  FITC anti-rabies conjugate;

  Cells: BHK-21 C13 (ATCC CCL-10);

  Virus: CVS-11 (ATCC VR 959) strain is provided by the ATCC to the OIE Reference Laboratory for Rabies, Nancy, France (see Table given in Part 4 of this *Manual*). Vials are stored at –80°C;

  WHO standard for rabies immunoglobulin (human) No. 2, 30 IU per ampoule[2] (reconstituted with 5 ml of sterile deionised or distilled water, stored at –20°C, and diluted to 0.5 IU/ml with deionised water before use), or preferably OIE serum of dog origin (OIE Reference Laboratory for Rabies, Nancy, France [see Table given in Part 4 of this *Manual*] stored at –20°C and diluted to 0.5 IU/ml with sterile deionised or distilled water according to the titre of the batch). Moreover, for internal routine control,

2 National Institute for Biological Standards and Control (NIBSC), Blanche Lane, South Mimms, Potters Bar, Hertfordshire EN6 3QG, United Kingdom (UK).

laboratories should use a positive serum or a pool of dog origin that has been calibrated against the OIE International Standard Serum;

Naive serum: This lyophilised pool of ten negative dog sera, is stored at 4°C, and reconstituted with 0.5 ml of sterile deionised or distilled water.

- **CVS production**

i) *Cell growth:* the BHK-21 C13 cells (ATCC CCL-10) used to produce the CVS virus (ATCC VR 959 CVS-11) are trypsinised from a cell layer that is still growing, i.e. cells are in the exponential phase of their kinetic growth. If the confluence of the layer is complete, a new passage should be made. In the cell suspension, the cells must not be aggregated. 2×10^7 cells are used for a 75 cm^2 cell culture flask. Cells are collected within a volume of 20–30 ml in cell culture medium.

ii) *Infection of cells:* the multiplicity of infection (number of infective particles per cell) is adjusted to between 0.1 and 0.5. The glass bottle containing the virus/cell suspension is incubated for 60 minutes at 35.5–37°C. The contents of the bottle are gently stirred every 10–15 minutes.

iii) *Virus growth:* the virus/cell suspension is then centrifuged at 800 ***g*** for 15 minutes and the cell pellet is resuspended in cell culture medium mixed with 10% heat-inactivated FCS. Virus is harvested 2 days later.

iv) *Harvest and storage:* the supernatant is centrifuged at 800 ***g*** for 15 minutes at 4°C. If several flasks have been used, the different centrifuged supernatants are mixed and then aliquoted and frozen at –80°C. The infective titre of the harvest is established at least 3 days after freezing.

- **Titration of virus in $TCID_{50}$ (50% tissue culture infective dose)**

This titration method uses BHK-21 C13 cells (ATCC CCL-10) in microtitre plates.

Different steps of this procedure may be adapted according to the safety requirements and to the working practices of the laboratory, but the following must not be changed:

- inoculation of a 24-hour cell layer
- tenfold dilutions prepared using 0.9 ml of diluent and 0.1 ml of virus suspension
- six 50 µl replicates per dilution
- incubation for 72 hours
- qualitative reading
- calculation according to neoprobit graphic or Spearman–Kärber methods.

i) *Cell suspension:* the day before titration, a cell suspension containing 10^5 cells/ml is prepared in cell culture medium containing 10% heat-inactivated FCS. 200 µl per well is distributed into 96-well microtitre plates. The plates are then incubated for 24 hours at 35.5°C–37°C with 5% CO_2.

ii) *Dilution of the virus:* the serial dilutions are performed in 5 ml tubes using a cell culture medium without FCS as diluent. The dilution step is 10 (0.9 ml of diluent with 0.1 ml of the previous dilution). The range of dilutions is from 10^{-1} to 10^{-12}.

iii) *Infection of the cells:* the medium in the microtitre plates prepared at day 1 is discarded using an aspiration system. 50 µl of each virus dilution is distributed per well. Six replicates are used per dilution. The microtitre plate is then incubated for 1 hour at 35.5–37°C with 5% CO_2. Then 200 µl of cell culture medium containing 5% FCS is added.

iv) *Incubation:* incubation is for 3 days at 35.5–37°C in 5% CO_2.

v) *Staining and calculation of titre:* the staining procedure is the one classically used in the laboratory. Reading is qualitative, every well that shows specific fluorescence is considered to be positive. The titre calculation is made using:

- the neoprobit graphic method or
- the Spearman–Kärber formula:

$$\log_{10} \text{(end-point dilution)} = -\left(x0 - \frac{d}{2} + d \sum \frac{ri}{ni} \right)$$

x0 = – ($\log_{10}$ of the lowest dilution with all wells positive)
d = $\log_{10}$ of the dilution step, one in this case
ni = number of replicates, six in this case
ri = number of positive wells

Fig. 1. Proposed use of microplates for the fluorescent antibody virus neutralisation test. Wells to which undiluted sera must be added are filled with the indicated '50 µl'. Wells to which 50 µl of diluted challenge virus standard must be added are shaded . Dilutions are given in log_{10}.

Plate 1: Controls

	H	G	F	E	D	C	B	A		
Challenge virus									1	
standard									2	
titration									3	
									4	
WHO or OIE	50 µl					50 µl			5	Naive dog
standard serum	50 µl					50 µl			6	serum
(0.5 IU/ml)	50 µl					50 µl			7	(negative)
	50 µl					50 µl			8	
	50 µl								9	
Internal	50 µl								10	
positive control	50 µl								11	
	50 µl								12	
log (dilution)	0.48	0.95	1.43	1.91	2.39	2.87	3.35	Cells		

Plate 2: Sera to be tested

log dilution		0.48	0.95	1.43	1.91	2.39	*4.23*	0.48	0.95	1.43	1.91	2.39	*4.23*	
		1	2	3	4	5	6	7	8	9	10	11	12	
	A	50 µl						50 µl						
Serum 1	B	50 µl						50 µl						Serum 3
	C	50 µl						50 µl						
	D	50 µl						50 µl						
	E	50 µl						50 µl						
Serum 2	F	50 µl						50 µl						Serum 4
	G	50 µl						50 µl						
	H	50 µl						50 µl						

- **Test procedure**

i) The microplates are used according to the pattern shown in Figure 1. Plate No. 1 is used for the titration of CVS (rows 1 to 4), and for the controls, standard sera and naive dog serum are used. Plate No. 2 and others are used for the sera to be tested.

ii) Medium is added to the wells as follows: plate 1, rows 1 to 4 and cells A9 to A12: add 150 µl per well; plate 2 and others, rows 6 and 12: add 200 µl per well; all other wells: add 100 µl.

iii) Sera to be tested are heat inactivated for 30 minutes at 56°C. As indicated in Figure 1, 50 µl of each undiluted serum to be tested is added to four adjacent wells.

iv) Dilutions of sera are conducted in the microplates as follows:

OIE serum, the WHO serum, the internal control and the naive dog serum: with a 50–200 µl multichannel pipette, mix the first dilution wells by sucking in and out at least eight times, transfer 50 µl from one row to the next one, until the last one is reached. Discard 50 µl from the last row.

Sera being tested (plate 2 and others): as above, transfer successively 50 µl from one row to the following one until rows 5 and 11 (dil. $10^{-2.39}$) are reached. With a 5–50 µl multichannel pipette, transfer 10 µl from rows 5 and 11 to rows 6 and 12, respectively (from dil. $10^{-2.39}$ to dil. $10^{-4.23}$). Using a multichannel pipette adjusted to 100 µl, mix rows 6 and 12 and discard 180 µl. Then add 70 µl of medium to these rows. This procedure does not lend itself to high throughput testing. To attain or exceed the recommended final dilution alternative procedures may be used. These may require modifications to the plate layout.

- **Addition of challenge virus standard**

i) Stock CVS is stored in 1 ml microtubes at –80°C. One tube is thawed rapidly under cold running water, and placed in melting ice.

ii) One dilution from this tube is prepared in order to obtain 100 $TCID_{50}$ in 50 µl. Of this dilution, 50 µl is added to each serum-filled well (see Figure 1). For virus titration, 50 µl is added to wells H1 to H4 (plate 1). Next, transfer 50 µl from row to row (plate 1, lines 1–4). Discard 50 µl from the last row (plate 1, wells A1 to A4). No virus is added to wells A9 to A12 of plate 1 (controls).

iii) Incubate the microplates at 37°C in a humid incubator with 5% CO_2 for 1 hour.

iv) *Addition of cells:* trypsinise a subconfluent culture of 3-day-old BHK-21 cells. Resuspend the cells to obtain a 4×10^5 cells/ml suspension in DMEM supplemented with 10% complement inactivated FCS. Add 50 µl of the cell suspension to each well.

v) Incubate the microplates for 48 hours at 37°C in a humid incubator with 5% CO_2.

- **Fixation and staining**

i) After the 48-hour incubation period, the medium is discarded, and the microplates are rinsed once in PBS, pH 7.2, and once in 80% acetone. The microplates are then fixed in 80% acetone at room temperature for 30 minutes (without a lid), and are dried at room temperature for at least 1 hour.

ii) Add 50 µl of the FITC anti-rabies conjugate, at the working dilution, to each well, gently rock the microplates and incubate at 37°C for 30 minutes. Discard the fluorescent conjugate and rinse the microplates twice with PBS. Excess PBS is removed by briefly inverting the microplates on absorbent paper.

- **Reading and interpreting the results**

i) The total surface of each well is observed. The reading evaluation is qualitative (plus or minus): no fluorescent cell – a minus score is recorded for the well; fluorescent cells (one cell or more) – a plus score is recorded for the well.

ii) Controls are read first. For control cells, titration of CVS, naive serum, and standard sera (WHO standard and/or OIE standard serum), titres are calculated according to the Spearman–Kärber method or the neoprobit graphic method (2).

iii) Results of titration of CVS ($TCID_{50}$), naive serum (D_{50} [median dose]) and positive standard (D_{50}) are reported on a control card for each of these three controls. The control results of the current test are compared with the accumulated control test results from previous tests. The test is validated if the values obtained for the three controls in the current test are not statistically different from the mean of all the values obtained in the tests conducted previously according to this technique.

iv) The D_{50} of tested sera are compared with that of the positive standard serum in the same test:

  - If D_{50} of tested serum is $<D_{50}$ of the positive standard serum diluted to 0.5 IU/ml, the titre is <0.5 IU/ml
  - If D_{50} of tested serum is $\geq D_{50}$ of the positive standard serum diluted to 0.5 IU/ml, the titre is ≥0.5 IU/ml

b) The rapid fluorescent focus inhibition test (RFFIT) for determining rabies virus-neutralising antibody (a prescribed test for international trade)

- **Standard procedure (from WHO Laboratory Techniques in Rabies, 1996)**

- **Preparation of seed virus suspension**

i) Trypsinise one 3-day-old 150 ml flask culture of mouse neuroblastoma (MNA) cells[3]. These cells prefer an acidic medium, supplemented with vitamins (34). A similar cell line (CCL-131) may be obtained on request from the ATCC (see footnote 1).

---

3 Available on request from the Rabies Laboratory, Division of Viral and Rickettsial Diseases, Centres for Disease Control and Prevention, Atlanta, Georgia, USA.

ii) Resuspend 3×10^7 cells in a 50 ml conical centrifuge tube in 2.7 ml of Eagle's minimal essential medium supplemented with 10% fetal bovine serum (EMEM-10).

iii) Using standard rabies safety procedures, add 1×10^7 infectious units of CVS-11 rabies virus (ATCC, VR959) and vortex/mix once. Incubate the cells and virus for 15 minutes at 37°C; vortex/mix the cells once during this time.

iv) Add 10 ml EMEM-10, vortex/mix, and centrifuge the cells at 500 ***g*** for 10 minutes.

v) Discard the supernatant. Resuspend the cells in 30 ml of growth medium and transfer to a 150 ml flask.

vi) Gently rock the flask to mix the cell suspension, and then prepare three eight-well tissue-culture chamber slides by pipetting 0.2 ml of the cell suspension into one well of each slide.

vii) Incubate the flask and slides at 37°C in a humidified incubator with 0.5% carbon dioxide (CO_2). The flask should be incubated as a closed culture (tighten the cap).

viii) At 20, 40 and 64 hours after infection, acetone fix and stain one slide using an immunofluorescence technique (23) to determine the virus infectivity. The supernatant should be harvested 24 hours after the cells reach 100% infectivity (typically 40 hours after infection).

ix) Transfer the supernatant to a 50 ml centrifuge tube and centrifuge at 4000 ***g*** for 10 minutes.

x) Distribute the supernatant into 0.5 ml aliquots and store at –70°C.

- **Titration of seed virus suspension**

i) Thaw one aliquot of the seed virus and prepare serial tenfold dilutions (10^{-1}–10^{-8}) in EMEM-10.

ii) Distribute 0.1 ml of each virus dilution into one well of an eight-well tissue-culture chamber slide. Add 0.2 ml of MNA cells suspended in EMEM-10 (concentration 5×10^4 cells per 0.2 ml) to each well.

iii) Mix the cells and virus by gently rocking the slide, then incubate at 37°C in a humidified incubator with 0.5% CO_2 for 40 hours.

iv) Acetone fix and stain the slide using an immunofluerescence technique. Evidence of virus infection should be observed at the 10^{-6} dilution of virus, indicating a virus stock suspension containing at least 1×10^6 infectious units per 0.1 ml. Prepare sufficient seed virus so that frequent serial passage of the virus is unnecessary.

- **Preparation of stock virus suspension**

i) Infect 3×10^7 MNA cells with 1×10^7 infectious units of the seed virus preparation (see above).

ii) Harvest the supernatant 24 hours after the cells reach 100% infectivity (typically 40 hours after infection).

iii) Distribute the supernatant into 0.5 ml aliquots and store at –70°C.

- **Titration of stock virus suspension**

i) Thaw one aliquot of the stock virus and use this to prepare serial tenfold dilutions (10^{-1}–10^{-6}) in EMEM-10.

ii) Distribute 0.1 ml of each virus dilution into one well of an eight-well tissue-culture chamber slide. Add 0.2 ml of MNA cells suspended in EMEM-10 (concentration 1×10^5 cells per 0.2 ml) to each well.

iii) Mix the cells and virus suspension by gently rocking the slide, then incubate at 37°C in a humidified incubator with 0.5% CO_2 for 20 hours.

iv) Acetone fix and stain the slide using an immunofluorescence technique.

Each well of an eight-well tissue-culture chamber slide contains 25–50 distinct microscopic fields when observed at ×160–200 magnification. One unit of virus for the RFFIT is determined as the dilution at which 50% of the observed microscopic fields contain one or more foci of infected cells (the focus-forming dose, FFD_{50}). The stock virus suspension should contain at least 1×10^4 FFD_{50} per 0.1 ml (i.e. the well with cells infected with the 10^{-4} dilution of the virus should contain at least one focus of infected cells in 50% of the observed microscopic fields). A stock virus suspension of this titre can then be diluted to $10^{-2.3}$ to obtain a challenge virus containing 50 FFD_{50}.

- **Reference sera**

A national or international reference serum standard diluted to a potency of 2.0 IU/ml should be included in each test. The reference serum used at the Centres for Disease Control and Prevention is the first international standard for rabies immunoglobulin (36), which may be obtained from the NIBSC (see footnote 2). The reference serum should be maintained as frozen aliquots in amounts sufficient for 1 week of tests. A positive serum control standard diluted to a potency of 0.5 IU/ml and a negative serum control standard with a potency of <0.1 IU/ml should also be prepared by the laboratory and included in each test.

- **Test sera**

Serum samples should be heated at 56°C for 30 minutes before testing in order to inactive complement. If sera are frozen, they should be reheated after thawing. Serial dilutions of test sera may be prepared in an eight-well tissue-culture chamber slide. Screening dilutions of 1/5 and 1/50 are sufficient for routine evaluation of vaccination efficacy and may be made as follows:

i) Prepare a 1/2.5 dilution by adding 0.1 ml of inactivated serum and 0.15 ml of EMEM-10 to one of the slides. Mix by gently rocking the slide.

ii) Transfer 0.05 ml of the 1/2.5 dilution to a second well containing 0.45 ml of EMEM-10. Discard all but 0.1 ml from the well containing the 1/2.5 dilution.

iii) Mix the second well and discard all but 0.1 ml.

iv) Add 0.1 ml of the challenge virus preparation (containing 32–100 FFD_{50}) to all serum dilutions.

v) Mix and incubate at 35°C in a humidified incubator with 0.5% CO_2 for 90 minutes.

- **Addition of cells**

i) During the incubation period, trypsinise a stock culture of 3–5-day-old MNA cells.

ii) Resuspend the cells in EMEM-10 to give a final concentration of 1×10^5 cells per 0.2 ml.

iii) Distribute 0.2 ml of the cell suspension into each well of the slide and incubate at 35°C in a humidified incubator with 0.5% CO_2 for a further 20 hours.

- **Acetone fixation and staining by immunofluorescence**

i) After 20 hours, remove the slides from the incubator and pour off the medium into a virucidal solution.

ii) Rinse the slides once in PBS and then fix for 10 minutes at room temperature in cold acetone (–20°C).

iii) Leave the slides to dry for 10 minutes before adding FITC-conjugated anti-rabies serum. The conjugate may be prepared in EMEM-10 or PBS; there is no need to adsorb the conjugate with tissue or cells. The working dilution of the conjugate should be determined by titration. The slides should be stained for 20–30 minutes at 37°C and then rinsed in PBS and distilled water, respectively.

iv) Observe the slides under a fluorescence microscope.

- **Calculation of virus-neutralising antibody titres**

Residual virus is detected using a standard fluorescence microscope. The serum neutralisation end-point titre is defined as the dilution factor of the highest serum dilution at which 50% of the observed microscopic fields contain one or more infected cells (i.e. a 97% reduction in the virus inoculum). This value may be obtained by mathematical interpolation. Alternatively, a 100% neutralisation titre may be determined by recording the highest serum dilution at which 100% of the challenge inoculum is neutralised and there are no infected cells in any of the observed fields. For both titration methods, the titre of antibody in the test serum (in IU/ml) can be obtained by comparison with the titre of the national reference standard included in each test. It should be noted that it is also valid to perform the RFFIT using BHK-21 cells instead of neuroblastoma cells. A modified protocol for this has been published (38).

c) Virus neutralisation in mice

The principle of this test is the neutralisation *in vitro* of a constant amount of rabies virus (50 LD_{50} [50% lethal dose]/0.03 ml of CVS strain) by varying quantities of the serum to be titrated, during an incubation of 90 minutes at 37°C. The virus/serum mixture (0.03 ml) is inoculated into the brain of 3-week-old mice. The serum titre is the final dilution of serum in the virus/serum mixture that protects 50% of the mice (mortality is 100% in the absence of neutralisation). This titre can be expressed in IUs by comparing it with the neutralising dilution of a standard serum under the same experimental conditions.

To perform the test, thaw an ampoule of CVS virus and prepare a suspension containing 100 LD_{50}/0.03 ml (taking into account that it will be diluted twofold by the addition of the same volume of test serum before being injected). The amount of virus actually used during the test (permissible limits: 30–300 LD_{50}/0.03 ml) is checked by titrating four dilutions of the viral preparation, each of which are inoculated into five mice. The test sera are heated at 56°C for 30 minutes to inactivate any complement.

- A standard serum must be included in order to check the titration conditions. The maximum allowable difference between its expected neutralising capacity and that measured during the titration is $10^{0.5}$. The greatest dilution must not neutralise the virus. The diluent is the same as that used for the viral preparation.

  To each serum dilution an equal volume of the viral preparation containing 100 LD_{50}/0.03 ml is added. The mixtures are incubated in a 37°C water bath for 90 minutes, then placed in melting ice to reduce virus inactivation due to temperature. The reaction is stopped by immersion in melting ice. During inoculation, the tubes that are not used immediately are kept at 4°C.

  For each dilution, five mice are inoculated intracerebrally with 0.03 ml of the serum/virus mixture. Mortality is recorded during 21 days after inoculation, although deaths occurring during the first 4 days are regarded as nonspecific (due to shock, infection, etc.). The serum titre can be calculated in IUs by comparison with an international standard serum.

B. REQUIREMENTS FOR VACCINES AND DIAGNOSTIC BIOLOGICALS

Rabies vaccines prepared from Pasteur's original 1885 strain and its derivative strains (Pasteur Virus, Challenge Virus Standard, Pitman-Moore, etc.), and strains isolated more recently (Flury, Street-Alabama-Dufferin [SAD], Vnukovo and Kelev), protect against all strains of genotype 1 isolated so far. With the exception of genotype 3, there appears to be a degree of immunological cross-protection among all the lyssaviruses. However, conventional rabies virus vaccines may not provide adequate cross-protection against other lyssaviruses, particularly Mokola virus (32). The principles governing the preparation of inactivated rabies vaccines are identical whether they are to be used in humans or animals, although an adjuvant may be added to vaccines for animal use.

For animals, live vaccines are also effective by the oral route and can be distributed in baits in order to immunise wild (or domestic) animals. Live recombinant vaccine (e.g. vaccinia rabies-glycoprotein recombinant) has also proved to be effective (25).

Different standards apply to vaccines containing live virus modified by passage in animals, eggs or cell cultures to reduce its virulence for the target animal, and to vaccines prepared from inactivated virus. Both types of vaccine have their advantages and disadvantages (5), but they can both be used to immunise animals for periods of between 1 and 3 years. Live attenuated rabies vaccines are not accepted in some countries. They are not to be relied on to protect previously unvaccinated animals that have been exposed to infection (12). Only in humans has the efficiency of post-exposure treatment with vaccine alone been proven and even in these cases there is an additional strong recommendation to administer anti-rabies immunoglobulin. Post-exposure prophylaxis using vaccine and hyperimmune serum has been demonstrated in dogs (17).

All handling of the virus during manufacture and testing of vaccines must conform to the strict safety precautions specified by WHO (37, 38) and to national guidelines and regulations.

1. Seed management

a) Characteristics of the seed

Any strain belonging to serotype 1, which has been proved to protect against field rabies viruses (currently found in the country where the vaccine is to be used), is suitable. The strain of virus used must have well-known biological (e.g. pathogenicity) and antigenic properties (typing by MAbs). If it is to be used as a live vaccine, the master seed virus must be shown not to cause clinical rabies. At least two animals (preferably five to six per group) of each of the species for which the vaccine is intended and, so far as possible, any species that might be in contact with vaccine or vaccinated animals should be tested. This can be done by inoculating in or adjacent to a major nerve, a dose equivalent to ten times the intended viral titre in one dose of the proposed final product. Animals should be observed for at least 90 days for any adverse effect attributable to the master seed.

b) Method of culture

A master cell stock of the seed virus should be prepared and kept at or below –70°C. Subculture from this stock will be used for vaccine production. Virus multiplication is verified by titration during growth of the seed virus.

c) **Validation as a vaccine**

Before a vaccine is licensed, evidence of efficacy should be established by the challenge of vaccinated and control animals of each target species. The challenge should be performed at the end of the period after vaccination for which the manufacturer claims maintenance of immunity. Antibody kinetics must also be determined in order to establish the correlation between antibody titre and resistance to challenge.

The efficacy of the produced vaccine is assessed by studies on every target species previously vaccinated as recommended. Protection at the end of the period of immunity is monitored by a measurement of specific neutralising antibodies and by challenge with rabies virus. The experimental conditions of this challenge should mimic the natural conditions of infection, but, from a practical point of view, it could be easier to obtain 100% mortality of the control animals with a well-known rabies virus strain than with a locally isolated one. In animals vaccinated with inactivated vaccines, the percentage of seroconversion and the mean level of antibody allow a good prognosis for survival to challenge (3).

The correlation between potency in the target species and antigenic value as estimated in mice should be established (see Section B.4.c. below).

For the purposes of licensing a vaccine, safety tests should be conducted in the target species. In the case of live virus vaccines (including recombinant vaccines) used in oral vaccination campaigns, safety tests should also be carried out on those other species that live in the area of vaccination and could become exposed to the vaccine (5).

Vaccine stability is ascertained by testing batches after prolonged storage, usually 1–2 years. A process of accelerated ageing, by storage at 37°C for 1 week, is sometimes used. The storage life claimed by the manufacturer is checked by the national licensing authority. In general, it is 12–18 months for fluid vaccines, and possibly 24 months for lyophilised vaccines.

2. Method of manufacture

Whatever method is adopted, close attention must be paid to the quality of the substrate. Both animals and eggs should be of SPF origin, and the cell cultures, such as BHK cell lines, must conform to international standards of sterility and innocuity.

a) **In animals**

The virus is inoculated intracerebrally and the nervous tissue is harvested when the animal has been killed in the terminal stages of rabies. The virus is inactivated by physical methods, such as irradiation with ultraviolet light, or by chemical methods, such as the addition of phenol or beta-propiolactone. Vaccines should be prepared in young animals (mice, lambs, etc.) for high yield of virus and to reduce the myelin content of vaccine and associated adverse events. In certain cases, the virus is not inactivated entirely, as for example in the phenol-treated vaccines of the Fermi type, but such vaccines are no longer recommended.

b) **In eggs**

A modified egg-adapted strain of virus is inoculated into SPF-embryonated chicken eggs, which are then incubated at 38°C for 5–6 days. The virus is harvested in the form of infective embryo tissues, and is usually lyophilised and used as a live vaccine. Examples of such vaccines include those that contain the Flury low egg passage (LEP), or the more desirable high egg passage (HEP) variant strain, which is safer for some animal species such as the cat.

c) **In cell cultures**

Cultures are infected with cell-culture-adapted strains of rabies virus and incubated at 35–36°C. These may then be used as live virus vaccines (as in Flury and SAD vaccines), or as inactivated vaccines after the addition of phenol (Semple vaccine) or some other chemical, such as beta-propiolactone.

Cell culture can also be used to grow the vector viruses (e.g. vaccinia virus) harbouring the gene coding for the expression of rabies virus glycoprotein (25).

During manufacture, the multiplication of the virus in one of the substrates mentioned above is monitored, followed by harvesting at the most appropriate time, usually 4–6 days after inoculation of animals, eggs or cell cultures. The virus harvest is suspended in a buffer solution at a dilution that will provide an optimum antigenicity of the end-product. If required, the suspension is either inactivated or lyophilised. An adjuvant is recommended for vaccines prepared from inactivated virus, as well as for other vaccine antigens that may be incorporated in polyvalent vaccines.

3. In-process control

This consists of monitoring virus growth to provide an optimum titre and ensure the absence of undesirable microbial contamination.

In live virus vaccines, kinetics of virus growth should be established in order to ensure a final titre of virus correlated to the desired protection in target species.

In inactivated virus vaccines, immunogenic properties of the final product may be evaluated by *in-vitro* techniques (e.g. ELISA, agar gel immunodiffusion, antibody-binding tests or infected cell staining). These evaluations will indicate the best time for harvesting the virus in cell cultures.

4. Batch control

a) Sterility

Tests for sterility and freedom from contamination of biological materials may be found in Chapter I.4.

b) Safety

Safety tests for batches of inactivated virus vaccines are carried out by inoculation of cell culture or intracerebrally into mice to detect viable virus. A suitable safety test for live rabies vaccines should be carried out on each lot of vaccine, in the intended host species. At least three, preferably five to six, animals of the intended host species should be given a dose equivalent to ten times the recommended field dose, by the recommended route of administration. The animals should be observed for 90 days for adverse reactions attributable to the vaccine.

c) Potency

For live virus vaccines, including recombinant vaccines, potency tests are carried out by titrating the amount of virus present in the vaccine. Once a correlation has been established between the activity of the vaccine in the target species and virus titres, virus titrations become reliable indicators of vaccine efficacy. This is carried out using cell cultures or by the intracerebral inoculation of unweaned mice (in mice it is only possible with a few attenuated viruses). Recombinant vaccines should be monitored for the expressed rabies protein until assured that expression stablity is maintained in the manufacturing process. Titre of the vector can then be used as a reliable indicator of vaccine efficacy.

For inactivated virus vaccines, correlation between potency in the target species and antigenic value as estimated in mice provides a reliable indicator of vaccine activity. The potency of the vaccine is established in the USA by the National Institutes of Health (NIH) test. Elsewhere, the European Pharmacopoeia test is widely adopted.

Groups of at least ten mice, aged 3–4 weeks, are inoculated with single, decreasing doses of vaccine in accordance with the European Pharmacopoeia (20), or with two doses, 1-week apart, according to the NIH test (38). A sufficient number of dilutions of vaccine are compared to estimate the dilution at which 50% of the mice are protected against intracerebral challenge 14 days later (20, 38).

A WHO international standard vaccine is available (see footnote 2) for calibration of national standards, so that the results of testing for antigenicity can be expressed in IUs. The test is not valid unless:

i) For both the vaccine to be examined and the standard preparation, the PD_{50} (50% protective dose) lies between the largest and smallest doses given to the mice.

ii) The titration of the challenge virus suspension shows that 0.03 ml of the suspension contained at least 10 LD_{50}. The LD_{50} should be in the range 12–50 for a valid test.

iii) The confidence interval ($p = 0.95$) for the test must not be less than 25% and not more than 400% of the estimated potency: statistical analysis must show a significant slope and no significant deviations from linearity or parallelism of the dose–response lines.

The vaccine passes the test if the estimated potency is not less than 1 IU per dose, or the potency demonstrated in the duration of immunity test used to licence the product, in the smallest prescribed dose.

A simplified test can also be used for the purpose of anticipating which vaccines are likely to be of an antigenic value ≥1 IU per dose (4).

d) Duration of immunity

Duration of immunity is not tested for every batch, but is usually deduced from the antigenic value for inactivated vaccines, or from the virus titre for live vaccines (see Section B.4.c. above).

e) Stability

The proposed shelf life must be verified by appropriate tests. These experiments include biological and physico–chemical stability tests, and should be performed on a sufficient number of batches of vaccine stored under recommended conditions.

The thermostability of live virus vaccines in liquid form is generally poor. For freeze-dried inactivated virus vaccines, stability is generally granted for 2 years at 4°C.

f) Preservatives

Inactivated virus vaccines may contain preservatives (formalin, merthiolate). The nature and quantity of these preservatives must comply with national control regulations.

5. Tests on the final product

a) Safety

See Section B.4.b.

b) Potency

See Section B.4.c.

REFERENCES

1. AUBERT M.F.A. (1982). Sensibilité et fidélité du diagnostic de rage au laboratoire. *Comp. Immunol. Microbiol. Infect. Dis.*, **5**, 369–376.

2. AUBERT M.F.A. (1982). Une méthode simple de calcul des titres des suspensions virales, vaccinales ou séroneutralisantes: la méthode graphique. (A simple method for calculating titres of virus, vaccine or serum-neutralising suspensions: the graphic method.) *Rev. sci. tech. Off. int. Epiz.*, **1**, 828–833.

3. AUBERT M.F.A. (1992). Practical significance of rabies antibodies in cats and dogs. *Rev. sci. tech. Off. int. Eplz.*, **11**, 735–760.

4. AUBERT M.F.A. & BLANCOU J. (1982). Test simplifié de contrôle d'activité des vaccins antirabiques à virus inactivés. *Rev. sci. tech. Off. int. Epiz.*, **1**, 811–822.

5. BAER G.M. (1991). The Natural History of Rabies, Second Edition. CRC Press, Boca Raton, Florida, USA, 620 pp.

6. BARNARD B.J.H. & VOGES S.F. (1982). A simple technique for the diagnosis of rabies in formalin-preserved brain. *Ondersterpoort J. Vet. Res.*, **49**, 193–194.

7. BARRAT J. (1992). Experimental diagnosis of rabies. Adaptations to field and tropical conditions. Proceedings of the International Conference on Epidemiology, Control and Prevention of Rabies in Eastern and Southern Africa. Lusaka, Zambia, 2–5 June 1992, 72–83.

8. BARRAT J. (1993). ELISA systems for rabies antigen detection. Proceedings of the Southern and Eastern African Rabies Group International Symposium. Pietermaritzburg, South Africa, 29–30 April 1993, 152–155.

9. BARRAT J. & AUBERT M.F.A. (1995). Diagnostic de la rage animale en France de 1991 à 1993, bilan de CNEVA laboratoire d'études sur la rage et la pathologie des animaux sauvages en France. *Revue Méd. Vét.*, **146**, 561–566.

10. BARRAT J., BARRAT M.J., PICARD M. & AUBERT M.F.A. (1986). Diagnostic de la rage sur culture cellulaire, comparaison des résultats de l'inoculation au neuroblastome murin et de l'inoculation à la souris. *Comp. Immunol. Microbiol. Infect. Dis.*, **11**, 207–214.

11. BARRAT J. & BLANCOU J. (1988). Technique simplifiée de prélèvement, de conditionnement et d'expédition de matière cérébrale pour le diagnostic de rage. *Doc. WHO/Rab. Res.*/88.27.

12. BLANCOU J., SORIA BALTAZAR R., MOLLI I. & STOLTZ J.F. (1991). Effective postexposure treatment of rabies-infected sheep with rabies immune globulin and vaccine. *Vaccine*, **9**, 432–437.

13. BOURHY H., KISSI B. & TORDO N. (1993). Molecular diversity of the lyssavirus genus. *Virology*, **194**, 70–81.

14. BOURHY H., ROLLIN P.E., VINCENT J. & SUREAU P. (1989). Comparative field evaluation of the fluorescent antibody test, virus isolation from tissue culture, and enzymes immunodiagnosis for rapid laboratory diagnosis of rabies. *J. Clin. Microbiol.*, **27**, 519–523.

15. BOURHY H. & SUREAU P. (1991). Méthodes de laboratoire pour le diagnostic de la rage; Metodos de laboratorio para el diagnostics de la rabia; Laboratory methods for rabies diagnosis. Commission des Laboratoires de référence et d'Expertise de l'Institut Pasteur, Paris, France, 197 pp.

16. BRIGGS D.J., SMITH J.S., MUELLER F.L., SCHWENKE J., DAVIS R.D., GORDON C.R., SCHWEITZER K., ORCIARI L.A., YAGER P.A. & RUPPRECHT C.E. (1998). A comparison of two serological methods for detecting the immune response after rabies vaccination in dogs and cats being exported to rabies-free areas. *Biologicals*, **26**, 347–355.

17. CHO H.C. & LAWSON K.F. (1989). Protection of dogs against death from experimental rabies by postexposure administration of rabies vaccine and hyperimmune globulin (human). *Can. J. Vet. Res.*, **53,** 43–47.

18. CLIQUET F., AUBERT M. & SAGNE L. (1998). Development of a fluorescent antibody virus neutralisation test (FAVN test) for the quantitation of rabies-neutralising antibody. *J. Immunol. Methods*, **212**, 79–87.

19. CLIQUET F., SAGNE L., SCHEREFFER J.L. & AUBERT M.F.A. (2000). ELISA tests for rabies antibody titration in orally vaccinated foxes sampled in the fields. *Vaccine*, **18**, 3272–3279.

20. COUNCIL OF EUROPE (1997). Vaccinum rabiei inactivatum ad usum veterinarium. Inactivated Rabies Vaccine for Veterinary Use. European Pharmacopoeia, Third Edition. Monograph 0451. Editions of the Council of Europe, Strasbourg, France, 1776–1777.

21. FEKADU M., SHADDOCK J.H., SANDERLIN D.W. & SMITH J.S. (1988). Efficacy of rabies vaccines against Duvenhage virus isolated from European house bats *(Eptesicus serotinus)*, classic rabies virus and rabies-related viruses. *Vaccine*, **6**, 533–539.

22. GENOVESE M.A. & ANDRAL L. (1978). Comparaison de deux techniques utilisées pour le diagnostic de la rage: l'immunofluorescence et l'immunoperoxydase. *Rec. Med. Vet.*, **154** (7–8), 667–671.

23. GOLDWASSER R.A. & KISSLING R.E. (1958). Fluorescent antibody staining of street and fixed rabies virus antigens. *Proc. Soc. Exp. Biol. Med.*, **98**, 219–223.

24. HOOPER P.T., LUNT R.A., GOULD A.R., SAMARATUNGA H., HYATT A.D., GLEESON L.J., RODWELL B.J., RUPPRECHT C.E., SMITH J.S. & MURRAY P.K. (1997). A new lyssavirus – the first endemic rabies-related virus recognised in Australia. *Bull. Inst. Pasteur*, **95**, 209–218.

25. KIENY M.P., LATHE R., DRILLIEN R., SPEHNER D., SKORY S., SCHMITT D., WIKTOR T., KOPROWSKI H. & LECOCQ J.P. (1984). Expression of rabies virus glycoprotein from a recombinant vaccinia virus. *Nature*, **312**, 163–166.

26. MONTANO HIROSE J.A., BOURHY H. & SUREAU P. (1991). Retro-orbital route for brain specimen collection for rabies diagnosis. *Vet. Rec.*, **129**, 291–292.

27. PERRIN P., GONTIER C., LECOCQ E. & BOURHY H. (1992). A modified rapid enzyme immunoassay for the detection of rabies and rabies related viruses: RREID-Lyssa. *Biologicals*, **20**, 51–58

28. PERRIN P., LAFON M., VERSMISSE P. & SUREAU P. (1985). Application d'une méthode immunoenzymatique au titrage des anticorps antirabiques neutralisants en cultures cellulaires. *J. Biol. Stand.*, **13**, 35–42.

29. PERRIN P., ROLLIN P.E. & SUREAU P. (1986). A rapid rabies enzyme immuno-diagnosis (RREID) useful and simple technique for the routine diagnosis of rabies. *J. Biol. Stand.*, **14**, 217–222.

30. RUDD R.J. & TRIMACHI C.V. (1987). Comparison of sensitivity of BHK-21 and murine neuroblastoma cells in the isolation of a street strain rabies virus. *J. Clin. Microbiol.*, **25**, 145–168.

31. SMITH J.S., YAGER P.A. & BAER G.C. (1973). A rapid reproducible test for determining rabies neutralizing antibody. *Bull. WHO*, **48**, 535–541.

32. VON TEICHMAN B.F., DE KOKER W.C., BOSCH S.J., BISHOP G.C., MERIDITH C.D. & BINGHAM J. (1998). Mokola virus infection: description of recent south African cases and a review of the virus epidemiology. *J. S. Afr. Vet. Assoc.*, **69**, 169–171.

33. UMOH J.U. & BLENDEN D.C. (1981). Immunofluorescent staining of rabies virus antigen in formalin fixed tissue after treatment with trypsin. *Bull. WHO*, **59**, 737–744.

34. WIKTOR T.J., DOHERTY P.C. & KOPROWSKI H. (1977). In vitro evidence of cell-mediated immunity after exposure of mice to both live and inactivated rabies virus. *Proc. Natl Acad. Sci. USA*, *74*, 334–338.

35. WARNER C.K., WHITFIELD S.G., FEKADU M. & HO H. (1997). Procedures for reproducible detection of rabies virus antigen mRNA and genome *in situ* in formalin-fixed tissues. *J. Virol. Methods*, **67**, 5–12.

36. WORLD HEALTH ORGANIZATION EXPERT COMMITTEE ON BIOLOGICAL STANDARDS. THIRTY-FIFTH REPORT (1985). World Health Organisation Technical Report Series No. 725. WHO, Geneva, Switzerland.

37. WORLD HEALTH ORGANIZATION EXPERT COMMITTEE ON RABIES. EIGHTH REPORT (1992). World Health Organisation Technical Report Series No. 824, 84 pp.

38. WORLD HEALTH ORGANISATION (1996). Laboratory Techniques in Rabies, Fourth Edition, Meslin F.-X., Kaplan M.M. & Koprowski H., eds. WHO, Geneva, Switzerland.

39. ZALAN E., WILSON C. & PUKITIS (1979). A microtest for quantitation of rabies virus. *J. Biol. Stand.*, **7**, 213–220.

*
* *

CHAPTER 2.2.6.

PARATUBERCULOSIS (Johne's disease)

SUMMARY

Paratuberculosis (Johne's disease) is a chronic enteritis of ruminants caused by Mycobacterium avium *subsp.* paratuberculosis *(31).*

Identification of the agent: *The diagnosis of paratuberculosis is divided into two parts: the diagnosis of clinical disease and the detection of subclinical infection, which is essential for control of the disease at farm, national or international level.*

Diagnosis of paratuberculosis is made on clinical grounds confirmed by the demonstration of M. paratuberculosis *in the faeces by microscopy, culture, or by the use of DNA probes and the polymerase chain reaction. Diagnosis is made at necropsy by the finding of the pathognomonic lesions of the disease in the intestines, either grossly or histologically and by isolation of* M. paratuberculosis *in culture.*

The detection of subclinical infection depends on the demonstration of delayed-type hypersensitivity to johnin or to avian tuberculin, detection of specific antibodies by serology, or culture of M. paratuberculosis *from faeces. The choice of test depends on the circumstances and the degree of sensitivity required at individual animal or herd level.*

Cultures of M. paratuberculosis *may be obtained from faeces or tissues, after treatment to eliminate contaminants, by inoculation into artificial media with and without the specific growth factor – mycobactin – that is essential for the growth of* M. paratuberculosis.

Serological tests: *The single largest problem in paratuberculosis control is the difficulty of detecting subclinically infected cattle. The serological tests commonly used for paratuberculosis in cattle are complement fixation (CF), absorbed enzyme-linked immunosorbent assay (ELISA) and gel immunodiffusion. Sensitivity and specificity are often determined by reference to results of faecal culture, which itself has unknown sensitivity in subclinically infected cattle. When used to confirm diagnosis of paratuberculosis in cows with typical clinical signs, some tests, for example CF and absorbed ELISA, perform very well.*

Requirements for vaccines and diagnostic biologicals: *Vaccines for paratuberculosis may be live attenuated or killed bacteria either incorporated with an adjuvant or lyophilised and adjuvanted on reconstitution. Bacterial counting is difficult and bacterial content of vaccines may be based on weight, while vaccine potency may be judged by batch tests for sensitising ability in guinea-pigs.*

Vaccine safety or abnormal toxicity may also be tested in guinea-pigs.

For diagnostic skin tests, Johnin and avian tuberculin are purified protein derivatives (PPD) of a heat-treated culture of M. paratuberculosis *or* M. avium, *respectively. Johnin is standardised for content of PPD by chemical assay and its biological activity is identified in guinea-pigs sensitised with* M. paratuberculosis. *Avian tuberculin activity is determined in guinea-pigs sensitised with* M. avium *by comparison with a reference preparation calibrated in international units.*

A. DIAGNOSTIC TECHNIQUES

Mycobacterium paratuberculosis is an organism first observed by Johne & Frothingham in 1895. *Mycobacterium paratuberculosis* causes paratuberculosis or Johne's disease, a chronic intestinal granulomatous infection. First recognised in cattle, then in sheep and later in goats, paratuberculosis is found most often among domestic and wild ruminants and has a global distribution. The disease has also been reported in horses, pigs, deer and alpaca. Under natural conditions, the disease in cattle spreads by ingestion of *M. paratuberculosis* from the contaminated environment. The disease persists in breeding stocks after the introduction of infected animals. A potential source of infection in calves is milk from infected cows or milk that is contaminated with the faeces of diseased cattle.

The identification of *M. paratuberculosis* is based on its mycobactin requirement and its pathogenicity in the host. Mycobactin dependence has long been used as a taxonomic characteristic for *M. paratuberculosis* because most mycobacteria are able to make mycobactin for themselves. *Mycobacterium paratuberculosis, M. silvaticum* and some primary isolates of *M. avium* lack this capacity, however, and require mycobactin to grow in the laboratory. Thus, the mycobactin requirement is not confined to *M. paratuberculosis;* this characteristic exists to various degrees within the *M. avium* group (30).

Clinical signs of paratuberculosis are a slowly progressive wasting and diarrhoea, which is intermittent at first, becoming progressively more severe until it is constantly present (8). Diarrhoea is less common in small ruminants.

Intrauterine infection occurs in the offspring of a proportion of infected dams. Early lesions occur in the walls of the small intestine and the draining mesenteric lymph nodes, and infection is confined to these sites at this stage. As the disease progresses, gross lesions occur in the terminal small intestine, caecum and colon, and in the mesenteric lymph nodes. *Mycobacterium paratuberculosis* is present in the lesions and, terminally, throughout the body. The intestinal lesions are responsible for a protein leak and a protein malabsorption, which lead to muscular wasting. Clinical signs usually first appear in young adulthood, but the disease can occur in animals at any age over 1–2 years.

Within a few weeks of infection, a phase of multiplication of *M. paratuberculosis* begins in the small intestinal walls. Depending on the resistance of the individual, this infection is eliminated or the animal remains infected as a healthy carrier. The proportion of animals in these categories is unknown. A later phase of multiplication of the organisms in a proportion of carriers leads to the extension of lesions, interference with gut metabolism and clinical signs of disease. Subclinical carriers excrete variable numbers of *M. paratuberculosis* in the faeces. In most cases larger numbers of organisms are excreted as clinical disease develops.

Delayed-type hypersensitivity (DTH) is detectable early in the infection and remains present in a proportion of the subclinically infected carriers, but as the disease progresses, DTH wanes and may be absent in clinical cases. Serum antibodies are detectable later than DTH. They may also be present in carriers that have recovered from infection. Serum antibodies are present more constantly and are of higher titre as lesions become more extensive, reflecting the amount of antigen present.

Other mycobacterial diseases and infections, including mammalian and avian tuberculosis, cause DTH and the presence of serum antibodies. It follows therefore that these diseases need to be differentiated from *M. paratuberculosis* infection and paratuberculosis, both clinically and by the use of specific diagnostic tests. Exposure to environmental saprophytic mycobacteria may also sensitise livestock, resulting in nonspecific DTH reactions.

Animals vaccinated against paratuberculosis develop both DTH and serum antibodies. Vaccination prevents clinical disease but does not necessarily prevent infection. Thus, if it is necessary to attempt a diagnosis of infection in vaccinates, only tests to detect *M. paratuberculosis* in the faeces can be used (13).

In individual animals, especially from a farm in which the disease has not previously been diagnosed, a tentative clinical diagnosis must be confirmed by laboratory tests. However, a definitive diagnosis may be warranted on clinical grounds alone if the clinical signs are typical and the disease is known to be present in the herd. Confirmation of paratuberculosis depends on the finding of either gross or microscopic pathognomonic lesions and the isolation in culture of *M. paratuberculosis*.

To diagnose the presence of paratuberculosis in an individual clinically suspect animal, a number of laboratory tests can be used including: faecal smears, faecal culture, DNA probes using faeces or tissues, serology, necropsy and histology.

Herd tests to detect subclinical infection are carried out to determine the prevalence of the infection, usually so that control measures can be instituted. As no test is 100% sensitive, control of the disease by the disposal of positive reactors depends on repeated tests at 6-month or yearly intervals over a number of years and the elimination of reactors to serological tests or faecal shedders. Even these procedures are not always successful without changes in hygiene and livestock management to reduce the transmission of infection within a herd (2).

1. Identification of the agent

a) Necropsy

Paratuberculosis cannot be diagnosed on superficial examination of the intestines for signs of thickening. The intestines should be opened from the duodenum to the rectum to expose the mucosa. There is not a close correlation between the severity of clinical signs and the extent of intestinal lesions. The mucosa, especially of the terminal ileum, is inspected for pathognomonic thickening and corrugation. Early lesions are seen by holding the intestine up to the light, when discrete plaques can be visualised. The mesenteric lymph nodes may be enlarged and oedematous. Smears from the affected mucosa and cut surfaces of lymph nodes should be stained by Ziehl–Neelsen's method and examined microscopically for acid-fast organisms that have the morphological characteristics of *M. paratuberculosis*. However, acid-fast organisms are not present in all cases. Diagnosis is therefore best confirmed by the collection of multiple intestinal wall and mesenteric lymph node samples into fixative (10% formol saline) for subsequent histology. Both haematoxylin-and-eosin-stained sections and Ziehl–Neelsen-stained sections should be examined. The pathognomonic lesions consist of infiltration of the lamina propria, Peyer's patches and the cortex of the mesenteric lymph nodes with large, pale-staining epithelioid cells and multinucleated Langhans' giant cells, in both of which clumps or singly disposed acid-fast bacilli are usually, but not invariably, found. Langhans' giant cells are not uncommon and contain few organisms.

Lesions in sheep and goats are similar to those observed in cattle. There is often only slight thickening of the mucosa, but nodules of caseation and calcification sometimes form in the intestine and in associated lymph nodes. Enlargement of the mesenteric lymph nodes is seen in alpaca.

b) Bacteriology (microscopic)

Ziehl–Neelsen-stained smears of faeces are examined microscopically. A diagnosis of paratuberculosis can be made if clumps (three or more organisms) of small, strongly acid-fast bacilli are found. The presence of single acid-fast bacilli in the absence of clumps does not indicate a definitive diagnosis. The disadvantages of this test are that only about one-third of cases can be confirmed on microscopic examination of a single faecal sample, and that other acid-fast objects occur in faeces.

c) Bacteriology (culture)

Mycobacterium paratuberculosis infection mainly involves the intestinal canal and adjacent caecum. *Mycobacterium paratuberculosis* organisms are vastly outnumbered by other bacteria in faecal and intestinal tissue specimens.

Primary colonies of *M. paratuberculosis* may be expected to appear any time from 5 to 14 weeks after inoculation. Primary colonies on Herrold's medium containing mycobactin[1] are very small (1 mm in diameter), colourless, translucent and hemispherical. Their margins are round and even, and their surfaces are smooth and glistening. The colonies become more opaque and increase in size (4 or 5 mm) as incubation continues. The colonial morphology changes with age from smooth to rough, and from hemispherical to mammilate (29).

The uncommon, bright yellow pigmented sheep strain is difficult to grow on artificial media. It has been reported that unpigmented sheep strains grow less well than cattle strains, and no cultures should be discarded as negative without prolonged incubation.

For identification of *M. paratuberculosis,* <u>small</u> inocula of suspect colonies should be subcultured on the same medium with and without mycobactin, to demonstrate mycobactin dependency. (The test is not reliable if large numbers of bacilli are present.)

- **Media**

Examples of suitable media are:

i) *Herrold's egg yolk medium with mycobactin (12, 17)*

For 1 litre of medium: 9 g peptone; 4.5 g sodium chloride; 2.7 g beef extract; 27 ml glycerol; 4.1 g sodium pyruvate; 15.3 g agar; 2 mg mycobactin; 870 ml distilled water; six egg yolks (120 ml); and

1 Mycobactin can be obtained commercially (mycobactin J) from Allied Monitor, P.O. Box 71, 201 Golden Drive, Fayette, MO 65248, United States of America (USA), or Symbiotic Society, 299 av. Jean Jaurès, 69007 Lyon, France.

5.1 ml of a 2% aqueous solution of malachite green. Measure the first six ingredients and dissolve by heating in distilled water. Adjust the pH of the liquid medium to 6.9–7.0 using 4% NaOH, and test to ensure the pH of the solid phase is 7.2–7.3. Add the mycobactin dissolved in 4 ml ethyl alcohol. Autoclave at 121°C for 25 minutes. Cool to 56°C and aseptically add six sterile egg yolks[2] and sterile malachite green solution. Blend gently and dispense into sterile tubes.

It is possible to add 50 mg chloramphenicol, 100,000 U penicillin and 50 mg amphotericin B.

ii) *Modified Dubos's medium (26)*

For 1 litre of medium: 2.5 g Difco casamino acids; 0.3 g asparagine; 2.5 g anhydrous disodium hydrogen phosphate; 1 g potassium dihydrogen phosphate; 1.5 g sodium citrate; 0.6 g crystalline magnesium sulphate; 25 ml glycerol; 50 ml of a 1% solution of Tween 80; and 15 g agar. Dissolve each salt in distilled water with minimum heat and make up to 800 ml. Add mycobactin in alcoholic solution at 0.05% (2 mg dissolved in 4 ml ethyl alcohol), heat the medium to 100°C by free-steaming, and then sterilise by autoclaving at 115°C for 15 minutes. Cool to 56°C in a water bath, add antibiotics (100,000 U penicillin; 50 mg chloramphenicol; and 50 mg amphotericin B) and serum (200 ml of bovine serum sterilised by filtering through a Seitz 'EX' pad and inactivated by heat at 56°C for 1 hour). The medium is kept thoroughly mixed and then dispensed into sterile tubes. An advantage of this medium is that it is transparent, which facilitates the early detection of colonies.

iii) *Middlebrook 7H9, 7H10 and 7H11 media (Difco)* enhanced with mycobactin in the same proportion as for Herrold's medium can also be used.

- **Sample preparation**

Although faecal culture is technically difficult and time-consuming to carry out, it is still a good method for diagnosis of paratuberculosis in live animals. It is the only test that does not produce false-positive results (100% specificity). It will detect infected animals 6 months or more before they develop clinical signs, and during the clinical stage its sensitivity approaches 100%.

- *Processing tissue specimens*

Chemical preservatives should not be used. The tissues can be frozen.

To avoid contamination, the faeces should be rinsed from portions of intestinal tract before shipment to the laboratory.

i) *Digestion of tissues*

Approximately 4 g of mucosa are scraped from the ileocaecal valve and mesenteric node or other areas showing pathological change and placed in a sterile blender jar containing 50 ml of trypsin (2.5%). The mixture is adjusted to neutrality using 4% NaOH and pH paper, and stirred for 30 minutes at room temperature on a magnetic mixer. The digested mixture is filtered through gauze. The filtrate is centrifuged at approximately 2000–3000 *g* for 30 minutes. The supernatant fluid is poured off and discarded.

ii) *Decontamination of inoculum*

The sediment is resuspended in 20 ml of 0.75% hexadecylpyridinium chloride (HPC) and allowed to stand undisturbed for 18 hours at room temperature. The particles that settle to the bottom of the tube are referred to as the inoculum and are removed by pipette without disturbing the supernatant fluid.

iii) *Inoculation of culture media and incubation*

Approximately 0.1 ml of inoculum is transferred to each of three slants of Herrold's medium containing mycobactin and to one slant of Herrold's medium without mycobactin. The inoculum is distributed evenly over the surface of the slants. The tubes are allowed to remain in a slanted position at 37°C for approximately 1 week with screw caps loose.

The tubes are returned to a vertical position when the free moisture has evaporated from the slants. The lids are tightened and the tubes are placed in baskets in an incubator at 37°C.

The egg in Herrold's medium contributes sufficient phospholipids to neutralise the bactericidal activity of residual HPC in the inoculum. The other media (Modified Dubos and Middlebrook) do not have this property. Other treatments can be used for sample decontamination, for example oxalic acid at 5%.

2 Use fresh eggs not more than 2 days old from a flock that is not receiving antibiotics. With a brush, scrub the eggs with water containing a detergent. Rinse with water and place the eggs in 70° alcohol for 30 minutes. Dry by inserting between two sterile towels. With sterile rat-tooth forceps, crack one end of the eggshell, making a hole of approximately 10 mm, and remove the egg white with the forceps and gravity. Make the hole larger and break the yolk. Mix the egg yolk by twirling the forceps and remove the yolk sac. Pour the mixed egg yolk into media.

HPC is relatively ineffective in controlling the growth of contaminating fungi. Amphotericin B (fungizone) was found by Merkal & Richards (20) to control effectively fungal overgrowth of inoculated media. Fungizone may be incorporated in the Herrold's medium at a final concentration of 50 µg per ml of medium. Due to loss of antifungal activity, storage of Herrold's medium containing fungizone should be limited to 1 month at 4°C.

The slants are incubated for 15–20 weeks and observed weekly from the sixth week onwards.

- *Processing faecal specimens*

No refrigerant or chemical preservative is used.

i) *Suspension and decontamination of faeces*

1 g of faeces is transferred to a 50 ml tube containing 20 ml of sterile distilled water. The mixture is shaken for 30 minutes at room temperature. The larger particles are allowed to settle for 30 minutes. The uppermost 5 ml of faeces suspension is transferred to a 50 ml tube containing 20 ml of HPC. The tube is inverted several times to assure uniform distribution and allowed to stand undisturbed for 18 hours at room temperature.

ii) *Inoculation of culture media*

0.1 ml of the undisturbed sediment is transferred to each of four slants of Herrold's medium, three with mycobactin and one without mycobactin. A smear may be made from the sediment and stained by the Ziehl–Neelsen method.

iii) *Incubation and observation of slants*

The same as for tissue specimens.

Variations in the above methods have been described (3, 14, 19, 22, 25, 35, 36). The sensitivity of culture may be enhanced using liquid media and with centrifugation rather than sedimentation techniques. The double incubation method assists with decontamination of the inoculum (28)

d) DNA probes

DNA probes are being developed that offer a means of detecting *M. paratuberculosis* in diagnostic samples and of rapidly identifying bacterial isolates (7, 18). Because of their unique specificity, they can distinguish between *M. paratuberculosis* and other mycobacteria, especially those of the *M. avium* group.

McFadden *et al.* have identified a sequence (15, 16), termed IS900, which is an insertion sequence specific for *M. paratuberculosis.* It has been reported that a small number of isolates other than *M. paratuberculosis* have produced amplified products the same size as expected from *M. paratuberculosis.* A restriction enzyme digest may be applied to positive IS900 products to confirm that their sequence is consistent with *M. paratuberculosis* (4). The use of IS900 as a DNA probe for specific identification of *M. paratuberculosis* in faecal samples from cattle by enzymatic amplification of DNA using the polymerase chain reaction (PCR) has been reported (33). A commercial diagnostic test based on the detection of IS900 sequences following isolation of mycobacteria from faecal samples and enrichment of a DNA fraction from IS900 sequences by PCR has been developed. The test is available in kit form[3] suitable for use in laboratories. It has poor diagnostic sensitivity compared with faecal culture.

2. Serological tests

The serological tests commonly used for paratuberculosis in cattle are complement fixation (CF), enzyme-linked immunosorbent assay (ELISA) and agar gel immunodiffusion (AGID) (27) corresponding to humoral immunity, and the gamma interferon assay corresponding to cellular immunity.

a) Complement fixation test

The CF test has been the standard test used for cattle for many years. The CF test works well on clinically suspect animals, but does not have sufficient specificity to enable its use in the general population for control purposes. Nevertheless, it is often demanded by countries that import cattle. A variety of CF test procedures are used internationally. An example of a microtitre method for performing the CF test is as follows (9):

3 IDEXX DNA Probe test kit for the detection of *Mycobaterium paratuberculosis.*

i) The antigen is an aqueous extract of bacteria from which lipid has been removed (strain *M. paratuberculosis* 316F). *Mycobacterium avium* D9 may also be used.

ii) All sera are inactivated in the water bath at 60°C for 30 minutes and diluted at 1/4, 1/8 and 1/16. A positive control serum and a negative control serum should be included on each plate. The following controls are also prepared: antigen control, complement control and haemolytic system control.

iii) Reconstituted, freeze-dried complement is diluted to contain six times H_{50} (50% haemolysing dose) as calculated by titration against the antigen.

iv) Sheep erythrocytes, 2.5%, are sensitised with 2 units of H_{100} haemolysin.

v) All dilutions and reagents are prepared in calcium/magnesium veronal buffer; 25 µl volumes of each reagent are used in 96-well round-bottom microtitration plates.

vi) Primary incubation is at 4°C overnight and secondary incubation is at 37°C for 30 minutes.

vii) *Reading and interpreting the results:* Plates may be left to settle or centrifuged and read as follows: 4+ = 100% fixation, 3+ = 75% fixation, 2+ = 50% fixation, 1+ = 25% fixation and 0 = complete haemolysis. The titre of test sera is given as the reciprocal of the highest dilution of serum giving 50% fixation. A reaction of 2+ at 1/8 is regarded as positive. Results should be interpreted in relation to clinical signs and other laboratory findings.

b) Enzyme-linked immunosorbent assay

The ELISA is, at present, the most sensitive and specific test for serum antibodies to *M. paratuberculosis*. Its sensitivity is comparable with that of the CF test in clinical cases, but is greater than that of the CF test in subclinically infected carriers. The specificity of the ELISA can be increased by *M. phlei* absorption of sera.

The absorbed ELISA, designed by Yokomizo *et al.* (39) and modified by Milner *et al.* (21), was developed into a commercial kit by Cox *et al.* (5). This kit was evaluated by Ridge *et al.* (23), and was found to have a sensitivity in clinical cases of 88.3%, and in subclinical cases of 48.8%, and a specificity of 99.8%, in cattle.

The absorbed ELISA combines the sensitivity of ELISA with the added specificity of an absorption step. Sera to be tested are diluted with buffer containing soluble *M. phlei* antigen prior to testing in an indirect ELISA. This procedure eliminates nonspecific cross-reacting antibodies. In early versions, sera were absorbed with whole *M. phlei*, which were removed by centrifugation prior to testing.

A microtitre plate format has been developed in which *M. paratuberculosis* antigens are coated on 96-well plates. Samples are diluted in sample diluent containing *M. phlei* to remove cross-reacting antibodies. On incubation of the diluted sample in the coated well, antibody specific to *M. paratuberculosis* forms a complex with the coated antigens. After washing away unbound materials from the wells, horseradish peroxidase (HPRO)-labelled anti-bovine immunoglobulin is added. This reacts with immunoglobulins bound to the solid-phase antigen. The rate of conversion of substrate is proportional to the amount of bound immunoglobulin. Subsequent colour, measured (at 450 nm) spectrophotometrically is proportional to the amount of antibody present in the test sample.

The antigen used to coat the ELISA plates are available commercially (e.g. IDEXX, CSL, Pourquier, etc.).

An anti-bovine IgG labelled with HRPO is used as conjugate. The substrate chromogen solution is hydrogen peroxide tetramethyl benzidine. A solution of 0.5 M H_2SO_4 is used to stop the reaction when the absorbance of the positive control serum reaches a predetermined point.

The method and test materials needed, the interpretation of the results and calculations are fully described in the instructions accompanying the commercial kit. The procedure is the same as for any routine ELISA. Screening tests are usually performed in one well per serum, but are unreliable, and diagnostic tests should be performed in duplicate wells.

c) Agar gel immunodiffusion test

The AGID test is useful for the confirmation of the disease in clinically suspect cattle, sheep and goats (24). Several variations of the method are in use.

The antigen employed is a crude protoplasmic extract of laboratory strain *M. avium* 18 (formally *M. paratuberculosis* 18) prepared by disruption of cells in a hydraulic press cell fractionator. Disrupted cells are centrifuged at 40,000 ***g*** for 2 hours to remove cell wall debris, and the supernatant fraction is retained and lyophilised. This antigen is resuspended in water at a concentration of 10 mg/ml.

Agarose is dissolved in barbital buffer, pH 8.6, containing sodium azide, to give a final agarose concentration of 0.75%. Agarose may be poured into Petri dishes or on to glass slides. Wells are cut in a hexagonal pattern. Wells are 4 mm in diameter, 4 mm apart, and the agar should be 3–4 mm deep. Antigen is added to centre wells. Test, positive and negative control sera are added to alternate peripheral wells.

Plates are incubated in a humid chamber at room temperature. Gels are examined for precipitation lines after 24 and 48 hours' incubation. The appearance of one or more clearly definable precipitation line(s), showing identity with that of a control positive serum, before or at 48 hours, constitutes a positive test result. Absence of any precipitation lines is recorded as a negative test result. Nonspecific lines may occur.

d) Gamma interferon assay

The assay is based on the release of gamma interferon from sensitised lymphocytes during a 18–36-hour incubation period with specific antigen (avian purified protein derivative [PPD] tuberculin or johnin) (38). The quantitative detection of bovine gamma interferon is carried out with a sandwich ELISA that uses two monoclonal antibodies to bovine gamma interferon. The sensitivity and specificity may be comparable with the tuberculin skin test. A commercial diagnostic test based on the detection of the gamma interferon has been developed. The method and test materials needed, the interpretation of results, and calculations, are fully described in the instruction accompanying the commercial kit[4].

3. Delayed-type hypersensitivity

The test is carried out by the intradermal inoculation of 0.1 ml of avian PPD tuberculin or johnin (avian tuberculin[5] and johnin are of comparable sensitivity and specificity) into a clipped or shaven site, usually on the side of the middle third of the neck. The skin thickness is measured with calipers before and 72 hours after inoculation. Increases in skin thickness of over 2 mm should be regarded as indicating the presence of DTH. It should be noted that positive reactions in deer may take the form of diffuse plaques rather than discrete circumscribed swellings, thus making reading of the test more difficult. The presence of any swelling should be regarded as positive in this species. Tests for DHT are of limited value. Sensitisation to the *M. avium* complex is widespread in animals, and neither avian tuberculin nor johnin are highly specific (11). A herd test gives only an indication of the number of sensitised animals and may thus be used only as a preliminary test prior to the initiation of a control programme.

B. REQUIREMENTS FOR VACCINES AND DIAGNOSTIC BIOLOGICALS

Vaccines: Vaccines used against paratuberculosis are: live, attenuated, incorporated with oil and pumice; lyophilised, live, attenuated, which may be adjuvanted with, for example, oil after reconstitution; and heat-killed bacterins. Vaccines may be prepared from one strain of *M. paratuberculosis* 316F or 2E (Weybridge) or *M. paratuberculosis* 3 and 5 or II (Canadian strains), or as many as three strains may be used. The information below applies to a live, attenuated vaccine adjuvanted with oil and pumice (6, 32, 37). Vaccination may cause a reaction at the site of injection. Vaccination may also interfere with eradication programmes based on elimination of infected animals and can interfere with the interpretation of DTH skin tests for bovine tuberculosis.

Diagnostic products: Johnin PPD is a preparation of the heat-treated products of growth and lysis of *M. paratuberculosis*. Avian tuberculin PPD is a preparation of heat-treated products of growth and lysis of *M. avium* D4ER or TB 56. Details of avian tuberculin PPD are in Chapter 2.7.8. Avian tuberculosis. These two preparations are used, by intradermal injection, to reveal DTH as a means of identifying animals infected or sensitised with *M. paratuberculosis*.

1. Seed management

a) Characteristics of the seed

Vaccine: Seed strains should be of a prevalent type, which may be checked by biotyping or genetic analysis. They should have been demonstrated to be innocuous when administered by the recommended route of vaccination to intended target species.

4 *Mycobacterium paratuberculosis* gamma-interferon test kit, CSL Limited (Veterinary), 45 Poplar Road, Parkville, Victoria 3052, Australia.

5 Avian tuberculin can be obtained from VLA Weybridge, New Haw, Addlestone, Surrey KT15 3NB, United Kingdom, or from Symbiotic Society, 299 av. Jean Jaurès, 69007 Lyon, France.

Johnin: Strains of *M. paratuberculosis* used to prepare seed cultures should be identified by biotyping or genetic tests. They should be shown to be free from contaminating organisms.

b) Method of culture

Vaccine: Seed cultures may be made on potato slants partly immersed in a suitable medium, such as Reid's synthetic medium[6] (34). Cultures may be stored lyophilised. Active cultures are normally incubated at 37°C.

Johnin: The culture substrate should be shown to be capable of producing a product free from substances known to cause toxic or allergic reactions. A suitable medium for seed culture is that of Reid, solidified with 1.75% agar, in screw cap tubes. Cultures may also be stored lyophilised.

c) Validation as a vaccine

Vaccine: Purity tests should be carried out on seed cultures and final harvest by stained smears.

The vaccine should be used as part of a control programme and will not on its own provide complete protection against disease caused by *M. paratuberculosis* (37). There is usually good control of clinical disease, but subclinical infection persists in vaccinated herds, albeit at a reduced level. Vaccine should be administered to animals in early life only, e.g. calves in their first month of life. It should be inoculated subcutaneously and causes a small inflammatory swelling. This is gradually replaced by a cold, painless, fibro-caseous nodule, which varies in size and which may persist for years.

The use of vaccines may interfere with the outcome of diagnostic skin tests for tuberculosis, and this should be remembered when planning a control programme (10).

Johnin: Cultures should be checked by staining smears for the presence of contaminating organisms.

To test for lack of sensitising effect, three guinea-pigs that have not previously been treated with any material that could interfere with the test, are each injected intradermally on each of three occasions at 5-day intervals, with 0.01 mg of the preparation under test in a volume of 0.1 ml. Each guinea-pig, together with each of three control guinea-pigs that have not been injected previously, is injected intradermally 15–21 days after the third injection with the same dose of the same johnin. The reactions of the two groups of guinea-pigs should not be significantly different when measured 24–48 hours later.

2. Method of manufacture

Vaccine: For vaccine batches, the organisms may be grown on a liquid synthetic medium, such as Formula A. The organisms grow as a pellicle on the liquid surface. To ensure a good surface area, it is convenient to use vessels such as conical flasks containing one-third of their nominal volume of liquid medium. These flasks may be seeded directly from potato slant cultures, but with some strains, one or more passages on liquid medium may be necessary to ensure adequate pellicle growth for the final, vaccine batch passage. Such passaging should usually take place at 2-week intervals as longer periods may result in over-maturation and sinking of the pellicle. Incubation is at 37°C.

To prepare the vaccine, the pellicle growth from 2-week-old cultures of each strain to be included may be separated from the liquid medium by decantation, filtration and pressing between filter paper pads. The moist *M. paratuberculosis* culture is blended with an adjuvant, such as liquid paraffin, olive oil and pumice (6).

Johnin: Johnin for skin test diagnosis is a PPD prepared from one or more strains of *M. paratuberculosis* (available from VLA Weybridge or CDI, Lelystad, the Netherlands). It may be prepared by the following method.

---

6 L-Asparagine, 5.0 g
Potassium dihydrogen phosphate (KH_2PO_4, anhydrous), 2.0 g
Magnesium sulphate ($MgSO_4$-$7H_2O$), 1.0 g
Ammonium citrate ($[NH_4]_3\ C_6H_5O_7$), 2.0 g
Sodium chloride, 2.0 g
Ferric ammonium citrate, 0.075 g
Dextrose monohydrate B.P., 10 g
Glycerol B.P. (48 ml), 60 g
Distilled water to 1000 ml
pH (not adjusted) 5.6–5.8
When required, the above medium is solidified by the addition of 1.5% granulated agar (Difco). Sterilised at 121°C for 15 minutes.

Mycobacterium paratuberculosis strains are grown as a pellicle on liquid Reid's medium. Production cultures are usually inoculated from liquid seeding cultures rather than directly from seed on solid medium (Reid's synthetic medium). Production cultures may be grown in penicillin flasks containing half of their nominal volume of medium. These are incubated at 37°C for 10 weeks.

At the end of the incubation period, the culture medium has a pH of about 5 and little or no johnin will be obtained unless the pH is raised, using sodium hydroxide, to about 7.3 before steaming. After thorough mixing, the cultures are free steamed. The bulk of the killed organisms is removed by coarse filtration and the filtrate is clarified by further filtration. Protein in the filtrate is precipitated chemically, washed and redissolved. The product is sterilised by filtration. An antimicrobial preservative that does not give rise to false-positive reactions, such as phenol (not more than 0.5% [w/v]), may be added. Glycerol (not more than 10% [w/v]) may be added as a stabiliser. The product is dispensed aseptically into sterile glass containers, which are then sealed.

3. In-process control

Vaccine: Adequate growth of culture and cultural purity need to be checked. Presence of contaminating organisms may be detected by conventional sterility tests on harvests. Tests for pathogenic mycobacteria are carried out by injection of moist culture, taken prior to blending with adjuvant and diluted tenfold in saline, into two guinea-pigs, each receiving 1 ml. These are observed for 8 weeks, killed humanely, and examined for any abnormal lesions.

Johnin: After final filtration the sterility of each filtrate of the PPD solution is checked.

Sterile filtrates are tested for protein content by a Kjeldahl method (1). The protein content is adjusted to give between 0.475 and 0.525 mg/ml of protein in the final product. The pH is adjusted to the range 6.5–7.5.

4. Batch control

a) Sterility

Tests for sterility and freedom from contamination may be found in Chapter I.4. The vaccine organism will not normally grow to a detectable level in conventional sterility tests.

b) Safety

Vaccine: These tests are normally performed in laboratory animals, although multidose tests in target animals would also be satisfactory. A typical laboratory animal test would be as follows. Each of two guinea-pigs is inoculated, subcutaneously, with an acceptable batch of vaccine at a fraction of the cattle dose previously determined to give a nodule but no overt necrosis at the injection site. Animals are observed for 8 weeks, killed humanely and examined for any abnormal lesions.

Johnin: Two guinea-pigs should each be injected subcutaneously with 0.5 ml of the johnin under test. No significant local or systemic lesions should be seen within 7 days (1).

Tests on johnin for living mycobacteria may be performed either on the material immediately before it is dispensed into final containers or on samples taken from final containers themselves. A sample of at least 10 ml should be taken, and this should be injected intraperitoneally or subcutaneously into at least two guinea-pigs, dividing the volume to be tested equally between the guinea-pigs. It is desirable to take a larger sample, say 50 ml, and to concentrate any residual mycobacteria by centrifugation or membrane filtration. The guinea-pigs are observed for at least 42 days and post-mortem examinations are carried out. Any macroscopic lesions are examined microscopically and culturally.

c) Potency

Vaccine: As protection tests appear to be impractical, a test of sensitising ability may be used. This may then be related to bacterial content based on weight. A typical test would be as follows: guinea-pigs are sensitised by intramuscular injection of 0.5 ml of a 100-fold dilution in liquid paraffin of the vaccine under test. Skin tests are performed 6 weeks after sensitisation using intradermal inoculations of 0.2 ml of at least three serial dilutions of a *M. paratuberculosis* antigen, such as johnin PPD, the dilutions being chosen to give expected skin reactions of from 8 mm to 25 mm diameter. Each guinea-pig receives several dilutions per flank, their distribution being chosen by a Latin square design. After 24–48 hours, skin reactions are measured. A reference preparation for tests of this type has not yet been fully established. Avian tuberculin PPD of known international unitage may be used as a skin test antigen in tests of this type to ensure that the vaccine is capable of producing adequate sensitisation (corresponding to the vaccination).

Johnin: The potency of johnin is currently determined by chemical assay for protein using a Kjeldahl method. A PPD content of 0.5 + 0.025 mg/ml of final product is recommended (1).

The identity of the material should be confirmed by injecting small doses intradermally into guinea-pigs sensitised by injections of killed *M. paratuberculosis* 6 weeks previously.

It is possible to perform a potency test using dilutions of johnin in guinea-pigs sensitised with *M. paratuberculosis*, similar to such tests for the potency of bovine and avian tuberculin, but a standard preparation for this type of test has not yet been fully established.

d) Duration of immunity

Vaccine: After vaccination at the age of 14–30 days, the vaccination effect is expressed as the reduction in the rate of excretors among vaccinated animals as compared to nonvaccinated bovines (13).

The favourable vaccination results probably reflect a diminishing exposure to infection resulting from a reduction in the number of heavy excretors. Infection is not prevented in all vaccinated bovines.

e) Stability

Vaccine: The vaccine may be stored at 2–8°C for 9–12 months without loss of potency. It should not be frozen.

Johnin: Johnin should be protected from light and stored at 2–8°C. Under these conditions it should retain its potency for at least 5 years.

f) Preservatives

A preservative is normally included for vaccine in multidose containers. For johnin, the phenol used is no more than 0.5% (w/v). The concentration of the preservative in the final product and its persistence through shelf life should be checked.

g) Precautions (hazards)

Vaccine: The vaccine causes some side-effects, nodule formation and sensitisation of animals to the tuberculin test (10). In humans, accidental injection of vaccine has resulted in chronic inflammatory reactions requiring surgical treatment (13).

5. Tests on the final product

a) Safety

See Section B.4.b.

b) Potency

See Section B.4.c.

REFERENCES

1. ANON (1985). Johnin purified protein derivative. British Pharmacopoeia (Veterinary), 184–185.

2. ARGENTE G. (1988). Utilisation de la culture fécale dans un plan de prevention de la paratuberculose dans 500 troupeaux; justifications techniques et économiques. *In:* Second International Colloquium on Paratuberculosis. Laboratoire Central de Recherches Vétérinaires, 94703 Maisons-Alfort Cedex, France, 30–35.

3. COLLINS M.T., KENEFICK K.B., SOCKETT D.C., LAMBRECHT R.S., MCDONALD J. & JØRGENSEN J.B. (1990). Enhanced radiometric detection of *Mycobacterium paratuberculosis* by using filter-concentrated bovine fecal specimens. *J. Clin. Microbiol.*, **28**, 2514–2519.

4. COUSINS D., WHITTINGTON R., MASTERS A., EVANS R. & KLUVER P. (1999). Investigation of false positives in the IS900 PCR for identification of *M. paratuberculosis*. Proceedings of the Sixth International Colloquium on Paratuberculosis, Melbourne, Australia. International Association for Paratuberculosis, 259–264.

5. COX J.C., DRANE D.P., JONES S.L., RIDGE R. & MILNER A.R. (1991). Development and evaluation of a rapid absorbed enzyme immunoassay test for the diagnosis of Johne's disease in cattle. *Aust. Vet. J.*, **68**, 157–160.

6. DOYLE T.M. (1945). Vaccination against Johne's disease. *Vet. Rec.*, **57**, 385–387.

7. ELLINGSON J.L.E., BOLIN C.A. & STABEL J.R. (1998). Identification of a gene unique to *Mycobacterium avium* subspecies *paratuberculosis* and application to diagnosis of paratuberculosis. *Mol. Cell. Probes*, **12**, 133–142.

8. GILMOUR N.J.L. (1954). *Mycobacterium paratuberculosis. In:* Handbuch der Bakteriellen Infektionen bei Tieren, Blobel H. & Schliesser T., eds. Gustav Fischer Verlag, Jena, Germany, 281–313.

9. GROUPE DE TRAVAIL IMMUNO-SÉROLOGIE ANIMALE DE LA CSSA DU RNE (1993). Recherche des anticorps contre la paratuberculose des ruminants dans le sérum par l'épreuve de fixation du complément. Pr 109/00IS 310/00. CNEVA, 94701 Maisons-Alfort Cedex, France.

10. HALGAARD C. (1984). Adverse effects of vaccination against paratuberculosis: tuberculin sensitization and nodule formation. *In:* Paratuberculosis: Diagnostic Methods, Their Practical Application and Experience with Vaccination. Commission of the European Communities Agriculture Publication, Luxembourg, 145–153.

11. INDERLIED C.B., KEMPER C.A. & BERMUDES L.E.M. (1993). The *Mycobacterium avium* complex. *Clin. Microbiol. Rev.*, **6**, 266–310.

12. JORGENSEN J.B. (1982). An improved medium for the culture of *Mycobacterium paratuberculosis* from faeces. *Acta Vet. Scand.*, **23**, 325–335.

13. JORGENSEN J.B. (1984). The effect of vaccination on the excretion of *Mycobacterium paratuberculosis. In:* Paratuberculosis: Diagnostic Methods, Their Practical Application and Experience with Vaccination. Commission of the European Communities Agriculture Publication, Luxembourg, 131–136.

14. LAGADIC M., LE MENEC M. & ARGENTE G. (1983). Techniques de culture de *Mycobacterium paratuberculosis* : leur utilisation en routine dans un laboratoire de diagnostic. *Recueil Med. Vet.*, **159**, 801–807.

15. MCFADDEN J.J., BUTCHER P.D., CHIODINI R. & HERMON-TAYLOR J. (1987). Crohn's disease – isolated mycobacteria are identical to *Mycobacterium paratuberculosis,* as determined by DNA probes that distinguish between mycobacterial species. *J. Clin. Microbiol.*, **25**, 796–801.

16. MCFADDEN J.J., BUTCHER P.D., THOMPSON J., CHIODINI R. & HERMON-TAYLOR J. (1987). The use of DNA probes identifying restriction fragment length polymorphisms to examine the *Mycobacterium avium* complex. *Mol. Microbiol.*, **1**, 283–291.

17. MERKAL R.S. (1970). Diagnostic methods for the detection of paratuberculosis (Johne's disease). *In:* Proceedings of the 74th Annual Meeting of the US Animal Health Association, 620–623.

18. MERKAL R.S. (1984). Paratuberculosis. *In:* The Mycobacteria: A Sourcebook, Kubica G.P. & Wayne L.G., eds. Marcel Dekker, New York, USA, 1237–1249.

19. MERKAL R.S., LARSEN A.B., KOPECKY K.E. & NESS R.D. (1968). Comparison of examination and test methods for early detection of paratuberculosis in cattle. *Am. J. Vet. Res.*, **29**, 1533–1538.

20. MERKAL R.S. & RICHARDS W.D. (1972). Inhibition of fungal growth in the cultural isolation of mycobacteria. *Appl. Microbiol.*, **24**, 205–207.

21. MILNER A.R., MACK W.N., COATES K., WOOD P.R., SHELDRICK P., HILL J. & GILL I. (1988). The absorbed ELISA for the diagnosis of Johne's disease in cattle. *In:* Johne's Disease, Milner A. & Wood P., eds. CSIRO Publications, Melbourne, Australia, 158–163.

22. RIDGE S.E. (1993). Cultivation of *Mycobacterium paratuberculosis* from bovine fecal samples by using elements of the Roche MB Check system. *J. Clin. Microbiol.*, **31**, 400–405.

23. RIDGE S.E., MORGAN I.R., SOCKETT D.C., COLLINS M.T., CONDRON R.J., SKILBECK N.W. & WEBBER J.J. (1991). Comparison of the Johne's absorbed EIA and the complement fixation test for the diagnosis of Johne's disease in cattle. *Aust. Vet. J.*, **68**, 253–257.

24. SHERMANN D.M., MARKHAM R.J.F. & BATES F. (1984). Agar gel immunodiffusion test for the diagnosis of clinical paratuberculosis in cattle. *J. Am. Vet. Med. Assoc.*, **185**, 179–182.

25. SINGH S.N., MADDUX R.L. & KADEL W.L. (1991). Comparative evaluation of conventional sedimentation versus new double incubation culture method for the isolation of *Mycobacterium paratuberculosis* from bovine fecal samples. *In:* Proceedings of the Third International Colloquium on Paratuberculosis. International Association for Paratuberculosis, Providence, USA, 84–93.

26. SMITH H.W. (1953). Modification of Dubos's media for the cultivation of *Mycobacterium johnei. J. Pathol. Bacteriol.*, **66**, 375–381.

27. SOCKETT D.C., CONRAD T.A., THOMAS C.D. & COLLINS M.T. (1992). Evaluation of four serological tests for bovine paratuberculosis. *J. Clin. Microbiol.*, **30**, 1134–1139.

28. STABEL J.R. (1997). An improved method for the cultivation of *Mycobacterium paratuberculosis* from bovine fecal samples and comparison to three other methods. *J. Vet. Diagn. Invest.*, **9**, 357–380.

29. THOREL M.F. (1984). Identification of *Mycobacterium paratuberculosis. In:* Paratuberculosis: Diagnostic Methods, Their Practical Application and Experience with Vaccination. Commission of the European Communities Agriculture Publication, Luxembourg, 61–64.

30. THOREL M.F. (1991). Taxonomic and genomic research on mycobactin-dependent mycobacteria. *In:* Paratuberculosis: Diagnostic Methods, Their Practical Application and Experience with Vaccination. Proceedings of the Third International Colloquium on Paratuberculosis. International Association for Paratuberculosis, Orlando, Florida, USA, 222–235.

31. THOREL M.F, KRICHEVSKY M. & VINCENT LEVY-FREBAULT V. (1990). Numerical taxonomy of mycobactin-dependent mycobacteria, emended description of *Mycobacterium avium* subsp. *avium* subsp. nov., *Mycobacterium avium* subsp. *paratuberculosis* subsp. nov., and *Mycobacterium avium* subsp. *silvaticum* subsp. nov. *Int. J. Syst. Bacteriol.*, **40**, 254–260.

32. VALLEE H., RINJARD P. & VALLEE M. (1941). Sur la prémunition de l'entérite paratuberculeuse due au bacille de Johne. *Bull. Acad. Méd.*, **125**, 195–198.

33. VARY C.P.H., ANDERSON P.R., GREEN E., HERMON-TAYLOR J. & MCFADDEN J.J. (1990). Use of highly specific DNA probes and the polymerase chain reaction to detect *Mycobacterium paratuberculosis* in Johne's disease. *J. Clin. Microbiol.*, **28**, 268–275.

34. WATSON E.A. (1935). Tuberculin, johnin and mallein derived from non-protein media. *Can. J. Public Health*, **26**, 268–275.

35. WHIPPLE D.L., CALLIHAN D.R. & JARNAGIN J.L. (1991). Cultivation of *Mycobacterium paratuberculosis* from bovine fecal specimens and a suggested standardised procedure. *J. Vet. Diagn. Invest.*, **3**, 368–373.

36. WHITLOCK R.H., ROSENBERGER A.E., SWEENEY R.W., HUTCHINSON L.J. (1991). Culture techniques and media constituents for the isolation of *Mycobacterium paratuberculosis* from bovine fecal samples. Proceedings of the Third International Colloquium on Paratuberculosis. International Association for Paratuberculosis, Providence, USA, 94–111.

37. WILESMITH J.W. (1982). Johne's disease: A retrospective study of vaccinated herds in Great Britain. *Br. Vet. J.*, **138**, 321–331.

38. WOOD P.R., BILLMAN-JACOBE H., MILNER A.R. & CARRIGAN M. (1990). Serology and cellular assays for the diagnosis of mycobacterial infections in cattle. Proceedings of the Third international Colloquium on paratuberculosis. International Association for Paratuberculosis, Providence, USA, 12–19.

39. YOKOMIZO Y., MERKAL R.S. & LYLE P.A.S. (1983). Enzyme-linked immunosorbent assay for detection of bovine immunoglobulin G antibody to a protoplasmic antigen of *Mycobacterium paratuberculosis. Am. J. Vet. Res.*, **44**, 2205–2207.

*

* *

CHAPTER 2.2.7.

HEARTWATER

SUMMARY

Heartwater (also known as cowdriosis) is a rickettsial disease of ruminants caused by Cowdria ruminantium *and transmitted by* Amblyomma *ticks. It occurs in nearly all of sub-Sahelian countries of Africa and in Madagascar, and also in the Caribbean, threatening the American mainland.*

Clinically, the disease is characterised by a sudden high fever, often hydropericardium, lung oedema and, in acute and peracute forms, by nervous signs and a high mortality. Subacute heartwater also occurs, and has a higher recovery rate.

Identification of the agent: *The specific diagnosis of heartwater is based on the observation of colonies of* C. ruminantium *in capillary endothelial cells of the brain. In the absence of adequate tools, a piece of cerebellum can easily be removed with a curette through the foramen magnum after cutting off the head, while a sample of cerebral cortex can be obtained through a hole made in the skull with a hammer and a large nail. Brain smears are prepared by crushing a small piece of cerebral or cerebellar cortex between two microscope slides. The capillaries are spread out in a single cell layer by drawing one slide across the other. The smears are air-dried, fixed with methanol and stained with Giemsa. With fast stains, the smears can be fixed and stained in under 1 minute. The colonies (clusters) are reddish-purple to blue, and very often close to the nucleus of the infected endothelial cell. They can be scanty and difficult to find, particularly in peracute cases, but they are always present in the brain of a ruminant that died from heartwater and was not specifically treated.*

The colonies are still visible 2 days after death in a brain that has been stored at room temperature and up to 34 days in a brain that has been stored in a refrigerator.

Fresh whole blood collected from suspect animals can be inoculated intravenously into a susceptible sheep or goat. The development of clinical signs and the demonstration of Cowdria *in the brain of the inoculated animal are diagnostic for heartwater.*

Cowdria ruminantium *can be isolated from the blood of an infected host using cultivation on ruminant endothelial cells. When a cytopathic effect consisting of plaques of cell lysis appears, the presence of characteristic morulae is confirmed by staining the cell monolayer with eosin-methylene blue or by immunofluorescence or immunoperoxidase techniques using a specific antiserum.*

DNA probes and especially the more sensitive polymerase chain reaction (PCR) techniques are available to reveal the presence of C. ruminantium *in the blood of actively infected animals, to a lesser extent in the blood or bone marrow of carrier animals, and in the tick vectors. Apart from diagnosis, PCR is widely used for research on the* Cowdria *genome and for epidemiological studies.*

Serological tests: *Serological tests include indirect fluorescent antibody tests, enzyme-linked immunosorbent assays (ELISAs) and Western blotting. However, when the whole* Cowdria *is used as antigen, cross-reactions with* Ehrlichia *spp. occur in all of these tests.*

Two recently developed ELISAs that use recombinant major antigenic protein 1 (MAP1) antigens – the MAP1-B ELISA and the MAP1 competitive ELISA – have shown a dramatic improvement in specificity compared with previous tests, making the interpretation of serological results in regions where Ehrlichia *infections occur in ruminants more reliable. These tests can help to monitor experimental infections, to check the infection of immunised animals, and to screen animals prior to importation.*

Requirements for vaccines and diagnostic biologicals: *The immunisation against heartwater by the 'infection and treatment' method using infected blood or homogenised pre-fed* Amblyomma *ticks is still in use in some countries. A first generation vaccine consisting of inactivated purified elementary bodies of* C. ruminantium *emulsified in Montanide ISA 50 adjuvant has given promising results in experimentally controlled conditions, and is being evaluated in the field in endemic areas. In the near future, it could replace the infection and treatment method, which has practical difficulties.*

A. DIAGNOSTIC TECHNIQUES

Heartwater (cowdriosis) is a rickettsial disease of domestic and wild ruminants caused by *Cowdria ruminantium* and transmitted by *Amblyomma* ticks. It is also known by the synonyms malkopsiekte (Afrikaans), péricardite exsudative infectieuse (French), hidrocarditis infecciosa (Portuguese), idropericardite dei ruminanti (Italian), and a variety of names in different African languages (7).

Heartwater occurs in nearly all the Sub-Sahelian countries of Africa where *Amblyomma* ticks are present and in the surrounding islands: Madagascar, Reunion, Mauritius, Zanzibar, the Comoros Islands and Sao Tomé. The disease is also reported in the Caribbean (Guadeloupe, Marie-Galante and Antigua) (5, 25), from where it threatens the American mainland. All domestic and wild ruminants can be infected, but the former appear to be the most susceptible. Indigenous domestic ruminants are usually more resistant to the disease.

The average natural incubation period is 2 weeks, but can vary from 10 days to 1 month (1). In most cases, heartwater is an acute febrile disease, with a sudden rise in body temperature; temperature may exceed 41°C within 1–2 days. It remains high with small fluctuations and drops shortly before death.

Fever is followed by inappetence, sometimes listlessness, diarrhoea, particularly in cattle (4) (common in cattle but not in small ruminants), and dyspnoea indicative of lung oedema. Nervous signs develop gradually. The animal is restless, walks in circles, makes sucking movements and stands rigidly with tremors of the superficial muscles. Cattle may push their head against a wall or present aggressive or anxious behaviour. Finally, the animal falls to the ground, pedalling and exhibiting opisthotonos, nystagmus and chewing movements. The animal usually dies during or following such a nervous attack.

Subacute heartwater with less pronounced signs, and peracute heartwater with sudden death, can also occur, according to the breed of ruminant and to the strain of *Cowdria*.

The most common macroscopic lesions are hydropericardium, hydrothorax, pulmonary oedema, intestinal congestion, oedema of the mediastinal and bronchial lymph nodes (4), petechiae on the epicardium and endocardium, congestion of the brain, and moderate splenomegaly (1).

A tentative diagnosis of heartwater is based on the presence of *Amblyomma* vectors, of clinical nervous signs, and of transudates in the pericardium and thorax at post-mortem examination.

Extensive recent reviews are available (4, 7, 34).

1. Identification of the agent

Typical colonies of *C. ruminantium* can be observed in brain smears made after death.

The tedious task of opening the cranium is not necessary. One alternative method (29) is to cut off the head in front of the first cervical vertebra. Then, a curette is introduced through the foramen magnum, between the medulla and the meninges. The curette is turned over towards the brain and removed with a piece of cerebellum. Another simple method consists of making a hole in the skull with a hammer and a large nail and aspirating a sample of brain cortex with a needle attached to a syringe, using negative pressure (20). These methods also lessen the danger to the operator in cases where the nervous signs have been caused by rabies.

In the live animal, a brain biopsy may be obtained (31) aseptically and harmlessly after local anaesthesia, although with difficulty and appropriate restraint with large and especially with horned animals. Colonies of *Cowdria* are observed during the febrile period. This method is useful for experimental studies, but not suitable for routine diagnosis.

Colonies of *Cowdria* are still present 48 hours after death in a brain that has been stored at room temperature, and for up to 34 days in a brain that has been stored in a refrigerator (6, 33).

A small fragment of grey matter (approximately the size of a match head) is placed on a microscope slide, crushed by another slide and, while maintaining pressure, the slides are drawn over each other lengthwise to produce a single layer of cells. The slides are air-dried, fixed in methanol, stained with Giemsa diluted with Sörensen buffer (2.54 g KH_2PO_4; 8.55 g $Na_2HPO_4.H_2O$; *q.s.* to 5 litres with distilled water), pH 7.2, and washed with tap water. Fast Giemsa stains give quicker results, but the colour contrast is usually poorer (DiffQuick, RAL555, Field's stain, CAM's Quick stain).

The slides are examined under a microscope at a low magnification (×10 objective) to locate the cerebral capillaries. An oil-immersion lens with a magnification of at least ×50 is useful for identifying the colonies of rickettsias. Experience is required to identify *Cowdria* colonies and to differentiate them from other haemoparasites *(Babesia bovis)*, certain blood cells (thrombocytes, granulocytes), normal subcellular structures (mitochondria, mast cell granules), or stain artefacts (stain precipitates), etc. The specificity of the reading can be improved by staining formalin-fixed brain sections using immunoperoxidase techniques (11).

Cowdria colonies are formed by clusters of granules (0.2–0.5 µm), sometimes arranged in the shape of a ring or a horseshoe (1–3 µm), and that are placed close to the nucleus inside the endothelial cell (8). The granules can be scanty, particularly in peracute cases, but they are always present in the brain of an animal that died from heartwater. However, if the animal has been specifically treated 48 hours before, the granules of *Cowdria* tend to fuse making the diagnosis very difficult, and sometimes impossible.

Fresh whole blood collected from suspect animals can be inoculated intravenously into a susceptible sheep or goat. The development of clinical signs and the demonstration of *Cowdria* in the brain of the inoculated ruminant is diagnostic for heartwater.

Transmission electron microscopy showed that the *Cowdria* organisms develop inside a vacuole-like structure, which is surrounded by a membrane in the endothelial cell's cytoplasm (27). Each organism is enclosed by a double membrane. Within the vacuole-like structure, *Cowdria* electron-dense (elementary bodies) as well as intermediate reticulate forms are identified.

a) Isolation of *Cowdria ruminantium* using *in-vitro* culture

Isolation of *C. ruminantium* in cell culture is not the first choice to confirm the diagnosis of cowdriosis, as it is a time-consuming laboratory procedure, although numerous cell lines support growth. However, *Cowdria* isolation is necessary for typing the strains present in a region for the purpose of vaccination programmes. *Cowdria* can be isolated from the blood of reacting animals by cultivation on ruminant endothelial cells. Endothelial cells from umbilical cord, aorta, or the pulmonary artery of different ruminant species (cattle, goat, sheep) are used most often for isolation, although other endothelial cell types (brain capillaries, circulating endothelial cells, etc.) have been described for the routine culture of the microorganism. Endothelial cell lines from sable, eland, buffalo, kudo and bush pig can also be used to grow *C. ruminantium* (30). No standard cell line has yet been designated for isolation.

- **Isolation procedure**

i) The blood of the reacting animal is collected in anticoagulant (heparin or sodium citrate) and diluted 1/2 in the culture medium consisting of Glasgow minimal essential medium (MEM) supplemented with 10% fetal bovine serum, tryptose phosphate broth, 200 mM L-glutamin, and antibiotics if necessary (penicillin 100 international units/ml, streptomycin 100 µg/ml).

ii) The culture medium is poured off the endothelial cell monolayer, and infective blood (approximately 2 ml for a 25 cm^2 flask) is added. The flask is incubated at 37°C on a rocking platform for 2 hours.

iii) After incubation, the blood is poured off and the monolayer is gently washed three times with prewarmed culture medium. Fresh culture medium is added and the flask is incubated at 37°C. The medium is changed twice weekly.

(The use of plasma instead of blood is more efficient when taken from an animal with a febrile reaction >41°C. In this case, steps ii and iii above may be replaced with the following:

- Seed 4 ml of plasma on to a susceptible endothelial cell culture and incubate for 1 hour at 37°C on a rocking platform.
- Wash off plasma with growth medium and then add 5 ml of growth medium (per 25 cm^3 flask) and observe for development of CPE.)

iv) The monolayer is inspected regularly for the appearance of small plaques of cell lysis. The first plaques generally appear after about 2 weeks. Passaging on uninfected cell monolayers is performed when the lysis reaches 80% of the cell layer. The remaining cells are stained with eosin–methylene blue and examined microscopically for the presence of *C. ruminantium* morulae. Alternatively, cells can be stained by an indirect fluorescent antibody (IFA) test or an immunoperoxidase test using a *Cowdria*-specific antiserum.

b) Isolation of *Cowdria ruminantium* using *in-vivo* culture

It is feasible to assess the presence of heartwater in a herd, a region or a country, or to isolate a strain of *Cowdria*, by inoculating blood or tick supernatant into a susceptible animal (3). Blood from individual animals, or pooled blood, is injected slowly at a dose of 10–100 ml intravenously into a susceptible sheep or goat. Another method consists of collecting and homogenising adult *Amblyomma* ticks, and after centrifuging the homogenate, inoculating the resulting supernatant. The latter method is more sensitive because the concentration of *Cowdria* is higher in the tick than in the blood. It should be remembered that the tick infection rate determined by this method can be as low as 1% (7), therefore, to detect an infection, at least 100 ticks are needed and as many as possible should be used. In both cases, the inoculum with 10% dimethyl suphoxide can be stored in liquid nitrogen for several years. Note that inoculation of tick homogenates into susceptible animals may cause anaphylaxis, which can be prevented by the simultaneous administration of adrenaline. The development of clinical signs and the demonstration of *Cowdria* in the brain of the inoculated ruminant is diagnostic for heartwater.

2. Molecular methods

A genomic DNA fragment specific for *C. ruminantium* has been cloned and used as a nucleic acid probe (37). It recognises all strains of *C. ruminantium* tested so far. This probe, designated pCS20, readily detects infection in clinically ill animals and experimentally infected *Amblyomma* ticks. However, it is not sufficiently sensitive to detect most carrier animals and/or low level infections in ticks. The pCS20 probe proved nevertheless to be more sensitive than 16S and MAP1 (major antigenic protein 1) probes for the detection of *C. ruminantium* in ticks when hybridised on a polymerase chain reaction (PCR)-amplified product of the homologous DNA fragment (2).

Two primers – AB128 and AB129 – have been designed from the DNA sequence of the pCS20 probe (19) for use in a PCR; this latter has been shown to have a sensitivity 350-fold more than the nucleic acid probe (15). It has a sensitivity and specificity of 98% and detects all 37 strains of *C. ruminantium* from all endemic areas. An easier to use PCR/enzyme-linked immunosorbent assay (ELISA) has also been described (26) with similar performance characteristics. Low levels of infection in animals and in ticks fed on carrier animals are detected by PCR, while hybridisation reaction with pCS20 probe usually remains negative (26). Nevertheless, although highly effective in detecting infection in ticks, this PCR appears to have significantly less ability to detect infection in ruminants. In one study (18) only between 3.3 and 26.7% of animals were positive whereas almost 100% of them had been infected with *Cowdria*.

Primers 32F1 and 32R1 designed from the sequence of the major antigenic protein gene (MAP1) of *C. ruminantium* were successfully used in a PCR to detect the pathogen in blood and bone marrow of carrier sheep and wild African ungulates (14).

- **Reading the results**

PCR is the molecular method of choice for the diagnosis of cowdriosis because it is easier to perform and more sensitive than DNA probes. With all PCRs, however, care must be taken to ensure that no cross-contamination occurs between samples. Negative and positive controls must be included in each test. As heartwater serology has several limitations (see below), the PCR could be used to confirm serological results when, for example, seronegative animals originating from an endemic area must be translocated to a heartwater-free area at risk (presence of potential vectors). However, despite promising experimental results in detecting asymptomatic carriers, no systematic comparison of the different PCR tests has been completed to identify the most sensitive one. Also, there is little available information on the reliability of carrier detection by PCR, and further research is needed before a standard test with known sensitivity can be designed. At present, PCR appears to be more reliable in detecting infection in ticks, and this could have epidemiological value in determining the geographical distribution of *Cowdria*.

3. Serological tests

Various serological tests for diagnosing heartwater have been described: an IFA test with *C.-ruminantium*-infected endothelial cell culture as antigen (CIFA test), indirect ELISA, a competitive ELISA (C-ELISA), and a Western blot. The IFA test using *C.-ruminantium*-infected mouse peritoneal macrophages (MIFA) is now seldom used.

One drawback of all of these tests is the detection of false-positive reactions due to common antigenic determinants between the *C. ruminantium* MAP1 and the presence of similar proteins in several *Ehrlichia* species. Almost all of these tests are no longer used for epidemiology or diagnosis. The CIFA test is still used in some places, but care must be taken when interpreting the results because of the problem of false-positive reactions.

To overcome the problem of cross-reactions with *Ehrlichia*, two ELISAs based on a recombinant MAP1 antigen (12, 35) have been developed. The first is an indirect ELISA that uses an immunogenic region of the MAP1 protein – called MAP1-B – that gives far fewer cross-reactions with *Ehrlichia spp.* (MAP1-B ELISA) (36). The second is a competitive ELISA that uses the MAP1 gene cloned in the baculovirus and monoclonal antibodies (MAbs) raised against the MAP1 protein (MAP1 C-ELISA) (13). Both tests have dramatically improved specificity, but they still show some reactivity with high titre sera against *E. canis*, *E. chaffeensis* and an unclassified white-tailed deer agent.

a) Indirect fluorescent antibody test with infected endothelial cell tissue culture as antigen (CIFA test) (23)

To prepare the antigen, a *C. ruminantium* strain is cultivated in ruminant endothelial cell cultures. When most cells are lysed, the remaining adherent cells are scraped and mixed with the supernatant. The cells are centrifuged three times with PBS at 200 ***g*** for 10 minutes. Of the washed cell suspension, 10 µl is placed in every well of an immunofluorescence slide. The antigen slides are dried, fixed in acetone and stored at –20°C.

- **Test procedure**

i) The sera to be tested are diluted 1/20 in PBS, added to the antigen wells and incubated for 30 minutes in a humid chamber at 37°C.

ii) The slides are then washed in buffer for 15 minutes.

iii) The appropriate anti-species conjugate, usually diluted 1/60, is added to cover the wells. The slides are incubated again for 30 minutes at 37°C.

iv) After a second washing, the slides are mounted in glycerine buffer under a cover-slip and examined under a fluorescence microscope.

v) Control positive and negative sera are included on each slide.

b) Indirect fluorescent antibody test with infected mouse peritoneal macrophages as antigen (MIFA test) (10)

Mice are injected intraperitoneally with 0.2 ml of Kümm strain stabilate stored in liquid nitrogen. Clinical signs – ruffled hair coat and lethargy – appear 12 days later, and several mice may die. The surviving mice are killed. The peritoneal cells containing some macrophages with morula colonies are removed by injecting 2 ml of phosphate buffered saline (PBS) into the peritoneal cavity and withdrawing the fluid. The pooled peritoneal fluid is centrifuged for 5 minutes at 2000 ***g*** and the pellet is resuspended in 0.3 ml of buffer.

A droplet of the cell suspension is placed in every well of an immunofluorescence slide to form a monolayer of cells. The antigen slides are air-dried, wrapped in tissue and tinfoil and stored: at 4°C for 21 days, at –18°C for 6–9 months, or at or under –70°C for over 1 year.

Just before use, the antigen slides are plunged into cold methanol for 1–3 seconds. A thick felt pen is used to separate the wells to avoid confluence of sera between wells.

The IFA procedure is the same as the previous test, but the initial serum dilution is 1/80.

c) MAP1-B enzyme-linked immunosorbent assay (36)

Using the vector pQE9, the PCR fragment MAP1-F2R2, which encodes the amino acids 47–152 of the MAP1 protein including the immunogenic region MAP1-B, is expressed in *Escherichia coli* M15[pREP4] as a fusion protein containing six additional histidine residues. The recombinant MAP1-B is purified using Ni^{2+}-NTA agarose (nitrilotriacetic acid agarose) under denaturing conditions as described by the manufacturer[1]. The antigen is preserved at 4°C and each batch is titrated.

The antigen is diluted at 0.5 µg/ml in 0.05 M sodium carbonate buffer, pH 9.6, and immobilised on to polystyrene plates by incubation for 1 hour at 37°C, and stored at 4°C until use.

1 Qiagen, Max-Volmer-Straße 4, 40724 Hilden, Germany.

- **Test procedure**

i) Plates are blocked for 30 minutes by adding 100 µl per well of 0.1 M PBS, pH 7.2, supplemented with 0.1% Tween 20 and 3% nonfat dry milk (PBSTM).

ii) The plates are washed three times with PBS supplemented with 0.1% Tween 20 (PBST) and twice with distilled water.

iii) 100 µl of test serum diluted 1/100 in PBSTM is added in duplicate to wells, which are then incubated for 1 hour at 37°C.

iv) Plates are washed three times in PBST and twice in distilled water.

v) Horseradish-peroxidase-conjugated anti-species IgG optimally diluted in PBSTM is added at 100 µl per well and the plate is incubated for 1 hour at 37°C.

vi) After washing as in step iv, each well is filled with 100 µl of 0.1 M citrate buffer, pH 5.5, containing 0.5 mg/ml orthophenylene-diamine and 3 µl/ml of 9% H_2O_2.

vii) The reaction is stopped after 30 minutes of incubation at room temperature by adding 50 µl of 2 N H_2SO_4. Absorbance is read at 495 nm. Positive and negative controls are included in each plate.

d) **MAP1 competitive enzyme-linked immunosorbent assay (13)**

Recombinant MAP1 antigen is prepared as follows: 8-day-old *Trichoplusia ni* insect larvae are infected by a baculovirus expressing the *map1* gene and moribund larvae are homogenised (10% [w/v]) in PBS supplemented with 0.001% (v/v) Triton X-100.

Anti-MAP1 MAb is prepared as follows: spleen cells of BALB/C mice previously inoculated with larval homogenate are fused to SP2/0 cells. Supernatant fluids from hybridoma cell cultures are screened for reactivity with MAP1 by immunoblotting and immunoperoxidase methods. A reactive cell culture is subcloned, isotyped and subsequently used for ascites production.

After a further 1/800 (v/v) dilution in PBS, the antigen is immobilised on to polystyrene plates (Nunc-Immuno Plates PolySorp) by incubation overnight at 4°C, and stored at –70°C

- **Test procedure**

i) Prior to use, the plates are blocked for 30 minutes by adding 100 µl per well of PBS, pH 7.2, supplemented with 0.05% Tween 20 and 5% nonfat dry milk.

ii) Plates are washed three times with PBS–Tween and 50 µl/well of test serum diluted 1/50 in PBS supplemented with 0.05% Tween 20 and 1% nonfat dry milk (PBSTM) is added in duplicate and the plates are incubated for 30 minutes at 37°C.

iii) Without an intervening washing step, 75 µl/well of the MAb diluted 1/4000 (v/v) in PBSTM is added and the plates are incubated for another 30 minutes at 37°C.

iv) Plates are washed three times in PBS–Tween and horseradish-peroxidase-conjugated anti-mouse IgG optimally diluted in PBSTM is added at 50 µl per well. The plate is incubated for 1 hour at 37°C.

v) After three washings as before, 100 µl of 0.1 M citrate buffer, pH 5.5, containing 0.5 mg/ml O-phenylene diamine and 3 µl/ml of 9% H_2O_2 are added to each well. After 30 minutes of incubation at room temperature in the dark, the reaction is stopped by adding 50 µl of 2N H_2SO_4 and the absorbance is read at 495 nm. Positive and negative controls are included in each plate.

- **Reading the results**

All serological tests based on nonrecombinant *Cowdria* antigens, such as CIFA, ELISAs, and Western blotting, are still used for experimental studies but are no longer used for seroepidemiological studies. The tests have been compared and applied to known positive and negative sera to *C. ruminantium* (9). No false-positive reactions were observed with any of the tests against the known negative sera. There is good correlation among tests, but the specificity of all five tests is low because cross-reactions occur with certain *Ehrlichia* spp.

The interpretation of results of the various tests applied to field surveys is thus difficult in areas where *Ehrlichia* infections occur in ruminants, which is probably the case in most of the heartwater-endemic regions of Africa. This situation has also been demonstrated in farms without *Amblyomma* but infected with tick species not known to be vectors of *C. ruminantium* (28).

Both the MAP1-B ELISA and the MAP1 C-ELISA, although still under evaluation in Africa, have shown a high specificity after evaluation in 3000 ruminant sera (goat, sheep and cattle) collected from 14 *A.-variegatum*-infested islands of the Lesser Antilles, among which only three are known to be infected by *C. ruminantium* (24). Overall specificity calculated from the 11 heartwater-free islands was 98.5% and 99.4% for the MAP1 C-ELISA and the MAP1-B ELISA, respectively. Although a few false-positive sera are still found, these tests are likely to solve much of the specificity problems of the earlier serological tests.

Serological tests are useful for the assessment of heartwater infection in vaccinated animals. The tests can also be used to screen animals prior to importation into heartwater-free areas. However, antibodies are maintained at detectable levels in naturally infected domestic ruminants for a few months only in the absence of new infective contact. Circulating antibodies disappear more rapidly in cattle than in small ruminants. It is possible that serologically negative animals may still be carriers of infection. Serology should therefore be regarded as a diagnostic method to be applied at the herd level, not at the individual level.

Molecular methods, such as PCR assay, could potentially help in detecting carrier animals without detectable antibodies, but this approach has not yet been evaluated extensively.

B. REQUIREMENTS FOR VACCINES AND DIAGNOSTIC BIOLOGICALS

Although promising research results have been obtained with attenuated and inactivated organisms, no vaccines are available at present. The only method of immunisation against heartwater remains the 'infection and treatment' method using infected blood or homogenised pre-fed infected ticks followed by treatment of reacting animals with tetracyclin. This method is still in use in several areas. However, it is likely to be replaced soon by vaccination with preparations of inactivated *C. ruminantium* elementary bodies emulsified in oil adjuvants, following the demonstration that susceptible goats can be protected by inactivated *Cowdria* in Freund's adjuvant (21). This vaccine also protected against challenge in sheep (16) using different strains of *C. ruminantium,* and in cattle (32) using the same strain as in goats. A first generation vaccine preparation of inactivated *Cowdria* in Montanide ISA 50 oil adjuvant (adjuvant licensed for animal use) was shown to be similarly effective to the Freund's adjuvant preparation on laboratory challenge of immunised goats (22).

Animals can be immunised with two subcutaneous injections of 250 µg of antigen emulsified (50/50) in Montanide ISA 50 adjuvant in a volume of 2 ml.

Evaluation of an inactivated vaccine adjuvanted with ISA50 has protected sheep against natural field challenge in Zimbabwe (17). Further studies on optimisation of vaccine production, quality control and efficiency in the different target species are being conducted.

REFERENCES

1. ALEXANDER R.A. (1931). Heartwater – The present state of our knowledge of the disease. *In:* 17th Report of the Director of Veterinary Services and Animal Industry, Union of South Africa, 89–150.

2. ALLSOPP M.T., HATTINGH C.M., VOGEL S.W. & ALLSOPP B.A. (1998). Comparative evaluation of 16S map 1 and pCS20 probes for the detection of *Cowdria* and *Ehrlichia* species in ticks. *Ann. N.Y. Acad. Sci.*, **849**, 78–84.

3. BARRE N., CAMUS E., BIRNIE E., BURRIDGE M.J. & UILENBERG G. (1984). Setting up a method for surveying the distribution of cowdriosis (heartwater) in the Caribbean. *In:* Proceedings of the 13th World Congress on Diseases of Cattle, Durban, South Africa, 1, 536–541.

4. BEZUIDENHOUT J.D., PROZESKY L., DU PLESSIS J.L. & VAN AMSTEL S.R. (1994). Chapter 35: Heartwater. *In:* Infectious Diseases of Livestock, with special reference to Southern Africa, Coetzer J.A.W., Thomson G.R., Tustin R.C. & Kriek N.P.J., eds. Oxford University Press, Oxford, UK, Vol. 1, 351–370.

5. BIRNIE E.F., BURRIDGE M.J., CAMUS E. & BARRE N. (1985). Heartwater in the Caribbean: isolation of *Cowdria ruminantium* from Antigua. *Vet. Rec.*, **116**, 121–123.

6. CAMUS E. & BARRE N. (1988). Le diagnostic de la cowdriose à partir d'écrasement de cerveau. *Rev. Elev. Med. Vet. Pays Trop.*, **41**, 247–252.

7. CAMUS E., BARRE N., MARTINEZ D. & UILENBERG G. (1996). Heartwater (cowdriosis). A Review, Second Edition. Office International des Epizooties, Paris, France, pp. 177.

8. COWDRY E.V. (1925). Studies on the etiology of heartwater. I. Observation of a *Rickettsia, Rickettsia ruminantium* (n.sp.), in the tissues of infected animals. *J. Exp. Med.*, **42**, 231–252.

9. DU PLESSIS J.L., BEZUIDENHOUT J.D., BRETT M.S., CAMUS E., JONGEJAN F., MAHAN S.M. & MARTINEZ D. (1993). The serodiagnosis of heartwater: a comparison of five tests. *Rev. Elev. Med. Vet. Pays Trop.*, **46**, 123–129.

10. DU PLESSIS J.L. & MALAN L. (1987). The application of the indirect fluorescent antibody test in research on heartwater. *Onderstepoort J. Vet. Res.*, **54**, 319–325.

11. JARDINE J.E., VOGEL S.W., VAN KLEEF M. & VAN DER LUGT J.J. (1995). Immunohistochemical identification of *Cowdria ruminantium* in formalin-fixed tissue sections from mice, sheep, cattle and goats. *Onderstepoort J. Vet. Res.*, **62**, 277–280.

12. JONGEJAN F. & THIELEMANS J.C. (1989). Identification of an immunodominant antigenically conserved 32-kilodalton protein from *Cowdria ruminantium. Infect. Immun.*, **57**, 3243–3246.

13. KATZ J.B., DEWALD R., DAWSON J.E., CAMUS E., MARTINEZ D. & MONDRY R. (1997). Development and evaluation of a recombinant antigen, monoclonal antibody-based competitive ELISA for heartwater serodiagnosis. *J. Vet. Diagn. Invest.*, **9**, 130–135.

14. KOCK N.D., VAN VLIET A.H.M., CHARLTON K. & JONGEJAN F. (1995). Detection of *Cowdria ruminantium* in blood and bone marrow samples from clinically normal, free-ranging Zimbabwean ungulates. *J. Clin. Microbiol.*, **33**, 2501–2504.

15. MAHAN S.M. (1995). Review of the molecular biology of *Cowdria ruminantium. Vet. Parasitol.*, **57**, 51–56.

16. MAHAN S.M., ANDREW H.R., N. TEBELE, BURRIDGE M.J. & BARBET A. (1995). Immunisation of sheep against heartwater with inactivated *Cowdria ruminantium. Res. Vet. Sci.*, **58**, 46–49.

17. MAHAN S.M., KUMBULA D., BURRIDGE M.J. & BARBET A.F. (1998). The inactivated *Cowdria ruminantium* vaccine for heartwater protects against heterologous strains and against laboratory and field tick challenge. *Vaccine*, **16**, 1203–1211.

18. MAHAN S.M., PETER T.F., SIMBI B.H. & BURRIDGE M.J. (1998). PCR detection of *Cowdria ruminantium* infection in ticks and animals from heartwater-endemic regions of Zimbabwe. *Ann. N.Y. Acad. Sci.*, **849**, 85–87.

19. MAHAN S.M., WAGHELA S.D., MCGUIRE T.C., RURANGIRWA F.R., WASSINK L.A. & BARBET A.F. (1992). A cloned DNA probe for *Cowdria ruminantium* hybridizes with eight heartwater strains and detects infected sheep. *J. Clin. Microbiol.*, **30**, 981–986.

20. MALIKA J., LAWRENCE J.A., WHITELAND A.P. & KAFUWA P.T. (1992). A simple method for collection of brain samples for the diagnosis of heartwater. *Bull. Anim. Health Prod. Afr.*, **40**, 157–159.

21. MARTINEZ D., MAILLARD J.C., COISNE S., SHEIKBOUDOU C & BENSAID A. (1994). protection of goats against heartwater acquired by immunisation with inactivated elementary bodies of *Cowdria ruminantium. Vet. Immunol. Immunopathol.*, **41**, 153–163.

22. MARTINEZ D., PEREZ J.M., SHEIKBOUDOU C., DEBUS A. & BENSAID A. (1996). Comparative efficacy of Freund's and Montanide ISA 50 adjuvants for the immunisation of goats against heartwater with inactivated *Cowdria ruminantium. Vet. Parasitol.*, **67**, 175–184.

23. MARTINEZ D., SWINKELS J., CAMUS E. & JONGEJAN F. (1990). Comparaison de trois antigènes pour le sérodiagnostic de la cowdriose par immunofluorescence indirecte. *Rev. Elev. Med. Vet. Pays Trop.*, **43**, 159–166.

24. MONDRY R., MARTINEZ D., CAMUS E., LIEBISCH A., KATZ J.B., DEWALD R., VAN VLIET A.H.M. & JONGEJAN F. (1998). Validation and comparison of three enzyme-linked immunosorbent assays for the detection of antibodies to *Cowdria ruminantium* infection. *Ann. N.Y. Acad. Sci.*, **849**, 262–272.

25. PERREAU P., MOREL P.C., BARRE N. & DURAND P. (1980). Existence de la cowdriose (heartwater) à *Cowdria ruminantium* chez les ruminants des Antilles françaises (La Guadeloupe) et des Macareignes (La Réunion et Ile Maurice). *Rev. Elev. Med. Vet. Pays Trop.*, **33**, 21–22.

26. PETER T.F., DEEM S.L., BARBET A.F., NORVAL R.A.I., SIMBI B.H., KELLY P.J. & MAHAN S.M. (1995). Development and evaluation of PCR assay for detection of low levels of *Cowdria ruminantium* infection in *Amblyomma* ticks not detected by DNA probe. *J. Clin. Microbiol.*, **33**, 166–172.

27. PIENAAR J.G. (1970). Electron microscopy of *Cowdria* (*Rickettsia*) *ruminantium* (Cowdry, 1926) in the endothelial cells of the vertebrate host. *Onderstepoort J. Vet. Res.*, **37**, 67–78.

28. SAVADYE D.T., KELLY P.J. & MAHAN S. (1998). Evidence to show that an agent cross-reacts serologically with *Cowdria ruminantium* in Zimbabwe is transmitted by ticks. *Exp. Appl. Acarol.*, **22**, 111–122.

29. SCHREUDER B.E.C. (1980). A simple technique for the collection of brain samples for the diagnosis of heartwater. *Trop. Anim. Health Prod.*, **12**, 25–29.

30. SMITH G.E., ANDERSON E.C., BURRIDGE M.J., PETER T.F. & MAHAN S.M. (1998). Growth of *Cowdria ruminantium* in tissue culture cell lines from wild African mammals. *J. Wildl. Dis.*, **34**, 297–304.

31. SYNGE B.A. (1978). Brain biopsy for the diagnosis of heartwater. *Trop. Anim. Health Prod.*, **10**, 45–48.

32. TOTTE P., MCKEEVER D., MARTINEZ D. & BENSAID D. (1997). Analysis of T-cell responses in cattle immunised against heartwater by vaccination with killed elementary bodies of *Cowdria ruminantium. Infect. Immun.*, **65**, 236–241.

33. UILENBERG G. (1971). Etudes sur la cowdriose à Madagascar. Première partie. *Rev. Elev. Med. Vet. Pays Trop.*, **24**, 239–249.

34. UILENBERG G. & CAMUS E. (1993). Heartwater (cowdriosis). *In:* Rickettsial and Chlamydial Diseases of Domestic Animals, Woldehiwet Z. & Ristic M., eds. Pergamon Press, Oxford, UK, 293–332.

35. VAN VLIET A.H.M., JONGEJAN F., VAN KLEEF M. & VAN DER ZEIJST B.A.M. (1994). Molecular cloning, sequence analysis, and expression of the gene encoding the immunodominant 32-kilodalton protein of *Cowdria ruminantium. Infect. Immun.*, **62**, 1451–1456.

36. VAN VLIET A.H.M., VAN DER ZEIJST B.A.M., CAMUS E., MAHAN S.M., MARTINEZ D. & JONGEJAN F. (1995). Use of a specific immunogenic region on the *Cowdria ruminantium* MAP1 protein in a serological assay. *J. Clin. Microbiol.*, **33**, 2405–2410.

37. WAGHELA S.D., RURANGIRWA F.R., MAHAN S.M., YUNKER C.E., CRAWFORD T.B., BARBET A.F., BURRIDGE M.J. & MCGUIRE T.C.(1991). A cloned DNA probe identifies *Cowdria ruminantium* in *Amblyomma variegatum* ticks. *J. Clin. Microbiol.*, **29**, 2571–2577.

*
* *

CHAPTER 2.2.8.

NEW WORLD SCREWWORM (*Cochliomyia hominivorax*) and OLD WORLD SCREWWORM (*Chrysomya bezziana*)

SUMMARY

The New World screwworm[1] (NWS), Cochliomyia hominivorax *(Coquerel) and the Old World screwworm[1] (OWS),* Chrysomya bezziana *Villeneuve, are both obligate parasites of mammals during their larval stages. Both species are in the subfamily Chrysomyinae of the family Calliphoridae of the order Diptera (true flies). Larvae feeding on the skin and underlying tissues of the host cause a condition known as wound or traumatic myiasis, which can be fatal. Infestations are generally acquired at sites of previous wounding, due to natural causes or to animal husbandry practices, but they may also occur in the mucous membranes of body orifices.*

Female flies are attracted to wounds at the edges of which they lay an average of 175 (OWS) to 340 (NWS) eggs. The larvae emerge within 12–24 hours and immediately begin to feed, burrowing head-downwards into the wound. After growth involving two moults, the larvae leave the wound and drop to the ground into which they burrow to pupate. The duration of the life cycle is temperature dependent, being shorter at higher temperatures, and may be completed in under 3 weeks in the tropics.

Treatment is generally effected by application of organophosphorous insecticides into infested wounds, both to kill larvae and to provide a residual protection against reinfestation. Preventive measures include the spraying or dipping of susceptible livestock with organophosphorous compounds and, more recently, use of avermectins as subcutaneous injections to animals 'at risk'. Strict control of the movement of animals out of affected areas also acts as a preventive measure.

Identification of the agent: *The larvae of NWS and OWS can be easily confused with each other and with the larvae of other agents of myiasis. Accurate diagnosis involves the identification of larvae extracted from the deepest part of an infested wound. The mature, third instar larvae are most reliable for this purpose and those of NWS can be identified by their darkly pigmented dorsal tracheal trunks, extending from the twelfth segment forward to the tenth or ninth. This pigmentation is unique to the larvae of NWS among the species encountered in wound myiasis. Confirmation of OWS relies on the recognition of a characteristic combination of spinulation, the number of lobes on the anterior spiracles (4–6) and pigmentation of secondary tracheal trunks.*

In the adult stage, species in the genus Cochliomyia *may be separated from other genera involved in wound myiasis by confirmation of a body colour that is usually a metallic blue/green and with three dark longitudinal stripes always present on the thorax. The separation of NWS from the very similar* C. macellaria *and identification of adult OWS are discussed in this chapter.*

Serological tests: *At present there are no applicable serological tests, nor are they indicated in the identification of this disease. However, serology may have a future role in studies of the prevalence of myiasis.*

Requirements for vaccines and diagnostic biologicals: *There are no vaccines or biological products available except for the use of sterilised male flies in the sterile insect technique. In this technique, vast numbers of sterilised male flies are sequentially released into the environment*

1 In this chapter, the term 'New World' refers to the Americas and the term 'Old World' refers to Europe, Africa and Asia.

where their matings with wild females produce infertile eggs, leading to an initial population reduction and, progressively, eradication.

A. DIAGNOSTIC TECHNIQUES

The New World screwworm fly (NWS), *Cochliomyia hominivorax* (Coquerel) and the Old World screwworm fly, *Chrysomya bezziana* Villeneuve, are members of two genera of the subfamily Chrysomyinae of the Dipteran family Calliphoridae (blowflies). Both species are obligate parasites of mammals and, rarely, birds. Despite being in different genera and geographically separated, the two species have evolved in remarkable parallel. They have almost identical life histories because they fill identical parasitic niches in their geographical zones. The following discussion will relate to both species except where indicated.

Unlike most other species of blowfly, adult female screwworms do not lay their eggs on carrion. Instead, they lay them at the edges of wounds on living, injured mammals or at their body orifices. Virtually any wound is attractive, whether natural (from fighting, predators, thorns, disease, and/or tick and insect bites) or man made (from shearing, branding, castrating, de-horning, docking and/or ear-tagging). Commonly infested natural wounds are the navels of newborn animals and the vulval and perineal regions of their mothers, especially if traumatised. If eggs are deposited on mucous membranes, the larvae can invade natural body openings such as the nostrils and associated sinuses, the eye orbits, mouth, ears and genitalia.

Within 12–24 hours of the eggs being laid, larvae emerge and immediately begin to feed on the underlying tissues, burrowing gregariously head-downwards into the wound in a characteristic screwworm fashion. As they feed, tearing the tissue with their hook-like mouthparts, the wound is enlarged and deepened, resulting in extensive tissue destruction. Infested wounds often emit a characteristic odour, which can be the first indication that at least one animal in a group is infested. Although the odour is not always apparent to humans, it is obviously highly attractive to gravid females (12), which lay further batches of eggs so increasing the extent of the infestation. A severe infestation that is left untreated may result in the death of the host.

Following two moults, the larvae reach maturity about 5–7 days after hatching. They stop feeding and leave the wound, falling to the ground into which they burrow and pupariate. The pupa develops within the puparium, a barrel-shaped protective structure formed by hardening and darkening of the cuticle of the mature larva. On completion of development, adult flies usually emerge from the puparium in the morning and work their way up to the soil surface where they extend their wings for hardening prior to flight. Males become sexually mature and able to mate within 24 hours, but females mature their ovaries, become responsive towards males and mate only when about 3 days old. About 4 days after mating, female flies are ready to oviposit. They seek a suitable host and lay their eggs, all oriented in the same direction, firmly attached to each other and to the oviposition substrate. The numbers of eggs laid per batch varies depending on many factors (e.g. fly strain, disturbance during oviposition), but the average first batch has in the order of 175 eggs for OWS and 340 for NWS (27). Following the first egg batch, further batches are laid at intervals of 3–4 days (33). Adult flies live on average for 2–3 weeks in the field.

The rate of development of the immature stages is influenced by environmental and wound temperatures, being slower at low temperatures although true diapause does not occur. This effect is most pronounced in the pupal stage that can vary from 1 week to 2 months' duration depending on the season (16). Thus, the complete life cycle of NWS may take 2–3 months in cold weather (23), while in temperate conditions with an average air temperature of 22°C it is completed in about 24 days (16), and in tropical conditions of about 29°C it is completed in about 18 days (33).

The degree to which NWS and OWS can tolerate cold has had a major influence on their distributions, best documented for NWS. Historically, the range of NWS extended from the southern states of the United States of America (USA), through Mexico, Central America, the Caribbean islands and northern countries of South America to Uruguay, northern Chile and northern Argentina (14). This distribution contracted during the winter months but expanded during the summer months, producing a seasonality at its edges and year round populations in the central areas of its distribution - the New World tropics. Use of the sterile insect technique (SIT) in major programmes has resulted in eradication of NWS from the USA, Mexico (11), Curacao, Puerto Rico and the Virgin Islands and, in Central America, from Guatemala, Belize, Honduras and El Salvador. An eradication programme is continuing in Central America, in Nicaragua, Costa Rica and Panama. The first sterile flies were released in Panama in July 1998. The ultimate objective is to establish a barrier zone in Panama that will become the future northern limit of NWS in the Americas. A NWS eradication programme was also officially launched in Jamaica in July 1998, as part of a plan to eradicate the species from the entire Caribbean. Although NWS is a New World species, in 1988 it was detected in Libya in North Africa where it threatened to become firmly established. However, it was eradicated in 1991 by an intensive SIT campaign (8, 17).

The distribution of OWS is confined to the Old World as the name suggests, throughout much of Africa (from south of the Sahara to northern South Africa, although also reported from Algeria [1]), the Gulf countries, the Indian subcontinent, and South-East Asia (from southern China through the Malay peninsula and the Indonesian and Philippine islands to Papua New Guinea) (14, 27, 31, 35). The situation in the Gulf area and surrounding regions is dynamic with recent reports confirmed from Iran (22) and Iraq. The climatic requirements of the two screwworm species are very similar and their potential distributions, if unrestrained, would overlap considerably (31).

Organophosphorous insecticides, such as dichlofenthion, fenchlorphos and, in particular, coumaphos, are recommended for the treatment of wounds infested with OWS and NWS (10, 24, 29). They have the effect of expelling the larvae, which die on the ground. To provide residual protection against reinfestation, they must be applied at 2–3-day intervals until the wound has healed. The contents of individual wound treatment sachets, e.g. 5 g of 5% coumaphos (wettable powder), should be either sprinkled directly on to a wound or, more effectively, brushed into the wound as a paste after first being mixed with ordinary cooking oil (33 ml). Organophosphorous compounds may also be applied as aerosol sprays, in which marker dyes and bacteriostats are included, or as dusts, which are puffed into the wound from plastic squeeze bottles. Dichlofenthion is used in South America as a 1% aerosol to treat NWS cases and is also effective against OWS (24). Any larvae that die in the wound should be removed to prevent sepsis. Close attention should always be paid to the manufacturers' safety instructions.

Treatment and prevention of screwworm infestation can be achieved by spraying or dipping livestock with coumaphos (0.25% aqueous suspension of 50% wettable powder) or other organophosphorous insecticide at the maximum concentration prescribed for external parasite control. The effects of such treatment are twofold: first, the treatment kills larvae directly and provides residual protection; secondly, the treatment kills ticks and other external parasites, which means that there are fewer wounds available as sites for oviposition. Synthetic pyrethroids have potential for control of screwworm larvae in wounds, but there have been few reported trials of their effect on screwworms (e.g. Permethrin versus NWS, 25). Dipping or spraying of a group of animals would be indicated if any member of the group was found to be infested, or if animals were traversing or leaving an infested area, or following wound-inducing animal husbandry practices, e.g. shearing.

A single subcutaneous injection of ivermectin (200 µg/kg) was effective against OWS in preventing navel strike of newborn calves (24) and scrotal strike of castrated calves (28). Ivermectin also prevented re-strike of treated wounds of adult cattle. Early results suggested that ivermectin may be ineffective against NWS (Mackley & Brown in ref. 11), but more recent studies demonstrated that it produced a significant reduction in the incidence of navel and scrotal myiasis due to NWS (3). Abamectin (subcutaneous injection, 200 µg/kg) gave good, but not 100%, prevention of post-castration myiasis by NWS (2). Of particular note are the increasing number of publications reporting that a subcutaneous injection of doramectin (200 µg/kg) was 100% effective as a NWS prophylactic, preventing infestation of umbilical or castration wounds of calves and infestation of post-parturient cows, for at least 12–14 days post-treatment (20, 21). In one comparative trial of doramectin and ivermectin (both at 200 µg/kg subcutaneous injection), doramectin gave 100% protection from experimentally induced NWS myiasis up to 21 days post-treatment, and partial protection at 28 days, but ivermectin gave only incomplete protection from 2 hours post-treatment (19). There are early indications that fipronil (a phenyl-pyrazole) might be effective as a preventive of post-castration myiasis.

Indirect prevention of screwworm infestation includes the avoidance of wounding procedures at the time of year when screwworm are numerous, the careful handling of livestock to minimise wounding, the removal of sharp objects (e.g. wire strands) from livestock pens and the use of measures to reduce other wound-causing parasites, in particular ticks, e.g. by dipping and by insecticide-impregnated ear-tags.

To prevent the spread of the disease beyond present limits, strict observation of the requirements for international trade, as set out in the OIE *International Animal Health Code*, is necessary.

1. Identification of the agent

The identification of the eggs and first instar larvae of the agents of myiasis is difficult and as these stages are seldom encountered during the collection of specimens from infested wounds, they will not be considered further here.

Larvae being collected for diagnosis should be removed from the deepest part of the wound to reduce the possibility of collecting non-screwworm species, which may infest the shallower parts of the wound. Living specimens should first be examined for pigmentation of the dorsal tracheal trunks (Figure 1) and then be preserved in 80% ethanol and returned to the laboratory for examination under a dissecting microscope at up to ×50 magnification (for further techniques see refs 7, 13, 26, 35). Optimal preservation of larvae, in their natural extended state, is made by killing them by brief immersion in near-boiling water before placement in 80% ethanol.

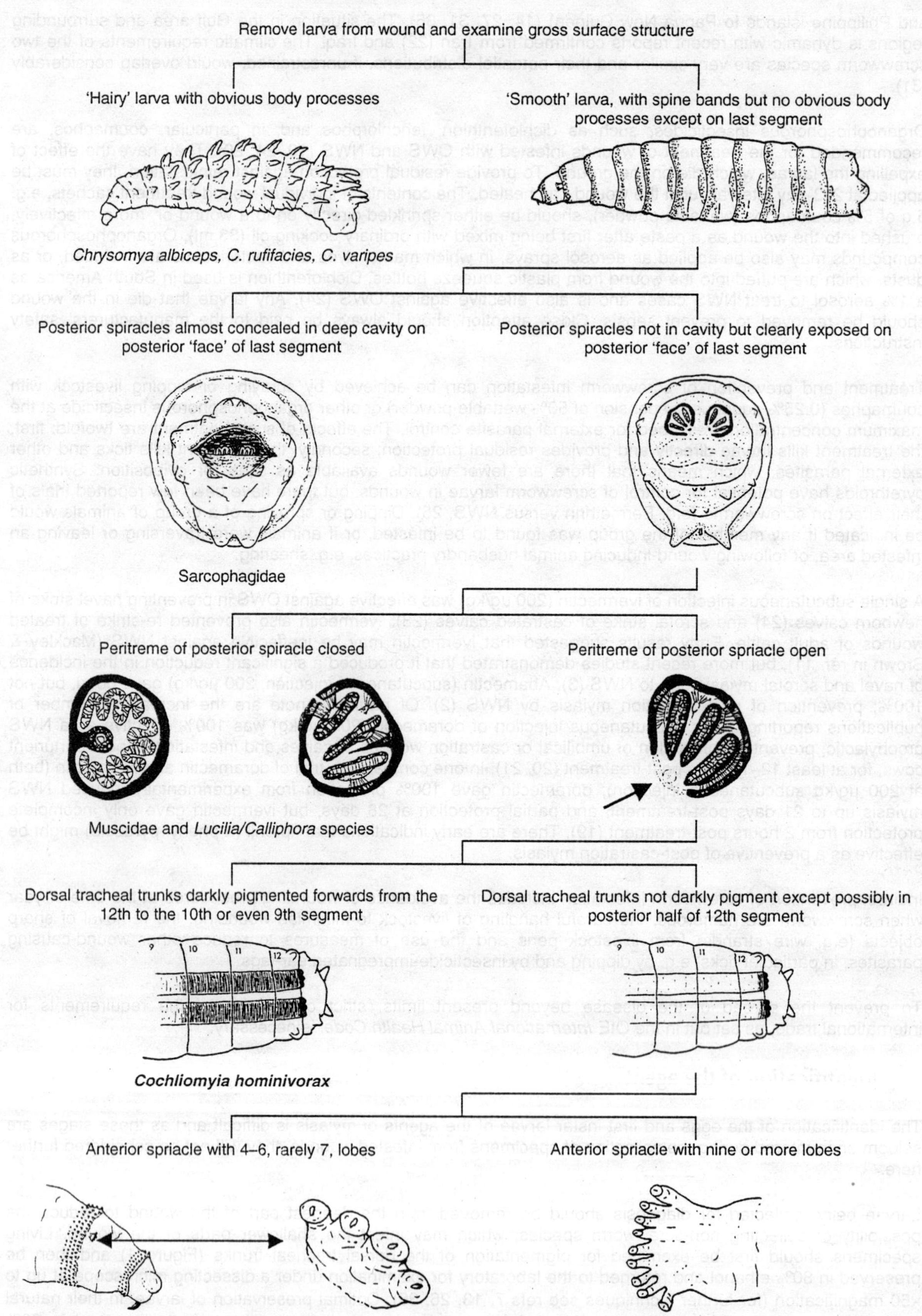

Fig. 1. *Key for the diagnosis of third instar larvae of* Cochliomyia hominivorax *and* Chrysomya bezziana *from cases of wound myiasis.*

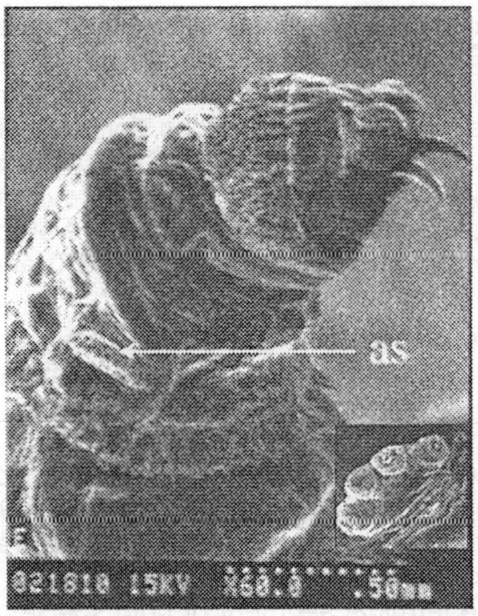

***Fig. 2.** Head and first two thoracic segments of third instar larva of* Cochliomyia hominovorax *(as = anterior spiracle; inset is the anterior spiracle of* Chrysomya bezziana*).*

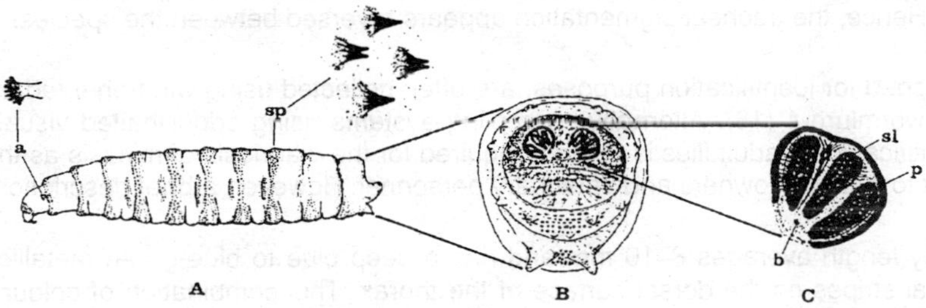

***Fig. 3.** Characteristics of third instar larva of* Cochliomyia hominivorax*: (A) whole larva, lateral aspect; (B) posterior face of terminal segment; (C) posterior spiracular plate; a = anterior spiracle; b = button adjacent to opening in peritreme; p = peritreme; sl = spiracular slit; sp = spines). (After Laake* et al. *[16].)*

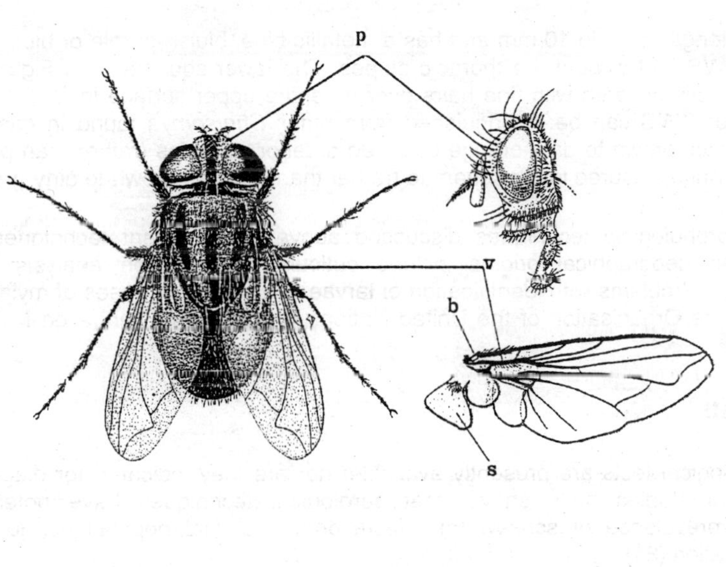

***Fig. 4.** Characteristics of adult* Cochliomyia hominivorax*; note longitudinal thoracic stripes; b = basicosta; p = fronto-orbital plate, indicated from above on whole* C. hominivorax *and laterally on head of typical calliphorid fly; s = lower squama, surface hairless except at base; v = stem vein with hairs on dorsal posterior surface.*

Second instar larvae: Second instar larvae have only two slits in the posterior spiracles compared with the three slits of the third instar larvae (Figures 2 and 3). Second instars of NWS can be diagnosed by the presence of dark pigmentation of the dorsal tracheal trunks for over half their length in the terminal segment. Other species have less marked pigmentation of the dorsal tracheal trunks, for example, these trunks are pigmented for no more than one-third of their length in the twelfth segment of OWS. The anterior spiracles of the second instar NWS have from seven to nine branches compared with about four branches in OWS (15). More positive identification may be gained by rearing living larvae to third instar on a medium of 1 litre water, 1 kg ground meat, 70 g dried blood and 1.5 ml formalin, mixed and maintained at 35–38°C and 70% relative humidity.

Third instar larvae: Third instar larvae of both NWS and OWS have a robust, typical maggot shape, with a cylindrical body from 6 to 17 mm long and from 1.1 to 3.6 mm in diameter, pointed at the anterior end (16, 26). Fully mature larvae of NWS develop a reddish tinge over the creamy white colour of younger larvae. Both screwworm species have prominent rings of spines around the body and these spines appear large and conspicuous under a microscope when compared with non-screwworm species, the longest averaging 130 µm. In NWS the spines can be either single or double pointed, but in OWS they are always single pointed. The anterior spiracles of NWS each have from six to eleven well separated branches, but usually from seven to nine (Figure 2). In OWS, the anterior spiracles each have from three to seven branches, but usually from four to six (Figure 2). On the posterior face of the terminal segment of both species, the posterior spiracles have a darkly pigmented, incomplete peritreme enclosing three straight, slightly oval-shaped slits, which point towards the break in the peritreme. The diagnostic features mentioned above are illustrated in Figure 3. Of greatest diagnostic value are the dorsal tracheal trunks, which extend forwards from the posterior spiracles and are darkly pigmented up to the tenth or ninth segment in NWS (Figure 1; see also refs 7, 9, 13, 14, 26, 35 for identification keys). This is seen most easily in living larvae. Those in preservative may need dissection to remove opaque tissues covering the trunks. The dorsal tracheal trunks of OWS are darkly pigmented only in the twelfth segment, but in this species the trachea branching off the dorsal tracheal trunks are pigmented, whereas they are not pigmented in NWS. Hence, the tracheal pigmentation appears reversed between the species.

Adult: Adult flies, needed for identification purposes, are often collected using wind-oriented traps (4) baited with a synthetic odour, swormlure-4 (18). Alternative sampling systems using odour-baited visual targets are being developed (12). Identification of adult flies is seldom required for the diagnosis of myiasis as the larval stages are those most apparent to livestock owners and veterinary personnel. However, a brief description follows.

a) **NWS:** The body length averages 8–10 mm and has a deep blue to blue-green metallic colour, with three dark longitudinal stripes on the dorsal surface of the thorax. This combination of colour and pattern is not shared by any other species involved in wound myiasis except the secondary screwworm of the New World, *Cochliomyia macellaria* (Fabricius). These two *Cochliomyia* species can be separated by the presence of black setulae on the fronto-orbital plates of the head of NWS compared with only light yellow hairs on the fronto-orbital plates of *C. macellaria.* The fifth (= fourth visible) abdominal tergite of NWS has only a very slight lateral dusting, whereas that of *C. macellaria* has a dense dusting, producing a pair of distinct, lateral, silvery-white spots. In addition, females of NWS have a dark brown-black basicosta whereas those of *C. macellaria* have a yellow basicosta (Figure 4; see also refs 6, 9, 16, 26).

b) **OWS:** The body length is up to 10 mm and has a metallic blue, bluish-purple or blue-green colour, i.e., it is very similar to NWS, but without the thoracic stripes. The lower squama (s in Figure 4) also differs from NWS, being distinctly covered with fine hairs over its entire upper surface in OWS and other *Chrysomya* species. Adults of OWS can be distinguished from other *Chrysomya* found in cases of myiasis by the combination of black-brown to dark-orange coloured anterior spiracles (rather than pale yellow, creamy or white) with waxy-white coloured lower squamae (rather than blackish-brown to dirty-grey) (26, 35).

In addition to the morphological techniques discussed above, more recent techniques for identification of screwworms and their geographical origins include cuticular hydrocarbon analysis (5) and analysis of mitochondrial DNA (32). Problems with identification of larvae or adults from cases of myiasis can be referred to the Food and Agriculture Organisation of the United Nations Collaborating Centre on Myiasis Causing Insects and their Identification[2].

2. Serological tests

No standardised serological tests are presently available, nor are they indicated for diagnosis of this disease. However, experimental studies have shown that serological techniques have potential value in future investigations of the prevalence of screwworm infestations in animal populations, to detect antibodies to screwworm post-infestation (34).

2 Department of Entomology, The Natural History Museum, Cromwell Road, London SW7 5BD, United Kingdom. Fax: +44 (0)207-942-5229. E-mail: m.hall@nhm.ac.uk

B. REQUIREMENTS FOR VACCINES AND DIAGNOSTIC BIOLOGICALS

There are no biological products such as vaccines available currently. However, the only proven method of eradication of NWS does rely on a biological technique, the sterile insect technique, SIT (11, 17), which has also been applied experimentally to OWS (30). In this technique, male flies sterilised in their late pupal stage by gamma irradiation are sequentially released into the wild in vast numbers. Any of their matings with wild females result in infertile eggs only, leading to a progressive population reduction and, eventually, eradication. In operational situations, SIT is supported by the treatment with insecticide of screwworm-infested wounds in livestock, by strict control of livestock movement, by the quarantining of infested animals and by an active publicity campaign. SIT is very expensive because of the cost of continuous production and aerial dispersion of sterile flies. It is considered to be cost-effective only when it is used as an eradication strategy in situations where the geography would favour such a programme (e.g. refs 8, 17). Presently only one New World sterile screwworm production facility exists, at Tuxtla Gutiérrez in the south of Mexico. Another will be built in Panama[3]. An experimental facility to produce sterile OWS opened in Malaysia in 1998[4].

REFERENCES

1. ABED-BENAMARA M., ACHIR I., RODHAIN F. & PEREZ-EID C. (1997). Premier cas algérien d'otomyiase humaine à *Chrysomya bezziana. Bull. Soc. Pathol. Exot. Filiales,* **90**, 172–175.

2. ANZIANI O.S., GUGLIELMONE A.A. & AGUIRRE D.H. (1995). Administracion de abamectina para la prevencion de miasis (*Cochliomyia hominivorax*) post castracion en bovinos. *Veterinaria Argent.*, **12**, 233–236.

3. BENITEZ USHER C., CRUZ J., CARVALHO L., BRIDI A., FARRINGTON D., BARRICK R.A. & EAGLESON J. (1997). Prophylactic use of ivermectin against cattle myiasis caused by *Cochliomyia hominivorax* (Coquerel, 1858). *Vet. Parasitol.*, **72**, 215–220.

4. BROCE A.B., GOODENOUGH J.L. & COPPEDGE J.R. (1977). A wind-oriented trap for screwworm flies. *J. Econ. Entomol.*, **70,** 413–416.

5. BROWN W.V., MORTON R., LACEY M.J., SPADBERY J.P. & MAHON R.J. (1998). Identification of the geographical source of adults of the Old World screw-worm fly, *Chrysomya bezziana* Villeneuve (Diptera: Calliphoridae), by multivariate analysis of cuticular hydrocarbons. *Comp. Biochem. Physiol.*, **119 B**, 391–399.

6. DEAR J.P. (1985). A revision of the New World Chrysomyini (Diptera: Calliphoridae). *Rev. Bras. Zool.*, **3**, 109–169.

7. FOOD AND AGRICULTURE ORGANIZATION OF THE UNITED NATIONS (FAO) (1991). Manual for the Control of the Screwworm Fly, Cochliomyia hominivorax *(Coquerel)*. FAO, Rome, Italy, 93 pp.

8. FOOD AND AGRICULTURE ORGANIZATION OF THE UNITED NATIONS (FAO) (1992). The New World Screwworm Eradication Programme. FAO, Rome, Italy, 192 pp.

9. FOOD AND AGRICULTURE ORGANIZATION OF THE UNITED NATIONS (FAO) (1993). Manual for the Control of the Screwworm Fly, *Cochliomyia hominivorax* (Coquerel). Volume 2. Guide for the Identification of Flies in the genus *Cochliomyia* (Diptera: Calliphoridae). FAO, Rome, Italy, 18 pp.

10. GRAHAM O.H. (1979). The chemical control of screwworms: a review. *Southwest. Entomol.*, **4**, 258–264.

11. GRAHAM O.H., ed. (1985). Symposium on eradication of the screwworm from the United States and Mexico. *Miscell. Pub. Entomol. Soc. Am.*, **62**, 1 68.

12. HALL M.J.R. (1995). Trapping the flies that cause myiasis: their responses to host-stimuli. *Ann. Trop. Med. Parasitol.*, **89**, 333–357.

13. HALL M.J.R. & SMITH K.G.V. (1993). Diptera causing myiasis in man. *In:* Medical Insects and Arachnids, Lane R.P. & Crosskey R.W., eds. Chapman & Hall, London, UK, 429–469.

3 For further information contact: United States Department of Agriculture/Animal and Plant Health Inspection Service (USDA/APHIS), 4700 River Road, Riverdale, Maryland 20737, USA.

4 For further information contact: Institut Haiwan, Box 520, 86009 Kluang, Johor, Malaysia.

14. JAMES M.T. (1947). The Flies that Cause Myiasis in Man. United States Department of Agriculture Miscellaneous Publication No. 631, USA, 175 pp.

15. KITCHING R.L. (1974). The immature stages of the Old-World screw-worm fly, *Chrysomya bezziana* Villeneuve, with comparative notes on other Australasian species of *Chrysomya* (Diptera, Calliphoridae). *Bull. Entomological Res.*, **66**, 195–203.

16. LAAKE E.W., CUSHING E.C. & PARISH H.E. (1936). Biology of the Primary Screwworm Fly, *Cochliomyia americana*, and a Comparison of its Stages with those of *C. macellaria*. United States Department of Agriculture, Technical Bulletin No. 500, USA, 24 pp.

17. LINDQUIST D.A., ABUSOWA M. & HALL M.J.R. (1992). The New World screwworm fly in Libya: a review of its introduction and eradication. *Med. Vet. Entomol.*, **6**, 2–8.

18. MACKLEY J.W. & BROWN H.E. (1984). Swormlure-4: a new formulation of the Swormlure-2 mixture as an attractant for adult screwworms, *Cochliomyia hominivorax* (Diptera: Calliphoridae). *J. Econ. Entomol.*, **80**, 629–635.

19. MOYA-BORJA G.E., MUNIZ R.A., UMEHARA O., GONCALVES L.C.B., SILVA D.S.F. & MCKENZIE M.E. (1997). Protective efficacy of doramectin and ivermectin against *Cochliomyia hominivorax. Vet. Parasitol.*, **72**, 101–109.

20. MOYA-BORJA G.E., OLIVEIRA C.M.B., MUNIZ R.A. & GONCALVES L.C.B. (1993). Prophylactic and persistent efficacy of doramectin against *Cochliomyia hominivorax* in cattle. *Vet. Parasitol.*, **49**, 95–105.

21. MUNIZ R.A., CORONADO A., ANZIANI O.S., SANVARIA A., MORENO J., ERRECALDE J. & GONCALVES L.C.B. (1995). Efficacy of injectable doramectin in the protection of castrated cattle against field infestations of *Cochliomyia hominivorax. Vet. Parasitol.*, **58**, 327–333.

22. NAVIDPOUR SH., HOGHOOGHI-RAD N., GOODARZI H & POOLADGAR A.R. (1996). Outbreak of *Chrysomyia bezziana* in Khoozestan province, Iran. *Vet. Rec.*, **139**, 217.

23. PARMAN D.C. (1945). Effect of weather on *Cochliomyia americana* and a review of methods and economic applications of the study. *J. Econ. Entomol.*, **38**, 66–76.

24. PERKINS I.D. (1987). Use of insecticides to control screwworm fly strike by *Chrysomya bezziana* in cattle. *Aust. Vet. J.*, **64**, 17–20.

25. SILVA D.J., VIANNA W.O., LOMBA F. & DA SILVA D.J. (1991). Insecticidas no controle de larvas de mosca da especie *Cochliomyia hominivorax* (Coquerel). *Bol. Indust. Anim.*, **48**, 1–6.

26. SPRADBERY J.P. (1991). A Manual for the Diagnosis of Screw-worm Fly. Commonwealth Scientific and Industrial Research Organization (CSIRO) Division of Entomology, Canberra, Australia, 64 pp.

27. SPRADBERY J.P. (1994). Screw-worm fly: a tale of two species. *Agric. Zoo. Rev.*, **6**, 1–62.

28. SPRADBERY J.P., TOZER R.S., DREWETT N. & LINDSEY M.J. (1985). The efficacy of ivermectin against larvae of the screwworm fly *(Chrysomya bezziana). Aust. Vet. J.*, **62**, 311–314.

29. SPRADBERY J.P., TOZER R.S. & POUND A.A. (1991). The efficacy of insecticides against the screw-worm fly *(Chrysomya bezziana). Aust. Vet. J.*, **68**, 338–342.

30. SPRADBERY J.P., TOZER R.S., ROBB J.M. & CASSELLS P. (1989). The screw-worm fly, *Chrysomya bezziana* Villeneuve (Diptera: Calliphoridae) in a sterile insect release trial in Papua New Guinea. *Res. Pop. Ecol.*, **31**, 353–366.

31. SUTHERST R.W., SPRADBERY J.P. & MAYWALD G.F. (1989). The potential geographical distribution of the Old World screwworm fly, *Chrysomya bezziana. Med. Vet. Entomol.*, **3**, 273–280.

32. TAYLOR D.B., SZALANSKI A.L. & PETERSON R.D. II (1996). Identification of screwworm species by polymerase chain reaction-restriction fragment length polymorphism. *Med. Vet. Entomol.*, **10**, 63–70.

33. THOMAS D.B. & MANGAN R.L. (1989). Oviposition and wound-visiting behaviour of the screwworm fly, *Cochliomyia hominivorax* (Diptera: Calliphoridae). *Ann. Entomol. Soc. Am.*, **82**, 526–534.

34. THOMAS D.B. & PRUETT J.H. (1992). Kinetic development and decline of antiscrewworm (Diptera: Calliphoridae) antibodies in serum of infested sheep. *J. Med. Entomol.*, **29**, 870–873.

35. ZUMPT F. (1965). Myiasis in Man and Animals in the Old World. Butterworths, London, 267 pp.

*

* *

CHAPTER 2.2.9.

TRICHINELLOSIS

SUMMARY

Trichinellosis is mainly important because of its public health significance. The adults of Trichinella *species may be found in the small intestine of humans, pigs, rats, bears and many other flesh-eating mammals, but may also occur in horses that have eaten fodder containing dead infected rodents. Their larvae form cysts in the voluntary muscles of their hosts.*

Diagnostic tests for Trichinella *infection fall into two categories: 1) direct detection of first-stage larvae encysted or free in striated muscle tissue, and 2) indirect detection of parasitism by tests for specific antibodies.*

For ante-mortem tests, serodiagnostic methods are preferable to biopsy. The sensitivity of serological methods is equal to or better than direct methods. In light or moderate infections in pigs, a serological response is often not detected for 3 weeks or longer after muscle larvae become infective. In such cases, a false-negative serological result might be obtained. However, infections under three larvae/gram of tissue are not detected reliably by conventional direct methods. A low rate of false-positive results has been reported for serological tests.

Identification of the agent: *Two general methods, compression or digestion of muscle tissue, are used for the direct detection of* Trichinella *infection. Both methods test for the presence of parasites in tissues where infection is heaviest, these being in descending order of incidence in pigs: the diaphragm (crus), tongue, masseter and abdominal muscles, although this partially depends on the degree of infection. In horses, muscles of the tongue and masseter harbour the most worms, followed by the diaphragm and muscles in the neck. The selection of an appropriate method for direct inspection for* Trichinella*-infection depends on the facilities available and the number of samples to be tested.*

The first method is by visual inspection of compressed pieces of muscle tissue for the presence of larvae in situ. *This requires a specialised microscope, the trichinoscope, which has an estimated efficiency of detecting as few as three to five larvae/gram of tissue. It has the disadvantage of requiring considerable time for the inspection of multiple samples from each carcass. It is also very difficult to detect the larvae of* T. pseudospiralis, *which are free in muscle cells. In recent years this species has been reported from several countries, in domestic and wild pigs and in humans.*

The second method involves the digestion of individual or pooled muscle tissue samples, followed by selective screening, filtration, or sedimentation procedures. Finally these samples are inspected microscopically for the presence of larvae. Digestion methods may be mechanically assisted by stirring or homogenising the digest mixture. Digestion methods have an efficiency of approximately three larvae/gram of tissue examined when the tissue sample size is 1 gram.

Serological tests: *The enzyme-linked immunosorbent assay (ELISA) is the best method for the ante-mortem detection of* Trichinella *infection. It is comparable in sensitivity to the best direct methods. Infection levels as low as one larva/100 g of tissue have been detected. The specificity of ELISA for* Trichinella *infection is directly linked to the type and quality of the antigen employed in the test. Secretory antigens collected by short-term maintenance of* T. spiralis *muscle larvae* in vitro *currently provide the most specific and economical source. There are no known cross-reactions using these antigens, although a low rate of false-positive results has been obtained in some studies.*

The use of secretory antigens is recommended for surveillance programmes by ELISA. As a confirmatory test, the digestion of up to 100 g of tissue will ensure an accurate diagnosis. A low rate of false-negative ELISA results may be obtained with recently infected animals that have low grade infections.

Requirements for vaccines and diagnostic biologicals: *At the present time, the immunoprophylaxis of* Trichinella *infection in pigs is under study, but so far there is no widespread use of vaccines.*

A. DIAGNOSTIC TECHNIQUES

Trichinellosis is mainly important because of its public health significance. The adults of *Trichinella* sp. may be found in the small intestine of humans, pigs, rats, bears and many other flesh-eating mammals, but may also occur in horses that have eaten fodder containing infected rodents or other infected materials. The parasite has a direct life history. The females are ovo-viviparous. The larvae are shed into the lacteals, enter the lymph, reach the venous blood, and though many die out, others survive to settle in voluntary muscles, especially those of the diaphragm and tongue in pigs and tongue and masseters in horses.

Seven species of *Trichinella* are recognised. *Trichinella spiralis* (also called T-1) is distributed in temperate regions world-wide and is commonly associated with domestic pigs. It is highly infective for pigs, mice and rats. *Trichinella nativa* (T-2) is a cold-climate-adapted species. It has limited infectivity for pigs, but is commonly found in wild canids, bear, and walrus; it is further distinguished by its resistance to freezing. *Trichinella britovi* (T-3) is found predominantly in wild animals, although it may occasionally be found in pigs or horses. It occurs in temperate regions of Europe and Asia. *Trichinella britovi* has some intermediate characteristics of other species, including some resistance to freezing, moderate infectivity for swine and slow capsule formation (larvae have been confused for nonencapsulating species in some cases. *Trichinella murrelli* (T-5) is a North American species found in wildlife and occasionally horses and humans. It has low infectivity for domestic pigs, but poses a risk to humans who eat game meat. *Trichinella nelsoni* (T-7) has been isolated sporadically from wildlife in Africa. It is characterised by greater resistance to elevated temperatures as compared with other species of *Trichinella.* Two species of *Trichinella* do not form a capsule in muscle. *Trichinella pseudospiralis* (T-4) is cosmopolitan in distribution and has been recovered from raptorial birds, wild carnivores, rats and marsupials in Asia, North America and the Australian subcontinent. *Trichinella papuae* (T-10) is a second species that does not form a capsule. To date, it has only been reported from Papua New Guinea. In addition to the species described, several other isolates are recognised. *Trichinella* T-6 is found in North America. It is resistant to freezing, has low infectivity for pigs, is found in a variety of wild mammals and has been implicated in human disease. *Trichinella* T-8 is an isolate from Africa that is similar to *T. britovi,* but is found to differ using molecular markers. *Trichinella* T-9 from Japan is similar to *T. britovi,* but is found to differ by molecular analysis. As molecular techniques are refined and further comparative studies are performed on *Trichinella* isolates, further taxonomic resolution should be applied to this genus. Several excellent reviews of the current status of *Trichinella* species are available (11, 14). All species and types of *Trichinella* cause disease in humans.

Human trichinellosis is a serious disease that can cause much suffering and may result in death. The worms may have little effect within the intestine, but severe signs and symptoms may result from the migration of the larvae and their presence in voluntary muscle. The disease is transmitted by eating infected meat that has not been sufficiently cooked (or otherwise made safe). Control is accomplished by meat inspection, by processing (cooking, freezing, or curing of meat) (4), and by prevention of exposure of animals to infected meat including uncooked food waste, rodents and other wildlife. Game meats should always be considered a potential source of infection, and therefore game meats should be tested or cooked thoroughly. *Trichinella* found in game meats (*T. nativa* or T-2 and T-6) may be resistant to freezing and therefore frozen meat may still pose a public health risk.

A number of diagnostic tests are available for the detection of *Trichinella* infection (trichinellosis) in pigs and other species. These are either: (a) the direct demonstration of the parasite in tissue samples or digests; or (b) the indirect demonstration of the parasite by the detection of specific antibodies using serological methods.

1. Identification of the agent (the prescribed test for international trade)

The direct demonstration of the parasites is generally limited to post-mortem inspection of carcasses, although methods of ante-mortem biopsy have been reported (10). The sensitivity of direct testing depends on the amount of tissue examined and the site from which it was obtained. Current methods for testing by digestion employing a 1 g sample (1, 2) have a sensitivity of approximately three larvae/gram of tissue (3, 6). Direct methods will identify infected pigs or horses as early as 17 days after exposure, coincident with the time that muscle larvae become infective for a new host. Direct methods remain effective as long as muscle larvae remain viable. Where large quantities of tissue (up to 100 g) are available for digestion, the sensitivity of this test is greatly increased. The disadvantages of direct inspection methods, particularly by trichinoscopy, are the time and labour required.

Two methods are generally employed for the direct diagnosis of trichinellosis:

a) The trichinoscope or compression method

Trichinoscopy for the inspection of pork has been described elsewhere (1, 2). Samples are taken for examination from the pillars of the diaphragm (crus) and cut into at least 28 pieces, each about 2 × 10 mm in size. Alternative sites for tissue collection include the tongue, masseter and abdominal muscles, but larger samples are required for comparable sensitivity. (The predeliction sites of muscle larvae vary with host species and have only been well established in pigs and horses.) The tissues are compressed between glass plates (compressorium; Hauptner Herberholz, Solingen, Germany) until they become translucent. They are then examined for larvae through a specially constructed projection microscope, the trichinoscope, or a conventional microscope at ×15–40 magnification. Larvae will appear coiled within an individual muscle cell, and the muscle cell typically appears oval in shape as a result of the formation of the capsule. In heavy infections, multiple larvae may be seen in a single cell. Nonencapsulating *Trichinella*, including *T. pseudospiralis* and related types, may be seen outside of muscle cells and typically are not coiled.

b) The digestion method

Muscle tissue can be digested with artificial digestive fluid. This releases live trichinae from the muscle capsules. Four digestion procedures are recommended within the European Union (EU) (1, 2), and EU Directives should be consulted for more complete details. The procedures include:

i) The artificial digestion method for individual or pooled samples,

ii) The mechanically assisted pooled sample digestion sedimentation technique,

iii) The mechanically assisted pooled sample digestion method on filter isolation technique,

iv) The magnetic stirrer method for pooled samples.

The magnetic stirrer method for pooled samples can be employed in a variety of circumstances with a minimum of equipment. A general example of the principles of this method is as follows:

- **Sampling**

Muscle samples are taken from the diaphragm pillars or tongue of pigs, or tongue or masseter muscle of horses; other sites generally have lower numbers of larvae. Sample sizes can vary; individual samples of 100 g may be taken from one animal, or multiple samples may be collected from a number of animals to make a 100 g pool. The size of the samples that make up the latter will determine the sensitivity of the method. EU Directives require 1 g samples in 100 g pools for testing pig carcasses. For testing horsemeat, the EU requires at least 5 g samples. In the USA, 5 g samples are required for pigs. For endemic areas, a minimum sample size of 5 g is recommended, with 20 animals involved in each 100 g pool. The samples are ground, blended or diced to facilitate digestion.

- **Digestion and recovery**

Each 100 g of tissue is digested in 1–2 litres of artificial gastric fluid containing 1% (w/v) pepsin (1/10,000 National Formulary) and 1% (v/v) hydrochloric acid (0.12 N final). The ground or diced sample is added to the digestion fluid and the mixture is stirred on a magnetic stirrer for 3 hours at 37°C (or for shorter periods of time at higher temperatures (e.g. 30–60 minutes at 44–46°C). At the conclusion of stirring, the digest is allowed to settle for 15–20 minutes and the upper two-thirds of the fluid is decanted. The remaining fluid and deposit are poured through a 355 µm mesh screen into a conical settling glass and allowed to settle for a further 15–20 minutes. The maximum possible supernatant fluid is aspirated without disturbing the sediment: the latter is washed with warm (37°C) tap water and allowed to settle for another 15–20 minutes; if necessary, the washing step is repeated until the supernatant fluid is clear. The washed sediment is transferred to a 50 ml tube, allowed to settle, and aspirated down to a final volume of 10 ml. For enumeration purposes, all 10 ml are poured into a gridded Petri dish and examined for *Trichinella* larvae with a dissecting microscope (×15–40 magnification). First stage larvae, digested free from muscle cells, are approximately 1 mm in length and 0.03 mm in width. The most distinguishing feature of *Trichinella* larvae is the stichosome, which consists of a series of discoid cells lining the oesophagus and occupying the anterior half of the worms body. *Trichinella* larvae may appear coiled (when cold), motile (when warm) or C-shaped (for dead larvae). In case of doubt, worms should be examined at higher magnification and further tissues should be examined. If the counts are high, appropriate dilutions must first be made. When larvae are detected in pooled sample digests, the entire procedure must be repeated on the individual samples comprising the pool.

Use of a thermostatically controlled tissue blender (Stomacher) shortens the time required for digestion to about 12–15 minutes. Details of other methods using a Stomacher Lab Blender 3500T (Seward, London, United Kingdom) have been described (2) and an alternative protocol for the magnetic stirrer method for pooled samples, approved by the EU (84/319/EEC), can also be recommended (2).

c) Species identification

Identification of the species/type of *Trichinella* recovered from muscle tissue can be valuable in understanding the epidemiology of the parasite and in assessing the relative risk of human exposure. Requests for speciation/typing can be made through the OIE Reference Laboratory in Rome, Italy (see Table given in Part 4 of this *Manual*).

2. Serological tests

The use of enzyme-linked immunosorbent assay (ELISA) to detect the presence of parasite-specific antibodies provides a rapid method that can be performed on blood or serum collected before or after slaughter. Infections as low as one larva/100 g of tissue have been detected by ELISA. Several antigen preparations have been developed that provide a high degree of specificity for *Trichinella* infection in pigs and horses (5–7, 15). In abattoir testing, the ELISA yielded less than 0.3% false-positive results and was nearly 100% sensitive in detecting infected pigs with more than one larva/gram of tissue (12). The *T. spiralis* excretory–secretory (ES) antigens used in the ELISA are conserved in all species/types of *Trichinella* (13), and therefore infection may be detected in pigs or other animals harbouring any of the seven species or types. Serological tests other than ELISA (e.g. indirect immunofluorescence tests) lack specificity and are not suitable for detection of *Trichinella* infection.

A disadvantage of serology for detection of *Trichinella* infection is the occurrence of a low rate of false-negative results in the case of infected animals. Such results are due to a lag in the kinetics of antibody responses in animals lightly or moderately infected with *T. spiralis* or infected with sylvatic *Trichinella* species (5). This slow rate of antibody production means that infected animals cannot be detected for several weeks following exposure. Serological responses in pigs persist for at least 6 months after infection with no decline (3), however, antibody has been reported to decline in horses within a few months following infection, coincident with a decline in muscle larvae. Thus, serological evaluation of *Trichinella* in horses may be of limited value. Little is known of antibody responses to *Trichinella* infection in game species.

Serological testing by ELISA has an advantage of increased sensitivity over digestion methods for detecting *Trichinella* infection in lightly infected animals; this sensitivity is useful for detecting ongoing transmission at the farm. While digestion testing, using a 1 g sample, will only detect infections greater than three larvae/gram, some animals with infection greater than three larvae/gram will remain seronegative until 21–35 days following infection (3, 6). Thus, serology is of particular value for surveillance programmes, especially in pigs, and is an alternative to digestion for slaughter testing. Because *Trichinella* infection is usually rare in animals, a surveillance programme cannot be based on random sampling, but will often have to rely on whole-herd testing. This may have very great economic implications for a surveillance programme.

- **Enzyme-linked immunosorbent assay**

Diagnosis of *Trichinella* infection by ELISA can be accomplished by using secreted stichosome antigens collected from *T. spiralis* larvae (5). The antigens recognised in worm secretions consist of a group of structurally related glycoproteins with molecular weights of 45–55 kDa (7).

- **Antigen production**

The specificity and sensitivity of ELISA is largely dependent on the quality of the antigen used in the test. Antigens that are specifically secreted from the stichocyte cells of living L1 larvae and bear the TSL-1 carbohydrate epitope are those antigens that are recognised by *Trichinella*-infected animals. These antigens are found in all species/types of *Trichinella*, and therefore these antigens can detect infections with any of these *Trichinella* parasites. The parasite used to prepare antigens should be *T. spiralis*, designated T-1 by the International Trichinellosis Reference Centre, Rome, Italy. The parasite may be maintained by serial passage in mice or rats prior to use for preparing diagnostic antigens.

To prepare antigen for use in the ELISA (9), *T. spiralis* (T-1) muscle-stage larvae are recovered from skinned, eviscerated, ground rat carcasses by digestion in 1% pepsin with 1% HCl for 3 hours at 37°C (as described above). These larvae are washed (three times for 20 minutes each) in Dulbecco's modified Eagle's medium (DMEM) with penicillin (500 units/ml) and streptomycin (500 units/ml), and then placed (at a density of 5000 L1/ml) into DMEM supplemented with HEPES (N-2-hydroxyethylpiperazine, N-2-ethanesulphonic acid) (10 mM), glutamine (2 mM), pyruvate (1 mM), and penicillin (250 units/ml)–

streptomycin (250 µg/ml) (complete DMEM) at 37°C in 10% CO_2 in air. Culture medium is recovered, after 18–20 hours, worms are removed by filtration, and the fluid is concentrated under pressure with a 3000 Da molecular weight retention. Secretory antigens thus recovered may be stored frozen for short periods at –20°C or for longer at –70°C; they comprise approximately 25 protein components as determined by SDS-PAGE (sodium dodecyl sulphate-polyacrylamide gel electrophoresis), many of which bear the diagnostic TSL-1 carbohydrate antigen epitope.

The quality of antigen is critical to the specificity of the ELISA. Steps should be taken to monitor growth of bacteria either visually, by phase microscopy, or by plating a sample of media. Cultures showing any bacterial growth should be discarded. Larvae should not be maintained longer than 20 hours; worm deterioration after this time contributes to leaking of somatic antigens that reduce test specificity. Antigen, produced as described, should have a 280/260 nm absorbance ratio of >1.0. The antigens obtained from *in vitro* maintenance of *Trichinella* larvae should be tested against a panel of known negative and positive sera.

- **Test procedure**

  An example of an ELISA for detecting *Trichinella* infection in pigs is given below. It is essential that all reagents used in the assay be standardised for optimal concentration to obtain reliable results. Typical values are indicated in the example.

i) Coat 96-well microtitre plates with 100 µl/well of *T. spiralis* excretory–secretory antigens diluted to 5 µg/ml in coating buffer (50 mM carbonate/bicarbonate buffer, pH 9.6). Coating is performed for 60 minutes at 37°C or overnight at 4°C.

ii) Wash antigen-coated wells three times with wash buffer containing 50 mM Tris, pH 7.4, 150 mM NaCl, 5.0% nonfat dry milk and 1.0% Triton X-100. Following each washing, plates are blotted dry.

iii) Dilute pig sera 1/10 or 1/100 in wash buffer. Alternative sources of antibodies that may be used in place of sera include whole blood or tissue fluids (8). Add 100 µl of diluted sera to antigen-coated wells. A known positive and known negative serum sample should be used on each plate at the same dilution as the test sera. Incubate at room temperature for 30 minutes.

iv) Wash wells three times as in step ii.

v) Add 100 µl/well of an affinity-purified rabbit anti-swine IgG–peroxidase conjugate at an appropriate dilution in wash buffer, e.g. a 1/1000 dilution of rabbit anti-swine IgG (0.1 mg/ml) produced by Kirkegaard and Perry Laboratories, Gaitherburg, Maryland, USA. Following the addition of the second antibody, incubate the plates for 30 minutes at room temperature.

vi) Wash wells three times as in step ii. Rinse one time with distilled water.

vii) Add 100 µl of a suitable peroxidase substrate (e.g. 5'-aminosalicylic acid [0.8 mg/ml] with 0.005% hydrogen peroxide, pH 5.6–6.0).

viii) After 5–15 minutes, read plates for colour density at 450 nm on an automated microplate reader. Values obtained in the ELISA four times that of normal serum pool controls are considered to be positive. Values three times higher than normal are classified as suspect. However, the cut-off value is influenced by the breed of pig.

Commercial adaptations of the ELISA are available in a shorter format, taking less than 1 hour for completion.

B. REQUIREMENTS FOR VACCINES AND DIAGNOSTIC BIOLOGICALS

At the present time the immunoprophylaxis of *Trichinella* infection in pigs is under study, but so far there is no widespread use of vaccines.

REFERENCES

1. European Economic Community (1977). Commission Directive 77/96/EEC. *Off. J. European Communities*, **26**, 67–77.

2. European Economic Community (1984). Commission Directive 84/319/EEC. *Off. J. European Communities*, **167**, 34–43.

3. Gamble H.R. (1996). Detection of trichinellosis in pigs by artificial digestion and enzyme immunoassay. *J. Food Prot.*, **59**, 295–298.

4. GAMBLE H.R. (1997). Parasites associated with pork and pork products. *Rev. sci. tech. Off. Int. Epiz.*, **16**, 496–506.

5. GAMBLE H.R., ANDERSON W.R., GRAHAM C.E. & MURRELL K.D. (1983). Serodiagnosis of swine trichinosis using an excretory-secretory antigen. *Vet. Parasitol.*, **13**, 349–361.

6. GAMBLE H.R., GAJADHAR A.A. & SOLOMON M.B. (1996). Methods for the detection of trichinellosis in horses. *J. Food Prot.*, **59**, 420–425.

7. GAMBLE H.R. & GRAHAM C.E. (1984). Monoclonal antibody-purified antigen for the immunodiagnosis of swine trichinosis. *Am. J. Vet. Res.*, **45**, 67–74.

8. GAMBLE H.R. & PATRASCU I.V. (1996). Whole blood, serum, and tissue fluids in an enzyme immunoassay for swine trichinellosis. *J. Food Prot.*, **59**, 1213–1217.

9. GAMBLE H.R., RAPIC D., MARINCULIC A. & MURRELL K.D. (1988). Influence of cultivation conditions on specificity of excretory-secretory antigens for the immunodiagnosis of trichinellosis. *Vet. Parasitol*, **30**,131–137.

10. KAZACOS K.R., LITTLE A.S., ROHE F.J., WADE W.F. & GAAFAR S.M. (1986). A tongue biopsy technique for the detection of trichinosis in swine. *Vet. Parasitol.*, **19**, 151–156.

11. MURRELL K.D., LICHTENFELS J.R., ZARLENGA D.S. & POZIO E. (2000). The systematics of the genus *Trichinella* with a key to species. *Vet. Parasitol.*, (in press).

12. OLIVER D.G., SINGH P., ALLISON D.E., MURRELL K.D. & GAMBLE H.R. (1989). Field evaluation of an enzyme immunoassay for detection of hogs in a high volume North Carolina abattoir. *In:* Trichinellosis, Tanner C.E., ed. Consejo Superior de Investigaciones Press, Madrid, Spain, 439–444.

13. ORTEGA-PIERRES M.G., YEPEZ-MULIA L., HOMAN W., GAMBLE H.R., LIM P., TAKAHASHI Y., WASSOM D.L. & APPLETON J.A. (1996). Workshop on a detailed characterization of *Trichinella spiralis* antigens: A platform for future studies on antigens and antibodies to this parasite. *Parasite Immunol.*, **18**, 273–284.

14. POZIO E. (2000). Factors affecting the flow among domestic, synanthropic and sylvatic cycles of *Trichinella*. *Vet. Parasitol.*, (in press).

15. SEAWRIGHT G.L., DESPOMMIER D.D., ZIMMERMAN W. & ISENSTEIN R.S. (1983). Enzyme immunoassay for swine trichinellosis using antigens purified by immunoaffinity chromatography. *Am. J. Trop. Med. Hyg.*, **32**, 1275–1284.

*

* *

SECTION 2.3.

BOVINE DISEASES IN LIST B

CHAPTER 2.3.1.

BOVINE BRUCELLOSIS

SUMMARY

Bovine brucellosis is usually caused by Brucella abortus, *less frequently by* B. melitensis, *and rarely by* B. suis. *It is manifested by abortion, with excretion of the organisms in uterine discharges and in milk. Diagnosis depends on the isolation of* Brucella *from abortion material, udder secretions or from tissues removed at post-mortem. Alternatively, specific cell-mediated or serological responses to* Brucella *antigens can be demonstrated.*

Brucella abortus, B. melitensis and B. suis *are highly pathogenic for humans, and all infected tissues, cultures and potentially contaminated materials must be handled under containment level 3 (biosafety 3) conditions.*

Identification of the agent: *The demonstration by modified acid-fast or immunospecific staining of organisms of* Brucella *morphology in abortion material or vaginal discharges provides presumptive evidence of brucellosis, especially if supported by serological tests. After isolation, the species and biovar should be identified by phage lysis and/or oxidative metabolism tests, cultural, biochemical and serological criteria. The recently developed polymerase chain reaction and DNA probe methods provide additional means of detection.*

Serological tests: *The buffered* Brucella *antigen tests, i.e. rose bengal test and buffered plate agglutination test, the enzyme-linked immunosorbent assay or the fluorescence polarisation assay are suitable tests for screening herds and individual animals. The reactivity of samples that are positive in screening tests should be retested using established confirmatory tests such as the complement fixation test or enzyme-linked immunosorbent assay. The serum agglutination test is inferior to other tests in specificity and sensitivity, and is not recommended if other procedures are available. The indirect enzyme-linked immunosorbent assay or milk ring test performed on bulk milk samples are effective for screening and monitoring dairy cattle for brucellosis, but the milk ring test is less reliable in large herds and is less sensitive with* B. melitensis. *Another immunological test is the brucellin skin test, which can be used as a screening or as a confirmatory herd test when positive serological reactors occur in the absence of obvious risk factors in unvaccinated herds. A purified, standardised antigen preparation is available.*

Requirements for vaccines and diagnostic biologicals: Brucella abortus *strain 19 (S19) live vaccine should be prepared from US-derived seed cultures*[1]*, and each batch must conform to minimum standards for viability, smoothness, pathogenicity and ability to immunise guinea-pigs and/or mice against challenge with a virulent strain of* B. abortus. Brucella melitensis *strain Rev.1 vaccines may be used to immunise cattle at risk of infection with* B. melitensis. *They should be prepared from an approved Elberg seed strain, and each batch must conform to minimum standards (see Chapter 2.4.2. Caprine and ovine brucellosis [excluding* B. ovis *infection]).* Brucella abortus *strain RB51 vaccine was produced from a laboratory-derived rough mutant of smooth*

1 Obtainable from the United States Department of Agriculture (USDA), National Veterinary Services Laboratories (NVSL), 1800 Dayton Road, Ames, Iowa 50010, United States of America (USA).

B. abortus strain 2308 and is the latest development in vaccination in the USA. Brucellin preparations for the intradermal test must be free from smooth lipopolysaccharide and must not produce nonspecific inflammatory reactions or interfere with serological tests. Diagnostic antigens must be prepared from approved smooth strains of B. abortus and comply with minimum standards for identity, purity, sensitivity and specificity.

A. DIAGNOSTIC TECHNIQUES

Brucellosis in cattle is usually caused by biovars of *Brucella abortus*. In some countries, particularly in southern Europe and western Asia, where cattle are kept in close association with sheep or goats, infection can also be caused by *B. melitensis*. *Brucella suis* rarely causes infection in cattle. The disease is usually asymptomatic in nonpregnant females, but adult male cattle may develop orchitis. Following infection with *B. abortus* or *B. melitensis*, pregnant adult females develop a placentitis usually resulting in abortion between the fifth and ninth month of pregnancy. Even in the absence of abortion, profuse excretion of the organism occurs in the placenta, fetal fluids and vaginal discharges. The mammary gland and associated lymph nodes may also be infected, and organisms may be excreted in the milk. Subsequent pregnancies are usually carried to term, but uterine and mammary infection recurs, with reduced numbers of organisms in cyetic products and milk. In acute infections, the organism is present in most major body lymph nodes. Brucellosis may be a cause of infertility and returns to service. Hygromas, usually involving leg joints, are a common manifestation of brucellosis in some tropical countries and may be the only obvious indicator of infection; the hygroma fluid is often infected with *Brucella*. An arthropathy, usually affecting the femoro-tibial joint, has been recognised as an infrequent complication of vaccination with *Brucella abortus* strain 19 (S19) vaccines (3, 7).

Brucellosis has also been reported in the one-humped camel *(Camelus dromedarius)* and in the two-humped camel *(C. bactrianus)*, related to contact with large and small ruminants infected with *B. abortus* or *B. melitensis*. In addition, brucellosis has been observed in the domestic buffalo *(Bubalus bubalus)*, bison *(Bison bison)*, yak *(Bos grunniens)*, elk *(Cerves canadensis)* and also occurs in the African buffalo *(Syncerus caffer)* and various African antelope species. The manifestations of brucellosis in these animals are similar to those in cattle.

Brucellosis is readily transmissible to humans, causing an acute febrile illness (*B. abortus:* undulant fever or *B. melitensis:* Malta fever), which may progress to a more chronic form, and can produce serious complications affecting the musculo-skeletal, and other organ systems. Infection is often due to occupational exposure and may be via the conjunctiva or abraided skin, but ingestion of dairy products constitutes the main risk to the public. Laboratory manipulation of live cultures or contaminated material from infected animals is hazardous and must be done under containment level 3 (biosafety 3) conditions to minimise occupational exposure to this zoonotic agent.

1. Identification of the agent

All abortions in cattle should be treated as suspected brucellosis and should be investigated. The clinical picture is not pathognomonic, although the herd history may be helpful. Smears of placental cotyledon, vaginal discharge and fetal lung, liver and abomasal contents should be fixed with heat or ethanol and stained by the modified Ziehl–Neelsen (Stamp's), Kösters', Gram or Macchiavello methods, or with a fluorochrome or peroxidase-labelled antibody conjugate (22). The presence of large aggregates of intracellular, weakly acid-fast organisms of *Brucella* morphology or immuno-specifically stained organisms is presumptive evidence of brucellosis. Care must be taken in the interpretation of results as other infectious agents may have similar morphology (e.g. *Coxiella burnetii, Chlamydia psittaci*) or immunological cross-reactivity (e.g. *Yersinia enterocolitica*). DNA probes or polymerase chain reaction (PCR) methods are currently under development that can be used to demonstrate the agent in various biological samples (8, 21).

Genetic evidence indicates that all members of the *Brucella* genus are closely related and probably should be considered variants of a single species. Nevertheless, there are real differences in host preference and epidemiology displayed by the major variants, as well as molecular evidence of genomic variation. From a practical point of view, it is convenient to maintain the classification into six nomenspecies: *Brucella abortus, B. melitensis, B. suis, B. neotomae, B. ovis* and *B. canis*. The first three of these are subdivided into biovars based on cultural and serological properties. Strains of *Brucella* have recently been isolated from marine mammals (23) that cannot be ascribed to any of the above-recognised species. Investigations are continuing to establish their correct position in the taxonomy of the genus. *Brucella* is not closely related to any other known animal pathogens, but shows close genetic relatedness to some plant pathogens and symbionts of the genera *Agrobacterium, Ochrobactrum* and *Rhizobium*.

Culture of placental cotyledon, vaginal discharge, fetal tissues or abomasal contents, or hygroma fluid should be made on solid media of appropriate selectivity. There are many varieties of suitable media, such as serum dextrose agar (SDA), trypticase soy agar (TSA) and blood agar (base #2, Oxoid) and these may be supplemented with bacitracin (25 µg/ml = 25,000 U), natamycin (50 mg), polymyxin B (5 µg/ml = 5000 U), and vancomycin (20 µg/ml). SDA with the addition of these antibacterials is also known as Farrell's modified SDA (6,

9). The addition of extra serum to the medium enhances the growth of some *Brucella* strains. Cultures can also be made from milk or colostrum, and from samples of tissues collected at post-mortem, such as mammary gland, uterus, supramammary, and internal iliac lymph nodes from females, and testes, epididymides, seminal vesicles, accessory glands, external inguinal, and internal iliac lymph nodes from males. The parotid, mandibular and retropharyngeal lymph nodes, from either males or females, are good sources of the organism. Tissues should be removed as aseptically as possible and are best prepared for culture by maceration in a Colworth Stomacher or similar equipment.

As the number of *Brucella* organisms is likely to be lower in milk, colostrum and some tissue samples than in abortion material, enrichment is advisable. (In the case of milk, results are improved by centrifugation and culture from the cream and the pellet.) This can be carried out in liquid medium consisting of serum–dextrose broth, tryptone soya broth or *Brucella* broth supplemented with an antibiotic mixture of amphotericin B (1 µg/ml) and vancomycin (20 µg/ml) (all final concentrations). The enrichment medium should be incubated at 37°C in air supplemented with 5–10% (v/v) CO_2 for up to 6 weeks, with weekly subcultures on to solid selective medium. If preferred, a biphasic system of solid and liquid selective medium in the same bottle (Castañeda technique) may be used to minimise subculture. All culture media should be subject to quality control and must support the growth of fastidious strains, such as *B. abortus* biovar 2, from small inocula.

Colonies of *Brucella* type are slow growing and fastidious, usually between 0.5 and 1 mm in diameter, raised, convex and with an entire edge. In transmitted light smooth colonies are shiny, pale yellowish in colour, but in reflected light appear bluish grey and slightly opalescent. Rough colonies are similar in size and shape but are less transparent and appear dull white or yellowish in reflected light. Suspect isolates should be checked by examining a Gram-stained or Stamp's stained smear. If organisms of *Brucella* morphology (small Gram-negative or Stamp's positive coccobacilli, or short rods with rounded ends and slightly convex sides) are seen, the colonies should be tested for agglutination with *Brucella*-specific antiserum after checking for dissociation. The latter is easily tested by suspending colonies in 0.1% (w/v) aqueous acriflavine: rough colonies form agglutinates, or by crystal violet staining: rough colonies stain red and smooth colonies stain pale yellow. If the colonies are smooth, they should be checked against antiserum to smooth *B. abortus*, or preferably antisera monospecific for the A and M surface antigens. In the case of nonsmooth colonies, isolates should be checked with antiserum to *Brucella* R antigen.

Positive agglutination with a *Brucella* antiserum provides presumptive identification of the isolate as *Brucella*. Subsequent full identification is best performed by a reference laboratory. Additional identification should be done by using either oxidative metabolism tests (quantitative measurement by Warburg manometry or Gilson respirometry under biosecurity level 3), PCR or phage lysis tests to identify the species (in the latter case the phage lysis pattern is dependent on the colonial phase of the isolate and it is essential that this be determined correctly) (1). Identification to biovar level depends on examination for growth in the presence of basic fuchsin (pararosanline) and thionin at final concentrations of 20 µg/ml, production of H_2S (detected by lead acetate papers), requirement of CO_2 for growth, and agglutination pattern with A-, M-, or R-specific antisera. Reference strains should be included in each series of tests to control the quality of reagents and techniques.

Identification of the vaccine strains *B. abortus* S19 or *B. melitensis* strain Rev.1, depends on further tests. In the first case, lack of requirement for CO_2, inhibition of growth by benzylpenicillin (3 µg/ml = 5 International Units [IU]/ml), thionin blue (2 µg/ml), and *i*-erythritol (1 mg/ml) (all final concentrations), a high utilisation of L-glutamate (1), and a low residual virulence for guinea-pigs, are characteristic of *B. abortus* S19. In the second case, *B. melitensis* strain Rev.1 has the normal properties of a biovar 1 strain of *B. melitensis,* but grows much more slowly on ordinary media, does not grow in the presence of basic fuchsin, thionin (20 µg/ml) or benzylpenicillin (3 µg/ml) (final concentrations), but does grow in the presence of streptomycin at 2.5 or 5 µg/ml, has very weak urease activity, and shows a reduced virulence for guinea-pigs and mice (1, 5, 6). *Brucella abortus* strain RB51 is identified by several characteristics; these are: rough morphology (by crystal violet staining and agglutination in acriflavin), resistance to growth in the presence of rifampicin (250 µg per ml of media), inability to produce O-polysaccharide (OPS), and by specific PCR (26, 30). The inability to produce OPS can be demonstrated by reacting RB51 colonies with OPS-specific monoclonal antibodies (MAbs), such as BRU38, in dot-blot assays or western blots (22, 26). An indirect way of demonstrating lack of OPS is by injecting 4×10^8 viable RB51 organisms into BALB/c mice and testing for the induction of OPS-antibodies; the serology will be negative (26). This characteristic of RB51 allows for multiple vaccinations with this vaccine without seroconversion (11, 28).

Both vaccine strains S19 and RB51 may be identified using specific PCRs (4, 8). The genetic basis of the S19 sensitivity to erythritol is a 702 base pair (bp) deletion in the ery locus. This genetic marker can be exploited in a PCR assay in which two oligonucleotide primers based on sequences flanking the deletion site are used to amplify the target DNA. S19 *Brucella* targets produce a single band of 361bp, whereas all other strains of *Brucella* (which do not have the deletion) produce a product of 1063 bp (25).

Brucella abortus strain RB51's *wboA* gene encoding a glycotransferase, an enzyme essential for the synthesis of OPS, is disrupted by an IS711 element. This stable mutation allowed for the development of an RB51-specific PCR (26). The nucleotide sequences of the primers to be used in the PCR for specific-strain RB51 identification are:

Primer 1: 5'-TTA-AGC-GCT-GAT-GCC-ATT-TCC-TTC-AC-3'

Primer 2: 5'-TTT-AGT-TTG-CCG-TAA-TAT-AGG-TCT-AGA-ACC-TGT-C-3'

Primer 3 5'-GCC-AAC-CAA-CCC-AAA-TGC-TCA-CAA-3'

Detailed information on antibiotic sensitivity and other biochemical characteristics of *B. abortus* strain RB51 can be found elsewhere (28).

2. Serological tests

No serological test is appropriate in each and all epidemiological situations. Consideration should be given to all factors that impact on the relevance of the test method and test results to a specific diagnostic interpretation or application. For the purposes of this chapter, the serological methods described represent standardised and validated methods with suitable performance characteristics to be designated as either prescribed or alternative tests for international trade. This does not preclude the use of modified or similar test methods or the use of different biological reagents. However, the methods and reagents described in this chapter represent a standard of comparison with respect to expected diagnostic performance.

It should be stressed that the serum agglutination test (SAT) is unsatisfactory for the detection of bovine brucellosis, and its use for the purposes of international trade should be discouraged. Despite this, some European Union (EU) member states still require that individual animals should not react in the SAT to a level exceeding 30 IU for purposes of international trade.

The EU also specifies an upper limit for the complement fixation test (CFT) of 20 ICFTU (international complement fixation test units). The CFT is diagnostically more sensitive and specific than the SAT, and also has a standardised system of unitage. The diagnostic performance characteristics of some enzyme-linked immunosorbent assays (ELISAs) and the fluorescence polarisation assay (FPA) are comparable with or better than that of the CFT, and as they are technically simpler to perform and more robust, their use may be preferred (16, 32).

For control of brucellosis at the national or local level, it is usually necessary to screen using a rapid and simple test with a more specific confirmatory test performed on positively reacting samples. The buffered *Brucella* antigen tests (BBATs), i.e. the rose bengal test (RBT) and the buffered plate agglutination test (BPAT), as well as the ELISA and the FPA, are suitable screening tests. Positively reacting samples should be retested using a suitable confirmatory test.

In other species, for example, buffaloes *(Bubalus bubalus)*, bison *(Bison bison)*, yak *(Bos grunniens)*, elk *(Cerves canadensis)*, and camels *(Camelus bactrianus* and *C. dromedarius)*, *B. abortus* infection follows a course similar to that in cattle. The same serological procedures may be used for these species (14), but each test should be validated in the species under study.

Primary reference sera have been developed and designated by the OIE as International Standard Sera[2]. The use of these promotes international harmonisation of diagnostic testing and antigen standardisation (32). For RBT and CFT the OIEISS (previously the WHO Second International anti-*Brucella abortus* Serum) which contains 1000 IU and ICFTU is used. In addition, three OIE ELISA Standard Sera are available for use. These consist of a strong positive, a weak positive and a negative standard. Primary reference standards are those against which all other standards are compared and calibrated. These reference standards are all available to national reference laboratories and should be used to establish secondary or national standards against which working standards can be prepared and used in the diagnostic laboratory for daily routine use.

- **Production of cells**

  Brucella abortus strain 99 (Weybridge) or *B. abortus* strain 1119-3 (USDA) should always be used for diagnostic antigen production[3]. The strains must be completely smooth and should not auto-agglutinate in saline and 0.1% (w/v) acriflavine. They must be pure cultures and conform to the characteristics of CO_2-independent strains of *B. abortus* biovar 1. The original seed cultures should be propagated to produce a seed lot that must conform to the properties of these strains, and should be preserved by lyophilisation or by freezing in liquid nitrogen.

2 OIEISS should be obtained from the OIE Reference Laboratory for Brucellosis at VLA Weybridge, New Haw, Addlestone, Surrey KT15 3NB, United Kingdom (UK).

3 Original seed should be obtained from the OIE Reference Laboratory for Brucellosis at VLA Weybridge, New Haw, Addlestone, Surrey KT15 3NB, United Kingdom (UK), or the NVSL of the USDA (see footnote 1).

For antigen production, the seed culture is used to inoculate a number of potato-infusion agar slopes that are then incubated at 37°C for 48 hours. SDA and trypticase soy agar (TSA), to which 5% equine or newborn calf serum and/or 0.1% yeast extract may be added, are satisfactory solid media provided a suitable seed is used as recommended above. The growth is checked for purity, resuspended in sterile phosphate buffered saline (PBS), pH 6.4, and used to seed layers of potato-infusion agar or glycerol–dextrose agar in Roux flasks. These are then incubated at 37°C for 72 hours with the inoculated surface facing down. Each flask is checked for purity by Gram staining samples of the growth, and the organisms are harvested by adding 50–60 ml of phenol saline (0.5% phenol in 0.85% sodium chloride solution) to each flask. The flasks are gently agitated, the suspension is decanted, and the organisms are killed by heating at 80°C for 90 minutes. Following a viability check, the antigen is stored at 4°C.

Alternatively, the cells may be produced by batch or continuous culture in a fermenter (10), using a liquid medium containing (per litre of distilled water) D-glucose (30 g), a high-grade peptone (30 g), yeast extract (Difco) (10 g), sodium dihydrogen phosphate (9 g) and disodium hydrogen phosphate (3.3 g). The initial pH is 6.6, but this tends to rise to pH 7.2–7.4 during the growth cycle. Care should be taken to check batches of peptone and yeast extract for capacity to produce good growth without formation of abnormal or dissociated cells. Vigorous aeration and stirring is required during growth, and adjustment to pH 7.2–7.4 by the addition of sterile 0.1 M HCl may be necessary. The seed inoculum is prepared as described above. The culture is incubated at 37°C for 48 hours. Continuous culture runs can be operated for much longer periods, but more skill is required to maintain them. In-process checks should be made on the growth from either solid or liquid medium to ensure purity, an adequate viable count and freedom from dissociation to rough forms. Cells for use in the preparation of all antigens should be checked for purity and smoothness at the harvesting stage.

The culture is harvested by centrifugation at 10,000 ***g*** to deposit the organisms, which are resuspended in phenol saline. The organisms are killed by heating at 80°C for 90 minutes and are stored at 4°C. They must form stable suspensions in physiological saline solutions and show no evidence of auto-agglutination. A viability check must be performed on the suspensions and no growth must be evident after 10 days' incubation at 37°C. The packed cell volume (PCV) of the killed suspensions can be determined by centrifuging 1 ml volumes in Wintrobe tubes at 3000 ***g*** for 75 minutes.

a) Enzyme-linked immunosorbent assay (a prescribed test for international trade)

- **Indirect ELISA**

Numerous variations of the indirect ELISA (iELISA) have been described employing different antigen preparations, antiglobulin-enzyme conjugates, and substrate/chromogens. Several commercial iELISAs are available that have been validated in extensive field trials and are in wide use. In the interests of international harmonisation, the three OIE ELISA Standard Sera should be used by national reference laboratories to check or calibrate the particular test method in question.

The assay should be calibrated such that the optical density of the strong positive OIE ELISA Standard Serum should represent a point on the linear portion of a typical dose–response curve just below the plateau. The weak positive OIE ELISA Standard Serum should give a reaction that lies on the linear portion of the same dose–response curve just above the positive/negative threshold. The negative serum and the buffer control should always give reactions that are always less than the positive/negative threshold (33).

The iELISA is a highly sensitive test but it is not capable of differentiating between antibody resulting from *B. abortus* S19 vaccination and that induced by pathogenic strains. The iELISA should therefore be considered more as a screening test than a confirmatory test in the testing of vaccinated cattle.

The protocol described below is quoted as an example of one which has been internationally validated and has been used extensively in internationally sponsored, technical cooperation and research collaboration projects world-wide.

The antigen-coating buffer is 0.05 M carbonate/bicarbonate buffer, pH 9.6, composed of sodium hydrogen carbonate (2.93 g) and sodium carbonate (1.59 g) (sodium azide [0.2 g/litre] is optional) in 1 litre of distilled water. The conjugate and test sera diluent buffer is 0.01 M PBS, pH 7.2, composed of disodium hydrogen orthophosphate (1.4 g), potassium dihydrogen phosphate (0.20 g), sodium chloride (8.500 g) and 0.05% Tween 20 dissolved in 1 litre of distilled water (PBST). This buffer is also used as wash buffer.

The conjugate used is an MAb specific for the heavy chain of bovine IgG_1 and conjugated to horseradish peroxidase (HRPO). The substrate stock solution is 3% hydrogen peroxide. The chromogen stock solution is 0.16 M 2,2'-azino-bis-(3-ethylbenzthiazoline-6-sulphonic acid) (ABTS) in distilled water. Substrate buffer is citrate buffer, pH 4.5, composed of trisodium citrate dihydrate (7.6 g) and citric acid (4.6 g) dissolved in 1 litre of distilled water. The enzymatic reaction-stopping solution is 4% sodium dodecyl sulphate (SDS).

- **Antigen production**

Smooth lipopolysaccharide (LPS) from *B. abortus* S1119-3 or S99 is prepared by heating 5 g dry weight (or 50 g wet weight) of cells suspended in 170 ml distilled water to 66°C followed by the addition of 190 ml of 90% (v/v) phenol at 66°C. The mixture is stirred continuously for 15 minutes and centrifuged at 10,000 ***g*** for 15 minutes at 4°C. The brownish phenol in the bottom layer is removed with a long cannula and large cell debris may be removed by filtration (using a Whatman # 1 filter) if necessary.

The LPS is precipitated by the addition of 500 ml cold methanol containing 5 ml methanol saturated with sodium acetate. After 2 hours' incubation at 4°C, the precipitate is removed by centrifugation at 10,000 ***g*** for 10 minutes. The precipitate is stirred with 80 ml of distilled water for 18 hours and centrifuged at 10,000 ***g*** for 10 minutes. The supernatant solution is kept at 4°C. The precipitate is resuspended in 80 ml distilled water and stirred for an additional 2 hours at 4°C. The supernatant solution is recovered by centrifugation as above and pooled with the previously recovered supernatant.

Next, 8 g of trichloroacetic acid is added to the 160 ml of crude LPS. After stirring for 10 minutes, the precipitate is removed by centrifugation and the translucent supernatant solution is dialised against distilled water (two changes of at least 4000 ml each) and then freeze dried.

The freeze-dried LPS is weighed and reconstituted to 1 mg/ml in 0.05 M carbonate buffer, pH 9.6, and sonicated in an ice bath using approximately 6 watts three times for 1 minute each. The LPS is then freeze dried in 1 ml amounts and stored at room temperature.

- **Test procedure**

i) The freeze-dried LPS is reconstituted to 1 ml with distilled water and further diluted 1/1000 with 0.05 M carbonate buffer, pH 9.6. To coat the microplates, 100 µl volumes of LPS solution are added to all wells, the plates are covered and incubated for 18 hours at 4°C. After incubation, the plates may be used or sealed, frozen and stored at –20°C for up to a year. Frozen plates are thawed for 30–45 minutes at 37°C before use.

ii) Unbound antigen is removed by washing all microplate wells with PBST four times. Volumes (100 µl) of serum diluted 1/50 in PBST, pH 6.3, containing 7.5 mM each of ethylene diamine tetra-acetic acid (EDTA) and ethylene glycol tetra-acetic acid (EGTA) (PBST/EDTA) are added to specified wells and incubated at ambient temperature for 30 minutes.

iii) The following are included (in duplicate) on each plate: a strong positive, a weak positive, a negative control serum, and a duplicate set of wells to which buffer only is added. Test sera may be tested as singles or duplicates, resulting in 40 or 88 tests per plate.

iv) Unbound serum is removed by washing four times with PBST. Volumes (100 µl) of an MAb[4] (M23) specific for a heavy chain epitope of bovine IgG_1 conjugated with HRPO and diluted in PBST are added to each well and the plates are incubated at ambient temperature for 30 minutes.

v) Unbound conjugate is removed by four washing steps. Volumes (100 µl) of substrate/chromogen (1.0 mM H_2O_2 [100 µl/20 ml citrate buffer] and 4 mM ABTS [500 µl/20 ml citrate buffer]) are added to each well, the plate is shaken for 10 minutes and colour development is assessed in a spectrophotometer at 414 or 405 nm. If required, 100 µl volumes of 4% SDS may be added directly to all wells as a stopping reagent.

vi) The control wells containing the strong positive serum are considered to be 100% positive and all data are calculated from these absorbance readings (between 1.000 and 1.800) using the equation:

% positivity (%P) = absorbance (test sample)/absorbance (strong positive control) × 100

Using this iELISA protocol calibrated against the OIE ELISA Standard Sera, the diagnostic sensitivity should be equal to or greater than the BBATs in the testing of infected cattle, and the diagnostic specificity should be equivalent to the CFT in the testing of unvaccinated cattle. It can be expected that the diagnostic specificity in the testing of vaccinated cattle will be significantly lower than for the CFT depending on where the iELISA positive/negative threshold is set.

- **Competitive ELISA**

The competitive ELISA (cELISA) using an MAb specific for one of the epitopes of the *B. abortus* OPS has been shown to have higher specificity than the iELISA (12, 17, 27). This is accomplished by selecting an MAb that has higher affinity than cross-reacting antibody, usually IgM of lower affinity. The cELISA is also

4 MAbs M23 and M84 may be obtained for research or standardisation purposes from the OIE Reference Laboratory for Brucellosis at the Animal Diseases Research Institute, 3851 Fallowfield Road, Nepean, Ontario K2H 8P9, Canada.

capable of eliminating most reactions due to residual antibody produced in response to vaccination with *B. abortus* S19. The choice of MAb and its unique specificity and affinity will have a distinct influence on the diagnostic performance characteristics of the assay. As with any MAb-based assay, the availability of the MAb or the hybridoma must also be considered with respect to international acceptance and widespread use.

Several variations of the cELISA have been described. In the interests of international harmonisation, the three OIE ELISA Standard Sera should be used by national reference laboratories to check or calibrate the test method in question.

The assay should be calibrated such that the OD of the strong positive OIE ELISA Standard Serum should represent a point on the linear portion of a typical dose–response curve just above the plateau (i.e. close to maximal inhibition). The weak positive OIE ELISA Standard Serum should give a reaction that lies on the linear portion of the same dose–response curve just above the positive/negative threshold (i.e. moderate inhibition). The negative serum and the buffer/MAb control should give reactions that are always less than the positive/negative threshold (i.e. minimal inhibition).

The protocol described below is quoted as an example of one which has been internationally validated and has been used extensively in internationally sponsored, technical cooperation and research collaboration projects world-wide.

The buffer systems are the same as those described for the iELISA.

- **Antigen production**

Smooth LPS from *B. abortus* S1119-3 is prepared and used as for the iELISA.

- **Test procedure**

i) The freeze-dried LPS is reconstituted to 1 ml with distilled water and further diluted 1/1000 with 0.05 M carbonate buffer, pH 9.6. To coat the microplates, 100 µl volumes of LPS solution are added to all wells and the plates are covered and incubated for 18 hours at 4°C. After incubation, the plates may be used or sealed, frozen and stored at –20°C for up to 1 year. Frozen plates are thawed for 30–45 minutes at 37°C before use.

ii) Unbound antigen is removed by washing all microplate wells four times with PBST. Volumes (50 µl) of MAb (M84) diluted appropriately in PBST/EDTA are added to each well, followed immediately by 50 µl volumes of serum diluted 1/10 in PBST/EDTA. Plates are incubated for 30 minutes at ambient temperature with shaking for at least the initial 3 minutes.

iii) The following are included (in duplicate) on each plate: a strong positive, a weak positive, a negative control serum, and a duplicate set of wells to which MAb and buffer are added. Sera may be tested as singles or duplicates, resulting in 88 or 40 tests per plate.

iv) Unbound serum and MAb are removed by washing the microplate four times with PBST. Volumes (100 µl) of commercial goat anti-mouse IgG (H and L chain) HRPO conjugate diluted in PBST are added to each well and the plates are incubated at ambient temperature for 30 minutes.

v) Unbound conjugate is removed by four washing steps. Volumes (100 µl) of substrate/chromogen (1.0 mM H_2O_2 and 4 mM ABTS) are added to each well, the plates are shaken for 10 minutes and colour development is assessed in a spectrophotometer at 414 or 405 nm. If required, 100 µl volumes of 4% SDS may be added directly as a stopping reagent.

vi) The control wells containing MAb and buffer (no serum) are considered to be 0% inhibition and all data are calculated from these absorbance readings (between 1000 and 1800) using the equation:

% inhibition (%I) = 100 – (absorbance [test sample]/absorbance [buffer control] × 100).

The LPS antigen, small amounts of the MAb M84, software for generation of data using particular spectrophotometers and a standard operating procedure for the cELISA are available for research and standardisation (see footnote 4 for address).

Using this cELISA protocol calibrated against the OIE ELISA Standard Sera, the diagnostic sensitivity should be equal to or greater than the BBATs and equivalent to the iELISA in the testing of infected cattle (15–17). The diagnostic specificity of the cELISA should be equivalent to or greater than the CFT and the iELISA in the testing of unvaccinated cattle. The diagnostic specificity of the cELISA in the testing of *B. abortus* S19 vaccinated cattle will be somewhat lower. Nonetheless, the diagnostic specificity of cELISA will be very much superior to that of the iELISA in the testing of vaccinated animals.

b) **Buffered *Brucella* antigen tests (prescribed tests for international trade)**

- **Rose bengal test**

- **Antigen production**

Antigen for the RBT is prepared by depositing killed *B. abortus* strain 99 or 1119-3 cells by centrifugation at, for example, 23,000 ***g*** for 10 minutes at 4°C, and uniformly resuspending in phenol saline at the rate of 1 g to 22.5 ml. (Note: if sodium carboxymethyl cellulose is used as the sedimenting agent during preparation of the cell concentrate, insoluble residues must be removed by filtering the suspension through an AMF-CUNO Zeta-plus prefilter [Type CPR 01A] before staining.) To every 35 ml of this suspension, 1 ml of 1% (w/v) rose bengal (CI No. 45440) in distilled water is added, and the mixture is stirred for 2 hours at room temperature. The mixture is filtered through cotton wool, and centrifuged at 10,000 ***g*** to deposit the stained cells, which are then uniformly resuspended at the rate of 1g cells to 7 ml of diluent (21.1 g of sodium hydroxide dissolved in 353 ml of phenol saline, followed by 95 ml of lactic acid, and adjusted to 1056 ml with phenol saline). The colour of this suspension should be an intense pink and the supernatant of a centrifuged sample should be free from stain; the pH should be 3.65 ± 0.05. After filtration through cotton wool, the suspension is filtered twice through a Sartorius No. 13430 glass fibre prefilter, adjusted to a PCV of approximately 8%, pending final standardisation against serum calibrated against the OIEISS, and stored at 4°C in the dark. The antigen should never be frozen.

When used in the standard test procedure, the RBT antigen should give a clearly positive reaction with 1/45 dilutions, but not 1/55 dilutions, of the OIEISS diluted in 0.5% phenol saline. It may also be advisable to compare the reactivity of new and previously standardised batches of antigen using a panel of defined sera.

- **Test procedure**

Serum samples may be screened using the RBT. Serum (20–30 µl) is mixed with an equal volume of antigen on a white tile or enamel plate to produce a zone approximately 2 cm in diameter. The mixture is rocked gently for 4 minutes at ambient temperature, and then observed for agglutination (13). Any visible reaction is considered to be positive. The test is very sensitive, especially in vaccinated animals, and positive samples should be retested by a confirmatory test such as the CFT or ELISA. False-negative reactions may occur and can be detected by retesting animals at intervals over a period of at least 3 months.

- **Buffered plate agglutination test**

- **Antigen production**

Antigen for the BPAT is prepared from *B. abortus* strain 1119-3 according to the procedure described by Angus & Barton (2).

Two staining solutions are required: a solution of brilliant green certified biological stain in distilled water (2 g/100 ml) and a solution of crystal violet certified biological stain in distilled water (1 g/100 ml). Once prepared, the two solutions should be stored separately for a period of 24 hours, and then mixed together in equal volumes in a dark bottle and stored in a refrigerator for a period of no fewer than 6 months before use. The mixed stain may be used between 6 and 12 months after initial preparation, after which it should be discarded.

Buffered diluent is prepared by slowly dissolving sodium hydroxide (150 g) in 3–4 litres of sterile phenol saline. Lactic acid (675 ml) is added to this solution, and the final volume is adjusted to 6 litres by adding sterile phenol saline. The pH of the solution should be between 3.63 and 3.67.

Brucella abortus packed cells are diluted to a concentration of 250 g/litre in phenol saline; 6 ml of stain is added per litre of the cell suspension, and the mixture is shaken thoroughly before being filtered through sterile absorbent cotton. The cells are centrifuged at 10,000 ***g*** at 4°C, and the packed cells are then resuspended at a concentration of 50 g/100 ml in buffered diluent (as described above). This mixture is shaken thoroughly for 2 hours, and is then further diluted by the addition of 300 ml of buffered diluent per 100 ml of suspended cells (i.e. final concentration of 50 g packed cells/400 ml buffered diluent). The mixture is stirred at room temperature for 20–24 hours before the cell concentration is adjusted to 11% (w/v) in buffered diluent. This suspension is stirred overnight before testing. Pending final quality control tests, the antigen is stored at 4°C until required for use. The antigen has a shelf life of 1 year and should not be frozen.

The pH of the buffered plate antigen should be 3.70 ± 0.03 and the pH of a serum:antigen mixture of ratio 8:3 should be 4.02 ± 0.04. The 11% stained-cell suspension should appear blue-green. Each batch of buffered plate antigen should be checked by testing at least 10 weakly reactive sera and comparing the results with one or more previous batches of antigen. If possible, the antigen batches should be compared with the standard antigen prepared by the NVSL of the USDA (see footnote 1 for address).

- **Test procedure**

Serum samples may also be screened using the BPAT. Serum (80 µl) is mixed with a 30 µl volume of antigen on a glass plate marked in 4 × 4 cm squares. After the initial mixing, the plate should be rotated three times in a tilting motion to ensure even dispersion of the reagents, and then incubated for 4 minutes in a humid chamber at ambient temperature. The plate should be removed and rotated as above, and then returned for a second 4-minute incubation. At this point, the plate should be removed, rotated, and observed for agglutination (1). Any visible reaction is considered to be positive. Like the RBT, the test is very sensitive, especially in vaccinated animals, and positive samples should be checked by the ELISA or CFT. False-negative reactions occur and can be detected by retesting animals at intervals over at least 3 months.

c) Complement fixation test (a prescribed test for international trade)

The CFT is a widely used and accepted confirmatory test although it is complex to perform, requiring good laboratory facilities, and adequately trained staff to accurately titrate and maintain the reagents. Numerous variations of the test occur, but each may be most conveniently carried out using microtitration plates. Either warm or cold fixation may be used for the incubation of serum, antigen and complement; either 37°C for 30 minutes or 4°C for 14–18 hours.

All dilutions are made in veronal buffered saline prepared from a stock solution of sodium chloride (42.5 g), barbituric acid (2.875 g), sodium diethyl barbiturate (1.875 g), magnesium sulphate (1.018 g), and calcium chloride (0.147 g) in 1 litre of distilled water and diluted by the addition of four volumes of 0.04% gelatine solution before use. The indicator system is a 3% suspension of fresh sheep red blood cells (SRBC) sensitised with an equal volume of rabbit anti-SRBC serum (haemolysin). This is prepared at a dilution previously determined to contain five times the minimum haemolysin concentration required to produce 100% lysis of the SRBC in the presence of a 1/10 dilution of fresh guinea-pig complement. The latter is independently titrated to determine the minimum concentration required to produce 100% lysis of the sensitised SRBC suspension; this is defined as the minimum haemolytic dose (MHD). The complement is used at 1.25 MHD in the test.

- **Antigen production**

Numerous variations of the test exist but, which ever procedure is selected, the test must use an antigen that has been prepared from an approved smooth strain of *B. abortus*, such as strain 99 or 1119-3, and standardised against the OIEISS. Antigen for the CFT can be prepared by special procedures (1, 10) or a whole cell antigen can be used after diluting the stock suspension such that the PCV of the concentrated antigen suspension for CFT should be approximately 2% before standardisation against the OIEISS. The antigen should be standardised to give 50% fixation at a dilution of 1/200 of the OIEISS and must also show complete fixation at the lower serum dilutions, because too weak (or too strong) a concentration of antigen may not produce 100% fixation at the lower dilutions of serum. When two dilutions of antigen are suitable, the more concentrated antigen suspension must be chosen in order to avoid prozone occurrence.

The appearance of the antigen when diluted 1/10 must be that of a uniform, dense, white suspension with no visible aggregation or deposit after incubation at 37°C for 18 hours. It must not produce anticomplementary effects at the working strength for the test. The antigen is stored at 4°C and should not be frozen.

- **Test procedure**

i) Test sera and appropriate working standards (see above) are diluted with an equal volume of veronal buffered saline in small tubes and incubated at 58°C for 50 minutes in order to inactivate the native complement.

ii) Using standard 96-well U-bottom microtitre plates, 25 µl volumes of diluted test serum are placed in the wells of the first and second rows, and 25 µl volumes of veronal buffered saline are added to all wells except those of the first row.

iii) Serial doubling dilutions are then made by transferring 25 µl volumes of serum from the second row onwards continuing for at least four dilutions.

iv) Repeat steps ii and iii above for each serum to act as anticomplementary serum controls (see below).

v) Volumes (25 µl) of complement at 1.25 MHD, are added to each well and 25 µl of antigen, diluted to working strength, is added to all wells excluding those of the anticomplementary controls. These latter wells receive 25 µl of veronal buffered saline instead.

vi) Control wells containing: diluent only, negative serum + complement + diluent, antigen + complement + diluent, and complement + diluent, are set up to contain 75 µl total volume in each case.

vii) The plates are incubated at 37°C for 30 minutes with agitation at least for the initial 10 minutes, or at 4°C for 14–18 hours.

viii) Volumes (50 µl) of sensitised SRBC suspension are added to each well, and the plates are reincubated at 37°C for 30 minutes with agitation at least for the first 10 minutes.

ix) The results are read after the plates have been left to stand at 4°C for up to 1 hour to allow unlysed cells to settle or the plates are centrifuged to deposit the cells.

The degree of haemolysis is compared with standards corresponding to 0, 25, 50, 75 and 100% lysis. Results should always be expressed in ICFTU, calculated in relation to those obtained in a parallel titration with a working or national standard serum calibrated against the OIEISS, which contains 1000 ICFTU. In general, sera giving positive fixation at a titre equivalent to 20 ICFTU or greater, are considered to be positive.

False-positive reactions may arise in the testing of *B. abortus* S19 vaccinated animals. Females that have been vaccinated with *Brucella abortus* S19 vaccine at the age of between 3 and 6 months, are considered to be positive if the sera gives a positive fixation at a titre of 30 ICFTU/ml when the animals are tested at an age of 18 months or older.

d) Fluorescence polarisation assay

The fluorescence polarisation assay (FPA) has received very promising reports in the literature. It may be applicable in appropriate circumstances. It is a simple technique for measuring antigen/antibody interaction and may be performed in a laboratory setting or in the field. It is a homogeneous assay in which analytes are not separated and it is therefore very rapid.

The mechanism of the assay takes into account that a molecule in solution randomly rotates. Molecular size is the main factor influencing the rate of rotation that is inversely related. Thus a small molecule rotates faster than a large molecule. If a molecule is labelled with a fluorochrome, the time of rotation through an angle of 68.5° is determined by measuring polarised light intensity in vertical and horizontal planes. Thus a large molecule is confined to emitting more light to a single plane (more polarised) than a small molecule rotating faster and emitting more depolarised light.

For most FPAs, an antigen of small molecular weight, less than 50 kD, is labelled with fluorescein and added to serum or other fluid to be tested for the presence of antibody. If antibody is present, attachment to the labelled antigen will cause its rotational rate to decrease and this decrease may be measured.

For the diagnosis of brucellosis, a small molecular weight fragment (average 22 kD) of the OPS of *B. abortus* smooth LPS is labelled with fluorescein isothiocyanate and used as the antigen. This antigen is added to diluted serum or whole blood and a measure of the antibody content is obtained in about 2 minutes using a fluorescence polarisation analyser (15).

The FPA can be performed in glass tubes or a 96-well plate format. The bovine serum is diluted 1/100 or, if EDTA-treated blood is used (heparin-treated blood tends to increase assay variability), 1/50 in 0.1 M phosphate buffer, pH 7.2, containing 0.15 M sodium chloride, 0.1% sodium azide and 0.05% lithium dodecyl sulphate (PBSAL). An initial reading to assess light scatter is obtained with the fluorescence polarisation analyser (FPM) after mixing. Suitably titrated, labelled antigen is added, mixed and a second reading is obtained in the FPM about 2 minutes later. An FPM reading (in millipolarisation units, mP) over the established threshold level is indicative of a positive reaction. A typical threshold level is 90 mP units, however, the test should be calibrated locally against standard reference sera. Control sera of strong positive, weak positive and negative, as well as S19 vaccinate serum, should be included.

- **Antigen production**

OPS from 5 g dry weight (or 50 g wet weight) of *B. abortus* strain 1119-3 is prepared by adding 400 ml of 2% (v/v) acetic acid, autoclaving the suspension for 15 minutes at 121°C and removing the cellular debris by centrifugation at 10,000 ***g*** for 10 minutes at 4°C. The supernatant solution is then treated with 20 g of trichloroacetic acid to precipitate any proteins and nucleic acids. The precipitate is again removed by centrifugation at 10,000 ***g*** for 10 minutes at 4°C. The supernatant fluid is dialised against at least 100 volumes of distilled water and freeze dried.

3 mg of OPS is dissolved in 0.6 ml of 0.1 M sodium hydroxide (4 g NaOH/litre) and incubated at 37°C for 1 hour, followed by the addition of 0.3 ml of fluorescein isothiocyanate isomer 1 at a concentration of 100 mg/ml in dimethyl sulphoxide and a further incubation at 37°C for 1 hour. The conjugated OPS is applied to a 1 × 10 cm column packed with diethylaminoethyl Sephadex A 25 equilibrated in 0.01 M phosphate buffer, pH 7.4. The first fraction (after 10–15 ml of buffer) is bright green, after which the buffer is switched to 0.1 M phosphate, pH 7.4. This results in the elution of 10–15 ml of buffer followed by 25–40 ml of green fluorescent material. The latter material is the antigen used in the FPA. Antigen preparation may be scaled up proportionally.

The amount of antigen used per test is determined by diluting the material derived above until a total fluorescence intensity of 250,000–300,000 is achieved using the FPM.

The antigen is stored as a liquid for several years at 4°C in a dark bottle or it may be freeze dried in dark bottles.

Small quantities of labelled antigen for research and standardisation purposes and standard operating procedures for antigen preparation and the FPA may be obtained (see footnote 4 for address).

- **Test procedure**

i) 1 ml of PBSAL buffer is added to a 10 × 75 mm borosilicate glass tube. 10 µl of serum or 20 µl of EDTA-treated blood is added to the tube and mixed well. A reading is obtained on the FPM to determine light scatter.

ii) A volume of antigen that results in a total fluorescence intensity of 250–300 × 10^3 is added to the tube and mixed well. This volume will vary from batch to batch, but is generally in the range of about 10 µl. A second reading is obtained on the FPM after incubation at ambient temperature for approximately 2 minutes.

iii) A reading above the predetermined threshold is indicative of a positive reaction.

iv) The following are included in each batch of tests: a strong positive, a weak positive, a negative working standard serum (calibrated against the OIE ELISA Standard Sera).

The diagnostic sensitivity and specificity of the FPA for bovine brucellosis are almost identical to those of the cELISA. The diagnostic specificity for cattle recently vaccinated with *B. abortus* S19 is over 99% (15).

3. Other tests

An extremely efficient means of screening dairy herds is by testing milk from the bulk tank. Milk from this source can be obtained cheaply and more frequently than blood samples and is often available centrally at dairies. When a positive test result is obtained, all cows contributing milk should be blood tested. The milk iELISA is the most sensitive and specific test, and is particularly valuable for the testing of large herds. The milk ring test (MRT) is a suitable alternative if the ELISA is not available. The iELISA can also be used for testing individual animals.

An alternative immunological test is the brucellin skin test, which can be used for screening unvaccinated herds, provided that a purified, standardised antigen preparation (e.g. brucellin INRA, see Chapter 2.4.2. for address) is used.

a) Milk iELISA

As with the serum iELISA numerous variations of the milk iELISA are in use. Several commercial iELISAs are available that have been validated in extensive field trials and are in wide use. In the interests of international harmonisation, the three OIE ELISA Standard Sera should be used by national reference laboratories to check or calibrate the particular test method in question. Milk samples are generally tested at much lower dilutions than sera, i.e. undiluted to 1/10 in diluent buffer. The cELISA should not be used to test milk.

b) Milk ring test

In lactating animals, the MRT can be used for screening herds for brucellosis. In large herds (>100 lactating cows), the sensitivity of the test becomes less reliable. False-positive reactions may occur in recently vaccinated cattle (less than 4 months post-vaccination) or in samples containing abnormal milk, such as colostrum or that due to mastitis.

- **Antigen production**

MRT antigen is prepared from concentrated, killed *B. abortus* strain 99 or 1119-3 cell suspension, grown as described previously. It is centrifuged at, for example, 23,000 ***g*** for 10 minutes at 4°C, followed by resuspension in haematoxylin-staining solution. Various satisfactory methods are in use; one example is as follows: 100 ml of 4% (w/v) haematoxylin (CI No. 75290) dissolved in 95% ethanol is added to a solution of ammonium aluminium sulphate (5 g) in 100 ml of distilled water + 48 ml of glycerol. 2 ml of freshly prepared 10% (w/v) sodium iodate is added to the solution. After standing for 30 minutes at room temperature, the deep purple solution is added to 940 ml of 10% (w/v) ammonium aluminium sulphate in distilled water. The pH of this mixture is adjusted to 3.1, and the solution must be aged by storage at room temperature in the dark for 45–90 days.

Before use, the staining solution is shaken and filtered through cotton wool. The packed cells are suspended in the staining solution at the rate of 1 g per 30 ml stain, and held at room temperature for 48 hours (some laboratories prefer to heat at 80°C for 10 minutes instead). The stained cells are then deposited by centrifugation, and washed three times in a solution of sodium chloride (6.4 g), 85% lactic acid (1.5 ml) and 10% sodium hydroxide (4.4 ml) in 1.6 litres of distilled water, final pH 3.0. The washed cells are resuspended at the rate of 1 g in 27 ml of a diluent consisting of 0.5% phenol saline, adjusted to pH 4.0 by the addition of 0.1 M citric acid (approximately 2.5 ml) and 0.5 M disodium hydrogen phosphate (approximately 1 ml) and maintained at 4°C for 24 hours. The mixture is filtered through cotton wool, the pH is checked, and the PCV is determined and adjusted to approximately 4%.

The sensitivity of the new batch should be compared with a previously standardised batch using a panel of samples of varying degrees of reaction prepared by diluting a positive serum in milk. A 1/500 dilution of the OIEISS in negative milk should be positive, while a 1/1000 dilution should be negative. The antigen must be stored at 4°C and not frozen.

The pH of the antigen should be between 3.3 and 3.7 and its colour should be dark blue. There might be a little free stain in the supernatant of a centrifuged sample. When diluted in milk from a brucellosis-free animal, the antigen must produce a uniform coloration of the milk layer with no deposit and no coloration of the cream layer.

- **Test procedure**

The test is performed by adding 30 µl of antigen to a 1 ml volume of whole milk that has been stored for at least 24 hours at 4°C. The height of the milk column in the tube must be at least 25 mm. The milk samples must not have been frozen, heated or subjected to violent shaking. The milk/antigen mixtures are normally incubated at 37°C for 1 hour, together with positive and negative working standards. However, overnight incubation at 4°C increases the sensitivity of the test and allows for easier reading of the tests. A strongly positive reaction is indicated by formation of a dark blue ring above a white milk column. Any blue layer at the interface of milk and cream should be considered to be positive as it might be significant, especially in large herds. The test is considered to be negative if the colour of the underlying milk exceeds that of the cream layer.

c) Brucellin skin test

The relatively low sensitivity of the Brucellin test limits the detection of individual infected animals. Therefore this test alone cannot be recommended as the sole diagnostic test or for the purposes of international trade. However, it has a very high specificity, such that serologically negative animals that are positive reactors to the Brucellin test should be regarded as infected animals (19, 20). Also, results of this test may aid the interpretation of serological reactions thought to be due to infection with cross-reacting bacteria, especially in brucellosis-free areas (24). It is essential to use a standardised, defined Brucellin preparation that does not contain smooth LPS antigen, as this may provoke nonspecific inflammatory reactions or interfere with subsequent serological tests. One such preparation is Brucellin INRA prepared from a nonsmooth strain of *B. melitensis*. The requirements for its production are detailed in Chapter 2.4.2., Section B2. Brucellin.

- **Test procedure**

A volume of 0.1 ml of Brucellin is injected intradermally into the caudal fold, the skin of the flank, or the side of the neck. The test is read after 48–72 hours, and a positive reaction is indicated by local swelling and induration. It is recommended that the skin thickness at the injection site should be measured with vernier callipers before injection and at re-examination. Strong reactions are easily recognised, but borderline reactions require careful interpretation. Although the Brucellin intradermal test is one of the most specific tests in brucellosis (in nonvaccinated animals), diagnosis should not be made solely on the basis of positive intradermal reactions given by a few animals in the herd, but should be supported by a reliable serological test, such as the ELISA.

B. REQUIREMENTS FOR VACCINES AND DIAGNOSTIC BIOLOGICALS

Brucella abortus strain 19 vaccine

The most widely used vaccine for the prevention of brucellosis in cattle is prepared from *B. abortus* S19. It is used as a live vaccine and is normally given to female calves aged between 3 and 6 months as a single subcutaneous dose of 5–8 × 10^{10} viable organisms. A reduced dose of from 3 × 10^8 to 3 × 10^9 organisms can be administered to beef or dairy cattle aged between 4 and 12 months, but 5–10% of the animals will develop persistent antibody titres. Alternatively, it can be administered to cattle of any age as two doses of 5–10 × 10^9 viable organisms, given by the conjunctival route; this produces protection without a persistent antibody response. Requirements for *B. abortus* S19 vaccine have been defined by the World Health Organization (31).

Brucella abortus S19 vaccine induces good immunity to moderate challenge by virulent organisms. The vaccine must be prepared from USDA-derived seed (see footnote 1) and each batch must be checked for purity, viability, smoothness, and absence of toxicity or virulence.

Brucella abortus strain RB51

Since 1996, *B. abortus* strain RB51 has become the official USA vaccine for prevention of brucellosis in cattle. Use of *B. abortus* S19 is now prohibited in the USA. Other countries where the vaccine is officially approved and used at this time are: Argentina, Chile, Colombia, Costa Rica, Mexico, Paraguay, and Venezuela. Each country is using slightly different methods to adminster the vaccine. In the USA, calves are vaccinated subcutaneously between the ages of 4 and 12 months with 1–3.4 × 10^{10} viable strain RB51 organisms. Vaccination of cattle over 12 months of age is carried out only under authorisation from the State or Federal Animal Health Officials, and the recommended dose is 1 × 10^9 viable strain RB51 organisms. In other countries, it is recommended to vaccinate cattle as calves (4–12 months of age) with a 1–3.4 × 10^{10} dose, with revaccination from 12 months of age onwards with a similar dose to elicit a booster effect and increase immunity. Details on the recommendations of use vary somewhat from country to country. Although experimental work has demonstrated that *B. abortus* strain RB51 vaccination of pregnant cattle does not induce abortions, field experience indicates that it can induce a small percentage of abortions if applied to pregnant cattle. This is particularly true if cattle did not receive calfhood vaccination with *B. abortus* S19 or *B. abortus* strain RB51. It appears nevertheless, that *B. abortus* strain RB51 has a lesser abortafecient effect than S19 (18). Due to these observations, vaccination of pregnant cattle should be avoided. The vaccine can be administered multiple times if desired without inducing antibodies reactive in any serological test using whole cells or smooth LPS as antigen.

Control procedures for these two vaccines follow. The control procedure detailed in Chapter 2.4.2. for *B. melitensis* Rev.1 is also applicable to S19 vaccine.

1. Seed management

a) Characteristics of the seed

Brucella abortus S19 original seed for vaccine production must be obtained from the USDA (see footnote 1), and used to produce a seed lot that is preserved by lyophilisation or by freezing at liquid nitrogen temperature. The properties of this seed lot must conform to those of a pure culture of a CO_2-independent *B. abortus* biovar 1 that is also sensitive to benzylpenicillin, thionin blue and *i*-erythritol at recommended concentrations, and that displays minimal pathogenicity for guinea-pigs.

Brucella abortus RB51 original seed for vaccine production is available commercially[5]. These companies have legal rights to the vaccine.

b) Method of culture

Brucella abortus S19 for vaccine production is grown on medium free from serum or other animal products, under conditions similar to those described for *B. abortus* strain 99 or 1119-3.

Brucella abortus strain RB51 follows similar culture methods.

5 Colorado Serum Company, 4950 York Street, P.O. Box 16428, Denver, Colorado 80216-0428, USA; or Veterinary Technologies Corporation, 1872 Pratt Drive, Suite 1100B, Blacksburg, Virginia 24060, USA.

c) Validation as a vaccine

Numerous independent studies have confirmed the value of *B. abortus* S19 as a vaccine for protecting cattle from brucellosis. The organism behaves as an attenuated strain when given to sexually immature cattle. In rare cases, it may produce localised infection in the genital tract. Antibody responses persisting for 6 months or longer are likely to occur in a substantial proportion of cattle that have been vaccinated with the standard dose as adults. Some of the cattle vaccinated as calves may later develop arthropathy, particularly of the femoro-tibial joints (3, 7). The vaccine is safe for most animals if administered to calves between 3 and 8 months of age. It may also be used in adult animals at a reduced dose. It produces lasting immunity to moderate challenge with virulent strains, but the precise duration of this is unknown. Protection against *B. melitensis* is less evident. The vaccine strain is stable and reversion to virulence is extremely rare. It has been associated with the emergence of *i*-erythritol-using strains when inadvertently administered to pregnant animals. The organism behaves as an attenuated strain in the guinea-pig, and even large inocula are rapidly cleared from the tissues. It has some virulence for humans, and infections have occasionally followed accidental inoculation with the vaccine. Care should be taken in its preparation and handling, and a hazard warning should be included on the label of the final containers.

Both experimental challenge studies and field studies have confirmed the value of *B. abortus* strain RB51 for protecting cattle from brucellosis. The organism is attenuated in calves and adults. As *B. abortus* strain RB51 does not contain smooth LPS, it does not induce antibodies to the OPS antigen and therefore, there is no serological conversion of vaccinated animals. As with *B. abortus* S19, it produces lasting immunity to moderate challenge with virulent strains, but the precise duration of this is unknown. The vaccine is very stable and no reversion to smoothness has been described *in vivo* or *in vitro*. The organism behaves as an attenuated strain in a variety of animals including guinea-pigs where it is rapidly cleared from the tissues and does not induce abortions. It may have some virulence for humans, and infections may follow accidental inoculation with the vaccine, although no such infections have yet been reported. In any case, accidental inoculations should be treated with tetracyclines.

2. Method of manufacture

For production of *B. abortus* S19 vaccine, the procedures described above (in Section A.2.) can be used, except that the cells are collected in PBS, pH 6.3, and deposited by centrifugation or by the addition of sodium carboxymethyl cellulose at a final concentration of 1.5 g/litre. The yield from one fermenter run or the pooled cells from a batch of Roux flask cultures that have been inoculated at the same time from the same seed lot, constitutes a single harvest. More than one single harvest may be pooled to form a final bulk, which is used to fill the final containers of a batch of vaccine. Before pooling, each single harvest must be checked for purity, cell concentration, dissociation and identity. A similar range of tests must be done on the final bulk, which should have a viable count of between 8 and 24 × 10^9 colony forming units/ml. Adjustments in concentration are made by the addition of PBS for vaccine to be dispensed in liquid form, or by the addition of stabiliser for lyophilised vaccine. If stabiliser is to be used, loss of viability on lyophilisation should be taken into account, and should not be in excess of 50%. The final dried product should not be exposed to a temperature exceeding 35°C during drying, and the residual moisture content should be 1–2%. The contents must be sealed under vacuum or dry nitrogen immediately after drying, and stored at 4°C.

The production of *B. abortus* strain RB51 is very similar to the one used for *B. abortus* S19.

3. In-process control

Brucella abortus S19 vaccine should be checked for purity and smoothness during preparation of the single harvests. The cell concentration of the bulks should also be checked. This can be done by opacity measurement, but a viable count must be performed on the final filling lots. The identity of these should also be checked by agglutination tests with antiserum to *Brucella* A antigen. The viable count of the final containers should not be less than 50 × 10^9 per dose after lyophilisation, if this is to be done, and at least 95% of the cells must be in the smooth phase.

Brucella abortus strain RB51 vaccine should be checked for purity and roughness during preparation of the single harvests. The cell concentration of the bulks should also be checked. A viable count must be performed on the final filling lots. The viable count of the final containers should be 1–3.4 × 10^{10} viable colony forming units of RB51 per dose (dose of 2 ml to be applied subcutaneously) and 100% of the cells must be in the rough phase. All colonies should be negative on dot-blot assays with MAbs specific for the OPS antigen.

4. Batch control

a) Sterility

Tests for sterility and freedom from contamination of biological materials may be found in Chapter I.4.

b) Safety

A safety test on *B. abortus* S19 vaccine may be performed in guinea-pigs. Groups of at least 10 animals are given intramuscular injections of doses of vaccine diluted in PBS, pH 7.2, to contain 5×10^9 viable organisms. The animals should show no obvious adverse effects and there must be no mortality. After 10 days, the animals are killed, and spleens and blood samples collected. The spleen tissue must not contain more than 5×10^5 *Brucella* organisms/g and the CFT titre must not exceed 1000 ICFTU. In practice, batches of vaccine that fail this test are encountered extremely infrequently.

A safety test on *B. abortus* strain RB51 vaccine is not routinely done. If desired, BALB/c, 4–6-week-old female mice can be injected intraperitoneally with 1×10^8 colony forming units and the spleen cultured at 6 weeks post-inoculation. Spleens should be free from RB51 and the mice should not develop anti-OPS antibodies.

c) Potency

The potency of *B. abortus* S19 vaccine is determined routinely in guinea-pigs or mice. Groups of guinea-pigs are injected subcutaneously with 1/15 of the standard subcutaneous cattle dose of the test vaccine or a reference preparation, followed 6 weeks later with an intramuscular challenge of a virulent *B. abortus* strain, such as 544 or 2308. This can be given at the single dose level of 5×10^3 viable organisms, but it is preferable to use a graded challenge of 5×10^2, 5×10^3 and 5×10^4 organisms. After a further 6 weeks, the animals are killed and the spleen counts of viable *B. abortus* organisms are determined. The protection index (organisms/g of spleen in vaccinated compared with unvaccinated animals) relative to the reference preparation is then calculated (29). The virulence and infectivity of the challenge strain must be such that the ID_{50} (50% infective dose) is less than 10^2 organisms, and that 5 weeks after inoculating guinea-pigs with 5000 organisms, the mean spleen:body weight ratio is not less than 0.30% and the mean CFT titre is not less than 600 ICFTU.

In the mouse potency assay, graded doses of vaccine are injected into 5-week-old mice (preferably CD1) weighing 21–25 g. The mice are challenged 30 days later by the intraperitoneal injection of 2×10^5 viable *B. abortus* strain 544 organisms, and 15 days later the spleen counts are determined. Parallel tests are conducted with a reference vaccine and the protection index is calculated.

There is some dispute as to the validity of mouse or guinea-pig assays for determining the potency of *Brucella* vaccines. However, provided that statistically valid numbers of animals are used (at least 30 per group) and simultaneous comparison is made with a reference vaccine, the results appear to differentiate between effective and ineffective vaccines.

A potency test on *B. abortus* strain RB51 vaccine is not routinely carried out. It could be carried out in BALB/c female mice if desired using 1×10^4 *B. abortus* strain 2308 organisms as the challenge strain. The usefulness of this test to predict protection in cattle is questionable.

d) Duration of immunity

Vaccinating calves with a full dose of *B. abortus* S19 vaccine is considered to give long-lasting immunity, and subsequent doses are not recommended. Use of reduced doses, whether given by intradermal or conjunctival routes, produces less durable immunity, and repeated doses may need to be given annually. This can lead to antibody responses that may interfere with serological tests.

Vaccination of calves with *B. abortus* strain RB51 is believed to stimulate an immunity that will last for a period similar to the one induced with *B. abortus* S19 although there are no specific studies to demonstrate this. Field studies carried out where challenge occurred 1 year post-vaccination, suggest that *B. abortus* strain RB51-induced immunity in cattle is stronger than immunity induced by *B. abortus* S19 (11).

e) Stability

Brucella abortus S19 vaccine prepared from seed stock from appropriate sources is stable in characteristics and shows no tendency to reversion to virulence. The lyophilised vaccine shows a gradual loss of viable count, but should retain its potency for the recommended shelf life. Allowance for this phenomenon is normally made by ensuring that the viable count immediately following lyophilisation is well in excess of the minimum requirement. Maintenance of a cold chain during distribution of the vaccine will ensure its viability.

Brucella abortus strain RB51 has shown no tendency to revert to virulent smooth organisms after many passages *in vitro* or *in vivo*. This is probably due to the nature and place of the mutations found in this strain. *Brucella abortus* strain RB51 has its *wboA* gene disrupted by an IS711 element impeding synthesis of OPS. Unpublished data indicate that it also contains a second mutation affecting either the export of OPS to the bacterial surface, the coupling of OPS to the core of the LPS, or both.

f) Preservatives

Antimicrobial preservatives must not be used in live *B. abortus* S19 or *B. abortus* strain RB51 vaccines. For preparation of the lyophilised vaccine, a stabiliser containing 2.5% casein digest, e.g. Tryptone (Oxoid), 5% surcrose and 1% sodium glutamate, dissolved in distilled water and sterilised by filtration is recommended.

g) Precautions (hazards)

Brucella abortus S19, although an attenuated strain, is still capable of causing disease in humans. The cell cultures and suspensions must be handled under appropriate conditions of biohazard containment. Reconstitution and subsequent handling of the reconstituted vaccine should be done with care to avoid accidental injection or eye or skin contamination. Vaccine residues and injection equipment should be decontaminated with a suitable disinfectant (phenolic, iodophor or aldehyde formulation) at a recommended concentration. Medical advice should be sought in the event of accidental exposure.

There is not enough information available to assess the virulence of *B. abortus* strain RB51 for humans although no accidental infections have been described. It is advisable to handle strain RB51 with the same precautions as *B. abortus* S19. *Brucella abortus* strain RB51 is highly sensitive to tetracyclines and those accidentally inoculated should consider preventive treatment with this antibiotic.

5. Tests of the final product

a) Safety

See Section B.3.b.

b) Potency

For the lyophilised vaccine, potency must be determined on the final product. The procedure is as described in Section B.4.c.

c) Brucellin

See Chapter 2.4.2. Section B2.

REFERENCES

1. ALTON G.G., JONES L.M., ANGUS R.D. & VERGER J.M. (1988). Techniques for the Brucellosis Laboratory. Institut National de la Recherche Agronomique, Paris, France.

2. ANGUS R.D. & BARTON C.E. (1984). The production and evaluation of a buffered plate antigen for use in a presumptive test for brucellosis. *Dev. Biol. Stand.*, **56**, 349–356.

3. BRACEWELL C.D. & CORBEL M.J. (1980). An association between arthritis and persistent serological reactions to *B. abortus* in cattle from apparently brucellosis-free herds. *Vet. Rec.*, **106**, 99.

4. BRICKER B.J. & HALLING S.M. (1995). Enhancement of the *Brucella* AMOS PCR assay for differentiation of *Brucella abortus* vaccine strains S19 and RB51. *J. Clin. Microbiol.*, **33**, 1640–1642.

5. CORBEL M.J., BRACEWELL C.D., THOMAS E.L. & GILL K.P.W. (1979). Techniques in the identification of *Brucella* species. *In:* Identification Methods for Microbiologists, Second Edition. Skinner F.A. & Lovelock D.W., eds. Academic Press, London, UK and New York, USA, 86–89.

6. CORBEL M.J. & HENDRY D.M.F.D. (1983). Methods for the identification of *Brucella*. Booklet 2085. Ministry of Agriculture, Fisheries and Food, Lion House, Alnwick, Northumberland, UK.

7. CORBEL M.J., STUART F.A., BREWER R.A., JEFFREY M. & BRADLEY R. (1989). Arthropathy associated with *Brucella abortus* Strain 19 vaccination in cattle. 1. Examination of field cases. *Br. Vet. J.*, **145**, 337.

8. EWALT D.R. & BRICKER B.J. (2000). Validation of the abbreviated *Brucella* AMOS PCR as a rapid screening method for differentiation of *Brucella abortus* field strain isolates and the vaccine strains, 19 and RB51. *J. Clin. Microbiol.*, **38**, 3085–3086.

9. FARRELL I.D. (1974). The development of new selective medium for the Isolation of *Brucella abortus* from Contaminated Sources. *Res. Vet. Sci.*, **16**, 280–286.

10. HENDRY D.M.F.D., CORBEL M.J., BELL R.A. & STACK J.A. (1985). *Brucella* antigen production and standardisation. Booklet 2499. Ministry of Agriculture, Fisheries and Food, Lion House, Alnwick, Northumberland, UK.

11. LORD V.R., SCHURIG G.G., CHERWONOGRODSKY J.W., MARCANO M.J. & MELENDEZ G.E. (1998). Vaccination of cattle with *Brucella abortus* strain RB51 and 19: A field study under high and low disease prevalence. *Am. J. Vet. Res.*, **59**, 1016–1020.

12. MACMILLAN A.P., GREISER-WILKE I., MOENNIG V. & MATHIAS L.A. (1990). A competition enzyme immunoassay for brucellosis diagnosis. *Dtsch Tierarztl. Wochenschr.*, **97**, 83–85.

13. MORGAN W.J.B., MACKINNON D.J., LAWSON J.R. & CULLEN G.A. (1969). The rose bengal plate agglutination test in the diagnosis of brucellosis. *Vet. Rec.*, **85**, 636–641.

14. NICOLETTI P. (1992). An evaluation of serologic tests used to diagnose brucellosis in buffaloes *(Bubalus bubalis). Trop. Anim. Health Prod.*, **24**, 40–44.

15. NIELSEN K., GALL D., JOLLEY M., LEISHMAN G., BALSEVICIUS S., SMITH P., NICOLETTI P. & THOMAS F. (1996). A homogenous fluorescence polarisation assay for detection of antibody to *Brucella abortus*. *J. Immunol. Methods*, **195**, 161–168.

16. NIELSEN K., KELLY L., GALL D., BALSEVICIUS S., BOSSE J., NICOLETTI P. & KELLY W. (1996). Comparison of enzyme immunoassays for the diagnosis of bovine brucellosis. *Prev. Vet. Med.*, **26**, 17–32.

17. NIELSEN K., KELLY L., GALL D., NICOLETTI P. & KELLY W. (1995). Improved competitive enzyme immunoassay for the diagnosis of bovine brucellosis. *Vet. Immunol. Immunopathol.*, **46**, 285–291.

18. PALMER M.V., OLSEN S.C. & CHEVILLE N.F. (1997). Safety and immunogenicity *of Brucella abortus* strain RB51 vaccine in pregnant cattle. *Am. J. Vet. Res.*, **58**, 472–477.

19. POUILLOT R., GARIN-BASTUJI B., GERBIER G., COCHE Y., CAU C., DUFOUR B. & MOUTOU F. (1997). The brucellin skin test as a tool to differentiate false positive serological reactions in bovine brucellosis. *Vet. Res.*, **28**, 365–374.

20. REPORT OF THE SCIENTIFIC COMMITTEE ON ANIMAL HEALTH AND ANIMAL WELFARE (1999). The modification of technical annexes of Council Directive 64/432/EEC to take account of Scientific Developments regarding Tuberculosis, Brucellosis and Enzootic Bovine Leucosis. Sanco/B3/R10, 11 October.

21. ROMERO C. & LOPEZ-GONI L. (1999). Improved method for purification of bacterial DNA from bovine milk for detection of *Brucella* spp. By PCR. *Appl. Environ. Microbiol.*, **65**, 3735–7373.

22. ROOP II, R.M., PRESTON-MOORE D., BAGCHI T. & SCHURIG G.G. (1987). Rapid Identification of smooth *Brucella* species with a monoclonal antibody. *J. Clin. Microbiol.*, **25**, 2090–2093.

23. ROSS H, FOSTER G, JAHANS K. & MACMILLAN A. (1996). Isolation of *Brucella* from seals and small cetaceans. *Vet. Rec.*, **138**, 587–589.

24. SAERGERMAN C., VO T.-K.O., DE WAELE L., GILSON D., BASTIN A., DUBRAY G., FLANAGAN P., LIMET J.N., LETESSON J.J. & GODFROID J. (1999). Diagnosis of bovine brucellosis by skin test: conditions for the test and evaluation of its performance. *Vet. Rec.*, **145**, 214–218.

25. SANGARI F.J., GARÇIA-LOBO J.M. & AGUERO J. (1994). The *Brucella abortus* vaccine strain B19 carries a deletion in the erythritol catabolic genes. *FEMS Microbiol. Lett.*, **121**, 337–342.

26. SCHURIG G.G., ROOP R.M., BUHRMAN D., BOYLE S., BAGCHI T. & SRIRANGANATHAN N. (1991). Biological Properties of RB5l, a stable, O-chain deficient mutant of *Brucella abortus*. *Vet. Microbiol.*, **28**, 171–188.

27. STACK J.A., PERRETT L.L., BREW S.D., MACMILLAN A.P. (1999). cELISA for bovine brucellosis suitable for testing poor quality samples. *Vet. Record,* **145**, 735–736.

28. STEVENS M.G., HENNAGER S.G., OLSEN S.C. & CHEVILLE N.F. (1994). Serologic responses in diagnostic tests for brucellosis in cattle vaccinated with *Brucella abortus* 19 or RB51. *J. Clin. Microbiol.*, **32**, 1065–1066.

29. THORNTON D.H. & MUSKETT J.C. (1972). The use of laboratory animals in the potency test of *Brucella abortus* S19 vaccine. *J. Comp. Pathol.*, **82**, 201–208.

30. VEMULAPALLI R., MCQUISTON J.R., SCHURIG G.G., SRIRANGANATHAN N., HALLING S.M. & BOYLE S.M. (1999). Identification of an IS711 element interrupting the wboA gene of *Brucella abortus* vaccine strain RB51 and a PCR assay to distinguish strain RB51 from other *Brucella* species and strains. *Clin. Diagn. Lab. Immunol.*, **6**, 760–764.

31. WORLD HEALTH ORGANIZATION (WHO) (1970). Report 1970. WHO Expert Committee on Biological Standardisation. Annex 2. Requirements for *Brucella abortus* strain 19 vaccine (Live – for veterinary use). (Requirements for biological substances No. 20). WHO Technical Report Series, No. 464, 58.

32. WRIGHT P.F., NILSSON E., VAN ROOIJ E.M.A., LELENTA M. & JEGGO M.H. (1993). Standardisation and validation of enzyme-linked immunosorbent assay techniques for the detection of antibody in infectious disease diagnosis. *Rev. sci. tech. Off. int. Epiz.*, **12**, 435–450.

33. WRIGHT P.F., TOUNKARA K., LELENTA M. & JEGGO M.H. (1997). International reference Standards: antibody standards for the indirect enzyme-linked immunosorbent assay. *Rev. Sci. Tech.*, **3**, 824–832.

*

* *

CHAPTER 2.3.2.

BOVINE GENITAL CAMPYLOBACTERIOSIS

SUMMARY

Bovine genital campylobacteriosis is a venereal disease characterised by infertility, early embryonic mortality, and abortion. The causal agent of this sexually transmissible disease is Campylobacter fetus *subsp.* venerealis. *The prepuce of healthy carrier bulls is the natural reservoir of this bacterium.* Campylobacter fetus *is divided into two subspecies:* C. fetus *subsp.* venerealis *and* C. fetus *subsp.* fetus.

Bovine genital campylobacteriosis is caused by C. fetus *subsp.* venerealis, *a bacterium with pronounced tropism for the genital system of cattle. Transmission of the causal agent takes place mainly during natural mating, but the presence of* C. fetus *subsp.* venerealis *in the semen of chronic carrier bulls creates the risk of spread of the disease through artificial insemination.* Campylobacter fetus *subsp.* fetus *is usually recovered from the intestinal tract of cattle. Its pathogenic role is minor compared with* C. fetus *subsp.* venerealis, *though it can produce sporadic abortions. It has been shown to persist in virgin heifers, after experimental infection, for at least several weeks and up to 10 months or more.*

Bovine genital campylobacteriosis can be diagnosed from samples taken from bulls, cows or aborted fetuses. Diagnosis is made by demonstration either of the causal organism or of a specific immune response to it. In the case of bulls, samples of semen or of preputial smegma secretions can be collected. In cows, mucus samples are obtained by suction, vaginal lavage, or by use of tampons. Aborted fetuses can also be examined by similar techniques, and wet preparations of the stomach contents can be examined for the organism by dark-field and phase-contrast microscopy.

Identification of the agent: *The organism is a Gram-negative, spirally curved rod, approximately 1.5 µm long and 0.5 µm wide. It can be cultured when incubated microaerobically at 37°C for at least 3 days. Confirmation of the isolate and discrimination between the subspecies of* C. fetus *can be performed by biochemical or molecular methods.*

Immunofluorescence may also be used to identify the organism.

Serological tests: *Agglutination tests on vaginal mucus provide a useful herd test, but are not useful for identifying individual infected animals. The animals to be tested should be selected carefully, as even in infected herds some animals may have escaped infection. After infection, there is a lag phase before antibodies develop. Also, agglutinins tend to disappear at the time of oestrus.*

The enzyme-linked immunosorbent assay is a more sensitive test, but should also be used as a herd test rather than to test individuals.

Requirements for vaccines and diagnostic biologicals: *A vaccine may be prepared from* C. fetus *subsp.* venerealis *or* C. fetus *subsp.* fetus *that shares antigens with* C. fetus *subsp.* venerealis. *This vaccine is inactivated with formalin, and may be administered in an oil-emulsion adjuvant.*

A. DIAGNOSTIC TECHNIQUES

The genus *Campylobacter* (formerly included in the genus *Vibrio*) (40) comprises many species, among which the following are often isolated from domestic animals: *C. fetus, C. sputorum, C. jejuni* and *C. coli.* There are two subspecies of *C. fetus: Campylobacter fetus* subsp. *venerealis* and *C. fetus* subsp. *fetus.* It is *C. fetus* subsp.

venerealis that causes bovine genital campylobacteriosis (14, 42). Glycine-tolerant variants of *C. fetus* subsp. *venerealis* have been described and are designated *C. fetus* subsp. *venerealis* biovar *intermedius* (35).

On the basis of protein-banding patterns using polyacrylamide gel electrophoresis (PAGE) of whole cell proteins, no discrimination can be made between the two *C. fetus* subspecies (12, 39). However, on the basis of antigenic differences, several serotypes of *C. fetus* have been described (4, 34)

Studies of DNA homology have failed to reveal any major difference between the *venerealis* and *fetus* subspecies (18, 30, 44). However, on the basis of numerical analysis of pulsed-field gel electrophoresis (PFGE) patterns, division of *C. fetus* into two subspecies clusters has been possible (29). Considerable agreement is seen between the clusters and identification based on phenotypic and polymerase chain reaction (PCR) methods. The recently developed amplified fragment length polymorphism analysis (AFLP) also discriminates between both subspecies (43), as does a recently described PCR assay (21). However, a small percentage of strains are not correctly subspeciated by this PCR assay as described in the original paper (21), and this observation was confirmed in a later study (43). 'Taxonomic' differentiation of *C. fetus* into two subspecies is still justified because of the clinical and epidemiological differences between them. Epidemiologically, *C. fetus* subsp. *venerealis* is the most important of the two because of its genital tropism. *Campylobacter fetus* subsp. *fetus* is usually recovered from the intestinal tract of cattle. Its pathogenic role is minor compared with *C. fetus* subsp. *venerealis*, though it can produce sporadic abortions. It has been shown to persist in virgin heifers, after experimental infection, for at least several weeks and up to 10 months or more (27, 31, 36).

1. Identification of the agent (the prescribed test for international trade)

Campylobacteriosis is diagnosed bacteriologically by isolating *C. fetus* in culture, or by immunofluorescence. Bacteriological culture may be done directly from samples, or after transport and/or enrichment of samples. The use of a transport medium is essential if the samples are not to be processed in the laboratory within 6 hours or more after collection. For dispatch to the laboratory, if the samples are not in transport medium, the samples must be placed in an insulated container (within the temperature range 4–30°C), and protected from light.

a) Collection of samples

i) *In the male: preputial mucus or secretions, and semen*

In bulls, preputial mucus or smegma may be obtained by scraping (37), by suction (with Bartlett's pipette) (3), or by preputial washing (9). Preputial smegma can also be collected from the artificial vagina after semen collection, by washing the artificial vagina with 20–30 ml of phosphate buffered saline (PBS).

For preputial washing, 20–30 ml of sterile PBS, pH 7.2, is introduced into the preputial sac. After vigorous massage for 15–20 seconds, the infused liquid is collected in a sterile flask, which is sealed immediately and then sent to the laboratory.

Semen is collected under conditions that are as aseptic as possible. The semen is transferred to a sterile tube, which is sealed immediately after filling. Samples of smegma, obtained by scraping or suction, and semen samples may be diluted with PBS, or sown directly on to culture media or enrichment media (transport and enrichment media [TEM], Stuart's or SBL medium). Dishes containing transport medium are sealed, and then sent to the laboratory in an insulated container (preferably at 4–18°C), protected from light (13).

ii) *In the female: vaginal mucus, cervicovaginal mucus*

Samples may be obtained by swabbing, suction (Bartlett's pipette), or by washing the vaginal cavity. The use of a sterile speculum, preferably of a disposable type, is vital for obtaining samples of good quality (38).

After cleaning the vulval region, the vaginal cavity is washed by infusing 20–30 ml of sterile PBS into the cavity through a syringe attached to a sterile catheter. The fluid is sucked out and reinfused four to five times before being collected in a sterile flask, which is then sealed immediately and sent to the laboratory. Washing fluid in the vaginal cavity may also be collected by a tampon of sterile gauze held inside the vagina for 5–10 minutes after PBS infusion. Samples of vaginal mucus obtained by suction may be diluted with PBS, or sown directly on to culture or enrichment medium.

iii) *Aborted fetuses, placentas*

When abortion occurs, the placenta, and the stomach contents, lungs and liver of the fetus provide the best samples. They are removed under conditions that are as aseptic as possible, and sent to the laboratory in a cooled insulated container (at 4–8°C).

b) Treatment of samples

On arrival at the laboratory, samples should be sown directly on to culture medium, or processed further if required, for example by passing through a membrane filter to reduce contamination.

i) *Genital tract samples*

As vaginal mucus can be very viscous, it may be necessary to liquefy it by adding an equal volume of cysteine solution (aqueous solution of cysteine hydrochloride at 0.25 g/100 ml, pH 7.2, sterilised by membrane filtration). After 15–20 minutes of contact, the diluted and liquefied mucus can then be sown on to isolation medium. If the mucus is not very viscous, it can be sown directly or diluted with an equal volume of PBS, pH 7.2.

Preputial washings may be centrifuged (3500 *g*) to concentrate the sample. The final sample (reduced to 250 µl) may be sown on to the culture medium (directly or using the filter method).

ii) *Aborted fetuses, placentas*

Fetal stomach contents are sown directly on to suitable culture medium. Internal organs or pieces of organs are flamed to sterilise the surface, and then homogenised. The homogenate is sown on to culture medium.

After washing placental membranes with sterile normal saline or PBS, to eliminate most of the surface contamination, the chorionic villi are scraped and the scrapings are transferred to culture media.

iii) *Transport and enrichment media*

Various transport and enrichment media are available, such as Clark's (Australia), Lander's (United Kingdom [UK]), SBL medium (France), and Foley's and Clark's media (used in the United States of America) (16, 20, 24–26).

All the transport and enrichment media mentioned above contain cycloheximide. Because of its potential toxicity, this antifungal agent will no longer be available in the near future. Isolation of *C. fetus* subsp. *fetus* has been shown to be possible on amphotericin B containing media (1).

- *Australian transport and enrichment medium*

The Australian transport and enrichment media is an excellent medium, but its preparation is long and difficult, and this hampers its routine use when many samples have to be processed. It contains sterile bovine serum plus 5-fluorouracil (300 µg/ml), polymyxin B sulphate (100 International Units (IU)/ml), brilliant green (50 µg/ml), nalidixic acid (3 µg/ml), and cycloheximide (100 µg/ml). This mixture is distributed into 10 ml bottles provided with a rubber stopper and a screwed metal lid that has a hole in the top through which a needle can be inserted into the stopper. The filled bottles are placed in a water bath at 100°C. When the medium has solidified, the rubber stopper is pierced with a hypodermic needle, and the air inside is replaced by a mixture of 5% oxygen, 5% carbon dioxide and 90% nitrogen. This step is performed inside an anaerobic jar. The prepared medium must be stored in a refrigerator for 1 week before use. Its storage life is 3 months at 4°C.

Approximately 1 ml of the sample under test is injected into the medium using a syringe, with the needle passing through the rubber stopper. The bottle is stored at approximately 18°C and sent to the laboratory. The time taken for transport to the laboratory should not exceed 48 hours.

When the bottle is received at the laboratory, it is incubated at 37°C for 4 days, and then 3 ml of normal saline is introduced. After the medium has been shaken vigorously, 1 ml of fluid is withdrawn for further testing for *Campylobacter* by isolation in culture or by immunofluorescence.

- *Lander's medium (United Kingdom)*

This is a Mueller–Hinton broth with 5 g of bacteriological charcoal/litre, added before sterilisation. When required for use, the following are added to each litre, under sterile conditions: two bottles of '*Campylobacter* growth supplement' (Oxoid), haemolysed horse blood (70 ml), vancomycin (40 mg), polymyxin B sulphate (10,000 IU), cycloheximide (100 mg), trimethoprim (20 mg) and 5-fluorouracil (500 mg). The medium is distributed into 28 ml universal containers in 10 ml volumes. It can be stored for at least 3 weeks at 4°C.

This medium is inoculated with samples under test, volumes of which may have been passed through a filter of 0.65 µm pore size. After incubation at 37°C for 3 days, the medium is distributed into culture and isolation media.

- *Modified SBL medium (France)*

SBL medium, as modified by Clark (8), contains in each litre: Agar (8 g), sodium thioglycollate (0.5 g), sodium glycerophosphate (10 g), 1% aqueous calcium chloride (10 ml), cysteine hydrochlorhydrate (250 mg), and 0.1% aqueous methylene blue solution (2 ml). After sterilisation by autoclaving, the medium is rendered selective by adding, to each 1 ml, polymyxin (1 IU), novobiocin (5 µg), bacitracin (15 units), and cycloheximide (20 µg). The medium is then distributed under sterile conditions into completely filled anaerobic tubes.

Swabs soaked in various samples are placed in this transport medium and dispatched in an insulated container (at 18–30°C), to reach the laboratory within 24–48 hours.

c) Isolation of *Campylobacter fetus*

i) *Culture media for isolation*

Many media are in current use for the bacteriological diagnosis of bovine genital campylobacteriosis (7). Most culture media contain cycloheximide. Because of its potential toxicity, this antifungal agent will no longer be available in the near future. Isolation of *C. fetus* subsp. *fetus* has been shown to be possible on amphotericin B containing media (1).

Examples of media are the following:

- *Skirrow's medium (basic medium 1)*

Basic blood agar No. 2 (Oxoid) (40 g), and distilled water (1000 ml). Dissolve while boiling and distribute into bottles sterilised by autoclaving at 121°C for 15 minutes. Cool to 55°C and, under sterile conditions, add: haemolysed horse blood (50 ml), and two bottles of growth supplement (Skirrow's mixture) (32).

- *Brain–heart agar (basic medium 2)*

Calf brain infusion (200 g), ox heart infusion, (250 g), peptone proteose (10 g), glucose (2 g), sodium chloride (5 g), anhydrous disodium hydrogen phosphate (2.5 g), thiol medium (3 g), agar (20 g), and distilled water (1000 ml). Sterilise by autoclaving at 121°C for 15 minutes.

This medium can be made up as required, or stored at 4°C for approximately 15 days.

- *Brain–heart agar with blood*

Basic medium 2 (cooled to approximately 63°C after sterilisation, or warmed from cold for 30 minutes in a water bath); and sheep blood heated to 63°C for 3 minutes (7–10% by volume).

- *Selective medium*

Basic medium 1 or 2 (100 ml) cooled to approximately 63°C after sterilisation, or warmed from oold for 30 minutes in a water bath, sheep blood (7–10% by volume), and

EITHER inhibitory mixture No. 1 (final concentrations): bacitracin (15 IU/ml), novobiocin (50 µg/ml), polymyxin B sulphate (1 IU/ml), and cycloheximide (20 µg/ml).

OR inhibitory mixture No. 2 (final concentrations): vancomycin (20 µg/ml), trimethoprim (10 µg/ml), polymyxin B sulphate (5 IU/ml), and cycloheximide (100 µg/ml).

The antibiotic solutions must be sterilised by filtration before adding to the culture medium.

- *Clark's selective medium*

Peptone (10 g), sodium chloride (5 g), beef extract (5 g), agar (15 g), and distilled water (1000 ml). Dissolve the ingredients, except the agar, in water by shaking if necessary. Adjust the pH to 7.4–7.6, then add the agar and bring to the boil. Sterilise by autoclaving (121°C for 15 minutes). Cool to 55°C and add 10% sterile, defibrinated ovine or bovine blood, then bacitracin (15 IU/ml), polymyxin B sulphate (1 IU/ml), novobiocin (sodium salt) (5 µg/ml) and cycloheximide (10 µg/ml).

ii) *Sowing the media and incubation*

Each sample is sown directly, or after passage through a 0.65 µm pore size filter, on to one or two plates of basic medium, and one or two plates of selective medium. After sowing, the material is spread out with a wire loop to facilitate isolation of single colonies.

The plates are incubated at 37±1°C in an atmosphere of 5% O_2, 8% CO_2 and 87% N_2 for 5–7 days. The best culture conditions are provided by a triple gas incubator with controlled humidity (minimum 70%). If this is not available, a jar or similar tested container can be used by introducing, under a vacuum of 56 mmHg, a mixture of 10% CO_2 and 90% N_2 until a maximum pressure of 0.2 bar is obtained. If possible, the gases introduced should be sterilised by membrane filtration.

Conditions of culture and incubation are systematically verified by sowing control strains of *C. fetus* subsp. *fetus* and *C. fetus* subsp. *venerealis*. Such controls should be set up for each isolation attempt. However, it is unnecessary to set up more than one control per day, unless different batches of medium are used, in which case each batch has to be tested.

iii) *Reading the results:* Colonies of *C. fetus* usually appear in the recommended media after 2–5 days. Growth may be slow, particularly in the presence of contaminating bacteria in the samples. After 3–5 days of incubation, colonies measure 1–3 mm in diameter. They are slightly pink, round, convex, smooth and shiny, with a regular edge.

d) Identification tests

A pure culture is required for identification tests. However, the tests can be applied directly to colonies removed from isolation plates if there are many suspect colonies that have been correctly isolated. In the latter case, the test must be repeated after reinoculation of the colonies tested, to obtain a pure culture.

Identification tests are as follows: appearance and motility, if living; Gram staining, oxidase test and catalase test. A phase-contrast microscope is recommended for examining colonies in the living state.

Campylobacter fetus often takes the form of a thin, curved bacillus, 0.3–0.4 µm wide and 0.5–8.0 µm long. Short forms (comma-shaped), medium forms (S-shaped), and long forms (helical with several spirals) may be observed simultaneously in the living state. The bacteria are invariably separated from each other.

Campylobacter fetus is motile. The typical motility is of the polar amphitrichous type. It often disappears on subculture.

e) Confirmatory tests

These tests (see Table 1) must be done on pure cultures. Ideally, they should be performed using a standardised suspension with turbidity no greater than a McFarland No. 1, or equivalent.

Table 1. *Differential characteristics of the genus* Campylobacter

	Respiratory metabolism			Growth test			
	Oxidase	Catalase	H_2S(a)	25°C	42°C	Glycine 1%	NaCl 3.5%
C. fetus subsp. *venerealis*	+	+	–	+	±(b)	–	–
C. fetus subsp. *fetus*	+	+	–	+	±(b)	+	–
C. jejuni	+	+	–	–	+	+	–
C. sputorum biovar *faecalis*	+	+	++	–	+	+	±
C. sputorum biovar *bubulus*	+	–	++	–	+	+	+

(a) = On triple sugar iron agar medium; (b) = Although *C. fetus* does not belong to the thermophilic *Campylobacter* spp., growth of this species at 42°C has been reported (2, 11, 41);
(+) = growth and (–) = absence of growth of the strain on an appropriate medium under specified conditions.

i) *Test for growth in the presence of glycine*

The test is done on each suspect strain by preparing a suspension in buffer solution at pH 7.2. This is inoculated on to a glycine medium (15 ml of blood medium + precisely 1.65 ml of 10% aqueous solution of glycine), and on to basic blood medium. Incubation is performed under the specified atmospheric conditions. Two control strains (of subspecies *venerealis* and *fetus*) are tested in parallel. As all strains are fastidious, small changes in media can be important, and lack of growth in glycine should be considered to be a presumptive test for *C. fetus* subsp. *venerealis*. The reproducibility of the assay is poor and intermediate strains have been described (35).

ii) *Test for growth in the presence of sodium chloride*

A suspension of the suspect strain in buffer solution, pH 7.2, is inoculated on to blood medium containing 3.5% NaCl (15 ml of blood medium + 2.04 ml of 5 M sodium chloride solution), and on to plain blood medium. Incubation is performed under the specified atmospheric conditions. Two control strains are tested in parallel.

iii) *Test for hydrogen sulphide production*

The hydrogen sulphide (H_2S) test is done on triple sugar iron agar (TSI) medium containing peptone (20 g/litre), meat extract (2.5 g/litre), yeast extract (3 g/litre), sodium chloride (5 g/litre), ferric citrate (0.5 g/litre), sodium thiosulphate ($Na_2S_2O_3$) (0.5 g/litre), lactose (10 g/litre), sucrose (10 g/litre), glucose (1 g/litre), phenol red (0.024 g/litre), agar (11 g/litre), and distilled water (to 1000 ml). This medium is sterilised after distribution into tubes by autoclaving at 115°C for 15 minutes. It can be prepared as required, or can be made and kept under the usual storage conditions for approximately 3 weeks.

Just before use, melt the medium in a bath of boiling water and incline the tubes in order to obtain a slope with a depth of 3 cm. This ready-to-use medium can be stored under the usual conditions for 8–10 days before use.

iv) *Test for sensitivity to triphenyltetrazolium, cefalotin (cephalothin) and nalidixic acid*

Sensitivity to triphenyltetrazolium (TTC), cefalotin (also known as cephalothin) (CN), and nalidixic acid (NA) is tested by the disk technique (33). Disks, each containing TTC (200 µg), CN (30 µg) or NA (30 µg) are prepared in the laboratory by soaking filter paper disks in solutions of TTC (30 mg/ml), CN (3 mg/ml), and NA (3 mg/ml). The disks are then dried and stored until required.

For the test, 72-hour cultures of the strains under test are suspended in PBS, pH 7.2, at a concentration of 10^9 bacteria/ml. Using this suspension, 100 µl portions are placed as an even layer on to basic blood medium. The culture dishes are dried before the culture medium is deposited on the surface. The sensitivity disks are then placed on top. These cultures are incubated at 37°C in an appropriate atmosphere, and examined after 48 and 96 hours. A zone of inhibition of at least 3 mm around a disk indicates that the strain under test is sensitive to that antibiotic. All *C. fetus* subsp. *fetus* strains and most of the *C. fetus* subsp. *venerealis* strains are resistant to NA (28). All *C. fetus* strains, except for a small percentage of the *C. fetus* subsp. *fetus* strains are sensitive to CN (2).

Bacteriological identification depends on: absence of contamination of culture plates; satisfactory growth of control strains from the second day of incubation until reading, and results that are similar to those expected for tests with the control strain.

A negative result cannot be accepted before at least 6 days of incubation in the required conditions.

Any bacterium that presents the following characteristics is considered to belong to the species *C. fetus*:

- Characteristic appearance of colonies on the culture media described above,
- Slow growth (2–3 days) at 37±1°C in the special atmosphere (reduced oxygen tension),
- Characteristic morphology of a spiral bacterium,
- Motility of the amphitrichous type,
- Gram negative,
- Positive oxidase test,
- Positive catalase test,
- Characteristic respiratory requirements and biochemical properties.

f) Immunofluorescence

This test can be applied to identify the organism by the direct technique or to confirm the identification of a strain after isolation. It will not differentiate between different subspecies (32).

i) *Preparation of immune sera*

Campylobacter strains, preferably standard strains from recognised culture collections, *(C. fetus* subsp. *venerealis* biotype *venerealis*, *C. fetus* subsp. *venerealis* biotype *intermedius* or *C. fetus* subsp. *fetus)* are grown separately on blood agar medium microaerobically at 37°C for 3 days. The organisms are harvested into PBS, pH 7.2, and washed twice by centrifugation. Rabbits aged 3 months are inoculated intramuscularly with 2 ml of 10^{11} organisms/ml of a *C. fetus* subspecies resuspended in PBS and Freund's incomplete adjuvant. The inoculum is administered at four sites, 0.5 ml at each site. The animals are bled before inoculation, and at weekly intervals thereafter. When the serum titres reach high levels, as estimated by the immunofluorescence test or agglutination test, 0.1–1.0 ml of 10^{10} viable organisms/ml are injected intravenously. The rabbits are bled for serum 7 days later. Heterologous sera are pooled.

ii) *Preparation of conjugates*

The IgG fraction is separated by precipitation with sodium sulphate. The serum is adjusted to pH 8.0 with 0.1 M PBS, and 18 g of anhydrous sodium sulphate is added to each 100 ml. The precipitate is collected by centrifugation and redissolved in distilled water to its original volume. It is reprecipitated by the addition of 12 g of sodium sulphate/100 ml. The precipitate is collected, dissolved in distilled water to half its volume, and dialysed against PBS, pH 7.2, at 4°C until free of sulphate. The protein content is determined and the concentration is adjusted to 1.0–1.5 g protein (e.g. bovine serum albumin) per 100 ml with PBS. This solution is adjusted to pH 9.0 with 1 M sodium carbonate. Fluorescein isothiocyanate isomer 1 (FITC) in a minimum volume of 0.1 M sodium carbonate is added to a final concentration of 15 mg FITC/1.0 g protein. This is stirred for 18 hours at 4°C. The mixture is adjusted to pH 7.0 with 0.1 M hydrochloric acid, and dialysed against frequent changes of PBS at 4°C. Traces of free FITC are removed by gel filtration on Sephadex G25, and the final product is stored at –20°C or lower in small aliquots.

The working dilution of the conjugate is determined by testing various dilutions in PBS against smears of a *C. fetus* culture, and selecting twice the lowest concentration that produces brilliant fluorescence with these test organisms. Under high-power microscopy, the organisms fluoresce with a typical morphology, and are most often concentrated at the edges of the smear.

iii) *Immunofluorescence test*

The samples are fixed on to glass slides, stained with the FITC-conjugated antiserum, and examined for the fluorescing organisms. Staining is carried out in a humid chamber at 37°C for 30 minutes. The slides are then rinsed free of conjugate, washed in two changes of PBS (10 minutes each wash) and mounted in buffered glycerol (80% [v/v] glycerol: 20% 0.1 M phosphate buffer, pH 8.0).

The cover-slips are sealed to prevent drying, and the slides are examined under ultraviolet light microscopy.

2. Serological tests

Tests for antibodies include the vaginal mucus agglutination test and the enzyme-linked immunosorbent assay (ELISA).

a) Vaginal mucus agglutination test

This test is useful in herds, but not for identifying individual animals with *C. fetus* infection. Only around 50% of infected animals are identified. The test is best done on vaginal mucus taken 37–70 days after infection, but the presence of antibodies may be delayed for up to 3–4 months. Some cows may remain positive for several years, while others become negative within 2 months. Approximately 50% of positive cows will become negative in 6 months (15).

Samples taken by vaginal lavage are assumed to have been diluted 1/5 with the saline wash. When samples are obtained by the use of tampons, the vaginal mucus is extracted with 7 ml of physiological saline, and left overnight at 4°C. The fluid is pressed from the tampon, and used as the test fluid for the vaginal mucus agglutination test.

The antigen for the vaginal mucus agglutination test is a 48-hour growth of *C. fetus* subsp. *venerealis* on fresh (less than 2 weeks old) 7% sheep blood agar, preferably containing 0.1% Actidione. This is either subcultured on to 20–30 blood agar plates, or a suspension of the bacteria in sterile PBS is pipetted into Roux flasks of blood agar and spread over the surface of the medium by gentle rocking. The cultures are incubated microaerobically for 2–3 days at 37°C in 85% nitrogen, 10% carbon dioxide and 5% oxygen. The growth is harvested and suspended in 0.5% formol saline. If Roux flasks are used, 10 ml of formol saline and a few glass beads are used to remove the growth. The suspension is filtered through muslin to remove coarse debris, washed three times by centrifugation at 6000 ***g*** for 20 minutes, and the final wash is resuspended in 0.25% formol saline and stored for 1 week. To titrate the antigen, a dilution series is prepared in formol saline. Each dilution is titrated against doubling dilutions of a suitable bovine antiserum to *C. fetus*. Each tube should contain 0.5 ml of serum and 0.5 ml of antigen. The tube contents are mixed well before incubation at 37°C for 18 hours. The antigen titre is determined by the highest dilution that gives at least 50% agglutination with the positive serum sample.

Vaginal mucus samples are homogenised with four volumes of PBS (or 5% phenol saline) using ground glass beads. If a vaginal lavage has been carried out, the sample is already suitable. For the homogenate, 2 ml is transferred to a test tube placed in a water bath at 57°C. Approximately 10 ml of molten Oxoid agar no. 1 (20 g/litre) is also placed in the same water bath. When the contents of both tubes have equilibrated to 57°C, 2 ml of the agar is pipetted into the homogenate. The mixture is shaken vigorously, and quickly poured into a 45 mm wide-mouth screw-cap container. When the mixture has solidified, 2 ml of 5% phenol saline is layered over the top of the agar before the lid is secured. The container is then incubated for 18 hours at 37°C to extract the antibody.

The clear fluid is aspirated off the agar surface and used as the test sample in a three-tube agglutination test. The first tube is left empty, while 0.5 ml of 0.5% phenol saline is pipetted into the others. Then, 0.5 ml of the test sample is put into both the first and second tubes. The contents of the second tube are mixed, and 0.5 ml is transferred into the third tube. The contents of the third tube are mixed and 0.5 ml is discarded. Next, 0.5 ml of a standardised dilution of the antigen is added to each tube and mixed well. After incubation at 37°C for 18 hours, the tests are read by oblique light against a dark background. Each dilution is scored as follows:

Water clear	=	++++
75% clearing	=	+++
50% clearing	=	++
25% clearing	=	+
No clearing	=	–

A positive control titration should be carried out at the same time, using the same method as that for determining the titre of the antigen against a known positive antiserum. The antigen is used at the same standardised dilution against dilutions of positive serum. The results can be validated if the expected titre is obtained using the positive control samples.

A positive result is one where 50% agglutination has occurred in the third tube (dilution 1/80), or beyond if more than three tubes are used. The reaction is inconclusive if there is less evidence of agglutination. It is generally agreed that the mucus test is valuable for the diagnosis of genital campylobacteriosis, but it must be emphasised that interpretation of the results should be made on a herd basis. To use the test to its best advantage, it is necessary to select the animals with care, as even in herds where widespread infection exists, it is probable that a variable proportion of the animals may have escaped infection. There is a variable lag period between infection and the development of agglutinins, and at the time of oestrus, agglutinins tend to disappear, either partially or entirely, from the mucus, although they may be present in high concentrations at other stages of the cycle. In any case, agglutination titres tend to decline with time.

b) Enzyme-linked immunosorbent assay

An ELISA is available to detect antigen-specific secretory IgA antibodies in the vaginal mucus following abortion due to *C. fetus* subsp. *venerealis* (17, 19). These antibodies are long lasting, and their concentration remains constant in the vaginal mucus for several months (22).

Initial sampling can be done after the early involution period (usually 1 week after abortion) when mucus becomes clear.

- **Antigen preparation and coating**

Campylobacter fetus subsp. *venerealis* is grown on 7–10% blood agar in microaerobic conditions at 37°C for 3 days. The plates are checked for purity, and colonies are transferred to 0.5% formol saline for 1 hour, centrifuged at 17,000 ***g***, washed twice with PBS, pH 7.5, and then resuspended in 0.05 M carbonate buffer, pH 9.6. The final absorbance is adjusted to 0.21 at 610 nm. Flat-bottomed polystyrene microtitre plates coated with 10 µl of antigen are left overnight at 4°C, and then stored at –20°C. Before use, the plates are rinsed twice with distilled water and then tapped gently to remove moisture.

- **Test procedure**

i) Diluted vaginal mucus (100 µl) is added to each well, and the plate is incubated at 37°C for 2 hours.

ii) The plates are then washed as before, and 100 µl of rabbit anti-bovine IgA is added (NB must be anti-IgA).

iii) After 2 hours' incubation at 37°C, the plates are washed and 100 µl of goat anti-rabbit IgG conjugated to horseradish peroxidase is added to each well.

iv) After a further 2 hours' incubation at 37°C, the plates are washed, and 100 µl of substrate is added (5 amino-salicylic acid [0.8 mg/µl], pH 6.0, immediately activated by the addition of 2% 1 M hydrogen peroxide [H_2O_2]).

v) The plates are left at room temperature for 30 minutes and the reaction is then stopped by the addition of 50 µl of 3 M sodium hydroxide (NaOH). The absorbance is measured on an ELISA reader at 450 nm.

vi) *Interpretation of the results:* Each sample is tested in duplicate, and positive and negative controls are included in each plate. The absorbance measurements yielded by the test sample are corrected for the absorbance measurement of positive and negative controls according to the formula:

$$\text{Result} = \frac{\text{Absorbance}_{\text{sample}} - \text{Absorbance}_{\text{negative control}}}{\text{Absorbance}_{\text{positive control}} - \text{Absorbance}_{\text{negative control}}} \times 100$$

The test is considered to be positive if the result is above 40. Vaccinated animals will not react to IgA ELISA as their vaginal mucus contains only IgG isotype antibodies.

B. REQUIREMENTS FOR VACCINES AND DIAGNOSTIC BIOLOGICALS

Campylobacter fetus subsp. *fetus* vaccine confers immunity against *C. fetus* subsp. *venerealis* because both strains share common antigens (6). Two groupings of antigens of *C. fetus* are recognised: the thermolabile 'H' flagellar antigens and the thermostable 'O' somatic antigens. In addition, a capsular or 'K' antigen is present (23). The vaccine must incorportate these antigens. It is an oil-emulsion vaccine of one or more strains that have been inactivated by formaldehyde. Other vaccine preparations have also been described (10).

The addition of a second strain of *C. fetus* subsp. *venerealis* to the biological product is widely practised. The presence of from four to five heat-labile glycoprotein immunogens, shared by many *C. fetus* subsp. *venerealis* and *C. fetus* subsp. *fetus* strains, is critical. The presence of such immunogens should be confirmed (5).

In infected herds, all breeding animals, including bulls, cows and heifers, are vaccinated following the diagnosis of bovine genital campylobacteriosis. Additional antibiotic treatment of an infected bull at the time of the second vaccination is recommended, because vaccine may not always be effective in terminating established infection. Antimicrobiol susceptibility should be tested.

The next year's bulls and replacement heifers are vaccinated, and from the third year, bulls are vaccinated annually. In noninfected herds, only the bulls are vaccinated, and this is done once a year.

1. Seed management

a) Characteristics of the seed

The seed consists of a large, homogeneous batch of a culture of *C. fetus* subsp. *fetus* or *C. fetus* subsp. *venerealis* that has been thoroughly characterised as to identity and purity, preserved in small aliquots.

b) Method of culture

The initial growth of the seed is accomplished in semisolid medium. This consists of basal medium with the addition of 0.16% Bacto agar. Basal medium is composed of 2.8% *Brucella* broth, 0.5% yeast extract, 1.2% sodium succinate, and 0.001% calcium chloride. The initial culture is maintained for 3 days at 37°C in an atmosphere of 5% CO_2, 5% O_2 and 90% N_2. The growth is transferred to additional tubes with semisolid medium and incubated for 48 hours. The resulting growth is used for vaccine production.

c) Validation as a vaccine

The seed must be free from contaminating organisms. The purity of the seed must be checked by a suitable culture method.

It is not practicable to test efficacy under laboratory conditions. It is determined in the field on the basis of epidemiological observations.

The vaccine should be stored at 4°C.

2. Method of manufacture

The working seed material is seeded into broth medium consisting of basal medium with the addition of 0.025% sodium thioglycollate. These cultures are incubated at 37°C for 24 hours while being shaken at a rate of 80 rpm. The fluids are harvested, and formaldehyde is added to a final concentration of 0.2%.

The vaccine is mixed with an oil-emulsion adjuvant to extend the period of immunity.

3. In-process control

The identity of the organism should be checked by culture and identification, as well as the absence of contaminating organisms.

4. Batch control

a) Sterility

Tests for sterility and freedom from contamination of biological material may be found in Chapter I.4.

b) Safety

The inactivation process must be complete. This is checked by inoculating the equivalent of one dose on to the same medium under the same conditions as those used in the production process. This culture is incubated under the same conditions for 72 hours, after which there should be no evidence of bacterial growth. The final product must be shown to be free from viable bacterial and fungal contaminants, using suitable culture methods.

Two guinea-pigs are inoculated with 2 ml of the product, either intramuscularly or subcutaneously. They must not have an adverse reaction attributable to the vaccine during a 7-day observation period following inoculation.

c) Potency

Potency of the vaccine may be measured by seroconversion in rabbits. Their serum titres are measured by immunofluorescence or by the tube agglutination test. Five rabbits, serologically negative at 1/100 serum dilution, are vaccinated subcutaneously with half the dose used in cattle, on two occasions at an interval of 14 days. Serum from at least four of the five rabbits, collected 14 days after the second vaccination, must show at least a four-fold increase in titre.

5. Tests on the final product

a) Safety

See Section B.4.b.

b) Potency

See Section B.4.c.

• Acknowledgement

Parts of this chapter were taken from or based on the chapter on bovine genital campylobacteriosis in previous editions of the *Manual*.

REFERENCES

1. Atabay H.I. & Corry J.E.L (1998). The isolation and prevalence of campylobacters from dairy cattle using a variety of methods. *J. Appl. Microbiol.*, **84**, 733–740.

2. Barrett T.J., Patton C.M. & Morris G.K. (1988). Differentiation of Campylobacter species using phenotypic characterisation. *Lab. Med.*, **19**, 96–102.

3. Bartlett D.E. (1949). Procedures for diagnosing bovine trichomoniasis and handling affected herds. *J. Am. Vet. Med. Assoc.*, **114**, 293–305.

4. Berg R.L., Jutila J.W. & Firehammer B.D. (1971). A revised classification for *Vibrio fetus. Am. J. Vet. Res.*, **32**, 11–22.

5. BORDER M.M. & FIREHAMMER B.D. (1980). Antigens of *Campylobacter fetus* subsp. *fetus* eliciting vaccinal immunity in heifers. *Am. J. Vet. Res.*, **41**, 746–750.

6. BOUTERS R., DE KEYSER J., VANDEPLASSCHE M., VAN AERT A., BRONE E. & BONTE P. (1973). *Vibrio fetus* infections in bulls: curative and preventive vaccination. *Br. Vet. J.*, **129**, 52–57.

7. BUTZLER J.P. (1984). Campylobacter Infection in Man and Animals. CRC Press, Boca Raton, Florida 33431, USA, 246 pp.

8. CLARKE B.L. (1985). Bovine Campylobacteriosis. Australian Standard Diagnostic Techniques for Animal Diseases, 3, No. 22. CSIRO, Melbourne, Australia.

9. CLARKE B.L. & DUFTY J.H. (1978). Isolation of *Campylobacter fetus* from bulls. *Aust. Vet. J.*, **54**, 262–263.

10. CLARKE B.L., DUFTY J.H. & MONSBOURGH M.J. (1972). Immunisation against bovine vibriosis. A. Comparison of the protective properties of bacterins prepared by two methods. 2. Studies on the immunisation of yearlings and calves. *Aust. Vet. J.*, **48**, 376–381 and 382–384.

11. EDMONDS P., PATTON C.M., BARRETT T.J., MORRIS G.K., STEIGERWALT A.G. & BRENNER D.J. (1985). Biochemical and genetic characteristics of atypical *Campylobacter fetus* subsp. *fetus* strains isolated from humans in the United States. *J. Clin. Micro.*, **21**. 936–940.

12. FERGUSON D.A. & LAMBE D.W. (1984). Differentiation of *Campylobacter* species by protein banding patterns in polyacrylamide slab gels. *J. Clin. Microbiol.*, **20**, 453–460.

13. FLATSCHER J. & HOLZMANN A. (1984). Genital diseases in bulls: importance for artificial insemination-control measures. *In:* Eleventh Conference of the Office International des Epizooties Regional Commission for Europe, Vienna, Austria, 25–28 September, 393–402.

14. FLORENT A. (1959). Les deux vibrioses génitales: la vibriose due à *V. fetus venerealis* et la vibriose d'origine intestinale due à *V. fetus intestinalis*. *Meded. Veeartschool. Gent 3*, N° 3, 1–60.

15. GARCIA M.M., EAGLESOME M.D. & RIGBY C. (1983). Campylobacters important to veterinary medicine. *Vet. Bull.*, **53**, 793–818.

16. GARCIA M.M., STEWART R.B. & RUCKERBAUER G.M. (1984). Quantitative evaluation of a transport-enrichment medium for *Campylobacter fetus*. *Vet. Rec.*, **115**, 434–436.

17. GROHN K. & GENIGEORGIS C. (1985). Adaptation of ELISA for the detection of *Campylobacter* antibodies and its application in seroepidemiological studies in sheep and cattle herds. *Act. Vet. Scand.*, **26**, 30–48.

18. HARVEY S.M. & GREENWOOD J.R. (1983). Relationship among catalase-positive Campylobacters determined by deoxyribonucleic acid-deoxyribonucleic acid hybridisation. *Int. J. Syst. Bacteriol.*, **33**, 275–284.

19. HEWSON P.I., LANDER K.P. & GILL K.P.W. (1985). Enzyme linked immunosorbent assay for antibodies to *Campylobacter fetus* in bovine vaginal mucus. *Res. Vet. Sci.*, **38**, 41–45.

20. HUM S., BRUNNER J., MCINNES A., MENDOZA G. & STEPHENS J. (1994). Evaluation of cultural methods and selective media for the isolation of *Campylobacter fetus* subsp. *venerealis* from cattle. *Aust. Vet. J.*, **71**, 184–186.

21. HUM S., QUINN K., BRUNNER J. & ON S.L.W. (1997). Evaluation of a PCR assay for identification and differentiation of *Campylobacter fetus* subspecies. *Aust. Vet. J.*, **75**, 827–831.

22. HUM S., STEPHENS L.R. & QUINN C. (1991). Diagnosis by ELISA of bovine abortion due to *Campylobacter fetus*. *Aust. Vet. J.*, **68**, 272–275.

23. LAING J.A. (1960). *Vibrio fetus* infection in cattle. Food and Agriculture Organization of the United Nations (FAO) Agricultural Studies, No. 51, 21–25 and 32–35. FAO, Rome, Italy.

24. LANDER K.P. (1985). Campylobacter. Proceedings of a Conference held in Brussels, 17–18 January. Commission of the European Communities, Luxembourg, 145 pp.

25. LANDER K.P. (1990). The application of a transport and enrichment medium to the diagnosis of *Campylobacter fetus* infection in bulls. *Br. Vet. J.*, **146**, 334–340.

26. LANDER K.P. (1990). The development of a transport and enrichment medium for *Campylobacter fetus*. *Br. Vet. J.*, **146**, 327–333.

27. MACLAREN A.P.C. & AGUMBAH G.J.O. (1988). Infertility in cattle in South-West Scotland caused by an 'intermediate' strain of *Campylobacter fetus* subspecies *fetus* (formerly *Campylobacter fetus intestinalis*). *Br. Vet. J.*, **144**, 29–44.

28. ON S.L.W. (1966). Identification methods for Campylobacters, Helicobacters and related organisms. *Clin. Microb. Rev.*, **9**, 405–422.

29. ON S.L.W. & HARRINGTON C.S. (2000). Evaluation of numerical analysis of PFGE-DNA profiles for differentiating *Campylobacter fetus* subspecies by comparison with phenotypic, PCR and 16s rDNA sequencing methods. *J. Appl. Microbiol.*, **90**, 285–293.

30. OWEN R.J., COSTAS M. & DAWSON C. (1989). Application of different chromosomal DNA restriction digest fingerprints to specific and subspecific identification of *Campylobacter* isolates. *J. Clin. Microbiol.*, **27**, 2338–2340.

31. PARK R.W.A., MUNRO B.I., MELROSE D.R. & STEWART D.L. (1962). Observations on the ability of two biochemical types of *Vibrio fetus* to proliferate in the genital tract of cattle and their importance with respect to infertility. *Br. Vet. J.*, **118**, 411–420.

32. PEARSON A.D., SKIRROW M.B., LIOR H. & ROWE B. (1985). Campylobacter. III. Proceedings of the Third International Workshop on Campylobacter Infections. Ottawa, Canada, 7–10 July.

33. PEFANIS S.M., VENTER C.G. & HERR S. (1989). The use of cephalothin and triphenyltetrazolium chloride impregnated filter paper strips in the identification of *Campylobacter* species. *Onderstepoort J. Vet. Res.*, **56**, 143–144.

34. PEREZ-PEREZ G.I., BLASER M.J. & BRYNER J.H. (1986). Lipopolysaccharide structures of *Campylobacter fetus* are related to heat-stable serogroups. *Infect. Immunol.*, **51**, 209–212.

35. SALAMA S.M., GARCIA M.M. & TAYLOR D.E. (1992). Differentiation of the subspecies of *Campylobacter fetus* by genomic sizing. *Int. J. Syst. Bact.*, **42**, 446–450.

36. SCHURIG G.D., HALL C.E., BURDA K., CORBEIL L.B., DUNCAN J.R. & WINTER A.J. (1973). Persistent genital tract infection with *Vibrio fetus intestinalis* associated with serotypic alteration of the infecting strain. *Am. J. Vet. Res,.* **34**, 1399–1403.

37. TEDESCO L.F., ERRICO F. & DEL BAGLIVI P.L. (1977). Comparison of three sampling methods for the diagnosis of genital vibriosis in the bull. *Aust. Vet. J.*, **53**, 470–472.

38. THORNBER P.M. (1981). Technique for collecting vaginal mucus from cattle. *Vet. Rec.*, **109**, 564.

39. VANDAMME P., POT B., FALSEN E., KERSTERS K. & DE LEY J. (1990). Intra- and interspecific relationships of veterinary *Campylobacters* revealed by numerical analysis of electrophoretic protein profiles and DNA:DNA hybridizations. *System. Appl. Microbiol.*, **13**, 295–303.

40. VANDAMME P., FALSEN E., ROSSAU R., HOSTE B., SEGERS P., TYTGAT R. & DE LEY J. (1991). Revision of *Campylobacter, Helicobacter* and *Wolinella* taxonomy: emendation of generic descriptions and proposal of Arcobacter gen. nov. *Int. J. Syst. Bact.*, **41**, 88–103.

41. VARGA J., MEZES B., FODOR L. & HAJTOS I. (1990). Serogroups of *Campylobacter fetus and Campylobacter jejuni* isolated in cases of ovine abortion. *J. Vet. Med. B.*, **37**, 148–152.

42. VERON M. & CHATELAIN R. (1973). Taxonomic study of the genus *Campylobacter* Sebald and Véron and designation of the neotype strain for the type species *Campylobacter fetus* (Smith and Taylor) Sebald and Véron. *Int. J. Syst. Bacteriol.*, **23**, 122–134.

43. WAGENAAR J.A., VAN BERGEN M.A.P., NEWELL D.G., GROGONO-THOMAS R. & DUIM B. (2000). Comparative study using AFLP fingerprinting, PCR genotyping and phenotyping for differentiation of *Campylobacter fetus* strains. *J. Clin. Microbiol.* (in press).

44. WESLEY I.V., WESLEY R.D., CARDELLA M., DEWHIRST F.E. & PASTER B.J. (1991). Oligodeoxynucleotide probes for *Campylobacter fetus* and *Campylobacter hyointestinalis* based on 16S rRNA sequences. *J. Clin. Microbiol.*, **29**, 1812–1817.

*

* *

CHAPTER 2.3.3.

BOVINE TUBERCULOSIS

SUMMARY

Bovine tuberculosis is a chronic bacterial disease of animals and humans caused by the acid-fast, slow-growing nonphotochromogenic rod-shaped Mycobacterium bovis. *The disease has a world-wide distribution. In many countries bovine tuberculosis is still a major infectious disease among cattle and other domesticated animals, and among certain wildlife populations, and transmission to humans constitutes a public health problem.*

Aerosol exposure to M. bovis *is considered to be the most frequent route of infection of cattle, but infection by ingestion of contaminated material also occurs. After infection, nonvascular nodular granulomas known as tubercles may develop. Characteristic tuberculous lesions occur most frequently in the lungs and the retropharyngeal, bronchial and mediastinal lymph nodes. Lesions can also be found in the mesenteric lymph nodes, liver, spleen, on serous membranes, and in other organs.*

Bovine tuberculosis infection in cattle is usually diagnosed in the live animal on the basis of delayed hypersensitivity reactions. Specificity of clinical signs is low. In the case of a less advanced infection, there may be no clinical signs of the disease. In advanced tuberculosis, the characteristic signs include weakness, anorexia, emaciation, dyspnoea, enlargement of lymph nodes, and cough, but these signs are also observed in other diseases. After death, it is diagnosed by post-mortem examination and histopathological and bacteriological techniques. DNA probe/polymerase chain reaction (PCR techniques) may also be used, although as these are demanding techniques, they cannot yet replace traditional bacteriological diagnosis.

Identification of the agent: *Bacteriological examinations may comprise: the demonstration of acid-fast bacilli by microscopical examination; the isolation of mycobacteria on selective culture media and their subsequent identification by cultural and biochemical tests. DNA probe and PCR techniques may also be used; on very rare occasions – due to contamination of cultures or other exceptional reasons – guinea-pig inoculation could be justified, followed by isolation and identification as described above.*

Delayed hypersensitivity test: *This test is the standard method for detection of bovine tuberculosis. It involves injecting bovine tuberculin intradermally and measuring the subsequent swelling at the site of injection 3 days later.*

The comparative intradermal tuberculin test with bovine and avian tuberculin is used mainly to differentiate between animals infected with M. bovis *and those sensitised to tuberculin due to exposure to other mycobacteria or related genera.*

The choice of which of the two tests to use generally depends on the prevalence of tuberculosis infection and on the environmental level of infection with other sensitising organisms. Due to their higher specificity and easier standardisation, purified protein derivative (PPD) products have replaced heat-concentrated synthetic medium tuberculins. The recommended dose of bovine PPD in cattle is at least 2000 International Units (IU) and in the comparative tuberculin test, the doses should be no lower than 2000 IU each. The reactions are interpreted on the basis of appropriate schemes.

Blood-based laboratory tests: *New diagnostic blood tests are now available, e.g. the lymphocyte proliferation assay, the gamma-interferon assay, and the enzyme-linked immunosorbent assay (ELISA). Both the sensitivity and specificity need further evaluation, and the logistics and laboratory execution of these tests may be a limiting factor. More comparative studies of these new* *tests and skin testing under different field conditions are required. The use of the gamma-interferon assay and ELISA can be advantageous, especially with intractable cattle, zoo animals and wildlife.*

Requirements for vaccines and diagnostic biologicals: *Vaccines are not yet available. There are standard methods for the production of bovine PPD tuberculins. PPD used for performing the tests specified should be prepared in accordance with the World Health Organization requirements, and should conform to these requirements in respect of source materials, production methods and precautions, added substances, freedom from contamination, identity, safety, potency, specificity and freedom from sensitising effect. The bioassays for biological activity are of particular importance, and the potency should be expressed in IUs.*

A. DIAGNOSTIC TECHNIQUES

Bovine tuberculosis is an infectious disease caused by *Mycobacterium bovis,* and is usually characterised by formation of nodular granulomas known as tubercles. Although commonly defined as a chronic debilitating disease, bovine tuberculosis can occasionally assume an acute, rapidly progressive course. Any body tissue can be affected, but lesions are most frequently observed in the lymph nodes, lungs, intestines, liver, spleen, pleura, and peritoneum.

Although cattle are considered to be the true hosts of *M. bovis*, the disease has been reported in several other species of both domestic and nondomestic animals. Isolations have been made from buffaloes, bison, sheep, goats, equines, camels, pigs, deer, antelopes, dogs, cats, foxes, mink, badgers, ferrets, rats, primates, llamas, kudus, elands, tapirs, elks, elephants, sitatungas, oryxes, addaxes, rhinoceroses, possums, ground squirrels, otters, seals, hares, moles, raccoons, coyotes and several predatory felines including lions, tigers, leopards and lynx (15).

Mycobacterium bovis has been identified in humans in most countries where isolates of mycobacteria from human patients have been fully typed. The incidence of pulmonary tuberculosis caused by *M. bovis* is higher in farm and slaughterhouse workers than in urban inhabitants. One of the results of bovine tuberculosis eradication programmes has been a reduction in disease and death from tuberculosis among the human population. Pasteurisation of milk and improved sanitation have also been of great importance. *Mycobacterium bovis* is a zoonotic organism and, during diagnostic examination, should be treated as a risk group III organism.

The rigorous application of tuberculin testing and culling of reactor cattle has eliminated *M. bovis* infection from farmed bovine populations of some countries, but this strategy has not been universally successful. Extensive investigations of sporadic *M. bovis* reoccurrence have shown that wildlife reservoirs exist in some countries. The detection of infection in a wildlife population requires bacteriological investigation or the use of a valid testing method for the species involved (the tuberculin test is not effective in all species) together with epidemiological analysis of information. The badger *(Meles meles)* in the United Kingdom (22) and the Republic of Ireland (19), the brush-tail possum *(Trichosurus vulpecula)* in New Zealand (2), and several wild living species in Africa have been shown to be capable of harbouring *M. bovis* infection. Control of transmission from the wildlife population to farmed species is complex and, to date, has relied on the eradication of the infected wildlife population. The use of vaccination to control the disease in some species continues to be investigated.

Mycobacterium bovis has been isolated from both farmed and free-living cervidae. The disease may be subacute or chronic, with a variable rate of progression. A small number of animals may become severely affected within a few months of infection, while others may take several years to develop clinical signs, which are related to lesions in the animal. The lesions produced may resemble those found in cattle (proliferative granuloma, caseation, granulation and calcification with ageing). The lesions may also be thin-walled abscesses with little calcification and containing purulent material. The lymph nodes affected are usually those of the head and chest. The mesenteric lymph nodes may be affected – large abscesses may be found at this site. The distribution of lesions will depend on the infecting dose, route of infection and the incubation period before examination.

The tuberculin test can be used in farmed deer. The test must be carried out very carefully, with hair clipping at the site of testing, accurate intradermal injection, and careful pre- and post-inoculation skin thickness measurement using callipers to obtain results that are valid (4).

Bovine tuberculosis in wildlife was first reported in 1929 in greater kudu *(Tragelaphus strepsiceros)* and common duiker *(Sylvicapra grimmi)* in South Africa. The existence of tuberculosis in wild animals living under natural conditions was considered unique since Calmette (1923) had stated that "wild animals...never contract tuberculosis spontaneously, but in captivity they are susceptible to it". During the 1940s greater kudu in the same region were found to be endemically infected. In the Queen Elizabeth National Park, Uganda, tuberculosis caused by *M. bovis* was confirmed in one and suspected in a number of African buffaloes *(Syncerus caffer)* during the annual dry seasons. Subsequently, in 1982, a prevalence of 10% in buffalo and 9% in warthog

(Phacochoerus aethiopicus) were found. In Zambia, *M. bovis* infection has been reported in Kafue lechwe *(Kobus leche kafuensis)* and in a single eland *(Traurotragus oryx)*. An outbreak of tuberculosis in wild olive baboons *(Papio cynocephalus anubis)* was reported in Kenya. *Mycobacterium bovis* infection has also been diagnosed in African buffalo in the Kruger National Park in South Africa (3), and more recently spill over to other species such as chacma baboon *(Papio ursinus)*, lion *(Panthera leo)* and cheetah *(Acynonyx jubatus)* as well as greater kudu has occurred.

Tuberculosis caused by *M. bovis* can cause severe economic losses in African buffalo both in nature reserves and on private game farms through deaths and movement restriction applicable to the infected population. The disease has a progressive nature in the individual animal as well as within a population. African buffalo form an integral part of the ecosystem they live in and infected herds must therefore be regarded as a source of infection to other species and the environment. From a conservation point of view, bovine tuberculosis poses a serious threat, specifically to endangered species.

In countries with tuberculosis eradication programmes, clinical evidence of tuberculosis in cattle is seldom encountered because the intradermal tuberculin test enables presumptive diagnosis and elimination of infected animals before signs appear. Prior to the national tuberculosis eradication campaigns, however, the signs associated with tuberculosis were commonly observed.

These signs vary with the distribution of tubercles in the body but, with few exceptions, the course of the disease is chronic. In many instances, characteristic signs are lacking, even in advanced stages of the disease when many organs may be involved. Lung involvement may be manifested by a cough, which can be induced by changes in temperature or manual pressure on the trachea.

Dyspnoea and other signs of low-grade pneumonia are also evidence of lung involvement. In advanced cases, lymph nodes are often greatly enlarged and may obstruct air passages, the alimentary tract, or blood vessels. Lymph nodes of the head and neck may become visibly affected and sometimes rupture and drain. Involvement of the digestive tract is manifested by intermittent diarrhoea and constipation in some instances. Extreme emaciation and acute respiratory distress may occur during the terminal stages of tuberculosis. Lesions involving the female genitalia may occur. Male genitalia are seldom involved.

Tubercles of cattle are most frequently seen at necropsy in bronchial, mediastinal, retropharyngeal, and portal lymph nodes, which may be the only tissue affected. In addition, the lung, liver, spleen, and the surfaces of body cavities are commonly affected. Other anatomical sites must be considered as having the potential to become infected.

At necropsy, a tuberculous granuloma usually has a yellowish appearance and is caseous, caseo-calcareous, or calcified in consistency. Occasionally, its appearance may be purulent. Some nontuberculous granulomas occur in which purulent content with a greenish lustre is replaced by granulation tissue, which may have a resemblance to tuberculous granulomas. The caseous center is usually dry, firm, and covered with a fibrous connective capsule of varying thickness. Fixed tissues in a tubercle are not easily removed intact, as is the case with some nontuberculous granulomas. A lesion may be small enough to be missed by the unaided eye, or so large that it involves the greater part of an organ.

1. Identification of the agent

In cattle, clinical evidence of tuberculosis is usually lacking. For this reason, its diagnosis in individual animals and an eradication programme were not possible prior to the development of tuberculin by Koch in 1890. Tuberculin, a concentrated sterile culture filtrate of tubercle bacilli grown on glycerinated beef broth and, more recently, on synthetic media, provides a means of detecting the disease in animals.

Immunological responses to *M. bovis* infections in cattle are being studied in an attempt to develop improved or alternative diagnostic methods, as skin testing sometimes has practical drawbacks. Currently, however, there is no universally accepted diagnostic blood test for tuberculosis in cattle or other animals.

The presence of *M. bovis* in clinical and post-mortem specimens may be demonstrated by examination of stained smears and confirmed by cultivation of the organism on primary isolation medium. Collection containers should be clean and preferably sterile; where feasible, one-use plastic, disposable containers, 50 ml in capacity, may be used for a variety of specimen types. Specimens that are to be sent to the laboratory by post must be cushioned and sealed to prevent leakage, and properly packaged to withstand breakage or crushing in transit. Prompt delivery of specimens to the laboratory greatly enhances the chances of cultural recovery of *M. bovis*, but if delays in delivery are anticipated, specimens should be refrigerated or frozen to retard the growth of contaminants and to preserve the mycobacteria. In warm ambient conditions, when refrigeration is not possible, boric acid may be added (0.5% [w/v] final concentration) as a bacteriostatic agent, but only for limited periods, no longer than 1 week. All procedures involving culture should be performed in a biological safety cabinet.

a) Microscopic examination

Mycobacterium bovis can be demonstrated microscopically on direct smears from clinical samples, and on prepared tissue materials. The acid fastness of *M. bovis* is normally demonstrated with the classic Ziehl–Neelsen stain, but a fluorescent acid-fast stain may also be used. Immunoperoxidase techniques may also give satisfactory results. The presumptive diagnosis of mycobacteriosis can be made if the tissue has acid-fast organisms and characteristic histological lesions (caseous necrosis, mineralisation, epithelioid cells, multinucleated giant cells and macrophages).

b) Culture of *Mycobacterium bovis*

For the confirmation of *M. bovis,* material is taken from abnormal lymph nodes and parenchymatous organs such as lungs, liver, spleen, etc. In those cases where the animal reacts positively to the tuberculin test but shows no pathological lesions, samples from the retropharyngeal, bronchial, mediastinal, supramammary, mandibular and some mesenteric lymph nodes and liver are collected for examination and culture.

In order to process specimens for culture, the tissue is first homogenised by grinding in a blender followed by decontamination with either acid or alkali, such as 5% oxalic acid or 2–4% sodium hydroxide. However, other concentrations and other chemicals may also be suitable for decontamination, depending on the local situation. The mixture is shaken for 10 minutes at room temperature, and then neutralised. The suspension is centrifuged for 15 minutes at 3000–5000 *g*, the supernatant fluid is discarded, and the fine top layer of the sediment is used for culture and microscopic examination. A sample of the homogenate should be stored at –20°C for future reference, until the case is completed.

For primary isolation, the sediment is usually inoculated on to a set of solid media consisting of egg-based media, such as Lowenstein–Jensen, Coletsos base and Stonebrink's media. These should contain either pyruvate or glycerol or both (1 or 2 slopes each), and an agar-based medium, such as Middlebrook 7H10 or 7H11.

Radiometric methods with a liquid, such as Middlebrook 7H12, can also be used. The principle is that radiolabelled carbon dioxide ($^{14}CO_2$), obtained from metabolism of ^{14}C-labelled palmitic acid, is measured in an ion chamber system. The radiometric method provides results significantly more rapidly, but is rather sensitive to contamination with either atypical mycobacteria or nonmycobacterial organisms (16).

Cultures are incubated for at least 8 weeks at 37°C with or without CO_2. The media should be in tightly closed tubes to avoid desiccation. Slopes are examined for macroscopic growth at 1, 3, 5 and 7 weeks or longer. When growth is visible, smears are prepared and stained by the Ziehl–Neelsen technique. In general, the best medium for isolation of *M. bovis* is Stonebrink's medium containing sodium pyruvate without glycerol. Growth of *M. bovis* generally occurs after 3–5 weeks' incubation.

If gross contamination of culture media occurs, or a specimen shows a negative culture result and a positive macroscopic and histopathology result, the culture process should be repeated using the reference sample. A frozen portion of the tissue may also be processed for inoculation into at lease two guinea-pigs, although this should be avoided if possible. The decontaminated sediment is mixed with a minimal quantity of phosphate buffer and 0.5 ml is injected intramuscularly into the medial aspect of the thigh of the hind leg. The guinea-pigs are tested after 4–5 weeks with 80 International Units (IU) avian and 80 IU bovine tuberculin. The diameters of induration are read 24 hours after injection. If the skin test is positive, a post-mortem examination is performed and abnormal lymph nodes and other tissues are collected for isolation by culture. If the tuberculin test is negative, a retest is carried out 4–6 weeks later.

Growth considered to be mycobacterial is subcultured on to egg media and Middlebrook 7H10 or into Tween albumin broth, and incubated until visible growth appears. In some laboratories, sterile ox bile is used before inoculation to facilitate the dispersion of the bacterial mass into small viable units.

Identification of isolates is usually carried out by determining cultural and biochemical properties. On a suitable pyruvate-based solid medium colonies of *M. bovis* are smooth and off-white (buff) in colour. The organism grows slowly at 37°C, but does not grow at 22°C or 45°C. *Mycobacterium bovis* is sensitive to thiophen-2-carboxylic acid hydrazide (TCH) and to isonicotinic acid hydrazide (INH). This can be tested for by growth on 7H10/7H11 Middlebrook agar medium or on egg-containing media. The egg medium should be prepared without glycerol, to permit good growth of *M. bovis,* and also without pyruvate because it inhibits INH and could have a similar effect on TCH (which is an analogue of INH) and thus give false-positive (resistant) results. *Mycobacterium bovis* strains are also sensitive to para-amino salicylic acid and streptomycin. Effective drug concentrations are different for agar or egg media. Results for niacin production and nitrate reduction are negative in *M. bovis*. In the amidase test, *M. bovis* is positive for urease and negative for nicotinamidase and pyrazinamidase. It is a microaerophillic and nonchromogenic bacterium. Additional tests may be used for identification, including DNA analysis techniques.

It is necessary to distinguish *M. bovis* from the other members of the 'tuberculosis complex', i.e. *M. tuberculosis* (the primary cause of tuberculosis in humans), *M. africanum* (occupies an intermediate phenetic position between *M. tuberculosis* and *M. bovis*), and *M. microti* (the 'vole bacillus', a rarely encountered organism). The above-mentioned tests will serve to separate *M. bovis* from the other species.

Sometimes *M. avium* can be isolated from tuberculosis-like lesions in cattle. In such cases, a careful identification of *M. avium* is needed, and a mixed infection with *M. bovis* should be excluded. *Mycobacterium tuberculosis* may sensitise cattle to bovine tuberculin without causing distinct tuberculous lesions.

c) Nucleic acid recognition methods

The polymerase chain reaction (PCR) has been widely evaluated for the detection of *M. tuberculosis* complex in clinical samples (mainly sputum) in human patients, but there are few reports of its use for the diagnosis of tuberculosis in animals. A number of commercially available kits and various 'in-house' methods have been evaluated for the detection of the *M. tuberculosis* complex. Various primers have been used, including primers that have amplified sequences from 16s rRNA, 16s rDNA, the insertion sequences IS6110 and IS1081, and genes coding for *M.-tuberculosis*-complex-specific proteins, such as MPB64 and the 38 kDa antigen b. Amplification products have been analysed by hybridisation with probes or by gel electrophoresis. Commercial kits and the in-house methods have shown variable and less than satisfactory results in interlaboratory comparisons (18). False-positive and false-negative results, particularly in specimens containing low numbers of bacilli, have reduced the reliability of this test. Variability in results has been attributed to decontamination methods, DNA extraction procedures, techniques for the elimination of polymerase enzyme inhibitors, internal and external controls and procedures for the prevention of cross-contamination. Improvement in the reliability of PCR as a practical test for the detection of *M. tuberculosis* complex in clinical specimens will require the development of standardised and more robust procedures. PCR has been used on formalin-fixed, paraffin-embedded tissues to detect the *M. tuberculosis* group and distinguish it from *M. avium*.

DNA analysis techniques may prove to be faster and more reliable than biochemical methods for the differentiation of *M. bovis* from other members of the *M. tuberculosis* complex. A mutation at nucleotide position 285 in the *oxy*R gene has been found to be specific for *M. bovis* in all *M. tuberculosis* complex isolates examined to date (7). It is of practical significance that the specific gene probe for hybridisation, needed for visualisation of the amplified segment, can be labelled with biotin or digoxigenin instead of isotopes.

Genetic fingerprinting allows laboratories to distinguish between different strains of *M. bovis* and will enable patterns of origin, transmission and spread of *M. bovis* to be described. The most widely used method is Spoligotyping (from 'spacer oligotyping'), which allows the differentiation of strains inside each species belonging to the *M. tuberculosis* complex, including *M. bovis*, and can also distinguish *M. bovis* from *M. tuberculosis* (13). Other new techniques are currently under development in order to differentiate more accurately the strains that have the same spoligotype. These include restriction fragment length polymorphism (RFLP) using the PGRS probe (poly G repeat sequence) and amplified fragment length polymorphism (AFLP) characterisation of the VNTR profile (variable number tandem repeat) (5, 6, 14).

2. Delayed hypersensitivity test

• The tuberculin test (the prescribed test for international trade)

The standard method for detection of bovine tuberculosis is the tuberculin test, which involves the intradermal injection of bovine tuberculin purified protein derivative (PPD) and the subsequent detection of swelling at the site of injection 3 days later.

The comparative intradermal tuberculin test is used to differentiate between animals infected with *M. bovis* and those sensitised to tuberculin due to exposure to other mycobacteria. This sensitisation can be attributed to the large antigenic cross-reactivity among mycobacterial species and related genera. The test involves the intradermal injection of bovine tuberculin and avian tuberculin into different sites, usually on the same side of the neck and measuring the responses 3 days later.

The tuberculin test is usually performed on the mid-neck, but the test can also be performed in the caudal fold of the tail. However, the skin of the neck is more sensitive to tuberculin than the skin of the caudal fold. To compensate for this difference, higher doses of tuberculin may be used in the caudal fold. Where the caudal fold site is used, a short needle, bevel edge outwards, is inserted obliquely into the deeper layers of the skin on the lateral aspect of the caudal fold, midway along the fold and midway between the hairline and the ventral aspect of the fold.

In the past, heat-concentrated synthetic medium (HCSM) tuberculin was used, but, in most countries, HCSM tuberculin has been replaced by PPD tuberculin. The HCSM tuberculins can have a good potency if correctly standardised for biological activity, but their specificity is inferior to PPD tuberculins. Moreover, it has been shown that bovine PPDs prepared with the *M. bovis* production strain AN5 are more specific for detecting bovine tuberculosis than human PPDs prepared with *M. tuberculosis*.

The potency of tuberculins must be estimated by biological methods, based on comparison with standard tuberculins, and potency is expressed in IU. In several countries, bovine tuberculin is considered to be of acceptable potency if its estimated potency guarantees per bovine dose at least 2000 IU (±25%) in cattle. In cattle with diminished allergic sensitivity, a higher dose of bovine tuberculin is needed, and in national eradication campaigns doses of up to 5000 IU are recommended. The volume of each injection dose must not exceed 0.2 ml.

In the intradermal comparative test, the dose of tuberculin injected must be no lower than 2000 IU of bovine tuberculin and no lower than 2000 IU of avian tuberculin. The distance between the two injections should be approximately 12–15 cm. In young animals in which there is no room to separate the sites sufficiently on one side of the neck, one injection must be made on each side of the neck at identical sites in the centre of the middle third of the neck.

- **Test procedure**

i) A correct injection technique is important. The injection sites must be clipped and cleansed. A fold of skin within each clipped area is measured with callipers. A short needle, bevel edge outwards and graduated syringe charged with tuberculin attached, is inserted obliquely into the deeper layers of the skin. The dose of tuberculin is then injected. A correct injection is confirmed by palpating a small pea-like swelling at each site of injection. The skin-fold thickness of each injection site is remeasured 72 hours after injection. The same person should measure the skin before the injection and when the test is read.

ii) The interpretation is based on observation and the recorded increases in skin-fold thickness. In the single intradermal test (which requires a single injection of bovine tuberculin), the reaction is considered to be negative if only limited swelling is observed, with an increase of no more than 2 mm and without clinical signs, such as diffuse or extensive oedema, exudation, necrosis, pain or inflammation of the lymphatic ducts in that region or of the lymph nodes. The reaction is considered to be inconclusive if none of these clinical signs is observed and if the increase in skinfold thickness is more than 2 mm and less than 4 mm. The reaction is considered to be positive if clinical signs, as mentioned above, are observed or if there is an increase of 4 mm or more in skin-fold thickness. Moreover, in *M.-bovis*-infected herds, any palpable or visible swelling should be considered to be positive. Sometimes a more stringent interpretation is used, particularly in a high risk population or in-contact animals. Animals that are inconclusive by the single intradermal test should be subjected to another test after an interval of 42 days. Animals that are not negative to this second test should be deemed to be positive to the test. Animals that are positive to the single intradermal test may be subjected to an intradermal comparative test. Retesting can be performed in accordance with the national or local control programmes.

iii) In the interpretation of the intradermal comparative test, a reaction is usually considered to be positive if the bovine reaction is positive and more than 4 mm greater than the avian reaction. The reaction is considered to be inconclusive if the bovine reaction is positive and from 1 to 4 mm greater than the avian reaction. The reaction is considered to be negative if the bovine reaction is negative or if the bovine reaction is positive, but equal to or less than a positive avian reaction. This interpretation scheme is used in European Union (EU) countries and is recommended in Council Directive 64/432/EEC (8). Sometimes a more stringent interpretation is used.

iv) In the caudal fold test, the standard interpretation is that any palpable or visible change is deemed to be a reaction. A modified interpretation is also in use: a positive test is any palpable or visible swelling at the site of the injection that has a caudal fold thickness difference of 4 mm when compared with the thickness of the opposite caudal fold. If an animal has only one caudal fold, the animal is considered to be test positive if the caudal fold thickness is 8 mm or more.

3. Blood-based laboratory tests

Besides the classical intradermal tuberculin test, a number of new diagnostic blood tests have become available (10). Corresponding to cellular immunity are the lymphocyte proliferation assay and the gamma-interferon assay, while the enzyme-linked immunosorbent assay (ELISA) corresponds to humoral immunity.

a) **Lymphocyte proliferation assay**

This type of *in-vitro* assay detects cellular reactivity to tuberculin PPD antigens in whole blood samples. The assay has scientific value, but is not used for routine diagnosis because the test is time-consuming and the logistics and laboratory execution are complicated (it requires long incubation times and the use of radio-active nucleotides). However, the test may be useful in wildlife and zoo animals.

b) **Gamma-interferon assay**

In this test, the release of a lymphokine in a whole-blood culture system is measured. The assay is based on the release of gamma-interferon from sensitised lymphocytes during a 16–24-hour incubation period with specific antigen (PPD-tuberculin). The quantitative detection of bovine gamma-interferon is carried out with a sandwich ELISA that uses two monoclonal antibodies to bovine gamma-interferon. The sensitivity and specificity of these assays may be comparable with, but not higher than, those of the intradermal tuberculin test. In animals that are difficult or dangerous to handle, such as excitable cattle or other bovidae, the advantage over the skin test is that the animals need only be captured once, but serious disadvantages include the relatively high costs and the fact that the examination of the blood samples should be started within 8 hours of collection. Moreover, this test only works with the family bovidae, and hence should only be used on cattle, buffalo, sheep, goats, etc. However, scientists have already cloned the badgers' gamma-interferon gene, which will be used to develop the test for badgers.

c) **Enzyme-linked immunosorbent assay**

There have been numerous unsuccessful attempts to develop clinically useful serodiagnostic tests for tuberculosis. The ELISA appears to be the best choice and can be a complement, rather than an alternative, to tests based on cellular immunity. It may be helpful in anergic cattle. An advantage of the ELISA is its simplicity, but both specificity and sensitivity are limited, mostly due to the late and irregular development of the humoral immune response in cattle during the course of the disease. Improvement may be possible by using different antigens, including proteins (e.g. MPB 70, which is very specific) and (peptido) glycolipids. Moreover, in *M.-bovis*-infected animals, an anamnestic rise has been described, resulting in better ELISA results 2–8 weeks after a routine tuberculin skin test. The ELISA may also be useful for detecting *M. bovis* infections in wildlife (for badgers, the BROCK ELISA has been developed) and zoo animals for the same reasons as mentioned for the gamma-interferon assay. In New Zealand, the ELISA is approved as an ancillary parallel test for farmed deer, carried out 17–33 days after the mid-cervical skin test.

B. REQUIREMENTS FOR VACCINES AND DIAGNOSTIC BIOLOGICALS

At present the only available vaccine against *M. bovis* infections is bacille-Calmette-Guerin (BCG), which is a live attenuated strain of *M. bovis*. This has shown variable efficacy in cattle trials, which may be attributable to various factors including vaccine formulation, route of vaccination, and the degree of exposure to environmental mycobacteria (21). The DNA of the tuberculosis organism is now being studied in detail and the entire genome sequence should be known soon. This may be particularly useful in identifying genes associated with virulence and in advancing towards a DNA vaccine. In infected countries where there is no test and slaughter control scheme, BCG vaccination may be used to reduce the spread of infection in cattle. Before embarking on a vaccination programme, the vaccination schedule must be optimised for local conditions. Typical dosage would be from 10^4 to 10^6 colony forming units given subcutaneously. Vaccine should be based on the standard reference strain, BCG Pasteur (24). It is important to recognise that use of vaccine will compromise tuberculin skin tests or other immunological tests. Cattle vaccination should not therefore be used in countries where control or trade measures based on such testing are in operation.

Tuberculins were preparations made from the heat-treated products of growth and lysis of *M. tuberculosis* or *M. bovis* (known as human and bovine tuberculins, respectively). At the beginning the culture medium used for their production was glycerol broth. In the 1940s, the 'heat concentrated synthetic medium tuberculins' or HCSM tuberculins, prepared from cultures in a synthetic liquid medium, replaced the 'old' tuberculins. Currently, both the old and HSCM tuberculins have been replaced, almost world-wide, with the purified protein derivatives or PPD.

BCG vaccines may also be used to reduce spread of *M. bovis* in wildlife reservoirs of infection. It is essential before doing so to validate the delivery system for the particular wildlife species.

- **Production of tuberculin**

1. Seed management

a) **Characteristics of the seed**

Strains of *M. bovis* used to prepare seed cultures must be identified as to species by appropriate tests. A record must be kept of their origins and subsequent history. The production strains *M. bovis* AN5 or Vallee are the most commonly used.

b) Method of culture

If the source culture was grown on solid medium, it is necessary to adapt the organism to grow as a floating culture (e.g. by incorporating a sterile piece of potato in the culture flasks of liquid media, such as Watson Reid's medium). When the culture has been adapted to liquid medium, it may be used to produce the master seed lot, which is preserved in freeze-dried form. This is used to inoculate media for the production of the secondary seed lots, which must not be more than four culture passages from the master seed. The secondary seed is used to inoculate production cultures (1, 11).

The production culture substrate must be shown to be capable of producing a product that conforms to recognised international standards (World Health Organization [WHO], European Pharmacopoeia or other recognised control authorities). It must be free from ingredients known to cause toxic or allergic reactions.

c) Validation

The strains of *M. bovis* used as seed cultures must be shown to be free from contaminating organisms.

Seed lots must be shown to be efficacious in producing tuberculin with sufficient potency. The necessary tests are described in Section B.4. below.

2. Method of manufacture

The organism is cultured in a synthetic medium, the protein in the filtrate is precipitated chemically (ammonium sulphate or trichloroacetic acid [TCA] are used), then washed and resuspended. PPD tuberculin is recommended as it can be standardised more precisely.

An antimicrobial preservative that does not give rise to false-positive reactions, such as phenol (not more than 0.5% [w/v]), may be added. Glycerol (not more than 10% [w/v]) or glucose (2.2% [w/v]) may be added as a stabiliser. Mercurial derivatives should not be used. The product is also dispensed aseptically into sterile, neutral glass containers, which are sealed so as to preclude contamination. The product may be freeze-dried.

3. In-process control

The production flasks, inoculated from suitable seed cultures, are incubated for the appropriate time period. Any flasks showing contamination or grossly abnormal growth should be discarded after autoclaving.

As incubation proceeds, the surface growth of many cultures becomes moist and may sink into the medium or to the bottom of the flask.

In PPD tuberculins, the pH of the dissolved precipitate (the so-called concentrated tuberculin) should be 6.6–6.7.

The protein level of the PPD concentrate is determined by the Kjeldahl or other suitable method. Total nitrogen and TCA precipitable nitrogen are usually compared.

The final product should be bioassayed in guinea-pigs. Potency and specificity assays are carried out in comparison with a reference tuberculin (PPD). Further dilutions are made with a buffer according to the protein content and the required final concentration, usually 1.0 mg/ml (1, 11).

4. Batch control

Samples should be taken from each batch and tested for sterility, safety, sensitising effect, pH, preservatives, protein content, potency and specificity.

a) Sterility

Sterility testing is generally performed according to international guidelines (see also Chapter I.4.).

b) Safety

Two guinea-pigs, each weighing not less than 250 g, that have not been treated previously with any material that will interfere with the test, are injected subcutaneously with 0.5 ml of the tuberculin under test. No abnormal effects should occur within 7 days.

Tests on tuberculin for living mycobacteria may be performed either on the tuberculin immediately before it is dispensed into final containers or on samples taken from the final containers themselves. A sample of at least 10 ml must be taken and this must be injected intraperitoneally into at least two guinea-pigs, dividing the dose between them. It is desirable to take a larger sample, such as 50 ml, and to concentrate any residual mycobacteria by centrifugation or membrane filtration. The guinea-pigs are observed for at least 42 days and are then examined macroscopically at post-mortem. Any lesions found are examined microscopically and by culture.

c) **Sensitising effect**

To test the sensitising effect, three guinea-pigs that have not been treated previously with any material that could interfere with the test are injected intradermally on each of three occasions with the equivalent of 500 IU of the preparation under test in a 0.1 ml volume. Each guinea-pig, together with each of three control guinea-pigs that have not been injected previously, is injected intradermally 15–21 days after the third injection with the same dose of the same tuberculin. The reactions of the two groups of guinea-pigs should not be significantly different when measured 24–28 hours later.

d) **Potency**

Potency is determined by comparison with a reference preparation of bovine tuberculin in guinea-pigs sensitised with *M. bovis*.

In the 1970s, countries in the then European Economic Community (EEC, now the EU) recognised a standard for bovine HCSM tuberculins. This EEC standard for bovine HCSM has a potency of 65,000 provisional Community tuberculin units per ml.

As early as the 1960s, the EEC recognised an EEC standard for bovine PPD, which was given a potency of 50,000 provisional Community tuberculin units per mg of PPD, and was dispensed in the lyophilised state. Unfortunately, the number of freeze-dried ampoules was not sufficient for the WHO's requirements and therefore it was decided to produce a new bovine PPD preparation that could be designated by the WHO as the new international standard for bovine PPD tuberculins.

This new bovine PPD standard had to be calibrated against the existing EEC standard. Based on international collaborative assays, both in guinea-pigs and cattle, it was found that the new bovine standard had a relative potency of 65% against the EEC standard. Therefore, in 1986, the WHO officially gave the international standard for bovine PPD tuberculins a unitage of 32,500 IU/mg. This means that the provisional Community tuberculin units are equipotent with the IUs. The European Pharmacopoeia has also recognised the WHO international standard for bovine PPD.

In order to save the stock of the actual international standard, it is desirable that the countries where bovine PPD tuberculin is produced, establish their own national reference preparations for bovine PPD as working standards. These national reference preparations must have been calibrated against the official international standard for bovine PPD, both in guinea pigs and cattle (17, 20, 23).

- **Standardisation in guinea-pigs**

A suitable assay for potency is as follows: The produced PPD tuberculins are bioassayed in homologously sensitised guinea-pigs against the standard for bovine PPD tuberculin by a six-point assay comprising three dilutions at five-fold intervals of each tuberculin. The dilutions of the tuberculin preparations are made in isotonic buffer solution containing 0.0005% (w/v) polysorbate 80 (Tween 80). Volumes of 0.001, 0.0002 and 0.00004 mg tuberculoprotein corresponding to the international standard for PPD of 32, 6.4 and 1.28 IU, respectively, are chosen because these amounts give good readable skin reactions with acceptable limits. The injection volume is 0.2 ml. In one assay, two test tuberculins are compared with the standard tuberculin in nine guinea-pigs, applying eight intradermal injections per animal and employing a balanced incomplete Latin square design (9).

The guinea-pigs are sensitised with a low dose (e.g. 0.001 or 0.0001 mg wet weight) of live bacilli of a virulent strain of *M. bovis* (e.g. 1 mg wet weight) 5–7 weeks prior to the assay. The bacilli are suspended in physiological saline, and a deep intramuscular injection of 1 ml is made on the medial side of the thigh. At the time of the assay, the guinea-pigs infected with the low dose of *M. bovis* should still be in good health and the results of numerous post-mortem examinations carried out shortly after the standardisation assays should show that the guinea-pigs do not suffer from open tuberculosis and thus are not excreting tubercle bacilli.

An alternative, but less reliable, potency test can be used that does not use live pathogenic mycobacteria and is more suitable for laboratories that do not have isolation areas for safe housing of infected guinea-pigs. This tuberculin potency test is performed as follows: the PPD tuberculin is bioassayed in homologously sensitised guinea-pigs against the standard for bovine PPD tuberculin by an eight-point assay comprising four dilutions corresponding to about 20, 10, 5 or 2.5 IU. The injection volume is 0.1 ml. In this assay, two test tuberculins are compared with standard tuberculin in eight guinea-pigs, applying eight intradermal injections per animal and employing a Latin square design. The guinea-pigs are sensitised with inactivated bacilli of *M. bovis,* 5–7 weeks before the assay. The bacilli are suspended in buffer and made into an emulsion with Freund's incomplete adjuvant. A deep intramuscular injection is made on the medial side of the thigh, using a dose of 0.5 ml.

Normally, the reading of the assays is done 24 hours after the injection of the tuberculins, but a second additional reading can be performed after 42 hours. The different diameters of erythema are measured with callipers in millimetres and recorded on assay sheets. The results are statistically evaluated using standard statistical methods for parallel-line assays according to Finney (9). The relative potencies of the two test tuberculins are calculated with their 95% confidence limits, the slopes of the log dose–response curves for each preparation (increase in mean reaction per unit increase in log dose) and the F ratios for deviations from parallelism.

According to the European Pharmacopoeia, the estimated potency for bovine tuberculins must be not less than 66% and not more than 150% of the potency stated on the label.

- **Standardisation of bovine tuberculin in cattle**

According to WHO Technical Report Series No. 384, potency testing should be performed in the animal species and under the conditions in which the tuberculins will be used in practice (23). This means that bovine tuberculins should be assayed in naturally infected tuberculous cattle. As this requirement is difficult to accomplish, routine potency testing is conducted in guinea-pigs. However, periodic testing in tuberculous cattle is necessary and standard preparations always require calibration in cattle. The frequency of testing in cattle can be reduced if it is certain that the standard preparations are representative of the routine issue tuberculins and that the production procedures guarantee consistency.

A suitable potency assay for bovine tuberculins in cattle is as follows: The test tuberculins are assayed against a standard for bovine PPD tuberculin by a four-point assay using two dilutions at five-fold intervals of each tuberculin. For the standard, 0.1 and 0.02 mg of tuberculoprotein are injected as these volumes correspond with about 3250 and 650 IU if the international standard for bovine PPD turberculin is used. The test tuberculins are diluted in such a way that the same weights of protein are applied. The injection volume is 0.1 ml, and the distance between the middle cervical area injection sites is 15–20 cm. In one assay, three test tuberculins are compared with the standard tuberculin in eight tuberculous cattle, applying eight intradermal injections per animal in both sides of the neck, and employing a balanced complete Latin square design. The thickness of the skin at the site of each injection is measured with callipers in tenths of a millimetre, as accurately as possible before and 72 hours after injection (12).

The results are statistically evaluated using the same standard methods for parallel-line assays as employed in the potency tests in guinea-pigs.

e) Specificity

A suitable assay for specificity is as follows: three bovine test tuberculins are assayed against the standard for avian PPD tuberculin (or three avian test tuberculins against the standard for bovine PPD tuberculin) by a four-point assay in heterologously sensitised guinea-pigs, comprising two dilutions at 25-fold intervals of each tuberculin. Quantities of 0.03 mg and 0.0012 mg of test tuberculoprotein, corresponding to approximately 1500 and 60 IU, are chosen because these doses give good readable skin reactions. The injection doses of the standard are lower, namely 0.001 mg and 0.0004 mg. In one assay, three test tuberculins are compared with the standard tuberculin in eight guinea-pigs by applying eight intradermal injections per animal and employing a balanced complete Latin square design. The reading of the results and the statistical evaluation are identical with the potency test.

f) Stability

Provided the tuberculins are stored at a temperature of between 2 and 8°C and protected from light, they may be used up to the end of the following periods subsequent to the last satisfactory potency test: Liquid PPD tuberculins: 2 years; Lyophilised PPD tuberculins: 8 years; and HCSM tuberculins diluted: 2 years.

g) pH control

The pH should be between pH 6.5 and 7.5.

h) Protein content

The protein content is determined as indicated in Section B.3. In-process control.

i) **Storage**

During storage, liquid bovine tuberculin should be protected from light and held at a temperature of 5±3°C. Freeze-dried preparations may be stored at higher temperatures (but not exceeding 25°C) and protected from light. Periods of exposure to higher temperatures or to direct sunlight in practical use should be kept at a minimum.

j) **Preservatives**

Antimicrobial preservatives or other substances that may be added to a tuberculin must have been shown not to impair the safety and effectiveness of the product.

The maximum permitted concentration for phenol is 0.5% (w/v), and for glycerol it is 10% (v/v).

k) **Precautions (hazards)**

Experience both in humans and animals led to the observation that appropriately diluted tuberculin, injected intradermally, results in a localised reaction at the injection site without generalised manifestations. Even in very sensitive individuals, severe, generalised reactions are extremely rare and limited. But experience has shown that a hypersensitive operator can acquire severe generalised signs after accidental intradermal contact (needle stab-wound) with bovine tuberculin. These individuals should be advised not to carry out the tuberculin skin test with the high dose of 2000–5000 IU tuberculin, which is about 1000 times the normal human dose of 5 IU.

5. Tests on the final product

a) **Safety**

A test for the absence of toxic or irritant properties must be carried out (see Section B.4.b.).

b) **Potency**

The potency of tuberculins must be estimated by biological methods. These methods must be used for HCSM and PPD tuberculins; they are based on comparison of the tuberculins to be tested with a standard reference preparation of tuberculin of the same type (see also Section B.4.d.).

REFERENCES

1. ANGUS R.D. (1978). Production of reference PPD tuberculins for veterinary use in the United States. *J. Biol. Stand.*, **6**, 221.

2. ANIMAL HEALTH DIVISION (NEW ZEALAND) (1986). Possum research and cattle tuberculosis. *Surveillance,* **13**, 18–38.

3. BENGIS R.G., KRIEK N.P.J., KEET D.F., RAATH J.P., DE VOS V. & HUCHZERMEYER H.F.A.K. (1996). An outbreak of tuberculosis in a free-living African buffalo (*Syncerus caffer*, Sparrman) population in the Kruger National Park: A preliminary report. *Onderstepoort. J. Vet. Res.*, **63**, 15.

4. CLIFTON-HADLEY R.S. & WILESMITH J.W. (1991). Tuberculosis in deer: a review. *Vet. Rec.,* **129**, 5–12.

5. DURR P.A., CLIFTON-HADLEY R.S. & HEWINSON R.G. (2000). Molecular epidemiology of bovine tuberculosis. II. Applications of genotyping. *Rev. sci. tech. Off. int. Epiz.,* **19**, 689–701.

6. DURR P.A., HEWINSON R.G. & CLIFTON-HADLEY R.S. (2000). Molecular epidemiology of bovine tuberculosis. I. *Mycobacterium bovis* genotyping. *Rev. sci. tech. Off. int. Epiz.,* **19**, 675–688.

7. ESPINOSA DE LOS MONTEROS L.E., GALAN J.C., GUTIERREZ M., SAMPER S., GARCIA MARIN J.F., MARTIN C., DOMINGUEZ L., DE RAFAEL L., BAQUERO F., GOMEZ-MAMPASO E. & BLAZQUEZ J. (1998). Allele-specific PCR method based on *pnsA* and *oxyR* sequences for distinguishing *Mycobacterium bovis* from *M. tuberculosis:* intraspecific *M. bovis pncA* sequence polymorphism. *J. Clin. Microbiol.*, **36**, 239–242.

8. EUROPEAN UNION. Directive 80/219, amending Directive 64/432, Annex B.

9. FINNEY D.J. (1964). Statistical Methods in Biological Assays, Second Edition. Charles Griffin, London, UK.

10. HAAGSMA J. (1993). Working Paper on Recent Advances in the Field of Tuberculosis Control and Research. World Health Organization Meeting on Zoonotic Tuberculosis with Particular Reference to *Mycobacterium bovis*, 15 November 1993, Geneva, Switzerland.

11. HAAGSMA J. & ANGUS R.D. (1994). Tuberculin production. *In: Mycobacterium bovis* Infections in Humans and Animals, Steele J.H. & Thoen C.O., eds. Iowa State University Press, Ames, Iowa, USA.

12. HAAGSMA J., O'REILLY L.M., DOBBELAAR R. & MURPHY T.M. (1984). A comparison of the relative potencies of various bovine PPD tuberculins in naturally infected tuberculous cattle. *J. Biol. Stand.*, **10**, 273.

13. HEIFETS L.B. & JENKINS P.A. (1998). Speciation of *Mycobacterium* in clinical laboratories. *In:* Mycobacteria I. Basic Aspects, Gangadharam P.R. & Jenkins P.A., eds. Chapman and Hall, New York, USA, 308–350.

14. KAMERBEEK J., SCHOULS L., KOLK A., VAN AGTERVELD M., VAN SOOLINGEN D., KUIJPER S., BUNSCHOTEN A., MOLHUIZEN H., SHAW R., GOYAL M. & VAN EMBDEN J. (1997). Simultaneous detection and strain differentiation of *Mycobacterium tuberculosis* for diagnosis and epidemiology. *J. Clin. Microbiol.*, **35**, 907–914.

15. KONYHA L.D., HIMES E.M. & THOEN C.O. (1980). Bovine tuberculosis. *In:* Handbook Series in Zoonoses. Steele J.H., Stoenner H. & Kaplan W., eds. CRC Press, Boca Raton, Florida, USA.

16. KUBICA G.P. (1984). Clinical microbiology. *In:* The Mycobacteria, a Source Book, Part A, Kubica G.P. & Wayne L.G., eds. Marcel Dekker, New York, USA.

17. MAXILD J., BENTZON M.W., MOLLER S. & ZACHARIASSEN P. (1976). Assays of different tuberculin products performed in guinea pigs. *J. Biol. Stand.*, **4**, 171.

18. NOREDHOEK G.T., VAN EMBDEN J.D.A. & KOLK A.H.J. (1996). Reliability of nucleic acid amplification for detection of *Mycobacterium tuberculosis*: an international collaborative quality control study among 30 laboratories. *J. Clin. Microbiol.*, **34**, 2522–2525

19. O'REILLY L.M. & DABORN C.J. (1995). The epidemiology of *Mycobacterium bovis* infections in animals and man: a review. *Tubercle Lung Dis.* (Supple. 1), **76**, 1–46.

20. SCHNEIDER W., DOBBELAER R., DAM A., JORGENSEN J.B., GAYOT G., AUGIER J., HAAGSMA J., REES W.H.G., LESSLIE I.W. & HEBERT C.N. (1979). Collaborative assay of EEC standards for bovine tuberculins. *J. Biol. Stand.*, **7**, 53.

21. SKINNER M.A., WEDLOCK D.N. & BUDDLE B.M. (2001). Vaccination of animals against *Mycobacterium bovis*. *Mycobacterial* Infections in Domestic and Wild Animals. *Rev. sci. tech. Off. int. Epiz.*, **20**, (in press).

22. WILESMITH J.W. (1991). Epidemiological methods for investigating wild animal reservoirs of animal disease. *Rev. sci. tech. Off. int. Epiz.*, **10**, 205–214.

23. WORLD HEALTH ORGANIZATION (WHO) (1987). Requirements for Biological Substances No. 16, Annex 1: Requirements for Tuberculins. Technical Report Series No. 745, WHO, Geneva, Switzerland, 31–59.

24. WORLD HEALTH ORGANIZATION (WHO)/FOOD AND AGRICULTURE ORGANIZATION OF THE UNITED NATIONS (FAO)/OFFICE INTERNATIONAL DES EPIZOOTIES (OIE) (1994). Report on Consultation on Animal Tuberculosis Vaccines. WHO, Veterinary Public Health Unit, Geneva. WHO/CDS/VPH/94.138.

*

* *

CHAPTER 2.3.4.

ENZOOTIC BOVINE LEUKOSIS

SUMMARY

Enzootic bovine leukosis (EBL) is a disease of adult cattle caused by the retrovirus, bovine leukaemia virus (BLV). Cattle may be infected at any age, including the embryonic stage. Most infections are subclinical, but a proportion of cattle (~30%) over 3 years old develop persistent lymphocytosis, and a smaller proportion develop lymphosarcomas (tumours) in various internal organs. Natural infection has also been recorded in buffaloes, sheep and capybaras. Clinical signs, if present, depend on the organs affected. Cattle with lymphosarcomas almost invariably die either suddenly, or weeks or months after the onset of clinical signs.

Identification of the agent: *Virus can be isolated by cultivation of peripheral lymphocytes, followed by demonstration of the virus by electron microscopy or by BLV antigen detection tests. Proviral DNA can be detected in peripheral blood or tumours by the polymerase chain reaction.*

Serological tests: *The methods most widely used are agar gel immunodiffusion (AGID) on serum and the enzyme-linked immunosorbent assay (ELISA) on serum or milk. These tests have formed the basis for successful eradication policies in many countries. Other tests, such as radio-immunoassay, can also be used. A number of AGID and ELISA kits are available commercially.*

Requirements for vaccines and diagnostic biologicals: *No vaccine against BLV is available.*

A. DIAGNOSTIC TECHNIQUES

There may be several causes of lymposarcomas in cattle, but the only definitely known cause is the retrovirus, bovine leukaemia virus (BLV), which causes enzootic bovine leukosis (EBL). The term sporadic bovine leukosis (SBL) is usually reserved for calf, cutaneous and thymic types of lymphoma, which are defined by the age of the animal affected and the distribution of the tumours. The cause or causes of SBL are not known. There may also be lymphosarcomatous conditions that do not fall into either the SBL or EBL categories, i.e. adult multicentric lymphoma with sporadic occurrence of unknown aetiology. Only lymphomas caused by BLV infection should be termed leukosis or enzootic bovine leukosis.

Although animals can become infected with BLV at any age, tumours (lymphosarcomas) are seen typically in animals over 3 years of age. Infections are usually subclinical; only 30–70% of infected cattle develop persistent lymphocytosis, and 0.1–10% develop tumours. Signs will depend on the site of the tumours and may include digestive disturbances, inappetance, weight loss, weakness or general debility and sometimes neurological manifestations. Superficial lymph nodes may be obviously enlarged and may be palpable under the skin and by rectal examination. At necropsy, lymph nodes and a wide range of tissues are found to be infiltrated by neoplastic cells. Organs most frequently involved are the abomasum, right auricle of the heart, spleen, intestine, liver, kidney, omasum, lung, and uterus. The susceptibility of cattle to persistent lymphocytosis, and perhaps also to tumour development, is genetically determined. There is conflicting evidence of the role of the virus as a cause of immunological deficiency or increased cull rate. In one study it was demonstrated that BLV-infected herds have lower milk production (2.5–3% on a herd level), an increased cull rate, and are more susceptible to other diseases with infectious aetiology, e.g. mastitis, diarrhoea and pneumonia, but the effect on fertility is only minor (9).

Virus can be detected by *in-vitro* cultivation of peripheral blood lymphocytes. The virus is present in blood lymphocytes and in tumour cells as provirus integrated into the DNA of the cell. Virus is also found in the cellular fraction of various body fluids (nasal and bronchial fluids, saliva, milk). Natural transmission depends on the transfer of infected cells, for example during parturition. Artificial transmission occurs, especially by blood-contaminated needles, surgical equipment, gloves used for rectal examinations, etc. Lateral transmission in the absence of these contributory factors is usually slow. In regions where blood-sucking insects occur in large numbers, especially tabanids, these may transmit the virus mechanically.

Although several species can be infected by inoculation of the virus, natural infection occurs only in cattle *(Bos taurus* and *Bos indicus)*, water buffaloes, and capybaras. Sheep are very susceptible to experimental inoculation and develop tumours more often and at a younger age than cattle. Persistent antibody can also be detected after experimental infection in deer, rabbits, rats, guinea-pigs, cats, dogs, sheep, rhesus monkeys, chimpanzees, antelope, pigs, goats and buffaloes.

BLV was probably present in Europe during the 19th century, from where it spread to the American continent in the first half of the 20th century. It may then have spread back into Europe and on into other countries for the first time, by the importation of cattle from North America (11). A number of countries are recognised as officially free from BLV infection.

Several studies have been carried out in an attempt to determine whether BLV causes disease in humans, especially through the consumption of milk from infected cows. There is, however, no conclusive evidence of transmission, and it is now generally thought that BLV is not a hazard to humans.

1. Identification of the agent

BLV is an exogenous retrovirus related structurally and functionally to human T-lymphotropic viruses 1 and 2 (HTLV-1 and HTLV-2). The major target cells of BLV are B lymphocytes. The virus particle consists principally of single-stranded RNA, nucleoprotein p12, capsid (core) protein p24, transmembrane glycoprotein gp30, envelope glycoprotein gp51, and several enzymes, including reverse transcriptase. Proviral DNA, which is generated by reverse transcription of most of the virus genome, integrates at random into the nuclear DNA of the host cell where it remains, but does not give rise to free virus *in vivo*. When infected cells are cultured *in vitro*, usually by co-cultivation of lymphocytes and an indicator cell line, infectious virus is produced, most readily through stimulation with mitogens (16).

a) Virus isolation

Mononuclear cells from 1.5 ml of blood in ethylene diamine tetra-acetic acid (EDTA) are separated out on a ficoll/sodium metrizoate density gradient, then cultured with 2×10^6 fetal bovine lung (FBL) cells, and grown for 3–4 days in 40 ml of minimal essential medium (MEM) containing 20% fetal calf serum. Virus causes syncytia to develop in the cell sheet. Short-term cultures can be prepared by culturing mononuclear cells in the absence of FBL cells in 24-well plastic trays for 3 days (13). The p24 and gp51 antigens can be detected in the supernatant of the cultures by radio-immunoassay (RIA), enzyme-linked immunosorbent assay (ELISA), immunoblot or agar gel immunodiffusion (AGID), and the presence of the BLV particles can be demonstrated by electron microscopy.

b) Sheep inoculation

Inoculation of sheep is sometimes used for virus detection as an alternative to cell culture. In this case, infection is confirmed by the detection of a specific antibody response after 6 weeks.

c) Polymerase chain reaction

The use of the polymerase chain reaction (PCR) to detect BLV provirus has been described by various workers (3–5, 19). Primers constructed to match the *gag, pol* and *env* regions of the genome have all been used with variable success. Double (nested) PCR followed by gel electrophoresis and staining is the most rapid and sensitive method (4, 12). The method described is based on primer sequences from the *env* gene, coding for gp51. This gene is highly conserved, and the gene and the antigen are generally present in all infected animals throughout the course of infection. The technique is restricted to those laboratories that have the facilities for molecular virology, and the usual precautions and control procedures must be in place to ensure validity of the test results (see Chapter I.7.).

The nested PCR is applicable to the detection of BLV infection in individual animals in the following circumstances:

- Young calves with colostral antibodies,
- Tumour cases, for differentiation between sporadic and infectious lymphoma,
- New infections, before development of antibodies to BLV,
- Cases of weak positive or uncertain results in ELISA,
- The systematic screening of cattle in progeny-testing stations (before introduction into artificial-insemination centres),
- Cattle used for production of vaccines, ensuring that they are BLV free.

PCR is not suitable for use as a herd test, but may be used as an adjunct to serology for confirmatory testing.

- **Sensitivity and reliability of the method**

i) *Analytical sensitivity*

Although the nested PCR assay has a theoretical sensitivity of one target molecule, in practice the analytical sensitivity is somewhat lower, around five to ten target molecules of proviral DNA per sample.

ii) *False-positive samples*

The high sensitivity of the nested PCR method may cause problems of false-positive samples due to contamination between samples. To minimise this several special procedures are adopted during the analysis, such as the use of laminar air-flow hoods, separate rooms for different steps of the analysis, new gloves or the use of special tube openers for each individual assay, negative controls (water blanks), etc. These precautions against contamination have been described (5).

iii) *False-negative samples*

It should be noted that only a small proportion of the peripheral lymphocytes can be infected, thus limiting the sensitivity of the assay. The presence of inhibitory substances in some samples may cause false-negative results. To detect this, at least one positive control is used on every test run. In addition, internal controls (mimics) are added to each sample. The mimic is a modified target molecule that is amplified with the same primers as the real target but generates a longer PCR-product, which can be visualised by agarose gel electrophoresis. The mimic is added at a low concentration, and this, together with its larger PCR-product size, favour an amplification of the real target (2). However, it is possible for the mimic to compete with the true target. It may therefore be necessary to analyse each sample with or without the mimic.

- **Sample preparation**

Peripheral blood lymphocytes (PBL) are separated from EDTA blood samples by using the Ficoll-Paque separation method (Pharmacia & Upjohn, Uppsala, Sweden). Alternatively buffy coat may be used, or even whole blood, e.g. where samples have been frozen.

Tumours or other tissues should be homogenised to a 10% suspension.

- **DNA extraction**

Purification of total DNA is a prerequisite for achieving optimal sensitivity. Various purification methods are commercially available, e.g. NucleoSpin (Macherey-Nagel) or Chelating resin treatment (BioRad).

The following method is based on studies by Singer-Sam *et al.* (17) and Walsh *et al.* (20). Special precautions should be taken during all steps to minimise the risk of contamination (5).

i) Approximately 100 µl chelating resin (Sigma C-7901 or Chelex from Bio-Rad) is added for each sample in a 1.5 ml eppendorf tube.

ii) 100 µl of the samples and 10 µl of the mimic are added to the tubes with chelating resin. The samples are vortexed.

iii) The eppendorf tubes are closed and incubated at 56–60°C for 20 minutes.

iv) The tubes are vortexed for 10 seconds.

v) The tubes are incubated at 98°C for 8–10 minutes.

vi) The tubes are vortexed for 10 seconds and immediately put on ice.

vii) Optional: all samples are equilibrated to a standard amount of DNA (500 ng/reaction) applying, for example, the Beta Globin-method (19).

viii) The tubes are centrifuged at 15,000 ***g*** for 2 minutes.

ix) 5 µl is used in the PCR assay.

- **Nested PCR procedure**

i) *Primer design and sequences*

Several PCR protocols for the detection of BLV provirus sequences have been published (3, 4, 19). As an example, a PCR assay based on the one developed by Ballagi-Pordany *et al.* (3) is described in detail. The BLV region used as target is the gp51 *(env)* gene. The sequence used for designing the primers is available from GenBank, accession no. K02120. The sequences of the primers are:

Oligo	Sequence	Position in K02120
OBLV1A	(5'-CTT-TGT-GTG-CCA-AGT-CTC-CCA-GAT-ACA-3')	5029
OBLV6A	(5'-CCA-ACA-TAT-AGC-ACA-GTC-TGG-GAA-GGC-3')	5442
OBLV3	(5'-CTG-TAA-ATG-GCT-ATC-CTA-AGA-TCT-ACT-GGC-3')	5065
OBLV5	(5'-GAC-AGA-GGG-AAC-CCA-GTC-ACT-GTT-CAA-CTG-3')	5376

PCR^{I}-product size: 440 bp; PCR^{II}-product size: 341 bp; Mimic-product size: 761 bp.

ii) *Reaction mixtures*

Reaction mixtures are blended (except sample and mimic) before adding to the separate reaction tubes. One negative control (double distilled H_2O) per five samples, and one positive control should be added. Total volumes of mixtures are calculated by multiplying the indicated volumes by the total number of samples, including controls, plus one. Taq polymerase is used in a premade 1/10 dilution.

DNA samples and mimic[1] (2) should be added in separate rooms in the laboratory: laboratory room 1 for DNA preparations and mimics, and laboratory room 2 for PCR^{II}-products, to minimise contamination.

a) Reagents added in clean laboratory room

This mixture may be prepared in advance and stored at 4°C for up to 1 month.

Reagents per reaction (conc.)	PCR^{I} reaction	PCR^{II} reaction
double-distilled H_2O (standardised)	21 µl	21 µl
10 × PCR buffer (Perkin Elmer)	5 µl	5 µl
dNTP (10 mM)	4 × 1 µl	4 × 1 µl
Bovine serum albumin (1 mg/ml)	5 µl	5 µl
<u>*Primers (10 pmol/µl):*</u>		
OBLV1A	1.5 µl	–
OBLV6A	1.5 µl	–
OBLV3	–	1.5 µl
OBLV5	–	1.5 µl
In total:	38 µl	38 µl

The following should be added just before starting the PCR

Reagents per reaction (conc.)	PCR^{I} reaction	PCR^{II} reaction
$MgCl_2$ (25 mM)	5 µl	5 µl
Taq polymerase (1 unit/reaction)	2 µl	2 µl
Mineral oil	2 drops	2 drops
In total:	45 µl	45 µl

1 Available from Dr S. Belák, Department of Virology, National Veterinary Institute, Box 585, Biomedical Centre, S-751 23, Uppsala, Sweden.

b) Reagents added in laboratory room 1 (DNA) or 2 (PCR^II^)

Reagents per reaction (conc.)	PCR^I^ reaction	PCR^II^ reaction
DNA sample* (or water*)	5 µl	–
PCR^I^ product	–	5 µl
In total:	50 µl	50 µl

iii) *PCR thermoprofiles*

PCR^I^-thermoprofile

5 ×	94°C/45 seconds, 60°C/60 seconds, 72°C/90 seconds
30 ×	94°C/45 seconds, 55°C/60 seconds, 72°C/90 seconds
1 ×	72°C/420 seconds = >20°C

PCR^II^-thermoprofile

5 ×	94°C/45 seconds, 58°C/60 seconds, 72°C/90 seconds
30 ×	94°C/45 seconds, 53°C/60 seconds, 72°C/90 seconds
1 ×	72°C/420 seconds = >20°C

iv) *Laboratory procedure*

Mix PCR^I^-reagents as described in step ii. Use separate gloves or tube openers for each individual tube when adding the DNA samples. Put the samples on ice. Heat the thermoblock to 80°C. Put samples in the thermoblock and start the PCR^I^-programme (step iii).

Mix PCR^II^-reagents as described in step ii. Use separate gloves or tube openers for each individual tube when adding the PCR^I^ -product. Put the samples on ice. Heat the thermoblock to 80°C. Put samples in the thermoblock and start the PCR^II^-programme (step iii).

- **Agarose gel electrophoresis**

Take the PCR^II^-products to the electrophoresis laboratory. Load approximately 8 µl of the samples and 2 µl loading buffer on a 2% agarose gel. Add a 100 bp ladder size standard. Voltage and time depend on size and thickness of gel and equipment used. Stain the gel for 2 minutes in ethidium bromide (or use ethidium-bromide-containing gel), rinse with water and photograph the gel.

- **Interpretation of the results**

i) *Positive samples*

Positive samples should have PCR products of the expected size (341 bp), similar to the positive control. The mimic product (761 bp) should be present in all samples except possibly in strongly positive samples.

ii) *Negative samples*

Negative samples should have no PCR products of the expected size (341 bp), but mimic product (761 bp) should be present.

iii) *Unclear results*

The assay must be repeated if the positive controls (mimic or external positive control) are negative, or if the negative water controls are positive.

- **Confirmatory testing**

For confirmatory identification, the PCR products can be sequenced, hybridised to a probe, or analysed by restriction fragment length polymorphism (RFLP) analysis (10).

2. Serological tests

Infection with the virus in cattle is lifelong and gives rise to a persistent antibody response. Antibodies can first be detected 3–16 weeks after infection. Maternally derived antibodies may take up to 6 or 7 months to disappear. There is no way of distinguishing passively transferred antibodies from those resulting from active infection. Active infection, however, can be confirmed by the PCR. Passive antibody tends to protect calves against infection. During the periparturient period, cows may have serum antibody that is undetectable by AGID because of a shift of antibody from the dam's circulation to her colostrum. Therefore, when using the AGID test, a negative test result on serum taken at this time (2–3 weeks pre- and post-partum) is not conclusive and the test should be repeated. However, the AGID can be performed at this stage with first phase colostrum.

The antibodies most readily detected are those directed towards the gp51 and p24 of the virus. Most AGID tests and ELISAs in routine use detect antibodies to the glycoprotein gp51, as these appear earlier. Methods of performing these tests have been published (6, 8).

In order to compare different AGID tests and ELISAs, a bovine serum sample, E4, has been produced. E4 is used as the OIE standard serum to gauge sensitivities of tests. These sera were first adopted by the European Union reference laboratories. The serum is available to OIE Member Countries[2]. National standards should be produced and calibrated against E4 so that a standard serum is available for routine use within countries. Weak positive (equivalent to E4 diluted 1/10) and negative international reference standard sera are available in freeze-dried, irradiated form from the OIE Reference Laboratory in the UK (see Table given in Part 4 of this *Manual*).

a) Agar gel immunodiffusion (a prescribed test for international trade)

The AGID test is a specific, but not very sensitive, test for detecting antibody in serum samples from individual animals. It is, however, unsuitable for milk samples because of lack of specificity and sensitivity. The AGID is simple and easy to perform and has proven to be highly useful and efficient as a basis for eradication schemes. Commercial kits are available. The minimum requirement in terms of sensitivity for all the AGID systems is that they be able to detect BLV antibody in a 1/10 dilution of E4.

i) *Agar gel:* A 0.8–1.2% solution of agar or agarose is prepared in 0.2 M Tris buffer, pH 7.2, with 8.5% NaCl. One method of preparing the agar is to dissolve 24.23 g of Tris methylamine in 1 litre of distilled water and adjust to pH 7.2 with 2.5 M HCl. Sodium chloride (85 g) is dissolved in 250 ml Tris/HCl and made up to 1 litre. Agarose (8 g) is added and the mixture is heated in a pressure cooker at 4.55 kg/sq.cm for 10 minutes. The mixture is dispensed in 15 ml aliquots, which can be stored at 4°C for up to approximately 6 weeks.

ii) *Antigen:* The antigen must contain specific glycoprotein gp51 of BLV. Antigen is prepared in a suitable cell culture system, such as permanently infected fetal lamb kidney (FLK) cell monolayers. The cells used to produce the BLV antigen should be free from noncytopathic bovine viral diarrhoea virus and of bovine retroviruses, bovine immunodeficiency-like virus (lentivirus), and bovine syncytial virus (spumavirus). After 3–4 days' culture at 37°C, the growth medium is replaced with maintenance medium. The cells are harvested after 7 days using standard trypsin/versene solution. The cell suspension is centrifuged at 500 *g* for 10 minutes. Cells are resuspended in growth medium; 30% of the cells are returned to the culture vessel and the remainder is discarded. All culture supernatants are collected. The supernatants are concentrated 50–100-fold by available methods. This can be done by concentration in Visking tubing immersed in polyethylene glycol, or by precipitation with ammonium sulphate followed by ultrafiltration, or by precipitation in polyethylene glycol followed by desalting and size separation on a polyacrylamide bead column. The antigen contains gp51 predominantly, but may also contain p24.

   The antigen may be standardised for glycoprotein gp51 by titration against E4 as follows: a twofold dilution of the antigen preparation is made. The highest dilution that, when tested against undiluted standard serum E4, gives a precipitation line equidistant between the antigen and the serum will contain one unit. Two units of antigen are used in the test.

iii) *Known positive control serum:* The positive control serum comes from a naturally or experimentally infected animal (cattle or sheep). The precipitation line formed should be a sharp distinct line midway between the antigen and the control serum wells. A dilution of the control positive serum that gives a weak positive result should be included in the test as an indicator of the test's sensitivity.

iv) *Known negative control serum:* Serum from uninfected animals (cattle, sheep) is used.

v) *Test sera:* Sera from any species of animal are suitable.

2 Obtainable from the National Veterinary Laboratory, P. O. Box 373, DK1503, Copenhagen, Denmark.

- **Test procedure**

i) The agar is melted by heating in a water bath and poured into Petri dishes (15 ml per Petri dish of diameter 8.5 cm). The poured plates are allowed to cool at 4°C for about 1 hour before holes are cut in the agar. A punch is used that cuts a hexagonal arrangement of six wells round a central well. Various dimensions of wells can be used; one satisfactory pattern has been produced using wells of 6.5 mm in diameter with 3 mm between wells. For best results, agar plates are used the same day that they are poured and cut.

ii) Antigen is placed in the central wells of the hexagonally arranged patterns. Test sera are placed alternately with positive control serum in the outer wells. There should be one control pattern per plate with positive control serum, weak positive control serum and negative control serum in the place of test sera.

iii) The test plates are kept at room temperature (20–27°C) in a closed humid chamber, and read at 24, 48 and 72 hours.

iv) *Interpretation of the results:* A test serum is positive if it forms a specific precipitation line with the antigen and forms a line of identity with the control serum. A test serum is negative if it does not form a specific line with the antigen and if it does not bend the line of the control serum. Nonspecific lines may occur; these do not merge with or deflect the lines formed by the positive control. A test serum is a weak positive if it bends the line of the control serum towards the antigen well without forming a visible precipitation line with the antigen; the reaction is inconclusive if it cannot be read either as negative or positive. A test is invalid if the controls do not give the expected results. Sera giving inconclusive or weak positive results can be concentrated and retested.

b) Enzyme-linked immunosorbent assay (a prescribed test for international trade)

Either an indirect or blocking ELISA may be used. Assays based on both of these are available commercially; different kits may be required for serum or milk samples. Some ELISAs are sufficiently sensitive to be used with pooled samples. ELISAs are carried out in solid-phase microplates. BLV antigen is used to coat the plates either directly or by the use of a capture polyclonal or monoclonal antibody (MAb). The antigen is prepared in a similar manner to the antigen used in the AGID test and is used at a predetermined dilution (e.g. 1/10) in phosphate buffered saline (PBS). In kit form, the plates are sometimes purchased precoated. Some preservatives may be added to milk samples to prevent souring. Preserved samples will not usually deteriorate significantly if stored for up to 6 weeks at 4°C.

- **Indirect enzyme-linked immunosorbent assay – Milk ELISA**

The following method is suitable for antibody detection in pooled milk samples.

- **Controls**

According to European Union legislation, (Directive 88/406) the BLV reference serum 'E4', must give a positive result when diluted 250 times more than the number of individual samples that form the 'pooled-sample' under test. Thus, for this test protocol, where the method is deemed sufficiently sensitive to detect a single positive individual sample in a pool composed of 60 individual samples, the 'E4' weak positive control comprises 'E4 sub-standard' diluted in BLV-negative milk, at the rate of 1 in 250 × 60, i.e. 1 in 15,000. A strong positive should be included and prepared by diluting E4 serum 1 in 2500 in milk. A negative milk and a diluent control should also be included. The milk used for diluting the E4 serum controls and the test samples should be unpasteurised, cream free and preserved. Controls should be inoculated on the plate as follows: add 100 µl of control sample to 100 µl wash buffer in the plate to make a 1/2 dilution, adding to control antigen wells and BLV antigen wells.

- **Test procedure**

i) Milk samples must be stored, undisturbed in a refrigerator until a definite cream layer has formed (24–48 hours), or alternatively, centrifuged at 2000 rpm for 10 minutes, the cream layer should be removed prior to testing.

ii) A BLV antigen and a control negative antigen are precoated in alternate columns in the plate. 100 µl of test sample is added to 100 µl wash buffer in the plate to make a 1/2 dilution, adding to two control antigen wells and two BLV antigen wells.

iii) The plate is sealed and mixed on a shaker.

iv) The plate is incubated between 14 and 18 hours at 2–8°C.

v) 300 µl per well of wash diluent is added and discarded, and then 200 µl per well wash diluent is added, shaken for 10 seconds and discarded. Finally, 300 µl of wash diluent is added and soaked for 3 minutes and discarded.

vi) 200 µl per well of anti-bovine IgG-horseradish peroxidase affinity-purified conjugate diluted in wash diluent is added and the plate is incubated for 90 minutes at room temperature.

vii) The plate is washed by adding 300 µl of wash diluent per well; this is then discarded and a further 300 µl of wash diluent is added. This is left to soak for 3 minutes and discarded. Steps vi and vii are repeated.

viii) 200 µl of ABTS (2,2'-Azino-bis-[3-ethylbenzothiazoline-6-sulphonic acid]) substrate (prewarmed to 25°C) is added and the plate is incubated for 20 minutes at room temperature in the dark. The reaction may be stopped by adding 50 µl of stopping solution.

- **Reading and interpreting the results**

The plate reader is blanked on air and the absorbance is read at 405 nm. All microplate wells must be read within 2 hours of addition of stopper. The absorbance readings of the wells containing negative antigen are subtracted from the readings of wells containing the positive antigen. The two net absorbance values for each test sample should be averaged. The same applies for the replicate weak positive controls. Replicates should be within 0.1 absorbance units of each other.

For the test to be considered valid, the averaged net absorbance of the weak positive (WP) controls should be 0.2–0.6 absorbance units. The net absorbance of the strong positive control should be >1.0 absorbance units. The net absorbance of the negative and diluent controls should be less than the lower limit of the inconclusive range.

Assuming that the above criteria are met:

i) Test samples are positive if their net absorbance value is greater than or equal to that of the WP control.

ii) Test samples are inconclusive if their net absorbance value is 75% or less of the net absorbance value of the WP control.

i.e. if the WP control net absorbance = 0.40

then the lower limit of the inconclusive range = 0.40 × 0.750= 0.30

the inconclusive range in this example would be 0.30–0.39

and samples of ≥0.40 are considered positive

iii) Test samples are negative if their net absorbance value is less than the lower limit of the 'inconclusive' range (<0.30 in the example).

- **Blocking enzyme-linked immunosorbent assay – Serum ELISA**

The following method is suitable for antibody detection in single or pooled serum samples.

- **Test procedure**

i) *Coating the plate*

All wells are coated with BLV antibody, prediluted in coating buffer (100 µl/well), the plate is sealed and incubated for 18 hours at 4°C. A wash cycle (standard wash) is performed, which is three washes filling wells to the top, with a 3-minute soak in between each wash, and then the plate is blotted. BLV antigen is added, prediluted in wash buffer (100 µl/well), the plate is sealed and incubated for 2 hours at 37°C. A standard wash cycle is performed.

ii) *Preparation and addition of samples and controls*

The positive and negative control sera are prediluted (1/2) in wash buffer and the solution is added to four wells per control (100 µl/well). For testing pooled samples, 80 sera may be bulked then diluted (1/2) using wash buffer and the solution is added to two wells (100 µl/well) per sample. Single samples should be diluted 1/100 using wash buffer and the solution added to two wells (100 µl/well) per sample. After plating out the samples, the plate is sealed and incubated for 18 hours at 4°C. A brief wash is performed by filling the wells and immediately emptying them.

iii) *Preparation and addition of conjugates and substrate*

Prediluted biotinylated antibody is added (100 µl/well) to all wells – predilute using wash buffer + 10% fetal calf serum – the plate is sealed and incubated on a rocking table for 1 hour at 37°C. A standard wash is performed as described earlier. The peroxidase-conjugated avidin is prediluted in wash buffer and the solution is added to all wells (100 µl/well). The plate is sealed and incubated on a rocking table for 30 minutes at 37°C. A standard wash is performed. 100 µl ortho phenylamine diamine substrate is added to all wells, the plate is covered and left in the dark for 9 minutes. The reaction is stopped with 100 µl of 0.5 M sulphuric acid per well.

- **Reading and interpretation of results**

The plate reader is blanked on air and the absorbance is read at 490 nm. For dual wave-length readers a reference filter between 620 nm and 650 nm is used. Results are read within 60 minutes after the addition of stop solution.

The absorbance of the negative control should be about 1.1 ± 0.4; if the absorbance is below 0.7 the colour development time in step iii above (preparation and addition of conjugates and substrate) should be increased. Conversely, the time should be shortened if the absorbance is above 1.5. The absorbance of the positive control should be less than the absorbance of the negative control × 0.25.

A sample is positive when the absorbance of each of the two test wells is identical with or less than the mean absorbance of the four negative wells × 0.5.

A sample is negative when the absorbance of each of the two test wells is identical with or higher than the mean absorbance of the four negative control wells × 0.65.

For samples giving values between the absorbance of the negative control × 0.5 and × 0.65 it is recommended to retest the animal, using a sample taken 1 month later.

- **Sensitivity of the enzyme-linked immunosorbent assay**

A useful guide to calibrating the sensitivities of assays may be found in Annex G to EEC directive 88/406/EEC governing the diagnosis of brucellosis and EBL.

Where individual serum samples are tested as a pool, E4 standard serum must test positive when diluted ten times more than the number of individual serum samples included in the pool (e.g. for a pool composed of 50 individual samples, E4 diluted 1 in 10 × 50, i.e. 1/500, must give a positive result). In assays where samples (serum or milk) are tested individually, E4 serum diluted 1/10 (in negative serum) or 1/250 (in negative milk) must be scored positive when tested in the same assay dilution as used for individual test samples.

B. REQUIREMENTS FOR VACCINES AND DIAGNOSTIC BIOLOGICALS

In young calves born to a BLV-infected mother, maternal antibodies to BLV gp51 are important in protection against BLV infection (12). However, experiments using inactivated BLV, fixed infected FLK cells, and purified gp51 have indicated that these give only short-term protection. It was also found that vaccination of cattle with live cells from a cell line BL3, established from an animal with sporadic bovine leukosis, resulted in short-term protection. The nature of the antigen conferring protection was possibly a tumour-associated transplantation antigen (18). Ovine cells synthesising only the *env* gene products gp51 and gp30 and the main structural protein p24, induced a serological response in cattle (1); cattle were protected after repeated vaccination with these cells.

Vaccination in sheep with a recombinant vaccinia virus expressing BLV gp51 induced protection (14). However, protection was achieved without production of detectable levels of neutralising antibodies. Also, Portetelle *et al.* found that vaccinia virus recombinants protected sheep even though anti-gp51 antibody waned (15). It is therefore thought that a cell-mediated immune response may play a role in protective immunity against BLV infection. Expression of gp51 has been obtained by recombinant vaccinia virus and yeast containing the coding sequence of BLV *env* gene. These have resulted in protection of sheep (7). Despite these advances in knowledge, there is as yet no vaccine available commercially for the control of EBL.

REFERENCES

1. ALTANER C., BARR J., ALTANEROVA V. & JANIK V. (1991). Protective vaccination against bovine leukaemia virus infection by means of cell-derived vaccine. *Vaccine,* **9**, 889–895.

2. BALLAGI-PORDANY A. & BELAK S. (1996). The use of mimics as internal standards to avoid false negatives in diagnostic PCR. *Mol. Cell. Probes,* **10**, 159–164.

3. BALLAGI-PORDANY A., KLINTEVALL K., MERZA M., KLINGEBORN B. & BELAK S. (1992). Direct detection of bovine leukaemia virus infection: practical applicability of a double polymerase chain reaction. *J. Vet. Med. [B],* **39**, 69–77.

4. BEIER D., BLANKENSTEIN P. & FECHNER H. (1998). Chances and limitations for the use of the polymerase chain reaction in the diagnosis of bovine leukemia virus (BLV) infection in cattle. *Dtsch Tierartzl. Wochenschr.,* **105**, 408–412.

5. BELAK S. & BALLAGI-PORDANY A. (1993). Experiences on the application of the polymerase chain reaction in a diagnostic laboratory. *Mol. Cell. Probes,* **7**, 241–248.

6. COMMISSION OF THE EUROPEAN COMMUNITIES (1991). Council Directive of Amending Directive 64/432/EEC as Regards the Diagnosis of Bovine Brucellosis and Enzootic Bovine Leukosis. *Off. J. European Communities Council*, 14 May 1991.

7. DANIEL R.C.W., GATEI M.H., GOOD M.F., BOYLE D.B. & LAVIN M.F. (1993). Recombinant viral vaccines for enzootic bovine leucosis. *Immunol. Cell Biol.,* **71**, 399–404.

8. DIMMOCK C.K., RODWELL B.J. & CHUNG Y.S. (1987). Enzootic bovine leucosis. Pathology, Virology and Serology. Australian standard diagnostic techniques for animal disease. No. 49. Australian Agricultural Council.

9. EMANUELSSON U., SCHERLING K. & PETTERSSON H. (1992). Relationships between herd bovine leukemia virus infection status and reproduction, disease incidence, and productivity in Swedish dairy herds. *Prev. Vet. Med.,* **12**, 121–131.

10. FECHNER H., BLANKENSTEIN P., LOOMAN A.C., ELWERT J., GEUE L., ALBRECHT C., KURG A., BEIER D., MARQUARDT O. & EBNER D. (1997). Provirus variants of the bovine leukemia virus and their relation to the serological status of naturally infected cattle. *Virology,* **237**, 261–269.

11. JOHNSON R. & KANEENE J.B. (1992). Bovine leukaemia virus and enzootic bovine leukosis. *Vet. Bull.,* **62**, 287–312.

12. KLINTEVALL K. (1995). Bovine Leukaemia Virus: Course of Infection and Means of Detection. Thesis, SLU Info/repro, Uppsala, Sweden, 1–38.

13. MILLER L.D., MILLER J.M., VAN DER MAATEN M.J. & SCHMERR M.J.F. (1985). Blood from bovine leukaemia virus-infected cattle: antigen production correlated with infectivity. *Am. J. Vet. Res.,* **46**, 808–810.

14. OHISHI K., SUZUKI H., YAMAMOTO T., MARUYAMA T., MIKI K., IKAWA Y., NUMAKUNAI S., OKADA K., OHSHIMA K. & SUGIMOTO M. (1991). Protective immunity against bovine leukaemia virus (BLV) induced in carrier sheep by inoculating with a vaccinia virus – BLV env recombinant: Association with cell mediated immunity. *J. Gen. Virol.,* **72**, 1887–1892.

15. PORTETELLE D., LIMBACH K., BURNY A., MAMMERICKX M., DESMETTRE P., RIVIERE M., ZAVADA J. & PAOLETTI E. (1991). Recombinant vaccinia virus expression of the bovine leukaemia virus envelope gene and protection of immunized sheep against infection. *Vaccine,* **9**, 194.

16. RESSANG A.A., MASTENBROEK N., QUAK J., VAN GRIENSVEN L.J.L.D., CALAFT J., HILGERS J., HAGEMAN C., SOUISSI T. & SWEN S. (1974). Studies on bovine leukaemia 1. Establishment of type C virus producing cell lines. *Zentralbl. Veterinarmed. [B].,* **21**, 602–617.

17. SINGER-SAM J., ET AL. (1989). Use of Chelex to improve the PCR signal from a small number of cells. *Amplifications: A forum for PCR users,* **3**, 11.

18. THEILEN G.H., MILLER J.M., HIGGINS J., RUPPANER R.N. & GARRETT W. (1982). Vaccination against bovine leukaemia virus infection. *Curr. Top. Vet. Med. Anim. Sci.,* **15**, 547–559.

19. VENABLES C., MARTIN T.C. & HUGHES S. (1997). Detection of bovine leukosis virus proviral DNA in whole blood and tissue by nested polymerase chain reaction. Fourth International Congress of Veterinary Virology, Edinburgh, UK, Abstracts, 202.

20. WALSH P.S., METZGER D.A. & HIGUCHI R. (1991). Chelex 100 as a medium for simple extraction of DNA for PCR-based typing from forensic material. *BioTechniques,* **10**, 506–513.

CHAPTER 2.3.5.

INFECTIOUS BOVINE RHINOTRACHEITIS/ INFECTIOUS PUSTULAR VULVOVAGINITIS

SUMMARY

Infectious bovine rhinotracheitis/infectious pustular vulvovaginitis, caused by bovine herpesvirus 1 (BHV1), is a disease of domestic and wild cattle. The virus is distributed world-wide, but has been eradicated from Denmark and Switzerland and control programmes have started in some other countries.

The disease is characterised by clinical signs of the upper respiratory tract, such as a (muco)purulent nasal discharge, and by conjunctivitis. Signs of general illness are fever, depression, inappetance, abortions and reduced milk yield. The virus can also infect the genital tract and cause pustular vulvovaginitis and balanoposthitis. Mortality is low. Many infections run a subclinical course. Secondary bacterial infections can lead to more severe respiratory disease.

***Identification of the agent:** The virus can be isolated from nasal swabs taken during the acute phase of the infection, and from various organs collected at post-mortem. Post-mortem examinations reveal a rhinitis, laryngitis, and tracheitis.*

For virus isolation, various cell cultures of bovine origin are used, for example, secondary lung or kidney cells or the Madin–Darby bovine kidney cell line. The virus produces a cytopathic effect in 2–4 days. It is identified by neutralisation or antigen detection methods using monospecific antisera or monoclonal antibodies. The BHV1 isolates can be further subtyped by DNA restriction enzyme analysis.

Viral DNA detection methods have been developed, and the polymerase chain reaction technique may prove to be particularly useful for testing semen samples.

***Serological tests:** The virus neutralisation test and various enzyme-linked immunosorbent assays (ELISA) are most widely used for antibody detection. Antibodies can be detected in milk with an ELISA.*

***Requirements for vaccines and diagnostic biologicals:** Attenuated and killed vaccines are available. The vaccines must protect cattle clinically in case of infection and markedly reduce the subsequent shedding of field virus. The vaccines must not induce disease, abortion, or any local or systemic reaction, and must be genetically stable. In 1995, genetically engineered (gE) deletion mutant marker vaccines became available. The use of a gE-ELISA makes it possible to distinguish infected cattle from cattle vaccinated with such a marker vaccine.*

A. DIAGNOSTIC TECHNIQUES

Infectious bovine rhinotracheitis/infectious pustular vulvovaginitis (IBR/IPV), caused by bovine herpesvirus 1 (BHV1), is a disease of domestic and wild cattle. BHV1 is a member of the genus *Varicellovirus* in the subfamily alphaherpesvirinae, which belongs to the Herpesviridae family. The viral genome consists of double-stranded DNA that codes for 30–40 structural proteins. The viral glycoproteins, which are located on the surface of the virion, play an important role in pathogenesis and immunity. Based on differences in DNA restriction enzyme analysis, BHV1 can be differentiated into subtypes 1, 2a and 2b (12). Subtype 2b virus is less virulent than subtype 1 virus (6). There is nevertheless only one antigenic type of BHV1.

The name of the disease indicates the most prominent clinical signs. After an incubation period of 2–4 days, a serous nasal discharge, salivation, fever, inappetance, and depression become evident. Within a few days the nasal and ocular discharges change to mucopurulent. The necrotic lesions in the nose may progress to pustules and ulcers covered by a pseudomembrane that obstructs the upper airways and leads to mouth breathing. The infection may also induce abortion and a reduction in milk yield. Where natural mating is practised, genital infection can lead to pustular vulvovaginitis or balanoposthitis. These are characterised by mild to severe necrotic lesions in vaginal or preputial mucosae. After artificial insemination with infected semen, endometritis can arise (9). In calves infected with BHV1, a systemic disease may develop, with focal necrotic lesions in viscera and possibly a prominent gastroenteritis. Many infections run a subclinical course (21). Meningoencephalitis usually appears to be the result of an infection with a related, but distinct, herpesvirus, recently proposed as BHV5 (16).

Uncomplicated cases of respiratory or genital disease caused by BHV1 last 5–10 days. Secondary bacterial infections with, for example, *Pasteurella* spp., can give rise to more severe clinical signs due to the deeper airways being affected.

The virus enters the animal via the nose and replicates to high titres in mucous membranes of the upper respiratory tract and in the tonsils. It subsequently disseminates to conjunctivae and by neuronal axonal transport reaches the trigeminal ganglion. A low level viraemia can occasionally occur. After genital infection, BHV1 replicates in mucous membranes of the vagina or prepuce, and becomes latent in sacral ganglia. The viral DNA remains in the neurons of the ganglia probably for the entire life of the host. Stress, such as transport and parturition, can induce reactivation of the latent infection. Consequently, the virus may be shed intermittently into the environment.

The primary lesion is a focal necrosis of nasal, laryngeal, tracheal or genital mucous membranes. This lesion is probably the direct sequel of virus replication and its subsequent cytopathic effect (CPE). The animal reacts with an intense inflammatory response. The lesions may coalesce to form large pustules that consist of massive infiltrates of leukocytes. When secondary bacterial infections are involved, a pneumonia may develop. In aborted fetuses, tiny necrotic foci are present in various tissues, particularly in the liver.

An infection normally elicits an antibody response and a cell-mediated immune response within 7–10 days. The immune response is presumed to persist for life, although it may fall below the detection limit of some tests. However, the protective immunity after infection is not lifelong: cattle can be reinfected. Maternal antibodies are transferred via colostrum to the young calf, which is consequently protected against BHV1-induced disease (11). Maternal antibodies have a biological half-life of about 3 weeks, but may be detected occasionally in animals up to 6 months old, and rarely in animals over this age.

The virus is distributed world-wide, paralleling the distribution of domestic cattle. Other ruminants may be infected with BHV1, but this probably has no influence on the spread of BHV1 among domestic cattle. Apart from ruminants, no other reservoir of BHV1 exists. The minimal infective dose of BHV1 is not known. After infection, nasal viral shedding is detected for 10–14 days, with peak titres of 10^8–10^{10} $TCID_{50}$ (50% tissue culture infective doses) per ml of nasal secretion. Airborne transmission of BHV1 is likely only over short distances. The semen of an infected bull may contain BHV1 and the virus can thus be transmitted by natural mating and artificial insemination (13).

The control of BHV1 is based on the normal hygienic measures taken on a farm. Ideally, a 2–3-week quarantine period is imposed for newly introduced cattle. Only cattle that are BHV1-seronegative are then admitted to the herd. Vaccination is a common preventive measure. Only vaccines whose efficacy and safety have been demonstrated convincingly should be used. Efficacy is primarily demonstrated in a vaccination challenge experiment in cattle in the laboratory. Vaccines usually prevent the development of clinical signs and reduce the shedding of virus after infection. However, one disadvantage of the use of conventional vaccines is the inability to distinguish between antibodies induced by vaccination or infection. This interferes with programmes to eliminate the virus from farms, regions or countries, that are based on serology. By using gene-deleted or subunit vaccines that lack a specified (glyco)protein, this problem can be overcome – examples include the BHV1 gE-negative vaccines that are available currently in various countries (8). A companion diagnostic test is used that detects only antibodies to the deleted glycoprotein, and thus enables differentiation between vaccinated animals and those infected with wild-type virus (or vaccinated with conventional vaccines). These tools allow the identification of infected cattle in vaccinated populations, and improves the prospects for widescale eradication of BHV1.

BHV1 infection may be suspected as the cause of disease on the basis of clinical, pathological and epidemiological signs. To make a definite diagnosis, however, laboratory examinations are required. A complete diagnostic procedure in the laboratory is aimed at detecting the causative virus (or viral components) and the specific antibodies they induce.

1. Identification of the agent

a) Collection and processing of samples

Nasal swabs are collected from several (from five to ten) affected cattle in the early phase of the infection. These cattle still have serous rather than mucopurulent nasal discharge. In case of vulvovaginitis or balanoposthitis, swabs are taken from the genitals. The swabs should be vigorously rubbed against the mucosal surfaces. The prepuce can also be washed with saline, and the washing fluid is then collected. The specimens are suspended in transport medium (cell culture medium containing antibiotics and 2–10% fetal bovine serum to protect the virus from inactivation), cooled at 4°C, and rapidly submitted to the laboratory.

During necropsy, mucous membranes of the respiratory tract, and portions of the tonsil, lung, and bronchial lymph nodes, are collected for virus detection. In case of abortion, the fetal liver, lung, spleen, kidney and a placental cotyledon are examined. Samples should be sent to the laboratory as quickly as possible, on ice.

After arrival at the laboratory, swabs are agitated in the transport medium to elute virus and left at room temperature for 30 minutes. Following removal of the swabs, the transport medium is clarified by centrifugation at 1500 ***g*** for 10 minutes. Tissues are homogenised to a 10–20% (w/v) suspension in cell culture medium before centrifugation at 1500 ***g*** for 10 minutes. The supernatants of these specimens are filtered through 0.45 µm filters and used for virus isolation.

The isolation of virus from semen needs some special adaptations, because the seminal fluid contains enzymes and other factors that are toxic to the cells and inhibit viral replication (see below).

b) Virus isolation

For virus isolation, various cell cultures can be used. Primary or secondary bovine kidney, lung or testis cells, cell strains derived from bovine fetal lung, turbinate or trachea, and established cell lines, such as the Madin–Darby bovine kidney cell line, are all suitable. Cell cultures can be grown in glass or plastic tubes, plates or dishes. When 24-well plastic plates are used, a 100–200 µl volume of the supernatants described above is inoculated into these cell cultures. After a 1-hour adsorption period, the cultures are rinsed and maintenance medium is added. The cell cultures are observed daily for CPE, which usually appears within 3 days after inoculation. It is characterised by grape-like clusters of rounded cells gathered around a hole in the monolayer; sometimes giant cells with several nuclei may be observed. Experience is needed to recognise this characteristic appearance. When, after 7 days, no CPE has appeared, a blind passage must be made. The cell culture is freeze–thawed and clarified by centrifugation, and the supernatant is used for inoculation of fresh monolayers.

To identify the virus that produces the CPE as BHV1, the supernatant of the culture should be neutralised with a monospecific BHV1 antiserum or monoclonal antibody (MAb). For this purpose, serial tenfold dilutions of the test supernatant are made, and to each dilution monospecific BHV1 antiserum or negative control serum is added. Following incubation at 37°C for 1 hour, the mixtures are inoculated into cell cultures; 3–5 days later, the neutralisation index is calculated. The neutralisation index is the virus titre (in $\log_{10}$) in the presence of negative control serum minus the virus titre in the presence of specific antiserum. If the neutralisation index is greater than 1.5, the isolate may be considered to be BHV1. To shorten the virus isolation procedure, two specimens may be inoculated into cell culture: one that has been preincubated with monospecific antiserum and another that has been preincubated with negative control serum. If the CPE is inhibited by the monospecific antiserum, the isolate can be considered to be BHV1.

An alternative method of virus identification is by direct demonstration of BHV1 antigen in cells around the CPE by an immunofluorescence or immunoperoxidase test (8) with conjugated monospecific antiserum or MAb.

- **Virus isolation from semen (a prescribed test for international trade)**

At least 0.05 ml of raw semen should be tested, with two passages in cell culture. For extended semen, an approximation should be made to ensure that the equivalent of 0.05 ml raw semen is examined. Raw semen is generally cytotoxic and should be prediluted before being added to cell cultures. A similar problem may sometimes arise with extended semen. A suitable test procedure is given below.

- **Test procedure**

i) Dilute 200 µl fresh semen in 2 ml fetal bovine serum (free of antibody against BHV1) with added antibiotics.

ii) Mix vigorously and leave for 30 minutes at room temperature.

iii) Inoculate 1 ml of the semen/serum mixture into a monolayer of susceptible cells (see virus isolation above) in a six-well tissue culture plate.

iv) Incubate the plates for 1 hour at 37°C.

v) Remove the mixture, wash the monolayer twice with 5 ml maintenance medium, and add 5 ml maintenance medium to each well.

vi) Include BHV1 negative and positive controls in the test. Extreme caution must be taken to avoid accidental contamination of test wells by the positive control, for example always handling the control last, and using separate plates.

vii) Observe plates under a microscope daily for the appearance of a CPE. If a CPE appears, confirmatory tests for BHV1 are made by specific neutralisation or immunolabelling methods (see above).

viii) If there is no CPE after 7 days, the cultures are frozen at –70°C, then thawed, clarified by centrifugation, and the supernatant is used to inoculate fresh monolayers.

ix) The sample is considered to be negative if there is no evidence of a CPE after 7 days' incubation of the passaged cultures.

c) Viral antigen detection

Nasal, ocular or genital swabs can be directly smeared on to glass cover-slips, or, following centrifugation, the cell deposit (see Section A.1.a.) may be spotted on to cover-slips. These cover-slips are subjected to a standard direct or indirect fluorescent antibody test. In a direct immunofluorescence test, the monospecific antiserum is conjugated to fluorescein isothiocyanate, whereas in the indirect procedure it is the anti-bovine immunoglobulin that is conjugated to fluorescein isothiocyanate. To obtain the best results, it is necessary to sample several animals in a herd that have fever and a slight, serous nasal discharge. Smears should be air-dried and fixed in acetone within 24 hours. Smears from nasal swabs from cattle with a purulent or haemorrhagic nasal discharge are often negative (17). The advantage of this antigen detection technique is that it can lead to a same-day diagnosis. However, the sensitivity of this procedure is lower than that of virus isolation (4). Positive and negative controls must be included in each test.

Tissues, collected at post-mortem, can be examined for the presence of BHV1 antigen by the immunofluoresence test on frozen sections. Immunohistochemistry may also be used. The advantage is that the location of the antigen can be determined. MAbs are increasingly being used for detecting BHV1 antigen, leading to enhanced specificity of the test. However, such MAbs must be carefully selected, because they must be directed against conserved epitopes that are present on all isolates of BHV1.

Another possibility for direct rapid detection of viral antigen is the use of an enzyme-linked immunosorbent assay (ELISA). Antigen can be captured by MAbs or polyclonal antibodies coated on a solid phase, usually the well of a microplate. Amounts of antigen equivalent to 10^4–10^5 $TCID_{50}$ of BHV1 are required in order to have a high rate of positive results (3). This may not be unrealistically high, because titres of 10^8–10^9 $TCID_{50}$/ml of nasal fluid can be excreted by cattle 3–5 days after infection with BHV1. Sensitivity can be increased by amplification systems (see ref. 5 for an example).

The advantages of antigen detection methods versus virus isolation are that no cell culture facilities are required and a laboratory diagnosis can be made in 1 day. The disadvantages are the lower sensitivity of direct antigen detection and the extra requirement to perform virus isolation, if the isolate is required for further study.

d) Nucleic acid detection

During the past decade, various methods of demonstrating BHV1 DNA in clinical samples have been described, including DNA–DNA hybridisation and the polymerase chain reaction (PCR). These have not as yet found widespread application in routine diagnostic work, but the PCR is increasing used. Compared with virus isolation, the PCR has the primary advantages of being more sensitive and more rapid: it can be performed in 1–2 days. It can also detect DNA in latently infected sensory ganglia (18). The disadvantage is that it is prone to contamination and therefore precautions have to be taken to prevent false-positive results.

So far the PCR has been used mainly to detect BHV1 DNA in artificially (25) or naturally (18, 19) infected semen samples. These workers found that it was important to thoroughly optimise the PCR conditions, including the preparation of the samples, the concentration of Mg^{2+}, primers and Taq polymerase, and the cycle programmes. The target region for amplification must be present in all BHV1 strains, and its nucleotide sequence must be conserved. The TK, gB, gC and gD genes have been used as targets for PCR amplification.

Experimentally, the PCR was found to be more sensitive than virus isolation: it detected five times as many positive samples as did virus isolation. In addition, it had a detection limit of only three molecules. Nevertheless, false-negative results cannot be excluded. To identify possible false-negative results, it is recommended to spike an internal control template into the reaction tube of the semen sample to be amplified by the same primers. Such a control template may be constructed by inserting, for example, an 100 base-pair fragment into the target region. This control template also makes it possible to semi-quantify the amount of DNA that is detected (18, 19).

PCR followed by Southern blot hybridisation is the most sensitive method for detecting BHV1 DNA. Before the PCR can be internationally recognised as a suitable diagnostic tool for animal trade, it would have to be validated by an interlaboratory comparative test.

e) Differentiation of bovine herpesvirus 1 subtypes

By using MAbs and an ELISA, immunofluorescence or immunoperoxidase tests, BHV1 subtype 1 and subtype 2b can be differentiated (24). Restriction endonuclease analysis makes it possible to differentiate among all the recognised BHV1 subtypes (12). The DNA is first extracted from virions or infected cells, then digested by restriction endonucleases, and the resulting fragments are separated by agarose gel electrophoresis. The number and size of the fragments indicates the subtype of the virus. Such techniques are of limited diagnostic value, but may be useful in epidemiological studies.

f) Interpretation of results

The isolation of BHV1 from an animal does not unequivocally mean that this virus is the cause of the disease outbreak. It may, for instance, be a latent virus that has been reactivated due to stressful conditions. A confirmatory laboratory diagnosis must be made from a group of animals and must be accompanied by seroconversion from negative to positive, or a four-fold or higher titre rise in antibodies to BHV1. Cattle from which the nasal swabs are to be collected must be bled twice, 2–3 weeks apart. These paired serum samples are examined together in one serological test.

2. Serological tests

Serological tests can be used for several purposes:

i) To diagnose an acute infection: serum samples from the acute and convalescent stages of infection in the same animals are examined in one test. A seroconversion from negative to positive or a four-fold or higher increase in antibody titre is considered to indicate infection.

ii) To demonstrate the absence of infection, for instance, for international trade purposes.

iii) To determine the prevalence of infection in seroepidemiological studies.

iv) To support eradication programmes and subsequent surveillance.

v) For research purposes, for instance, the evaluation of the antibody response after vaccination and challenge infection.

Virus neutralisation (VN) tests and various ELISAs (10) are usually used for detecting antibodies against BHV1 in serum. An alternative serological test is the indirect fluorescent antibody test (22). Because virus latency is a normal sequel to BHV1 infection, the identification of serologically positive animals provides a useful and reliable indicator of infection status. Any animal with antibody to the virus is considered to be a carrier and potential intermittent excretor of the virus. The only exceptions to this are young calves that have acquired passive colostral antibody from their dam, and noninfected cattle vaccinated with inactivated vaccines.

ELISAs, including the gE-ELISA, are increasingly used for the detection of antibodies in (bulk) milk samples, but have some limitations. A negative bulk milk test indicates that not more than 20% of the adult milking herd has antibodies to BHV1. Many individual seropositive cows have a milk antibody titre less than 1/5. Consequently, it is not possible to declare a herd to be free from BHV1 infection on the basis of bulk or pooled milk tests, and a negative bulk milk test should be followed up with individual serum samples from all cattle in the herd. For general surveillance purposes, bulk milk tank tests can give an estimate of BHV1 prevalence in an area or country. These should be supplemented by serum testing (individual or pooled) from nonmilking herds.

a) Virus neutralisation (a prescribed test for international trade)

VN tests are performed with various modifications. Tests vary with regard to the virus strain, the starting dilution of the serum, the virus/serum incubation period (1–24 hours), the type of cells used, the day of final reading and the reading of the end-point (50% versus 100%) (14). Of these variables, the virus/serum incubation period has the most profound effect on the antibody titre. A 24-hour incubation period may score up to 16-fold higher antibody titres than a 1-hour incubation period (1), and is recommended where maximum sensitivity is required (e.g. for international trade purposes). Various bovine cells or cell lines are suitable for use in the VN test, including secondary bovine kidney or testis cells, cell strains of bovine lung or tracheal cells, or the established Madin–Darby bovine kidney cell line.

A suitable protocol for a VN test is shown below.

i) Inactivate sera, including control standard sera, for 30 minutes in a water bath at 56°C.

ii) Make doubling dilutions of test sera in cell culture medium. Start with undiluted serum and continue to 1/1024 horizontally in a 96-well flat-bottomed cell-culture grade microtitre plate, at least two wells per dilution and 50 µl volumes per well. Dilutions of a positive control serum, and of weak positive and negative internal control sera, are also included in the test. An extra well with undiluted serum is used for toxicity control of sera.

iii) Add 50 µl per well of BHV1 stock at a dilution in culture medium calculated to provide 100–200 $TCID_{50}$ per well. In the toxicity control wells, add 50 µl of culture medium in place of virus. Add 100 µl of culture medium to ten empty wells for cell controls.

iv) Make at least four tenfold dilutions of the residual virus stock (back titration) in culture medium, using 50 µl per well and at least four wells per dilution.

v) Incubate the plates for 18–24 hours at 37°C.

vi) Add 100 µl per well of the cell suspension at 3×10^4 cells per well.

vii) Incubate the plates for 3–5 days at 37°C.

viii) Read the plates microscopically for CPEs. Validate the test by checking the back titration of virus (which should give a value of 100 $TCID_{50}$ with a permissible range of 30–300 $TCID_{50}$), the control sera and the cell control wells. The positive control serum should give a titre of ± 1 twofold dilution (±0.3 log_{10} units) from its target value. The weak positive serum should be positive. The negative serum should give no neutralisation when tested undiluted (equivalent to a final dilution of 1/2 at the neutralisation stage). In the cell control wells, the monolayer should be intact.

ix) The test serum results are expressed as the reciprocal of the dilution of serum that neutralised the virus in 50% of the wells. If 50% of the wells with undiluted serum neutralised the virus, the (initial dilution) titre is read as 1 (1/2 using the final dilution convention). If all the undiluted and 50% of the wells with 1/2 diluted serum neutralised the virus, the (initial dilution) titre is 2 (final dilution 1/4). For qualitative results, any neutralisation at a titre of 1 or above (initial dilution convention) is considered to be positive. If cytotoxicity is observed in the serum toxicity control wells, the sample is reported to be toxic (no result) unless neutralisation of the virus without cytotoxicity is observed at higher dilutions and a titre can be read without ambiguity. Where there is cytotoxicity with a serum from which it is critical to obtain a result, changing the medium in the wells of the lowest two or three dilutions 16–24 hours after the addition of cells will remove the cytotoxic effect with many problem sera.

b) Enzyme-linked immunosorbent assay (a prescribed test for international trade)

ELISAs for the detection of antibody against BHV1 appear to be gradually replacing VN tests. A standard procedure for ELISA has not been established. Several types of ELISA are available, including indirect and blocking ELISAs. Indirect ELISA procedures are more commonly used. Various ELISA kits are available commercially, most of which are also suitable for detecting antibodies in milk. For reasons of standardisation in a country or state, it may be desirable to compare the quality of the kits and to test each batch in one national reference laboratory, before it is used in other laboratories in the country.

There are a number of variations in the ELISA procedures. The most common are: antigen preparation and coating, the dilution of the test sample, the incubation period of antigen and test sample, and the substrate/chromogen solution. Before being used routinely, an ELISA should be validated with respect to sensitivity, specificity and reproducibility. For this purpose, a panel of strong positive, weak positive and negative sera should be tested.

- **Indirect enzyme-linked immunosorbent assay**

The general principle of an indirect ELISA is that antigen is coated to the solid phase of a microtitre plate and the test sample is subsequently added to the plate. If antibodies are present these will bind to the antigen. After a washing step to remove unbound antibodies, an anti-bovine immunoglobulin/enzyme conjugate is added. After a further washing step, the substrate/chromogen solution is added. If immunoglobulins are present in the well, a colour reaction develops and is measured by a photometer. The intensity of the colour reaction is related to the amount of antibodies in the test sample.

An example of an indirect ELISA procedure is given below:

i) Prepare the antigen by growing BHV1 in cell cultures. When extensive CPE is observed, cells and medium are frozen at –20°C. After thawing, the resulting cellular lysate is centrifuged for 4 hours at 8500 *g*. The virus-containing pellet is suspended in a small volume of phosphate buffered saline (PBS), cooled on ice and disrupted using an ultrasonic disintegrator. The antigen preparation is then centrifuged for 10 minutes at 800 *g*, and used at an appropriate dilution to coat the plates. Many alternative methods of antigen production may be found in the published literature.

ii) Coat the microtitre plate with antigen by adding 100 µl of diluted antigen (in 0.05 M carbonate buffer, pH 9.6) to each well of a microplate. Seal the plates with tape, incubate at 4°C overnight or 37°C for 1–2 hours, and store at –20°C.

iii) Before the test is performed, wash the plates. Add buffer, the serum sample and positive, weak positive and negative control sera. Usually, serum samples are diluted 1/10 to 1/100 in PBS with 0.05% Tween 20. Shake and seal the plates and incubate for 1 hour at 37°C.

iv) Wash the plates thoroughly, add anti-bovine immunoglobulin/horseradish peroxidase conjugate at a predetermined dilution, and incubate again for 1 hour at 37°C.

v) Add freshly prepared substrate/chromogen solution (e.g. 0.1 M citrate phosphate buffer, pH 4, containing 2,2'-Azino-bis-[3-ethylbenzothiazoline-6-sulphonic acid]).$2NH_4$ [0.5 mg/ml] and a 3% solution of freshly added H_2O_2 [2 µl/ml]), and incubate for the appropriate time.

vi) Measure the absorbance of the plates on a microplate photometer at the appropriate wavelength.

vii) A test sample is considered to be positive if it has an absorbance value of 0.2 higher than the negative control serum. The test is valid if the positive and weak positive sera are positive and if the negative serum has an absorbance value less than 0.2. Invalid tests should be repeated. The acceptable limits for control and cut-off values must be determined for the individual assay.

- **Blocking enzyme-linked immunosorbent assay**

The principle of a blocking or competitive ELISA is based on blocking the binding of antigen to an enzyme-labelled BHV1 antiserum or anti-BHV1 MAb by antibodies in the test sample. The presence of antibodies in the test sample will block binding, resulting in reduced colour development after addition of the substrate/chromogen solution. A comparison of indirect ELISAs and blocking ELISAs showed the latter to be generally more sensitive (14). Recently, gE-ELISAs have been described that can be used in conjunction with marker vaccines to detect infected cattle in vaccinated populations (20, 23). In one gE-ELISA, milk can replace serum (23).

c) Standardisation

In each serological test, appropriate controls of strong positive, weak positive and negative serum should be included. A scientific group in Europe, initiated by the group of artificial insemination veterinarians of the European Union (EU), has recently agreed on the use of a strong positive, a weak positive and negative serum for standardisation of BHV1 tests in laboratories that routinely examine samples from artificial insemination centres (15). These sera have been adopted as OIE international standards for BHV1 tests and are available at the OIE Reference Laboratories for IBR/IPV[1]. Prescribed tests for international trade purposes (VN or ELISA) must be capable of scoring both the strong and weak positive standards (or secondary national standards of equivalent potency) as positive.

B. REQUIREMENTS FOR VACCINES AND DIAGNOSTIC BIOLOGICALS

Several attenuated and inactivated BHV1 vaccines are available currently. The vaccines contain virus strains that have usually undergone multiple passages in cell culture. Some of the vaccine virus strains have a temperature-sensitive phenotype, i.e. they do not replicate at temperatures of 39°C or higher. Attenuated vaccines are administered intranasally or intramuscularly. Inactivated vaccines contain high levels of inactivated virus or portions of the virus particle (glycoproteins) supplemented with an adjuvant to stimulate an adequate immune response. Inactivated vaccines are given intramuscularly or subcutaneously.

Marker vaccines are now available in various countries. These attenuated or inactivated marker vaccines are based on deletion mutants or on a subunit of the virion, for instance glycoprotein D. The use of such marker vaccines in conjunction with companion diagnostic tests makes possible the distinction between infected and

1 Obtainable from Institute of Animal Science and Health, Virology Department, Edelhertweg 15, P.O. Box 65, 8200 AB Lelystad, The Netherlands, and AFSSA Lyon, Laboratoire de pathologie bovine, 31 avenue Tony Garnier, BP 7033, 69342 Lyon Cedex 07, France.

vaccinated cattle, and may thus provide the basis for novel eradication programmes of BHV1. Intensive vaccination programmes can reduce the prevalence of infected animals (2), which could be monitored by using a companion diagnostic test. In situations where it is economically justifiable, the residual infected animals could then be culled, resulting in a region free from BHV1. Some countries recently implemented such an eradication programme.

1. Seed management

a) Characteristics of the seed

The vaccine is prepared using a seed-lot system. The origin, passage history and storage conditions of the master seed virus (MSV) must be recorded. A virus identity test must be performed on the MSV. The seed lot contains BHV1 strains that have been attenuated to yield a live vaccine strain. The strains can be attenuated by multiple passages in cell cultures, by adapting virus to grow at low temperatures (temperature-sensitive mutants), or by genetic engineering, for example, by deleting one or more viral genes that are nonessential for replication. There should be some means of distinguishing the live vaccine virus from field viruses (for example temperature-specific growth patterns or restriction fragment length polymorphisms). Strains used for the preparation of inactivated vaccines need not be attenuated. The seed lot must be free from contaminants.

b) Method of culture

The cells used for vaccine production are prepared using a seed-lot system. The virus should be cultured on established cell lines that have been shown to be suitable for vaccine production, for example the Madin–Darby bovine kidney cell line. The history of the cell line must be known. The cell line must be free from extraneous agents and may be tested for tumorigenicity.

c) Validation as a vaccine

Irrespective of the method of preparation of the seed-lot vaccine virus, the seed-lot virus destined for incorporation in a live vaccine must be shown to be efficacious, safe and pure.

i) *Efficacy*

This must be shown in a vaccination challenge experiment under laboratory conditions. Example guidelines are given in a monograph of the European Pharmacopoeia (7). Briefly, the vaccine is administered to five 2–3-month-old BHV1 seronegative calves. Two calves are kept as controls. All the calves are challenged intranasally 3 weeks later with a virulent strain of BHV1 that gives rise to typical signs of a BHV1 infection. The vaccinated calves should show no or only mild signs. The maximum virus titre found in the nasal mucus of vaccinated calves should be at least 100 times lower than that found in control calves. The virus excretion period should be at least 3 days fewer in vaccinated than in control calves.

ii) *Safety*

A quantity of virus equivalent to ten doses of vaccine should (a) not induce significant local or systemic reactions in young calves; (b) not cause fetal infection or abortion, and (c) not revert to virulence during five serial passages in calves. For inactivated vaccine, a double dose is usually administered. The reversion to virulence test is not applicable to inactivated vaccines.

iii) *Purity*

The seed lot is tested for absence of extraneous viruses and absence from contamination with bacteria, fungi or mycoplasmas. The following extraneous viruses should be specifically excluded in BHV1 vaccines: adenovirus, Akabane virus, bovine coronavirus, bovine herpesviruses 1, 2 and 4, bovine parvovirus, bovine respiratory syncytial virus, bovine rotavirus, vaccinia virus, and the viruses of Aujeszky's disease, bluetongue, bovine ephemeral fever, bovine leukaemia, bovine papilloma, bovine papular stomatitis, bovine viral diarrhoea; cowpox, foot and mouth disease, lumpy skin disease, malignant catarrhal fever, parainfluenza 3, rabies, rinderpest, and vesicular stomatitis. As bovine viral diarrhoea virus has regularly been found to be a contaminant of vaccines, special attention should be paid to ensure that it is absent.

2. Method of manufacture

All substances used for the manufacture of vaccines must be free from contaminants. Cells should be used that are not further than 20 passages from the master cell seed. The seed virus should not be more than five passages from the MSV. Genetically engineered vaccine virus strains are treated in the same way as conventionally attenuated vaccine virus strains. When sufficient cells are grown, infection of the cell line with the vaccine virus takes place. The addition of antibiotics is normally restricted to cell culture fluids. The supernatant fluid is harvested at times when the virus (antigen) production peaks. For live vaccines, the supernatant is clarified, mixed with a stabiliser, freeze-dried and bottled. For the production of classical inactivated vaccines, the supernatant is homogenised before the inactivating agent is added in order to ensure proper inactivation. After the inactivation procedure, a test for detecting complete inactivation of the virus is carried out. The test should consist of at least two passages in cells. The inactivated virus suspension is then mixed with an adjuvant and bottled. The manufacture of vaccines must comply with guidelines for Good Manufacturing Practice (GMP).

3. In-process control

Working cell seed and working virus seed must have been shown to be free from contaminants. The cells must have their normal morphology before being inoculated with virus. They are checked for CPE during cultivation. Uninoculated control cells must have retained their morphology until the time of harvesting. A virus titration is performed on the harvested supernatant. During the production of inactivated vaccines, tests are performed to ensure inactivation. The final bulk should be tested for freedom from contaminants.

4. Batch control

The following tests must normally be performed on each batch. Example guidelines for performing batch control can be found in EU directives, the European Pharmacopoeia and the United States Department of Agriculture's Code of Federal Regulations.

a) Sterility

Bacteria, fungi, mycoplasmas and extraneous viruses must not be present. Tests for sterility and freedom from contamination of biological material may be found in Chapter I.4.

b) Safety

For inactivated vaccines, a twofold dose of vaccine, and for live vaccines, a tenfold dose of vaccine, must not produce adverse effects in young BHV1 seronegative calves.

c) Potency

It is sufficient to test one representative batch for efficacy, as described in Section B.1.c.i. In the case of live vaccine, the virus titre of each batch must be determined and must be not higher than 1/10 of the dose at which the vaccine has been shown to be safe, and no lower than the minimum release titre. In the case of inactivated vaccines, the potency is tested using another validated method, for instance, efficacy assessment in calves.

d) Duration of immunity

It is sufficient to test this on the seed lot of vaccine virus. An efficacious BHV1 vaccine should induce protective immunity for at least 1 year, although many existing vaccines have not been tested to this standard.

e) Stability

For live vaccines, virus titrations should be carried out 3 months beyond the indicated shelf life. In addition, tests for determining moisture content, concentrations of preservatives, and pH are performed. For inactivated vaccines, the viscosity and stability of the emulsion are also tested.

f) Preservatives

The efficacy of preservatives should be demonstrated. The concentration of the preservative and its persistence throughout shelf life should be checked. The concentration must be in conformity with the limits set for the preservative.

g) Precautions (hazards)

No special precautions need to be taken, because BHV1 is not pathogenic for humans.

5. Tests on the final product

a) Safety

Each product must be shown to be safe in at least two susceptible calves that receive a twofold (inactivated vaccine) or a tenfold (live vaccine) dose of vaccine.

b) Potency

See Section B.4.c.

REFERENCES

1. BITSCH V. (1978). The P37/24 modification of the infectious bovine rhinotracheitis virus serum neutralization test. *Acta Vet. Scand.*, **19**, 497–505.

2. BOSCH J.C., DE JONG M.C.M., FRANKEN P., FRANKENA K., HAGE J.J., KAASHOEK M.J., MARIS-VELDHUIS M.A., NOORDHUIZEN J.P.T.M., VAN DER POEL W.H.M., VERHOEFF J., WEERDMEESTER K., ZIMMER G.M. & VAN OIRSCHOT J.T. (1998). An inactivated gE-negative marker vaccine and an experimental gD-subunit vaccine reduce the incidence of bovine herpesvirus 1 infections in the field. *Vaccine*, **16**, 265–271.

3. COLLINS J.K., AYERS V.K. & CARMAN J. (1988). Evaluation of an antigen-capture ELISA for the detection of bovine herpesvirus type 1 shedding from feedlot cattle. *Vet. Microbiol.*, **16**, 101–107.

4. EDWARDS S., CHASEY D. & WHITE H. (1983). Experimental infectious bovine rhinotracheitis: comparison of four antigen detection methods. *Res. Vet. Sci.*, **34**, 42–45.

5. EDWARDS S. & GITAO G.C. (1987). Highly sensitive antigen detection procedures for the diagnosis of infectious bovine rhinotracheitis: amplified ELISA and reverse passive haemagglutination. *Vet. Micorobiol.*, **13**, 135–141.

6. EDWARDS S., NEWMAN R. H. & WHITE H. (1991). The virulence of British isolates of bovid herpesvirus 1 in relation to viral genotype. *Br. Vet. J.*, **147**, 216–231.

7. EUROPEAN PHARMACOPOEIA, 3RD EDITION (1997). Monograph 0696: Live freeze dried vaccine for infectious bovine rhinotracheitis. Council of Europe, Strasbourg, France.

8. KAASHOEK M.J., MOERMAN A., MADIC J., RIJSEWIJK F.A.M., QUAK J., GIELKENS A.L.J. & VAN OIRSCHOT J.T. (1994). A conventionally attenuated glycoprotein E-negative strain of bovine herpesvirus type 1 is an efficacious and safe vaccine. *Vaccine*, **12**, 439–444.

9. KENDRICK J.W. & MCENTREE K. (1987). The effect of artificial insemination with semen contaminated with IBR–IPV virus. *Cornell Vet.*, **57**, 3–11.

10. KRAMPS J.A., QUAK S., WEERDMEESTER K & VAN OIRSCHOT J.T. (1993). Comparative study on sixteen enzyme-linked immunosorbent assays for the detection of antibodies to bovine herpesvirus 1 in cattle. *Vet. Microbiol.*, **35**, 11–21.

11. MECHOR G.D., ROUSSEAUX C.G., RADOSTITS O.M., BABIUK L.A. & PETRIE L. (1987). Protection of newborn calves against fatal multisystemic infectious bovine rhinotracheitis by feeding colostrum from vaccinated cows. *Can. J. Vet. Res.*, **51**, 452–459.

12. METZLER A.E., MATILE H., GASSMANN U., ENGELS M. & WYLER R. (1985). European isolates of bovine herpesvirus 1: a comparison of restriction endonuclease sites, polypeptides, and reactivity with monoclonal antibodies. *Arch. Virol.*, **85**, 57–69,

13. PARSONSON I.M. & SNOWDON W.A. (1975). The effect of natural and artificial breeding using bulls infected with, or semen contaminated with, infectious bovine rhinotracheitis virus. *Aust. Vet. J.*, **51**, 365–369.

14. PERRIN B., BITSCH V., CORDIOLI P., EDWARDS S., ELOIT M., GUERIN B., LENIHAN P., PERRIN M., RONSHOLT L., VAN OIRSCHOT J.T., VANOPDENBOSCH E., WELLEMANS G., WIZIGMANN G. & THIBIER M. (1993). A European comparative study of serological methods for the diagnosis of infectious bovine rhinotracheitis. *Rev. sci. tech. Off. int. Epiz.*, **12**, 969–984.

15. PERRIN B., CALVO T., CORDIOLI P., COUDERT M., EDWARDS S., ELOIT M., GUERIN B., KRAMPS J.A., LENIHAN P., PASCHALERI E., PERRIN M., SCHON J., VAN OIRSCHOT J.T., VANOPDENBOSCH E., WELLEMANS G., WIZIGMANN G. & THIBIER M. (1994). Selection of European Union standard reference sera for use in the serological diagnosis of infectious bovine rhinotracheitis. *Rev. sci. tech. Off. int. Epiz.*, **13**, 947–960.

16. STUDDERT M.J. (1994). Bovine herpesvirus. *In:* Encyclopedia of Virology, Webster R.G. & Granoff A., eds. Academic Press, London, UK, 155–158.

17. TERPSTRA C. (1979). Diagnosis of infectious bovine rhinotracheitis by direct immunofluorescence. *Vet. Q.*, **1**, 138–144.

18. VAN ENGELENBURG F.A.C., MAES R.K., VAN OIRSCHOT J.T. & RIJSEWIJK F.A.M. (1993). Rapid and sensitive detection of bovine herpesvirus type 1 in bovine semen by a polymerase chain reaction based assay. *J. Clin. Microbiol.*, **31**, 3129–3135.

19. VAN ENGELENBURG F.A.C., VAN SCHIE F.W., RIJSEWIJK F.A.M. & VAN OIRSCHOT J.T. (1995). Excretion of bovine herpesvirus 1 in semen is detected much longer by PCR than by virus isolation. *J. Clin. Microbiol.*, **33**, 308–312.

20. VAN OIRSCHOT J.T., KAASHOEK M.J., MARIS-VELDHUIS M.A., WEERDMEESTER K. & RIJSEWIJK F.A.M. (1997). An enzyme-linked immunosorbent assay to detect antibodies against glycoprotein gE of bovine herpesvirus 1 allows differentiation between infected and vaccinated cattle. *J. Virol. Methods*, **67**, 23–34.

21. VAN OIRSCHOT J.T., STRAVER P.J., VAN LIESHOUT J.A.H., QUAK J., WESTENBRINK F. & VAN EXSEL A.C.A. (1993). A subclinical infection of bulls with bovine herpesvirus type 1 at an artificial insemination centre. *Vet. Rec.*, **132**, 32–35.

22. WELLEMANS G. & LEUNEN J. (1973). La rhinotrachéite infectieuse des bovins et sa serologie. *Ann. Med. Vet.*, **117**, 507–512.

23. WELLENBERG G.J., VERSTRATEN E.R.A.M., MARS M.H. & VAN OIRSCHOT J.T. (1998). Detection of bovine herpesvirus 1 glycoprotein E antibodies in individual milk samples by enzyme-linked immunosorbent assays. *J. Clin. Microbiol.*, **36**, 409–413.

24. WYLER R., ENGELS M. & SCHWYZER M. (1989). Infectious bovine rhinotracheitis/vulvovaginitis (BHV1). *In:* Herpesvirus Diseases of Cattle, Horses and Pigs, Wittmann G., ed. Kluwer Academic Publishers, Boston, USA, 1–72.

25. XIA J.C., YASON C.V. & KIBENGE F.S.B. (1995). Comparison of dot blot hybridisation, polymerase chain reaction, and virus isolation for detection of bovine herpesvirus-1 (BHV-1) in artificially infected semen. *Can. J. Vet. Res.*, **59**, 102–109.

*

* *

CHAPTER 2.3.6.

TRICHOMONOSIS[1]

SUMMARY

Bovine venereal trichomonosis is caused by Tritrichomonas foetus, *a flagellate protozoan. It is world-wide in distribution and at one time was of major economic importance as a cause of abortion and infertility, especially in dairy cattle. With the widespread use of artificial insemination, the prevalence is much reduced, though it may still be of importance in beef herds or where artificial insemination is not used.*

Three serotypes of the organism – belfast, manley *and* brisbane *– have been identified, although subsequent untyped strains have been isolated. Transmission is primarily by coitus, but mechanical transmission by insemination instruments or by gynaecological examination can occur. The organism can survive in whole or diluted semen at 5°C, or in deep-frozen semen. Bulls are the main reservoir of the disease as they tend to be long-term carriers, but most cows clear the infection spontaneously. For these reasons samples from bulls are usually preferred for diagnosing and controlling the disease.*

Identification of the agent: Tritrichomonas foetus *is a flagellate, pyriform eukaryotic protozoan with three anterior and one posterior flagellae and an undulating membrane, approximately 8–18 µm long and 4–9 µm wide. Organisms move with a jerky, rolling motion and are seen in preputial washings of infected bulls and vaginal washings, or sometimes, cervico–vaginal mucus of infected cows, or in aborted fetuses. Organisms can be cultured* in vitro *and may be stained with the Romanowsky stains. The standard diagnostic method for bulls involves the collection, examination and culture of smegma from the prepuce and penis. Smegma can be collected by a variety of means included preputial lavage or scraping the preputial cavity and glans penis at the level of the fornix with a dry insemination pipette. A number of* in-vitro *culture media exist, but more recently a commercially available field culture test*[2] *has been introduced that allows for trichomonad growth and direct microscopic examination.*

Serological tests: *An agglutination test using mucus collected from the cervix and an antigen made from cultured organisms has been used as a herd test. Similarly, an intradermal test using a trichloracetic acid precipitate of the organism has been used in herds. The infection may also be detected by a specific DNA probe and polymerase chain reaction amplification, which are both under development.*

Requirements for vaccines and diagnostic biologicals: *A partially efficacious, killed whole-cell vaccine is commercially available as either a monovalent, or part of a polyvalent vaccine containing* Campylobacter *and* Leptospira[3].

A. DIAGNOSTIC TECHNIQUES

Bovine venereal trichomonosis is caused by the flagellate protozoan *Tritrichomonas foetus*. The natural hosts of *T. foetus* are cattle *(Bos taurus, Bos indicus)* and possibly pigs, horses and roe deer. Nonpathogenic species of trichomonads occur in the intestine of cattle; *T. suis* of pigs is indistinguishable morphologically and serologically from *T. foetus*.

1 Nomenclature of parasitic diseases: see the note in Chapter X.6. Trypanosomosis (tsetse-transmitted).
2 InPouch™ TF Test, BioMed Diagnostics, San José, California, United States of America (USA).
3 Trich Guard or Trich Guard V5-L, Fort Dodge Laboratories, Fort Dodge, Iowa, USA.

Tritrichomonas foetus is pyriform, 8–18 µm long and 4–9 µm wide, with three anterior and one posterior flagellae, and an undulating membrane. Living organisms move with a jerky, rolling motion, and are best detected by phase-contrast or dark-field microscopy. Detailed morphological descriptions, including electron microscopy studies, have been published by Warton & Honigberg (37). It is important to differentiate *T. foetus* from other contaminant protozoa that may be present in the bovine reproductive tract (35).

The organism multiplies by longitudinal binary fission; there is no sexual reproduction and cysts have not been observed.

Historically, three serotypes based on agglutination studies are recognised (32). The *'belfast'* strain reportedly predominated in Europe, Africa and the USA (18); the *'brisbane'* strain in Australia (10); and the *'manley'* strain has been reported in only a few outbreaks (22). Other strains have subsequently been isolated throughout North America (13, 18, 21), but have not necessarily been serotyped.

Organisms may be cultured *in vitro*, preferably in Diamond's medium (8), Clausen's medium (23) or *Trichomonas* medium, which is available commercially (30). A field culture test (InPouch™ TF, see footnote 2) has been developed in the USA that allows for growth of the trichomonads and direct microscopic examination without aspiration of the inoculum (36).

Transmission of infection under natural conditions is by coitus, by artificial insemination, or by gynaecological examination of cows. In the bull, infection is primarily of the preputial cavity (1, 25), and little or no clinical manifestation occurs. In 4–5-year old bulls, spontaneous recovery rarely occurs, and the bull becomes a permanent source of infection. In bulls under 3–4 years old, infection may be transient.

In the bull, the organisms are present in small numbers, with some concentration in the fornix and around the glans penis (1). The chronically infected bull shows no gross lesions. In the cow, the initial lesion is a vaginitis, which can be followed in animals that become pregnant by invasion of the cervix and uterus. Various sequelae result, including a placentitis leading to early abortion (1–16 weeks), uterine discharge, and irregular oestrous cycles. In some cases, despite infection, pregnancy is not terminated by abortion and a normal, full-term calf is born. On a herd basis, cows exhibit irregular oestrous cycles, uterine discharge, pyometra, and early abortion. The cow usually recovers and generally becomes immune, at least for that breeding season, after infection or abortion (34).

1. Identification of the agent

a) Agent identification by direct samples or culture (the prescribed test for international trade)

A tentative diagnosis of trichomonosis is based on the clinical history, signs of early abortion, repeated returns to service, or irregular oestrous cycles. Confirmation depends on the demonstration of organisms in placental fluid, stomach contents of the aborted fetus, uterine washings, pyometra discharge, or vaginal mucus. In infected herds, the most reliable material for diagnosis is either preputial or vaginal washings, or preputial scrapings (31). In Western Europe, European Union (EU) Directives require collection of preputial washings, or in the case of female animals, a vaginal mucus agglutination test (11).

The number of organisms varies in different situations. They are numerous in the aborted fetus, in the uterus several days after abortion and, in recently infected cows, they are plentiful in the vaginal mucus 12–20 days after infection. Thereafter the number of organisms varies according to the phase of the oestrous cycle, being highest 3–7 days after ovulation. In the infected bull *Tritrichomonas foetus* organisms are present in highest numbers on the mucosa of the prepuce and penis, apparently not invading the submucosal tissues. It is generally recommended to allow 1 week to pass after the last service before taking a preputial sample. These may be obtained by a variety of methods including the use of artificial insemination pipettes or washings from the artificial vagina.

Samples from cows are collected by washing the vagina or irrigating the uterus with physiological saline using a plastic or glass pipette and a long rubber tube. The efficiency of different sampling methods has been compared (15, 24). Samples should be kept at 37°C. It is important to avoid faecal contamination, as this may introduce intestinal protozoa that may be confused with *T. foetus* (35). Where samples must be submitted to a laboratory and cannot be delivered within 24 hours, a transport medium should be used (e.g. Winters' medium, buffered saline solution with 5% fetal bovine serum, or skim milk with or without antibiotics [27]), or the field culture plastic pouch (36). During transportation, the organisms should be protected from extremes of temperature, which should remain above 5°C and below 38°C (4). In grossly contaminated samples, it may be necessary to sediment the material and to examine the sediment. Staining of preparations will not necessarily allow more detailed examination of the material or more accurate diagnosis, although some laboratories use methanol fixation and staining with iodine and a commercial Wright–Giemsa stain (20).

Where organisms are too few to allow accurate identification, cultures should be prepared. Culture of the organisms is usually required because, in most cases, the number of organisms is not large enough to make a positive diagnosis by direct examination. Several media can be used. The CPLM (cysteine/peptone/liver-infusion maltose) medium, BGPS (beef-extract/glucose/peptone serum) medium, Clausen's medium (Neopeptone-Lemco-liver extract glucose), Diamond's trichomonad medium, and Oxoid's *Trichomonas* medium, are the media of choice (9, 23, 30). It is important that aseptically collected samples be obtained for inoculation into the media and this should be done as soon as possible after collection. It is also important to make sure that the culture media are used before their established expiry date, as many media are not stable.

The organisms may be identified on the basis of characteristic morphological features. Samples may be examined with a microscope directly. Culture media may be examined microscopically at intervals from day 1 to day 10 after inoculation. The organisms may be seen under a standard light microscope using a magnification of ×100 or more. An inverted microscope may be useful for examining tubes containing (Diamond's) culture medium, and it is possible to view organisms through the plastic wall of the InPouch™ at low magnification. The pear-shaped organisms have three anterior and one posterior flagellae and an undulating membrane that extends nearly to the posterior end of the cell. They also have an axostyle that usually extends beyond the posterior end of the cell. Phase-contrast microscopy is very valuable in revealing these features. A recently developed rapid staining procedure may also be used (20).

- **Culture procedures**

- **Modified Diamond's medium**

Glassware used for culture should be washed in distilled water (avoiding the use of detergents). The modified Diamond's medium comprises: 2 g trypticase peptone, 1 g yeast extract, 0.5 g maltose, 0.1 g L-cysteine hydrochloride, and 0.02 g L-ascorbic acid and is made up with 90 ml distilled water containing 0.08 g each of K_2HPO_4 and KH_2PO_4, and adjusted to pH 7.2–7.4 with sodium hydroxide or hydrochloric acid. Following the addition of 0.05 g agar, the medium is autoclaved for 10 minutes at 121°C, allowed to cool to 49°C, and then 10 ml inactivated bovine serum (inactivated by heating to 56°C for 30 minutes), 100,000 units crystalline penicillin G and 0.1 g streptomycin sulphate are added aseptically. The medium is aseptically dispensed in 10 ml aliquots into sterile 16 × 125 mm screw-top vials and refrigerated at 4°C until use. Media should be cultured for up to 7 days, samples being examined at daily intervals (1, 14). The incorporation of agar into the medium confines contaminating organisms largely to the upper portion of the test tube, while helping to maintain microaerophillic conditions at the bottom of the tube where the trichomonads occur in largest numbers.

- **Field culture test (InPouch™ TF)**

Where a combination of convenience and sensitivity is required, a field culture test (InPouch™ TF system, see footnote 2) may be used. This consists of a clear flexible plastic pouch with two chambers. The upper chamber contains special medium into which the sample is introduced. Field samples for inoculation into the culture pouch would normally be collected by the preputial scraping technique (1, 31). Samples collected by preputial washing, require centrifugation before introduction of the sediment into the upper chamber. Following mixing, the medium is forced into the lower chamber, and the pouch is then sealed and incubated at 37°C. Microscopic examination for trichomonads can be done directly through the plastic pouch using an inverted microscope (3). Diagnostic results with samples from bulls using either Diamond's medium or the InPouch™ TF system have shown that the two methods give comparable results or some advantages (in convenience and in test results) with the InPouch™ system (3, 4, 19).

- **Overall sensitivity and specificity of the culture and identification test**

Any estimate of the diagnostic sensitivity and specificity of the culture and identification test will be dependent on efficacy of sample collection, handling and processing, as well as the composition and quality of the culture medium. In bulls, the sensitivity of the InPouch™ TF kit has been estimated to be 92% (95% confidence interval, 84–96%) (24). Estimates for Diamond's and related media have been variable, possibly due to variation in composition and preparation, but range from 78 to 99%. Until recently it has been assumed that the specificity of the culture test was 100%, but this is likely to be an overestimation.

Not every sample taken from a bull known to be infected will necessarily give a positive culture result. Even with optimum conditions of sampling, transport, culture and identification, more than one negative sample should be obtained before there is reasonable assurance that the animal is uninfected. To estimate the probability that an animal is uninfected, negative predictive values should be calculated using an estimate of diagnostic test sensitivity and the animal's pretest probability of infection (25). With samples from females, there are few estimates of the diagnostic sensitivity of the standard sample and culture method.

The infection in females is usually cleared within 90–95 days, so it may be difficult to isolate organisms from animals in the late stages of their infection. In experimentally infected young cows, using the InPouch™ TF method of culture, an apparent sensitivity of 88% was achieved through a 10-week period after infection (19).

The diagnosis of abortion induced by *T. foetus* is usually relatively easy because of the large number of organisms demonstrable in the fetal abomasal contents or placental fluids. Additionally, immunohistochemical techniques can be used to demonstrate tissue-invasive *T. foetus* organisms in aborted fetuses.

b) Polymerase chain reaction

Molecular-based techniques that use polymerase chain reaction (PCR) technology have been described for the identification of *T. foetus.* A specific DNA probe has been developed as a means of improving the diagnosis of *T. foetus* in culture medium, uterine material and preputial smegma (16). A 0.85 kb sequence has been found to be the best candidate probe on the basis of specificity. To improve sensitivity, a partial sequence of the probe is used to identify two oligonucleotide primers (TF1 and TF2), which can be used to amplify parasite-specific DNA by PCR. DNA is extracted using the IsoQuick Nucleic Acid Extraction Kit (MicroProbe Corp.), which has been found to be fast, easy and reliable and allows for the detection of a single *T. foetus* organism in culture or ten organisms in smegma samples. The presence of inhibitors of Taq DNA polymerase in bovine smegma lowers the sensitivity to that of the cultivation method, but offers the advantages of ease of performance, rapid detection (1 day), and an increased number of samples that can be handled. A more recent publication (12) used PCR and DNA enzyme immunoassay based on rRNA gene unit sequences, with comparable results. However, in some cases PCR failed to detect where culture was positive and conversely gave positive results where culture was negative. Therefore, although this technology shows much promise, further work needs to be done to evaluate its application in the diagnosis of *T. foetus* infection before it can replace the culture method as the routine diagnostic test.

2. Serological tests

In the 1940s, mucus agglutination tests and intradermal diagnostic tests were developed and are still in limited use, however, problems with sensitivity and specificity restrict their usefulness. Other serodiagnostic tests based on the antigen-trapping enzyme-linked immunosorbent assay are now being developed, although this method is more sensitive with organisms in culture than those in cervical or vaginal mucus (25). Immunohistochemical techniques using monoclonal antibodies have been shown to reveal *T. foetus* organisms in formalin-fixed tissues.

a) Mucus agglutination test

A mucus agglutination test was developed in the 1940s (26) that detects about 60% of naturally infected cows, antibody levels varying according to stage of oestrus. Mucus samples are collected from the cervical region of the vagina, preferably a few days after oestrus. Antibodies appear in cervical mucus about 6 weeks after infection, and persist for several months. Antibodies may also be found in preputial secretions (29, 33). The mucus agglutination test is most useful as a herd test, being capable of detecting latent or recently cleared infections. It is specific and does not cross-react with *Campylobacter foetus* or *Brucella abortus*, but lacks sensitivity.

A sterile glass tube, 30 cm in length, 9 mm in diameter, and bent at an angle of 150° approximately 9 cm from one end, or an artificial insemination pipette, should be used for taking the cervical sample. Any mucus containing blood should not be used and the animal should be resampled. Serum contains nonspecific antibodies and will cause agglutination to occur. The mucus is diluted 1/5 with physiological saline and emulsified in a Griffith's tube. Duplicate samples, diluted to 1/10 and 1/20, are prepared by pipetting 2 ml of mucus and 2 ml of melted agar (56°C in a water bath) into tubes for the 1/10 dilution, and 1 ml mucus, 1 ml saline and 2 ml melted agar for the 1/20 dilution. Duplicate controls containing 2 ml saline and 2 ml melted agar are also prepared. All tubes are kept in a water bath at 56°C during mixing and then poured individually into 5 cm Petri dishes and allowed to cool. The test antigen is made up by slowly adding a trichomonad culture to a 2/1 mixture of saline and 1% glucose broth to achieve a concentration of approximately 100,000 organisms/ml (approximately six trichomonads/microscope field at ×400). Then, 1.5 ml of antigen is added to each Petri dish, the dishes are incubated for 1.5 hours at 37°C and then left at room temperature for a further 1.5 hours. Agglutination at a dilution of 1/10 is considered to be positive.

b) Intradermal 'Tricin' test

An intradermal test for diagnosis of bovine trichomonosis has been reported (17). The injection site is in the skin of the neck, similar to the site used for the tuberculin test. A dose of 0.1 ml of the 'Tricin' antigen is injected intradermally and the reaction is measured 30–60 minutes later. The reaction consists of a shallow plaque observed visually and showing an increase of >2 mm in skin thickness.

The antigen 'Tricin' is produced by sedimenting a culture of trichomonads by centrifugation and washing twice in normal saline. The centrifuged organisms are then left in distilled water for 1 hour before re-centrifugation to remove debris and particulate bodies. The supernatant is treated with trichloroacetic acid to precipitate the antigen, which is washed in acetone, then twice in anhydrous ether. The precipitate can be dried and stored as a powder. 'Tricin' is extracted from the precipitate, following washing in alcohol, by incubating in a water bath at 40°C using 1 ml of precipitate (0.1 g of powder) with 25 ml of disodium phosphate (11.8 g/litre). The extract is centrifuged and neutralised in an acid phosphate solution (9.0 g/litre), and finally merthiolate is added to make a 1/40,000 dilution.

c) Immunohistochemistry on tissues

There are no specific macroscopic or microscopic lesions in the aborted fetus, and identification of the organisms is necessary for diagnosis. An immunohistochemical technique using a monoclonal antibody (MAb) to detect *T. foetus* in formalin-fixed paraffin-embedded placenta and fetal lungs from bovine abortions has been reported (28). Immunohistochemical staining is done using a commercially available labelled streptavidin–biotin system[4] and an MAb (34.7C4.4) to *T. foetus*. In the procedure, deparaffinised 4 µm sections are incubated with the MAb following blocking with nonimmune goat serum. After three rinses in buffer, the sections are incubated with biotinylated goat anti-mouse and anti-rabbit immunoglobulin for 30 minutes at 37°C. Following three additional rinses in buffer, peroxidase-labelled streptavidin is applied for 30 minutes at 37°C, and the enzyme activity is diluted with 3% AEC (3-amino-9-ethylcarbazole) in N,N dimethylformamide. Sections are counterstained with Gill II haematoxylin for 3 minutes, rinsed, and blued in buffer for 1 minute. This method has been used to diagnose abortions caused by *T. foetus*.

B. REQUIREMENTS FOR VACCINES AND DIAGNOSTIC BIOLOGICALS

Whole cell vaccines for cows have been shown to offer protection and are available commercially (7) as either a monovalent 'bacterin' or part of a polvalent vaccine also containing *Campylobacter* and *Leptospira* spp. (CL-vaccine) (1) (see footnote 3). These products show efficacy in the female but not in the bull (2). This is in contrast to earlier studies in Australia in which protection or even clearance was afforded to bulls receiving membrane or glycoprotein fractions of *T. foetus* (5, 6). Specific antibodies have been demonstrated in serum and vaginal mucus of young cows inoculated with a vaccine containing *T. foetus* (14). In this study a partially effective killed whole-cell vaccine did not prevent infection, but appeared to allow clearance of the infection from vaccinated females before the time in gestation when the fetus is generally most at risk of abortion. More effective vaccines, making use of cell-surface epitopes from *T. foetus* are being sought (7).

Whole cell vaccine is produced by growing *T. foetus* (culture VMC-84) in modified Diamond's medium (8) and freezing the culture at –20°C for 60 minutes. After thawing, a suspension of 5×10^7 organisms/ml in phosphate buffered saline is added to the CL-vaccine.

REFERENCES

1. BONDURANT R.H. (1997). Pathogenesis, diagnosis and management of trichomoniasis in cattle. *Vet. Clin. North Am. Food Anim. Pract.*, **13**, 345–361.

2. BONDURANT R.H., CORBEIL R.R. & CORBEIL L.B. (1993). Immunisation of virgin cows with surface antigen TF1.17 of *Tritrichomonas foetus. Infect. Immun.*, **61**, 1385–1394.

3. BORCHARDT K.A., NORMAN B.B., THOMAS M.W. & HARMON W.M. (1992). Evaluation of a new culture method for diagnosing *Tritrichomonas foetus. Vet. Med.*, **87**, 104–112.

4. BRYAN L.A., CAMBELL J.R. & GAJADHAR A.A. (1999). Effects of temperature on the survival of *Tritrichomonas foetus* in transport, Diamond's and InPouch™ TF media. *Vet. Rec.*, **144**, 227–232.

5. CLARK B.L., DUFTY J.H. & PARSONSON I.M. (1983). Immunisation of bulls against trichomoniasis. *Aust. Vet. J.*, **60**, 178–179.

6. CLARK B.L., EMERY D.L. & DUFTY J.H. (1983). Therapeutic immunisation of bulls with the membranes and glycoproteins of *Tritrichomonas foetus* var *brisbane. Aust. Vet. J.*, **61**, 65–66.

7. CORBEIL L.B. (1994). Vaccination strategies against *Tritrichomonas foetus. Parasitol. Today*, **10**, 103–106.

4 DAKO Corporation, Carpinteria, California, USA.

8. DIAMOND L.S. (1983). Lumen dwelling protozoa: entamoeba, trichomonads and giardia. *In: In Vitro* Cultivation of Protozoan Parasites, Jensen J.B., ed. CRC Press, Boca Raton, Florida, USA, 65–109.

9. EAGLESOME M.D. & GARCIA M.M. (1992). Microbial agents associated with bovine genital tract infections and semen. Part 1. *Brucella, Leptospira, Campylobacter fetus* and *Tritrichomonas foetus. Vet. Bull*, **62**, 743–775.

10. ELDER J.K. (1964). Examination of twelve strains of *Trichomonas foetus* (Reidmuller) isolated in Queensland and the description of a new serotype, *T. foetus* var. *brisbane. Queensl. J. Agric. Sci.*, **21**, 193–203.

11. EUROPEAN UNION (1988). Council Directive EEC 88/407 of 14th June 1988 laying down the animal health requirements applicable to intra-community trade in and imports of deep-frozen semen of domestic animals of the bovine species. *Off. J. European Communities Council*, **194**, 10–23.

12. FELLEISEN R.S.J., LAMBELET N., BACHMANN P., NICOLET J., MULLER N. & GOTTSTEIN B. (1998). Detection of *Tritrichomonas foetus* by PCR and DNA enzyme immunoassay based on rRNA gene unit sequences. *J. Clin. Microbiol.*, **36**, 513–519.

13. FITZGERALD P.R. (1986). Bovine trichomoniasis in parasites: Epidemiology and control. *Vet. Clin. N. Am. Food Anim. Pract.*, **2**, 277–282.

14. GAULT R.A., KVASNICKA W.G. HANKS D., HANKS M. & HALL M.R. (1995). Specific antibodies in serum and vaginal mucus of heifers inoculated with a vaccine containing *Tritrichomonas foetus. Am. J. Vet. Res.*, **56**, 454–459.

15. GREGORY M.W., ELLIS B. & REDWOOD D.W. (1990). Comparison of sampling methods for the detection of *Tritrichomonas foetus. Vet. Rec.*, **127**, 16.

16. HO M.S.Y., CONRAD P.A., CONRAD P.J., LEFEBVRE R.B., PEREZ B. & BONDURANT R.H. (1994). The detection of bovine trichomoniasis with a specific DNA probe and PCR amplification system. *J. Clin. Microbiol.*, **32**, 98–104.

17. KERR W.R. (1944). The intradermal test in bovine trichomoniasis. *Vet. Rec.*, **56**, 303–305.

18. KERR W.R. & ROBERTSON M. (1941). An investigation into the infection of cows with *Trichomonas foetus* by means of the agglutination reaction. *Vet. J.*, **97**, 351–363.

19. KITTEL D.R., CAMPERO C., VAN HOOSEAR K.A., RHYAN J.C. & BONDURANT R.H. (1998). Comparison of diagnostic methods for detection of active infection with *Tritrichomonas foetus* in beef heifers. *J. Am. Vet. Med. Assoc.*, **213**, 519–522.

20. LUN Z.-R. & GAJADHAR A.A. (1999). A simple and rapid method for staining *Tritrichomonas foetus* and *Trichomonas vaginalis. J. Vet. Diagn. Invest.*, **11**, 471–474.

21. LUN Z.-R., PARKER P. & GAJADHAR A.A. (2000). Comparison of growth rates in *Trichomonas foetus* isolates from various geographic regions using three different culture media. *Vet. Parasitol.*, **89**, 199–208.

22. MAHMOUD A.H. (1944). Isolation of *Trichomonas foetus* (Reidmuller 1928) in bacteria-free culture by the use of penicillin. *Ann. Trop. Med. Parasitiol.*, **38**, 219–222.

23. MINISTRY OF AGRICULTURE, FISHERIES AND FOOD (MAFF) (1986). Manual of Veterinary Parasitological Techniques, Reference Book 418. HMSO, London, UK.

24. PARKER S., CAMPBELL J.R., RIBBLE C. & GAJADHAR A.A. (1999). Comparison of two sampling tools for diagnosis of *Tritrichomonas foetus* in bulls and clinical interpretation of culture results. *J. Am. Vet. Med. Assoc.*, **215**, 231–235.

25. PARSONSON I.M., CLARK B.L. & DUFTY J.H. (1974). The pathogenesis of *Tritrichomonas foetus* infection of the bull. *Aust. Vet. J.*, **50**, 421–423.

26. PIERCE A.C. (1949). The mucus agglutination test for the diagnosis of bovine trichomoniasis. *Vet. Rec.*, **61**, 347–349.

27. Reece R.L., Dennett D.P. & Johnson R.H. (1983). Some observations on cultural and transport conditions for *Trichomonas* foetus var brisbane. *Aust. Vet. J.*, **60**, 62–63.

28. Rhyan J.C., Wilson K.L., Bengess D.E., Staokhouse L.L. & Quinn W.J. (1995). The immunohistochemical detection of *Tritrichomonas* foetus in formalin-fixed paraffin-embedded sections of bovine placenta and fetal lung. *J. Vet. Diagn. Invest.*, **7**, 98–101.

29. Rhyan J.C., Wilson K.L., Wagner B., Anderson M.L., BonDurant R.H., Burgess D.E., Mutwiri G.K. & Corbeil L.B. (1999). Demonstration of *Tritrichomonas foetus* in the external genitalia and of specific antibodies in preputial secretions of naturally infected bulls. *Vet. Pathol.*, **36**, 406–411.

30. Ribeiro L.M.M. (1990). An efficient medium for the isolation of *Tritrichomonas foetus. Onderstepoort J. Vet. Res.*, **57**, 209–210.

31. Shonmann M.J., BonDurant R.H., Gardner L.A., Van Hoosear K., Baltzer W. & Kachulis C. (1994). Comparison of sampling and culture methods for the diagnosis of *Tritrichomonas foetus* infection in bulls. *Vet. Rec.*, **134**, 620–622.

32. Skirrow S.Z. & BonDurrant R.H. (1988). Bovine trichomoniasis. *Vet. Bull.*, **58**, 591–603.

33. Soto P. & Parma A.E. (1989). The immune response in cattle infected with *Tritrichomonas foetus. Vet. Parasitol.*, **33**, 343–348.

34. Soulsby E.J.L. (1982). Helminths. Arrthropods and Protozoa of Domesticated Animals, Seventh Edition. Balliere Tindall, London, UK, 556–561.

35. Taylor M.A., Marshall R.N. & Stack M. (1994). Morphological differentiation of *Tritrichomonas foetus* from other protozoa of the bovine reproductive tract. *Br. Vet. J.*, **150**, 73–80.

36. Thomas M.W., Marmon W.M. & White C. (1990). An improved method for the detection of *Tritrichomonas foetus* infection by culture in bulls. *Agri-Practice,* **11**, 13–17.

37. Warton A. & Honigberg B.M (1979). Structure of trichomonads as revealed by scanning electron microscopy. *J. Protozoot.*, **26**, 56–62.

*

* *

CHAPTER 2.3.7.

BOVINE ANAPLASMOSIS

SUMMARY

Bovine anaplasmosis results from infection with Anaplasma marginale. *A second species,* A. centrale, *has long been recognised. Whether it truly represents a separate species is unclear.* Anaplasma marginale *is responsible for almost all outbreaks of clinical disease. The organism is classified in the genus* Anaplasma *belonging to the family Anaplasmataceae of the order Rickettsiales. Genetically,* A. marginale *clusters within genogroup II of the Ehrlichiae.*

Anaemia and jaundice are characteristic signs of anaplasmosis, but the clinical disease can only be confirmed by identifying the organism. Once infected, cattle may remain carriers for life, and identification of these animals depends on the detection of specific antibodies using serological tests, or of rickettsial DNA using specific nucleic acid probes or amplification techniques.

Identification of the agent: *Microscopic examination of blood or organ smears stained with Giemsa stain is the most common method of identifying* Anaplasma *in clinically affected animals. In these smears,* A. marginale *appear as dense, rounded, intraerythrocytic bodies approximately 0.3–1.0 µm in diameter with most situated on or near the margin of the erythrocyte.* Anaplasma centrale *is similar in appearance, but most of the organisms are situated away from the margin of the erythrocyte. Commercial stains that give very rapid staining of* Anaplasma *are available in some countries.*

It is important that smears be well prepared and free from foreign matter. Smears from live cattle should preferably be prepared from blood drawn from the jugular vein or another large vessel. For post-mortem diagnosis, smears should be prepared from internal organs (including liver, kidney, heart and lungs) and from blood retained in peripheral vessels. The latter are particularly desirable if post-mortem decomposition is advanced.

Serological tests: *The most widely used serological tests are the complement fixation (CF) and the card agglutination tests. There are conflicting reports on the sensitivity and specificity of these tests. However, it is clear that the CF test cannot consistently identify carrier animals. When used, these tests need to be carefully evaluated under local conditions. A recently developed competitive enzyme-linked immunosorbent assay (ELISA) has been demonstrated to have much improved sensitivity over the CF test in detecting carrier animals. Indirect ELISA, dot ELISA and indirect fluorescent antibody tests also are available.*

Nucleic-acid-based tests have recently been developed for experimental purposes, and have been shown to be capable of detecting the presence of low level infection in carrier cattle and in tick vectors. Currently, their main use is as research tools; however, the technique may be a future adjunct to serology in definitive identification of carrier cattle.

Requirements for vaccines and diagnostic biologicals: *Live vaccines are used in several countries to protect cattle against* A. marginale *infection. Vaccine consisting of live* A. centrale *is most widely used and gives partial protection against challenge with virulent* A. marginale.

Anaplasma centrale *vaccine is provided in chilled or frozen forms. Quality control is very important as other blood-borne agents that may be present in donor cattle can contaminate vaccines and be disseminated broadly. For this reason, frozen vaccine is recommended as it allows thorough post-production quality control, which limits the risk of contamination with other pathogens.*

Anaplasma centrale *vaccine is not entirely safe. A practical recommendation is to restrict its use, as far as possible, to calves, as nonspecific immunity will minimise the risk of some vaccine reactions that may require treatment with tetracycline or imidocarb. Partial immunity develops in 6–8 weeks and lasts for several years after a single vaccination.*

A. DIAGNOSTIC TECHNIQUES

Outbreaks of bovine anaplasmosis are usually due to infection with *Anaplasma marginale. Anaplasma centrale* is capable of producing a moderate degree of anaemia, but clinical outbreaks in the field are extremely rare. Appendages associated with the *Anaplasma* body have been observed in certain isolates of *A. marginale* (15); while this parasite has been termed *A. caudaturn,* it is not considered to be a separate species.

Anaplasma marginale occurs in most tropical and subtropical countries, and in some more temperate regions. *Anaplasma centrale* was first described from South Africa and has since been imported by some other countries – including Australia and some countries in South America, South-East Asia and the Middle East – for use as a vaccine against *A. marginale.*

Anaplasma species were originally regarded as protozoan parasites, but later research showed they had no significant attributes to justify this description. Since 1957 they have been classified in the family Anaplasmataceae of the order Rickettsiales. This family has four genera: *Anaplasma, Aegyptianella, Haemobartonella* and *Eperythrozoon* (29). Based on 16S ribosomal RNA gene analysis, *A. marginale* clusters within genogroup II of the Ehrlichiae (35).

Anaplasma species are transmitted either mechanically or biologically by arthropod vectors. A review based on a careful study of reported transmission experiments lists 14 different ticks as capable of transmitting *A. marginale* experimentally (16). These are: *Argas persicus, Ornithodoros lahorensis, Boophilus annulatus, B. decoloratus, B. microplus, Dermacentor albipictus, D. andersoni, D. occidentalis, D. variabilis, Hyalomma excavatum, Ixodes ricinus, Rhipicephalus bursa, R. sanguineus* and *R. simus.* The authors concluded that some of these reports, including those of *R. bursa, H. excavatum* and *O. lahorensis,* were not entirely convincing, and that the ticks identified as *A. persicus* were probably either *A. sanchezi* or *A. radiatus.* In addition, *Rhipicephalus e. evertsi* and *Hyalomma m. rufipes* have been listed as experimental vectors in South Africa (26). Intrastadial or transstadial transmission is the usual method of transmission, even in the one-host *Boophilus* species. Male ticks may be particularly important as vectors. Experimental demonstration of vector competence does not necessarily imply a role in transmission in the field. However, *Boophilus* species are clearly important vectors of anaplasmosis in countries such as Australia and countries in Africa, and there is good evidence that some species of *Dermacentor* are efficient vectors in the United States of America (USA).

Various other biting arthropods have been incriminated as mechanical vectors, particularly in the USA. Experimental transmission has been demonstrated with a number of species of *Tabanus* (horseflies), and with mosquitoes of the genus *Psorophora* (28). The importance of biting insects in the natural transmission of anaplasmosis has not been well documented, but appears to vary greatly from region to region. *Anaplasma marginale* can also be readily transmitted during vaccination against other diseases unless a fresh needle is used for injecting each animal. Similar transmission by means of unsterilised surgical instruments has been described.

The main biological vectors of *A. centrale* appear to be multihost ticks peculiar to Africa, including *R. simus.* The common cattle tick *(B. microplus)* has not been shown to be a vector. This is of relevance where *A. centrale* is used as a vaccine in *B.-microplus*-infested regions.

The most marked clinical signs of anaplasmosis are anaemia and jaundice, the latter occurring late in the disease. Haemoglobinaemia and haemoglobinuria are not present, and this may assist in the differential diagnosis of anaplasmosis from babesiosis, which is often endemic in the same regions. The disease can only be confirmed, however, by identification of the organism.

1. Identification of the agent

Samples from dead animals should include air-dried thin smears from the liver, kidney, heart and lungs and from a peripheral blood vessel. The latter is particularly recommended should there be a significant delay before post-mortem examination because, under these circumstances, bacterial contamination of organ smears often makes identification of *Anaplasma* equivocal. Brain smears, which are useful for the diagnosis of some forms of babesiosis, are of no direct value for diagnosing anaplasmosis (12), but should be included for differential diagnosis where appropriate.

Blood from organs, rather than organ tissues *per se*, is required for smear preparation, as the aim is to be able to examine microscopically intact erythrocytes for the presence of *Anaplasma*. Organ-derived blood smears will store satisfactorily at room temperature for several days (12).

Samples from live cattle should include thin blood smears and blood collected into an anticoagulant. Air-dried thin blood smears will keep satisfactorily at room temperature for at least 1 week. The blood sample in the anticoagulant should be held and transferred at 4°C, unless it can reach the laboratory within a few hours. This sample is useful for preparing fresh smears if those submitted are not satisfactory. In addition, a low packed cell volume and/or erythrocyte count can help to substantiate the involvement of *Anaplasma* when only small numbers of the parasites are detected in smears, such as may occur in the recovery stage of the disease.

In contrast to *Babesia bovis, Anaplasma* do not accumulate in capillaries, so blood drawn from the jugular or other large vessel is satisfactory. Because of the rather indistinctive morphology of *Anaplasma,* it is essential that smears be well prepared and free from foreign matter, as specks of debris can confuse diagnosis. Thick blood films as used for the diagnosis of babesiosis are not appropriate for the diagnosis of anaplasmosis, as *Anaplasma* are difficult to identify once they become dissociated from erythrocytes.

Both blood and organ smears are fixed in absolute methanol for 1 minute and stained in 10% Giemsa stain for 30 minutes. After staining, the smears are rinsed three or four times with tap water to remove adhering stain, and are then air-dried. Smears are examined under oil immersion at a magnification of ×700–1000.

In Giemsa-stained smears, *A. marginale* appear as dense, rounded and deeply stained intraerythrocytic bodies, approximately 0.3–1.0 µm in diameter. Most of these bodies are located on or near the margin of the erythrocyte. This feature distinguishes *A. marginale* from *A. centrale,* as in the latter most of the organisms have a more central location in the erythrocyte. Proprietary stains that give very rapid staining of *Anaplasma* are available in some countries[1].

The percentage of infected erythrocytes varies with the stage and severity of the disease. Maximum parasitaemias in excess of 50% may occur with *A. marginale.* Multiple infections of individual erythrocytes are common during periods of high parasitaemias.

The infection becomes visible microscopically 2–6 weeks following transmission. During the course of clinical disease, the parasitaemia approximately doubles each day for up to about 10 days, and then decreases at a similar rate. Quite severe anaemia may persist for some weeks after the parasites have become virtually undetectable in blood smears. Following recovery from initial infection, most cattle remain latently infected for life.

Fluorescent antibody staining may be used as an alternative staining technique for detecting *Anaplasma* in smears taken at post-mortem. A direct fluorescent antibody procedure for the post-mortem diagnosis of anaplasmosis has been described in detail by Johnston *et al.* (12). While it has been shown to be more sensitive than Giemsa staining for this purpose, nonspecific fluorescence can be a problem.

An expensive procedure, but one that may occasionally be justified to confirm infection, particularly in latently infected cattle, is the inoculation of blood from the suspect animal into a splenectomised calf. A quantity (up to 500 ml) of the donor's blood in anticoagulant is inoculated intravenously into the splenectomised calf, which is then tested by blood smear examination at least every 2–3 days. If the donor is infected, *Anaplasma* will be observed in smears from the splenectomised calf generally within 4 weeks, but this period may extend up to 8 weeks.

Nucleic-acid-based tests to detect *A. marginale* infection in carrier cattle have been developed recently (6, 7, 9, 10, 31). A radioactive RNA probe, which detected parasitaemias as low as 0.000025%, has been described (6). Infected ticks have also been identified using a cloned DNA probe (11). The analytical sensitivity of polymerase chain reaction (PCR)-based methods has been estimated at 0.0001% infected erythrocytes, but at this level only a proportion of carrier cattle would be detected (7, 9). Nested PCR has recently been used to sensitively and specifically identify *A. marginale* carrier cattle (31). This technique is capable of identifying as few as 30 infected erythrocytes per ml of blood, equivalent to a parasitaemia of approximately 0.0000001% (31). While posing significant quality control problems for routine use, nested PCR is capable of identifying carrier cattle at the lowest levels of parasitaemia (6, 31).

Nucleic-acid-based techniques, while currently used primarily for research purposes, hold promise for use in future diagnostic and epidemiological studies.

1 Proprietary stains include Camco-Quik and Diff-Quik, Baxter Scientific Products, McGaw Park, Illinois, USA, and Hema 3 and Hema-Quik, Curtin-Matheson, Houston, Texas, USA.

2. Serological tests

Anaplasma infections usually persist for the life of the animal. However, except for occasional small recrudescences, *Anaplasma* cannot readily be detected in blood smears after the acute parasitaemic episode. Thus, a number of serological tests have been developed with the aim of detecting latently infected animals.

A feature of the serological diagnosis of anaplasmosis is the highly variable results with regard to both sensitivity and specificity reported for many of the tests from different laboratories. This is due to inadequate evaluation of the tests using significant numbers of known positive and negative animals. Importantly, the capacity of several assays to detect known infections of long-standing duration has not been adequately addressed. An exception is the recently described competitive enzyme-linked immunosorbent assay (cELISA) (see below), which has been validated using true positive and negative animals defined by the nested PCR described above (31). Therefore, while most of the tests described in this section are useful for obtaining broad-based epidemiological data, caution is advised on their use for disease certification unless the test(s) has been properly evaluated and standardised under local conditions.

It should be noted that there is a high degree of cross-reactivity between *A. marginale* and *A. centrale* in serological tests. While the infecting species can sometimes be identified using antigens from homologous and heterologous species, equivocal results are obtained on many occasions.

a) Complement fixation test

This test is undertaken using standard complement fixation (CF) test procedures. Antigen consists of *Anaplasma* bodies that have been separated from erythrocytes by lysis, and then washed free from most haemoglobin and cellular debris. A microtitre technique is now most commonly used, as it requires only very small quantities of reagents. Detailed manuals for the conduct of both the standard (32) and the microtitre technique (33) for the CF test for anaplasmosis have been produced. While the CF test has been used extensively for many years, there is increasing evidence that it lacks sensitivity and fails to detect a significant proportion of carrier cattle.

b) Card agglutination test

The advantages of the card agglutination test (CAT) are that it is sensitive, may be undertaken either in the laboratory or in the field, and gives a result within a few minutes. Nonspecific reactions may be a problem. The CAT antigen is a suspension of *A. marginale* particles. Splenectomised calves are infected by intravenous inoculation with blood containing *Anaplasma*-infected erythrocytes. When the parasitaemia exceeds 50%, the animal is exsanguinated, the infected erythrocytes are washed, lysed, and the erythrocyte ghosts and *Anaplasma* particles are pelleted. The pellets are sonicated, washed, and then resuspended in a stain solution to produce the antigen suspension.

A test procedure that has been slightly modified from that originally described (1, 2) is as follows:

i) Ensure all test components are at a temperature of 25–26°C before use (this constant temperature is critical for the test).

ii) On each circle of the test card (a clear perspex/plastic or glass plate marked with circles that are 18 mm in diameter), place next to each other, but not touching, 10 µl of bovine serum factor (BSF), 10 µl of test serum, and 5 µl of CAT antigen[2]. Negative and low positive control sera must be tested on each card.

    BSF is serum from a selected animal with high known conglutinin level. If the conglutinin level is unknown, fresh serum from a healthy animal known to be free from *Anaplasma* can be used. The Jersey breed is often suitable. The BSF must be stored at –70°C in small aliquots, a fresh aliquot being used each time the tests are performed. The inclusion of BSF improves the sensitivity of the test.

iii) Mix well with a glass stirrer. After mixing each test, wipe the stirrer with clean tissue to prevent cross-contamination.

iv) Place the test card in a humid chamber and rock at 100–110 rpm for 7 minutes.

v) Read immediately against a backlight. Characteristic clumping of the antigen (graded from +I to +3) is considered to be a positive result. The test is considered to give a negative result when there is no characteristic clumping.

---

2 The test as conducted in the USA and Mexico uses larger volumes of reagents: antigen (15 µl), serum (30 µl), and bovine serum factor (30 µl), and a 4-minute reaction time (see step iv).

c) Competitive enzyme-linked immunosorbent assay

A competitive ELISA using a recombinant antigen termed rMSP5 and MSP5-specific monoclonal antibody (MAb) has proven very sensitive and specific for detection of *Anaplasma*-infected animals (14, 21, 31, 34). All *A. marginale* strains tested, *A. ovis* and *A. centrale*, express the MSP5 antigen, including the immunodominant epitope recognised by the MSP5-specific MAb. The test was 100% specific using 261 known negative sera from a nonendemic region, detecting acutely infected cattle as early as 16 days after experimental tick or blood inoculation, and was demonstrated to detect cattle that have been experimentally infected as long as 6 years previously (14). In detecting persistently infected cattle from an anaplasmosis endemic region of the USA that were defined as true positive or negative using a nested PCR procedure, the rMSP5-cELISA had a sensitivity of 96% and a specificity of 95% (31). A recently described indirect ELISA validates the use of rMSP5 as a diagnostic antigen (27). However, initial studies suggest that in its current format the indirect rMSP5 ELISA is less sensitive than the cELISA (27).

Test results using the rMSP5-cELISA are available in less than 2.5 hours. A test kit, soon to be commercially available[3], contains specific instructions. In general, however, it is conducted as follows.

- **Kit reagents**

A 96-well microtitre plate coated with rMSP5 antigen,

A 96-well coated adsorption/transfer plate for serum adsorption to reduce background binding,

100 × MAb–peroxidase conjugate,

10 × wash solution and ready-to-use conjugate-diluting buffer,

Substrate and stop solutions ready-to-use,

Positive and negative controls

- **Test Procedure**

i) Add 70 µl of undiluted serum sample to the coated adsorption/transfer plate and incubate at room temperature for 30 minutes.

ii) Transfer 50 µl per well of the adsorbed serum to the rMSP5-coated plate and incubate at room temperature for 60 minutes.

iii) Discard the serum and wash the plate twice using diluted washing solution.

iv) Add 50 µl per well of the 1 × diluted MAb–peroxidase conjugate to the rMSP5-coated plate, and incubate at room temperature for 20 minutes.

v) Discard the 1 × MAb–peroxidase conjugate and wash the plate four times using diluted wash solution.

vi) Add 50 µl per well of the substrate solution, cover the plate with foil, and incubate for 20 minutes at room temperature.

vii) Add 50 µl per well of stop solution to the substrate solution already in the wells and gently tap the sides of the plate to mix the wells.

viii) Read the plate in the plate reader at 620 nm.

- **Test validation**

The mean optical density (OD) of the negative control must range from 0.40 to 2.10. The per cent inhibition of the positive control must be ≥30%.

- **Interpretation of the results**

The % inhibition is calculated as follows:

$$100 - \frac{\text{Sample OD} \times 100}{\text{Mean negative control OD}} = \text{Per cent inhibition}$$

Samples with <30% inhibition are negative. Samples with ≥30% inhibition are positive.

3 Veterinary Medical Research and Development (VMRD), 4641 Pullman–Albion Rd., P.O. Box 502, Pullman, Washington 99163, USA. Tel.: (1.509) 334 58 15; Fax: (1.509) 332.53.56; http://www.vmrd.com

d) Indirect enzyme-linked immunosorbent assay

An indirect ELISA based on the use of a normal red blood cell antigen (negative antigen) and an *A.-marginale*-infected red blood cell antigen (positive antigen) has been found to be reliable for the detection of *A.-marginale*-positive sera (5). Although more cumbersome than tests using only one antigen, this test eliminates those sera that have high levels of nonspecific activity due to isoantibodies to normal red blood cell components. The test correctly identified all 100 known positive sera taken from cattle up to 3 years after infection, while 3% of negative sera, 2% of *Babesia bovis* and 4% of *B. bigemina* sera gave false-positive results.

The two antigen test is conducted as follows.

- **Negative antigen**

Blood is collected into Na_2-ethylene diamine tetra-acetic acid (EDTA) from a splenectomised calf. The cells are washed three times with phosphate buffered saline (PBS), and centrifuged at 5000 ***g*** for 10 minutes at 5°C. After the final centrifugation, white blood cells are removed by diluting the cells tenfold in PBS and passing them through a Whatman CFI 1 cellulose column. Following further centrifugation, one volume of cells is diluted in two volumes of PBS and stored as 2.5 ml aliquots in the vapour phase of liquid nitrogen. An aliquot is thawed at room temperature, as required, and sonicated for 30 seconds at 100 W with a small probe at 0°C. The whole sonicate is then diluted as required for use in the ELISA.

- **Positive antigen**

A calf previously used to produce negative antigen is infected with *A. marginale* by blood inoculation. When the parasitaemia reaches 80–85%, 500–1000 ml of blood is collected, processed and stored as described above. When required, aliquots are sonicated, as before, and diluted appropriately.

- **Test procedure**

Flat-bottomed 96-well micro-ELISA plates are used. Standard antigen checkerboard titrations are performed with each new batch of antigen, both positive and negative, to determine the working range, which is usually 1/400 (150–200 µg protein/ml). Diluted antigen (200 µl) is added to each well on the plate, one-half of the plate for positive antigen, the other half for negative antigen. The plates are sealed with plate sealers and incubated at 4°C overnight. After incubation, the antigen solution is removed and the plates are washed three times in PBS containing 0.1% Tween 20 (PBST), and then blocked with a 1% solution of normal horse serum in PBS for 60 minutes at 37°C.

After blocking, the plates are washed five times in PBST prior to the addition of 200 µl of test sera. (Test sera are diluted 1/400 to 1/800 in PBST containing 1% horse serum.) The plates are sealed with plate sealers and incubated for 2 hours at 37°C. The wells are then washed five times with PBST, and 200 µl of conjugated second antibody (goat anti-bovine IgG conjugated with horseradish peroxidase), at a dilution of 1/400 in PBS containing 1% horse serum, is added. The plates are then sealed and incubated for 2 hours at 37°C. After incubation, the conjugate is removed and the wells are washed five times in PBS prior to the addition of 200 µl of freshly prepared substrate.

Substrate is prepared as follows; recrystallised 5-amino salicylic acid is dissolved at 1 mg/ml in phosphate buffer, pH 6.8, at 37°C; 2 µl of 30% hydrogen peroxide is then added to each 1 ml of solution. After the addition of the substrate, the plates are sealed and gently agitated for 30 minutes at 22°C. Plates are then read immediately at 492 nm with a plate reader. Column one of each plate is always used as a blank.

Net readings are calculated for each sample by subtracting the negative antigen result from the positive antigen result. A group of 20 negative sera and a standard positive *A. marginale* serum are routinely tested with each batch of assays. A 'threshold' is calculated as the mean net absorbance reading (plus two standard deviations) of the 20 standard negative sera. Ratios of all other net absorbances are determined against the 'threshold' as unity. The positive serum is used to determine that each assay batch is performing normally.

e) Dot enzyme-linked immunosorbent assay

Compared with the ELISA, the dot ELISA has the potential advantages of being rapid, inexpensive and simple to perform. The dot ELISA described below has been reported to have a sensitivity of 93% and a specificity of 96% (19).

- **Antigen preparation**

i) High parasitaemic blood is collected in EDTA.

ii) Plasma is removed, and the erythrocytes are washed in 0.1 M glycine buffer, pH 3.0.

iii) The erythrocytes are washed in PBS, pH 7.4, in the presence of protease inhibitors (3.5 mM sodium tetrathionate) and 0.01% thimerosal.

iv) The buffy coat is removed after each wash.

v) The erythrocytes are resuspended in PBS at a 1/5 dilution, sonicated, subjected to three freeze–thaw cycles, and the lysate is resonicated.

vi) The material is mixed with an equal volume of 1% Nonidet P-40 in PBS, and incubated for 3 minutes at 25°C.

vii) *Anaplasma* bodies are recovered by differential centrifugation.

viii) The pellet is washed three times in cold buffer (155 mM choline chloride, 5 mM HEPES [N-2-hydroxyethylpiperazine, N-2-ethanesulphonic acid], pH 7.4).

ix) The pellet is resuspended in PBS, and the protein concentration is measured.

Antigen (1.0 µl/disc; 25 µg protein/ml) is dotted on to discs (6 mm in diameter) cut from nitrocellulose using a paper punch. The antigen-spotted discs are air-dried. Antigen on these discs remains stable for over 2 years when held at –20°C or at 4°C, and for at least 3 months when held at 25°C.

- **Test procedure**

i) The antigen-spotted discs are placed in wells in flat-bottomed microtitration plates.

ii) All procedures are undertaken at 25°C and using 200 µl reaction volumes.

iii) Known positive and negative sera and antigen controls are included.

iv) For blocking, PBS containing 0.5% Tween 20 is added to each of the wells, which are then incubated for 15 minutes.

v) Sera are tested at an initial concentration of 1/200 in PBS containing 0.05% Tween 20, and incubated for 1 hour.

vi) Three 10-minute washes with PBS containing 0.1% Tween 20, are performed.

vii) Alkaline phosphatase–protein A conjugate, diluted 1/500 in PBS containing 0.5% Tween 20, is added and the wells are incubated for 30 minutes, followed by washing as before, except that the last wash is in PBS alone.

viii) Nitroblue tetrazolium/5-bromo-4-chloro-indoxyl phosphate in 0.1M Tris buffer, pH 9.5, is added and the colour is allowed to develop for 10–20 minutes.

ix) A purple coloured dot of variable intensity indicates a positive reaction; no colour is seen on discs with negative reactions.

f) Indirect fluorescent antibody test

Because of the limitations on the number of indirect fluorescent antibody (IFA) tests that can be performed daily by one operator, other serological tests are generally preferred to the IFA test. The IFA test is performed as described for bovine babesiosis in Chapter 2.3.8., except that *A.-marginale*-infected blood is used for preparation of antigen smears. A serious problem encountered with the test is nonspecific fluorescence. Antigen made from blood collected as soon as adequate parasitaemia (5–10%) occurs is most likely to be suitable. Nonspecific fluorescence due to antibodies adhering to infected erythrocytes can be reduced by washing the erythrocytes in an acidic glycine buffer before antigen smears are prepared (20). Infected erythrocytes are washed twice in 0.1 M glycine buffer (pH 3.0, centrifuged at 1000 ***g*** for 15 minutes at 4°C) and then once in PBS, pH 7.4.

B. REQUIREMENTS FOR VACCINES AND DIAGNOSTIC BIOLOGICALS

Several immunisation methods have been used to protect cattle against anaplasmosis in endemic countries, but none is ideal (17). Use of the less pathogenic *A. centrale,* which gives partial cross-protection against *A. marginale,* is the most widely accepted method, although not used in North America. In Australia, approximately 700,000 doses of *A. centrale* vaccine are used annually. Another method involves the use of a strain of *A. marginale* attenuated by passage in nonbovine hosts, such as deer or sheep (30).

In this section, the production of live *A. centrale* vaccine is described. It involves infection of a susceptible, splenectomised calf and the use of its blood as a vaccine. Detailed accounts of the production procedure are available and reference should be made to these publications for details of the procedures outlined here (3, 8, 23).

Anaplasma centrale vaccine can be provided in either frozen or chilled form depending on demand, transport networks, and the availability of liquid nitrogen or dry ice supplies. Frozen vaccine is recommended in most instances, as it allows for thorough post-production quality control of each batch. It is, however, more costly to produce and more difficult to transport than chilled vaccine. The risk of contamination makes post-production control essential, but may be prohibitively expensive.

1. Seed management

a) Characteristics of the seed

Anaplasma centrale was isolated in 1911 in South Africa, and has been used as a vaccine in South America, Australia, Africa, the Middle East, and South-East Asia. It affords partial, but adequate, protection in regions where the challenging strains are of moderate virulence (e.g. Australia) (8). In the humid tropics where *A. marginale* appears to be a very virulent parasite, the protection afforded by *A. centrale* may be inadequate to prevent disease in some animals.

Anaplasma centrale usually causes benign infections, especially if used in calves under 9 months of age. Severe reactions following vaccination have been reported when adult cattle are inoculated.

Rapid passage of *A. centrale* in splenectomised calves appears to reduce its virulence (8).

b) Preparation and storage of stabilate

Infective material is readily stored as frozen stabilates of infected blood in liquid nitrogen or dry ice. Dimethyl sulphoxide (DMSO) is the recommended cryopreservative, as it allows for intravenous administration after thawing of the stabilate. A detailed account of the freezing technique is reported elsewhere (8), but briefly involves the following: infected blood is collected, chilled to 4°C, and cold cryoprotectant (4 M DMSO in PBS) is added slowly with stirring to a final blood:protectant ratio of 1:1, to give a final concentration of 2 M DMSO. The entire dilution procedure is carried out in an ice bath and the diluted blood is dispensed into suitable containers (e.g. 5 ml cryovials), and frozen, as soon as possible, in the vapour phase of a liquid nitrogen container.

c) Validation as a vaccine

The suitability of an isolate of *A. centrale* as a vaccine can be determined by inoculating susceptible cattle, monitoring the subsequent reactions, and then challenging the animals and susceptible controls with a virulent local strain of *A. marginale*. Both safety and efficacy can be judged by monitoring parasitaemias in stained blood films and the depression of packed cell volumes of inoculated cattle during the vaccination and challenge reaction periods. Evidence of purity of the isolate can be determined by serological testing of paired sera from the cattle used in the safety test for possible contaminants that may be present (24).

2. Method of manufacture

a) Production of frozen vaccine

Quantities of the frozen stabilate (5–10 ml) are thawed by immersing the vials in water preheated to 40°C. The thawed material is kept on ice and used as soon as possible (within 30 minutes) to infect a susceptible, splenectomised calf by intravenous inoculation.

The parasitaemia of the donor calf is monitored daily by examining stained films of jugular blood, and the blood is collected for vaccine production when suitable parasitaemias are reached. A parasitaemia of 1×10^8/ml (approximately 2% parasitaemia in jugular blood) is the minimum required for production of vaccine. If a suitable parasitaemia is not obtained, passage of the strain by subinoculation of 100–200 ml of blood to a second splenectomised calf may be necessary.

Blood from the donor is collected by aseptic jugular or carotid cannulation using heparin as an anticoagulant (5 International Units [IU] heparin/ml blood).

In the laboratory, the parasitised blood is mixed in equal volumes with 3 M glycerol in PBS supplemented with 5 mM glucose at 37°C (final concentration of glycerol 1.5 M). The mixture is then equilibrated at 37°C for 30 minutes and dispensed into suitable containers (e.g. 5 ml cryovials). The vials are cooled at approximately 10°C/minute in the vapour phase of liquid nitrogen and, when frozen, stored in the liquid phase (4).

DMSO can be used as a cryoprotectant in the place of glycerol. This is done in the same way as outlined for the preparation of stabilate (18, 22).

If glycerolised vaccine is to be diluted, the diluent should consist of PBS with 1.5 M glycerol and 5 mM glucose (13). Vaccine cryopreserved with DMSO should be diluted with diluent containing the same concentration of DMSO as in the original cryopreserved blood (25).

b) Production of chilled vaccine

Infective material for chilled vaccine is prepared in the same way as for frozen vaccine, but it must be issued and used as soon as possible after collection. The infective blood can be diluted to provide 1×10^7 parasites per dose of vaccine. A suitable diluent is 10% sterile bovine serum in a balanced salt solution containing the following quantities of salts per litre: NaCl (7.00 g), $MgCl_2.6H_2O$ (0.34 g), glucose (1.00 g), Na_2HPO_4 (2.52 g), KH_2PO_4 (0.90 g), and $NaHCO_3$ (0.52 g).

If diluent is not available, acid citrate dextrose (20% [v/v]) or citrate phosphate dextrose (20% [v/v]) should be used as anticoagulant to provide the glucose necessary for survival of the organisms.

c) Use of vaccine

In the case of frozen vaccine, vials should be thawed by immersion in water, preheated to 40°C, and the contents mixed with suitable diluent to the required dilution. If glycerolised vaccine is prepared, it should be kept cool and used within 8 hours (4). If DMSO is used as a cryoprotectant, the prepared vaccine should be kept on ice and used within 15–30 minutes (22). The vaccine is most commonly administered subcutaneously.

Chilled vaccine should be kept refrigerated and used within 6 days of preparation.

The strain of *A. centrale* used in vaccine is of reduced virulence, but is not entirely safe. A practical recommendation is, therefore, to limit the use of vaccine to calves, where nonspecific immunity will minimise the risk of vaccine reactions. When older animals have to be vaccinated, there is a risk of severe reactions. These reactions occur infrequently, but valuable breeding stock or pregnant animals obviously warrant close attention, and should be observed between weeks 4 and 6 post vaccination. Clinically sick animals should be treated with oxytetracycline or imidocarb at dosages recommended by the manufacturers.

Protective immunity develops in 6–8 weeks and usually lasts for several years.

Anaplasmosis and babesiosis vaccines are often used concurrently, but it is not advisable to use any other vaccines at the same time.

3. In-process control

a) Source and maintenance of vaccine donors

A source of calves free from natural infections of *Anaplasma* and other tick-borne diseases should be identified. If a suitable source is not available, it may be necessary to breed the calves under tick-free conditions specifically for the purpose of vaccine production.

The calves should be maintained under conditions that will prevent exposure to infectious diseases and to ticks and biting insects. In the absence of suitable facilities, the risk of contamination with the agents of infectious diseases present in the country involved should be estimated, and the benefits of local production of vaccine weighed against the possible adverse consequences of spreading disease (8).

b) Surgery

Donor calves should be splenectomised to allow maximum yield of organisms for production of vaccine. This is best carried out under general anesthesia in young calves. Details of the technique, including pre- and post-operative procedures, are reported elsewhere (8).

c) Screening of vaccine donors before inoculation

Donor calves should be examined for all blood-borne infections prevalent in the vaccine-producing country, including *Babesia, Anaplasma, Cowdria, Theileria* and *Trypanosoma*. This can be done by routine examination of stained blood films after splenectomy, and preferably also by serology. Any calves showing evidence of natural infections of any of these agents should be rejected. The absence of other infective agents should also be confirmed. These may include the agents of enzootic bovine leukosis, mucosal disease, infectious bovine rhinotracheitis, ephemeral fever, Akabane disease, bluetongue, foot and mouth disease, and rinderpest. The testing procedures will depend on the diseases prevalent in the country and the availability of tests, but should involve serology of paired sera at the very least and, in some cases, virus isolation (4, 22, 24).

d) Monitoring of parasitaemias following inoculation

It is necessary to determine the concentration of parasites in blood being collected for vaccine. There are accurate techniques for determining the parasite count (8) but, in the absence of these, the parasite concentration can be estimated from the erythrocyte count and the parasitaemia (percentage of infected erythrocytes).

e) Collection of blood for vaccine

All equipment should be sterilised before use (e.g. by autoclaving). Once the required parasitaemia is reached, the blood is collected in heparin using strict aseptic techniques. This is best done if the calf is sedated and with the use of a closed-circuit collection system.

Up to 3 litres of heavily infected blood can be collected from a 6-month-old calf. If the calf is to live, the transfusion of a similar amount of blood from a suitable donor is indicated. Alternatively, the calf should be killed immediately after collection of the blood.

f) Dispensing of vaccine

All procedures are performed in a suitable environment, such as a laminar flow cabinet, using standard sterile techniques. Use of a mechanical or magnetic stirrer will ensure thorough mixing of blood and diluent throughout the dispensing process.

4. Batch control

The potency, safety and sterility of vaccine batches cannot be determined in the case of chilled vaccine, and specifications for frozen vaccine depend on the country involved. The following are the specifications for frozen vaccine produced in Australia.

a) Sterility and freedom from contaminants

Standard tests for sterility are employed for each batch of vaccine and diluent (see Chapter I.4.).

The absence of contaminants is confirmed by inoculating cattle and monitoring them serologically for infectious agents that could potentially contaminate the vaccine. Cattle inoculated during the test for potency (see Section B.4.c.) are suitable for the purpose. Depending on the country of origin of the vaccine, these agents include the causative organisms of enzootic bovine leukosis, infectious bovine rhinotracheitis, mucosal disease, ephemeral fever, Akabane disease, Aino virus, bluetongue, parainfluenza, foot and mouth disease, lumpy skin disease, rabies, Rift Valley fever, rinderpest, contagious bovine pleuropneumonia, Jembrana disease, heartwater, pathogenic *Theileria* and *Trypanosoma* spp., *Brucella abortus, Coxiella,* and *Leptospira* (4).

b) **Safety**

Vaccine reactions of the cattle inoculated in the test for potency (see Section B.4.c.) are monitored by measuring parasitaemia and depression of packed cell volume. Only batches with pathogenicity levels equal to or lower than a predetermined standard are released for use.

c) **Potency**

Vaccine is thawed and diluted 1/50 with a suitable diluent (13). The diluted vaccine is then incubated for 8 hours at 30°C, and five cattle are inoculated subcutaneously with 2 ml doses. The inoculated cattle are monitored for the presence of infections by examination of stained blood smears. All should become infected for a batch to be accepted. A batch proving to be infective at 1/50 is recommended for use at a dilution of 1/5 with isotonic diluent.

d) **Duration of immunity**

Partial but long-lasting immunity results from one inoculation. There is no evidence that repeated vaccination will have a boosting effect.

e) **Stability**

The vaccine can be kept for 5 years when stored in liquid nitrogen. Once thawed, it rapidly loses its potency. Thawed vaccine cannot be refrozen.

f) **Preservatives**

No preservatives are added. Penicillin (500,000 IU/litre) and streptomycin (370,000 µg/litre) are added to the vaccine at the time of dispensing.

g) **Precautions (hazards)**

The vaccine is not infective for humans. When the product is stored in liquid nitrogen, the usual precautions pertaining to the storage, transportation and handling of deep-frozen material applies.

5. Tests on final product

a) **Safety**

See Section B.4.b.

b) **Potency**

See Section B.4.c.

REFERENCES

1. AMERAULT T.E. & ROBY T.O. (1968). A rapid card agglutination test for bovine anaplasmosis. *J. Am. Vet. Med. Assoc.*, **153**, 1828–1834.

2. AMERAULT T.E., ROSE J.E. & ROBY T.O. (1972). Modified card agglutination test for bovine anaplasmosis: evaluation with serum and plasma from experimental and natural cases of anaplasmosis. *Proc. U.S. Anim. Health Assoc.*, **76**, 736–744.

3. CALLOW L.L. (1984). Arthropod-borne Rickettsias of the blood. Part Three: Anaplasmosis. *In:* Animal Health in Australia, Vol. 5. Protozoal and Rickettsial Diseases. Australian Bureau of Animal Health, Australian Government Publishing Service, Canberra, Australia, 181–201.

4. DALGLIESH R.J., JORGENSEN W.K. & DE VOS A.J. (1990). New Australian vaccines for the control of babesiosis and anaplasmosis in the world cattle trade. *Trop. Anim. Health Prod.*, **22**, 44–52.

5. DUZGUN A., SCHUNTER C.A., WRIGHT I.G., LEATCH G. & WALTISBUHL D.J. (1988). A sensitive ELISA technique for the diagnosis of *Anaplasma marginale* infections. *Vet. Parasitol.*, **29**, 1–7.

6. ERIKS I.S., PALMER G.H., MCGUIRE T.C., ALLRED D.R. & BARBET A.F. (1989). Detection and quantitation of *Anaplasma marginale* in carrier cattle by using a nucleic acid probe. *J. Clin. Microbiol.*, **27**, 279–284.

7. FIGUEROA J.V., CHIEVES L.P., JOHNSON G.S. & BUENING G.M. (1993). Multiplex polymerase chain reaction based assay for the detection of *Babesia bigemina, Babesia bovis* and *Anaplasma marginale* DNA in bovine blood. *Vet. Parasitol.*, **50**, 69–81.

8. FOOD AND AGRICULTURE ORGANIZATION OF THE UNITED NATIONS (FAO) (1984). *In:* Ticks and Tick-borne Disease Control. A Practical Field Manual, Vol. 11. Tick-borne Disease Control. FAO, Rome, Italy, 621 pp.

9. GALE K.R., DIMMOCK C.M., GARTSIDE M., & LEATCH G. (1996). *Anaplasma marginale:* Detection of carrier cattle by PCR-ELISA. *Int. J. Parasitol.*, **26**, 1103–1109.

10. GE N-L., KOCAN K.M., EWING S.A., BLOUIN E.F., EDWARDS W.W., MURPHY G.L., & DAWSON L.J. (1997). Use of a non-radioactive DNA probe for detection of *Anaplasma marginale* infection in field cattle: comparison with complement fixation serology and microscopic examination. *J. Vet. Diagn. Invest.*, **9**, 39–43.

11. GOFF W., BARBET A., STILLER D., PALMER G., KNOWLES D., KOCAN K., GORHAM J. & MCGUIRE T. (1988). Detection of *Anaplasma marginale*-infected tick vectors by using a cloned DNA probe. *Proc. Natl Acad. Sci. USA,* **85,** 919–923.

12. JOHNSTON L.A.Y., TRUEMAN K.F., LEATCH G. & WILSON A.J. (1980). A comparison of direct fluorescent antibody and Giemsa staining for the post-mortem diagnosis of anaplasmosis. *Aust. Vet. J.*, **56**, 116–118.

13. JORGENSEN W.K., DE VOS A.J. & DALGLIESH R.J. (1989). Infectivity of cryopreserved *Babesia bovis, Babesia bigemina* and *Anaplasma centrale* for cattle after thawing, dilution and incubation at 30°C. *Vet. Parasitol.*, **31**, 243–251.

14. KNOWLES D., TORIONI DE ECHAIDE S., PALMER G., MCGUIRE T., STILLER D. & MCELWAIN T. (1996). Antibody against an *Anaplasma marginale* MSP5 epitope common to tick and erythrocyte stages identifies persistently infected cattle. *J. Clin. Microbiol.*, **34**, 2225–2230.

15. KREIER J.P. & RISTIC M. (1963). Anaplasmosis. X Morphological characteristics of the parasites present in the blood of calves infected with the Oregon strain of *Anaplasma marginale. Am. J Vet. Res.,* **24**, 676–687.

16. MARCHETTE N. & STILLER D. (1982). Chapter 11: The Anaplasmataceae, Bartonellaceae, and *Rochalimaea quintana. In:* Ecological Relationships and Evolution in the Rickettsiae, Vol. 11, Marchette N.J., ed. CRC Press, Boca Raton, Florida, USA, 98–106.

17. MCHAROY N. (1984). Immunization against anaplasmosis: a review. *Prev. Vet. Med.,* **2,** 135–146.

18. MELLORS L.T., DALGLIESH R.J., TIMMS P., RODWELL B.J. & CALLOW L.L. (1982). Preparation and laboratory testing of a frozen vaccine containing *Babesia bovis, Babesia bigemina* and *Anaplasma centrale. Res. Vet. Sci.*, **32**, 194–197.

19. MONTENEGRO-JAMES S., GUILLEN A.T., MA S.-J., TAPANG P., ABDEL-GAWAD A., TORI M. & RISTIC M. (1990). Use of the dot enzyme-linked immunosorbent assay with isolated *Anaplasma marginale* initial bodies for serodiagnosis of anaplasmosis in cattle. *Am. J. Vet. Res.*, **51**, 1518–1521.

20. MONTENEGRO-JAMES S., JAMES M.A. & RISTIC M. (1985). Modified indirect fluorescent antibody test for the serodiagnosis of *Anaplasma marginale* infections in cattle. *Am. J. Vet. Res.*, **46**, 2401–2403.

21. NDUNG'U L.W., AGUIRRE C., RURANGIRWA F.R., MCELWAIN T.F., MCGUIRE T.C., KNOWLES D.P. & PALMER G.H. (1995). Detection of *Anaplasma ovis* infection in goats by major surface protein 5 competitive inhibition enzyme-linked immunosorbent assay. *J. Clin. Microbiol.,* **33**, 675–679.

22. PIPANO E. (1981). Frozen vaccine against tick fevers of cattle. *In:* XI International Congress on Diseases of Cattle, Haifa, Israel. Mayer E., ed. Bregman Press, Haifa, Israel, 678–681.

23. PIPANO E. (1995). Live vaccines against hemoparasitic diseases in livestock. *Vet. Parasitol.*, **57**, 213–231.

24. PIPANO E. (1997). Vaccines against hemoparasitic diseases in Israel with special reference to quality assurance. *Trop. Anim. Health Prod.*, **29** (Suppl. 4), 86S–90S.

25. Pipano E., Krigel Y., Frank M., Markovics A. & Mayer E. (1986). Frozen *Anaplasma centrale* vaccine against anaplasmosis in cattle. *Br. Vet. J.*, **142**, 553–556.

26. Potgieter F.T. (1979). Epizootiology and control of anaplasmosis in South Africa. *J. S. Afr. Vet. Assoc.*, **50**, 367–372.

27. Reyna-Bello A., Cloeckaert A., Vizcaino N., Gonzatti M.I., Aso P.M., Dubray G. & Zygmunt M.S. (1998). Evaluation of an enzyme-linked immunosorbent assay using recombinant major surface protein 5 for serological diagnosis of bovine anaplasmosis in Venezuela. *Clin. Diagn. Lab. Immunol.*, **5**, 259–262.

28. Ristic M. (1968). Chapter 23: Anaplasmosis. *In:* Infectious Blood Diseases of Man and Animals, Vol. 11, Weinman D. & Ristic M., eds. Academic Press, New York, USA, 473–542.

29. Ristic M. & Kreier J.P. (1984). Family III. Anaplasmataceae Philip 1957. *In:* Bergey's Manual of Systematic Bacteriology, Vol. 1, Krieg N.R. & Holt J.G., eds. Williams & Wilkins, Baltimore, MD, USA, 719–729.

30. Ristic M., Sibinovic S. & Welter C.J. (1968). An attenuated *Anaplasma marginale* vaccine. *Proc. 72nd Meeting of the USA Livestock Sanitary Assoc.*, 56–69.

31. Torioni De Echaide S., Knowles D.P., McGuire T.C., Palmer G.H., Suarez C.E. & McElwain T.F. (1998). Detection of cattle naturally infected with *Anaplasma marginale* in a region of endemicity by nested PCR and a competitive enzyme-linked immunosorbent assay using recombinant major surface protein 5. *J. Clin. Microbiol.*, **36**, 777–782.

32. United States Department of Agriculture (USDA) (1958). A Manual for Conducting the Complement Fixation Test for Anaplasmosis. Agricultural Research Service, USDA, Beltsville, MD 20705, USA.

33. United States Department of Agriculture (USDA) (1974). A Microtiter Technique for the Complement Fixation Test for Anaplasmosis. Veterinary Services, Animal and Plant Health Inspection Service, US Department of Agriculture, Beltsville, MD 20705, USA.

34. Visser E.S., McGuire T.C., Palmer G.H., Davis W.C., Shkap V., Pipano E. & Knowles D.P. (1992). The *Anaplasma marginale* msp 5 gene encodes a 19-kilodalton protein conserved in all recognized *Anaplasma* species. *Infect. Immun.*, **60**, 5139–5144.

35. Walker D.H., & Dumler J.S. (1996) Emergence of the ehrlichioses as human health problems. *Emerg. Infect. Dis.*, **2**, 18–29.

*

* *

CHAPTER 2.3.8.

BOVINE BABESIOSIS

SUMMARY

Babesiosis is a tick-borne disease of cattle caused by the protozoan parasites Babesia bovis, B. bigemina, B. divergens *and others.* Boophilus *spp., the principal vectors of* B. bovis *and* B. bigemina, *are widespread in tropical and subtropical countries. The major vector of* B. divergens *is* Ixodes ricinus. *Other important vectors include* Haemaphysalis *and* Rhipicephalus *spp.*

Identification of the agent: *Smears of blood, brain, kidney, liver, and lung are suitable for demonstration of parasites in dead animals, provided decomposition is not advanced. The smears are fixed with methanol, stained with 10% Giemsa for 20–30 minutes, and examined at × 800–1000 magnification under oil immersion. In the case of live animals, thick and thin films of capillary blood should be taken from, for example, the tip of the tail.*

Serological tests: *The indirect fluorescent antibody (IFA) test is a widely used test for the detection of antibodies to* B. bovis *and* B. divergens, *but enzyme-linked immunosorbent assays are gaining popularity. The IFA test has been used for detection of antibodies to* B. bigemina, *but serological cross-reactions make species diagnosis difficult.*

Requirements for vaccines and diagnostic biologicals: *Vaccines consisting of live, attenuated strains of* B. bovis, B. bigemina *or* B. divergens *are produced in several countries from the blood of infected calves. The vaccines are provided in frozen or chilled forms. Production of frozen vaccine is usually recommended as it allows thorough post-production control of each batch. The risk of contamination of this blood-derived vaccine makes thorough quality control essential, but may be prohibitively expensive.*

Live Babesia *vaccines are not entirely safe. A practical recommendation is to limit their use to calves, when nonspecific immunity will minimise the risk of vaccine reactions. When older animals are to be vaccinated, the risk of reaction warrants close surveillance and treatment with a babesiacide if reactions occur.*

Protective immunity develops in 3–4 weeks and lasts for several years after a single vaccination.

A. DIAGNOSTIC TECHNIQUES

Bovine babesiosis is caused by protozoan parasites of the genus *Babesia,* order Piroplasmida, phylum Apicomplexa. Of the species affecting cattle, two – *Babesia bovis and B. bigemina* – are widely distributed and of major importance in Africa, Asia, Australia, and Central and South America. *Babesia divergens* is economically important in some parts of Europe.

The vector of *Babesia* is the tick (17). *Boophilus* spp. are the principal vectors of *B. bigemina* and *B. bovis* and is widespread in the tropics and subtropics. The vector of *B. divergens* is *Ixodes ricinus.* Other important vectors include *Haemaphysalis, Rhipicephalus* and other *Boophilus* spp. *Babesia bigemina* has the widest distribution.

Generally, *B. bovis* is more pathogenic than *B. bigemina* and *B. divergens.* Infections are characterised by high fever, ataxia, anorexia, general circulatory shock, and sometimes also nervous signs as a result of sequestration of infected erythrocytes in cerebral capillaries. In acute cases, the maximum parasitaemia (percentage of infected erythrocytes) in circulating blood is less than 1%. This is in contrast to *B. bigemina* infections, where the parasitaemia often exceeds 10% and may be as high as 30%. In *B. bigemina* infections, the major signs include fever, haemoglobinuria and anaemia. Intravascular sequestration of infected erythrocytes does not occur with *B. bigemina* infections. The parasitaemia and clinical appearance of *B. divergens* infections are somewhat similar to *B. bigemina* infections (19).

Infected animals develop a life-long immunity against subsequent reinfection with the same species. There is also evidence of a degree of cross-protection in *B.-bigemina*-immune animals against subsequent *B. bovis* infections. Calves rarely show clinical signs of disease after infection regardless of the *Babesia* spp. involved or the immune status of the dams (7, 9, 10,).

1. Identification of the agent

The traditional method of identifying the agent in infected animals is by microscopic examination of thick and thin blood films stained with, for example, Giemsa. The sensitivity of this technique is such that it can detect parasitaemias as low as 1 parasite in 10^7 red blood cells (RBCs) (10^{-7}) (5). Species differentiation is good in thin films but poor in the more sensitive thick films. This technique is usually adequate for detection of acute infections, but is not suitable for detection of carriers where the parasitaemias are usually well below levels detectable by this method. Parasite identification and differentiation can be improved by using a fluorescent dye, such as acridine orange instead of Giemsa (18). A quantitative buffy coat method using acridine orange to stain parasites in capillary tubes was developed to demonstrate *Plasmodium* in human blood and could potentially also detect low *Babesia* parasitaemias, but differentiation is likely to be poor (5).

Samples from live animals should preferably be taken from capillaries, such as those in the tip of the ear or tip of the tail, as *B. bovis* is more common in capillary blood. *Babesia bigemina* and *B. divergens* parasites are uniformly distributed through the vasculature. If it is not possible to make fresh smears from capillary blood, sterile jugular blood should be collected into an anticoagulant such as ethylene diamine tetra-acetic acid (EDTA) (e.g. 1 mg/ml). Heparin may affect the colour characteristics of the staining and is not recommended. The sample should be kept cool, preferably at 5°C, until delivery to the laboratory, again preferably within hours of collection. Thin blood films are air-dried, fixed in absolute methanol for 1 minute, and stained in 10% Giemsa stain for 20–30 minutes. It is preferable to stain blood films as soon as possible after preparation to ensure proper stain definition. Thick films are made by placing a small drop (approximately 50 µl) of blood on to a clean glass slide. This droplet is then air-dried, heat-fixed at 80°C for 5 minutes, and stained in 5% Giemsa for 20–30 minutes. Unstained blood smears should not be stored with formalin solutions as it may affect staining quality.

Samples from dead animals should consist of thin blood films, as well as smears from (in order of preference), cerebral cortex, kidney, liver, lung, and bone marrow. Organ smears are made by pressing a clean slide on to a freshly cut surface of the organ or by crushing a small sample of the tissue between two clean microscope slides drawn lengthwise to leave a film of tissue on each slide. The smear is then air-dried (assisted by gentle warming in humid climates), fixed for 5 minutes in absolute methanol, and stained for 20–30 minutes in 10% Giemsa. This method is especially suitable for the diagnosis of *B. bovis* infections, but is unreliable if death has occurred over 24 hours previously. However, parasites can often be detected in blood taken from veins in the lower limb region one or more days after death (1).

All stained smears are examined under oil immersion using (as a minimum) a ×8 eyepiece and a ×60 objective lens. *Babesia bovis* is a small parasite, usually centrally located in the erythrocyte. It measures approximately 1–1.5 µm long and 0.5–1.0 µm wide, and is often found as pairs that are at an obtuse angle to each other. *Babesia divergens* is also a small parasite and is very similar morphologically to *B. bovis*. However, obtuse-angled pairs are often located at the rim of the erythrocyte. *Babesia bigemina* is a much longer parasite, and is often found as pairs at an acute angle to each other. *Babesia bigemina* is typically pear-shaped, but many diverse single forms are found. It is 3–3.5 µm long and 1–1.5 µm wide, and paired forms often have two discrete red-staining dots in each parasite (*B. bovis* and *B. divergens* always have only one). In acute cases, the parasitaemia of *B. bovis* seldom reaches 1%, but with *B. bigemina* and *B. divergens* much higher parasitaemias are the norm. Thick blood films are especially useful for the diagnosis of low level *B. bovis* infections, as are organ smears (1).

Probes have been used to detect DNA of some *Babesia* spp., but generally are not more sensitive than direct microscopy and application in routine diagnostics is limited (18). Polymerase chain reaction (PCR) assays have proven to be very sensitive, particularly in detecting *B. bovis* and *B. bigemina* in carrier cattle (6, 10, 16). A full-scale comparison of available PCR tests with sensitive enzyme-linked immunosorbent assays (ELISAs) is needed to determine the usefulness of PCR assays in diagnostics. However, PCR assays generally do not lend themselves well to large-scale testing and are unlikely to supplant serological tests as the method of choice for epidemiological studies. PCR assays may be useful as confirmatory tests and in some cases for regulatory testing.

In-vitro culture methods have been used to demonstrate the presence of carrier infections of *Babesia* spp. (21), and *B. bovis* has also been cloned in culture. The minimum parasitaemia detectable by this method will depend, to a large extent, on the facilities available and the skills of the operator (5), but could be as low 10^{-10} (18), making it a very sensitive method for the demonstration of infection. An added benefit is that it is 100% specific.

Confirmation of infection in a suspected carrier animal can also be made by transfusing approximately 500 ml of jugular blood intravenously into a splenectomised calf known to be *Babesia*-free, and monitoring the calf for the presence of infection. This method is cumbersome and expensive, and obviously not suitable for routine diagnostic use. Mongolian gerbils *(Meriones unguiculatus)* can, however, be used to demonstrate the presence of *B. divergens*.

2. Serological tests

The indirect fluorescent antibody (IFA) test is widely used to detect antibodies to *Babesia* spp., but the *B. bigemina* test has poor specificity. Cross-reactions with antibodies to *B. bovis* in the *B. bigemina* IFA test are a particular problem in areas where the two parasites coexist. The IFA test has the disadvantages of low sample throughput and subjectivity. An internationally validated ELISA for the diagnosis of *B. bovis* infection has been developed (12, 27, 34) but, despite the efforts of several investigators in different laboratories, there is still no similarly validated ELISA for *B. bigemina*. ELISAs for antibodies to *B bigemina* typically have poor specificity. In one study (15), *B. bigemina* antiserum appeared to react nonspecifically with fibrinogen. However, an ELISA recently developed and validated in Australia (28) shows considerable promise. In the absence of any other workable test for *B. bigemina*, the procedure for that assay has been included here. ELISAs have also been developed for *B. divergens* (8) using antigen derived from culture, *Meriones* or cattle, but there does not appear to be one that has been validated internationally.

a) *Babesia bovis* enzyme-linked immunosorbent assay

Antigen preparation is based on a technique described by Waltisbuhl *et al.* (34). Infected blood (usually 5–10% parasitaemia) is collected from splenectomised calves into EDTA. The blood is washed three times in five volumes of phosphate buffered saline (PBS), and then infected cells are concentrated by differential lysis of uninfected cells in hypotonic saline solution. Infected cells are more resistant to lysis in hypotonic saline solutions than are uninfected cells. A series of hypotonic saline solutions are prepared, ranging from 0.35% to 0.50% NaCl, in 0.025% increments. To find the best concentration, five volumes of each saline solution is then added to one volume of packed RBCs, which are gently mixed and allowed to stand for 5 minutes.

The mixtures are then centrifuged and the supernatants are aspirated. An equal volume of plasma (retained from the original blood) is added to each tube containing packed RBCs, and the contents of the tubes are mixed. Thin blood films are prepared from each of these resuspended blood cell mixtures, fixed in methanol, and stained with Giemsa. These films are examined by microscope to determine which saline solution lyses most uninfected RBCs but leaves infected RBCs intact. It should be possible to achieve >95% infection in the remaining intact RBCs. The bulk of the packed RBCs is then differentially lysed with the optimal saline solution and centrifuged. The sediment (>95% infected RBCs) is lysed in distilled water at 4°C, and parasites are pelleted at 12,000 ***g*** for 30 minutes. The pellet is washed three times in PBS by resuspension and centrifugation at 4°C. It is then resuspended in one to two volumes of PBS at 4°C, and sonicated in appropriate volumes using medium power for 60–90 seconds. The sonicated material is ultracentrifuged, (105,000 ***g*** for 60 minutes at 4°C) and the supernatant is retained. The supernatant is mixed with an equal volume of glycerol and stored in 2–5 ml aliquots at –70°C. Short-term storage at –20°C is acceptable for the working aliquot.

- **Test procedure**

i) First, 100 µl of this antigen, diluted from 1/400 to 1/1600 in 0.1 M carbonate buffer, pH 9.6, is added to each well of a polystyrene 96-well microtitre plate, and incubated overnight, covered, at 4°C.

ii) Antigen is removed and the wells are then blocked for 2 hours at room temperature by the addition of 200 µl of a 2% solution of sodium caseinate in carbonate buffer.

iii) After blocking, the wells are rinsed briefly with PBS containing 0.1% Tween 20 (PBST) and 100 µl of bovine serum diluted 1/100 in PBST containing either 5% normal horse serum or 5% skim milk powder is added, and the plates are incubated for 2 hours at room temperature.

iv) The washing step consists of a brief rinse with PBST, followed by three 5-minute washes with the same buffer (during which the plate is shaken vigorously), and finally the plates are given a further brief rinse.

v) Next, 100 µl of peroxidase-labelled anti-bovine IgG diluted appropriately in PBST containing horse serum or skim milk (NB: some batches of skim milk powder may contain immunoglobulins that can interfere with anti-bovine IgG conjugates), is added and the plates are shaken for a further 30 minutes at room temperature.

vi) Wells are washed as described in step iv above, and 100 µl of peroxidase substrate (ABTS [2,2'-Azino-bis-(3-ethylbenzothiazoline-6-sulphonic acid)]) is added to each well. The substrate reaction is allowed to continue until the absorbance of a strong positive control serum included on each plate approaches 1. At this point the absorbance at 414 nm is read on a microtitre plate reader.

To control for inter-plate variation, known positive and negative serum controls are included in each plate (34). Test sera are then ranked relative to the positive control. ELISA results are expressed as a percentage of this positive control (percentage positivity). Positive and negative threshold values should be determined in each laboratory by testing as many known positive and negative sera as possible.

Each batch of antigen and conjugate should be titrated using a checkerboard layout. The most suitable enzyme label for the conjugate is horseradish peroxidase. ABTS or tetramethyl benzidine (TMB) are suitable substrates. With this test, it is possible to detect antibodies at least 4 years after a single infection. There should be 95–100% positive reactions with *B.-bovis*-immune animals, 1–2% false-positive reactions with negative sera, and <2% false-positive reactions with *B.-bigemina*-immune animals.

b) *Babesia bigemina* enzyme-linked immunosorbent assay

This ELISA is based on an immunodominant 58 kDa antigen identified by a number of groups in *B. bigemina* isolates from Australia, Central America and Texas, United States of America (USA), Egypt and Kenya (28). Two monoclonal antibodies (MAbs) (B9 and D6) directed against independent epitopes on this antigen have been used to develop the ELISA. MAb B9 is bound to microtitre plates to capture the 58 kDa antigen from a crude merozoite antigen preparation. The ability of bovine test sera to inhibit binding of peroxidase-labelled MAb D6 (HRP-D6) to the antigen is then measured in a competitive inhibition ELISA.

- **Antigen preparation**

First, 2–3 litres of blood are collected into heparin from a splenectomised calf infected with *B. bigemina* at peak parasitaemia (between 5 and 15% of erythrocytes infected). The calf must be sedated during this procedure and killed before recovery. The blood is centrifuged at 2000 ***g*** for 30 minutes and serum and buffy coat cells are removed by aspiration. The RBC pellet is then washed twice by resuspending in three volumes of PBS. The RBCs are then warmed to 37°C and lysed by addition of an equal volume of TEN buffer (20 mM Tris, 10 mM EDTA, 100 mM NaCl, pH 8.0) containing 1 mg/ml saponin, also prewarmed to 37°C. After 10 seconds of gentle mixing, four volumes of TEN are added to dilute the saponin. Intact RBCs are removed by centrifugation at 2000 ***g*** for 20 minutes. Parasites and RBC-membrane ghosts are then pelleted from the supernatant by centrifugation at 16,300 ***g*** for 30 minutes. This pellet is washed twice in PBS then resuspended in PBS to a final volume of 50–100 ml and stored at –20°C. To solubilise parasite antigens this material is extracted for 60 minutes at room temperature with an equal volume of 0.2% sodium laurylsarcosine (or 0.2% Nonidet P40). The soluble antigen is clarified by centrifugation at 100,000 ***g*** for 60 minutes, and then stored at –20°C until required. Typically this antigen can be diluted between 1/5 and 1/25 for use in the ELISA.

- **Test procedure**

i) MAb B9[1] is diluted in carbonate buffer, pH 9.6, to a concentration of 1.3 µg/ml and 100 µl is added to each well of a 96-well microtitre plate. The plates are incubated overnight at 4°C.

ii) Excess MAb is removed and wells are then blocked for 1 hour at room temperature by addition of 200 µl per well of 2% casein in carbonate buffer.

iii) Following a brief rinse (3 × 200 µl) with PBS containing 0.1% Tween 20 (PBST20), crude *B. bigemina* merozoite antigen diluted 1/5 to 1/25 (depending on the antigen batch) in PBST20 containing 2% bovine serum albumin (BSA), is added (100 µl per well) and the plates are incubated for a further 1 hour at room temperature with gentle shaking.

iv) The plates are then washed with PBST20 (3 × 200 µl rinse, 5-minute soak with shaking, 3 × 200 µl rinse), and 50 µl of undiluted bovine test serum followed by 50 µl of peroxidase-labelled MAb D6[1], diluted to a concentration of 0.03 µg/ml in PBST20 containing 2% BSA, are added to each well. The plates are then incubated at room temperature for 30 minutes with continuous gentle shaking.

v) Plates are washed again, 100 µl TMB peroxidase substrate is added to each well, and the plates are incubated in the dark until the absorbance of the negative control wells approaches 1. At this point the reaction is stopped by the addition of 50 µl of 1 M sulphuric acid and the absorbance is read at 450 nm. Positive and negative control sera should be included on each test plate.

The percent inhibition (PI) for test sera is calculated relative to the negative control serum (PI = 100 – [100 × test absorbance/negative control absorbance]). Positive and negative threshold values should be determined in each laboratory by testing as many known positive and negative sera as possible.

The specificity of the ELISA has been estimated at 97.0% and the sensitivity for detection of antibodies in experimentally infected cattle is 95.7% (28). Evaluation of this assay in the field is currently under way, but the sensitivity and specificity of this ELISA should be more than adequate for epidemiological studies.

c) Indirect fluorescent antibody test

- **Antigen preparation**

Antigen slides are made from jugular blood, ideally when the parasitaemia is between 2% and 5%.

---

1 Tick Fever Research Centre, 280 Grindle Road, Wacol, Queensland 4076, Australia.

Blood is collected into a suitable anticoagulant (sodium citrate or EDTA), and is then washed at least three times in from five to ten volumes of PBS to remove contaminating plasma proteins and, in particular, host immunoglobulins. After washing, the infected RBCs are resuspended in two volumes of PBS to which 1% BSA has been added. The BSA is used to adhere RBCs to the glass slide. By preference, single layered blood films are made by placing a drop of blood on to a clean glass slide, which is then spun in a cytocentrifuge. This produces very uniform smears. Alternatively, thin blood films may be made by the conventional technique. The films are air-dried and fixed for 5 minutes in an oven at 80°C. Fixed blood films are then wrapped (e.g. in aluminium foil) so as to be airtight, and stored at –70°C until required (for a maximum of 5 years).

- **Test procedure**

Test and control sera are diluted 1/30 in PBS. Sera may be used with or without heat inactivation at 56°C for 30 minutes. The slides are marked into 8–10 divisions with an oil pen to produce hydrophobic divisions. To each test square 5–10 µl of each serum dilution is added using a fine pipette. The preparations are then incubated at room temperature for 1 hour, in a humid chamber. For controls, dilutions of weak positive and negative sera are used on each test slide.

After incubation, the slides are gently rinsed twice with PBS and given two 10-minute washes with PBS. An appropriate dilution of anti-bovine IgG antibody labelled with fluorescein isothiocyanate (which is available commercially) is then added to each test square. Every new batch of conjugate must be titrated, the working range usually being between 1/400 and 1/1200. Conjugated rabbit and chicken antibodies are usually more suitable for this purpose than goat antibodies. The slides with the conjugate are incubated again at room temperature for 1 hour, and given three 5-minute washes in PBS. The wet slides are mounted with cover-slips in 10% glycerol in PBS, and examined by standard fluorescence microscopy. A competent operator can examine approximately 150 samples per day.

d) Other tests

Other serological tests have been described in recent years, and include a dot ELISA (29), a slide ELISA (24), latex and card agglutination tests (3, 25). These tests show acceptable levels of sensitivity and specificity for *B. bovis* and, in the case of the dot ELISA, also for *B. bigemina*. However, none of these tests appears to have been adopted for routine diagnostic use in laboratories other than those in which the original development and validation took place. Adaptability of these tests to routine diagnostic laboratories is therefore unknown.

B. REQUIREMENTS FOR VACCINES AND DIAGNOSTIC BIOLOGICALS

Cattle develop a durable, long-lasting immunity after a single infection with *B. bovis, B. divergens* or *B. bigemina.* This feature has been exploited in some countries to immunise cattle against babesiosis (1, 7, 13). Most of these live vaccines contain specially selected strains of *Babesia*, mainly *B. bovis* and *B. bigemina*, and are produced in government-supported production facilities as services to the livestock industries, in particular in Australia, Argentina, South Africa, Israel and Uruguay. An experimental *B. divergens* vaccine prepared from the blood of infected *Meriones* has also been used successfully in recent years in Ireland (20).

A killed *B. divergens* vaccine is prepared in Austria from the blood of infected calves (14), but little information is available on the level and duration of the conferred immunity. Experimental vaccines containing antigens produced *in vitro* have also been developed (2, 30), but the level and duration of protection against heterologous challenge are unclear. Parasite proteins have been characterised and there has been some progress towards the development of subunit vaccines (10, 31). No effective subunit vaccine is available commercially.

This section will deal with the production of live babesiosis vaccines, mainly those against *B. bovis* and *B. bigemina* infections in cattle. Production involves infection of calves with selected strains, and use of the blood as vaccine. Calves used for infection with these strains must be free of infectious agents that can be transmitted by products derived from their blood. Detailed accounts of the production procedures have been published (1, 7). Reference should be made to these publications for details of the procedures outlined here. In the case of *Babesia divergens,* blood of infected gerbils *(Meriones unguiculatus)* can be used instead of bovine blood. *In-vitro* culture methods have also been used to produce parasites for vaccine (23, 26). However, the relatively high cost of production from culture and evidence of possible antigenic drift during long-term maintenance in culture, make mass culture of *Babesia* impractical in most laboratories at present.

Babesia bovis and *B. bigemina* vaccines can be prepared in either frozen or chilled form depending on demand, transport networks and the availability of liquid nitrogen or dry ice supplies. Preparation of frozen vaccine is preferred (11, 13, 26, 32), as it allows for thorough post-production control of each batch. However, it is more costly to produce and more difficult to transport than chilled vaccine. The potential risk of contamination of this blood-derived vaccine makes post-production control essential, but may put production beyond the means of some countries in endemic regions (13). A production facility supplying an annual market of fewer than 50,000 doses is unlikely to operate without financial support.

1. Seed management

a) Characteristics of the seed

- **Internationally available strains**

Attenuated Australian strains of *B. bovis* and *B. bigemina* have been used effectively to immunise cattle in Africa, South America and South-East Asia (11, 13). Tick-transmissible and nontransmissible strains are available. A strain of *B. divergens* with reduced virulence for *Meriones* has also been developed (35).

- **Isolation and purification of local strains**

Strains of *B. bovis, B. divergens* and *B. bigemina* that are free from contaminants such as *Anaplasma, Eperythrozoon, Theileria, Trypanosoma* and various viral and bacterial agents, are most readily isolated by feeding infected ticks on susceptible splenectomised cattle (1). The vectors and modes of transmission of the species differ, and these features can be used to separate the species (17).

Babesia spp. can also be isolated from infected cattle by subinoculation of blood into susceptible splenectomised calves. A major disadvantage of this method is the difficulty of separating the *Babesia* spp. from contaminants such as *Anaplasma* and *Eperythrozoon*. Isolation of *B. divergens* is a relatively simple process because of the susceptibility of *Meriones* (20). Maintenance of isolated strains *in vitro* (22) can be used to eliminate most contaminants, but not to separate *Babesia* spp. Selective chemotherapy can be used to obtain pure *B. bovis* from a mixed *Babesia* infection, while rapid passaging in susceptible calves will allow isolation of *B. bigemina* (1).

- **Attenuation of strains**

Various ways of attenuating *Babesia* spp. have been reported. The most reliable way of reducing the virulence of *B. bovis* involves rapid passage of the strain through susceptible splenectomised calves. Attenuation is not guaranteed, but usually follows after from 8 to 20 calf passages (7).

The virulence of *B. bigemina* decreases during prolonged residence of the parasite in latently infected animals. This feature has been used to obtain avirulent strains by infecting calves, splenectomising them after 3 months and then using the ensuing relapse parasites to repeat the procedure (1).

Attenuation of *B. divergens* for *Meriones* followed long-term maintenance *in vitro* (35).

Attenuation of *Babesia* spp. with irradiation has been attempted, but the results were variable. Similarly, maintenance *in vitro* in modified media has been used experimentally.

Avirulent strains should be stored as stabilate for safety testing and for future use in the production of vaccine.

b) Preparation and storage of stabilate

Avirulent strains are readily stored as frozen stabilate of infected blood in liquid nitrogen or dry ice. Dimethyl sulphoxide (DMSO) (1) and polyvinylpyrrolidine MW 40,000 (33) are the recommended cryopreservatives, as they allow for intravenous administration after thawing of the stabilate. A detailed account of the freezing technique using DMSO is reported elsewhere (1). Briefly, it involves the following:

Infected blood is collected and chilled to 4°C. Cold cryoprotectant (4 M DMSO in PBS) is then added, while stirring slowly, to a final blood:protectant ratio of 1:1 with the final concentration of DMSO being 2 M. This dilution procedure is carried out in an ice bath, and the diluted blood is dispensed into suitable containers (e.g. 5 ml cryovials), and frozen, as soon as possible, in the vapour phase of a liquid nitrogen container. The vials are stored in the liquid phase in a designated tank to prevent possible contamination.

c) Validation as a vaccine

The suitability of a strain for use in a vaccine can be determined by inoculating susceptible cattle with vaccine prepared from it and then challenging them and susceptible controls with a virulent, heterologous strain. Both safety and efficacy can be judged by monitoring fever, parasitaemias in stained blood films, and depression of packed cell volumes. The purity of the isolate should be tested by performing serology for all potential contaminants that may be present on paired sera collected from the cattle used in the safety test.

2. Method of manufacture

a) Production of frozen vaccine concentrate

First, 5–10 ml quantities of frozen stabilate are rapidly thawed by immersing the vials in water preheated to 40°C. The thawed material is kept on ice and used as soon as possible (within 30 minutes) to infect a susceptible, splenectomised calf (free of potential vaccine contaminants) by intravenous inoculation.

Blood suitable for vaccine is obtained by monitoring films of jugular blood and collecting the required volume of blood when a suitable parasitaemia is reached. A parasitaemia of 1×10^8/ml (approximately 2% parasitaemia in jugular blood) is usually adequate for production of vaccine. If a suitable *B. bovis* parasitaemia is not obtained, passage of the strain by subinoculation of 100–500 ml of blood into a second splenectomised calf may be necessary. Passage of *B. bigemina* is not recommended.

Blood from the infected donor calf is collected by jugular or carotid cannulation using preservative-free heparin as anticoagulant (5 International Units [IU] heparin/ml blood).

In the laboratory, the parasitised blood is mixed in equal volumes with 3 M glycerol in PBS supplemented with 5 mM glucose (final concentration of glycerol 1.5 M) at 37°C. The mixture is then equilibrated at 37°C for 30 minutes, and dispensed into suitable containers (e.g. 5 ml cryovials). The vials are cooled at approximately 10°C/minute in the vapour phase of liquid nitrogen and, when frozen, stored in the liquid phase (11, 13).

DMSO can be used as cryoprotectant in the place of glycerol. This is carried out in the same way as outlined for the preparation of stabilate (32).

If glycerolised frozen vaccine is to be diluted, the diluent should be iso-osmotic and consist of PBS containing 1.5 M glycerol and 5 mM glucose. Similarly, the diluent used in vaccine cryopreserved with DMSO should be iso-osmotic, and should contain the same concentration of DMSO in PBS.

Frozen vaccine containing both *B. bovis* and *B. bigemina* can be prepared (26) by mixing equal numbers of the parasites obtained from different donors.

The dose of vaccine after reconstitution and dilution ranges from 1 to 2 ml depending on local practices and requirements.

b) Production of chilled vaccine

Infective material used in the production of chilled vaccine is obtained in the same way as for frozen vaccine but should be issued and used as soon as possible after collection. If it is necessary to obtain the maximum number of doses per calf, the infective material can be diluted to provide the required number of parasites per dose (usually from 2.5 to 10×10^7). A suitable diluent is 10% sterile bovine serum in a balanced salt solution containing the following ingredients per litre: NaCl (7.00 g), $MgCl_2.6H_20$ (0.34 g), glucose (1.00 g), Na_2HPO_4 (2.52 g), KH_2P0_4 (0.90 g), and $NaHCO_3$ (0.52 g).

Blood containing *B. divergens* may be diluted in Hanks' solution. If diluent is not required, sterile acid citrate dextrose or citrate phosphate dextrose should be used as the anticoagulant, at a rate of one part to four parts blood, to provide the glucose necessary for survival of the organisms.

3. In-process control

a) Sources and maintenance of vaccine donors

A source of donors free from natural infections with *Babesia*, other tick-borne diseases, and other infectious agents that can be transmitted with blood-derived products, should be identified. If a suitable source is not available, it may be necessary to breed donor calves under tick-free conditions specifically for the purpose of vaccine production.

Donor calves should be maintained under conditions that will prevent exposure to infectious diseases and to ticks and biting insects. In the absence of suitable facilities, the risk of contamination with the agents of infectious diseases present in the country involved should be estimated, and the benefits of local production of vaccine (as opposed to importation of a suitable product) should be weighed against the possible adverse consequences of spreading disease (1).

b) Surgery

Donor calves should be splenectomised to allow maximum yield of parasites for production of vaccine. This is best done under, general anaesthesia in young calves. Details of the technique, including pre- and post-operative procedures, are reported elsewhere (1).

c) Screening of vaccine donors before inoculation

Donor calves should be examined for agents of all blood-borne infections prevalent in the country, including *Babesia, Anaplasma, Theileria*, and *Trypanosoma*. This can be done by routine examination of stained blood films after splenectomy, and preferably also by serology. Calves showing evidence of natural infections of any of these agents should be rejected. The absence of other infective agents endemic in the country should also be confirmed. These may include the agents of enzootic bovine leukosis, mucosal disease, infectious bovine rhinotracheitis, Akabane disease, ephemeral fever, bluetongue, foot and mouth disease, and rinderpest. The test procedures will depend on the diseases prevalent in the country and the availability of tests, but should involve serology of paired sera and, in some cases, virus isolation (11, 32).

d) Monitoring of parasitaemias following inoculation

It is necessary to determine the concentration of parasites in blood collected for vaccine. There are accurate techniques for determining the parasite count (1), but the parasite concentration can be estimated from the RBC count and the parasitaemia (% infected RBCs).

e) Collection of blood for vaccine

All equipment should be sterilised before use (e.g. by autoclaving). The blood is collected in heparin using strict aseptic techniques when the required parasitaemia is reached. This is best done if the calf is sedated with, for example, xylacine and with the use of a closed-circuit collection system.

Up to 3 litres of heavily infected blood can be collected from a 6-month-old calf. If the calf is to live, the transfusion of a similar amount of blood from a suitable donor is indicated. Alternatively, the calf should be killed immediately after collection of the blood.

f) Dispensing of vaccine

All procedures are performed in a suitable environment, such as a laminar flow cabinet, using standard sterile techniques. Use of a mechanical or magnetic stirrer will ensure thorough mixing of blood and diluent throughout the dispensing process.

4. Batch control

The potency, safety and sterility of vaccine batches cannot be determined in the case of chilled vaccine, and specifications of frozen vaccine depend on the code of practice of the country involved. The following are the specifications for frozen vaccine produced in Australia.

a) Sterility and freedom from contaminants

Standard tests for sterility are employed for each batch of vaccine and diluent. The absence of contaminants is determined by doing appropriate serological testing of donor cattle and by inoculating donor lymphocytes into sheep and then monitoring them for evidence of viral infection. Potential contaminants include the agents of enzootic bovine leukosis, infectious bovine rhinotracheitis, mucosal disease, ephemeral fever, Akabane disease, Aino virus, bluetongue, and *Brucella abortus* and *Leptospira*, foot and mouth disease, lumpy skin disease, rabies, Rift Valley fever, rinderpest, contagious bovine pleuropneumonia, heartwater, Jembrana disease, and pathogenic *Theileria* and *Trypanosoma* spp. (11, 13).

b) Safety

Vaccine reactions of the cattle inoculated in the test for potency (see Section B.4.c.) are monitored by measuring parasitaemia, fever and depression of packed cell volume. Only batches with pathogenicity levels equal to or lower than a predetermined standard are released for use.

c) Potency

Glycerolised vaccine concentrate is thawed and diluted 1/5 with isotonic diluent (11, 13). The prepared vaccine is then incubated for 8 hours at 30°C, and five cattle are inoculated subcutaneously with 2 ml doses each. The inoculated cattle are then monitored for the presence of infections by examination of stained blood smears. Only fully infective batches are released for use at a working dilution of 1/5.

d) Duration of immunity

Long-lasting immunity usually results from one inoculation. Evidence of *B. bovis* vaccine failures have been reported (4) and are related to the choice of vaccine strains, the presence of heterologous field strains, and host factors. There is little evidence of time-related waning of immunity (7).

e) Stability

When stored in liquid nitrogen, the vaccine can be kept for 5 years. Sterile diluent can be kept for 2 years in a refrigerator. Thawed vaccine rapidly loses potency and cannot be refrozen.

f) Preservatives

Penicillin (500,000 IU/litre) and streptomycin (370,000 µg/litre) are added to the vaccine at the time of dispensing.

g) Use of vaccine

In the case of frozen vaccine, vials should be thawed by immersion in water preheated to 40°C. Glycerolised vaccine should be kept cool and used within 8 hours (8, 9), while vaccine with DMSO as cryoprotectant should be kept on ice and used within 15–30 minutes of thawing (32).

Chilled vaccine should be kept refrigerated and used within 4–7 days of preparation, depending on the viability of the parasites.

The strains of *B. bovis, B. divergens* and *B. bigemina* used in the vaccine may be of reduced virulence, but will not be entirely safe. A practical recommendation is, therefore, to limit the use of vaccine to calves, when nonspecific immunity will minimise the risk of vaccine reactions. If older animals are to be vaccinated, there is a risk of severe reactions. These reactions occur infrequently, but valuable breeding stock or pregnant animals obviously warrant due attention and should be observed daily for 3 weeks after vaccination. Ideally, rectal temperatures of vaccinated cattle should be taken and the animals should be treated if significant fever develops. Reactions to *B. bigemina* and *B. divergens* are usually seen by day 6–8 and those to *B. bovis* by day 10–16 (7).

Protective immunity develops in 3–4 weeks, and lasts at least 4 years in most cases.

Babesiosis and anaplasmosis vaccines are often used concurrently, but it is not advisable to use any other vaccines at the same time (7).

h) Precautions

Babesia bovis and *B. bigemina* vaccines are not infective for humans. However, cases of *B. divergens* have been reported in splenectomised individuals. When the vaccine is stored in liquid nitrogen, the usual precautions pertaining to the storage, transportation and handling of deep-frozen material applies.

5 Tests on the final product

a) Safety

See Section B.4.b.

b) Potency

See Section B.4.c.

REFERENCES

1. ANON (1984). Ticks and Tick-borne Disease Control. A Practical Field Manual, Vol. 11. Tick-borne Disease Control. Food and Agriculture Organisation of the United Nations (FAO), Rome, Italy.

2. BENITEZ M.T., MONTENEGRO-JAMES S., RAMOS P., APONTE J., OBREGON J.M. & ARENAS E.L. (1996). Produccion semi-industrial de vacuna anti-babesiosis origen cultivo *in vitro*. *Vet. Tropical*, 21, 59–74.

3. Blandino T., Alvarez M., Larramendi R., Gomez E. & Alonson M. (1991). Elaboracion y evaluacion de un antigeno de *Babesia bovis* para la prueba de aglutination en latex. *Rev. Salud Animal.,* **13**, 177–179.

4. Bock R.E., De Vos A.J., Lew A., Kingston T.G. & Fraser I.R. (1995). Studies on failure of T strain live *Babesia bovis* vaccine. *Aust. Vet. J.,* **72**, 296–300.

5. Bose R., Jorgensen W.K., Dalgliesh R.J., Friendhoff K.T. & De Vos A.J. (1995). Current state and future trends in the diagnosis of babesiosis. *Vet. Parasitol.,* **57**, 61–74.

6. Calder J.A.M., Reddy G.R., Chieves L., Courtney C.H., Littell R., Livengood J.R., Norval R.A.I., Smith C. & Dame J.B. (1996). Monitoring *Babesia bovis* infections in cattle by using PCR-based tests. *J. Clin. Microbiol.,* **34**, 2748–2755.

7. Callow L.L. (1984). Animal Health in Australia, Vol. 5. Protozoal and Rickettsial Diseases. Australian Bureau of Animal Health, Australian Government Publishing Service, Canberra, Australia.

8. Chauvin A., L'Hostis M., Valentin A., Precigout E., Cesbron-Zeggane N. & Gorenflot A. (1995). *Babesia divergens*: an ELISA with soluble parasite antigen for monitoring the epidemiology of bovine babesiosis. *Parasite,* **2**, 257–262.

9. Christensson D.A. (1987). Clinical and serological response after experimental inoculation with *Babesia divergens* of newborn calves with and without maternal antibodies. *Acta Vet. Scand.,* **28**, 381–392.

10. Dalgliesh R.J. (1993). Babesiosis. *In:* Immunology and Molecular Biology of Parasitic Infections, K.S. Warren, ed. Blackwell, Oxford, UK, 352–383.

11. Dalgliesh R.J., Jorgensen W.K. & De Vos A.J. (1990). New Australian vaccines for the control of babesiosis and anaplasmosis in the world cattle trade. *Trop. Anim. Health Prod.,* **22**, 44–52.

12. De Echaide S.T., Echaide I.E., Gaido A.B., Mangold A.J., Lugaresi C.I., Vanzini V.R. & Guglielmone A.A. (1995). Evaluation of an enzyme-linked immunosorbent assay kit to detect *Babesia bovis* antibodies in cattle. *Prev. Vet. Med.,* **24**, 277–283.

13. De Vos A.J. & Jorgensen W.K. (1992). Protection of cattle against babesiosis in tropical and subtropical countries with a live, frozen vaccine. *In:* Tick Vector Biology: Medical and Veterinary Aspects, Fivaz B., Petney T. & Horak I., eds. Springer-Verlag, Berlin, Germany, 159–174.

14. Edelhoffer R., Kanout A., Schuh M. & Kutzer E. (1998). Improved disease resistance after *Babesia divergens* vaccination. *Parasitol. Res.,* **84**, 181–187.

15. El-Gaysh A., Sundquist B., Christensson D.A., Hilali M. & Nasser A. M. (1996). Observations on the use of ELISA for detection of *Babesia bigemina* specific antibodies. *Vet. Parasitol.,* **62**, 51–61.

16. Figueroa J.V., Chieves L.P., Johnson G. S.& Buening G. M. (1992). Detection of *Babesia bigemina*-infected carriers by polymerase chain reaction amplification. *J. Clin. Microbiol.,* **30**, 2576–2582.

17. Friedhoff K.T. (1988). Transmission of *Babesia. In:* Babesiosis of Domestic Animals and Man, Ristic M., ed. CRC Press, Boca Raton, Florida, USA, 23–52.

18. Friedhoff K. & Bose R. (1994). Recent developments in diagnostics of some tick-borne diseases. *In:* Use of Applicable Biotechnological Methods for Diagnosing Haemoparasites, Ullenberg G., Permin A. & Hansen J.W., eds. Proceedings of the Expert Consultation, Merida, Mexico, 4–6 October 1993, Food and Agriculture Organisation of the United Nations (FAO), Rome, Italy, 46–57.

19. Friedhoff K.T., Ganse-Dumrath D., Weber C. & Muller I. (1989). Epidemiology and control of *Babesia divergens* infections in northern Germany. *In:* Proceedings of Eighth National Veterinary Haemoparasite Disease Conference, Hidalgo R.J., ed. Louisiana State University, Baton Rouge, USA, 441–449.

20. Gray J.S., Kaye B., Talty P.J. & McSweeney C. (1995). The field use of a gerbil-derived and drug controlled live vaccine against bovine babesiosis in Ireland. *Irish Vet. J.,* **48**, 358–362.

21. Holman P.J., Frerichs W.M., Chieves L. & Wagner G.G. (1993). Culture confirmation of carrier status of *Babesia* caballi-infected horses. *J. Clin. Microbiol.,* **31**, 698–701.

22. JORGENSEN W.K. & WALDRON N S.J. (1994). Use of *in vitro* culture to isolate *Babesia bovis* from *Theileria buffeli, Eperythrozoon wenyoni* and *Anaplasma* spp. *Vet. Parasitol.*, **53**, 45–51.

23. JORGENSEN W.K., WALDRON S.J., MCGRATH J., ROMAN R.J., DE VOS A.J. & WILLIAMS K.E. (1992). Growth of *Babesia bigemina* parasites in suspension cultures for vaccine production. *Parasitol. Res.*, **78**, 423–426.

24. KUNG'U M.W. & GOODGER B.V. (1990). A slide enzyme-linked assay (SELISA) for the diagnosis of *Babesia bovis* infections and for the screening of *Babesia*-specific monoclonal antibodies. *Int. J. Parasitol.*, **20**, 341–345.

25. MADRUGA C.R., KESSLER R.H., SCHENK M.A.M., HONER M.R. & MIQUITA M. (1995). Analise de testes de conglutinacao rapida para deteccao de anticorpos contra *Babesia bovis* e *Babesia bigemina*. *Arq. Bras. Med. Vet. Zoot.*, **47**, 649–657.

26. MANGOLD A.J., VANZINI V.R., ECHAIDE I.E., DE ESCHAIDE S.T., VOLPOGNI M.M. & GUGLIELMONE A.A. (1996). Viability after thawing and dilution of simultaneously cryopreserved vaccinal *Babesia bovis* and *Babesia bigemina* strains cultured *in vitro*. *Vet. Parasit.*, **61**, 345–348.

27. MOLLOY J.B., BOWLES P.M., BOCK R.E., TURTON J.A., KATSANDE T.C., KATENDE J.M., MABIKACHECHE L.G., WALDRON S.J., BLIGHT G.W. & DALGLIESH R.J. (1998). Evaluation of an ELISA for detection of antibodies to *Babesia bovis* in cattle in Australia and Zimbabwe. *Prev. Vet. Med.*, **33**, 59–67.

28. MOLLOY J.B., BOWLES P.M., JESTON P.J., BRUYERES A.G., BOWDEN J.M., BOCK R.E., JORGENSEN W.K., BLIGHT G.W. & DALGLIESH R.J. (1998). Development of an enzyme-linked immunosorbent assay for detection of antibodies to *Babesia bigemina* in cattle. *Parasitol. Res.*, **84**, 651–656.

29. MONTENEGRO-JAMES S., GUILLEN T. & TORO M. (1992). Dot-ELISA para diagnostico serologico de la anaplasmosis y babesiosis bovina. *Rev. Cientifica [FCV de Luz.]*, **2**, 23.

30. MONTENEGRO-JAMES S., TORO M., LEON E., GUILLEN A.T., LOPEZ R. & LOPEZ W. (1992). Immunisation of cattle with an inactivated polyvalent vaccine against anaplasmosis and babesiosis. *Ann. N.Y. Acad. Sci.*, **653**, 112–121.

31. MUSOKE A.J., PALMER G.H., MCELWAIN T.F., NENE V. & MCKEEVER D. (1996). Prospects for subunit vaccines against tick-borne diseases. *Br. Vet. J.*, **152**, 621–639.

32. PIPANO E. (1981). Frozen vaccine against tick fevers of cattle. *In:* XI International Congress on Diseases of Cattle, Mayer E., ed. Bregman Press, Haifa, Israel, 678–681.

33. STANDFAST N.F. & JORGENSEN W.K. (1997). Comparison of the infectivity of *Babesia bovis, Babesia bigemina* and *Anaplasma centrale* for cattle after cryopreservation in either dimethylsulphoxide (DMSO) or polyvinyl pyrrolidine (PVP). *Aust. Vet. J.*, **75**, 62–63.

34. WALTISBUHL D.J., GOODGER B.V, WRIGHT I.G., COMMINS M.A. & MAHONEY D.F. (1987). An enzyme linked immunosorbent assay to diagnose *Babesia bovis* infection in cattle. *Parasitol. Res.*, **73**, 126–131.

35. WINGER C.M., CANNING E.U. & CULVERHOUSE J.D. (1989). A strain of *Babesia divergens* attenuated after long-term culture. *Res. Vet. Sci*, **46**, 110–113.

*
* *

CHAPTER 2.3.9.

CYSTICERCOSIS

SUMMARY

Cysticercosis of farmed and wild animals is caused by the larval stages (metacestodes) of cestodes (tapeworms), the adult stages of which occur in the intestine of humans and dogs or wild Canidae. Bovine and porcine cysticercosis are caused by the metacestodes (cysticerci) of the human intestinal cestodes Taenia saginata *(in muscles) and* T. solium *(muscles and brain), respectively. Cysticerci of* T. solium *can also develop in the brain and musculature of humans. Bovine cysticercosis occurs virtually world-wide, but is at particularly high prevalence in Africa, less so in Caucasian and south/central Asian and eastern Mediterranean countries.* Taenia solium *is largely confined to Central and South America, southern Africa, parts of the Commonwealth of Independent States (CIS), the People's Republic of China and non-Islamic countries of Asia where there are free-ranging, scavenging pigs. In South-East Asia, the cysticerci of Asian* Taenia saginata asiatica *of humans occur in the liver of pigs.*

Cysticercosis of sheep and goats is caused by adult tapeworms that occur in the intestines of dogs and wild canids throughout the world. Cysticerci of T. ovis *occur in the muscles, those of* T. hydatigena *in the peritoneal cavity and on the liver. Metacestodes (coenuri) of* T. multiceps *occur mainly in the brain of sheep; it is present in most sheep-rearing areas, but has disappeared from the United States of America, New Zealand and Australia.*

Most adult and larval tapeworm infections cause little or no disease. Exceptions are severe, potentially fatal human neurocysticercosis caused by T. solium *and occasionally human neurocoenurosis caused by* T. multiceps. *These parasites also are occasional causes of muscle or ocular signs in humans. 'Gid' caused by* T. multiceps *in animals is frequently fatal. Acute cysticercosis due to* T. hydatigena *in sheep and goats is rare. Cysticercosis causes economic loss through condemnation of infected meat and offal.*

Chemotherapeutic agents are used for the treatment of adult tapeworm infections and neurocysticercosis; cysticercosis caused by T. multiceps *is treated largely by surgery.*

***Identification of the agent:** Adult* Taenia *tapeworms are dorsoventrally flattened, segmented and large, reaching from 20–50 centimetres (species in dogs) to several metres (species in humans). Anteriorly the scolex (head) has four muscular suckers and may have a rostellum often armed with two rows of hooks, the length and number of these being characteristic of a species. A notable exception is* T. saginata saginata, *which has an unarmed scolex. The scolex is followed by a neck, then immature, mature reproductive segments and finally gravid segments filled with eggs. Gravid segments break from the end of the tapeworm and they either migrate spontaneously through the anus or segments and free eggs are passed in the faeces.* Taenia *species cannot be differentiated on the basis of egg morphology.*

Cysticerci of T. saginata, T. ovis *and* T. solium *are about 0.5 cm long and are found in the musculature.* Taenia solium *can also occur in the brain. The metacestodes are grossly visible at post-mortem and meat inspection, but light infections are frequently missed at meat inspection.* Taenia hydatigena *cysticerci in the peritoneal cavity and on the liver are from 1–2 cm up to 6 cm in diameter. The coenuri of* T. multiceps *in the brain may reach 5 cm in diameter.*

Adult Taenia *infections in humans can be recognised by detection of* Taenia *coproantigen in faeces using antigen-capture enzyme-linked immunosorbent assay (AG-ELISA), but the test does not differentiate species. DNA probes and a polymerase chain reaction have been used experimentally to differentiate human* Taenia *spp. A number of immunological tests are under development for the diagnosis of cysticercosis, but remain experimental. For* T. solium *neurocysticercosis in humans, the enzyme-linked immunoelectrotransfer blot (EITB) test or immunoblot assay are hightly specific and commercially available. In animals, the experimental serum antigen-capture tests are insensitive in light infections. Palpation of tongues, particularly for the presence of* T. solium, *still remains widely used in surveys, but most diagnosis in animals continues to be done by meat inspection.*

Serological tests: *Tests for antibodies in serum are not used for the diagnosis of cysticercosis.*

Requirements for vaccines and diagnostic biologicals: *No biological products are in use. A recombinant* T. ovis *vaccine is registered in New Zealand, but is not commercially available. One for* T. saginata *is under commercial development.*

A. DIAGNOSTIC TECHNIQUES

Cysticercosis of farmed and wild animals is caused by the larval stages (metacestodes) of cestodes (tapeworms) of *Taenia* spp., the adult stages of which occur in the intestine of humans and dogs or wild Canidae. Adult tapeworms are found in the small intestine of carnivore definitive hosts: humans, dogs, and wild canids. Gravid segments that are shed by the tapeworms migrate spontaneously through the anus to fall to the ground and release eggs, or the segments and free eggs are passed in the faeces. Animals acquire infection from ingestion of segments and eggs in contaminated herbage, or in faeces. Humans may be infected by eggs on vegetables, etc., that have been contaminated by faeces or dirty hands or by faecal–oral transmission. In the case of *T. solium,* reinfection can occur through retroperistalisis and hatching of eggs internally. Diagnosis continues to be mainly parasitological based on the morphology of the adult tapeworm, the presence of eggs or segments in the faeces of infected definitive hosts, and the host and location of the metacestode.

1. Identification of the agent

Taenia saginata (the beef tapeworm): The adult is large, 4–8 metres long and can survive many years, usually singly, in the small intestine of humans. The scolex (or head) has four suckers and no rostellum or hooks. The ovary has two lobes. The gravid segments have a uterus that has 14–32 lateral branches. There is a vaginal sphincter muscle and the cirrus sac does not extend to the excretory vessels (27). Gravid segments usually leave the host singly and often migrate spontaneously from the anus.

Eggs are immediately infective when passed and are typical 'taeniid' eggs that cannot be differentiated from other *Taenia* or *Echinococcus* spp. eggs. Taeniid eggs measure about 30–45 µm in diameter; contain an oncosphere (or hexacanth embryo) bearing three pairs of hooks; have a thick, brown, radially striated embryophore or 'shell' composed of blocks; and there is an outer, oval, membranous coat, the true egg shell, that is lost in faecal eggs.

Metacestodes (or cysticerci) of *T. saginata* occur in the striated muscles of cattle (beef measles). They are oval, about 0.5 cm long, translucent and contain a single white scolex that is morphologically similar to the scolex of the future adult tapeworm. They may be viable in a thin fibrous capsule, or degenerate showing cream- or green-coloured caseation, or calcification.

Taenia solium (the pork tapeworm): The adult is similar to *T. saginata* but smaller, 3–5 metres. The scolex has an armed rostellum bearing two rows of hooks. The ovary has three lobes, there is no vaginal sphincter muscle and the cirrus sac extends to the excretory vessels. Gravid segments have 7–13 (<17) lateral branches and they do not usually leave the host spontaneously, but passively in chains with the faeces.

Metacestodes in the muscles and central nervous system of pigs, and the muscles, subcutaneous tissues and central nervous system of humans, are grossly similar to those of *T. saginata,* but have a scolex bearing a rostellum and hooks. Occasionally they reach up to 2 cm or more without a scolex in the brain of humans in a racemose form that may produce bullae.

Asian/Taiwan *Taenia:* Closely related to but genetically distinguishable from *T. saginata* (3), the adult in humans has an ovary, vaginal sphincter muscle and cirrus sac like those of *T. saginata*, but Asian *Taenia* does have a rostellum, posterior protuberances on segments and 11–32 uterine buds (7). Segments are passed singly and often spontaneously. The metacestodes are small and have a rostellum and two rows of primitive hooks, those of the outer row being numerous and tiny. They occur mainly in the liver of domesticated and wild pigs, occasionally in cattle, goats, and monkeys.

Taenia ovis: Adults in the intestine of dogs and wild carnivores reach 1–2 metres in length and have an armed rostellum and uterus with 11–20 branches. Metacestodes that occur in the musculature of sheep and less commonly goats are grossly similar to cysticerci of *T. saginata*, but both they and the adult have a rostellum with hooks. Often the cysticerci are degenerate with a cream caseous or calcified centre. *Taenia krabbei* is either a northern biotype of *T. ovis* or a separate species that occurs in wild carnivores and dogs with cysticerci in the muscles of reindeer and deer.

Taenia hydatigena: This is 0.5–2.5 metres long in the intestine of dogs and wild carnivores with an armed rostellum and 6–10 uterine branches. Metacestodes are large 1–2 cm, sometimes up to 6 cm in diameter and the scolex has a long neck. They are found attached to the omentum, mesenteries and occasionally on the liver, particularly in sheep, but also in domesticated and wild ruminants and pigs. A northern form or strain exists in a wolf and now in a dog and reindeer/deer cycle with metacestodes in the liver.

Taenia multiceps: Adults are 40–100 cm long in the intestine of carnivores and have an armed rostellum and 14–26 uterine branches. Metacestodes are coenuri, large, white fluid-filled cysts that have up to several hundred scolices invaginated on the wall in clusters. These reach 5 cm in diameter in the brain of sheep, the brain and intermuscular tissues of goats and also the brain of cattle, wild ruminants and occasionally humans. The cysts induce neurological signs that in sheep are called 'gid', 'sturdy', etc.

a) Diagnosis of adult parasites in humans or dogs

All parasite or faecal material from humans with possible *T. solium* infections must be handled with suitable safety precautions to prevent accidental infection with the eggs. *Taenia multiceps* and *Echinocccus* spp. also infect humans and, as taeniid eggs in dogs cannot be differentiated to species or genus level, in areas where these are endemic the same safety precautions apply. In addition to *Taenia* spp., humans may be infected by *Diphyllobothrium* and *Hymenolepis* spp. Also, six other species are recorded occasionally in humans. These are described by Lloyd (17) and all can be differentiated from *Taenia* spp. by egg/proglottid morphology. Recently, however, *T. taeniaeformis* with morphologically indistinguishable taeniid eggs was recorded in a child (6). In dogs and cats, *Echinococcus* spp. eggs cannot be distinguished from *Taenia* eggs, but the presence of the former can be determined by tapeworm size and *Echinococcus* genus-specific and, more recently, experimental *Echinococcus* species-specific antigen-capture enzyme-linked immunosorbent assay (AG-ELISA). Other worms, *Dipylidium, Diplopylidium, Mesocestoides* and *Diphyllobothrium* spp. have morphologically distinct eggs and proglottids (25).

Adult cestodes can be expelled from humans using an anthelmintic followed by a purgative and are identified on the basis of scolex and proglottid morphology. In animals, arecoline purgation has been useful; again the recovered taeniid or *Echinococcus* tapeworms are identified morphologically. Arecoline is no longer available as an anthelmintic, but can be obtained from chemical supply companies. As it has side-effects, old, infirm and pregnant animals should be excluded from treatment. A dose of 4 mg/kg should result in purgation in under 30 minutes. Walking and abdominal massage of recalcitrant cases or enema for constipated dogs may avoid the use of a second dose (2 mg/kg), which should be given only sparingly. Fortunately, arecoline purgation is being replaced rapidly by AG-ELISA for *Echinococcus* surveys and perhaps in the future this will also be true for *Taenia* spp.

Verster & Loos-Frank have given descriptions of parasitic diagnosis of all the *Taenia* spp. of humans and animals, their hosts and geographical distribution (19, 27). Methods for mounting, embedding, sectioning and staining the proglottids are given by Mayta *et al.* (20) and Loos-Frank (19). The following staining technique is that of Loos-Frank (19). Worms, after relaxation in water, can be stained directly, although small worms should be fixed in ethanol for a few minutes. Alternatively, worms can be fixed and stored in 70% ethanol containing 10% lactic acid, the scolex and worm being stored separately. The rostellar hooks of scolices or protoscolices should be cut off and mounted *en face* in Berlese's fluid (made by dissolving 15 g gum arabic in 20 ml distilled water and adding 10 ml glucose syrup and 5 ml acetic acid, the whole then being saturated with chloral hydrate, up to 100 g). The stain is lactic acid carmine: 0.3 g carmine is dissolved at boiling point in 42 ml lactic acid and 58 ml distilled water, 5 ml of 5% Iron chloride solution ($FeCl_2.4H_2O$) is added after cooling and can be used again to refresh older solutions. Specimens are left to sink in the stain within a vial and after several minutes are washed in 1-day-old tap water until blue. They are then fixed in 50–70% ethanol and dehydrated under the slight pressure of plastic foil. Salicylic acid methyl ester is used as clearant.

Spontaneous migration of *T. saginata* or Asian *Taenia* through the anus is likely to be noticed by the patient (>95%). When the segments migrate the sticky eggs are deposited in the perianal area and might be detected by application and examination of sticky tape. These signs are far less likely for chains of *T. solium* (2). Segments of all three may be found on the faeces, but are passed intermittently. Eggs are shed by segments into and on faeces, but are aggregated and not dispersed through the faeces. This is particularly true for the canine taeniids in that approximately 50% of the segments migrate from the anus spontaneously. The remainder are passed in the faeces, but commonly, the segments migrate and void the vast majority of their eggs. Even if all the eggs have been expelled by a migrating segment, segments can be identified as cestode in origin by the many concentric calcareous corpuscles contained within their tissues. Faeces, after mixing to reduce aggregation, can be examined for eggs. A variety of techniques are in use throughout the world and include ether or ethyl acetate extraction and flotation. For the latter, saturated sodium nitrate or Sheather's sugar solution (500 g sugar, 6.6 ml phenol, 360 ml water) with their higher specific gravity are superior to saturated NaCl as flotation media for taeniid eggs. Flotation can be carried out in commercially marketed chambers or by centrifugal flotation that includes a modified Wisconsin technique (faeces, diluted in water, are sieved, centrifuged and then resuspended in sugar or Sheather's solution, topped with a cover-slip, and centrifuged in sugar or Sheather's solution at 300 ***g*** for 4 minutes). Eggs adhering to the cover-slip can then be detected. Species cannot be determined from egg morphology, but DNA probes, the polymerase chain reaction (PCR), PCR restriction fragment length polymorphism (RFLP) and other similar techniques have proved useful for differentiation in the laboratory. These have been used largely experimentally to differentiate faecal eggs of *T. solium, T. saginata* and Asian *Taenia* (3, 8–10, 12). While equally applicable to differentiate species in dogs and cats, the same examinations have not been done for the taeniid cestodes. While the techniques for the human taeniids remain experimental, they could be carried out using the methodologies and equipment already available in many hospital laboratories after reading the literature and consultation with relevant scientists. However, eggs may be absent from or aggregated in the faeces. Adult cestodes may be expelled using an anthelmintic and identified on the basis of scolex and segment morphology. Details of morphology for parasitological diagnosis are given by references (10, 11, 16, 18).

An AG-ELISA to detect *Taenia* coproantigen in faeces is now available commercially (*Taenia* ELISA, Genzyme Virotech, Russelsheim, Germany) (2). The test is a solid-phase, microwell assay with wells coated with polyclonal, rabbit immunoglobulins against *Taenia*-specific antigens (TSA). After incubation of prepared samples and controls, the results are developed with horseradish-peroxidase-labelled rabbit anti-TSA, then the substrate tetramethyl benzidine is added and the reaction is stopped with citrate and read spectrophotometrically at 450 nm. Samples are tested in duplicate along with supplied controls: negative (normal human faecal material); cut-off (*Taenia*-positive human faecal material); and positive (*Taenia*-positive human faecal material) (all autoclaved). These controls serve as quantitative and qualitative controls and absorbance values for these should fall within the levels specified on the Quality Control Certificate supplied with the kit. The test on 56 *T. solium* positive humans gave a sensitivity of 98% and specificity of 99.2%. An additional 12 patients were coproantigen positive but noncompliant with subsequent parasitological confirmation, while 12 patients who passed no segments were considered to be false positives. While the *Taenia* ELISA technique does not differentiate *T. saginata* and *T. solium,* it supplies a very useful screening technique. An experimental AG-ELISA using similar technology to detect coproantigen of *T. hydatigena* in dogs has been described (5). Further, the AG-ELISA was developed experimentally in dogs (1) and, as it detects antigen with rabbit anti-AG antibodies, it could be used in dogs with appropriate controls. Both this and the *Echinococcus* AG-ELISA would have great use in differentiating these two genera in taeniid-egg-positive dogs. However, dogs have many *Taenia* spp. so immunological diagnosis to the *Taenia* genus is of limited value.

b) Diagnosis of metacestodes

In heavily infected animals, *T. saginata, T solium* and *T. ovis* metacestodes might be palpable in the tongue but, both in the living animal and on post-mortem examination or meat inspection, these will be difficult to differentiate from large sarcocysts. Light infections are easily missed on palpation and meat inspection: 78% of carcasses infected with >20 cysts were detected, but only 31% of those with fewer cysts (28). Metacestodes of *T. hydatigena* will be visible, viable or calcified on the omentum, mesenteries and liver surface. Those on and still migrating in the liver can be differentiated from *Echinococcus* by their scolex and by the presence of the PAS-positive (periodic acid-Schiff) laminated membrane that is present in *Echinococcus* cysts as small as <1 mm (18). *Taenia multiceps* in the brain induces neurological signs. Confirmation of the coenurus aetiology can be made by palpating softened bone on the skull over the coenurus or X-ray followed by surgical removal of the cyst. The most common presenting sign in humans of *T. solium* neurocysticercosis is seizures, but a range of signs are seen depending on the number, location and viability or level of degeneration (viable, transitional dying, calcification) of the cysticerci (4, 16). In humans, computerised tomography (CT) scan and magnetic resonance imaging (MRI) are used to detect the exact locations and viability of *T. multiceps* and *T. solium* metacestodes (4, 16). These remain the most efficient means of diagnosis, but availability of these diagnostic facilities can be problematical. Calcified cysts are detected by radiography. While PCR tests have been used largely for the differentiation of adult taeniids in humans, they could be usefully applied to unambiguously identify an actual metacestode. This would be useful in the finding of a new metacestode in a host species or geographical area from which, historically, the parasite was absent.

Experimental development of immunological tests to detect cysticercosis in humans and animals continues. Many of these tests show considerable promise for future commercialisation of tests to diagnose *T. solium* in humans. An AG-ELISA using polyclonal or monoclonal antibody (used to detect antigen in CSF) and enzyme-linked immunoelectrotransfer blot (EITB) assay (used to detect antibody in CSF) have had the most success, giving a specificity and sensitivity of 94 and 100%, respectively for EITB in 34 patients and sensitivity of 86% for AG-ELISA (11). The latter test gave false-negative results in patients with just one cyst or those with an enhancing CT lesion that probably represented a moribund parasite. However, antigen levels did correlate positively with parasite number and so the detection of viable parasites would have clinical use in relation to efficacy of drug treatment. For *T. solium* neurocysticercosis in humans, tests for serum antibody or serum antigen produce positive reactions that can be misleading in patients infected only in the musculature. Serological tests for animals have not reached the stage where commercialisation for individual diagnosis or large-scale detection of infected carcasses in slaughter houses is possible. Thus, all assays tested – AG-ELISA, antibody-ELISA, EITB and tongue inspection – showed low sensitivity in rural pigs infected naturally with low levels of *T. solium* (24). This contrasted with their high sensitivity and specificity when applied to commercially reared pigs free from infection and pigs experimentally infected with *T. solium* (23). The same has been true with *T. saginata* infections in cattle (17, 26). Thus, only a small percentage of cattle carrying fewer than 30–50 cysticerci were detected by AG-ELISA (17, 26). Conversely, antibody-based tests also detect nonviable cysts. Nonetheless, these AG-ELISAs do have use in field-based epidemiological studies. Thus far, tests for animals are at the experimental stage, using for example, laboratory-produced monoclonal antibodies.

2. Serological tests

Tests for antibodies in serum are not used for the diagnosis of cysticercosis.

B. REQUIREMENTS FOR VACCINES AND DIAGNOSTIC BIOLOGICALS

A *T. ovis* vaccine has been developed (22). The *T. ovis* 45W antigen is isolated as a recombinant protein from *Escherichia coli.* Potency control is by antibody-ELISA and *in vivo* immunogenicity, and the vaccine has given protection for a period of at least 1 year in field trials. The *T. ovis* vaccine was registered in 1994 by the New Zealand Animal Remedies Board. However, due to market changes in New Zealand the vaccine is not available commercially. A similar vaccine is under development for *T. saginata* (15). The *T. saginata* TSA-9 and TSA-18 antigens have been produced by isolation of recombinant protein from *E. coli.* They showed a high degree of homology to their low molecular weight homologues in *T. ovis.* When given in combination, the two antigens have given high levels of protection in experimental and field trials carried out in Australia, and the vaccine is currently under commercial development (15). Both the *T. ovis* and *T. saginata* vaccines have given >94% and 98% protection in cattle and sheep, respectively. A recombinant vaccine effective against *T. solium* cysticercosis in pigs has recently been described. Like *T. saginata*, the *T. solium* genome contains genes that encode protein homologues of the protective *T. ovis* antigens. As the *T. ovis* recombinant antigens were protective in pigs, it seems likely that the *T. solium* homologues will be available for control programmes in the near future (13, 14). Mass chemotherapy of human populations is also advocated as a control measure.

REFERENCES

1. ALLAN J.C., CRAIG P.S., GARCIA NOVAL J., MENCOS F., LIU D., WANG Y., WEN H., ZHOU P., STRINGER R., ROGAN M., ET AL. (1992). Coproantigen detection for immunodiagnosis of echinococcosis and taeniasis in dogs and humans. *Parasitology,* **104**, 347–356.

2. ALLAN J.C., VELASQUEZ-TOHOM M., TORRES-ALVAREZ R., YURRITA P. & GARCIA-NOVAL J. (1996). Field trial of the coproantigen-based diagnosis of *T. solium* taeniasis by enzyme-linked immunosorbent assay. *Am. J. Trop. Med. Hyg.*, **54**, 352–356.

3. BOWLES J. & MCMANUS D.P. (1994). Genetic characterisation of the Asian *Taenia*, a newly described taeniid cestode of humans. *Am. J. Trop. Med. Hyg.*, **50**, 33–44.

4. CARPIO A., PLACENCIA M., SANTILLAN F. & ESCOBAR A. (1994). A proposal for classification of neurocysticercosis. *Can. J. Neurol. Sci.*, **21**, 43–47.

5. DEPLAZES P. & ECKERT J. (1988). Untersuchungen zur Infektion des Hundes mit *Taenia hydatigena. Schweiz. Arch. Tierheilkd.*, **130**, 289–306.

6. EKANAYAKE S., WARNASURIYA N.D., SAMARAKOON P.S., ABEWICKRAMA H., KURUPPUARACHCHI N.D. & DISSANAIKE A.S. (1999). An unusual 'infection' of a child in Sri Lanka with *Taenia taeniaeformis* of the cat. *Ann. Trop. Med. Parasitol.*, **93**, 869–873.

7. FAN P.C., LIN C.Y., CHEN C.C. & CHUNG W.C. (1995). Morphological description of *Taenia saginata asiatica* (Cyclophyllidea: Taeniidae) from man in Asia. *J. Helminthol.*, **69**, 299–303.

8. GASSER R. & CHILTON N.B. (1995). Characterisation of taeniid cestode species by PCR-RFLP of ITS2 ribosomal DNA. *Acta Trop.*, **59**, 31–40.

9. GASSER R.B., ZHU X. & WOODS W. (1999). Genogyping *Taenia* tapeworms by single-strand confirmation polymorphism of mitochondrial DNA. *Electrophoresis*, **20**, 2834–2837.

10. GOTTSTEIN B., DEPLAZES P., TANNER I. & SKAGGS J.S. (1991). Diagnostic identification of *Taenia saginata* with the polymerase chain reaction. *Trans. R. Soc. Trop. Med. Hyg.*, **85**, 248–249.

11. GOTTSTEIN B., ZINI D. & SCHANTZ P.M. (1987). Species-specific immunodiagnosis of *Taenia solium* cysticercosis by ELISA and immunoblotting. *Trop. Med. Parasitol.*, **38**, 299–303.

12. HARRISON L.J., DELGADO J. & PARKHOUSE R.M. (1990). Differential diagnosis of *Taenia saginata* and *Taenia solium* with DNA probes. *Parasitology*, **100**, 459–461.

13. LIGHTOWLERS M.B. (1999). Eradication of *Taenia solium* cysticercosis: a role for vaccination of pigs. *Int. J. Parasitol.*, **29**, 811–817.

14. LIGHTOWLERS M.B., FLISSER A., GAUCI C.G., HEATH D.D., JENSEN O. & ROLFE R. (2000). Vaccination against cysticercosis and hydatid disease. *Parasitol. Today*, **16**, 191–196.

15. LIGHTOWLERS M.W., ROLFE R. & GAUCI C.G. (1996). *Taenia saginata*: vaccination against cysticercosis in cattle with recombinant oncosphere antigens. *Exp. Parasitol.*, **84**, 330–338.

16. LLOYD S. (1998). Cysticercosis and taeniosis *Taenia saginata, Taenia solium* and Asian *Taenia*. *In:* Zoonoses. Biology, Clinical Practice, and Public Health Control, Palmer S.R., Lord Soulsby E.J.L. & Simpson D.I.H., eds. Oxford University Press, Oxford, UK, 635–649.

17. LLOYD S. (1998). Other cestode infections. Hymenoleposis, diphyllobothriosis, coenurosis, and other adult and larval cestodes. *In:* Zoonoses. Biology, Clinical Practice, and Public Health Control, Palmer S.R., Lord Soulsby E.J.L. & Simpson D.I.H., eds. Oxford University Press, Oxford, UK, 651–663.

18. LLOYD S., MARTIN S.C., WALTERS T.M.H. & SOULSBY E.J.L. (1991). Use of sentinel lambs for early monitoring of the South Powys Hydatidosis Control Scheme: prevalence of *Echinococcus granulosus* and some other helminths. *Vet. Rec.*, **129**, 73–76.

19. LOOS-FRANK B. (2000). An up-date of Verster's (1969) 'Taxonomic revision of the genus *Taenia*' (Cestoda) in table format. *Syst. Parasitol.*, **45**, 155–183.

20. MAYTA H., TALLEY A., GILMAN R.H., JIMENEZ J., VERASTEGUI M., RUIZ M., GARCIA H.H. & GONZALEZ A.E. (2000). Differentiating *Taenia solium* and *Taenia saginata* infections by simple hematoxylin–eosin staining and PCR-restriction enzyme analysis. *J. Clin. Microbiol.*, **38**, 133–137.

21. ONYANGO ABUJE J.A., HUGHES G., OPICHA M., NGINYI K.M., RUGUTT M.K., WRIGHT S.H. & HARRISON L.J. (1996). Diagnosis of *Taenia saginata* cysticercosis in Kenyan cattle by antibody and antigen ELISA. *Vet. Parasitol.*, **61**, 221–230.

22. RICKARD M.D., HARRISON G.B., HEATH D.D. & LIGHTOWLERS M.W. (1995). *Taenia ovis* recombinant vaccine –'quo vadit'. *Parasitology*, **100**, S5–S9.

23. SCIUTTO E., HERNANDEZ M., GARCIA G., DE ALUJA A.S., VILLALOBOS A.N., RODARTE L.F., PARKHOUSE M. & HARRISON L. (1998). Diagnosis of porcine cysticercosis: a comparative study of serological tests for detection of circulating antibody and viable parasites. *Vet. Parasitol.*, **78**, 185–94.

24. SCIUTTO E., MARTINEZ J.J,. VILLALOBOS N.M., HERNANDEZ M., JOSE M.V., BELTRAN C., RODARTE F., FLORES I., BOBADILLA J.R., FRAGOSO G., PARKHOUSE M.E., HARRISON L.J. & DE ALUJA A.S. (1998). Limitations of current diagnostic procedures for the diagnosis of *Taenia solium* cysticercosis in rural pigs. *Vet. Parasitol.*, **79**, 299–313.

25. SOULSBY E.J.L. (1982). Helminths, Arthropods and Protozoa of Domesticated Animals, Seventh Edition. Balliere Tindall, London, UK, 809 p.

26. VAN KERCKHOVEN I., VANSTEENKISTE W., CLAES M., GEERTS S. & BRANDT J. (1998). Improved detection of circulating antigen in cattle infected with *Taenia saginata* metacestodes. *Vet. Parasitol.*, **76**, 269–274.

27. VERSTER A. (1969). A taxonomic revision of the genus *Taenia* Linnaeus 1758 s. str. *Onderstepoort J. Vet. Res.*, **37**, 3–58.

28. WALTHER M. & KOSKE J.K. (1980). *Taenia saginata* cysticercosis: a comparison of routine meat inspection and carcass dissection results in calves. *Vet. Rec.*, **106**, 401–402.

*

* *

CHAPTER 2.3.10.

DERMATOPHILOSIS

SUMMARY

Dermatophilosis (also known as streptothrichosis) is an exudative, pustular dermatitis that mainly affects cattle, sheep and horses, but also goats, many wild mammals, reptiles and, occasionally, humans. The severe disease in ruminants is promoted by immunomodulatory effects induced by infestation with the tick, Amblyomma variegatum.

Laboratory diagnosis of dermatophilosis depends on the demonstration of the bacterium Dermatophilus congolensis *in material from the skin or other organs. Sites other than the skin are rarely affected.*

Identification of the agent: Dermatophilus congolensis *normally affects the epidermis, causing the formation of scabs. It may be demonstrated in smears made from scabs emulsified or softened in water or in impression smears from the base of freshly removed adherent scabs. The organism is Gram positive but its morphology is more readily appreciated in smears stained with Giemsa. In stained smears, the organism is seen as branching filaments containing multiple rows of cocci. This characteristic appearance is diagnostic. In wet or secondarily infected scabs, only free cocci may be present, so that staining by immunofluorescence is necessary.* Dermatophilus congolensis *is demonstrated in histopathological sections by Giemsa staining or by immunofluorescence.* Dermatophilus chelonae *may be found in crocodiles.*

Isolation of D. congolensis *from freshly removed scabs is straightforward but the organism is readily overgrown by other bacteria. When cultured from contaminated sites, special techniques involving filtration, chemotaxis, or selective media are necessary.*

Demonstration and identification of D. congolensis *by immunofluorescence is a reliable and very sensitive method of diagnosis but requires that laboratories make their own diagnostic antisera as these are not available commercially. Although antigenic cross-reaction with* Nocardia *spp. has been reported, this is likely to give only weak fluorescence. Ideally, a monoclonal antibody specific to* D. congolensis *should be used.*

Serological tests: *A variety of serological tests has been used in studies of the epidemiology and pathogenesis of dermatophilosis. Antibody can be demonstrated in all but fetal blood in healthy ruminants but the elevated levels associated with clinical infection can be used to identify animals that have been infected with the disease.*

Requirements for vaccines and diagnostic biologicals: *No vaccines are available currently.*

A. DIAGNOSTIC TECHNIQUES

Dermatophilosis (also known as streptothrichosis, or in sheep as 'lumpy wool disease') is an exudative, pustular dermatitis that affects mainly cattle, sheep and horses, but also goats, many wild mammals, reptiles and, occasionally, humans. Dermatophilosis is caused by the bacterium *Dermatophilus congolensis,* the type species of the genus *Dermatophilus,* which is a member of the Actinomycetes (*Dermatophilus cheloniae* has been isolated from crocodiles). Typically, infection gives rise to the formation of dense scabs on the skin, but in certain areas, such as the perineum in ruminants and the pastern in horses, moist lesions with thickened, folded skin may occur. In such lesions, relatively thin scabs are found. Where lesions are exposed to prolonged wetting, with or without secondary infection, exudative lesions may be present.

The severe disease in ruminants is promoted by immunomodulatory effects induced by infestation with adults of the tick species *Amblyomma variegatum* (1).

It must be remembered that both scabs and cultures can cause human infections.

1. Identification of the agent

Diagnosis can usually be made by demonstrating the causal organism in scabs from the lesions or in exudate beneath the scabs. The organism has a characteristic microscopic appearance – its septate, branching filaments become longitudinally, as well as transversely, divided to form ribbons of spherical or ovoid cocci, each about 0.5 µm in diameter, in multiple rows. This appearance is diagnostic, provided that cocci are found in transverse rows of four or more, and is readily seen in stained preparations. However, the distinctive formation can be disrupted during the preparation of smears for examination if the material is spread too vigorously over the slide.

Impression smears may be made from the moist, concave undersurfaces of freshly removed scabs. Otherwise, thick smears are best prepared from scabs emulsified in sterile distilled water. Alternatively, scabs can be soaked overnight in sterile water or saline to sufficiently moisten them so that the undersurface of the scab can be used to make effective impression smears by firmly pressing this surface on to a microscope slide. Smears are then air-dried, fixed by heating or immersion in methanol for 5 minutes, and stained. The organism stains well in dilute carbol fuchsin or methylene blue stain, but Gram's stain or, preferably, a 1 in 10 dilution of Giemsa stain for 30 minutes, gives better differentiation in thick smears, the darkly stained *D. congolensis* contrasting with the paler or pink counterstained background of keratinocytes and neutrophils. Gram staining does not give as good results as Giemsa because it may overstain the background and does not clearly show the characteristic laddering of the coccoid forms.

Wet or secondarily infected scabs often contain few, if any, intact filaments, and the organism may not stain Gram positive. In such material, the cocci cannot be differentiated morphologically from other coccoid bacteria, so that staining by immunofluorescence is required. However, specific antisera for immunofluorescence are not commercially available. Thin, heat-fixed smears are used. In difficult cases and when infection of organs other than the skin is suspected, histopathological examination of biopsy or necropsy material is advisable. Giemsa stain or immunofluorescence is used.

The characteristic appearance of the lesions and of the organism in smears from typical bovine dermatophilosis makes culture unnecessary in most cases. However, in the rare cases in which a Giemsa-stained smear does not give a definitive result, confirmation of the diagnosis may be made by isolating the bacterium. Cultures are made on blood agar and incubated at 37°C. Growth is accelerated under microaerophilic conditions; rough, usually haemolytic, greyish-yellow colonies, about 1 mm in diameter, are seen pitting the medium after 24 hours. Incubation in air produces similar pinpoint colonies at 24 hours that grow to about 1 mm at 48 hours. The rough colonies are formed by the branching filaments, but continued growth in air stimulates the production of the cocci, which are commonly yellow in colour. Colonies take on a smooth, often yellowish, appearance. The cocci are normally vigorously motile when taken from young cultures. The colonies must be differentiated from *Nocardia* spp. and *Streptomyces* spp., neither of which produces filaments that break up into multiple rows of motile cocci.

For isolation, material can be streaked out directly from the moist undersurfaces of freshly removed, uncontaminated scabs or from scab emulsions, but the relatively slow-growing *D. congolensis* is readily overgrown by other bacteria. Special isolation techniques are thus required for contaminated specimens. In most specimens, free cocci, whether motile or not, will be present in emulsions of the material. Filtration of the emulsion through a 0.45 µm membrane filter is usually sufficient to reduce or eliminate contaminants and permits isolation from the filtrate, as described above. Alternatively, Haalstra's method (2) may be used. Small pieces of scab are placed in a bijou bottle containing 1 ml of sterile distilled water and allowed to stand at room temperature for 3–4 hours. The open bottle is then placed for 15 minutes in a candle jar. Samples of the surface liquid are removed with a bacteriological loop and cultured. The method depends on the release from the scab of the motile cocci of *D. congolensis* and their chemotropic attraction towards the carbon-dioxide-rich atmosphere of the candle jar. A selective medium consisting of 1000 units/ml of polymyxin B in blood agar can also be used, and is effective when the contaminants are sensitive to this antibiotic.

Immunofluorescence staining of smears or tissues is the most reliable and sensitive immunological technique for the identification of *D. congolensis* antigens and for the diagnosis of dermatophilosis. Polyclonal antibody obtained from animals inoculated with *D. congolensis* can be easily prepared using standard methods, but there is a risk of possible cross-reaction with some strains of *Nocardia* spp. Monoclonal antibody to species-specific antigen (3) is preferable. Thin, heat-fixed smears of scab emulsions, or impression smears, are stained. Known positive and negative control specimens should always be included.

When other diagnostic techniques fail, animal inoculation can be used to isolate *D. congolensis,* although this is rarely necessary and should be avoided if possible. Rabbits are clipped at the inoculation sites, which are swabbed with ether and then lightly scarified with a needle, while avoiding haemorrhaging. White skin should be used, if possible. A suspension of the specimen is applied to the prepared skin and observed daily. At sites inoculated with *D. congolensis*, erythema will be apparent after 48 hours. Some serous exudation may be seen, and scab formation will occur after approximately 72 hours. These lesions will normally be uncontaminated, and *D. congolensis* can be demonstrated in the scabs or isolated from them.

2. Serological tests

Clinical diagnosis is best performed using the methods described above rather than serological methods. Antibody can be demonstrated in all but fetal blood in healthy ruminants, but levels are raised following clinical infection. The enzyme-linked immunosorbent assay (ELISA) has proved to be a sensitive and convenient assay technique, and elevation of titres above baseline values can be used in epidemiological studies to identify animals that have had the disease (4). At present, the ELISA remains only suitable as a research and investigation method; it is not used for routine diagnosis.

B. REQUIREMENTS FOR VACCINES AND DIAGNOSTIC BIOLOGICALS

Vaccines are under development, but so far no commercial vaccines are available.

REFERENCES

1. AMBROSE N., LLOYD D.H. & MAILLARD J.C. (1999). Immune responses to *Dermatophilus congolensis* infections. *Parasitol. Today*, **15**, 295–300.

2. HAALSTRA R.T. (1965). Isolation of *Dermatophilus congolensis* from skin lesions in the diagnosis of streptothricosis. *Vet. Rec.*, 77, 824–825.

3. HOW S.J., LLOYD D.H. & LIDA J. (1988). Use of a monoclonal antibody in the diagnosis of infection by *Dermatophilus congolensis*. *Res. Vet. Sci.*, **45**, 416–417.

4. MARTINEZ D., AUMONT G., MOUTOUSSAMY M., GABRIEL D., TATAREAU J.C., BARRE N., VALLEE F. & MARI B. (1993). Epidemiological studies on dermatophilosis in the Caribbean. *Rev. Elev. Med. Vet. Pays Trop.*, **46**, 323–327.

*
* *

CHAPTER 2.3.11.

THEILERIOSIS

SUMMARY

The Theileria *parasites of cattle are important constraints to the improvement of the livestock industry throughout a large part of the world.* Theileria annulata *and* T. parva, *the most economically important species, are responsible for mortality and losses in production that can only be guessed at, but these species are consistently recorded as the cause of major disease entities. Control of theileriosis in many countries is by control of their vectors, often as part of a general tick-borne disease control strategy. Tick control has become less reliable because acaricides are expensive, resistance has developed to many of them, regulations regarding cattle movement and quarantine are not strictly enforced, and management and maintenance of dips and spray races are often poor. More reliable systems are desirable, and vaccination should provide better control of theileriosis.*

Identification of the agent: *Diagnosis of disease is based on clinical signs, a knowledge of the disease and vector distribution, and examination of Giemsa-stained blood and lymph node smears. The schizont is a characteristic diagnostic feature of infections with* T. parva *and* T. annulata *in lymph node biopsy or impression smears. Animals infected with* T. parva *show enlarged lymph nodes, fever, a gradually increasing respiratory rate, dyspnoea and/or diarrhoea, and various post-mortem lesions; parasitised cells may be found in impression smears from all tissues. The gross pathology caused by schizonts of* T. annulata *resembles that of* T. parva, *while the piroplasm stages may also be pathogenic, causing anaemia and jaundice.*

Serological tests: *Sero-epidemiology, particularly of* T. parva, *does not distinguish among the different immunogenic stocks. The most widely used diagnostic test for* Theileria *species is the indirect fluorescent antibody (IFA) test. For the IFA test, both schizont and piroplasm antigens may be prepared on slides or in suspension and preserved by deep freezing, except in the case of the piroplasm suspension that is stored at 4°C. Test sera are diluted with bovine lymphocyte lysate and incubated with the antigen in suspension, and anti-bovine immunoglobulin conjugate is then added. Using the test as described, the fluorescence is specific for the causative agent. The IFA test is sensitive, fairly specific, and usually easy to perform. However, because of the problems of cross-reactivity among some* Theileria *species, the test has limitations for large-scale surveys in areas where these species overlap. Developments in molecular biological techniques provide possibilities for new, more sensitive and specific tests.*

Requirements for vaccines and diagnostic biologicals: *Reliable vaccines of known infectivity are a recent development. For* T. annulata, *the vaccine is prepared from schizont-infected cell lines that have been isolated from cattle and attenuated during* in-vitro *culture. The vaccine contains schizont-infected cells and must remain frozen until shortly before administration. Vaccination against* T. parva *is based on a method of infection and treatment in which an aliquot of ground-up ticks infected with the nonattenuated viable sporozoite stage is inoculated subcutaneously and the animals are treated simultaneously with tetracyclines; usually a mild or inapparent reaction occurs and the immune response controls the infection. Safety precautions must be taken in the preparation and handling of* T. parva *vaccines to protect the workers involved and to avoid contaminating the stabilates. Consideration should also be given to the risk of introducing new isolates into an area where they may then become established through a carrier state.*

A. DIAGNOSTIC TECHNIQUES

Theileriae are obligate intracellular protozoan parasites that infect both wild and domestic Bovidae throughout much of the world (some species infect small ruminants). They are transmitted by ixodid ticks, and have complex life cycles in both vertebrate and invertebrate hosts. There are six *Theileria* spp. that infect cattle; the two most pathogenic and economically important are *T. parva*, causing East Coast fever, Corridor disease and Zimbabwean theileriosis; and *T. annulata*, causing tropical theileriosis. The parasite group referred to as *T. sergenti*, *T. buffeli*, *T. orienalis*, *T. taurotragi* and *T. mutans* generally cause no disease or only mild disease, and *T. velifera* is nonpathogenic, but they are common and complicate the epidemiology of theileriosis in cattle. The parasites referred to as *T. sergenti/T. buffeli/T. orientalis* are now thought to consist of two species – *T. sergenti* and *T. buffeli/T. orientalis* – and the name *T. buffeli* may have priority (13).

Most *Theileria* spp. produce a carrier infection in recovered cattle, but there are no data on the role of carriers in transmission under natural conditions. Indigenous cattle in enzootic areas may experience very mild disease or subclinical infection, while introduced indigenous or exotic cattle are susceptible and may die when infected.

The most widely used and most practical method for the control of theileriosis is the chemical control of ticks with acaricides. However, tick control has become less reliable because of acaricide resistance, the high cost of acaricides, poor management of tick control, and illegal cattle movement in many countries. Vaccination using attenuated schizont-infected cell lines has been widely used for *T. annulata*. For control of *T. parva*, a method of infection and treatment using ground-up infected ticks as stabilates and tetracycline treatment is being implemented in a number of countries in eastern, central and southern Africa.

Chemotherapy is also widely used. Parvaquone, buparvaquone and halofuginone are used to treat *T. parva* and *T. annulata*. These treatments do not sterilise the infections.

1. Identification of the agent (a prescribed test for international trade)

Theileria schizonts are a characteristic diagnostic feature in cattle with acute *T. parva* and *T. annulata* theileriosis. In the remaining *Theileria* species (*T. mutans, T. taurotragi, T. velifera* and the *T. sergenti, T. orientalis, T. buffeli* group), the schizonts are transitory and difficult to detect. For laboratory confirmation of acute theileriosis, thin smears are prepared from blood and from biopsy material of lymph nodes or liver, and stained with Giemsa. Schizonts are scarce in the peripheral blood in *T. annulata* sick animals, while a high rate of infected lymphocytes is usually seen in the lymphnodes of cattle with *T. parva* infection. The severity of lesions in animals that have died of *T. annulata* or *T. parva* infections depends on the course of the disease. In fulminating cases, lasting only a few days, lesions are limited mainly to hyperplasia of the lymphoid tissues and to disseminated haemorrhages. In typical less acute cases, numerous petechiae and large haemorrhages are seen in the subcutaneous tissues, especially in *T. annulata* infection. The spleen and the liver are enlarged, the latter having subcapsular haemorrhages. The myocardium is often degenerated, with epicardial and endocardial haemorrhagic areas. Ulceration of the abomasum and lymphocytic infiltration of the kidneys occur. Interstitial pneumonia and interlobular oedema are seen mainly in *T. parva* theileriosis. Post-mortem, schizont-parasitised cells are found in impression smears from most internal organs, but especially in smears from the lymph nodes, liver and spleen.

Piroplasms (erythrocytic stages) of most species of *Theileria* may persist for months or years in recovered animals, and may be detected intermittently in subsequent examinations. However, negative results of microscopic examination of blood films do not exclude latent infection. Relapse parasitaemia can be induced with some *Theileria* species by splenectomy. Piroplasms are also seen in post-mortem-prepared smears, but the parasites appear shrunken and their cytoplasm is barely visible.

The morphological features of the schizonts (except for those of *T. mutans*) or of the piroplasms do not represent a reliable indicator for differentiation among *Theileria* species. Indirect parasite identification by means of immunodiagnostic tests can be applied for the recognition of *Theileria*-infected cattle.

Polymerase chain reaction (PCR) and oligonucleotide probes have been used for direct detection of piroplasm infection and differentiation of *Theileria* species (2, 5, 11). These techniques, which may be much more sensitive than blood smear examination, have the potential to become internationally approved tests for trade, but at present only specialised laboratories possess the skills and the equipment needed for their performance. Great care must be taken when using these tests, to avoid carry-over or other causes of false-positive results.

Theileria-specific antibody has also been detected by the enzyme linked immunosorbent assay (ELISA) (18–20, 22).

2. Serological tests

The most widely used serological test for detecting anti-theilerial antibody is based on the indirect fluorescent antibody (IFA) technique using schizont or piroplasm antigen. This test may not differentiate between infections with some *Theileria* species when using serum that has not been diluted very much (7) and may not always be sufficiently sensitive to detect all infected cattle. Neither schizont nor merozoite IFA were able to detect antibodies in a few clinically healthy animals shown to be carrying *T. annulata* piroplasms in their peripheral blood (9). Despite this, the IFA test is the most widely used diagnostic test for *Theileria* spp.

- **The indirect fluorescent antibody test (a prescribed test for international trade)**

- **Preparation of schizont antigen**

i) *Schizont antigen slides*

The antigens used for the schizont IFA tests (7) are obtained from schizont-infected lymphoblastoid cell lines prepared as described below:

Cultures of from 200 ml to 1 litre of either *T. parva* or *T. annulata* schizont-infected cells containing 10^6 cells/ml, of which at least 90% of the cells are infected, are centrifuged at 200 ***g*** for 20 minutes at 4°C. The supernatant fluid is removed and the cell pellet is resuspended in 100 ml of cold (4°C) phosphate buffered saline (PBS), pH 7.2–7.4, and centrifuged as before. This washing procedure is repeated three times, and after the final wash the cell pellet is resuspended in PBS (approximately 100 ml) to give a final concentration of 10^7 cells/ml.

Thin smears of the cell suspension are made on Teflon-coated multispot slides[1], or on ordinary slides using nail varnish for separation into a number of enclosures. The smears should give between 50 and 80 intact cells per field of view when examined under ×40 objective lens. The antigens are distributed on to the slides using a 100 µl pipette. By dispensing and immediately sucking up the schizont or piroplasm suspension, a monolayer of schizonts or piroplasms remains on the slide within each enclosure. This is performed for each enclosure until the volume is exhausted. With this method, approximately 600 good quality slides containing a total of 6000 individual antigen spots can be obtained. The smears are air-dried, fixed in acetone for 10 minutes, individually wrapped in tissue paper and then in groups of five in aluminium foil, and stored in airtight, waterproof plastic containers at either –20°C or –70°C. The antigens keep for at least 1 year at –20°C and longer at –70°C.

ii) *Schizont antigen in suspension*

500 ml of *T.-parva-* or *T.-annulata*-infected cells containing 10^6 cells/ml are centrifuged at 200 ***g*** for 10 minutes at 4°C, and the cell pellet obtained is washed twice in 100 ml of cold PBS. The viability of the cells is determined by eosin or trypan blue exclusion (it should be greater than 90%). The cells are resuspended at 10^7/ml in cold saline. To this volume, two volumes of a cold fixative solution containing 80% acetone and 0.1% formaldehyde (0.25% formalin) in PBS are added drop by drop while the cell suspension is stirred gently and continuously. The cell suspension is kept at –20°C and allowed to fix for 24 hours. The fixed cells are then washed three times in cold saline and centrifuged at 200 ***g*** for 20 minutes at 4°C. After the last wash, the cells are resuspended at 10^7/ml saline. The fixed cells are distributed in aliquots of 0.5 ml. The antigen is stable at 4°C with 0.2% sodium azide as preservative for 2 weeks, and keeps indefinitely at –20°C. This method can also be used to prepare schizont antigen for *T. taurotragi.*

- **Preparation of piroplasm antigen**

i) *Piroplasm antigen slides*

The piroplasm stage of *Theileria* spp. cannot be maintained in culture, therefore the piroplasm antigen must be prepared from infected animals. Experimental infections are induced by infecting cattle subcutaneously with sporozoites or using ticks infected with either *T. parva, T. annulata* or *T. taurotragi.* Peak parasitaemias are of short duration and if animals survive the disease the percentage of infected red blood cells (RBCs) decreases considerably in a few days. Infections of the parasite group referred to as *T. sergenti/T. buffeli/T. orientalis, T. mutans* or *T. velifera* are usually induced by inoculating splenectomised cattle intravenously with blood from a carrier animal, or with a blood stabilate, or by application of infected ticks. When the piroplasm parasitaemia is 10% or higher, 100 ml of the infected blood is collected from the jugular vein in a heparinised or ethylene diamine tetra-acetic acid (EDTA) vacutainer, and gently mixed with 2 litres of PBS. The mixture is centrifuged at 500 ***g*** for 10 minutes at 4°C; the plasma and buffy coat are removed, the RBCs are again resuspended in 2 litres of PBS, and the centrifugation step is repeated. It is important to remove the buffy coat after each wash. This washing procedure is repeated four times. After the final wash, an aliquot of the packed RBCs is used to make doubling dilutions in PBS, and a 5 µl drop of each dilution is placed on slides. The dried spots are fixed in methanol and stained with Giemsa's stain, and the

1 Obtainable from, for example, Bellco Glass, Vineland, New Jersey, United States of America or Glaxo-Wellcome, United Kingdom.

concentration of RBCs examined using a light microscope. The dilution that gives a single layer of RBCs spread uniformly on the spot is then selected for large-scale preparation of piroplasm antigen slides. Approximately 10,000 antigen slides (100,000 antigen spots) can be prepared from 100 ml of infected blood. The antigen smears are allowed to dry at room temperature before fixing in cold (4°C) acetone for 10 minutes. The fixed smears can be stored as for the schizont antigen slides, and kept for similar periods.

ii) *Piroplasm antigen in suspension*

An alternative method of preparing antigens to that described above is available and has been tested for *T. parva*. In this procedure, 100 ml of blood is taken from an animal with a high piroplasm parasitaemia and prepared as described above, and the packed cell volume is adjusted to 5% in PBS.

One volume of the RBC suspension is added to two volumes of the fixative (see above schizont antigen in suspension) while stirring. The cells are allowed to fix at –20°C for 24 hours. The fixed cells are then washed three times with PBS and centrifuged at 1000 *g* for 30 minutes. The deposit is resuspended to the original volume of blood with PBS containing 0.2% sodium azide.

The piroplasm antigen is stable at 4°C when preserved with 0.2% sodium azide for a period of at least 3 years.

- **Standardisation of antigen**

Schizont or piroplasm antigens in suspension are mixed on a rotor mixer and titrated in PBS by doubling dilution starting from neat through to 1/16. The dilution giving a cell distribution of approximately 50–80 schizont-infected cells or 150–200 infected RBCs per field view when examined under a ×40 objective lens is taken to be the dilution recommended for use for that batch of antigen. Using this dilution, test antigen smears are prepared on slides. These antigen smears plus the antigen slides previously frozen (and thawed before use) are tested against a range of dilutions of a panel of known strong, intermediate and weak positive and negative control sera. If the positive control sera titrate to their known titres and the negative control sera give no fluorescence, the antigen is used in the routine IFA test.

Both types of antigen preparations, acetone-fixed smears stored at either –20°C or –70°C, and antigens fixed in suspension and stored at either 4°C or –20°C, are used routinely in many laboratories. The sensitivity of both types of antigen is comparable. In laboratories where adequate low temperature storage facilities and a reliable supply of electricity are available, the antigen slides can be used. However, such antigens can only be transported on dry ice or in liquid nitrogen. Antigens fixed in suspension have the advantage over antigen slides that the initial method of preparation is simpler and quicker. A large batch of this antigen can be stored in one container, and aliquots may be taken out as necessary, from which fresh smears are prepared for the IFA test. This way the need for a large storage facility is avoided. The antigens fixed in suspension can also be stored at 4°C and can be safely transported at room temperature without loss of antigenicity.

- **Preparation of bovine lymphocyte lysate**

A lymphocyte lysate is prepared according to the method described by Goddeeris *et al.* (14), for use in tests with antigens of *T. parva* in suspension. Briefly, a 3-month-old calf is splenectomised and maintained under conditions free from ticks and tsetse flies. To exclude the possibility of latent infection, blood smears from the animal are taken daily for a period of 4 weeks, stained with Giemsa's stain, and examined for parasites. The animal is killed and the thymus and all the accessible lymph nodes are removed. These tissues are sliced into small pieces in cold PBS containing 0.45% EDTA as anticoagulant. Cells are teased out of the tissue, separated from the debris by passing through a muslin cloth, and washed three times with PBS/EDTA by centrifugation at 200 *g* for 20 minutes at 4°C. The washed lymphocytes are resuspended in PBS without EDTA, to give a final concentration of 5×10^7 cells/ml. The cells are disrupted by sonication in 100 ml aliquots on ice for 5 minutes using the 3/8 probe. The sonicated material is centrifuged at 1000 *g* for 30 minutes at 4°C, and the supernatant, adjusted to 10 mg protein/ml, is stored at –20°C in 4 ml aliquots.

- **Test procedure**

Schizont and piroplasm antigen slides are removed from –20°C storage and allowed to thaw for 30 minutes at 4°C and for 30 minutes at room temperature, before being unpacked. The frozen schizont antigen, fixed in suspension and stored at –20°C, is thawed at room temperature, while the piroplasm antigen, kept at 4°C, is resuspended by agitation, passed through a 25-gauge needle to break the clumps (not necessary for schizont antigen), and diluted to previously standardised dilutions. The antigens are distributed on to the slides using a 100 µl pipette. By dispensing and immediately sucking up the schizont or piroplasm suspension, a monolayer of schizonts or piroplasms remains on each area of the slide. The slides are allowed to dry either at 37°C or at room temperature.

For initial screening using *T. parva* antigen in suspension, 1/40 dilutions of test and control sera are made in lymphocyte lysate (195 µl lymphocyte lysate + 5 µl serum), and incubated for 30 minutes at room temperature. For antigen slides, 1/40 and 1/60 dilutions are used. Further doubling or five-fold dilutions in PBS can be made if end-point antibody titre is desired. Of the diluted sera, 25 µl is then transferred to the antigen slides. For each slide, the positive and negative control sera, diluted 1/40, are included. The slides are incubated at room temperature in a humid chamber for 30 minutes, then washed twice in PBS for 15 minutes. To each enclosure, 20 µl of anti-bovine immunoglobulin fluorescein isothiocyanate conjugate at recommended optimal dilution, is added. Evans blue is incorporated into the conjugate at a final dilution of 1/10,000 as a counterstain. The slides are incubated for 30 minutes at room temperature in a humid chamber, washed, as before, mounted with a cover-slip in 50% glycerol in PBS, pH 8.0, and examined for fluorescence, for example, using a fluorescent microscope equipped with epi-Koem illumination (100 W mercury lamp), UV filter block, ×6.3 eyepieces and Phaco FL 40/1.3 oil objective lens.

- **Characteristics of the indirect fluorescent test**

Using the test as described, the fluorescence is generally specific for the particular *Theileria* species (see below). The incorporation of Evans blue provides a good contrast, making reading easy. Mounting the slides in 50% glycerol, at pH 8.0, reduces the rapid fading of fluorescein isothiocyanate and makes photography of the preparation possible. Once prepared, slides are stable and can be read for up to 72 hours after preparation when kept at 4°C in the dark.

Following infection with sporozoites, antibodies to *T. parva* and *T. annulata* are first detected between days 10 and 14 using the schizont antigen, while using the piroplasm antigen, antibodies are first detected between days 15 and 21. Antibodies last for a variable period of time after recovery, depending on such factors as the establishment of a carrier state, chemotherapeutic intervention, and presence or absence of rechallenge. Following recovery from either East Coast fever or tropical theileriosis, some animals may have low antibody titres in the IFA test after 4–6 months, but the antibodies may persist for more than 1 year following a single challenge.

The IFA test is useful for identifying herds that contain carriers of *T. annulata*, but is not always sufficiently sensitive to detect all infected individuals. Both schizont and merozoite IFA antigens have failed to detect antibody in some animals carrying patent infection with piroplasms (9).

In *T. mutans* infections induced by sporozoite inoculation, antibodies are first detected between days 10 and 15, after the appearance of piroplasms. Low titres are detectable for at least 12–24 months.

If the IFA test is used routinely for the detection of antibodies to one of the bovine *Theileria* spp., it is sensitive and requires little standardisation. However, if the test is used to detect antibodies where mixed infections of *Theileria* occur, the specificity of the test needs to be carefully evaluated. For example, *T. annulata* and *T. parva* cross-react, although these cross-reactions are four- to six-fold lower than with the homologous sera. This is not important in the field, as the diseases do not overlap. Such cross-reactivity does not seem to occur between *T. parva* and *T. mutans* or between *T. annulata* and *T. mutans*. There is low titre cross-reactivity between *T. parva* and *T. taurotragi*, which is a problem as the two infections overlap throughout much of the *T. parva* distribution.

- **Future tests for *Theileria* diagnosis**

The IFA test is reasonably sensitive, specific and usually easy to perform. However, because of the problems of cross-reactivity described above, the test has limitations for large-scale serological surveys in areas where these species overlap. The ELISA has been successfully adapted for the detection of anti-*T. annulata* antibodies (15), and has been shown to detect antibodies for a longer period of time than the IFA (18, 19). An ELISA for *T. mutans* has also been described (20). The use of two monoclonal antibodies (MAbs) specific for *T. mutans* has been described in the ELISA system for the detection of antibodies and antigens in acute, subacute and chronic infections. The test is more specific and sensitive than the IFA test. Significant progress is also being made with direct ELISAs for detection of *T. parva* and *T. mutans* antibodies using recombinant antigens. The antigens being validated are the p85 of *T. parva* and p32 of *T. mutans*, both expressed in *Escherichia coli* using pGEX as the expression vector. The expressed product is a fusion protein with glutathione S transferase, and is directly coated on to ELISA plates. These ELISAs provide higher sensitivity and specificity than the IFA tests, and are currently under validation in a number of countries (22).

A range of probes is available to detect all the *Theileria* species that are known to infect cattle, and are based on ribosomal RNA gene sequences and antigen genes (2, 5). DNA probes specific for *T. parva* (1, 8) and *T. mutans* (21), have also been developed. The technology of the PCR is available to amplify minute quantities of parasite DNA one-million-fold, thereby greatly increasing the sensitivity of the DNA probes (3). A specific PCR was developed to test whole blood samples from *T. annulata*-carrier cattle (11). It is hoped that a combination of ELISA, PCR and DNA probes will greatly enhance our present capacity to identify antibodies and parasites at various stages of *Theileria* infections, thus making possible accurate serological surveys of *Theileria* species. Eventually, the aim would be to develop these technologies for the diagnosis of all the vector-borne diseases.

B. REQUIREMENTS FOR VACCINES AND DIAGNOSTIC BIOLOGICALS

B1. Cell culture vaccines for *Theileria annulata*

Vaccination against *T. parva* and *T. annulata* has been attempted since the causal organisms were first recognised in the early part of the 19th century. However, the introduction of reliable live vaccines of known potency is a much more recent development. The most widely used are attenuated schizont cell culture vaccines against *T. annulata*. The procedures for production and safety testing have been described (12, 16, 23, 27), and the vaccine is widely used in Israel, Iran, Turkey, India, central Asia and the People's Republic of China.

1. Seed management

a) Characteristics of the seed

Primary cultures of *T.-annulata*-infected cells may be established from trypsinised lymph nodes, liver, or spleen taken aseptically from an infected animal after death, or from the buffy coat of heparinised peripheral blood separated on a density gradient (Ficoll Hypaque), or using lymphocytes harvested from lymph node biopsy material using a simple 'plastic syringe' method (12).

Seed cultures are prepared from cryopreserved cell lines that have been isolated from cattle and attenuated as described below. Cultivation for vaccine production is recommended from the seed culture following a maximum of 20–30 passages, because there is some uncertainty about the immunogenic stability of these cultures after long-term passage.

b) Method of culture

The infected cells are cultured initially in Eagle's minimum essential medium (MEM) supplemented with 20% calf serum and containing penicillin (100 µl/ml), streptomycin (50 µl/ml), and mycostatin (75 µl/ml) in 25 ml plastic screw-cap cell culture flasks. An alternative medium is RPMI 1640 with 10% fetal calf serum, 2 mM glutamine, penicillin and streptomycin, and is usually used with established cultures. Medium is replenished every 3–4 days. The presence of bright refractile cells free in the medium (on examination using a phase-contrast or inverted microscope) is indicative of infected cell growth. The cultures may establish as a monolayer or in suspension. Passage is effected by decanting the medium, adding 0.025% versene for 15 minutes to monolayer cultures, dispersing the cells, then counting and dispensing according to flask size. Approximately 10^6 cells are introduced into a 25 cm^2 flask, and the same seed rate in 100–200 ml is used in larger flasks. The general culture technique is as described by Brown (6).

Serum is essential for maintenance of these cultures, and is obtained either from calves up to the age of 6 months, or commercially, and is tested for toxicity through three passages in an established cell line before use.

c) Attenuation of virulence

Attenuation of *T. annulata* schizonts is achieved by prolonged growth and repeated passage in culture. The mechanism of attenuation is unknown, but the number of cell divisions is likely to be more important than time in culture or number of passages. Field isolates have required passage for periods of from 4 to 30 months for complete attenuation. Attenuation is assessed by the inoculation of the culture into susceptible calves every 20–30 passages. A sample of culture should be cryopreserved every ten passages in case of accidental loss or contamination. Complete attenuation is achieved when cultures do not cause fever or detectable schizonts and piroplasms in susceptible cattle. An attenuated culture will reliably infect cattle at 10^5 cells and induce a serological reaction, and will not produce disease at 10^9 cells. Cultures may be cryopreserved using either dimethyl sulphoxide (DMSO) or glycerol. Two methods of storing and delivering the vaccine are described below.

2. Method of manufacture

a) Differing methods of vaccine production are in use.

Before starting to produce vaccine, seed material with known characteristics is required (26). Three types of seed material are distinguished:

Master seed: Schizont-infected cells from a specific passage that have been selected and permanently stored and from which all other seed passages are derived.

To prepare Master seed, schizont-infected cells that have proved to be safe for cattle are propagated to obtain in a single culture passage approximately 5×10^8 cells. The cells are cryopreserved in about 100 cryotubes each containing 5×10^6 infected cells.

Working seed: Schizont-infected cells at a passage level between the Master seed and the Production seed. To prepare Working seed, the contents of a single cryotube of Master seed are transferred to a 10 ml centrifuge tube containing 8 ml complete medium. The tube is centrifuged at 600 ***g*** for 15 minutes at 4°C and the pellet is transferred into a 75 cm^2 culture flask containing 15–20 ml medium. The medium is replaced the next day, and 4 days later the cells are dispersed and subcultured in larger vessels. After 5–6 supplementary subcultivations, enough cells are available to start the production run.

Production seed: Schizont-infected cells from a specific passage level, which is used without further propagation, for preparation of a batch of vaccine.

The Production seed is obtained by propagating large numbers of cells in monolayers or suspension cultures. Monolayer cultures are grown in from 150 cm^2 to 175 cm^2 flasks that usually provide an average of 7×10^7 to 8×10^7 cells per vessel. About 80 ml of complete medium per flask is required. In a roller bottle culture system, $1.2–1.5 \times 10^8$ cells can be obtained in a conventional roller bottle (700 cm^2) containing 100–120 ml of medium. To obtain an optimal yield of cells from a given quantity of culture medium, flasks are incubated for 5 days and roller bottles for 6 days. The optimal initial concentration of cells for seeding the above vessels is about 2×10^5 cells/ml.

The schizont-infected cells from all vessels are harvested and pooled together and the total number is computed. Alternatively, about 20% of the cells may be seeded again to prepare another batch of vaccine. Several batches of vaccine can be produced using a portion of the Production seed as Working seed. As prolonged subcultivation may generate alterations in the features of the schizonts, such as immunogenic capacity, after several batches, subsequent vaccine is produced by making fresh Production seed from the Master seed.

Schizont-infected cells are mixed with dimethy sulphoxide (DMSO) at a final concentration of 7%, or glycerol (final concentration 10%) and dispensed in 1.8 ml aliquots in 2 ml plastic vials, each vial containing ten doses of concentrated vaccine. The proper number of schizont-infected cells per dose is a subject of controversy. Doses of $10^6–10^7$ infected cells are recommended in practical application in order to counteract variable environmental conditions in the field.

The vaccine is frozen by introducing the vials in an ultracold deep freezer (–70°C) and then transferred to liquid nitrogen after 24 hours. Alternatively vials can be introduced in liquid nitrogen vapours for 3 hours and then immersed in the liquid nitrogen for storage (24).

b) Cultured cells of two stocks (S11 and S15) are used in Iran (16). Each stock is concentrated in culture medium containing 9.5% glycerol to approximately 2×10^6 cells/ml, and 12 ml of concentrated cells are dispensed into 20 ml vials. These are cooled at –20°C for 1 hour, and then frozen to –70°C. The vaccine may be transferred to dry ice or liquid nitrogen storage. Vaccine is taken to the field in liquid nitrogen or dry ice; 20 ml of one vaccine stock is thawed at 37°C, and the animals are inoculated with 2 ml containing approximately 4×10^6 schizont-infected cells. The second stock is administered similarly within 30–60 days (16).

c) A fresh culture vaccine is used in Morocco, usually at a tenfold lower dose. However, there are problems with the quality control of vaccines of this kind.

3. Batch control

Before release the schizont vaccine is tested in Israel by the following procedure (26).

The frozen vaccine has a practically unlimited 'shelf life' in the frozen condition, but is usually produced in relatively small individual batches (5–10 thousand doses), which makes the full testing of each batch impracticable for economic reasons. It is recommended, therefore, that the Master seed be tested for safety and efficacy, while each batch be tested for sterility and potency only. This recommendation is based on the fact that once the cultured schizonts become attenuated, no reversion to virulence has ever been observed during further cultivation. As far as efficacy is concerned, no obvious alteration of the immunogenic properties has been detected during the limited number (20–30) of passages involved in producing the actual vaccine.

The procedures described for testing the vaccine are subject to approval by the veterinary authorities in the areas where the vaccine is used, and could be subject to modification if required by statutory regulations.

a) Safety

Freedom from properties causing undue local or systemic reactions: Despite the fact that the Master seed is prepared from attenuated schizonts, it is recommended for legal, as well as for practical reasons, to test the safety of a sample of actual vaccine that is produced from the particular Master seed. For this purpose, two to four susceptible calves, of the most sensitive stock available, are inoculated with a tenfold greater dose than is recommended for immunisation. This dose should not produce clinical signs beyond a transient rise in temperature. With completely attenuated Master seed, no schizonts or piroplasms will be seen in lymph node and liver smears or in blood films. However, different breeds of cattle may show different sensitivities to the vaccine. This should be borne in mind when vaccine from a partially attenuated Master seed is to be administered to high-grade cattle stocks.

Following a successful test for safety of a sample, all subsequent batches produced from the same Master seed can be released without further testing for safety. However, if parasites and clinical signs result from the vaccine in field cattle, the batch that has been involved, or another parallel one from the same Master seed, should be retested for safety.

b) Efficacy

Capacity to protect against naturally transmitted theileriosis. The batch of experimental vaccine used for the safety test can also be used for testing the efficacy of the culture-derived anti-theilerial vaccine. Three or four calves are vaccinated with a conventional dose of vaccine; 6 weeks later the vaccinated calves and the same number of unvaccinated calves are infected with sporozoites of *T. annulata*. Infection can be induced by infestation with live adult ticks issued from *T.-annulata*-infected preimaginal stages, or by inoculation of stabilate prepared from macerated infected ticks (for technique see Section B2.1). Experience shows that inoculation of stabilate (macerated ticks) generally induces a more severe response than an equivalent number of live infected ticks fed on cattle. However, in the long run, the results obtained by challenge with stabilate appear to be more reproducible than those obtained with different batches of live ticks, each infected under different conditions.

There are no internationally agreed standards for the size of a challenge dose used in testing the efficacy of *T. annulata* culture-derived vaccine. Five to ten female and the same number of male unfed infected *Hyalomma* ticks have been used for infection of cattle. Alternatively, stabilate equivalent to 2–4 macerated ticks inoculated subcutaneously in the neck area will invariably produce acute theileriosis. The responses to the challenge infection of the vaccinated and unvaccinated control calves are monitored through the following parameters: duration and severity of pyrexia, rate of schizont-infected cells in smears from lymph node or liver biopsy, rate of piroplasm infection in thin blood films, decrease in white and red blood cell counts, and severity of clinical manifestations such as anorexia, depression and recumbency.

The results of the efficacy test depends on factors such as the immunological characteristics of the *T. annulata* isolate grown and attenuated in culture, the virulence of the field isolate used for challenge, the species of infected ticks used to produce sporozoites, and the parasite dose used for challenge. Literature data (summarised by Pipano, 24) show that calves vaccinated with schizont vaccine may exhibit an apparently near total protection or may show a low level of parasitaemia, accompanied by mild fever and insignificant alteration of the remaining parameters from their prevaccination values. A lesser degree of protection was exhibited when cattle vaccinated with schizont vaccine were challenged with tick-derived parasites from a geographically remote area. In contrast, in most of the trials the nonvaccinated control calves exhibited high levels of parasitaemia and pancytopenia accompanied by severe clinical manifestations. In the absence of specific medication, a considerable portion of control animals succumbed to the infection.

Field observations have also been used for evaluation of the efficacy of anti-theileria vaccines (25). Susceptible indigenous cattle as well as high-grade exotic breeds were protected against clinical theileriosis and death in pastures on which nonvaccinated cattle succumbed to theileriosis. As completely attenuated schizont vaccine does not yield piroplasms, the presence of these theilerial stages in vaccinated cattle showing no clinical signs is considered to be the result of inapparent tick-induced infections.

c) Potency

Viability of schizont-infected cells: Frozen vaccine remains essentially stable during the storage period, even for long periods, but some loss of viability occurs during the freezing and thawing processes. Viability should be tested under conditions as similar as possible to those obtained when the vaccine is used in the field. For this reason, vaccine should be thawed and the diluted suspension of schizont-infected cells should be left at ambient temperature for 60 minutes before performing the viability tests. A simple test for evaluating viability of the infected cells is 'nigrosin dye exclusion counting' (30). Vaccine that, after being thawed and diluted and left at room temperature for 1 hour still contains 50% or more live cells can be released for use although in most cases 80–90% of live cells are found.

Viability of the schizonts is also reflected by the plating efficiency of the schizont-infected cells (30), as only cells containing viable schizonts multiply in culture. For this purpose, the thawed, diluted vaccine is transferred from the bottle to a centrifuge tube. A sample for counting is taken and the suspension is centrifuged for 15 minutes at 600 ***g***. Meanwhile, the total number of cells (live and dead) is determined in order to ascertain that the frozen vaccine had the necessary initial concentration of cells. After centrifugation, the supernatant is discarded and the cells are resuspended to the original volume using complete culture medium. Serial tenfold dilutions of cells in complete medium are performed in sterile 10 ml tubes so that the last two dilutions contain 5 × 10, and 5 cells per ml. Twelve replicates of 200 µl from each of the last two dilutions are introduced into a 96-well culture plate. The plates are incubated at 37°C in a 5% CO_2 atmosphere and cultures are checked with an inverted microscope 6 and 9 days after seeding. The number of wells theoretically containing 1 cell each in which growth is observed are counted. Vaccine showing a plating efficiency <2 (cells) are adequate for field use.

d) Sterility

Tests for sterility and freedom from contamination of biological materials may be found in Chapter I.4.

e) Method of use

These vaccines produce no adverse effects in healthy cattle (23). However, animals with existing infections, particularly viral infections, may not tolerate vaccination well. The administration of a viral vaccine, such as for foot and mouth disease, during the immunisation period (reaction period) should be avoided as the immune response to the *T. annulata* vaccine may be compromised (16). In Iran, it is recommended not to vaccinate cows that are over 5 months pregnant, although studies in Israel in pregnant cattle with similar vaccine stocks found no effect on pregnancy (24). The immunity engendered is long lasting.

In general, cattle should be immunised in the first few months of life, and tick challenge under natural conditions reinforces the immunity. Although antigenically different strains of *T. annulata* have been identified (24), it is generally considered that there is sufficient cross-protection among strains to provide adequate protection against field challenge throughout countries, such as Israel. In the vast infected areas in the region of the Caucasus mountains, a single stock has proved immunologically effective in 1.5 million cattle (10, 29). However, as described above, two stocks are used routinely in Iran (14).

B2. Infection and treatment vaccination for *Theileria parva*

Vaccination against *T. parva* is based on a method of infection and treatment in which an aliquot of ground-up ticks infected with nonattenuated, viable sporozoites is inoculated subcutaneously, and the animals are treated with tetracyclines (27). The tetracycline reduces the severity of the infection, and the resulting mild infection is usually controlled by the host's immune response, so that a carrier state is achieved. Precautions are necessary to prevent introduction of the disease, or new isolates of *T. parva*, to other areas. This method has also been applied effectively for *T. annulata*, but cell culture vaccination, which is not practical for immunisation against *T. parva*, is preferred. Some stabilates have been shown to infect cattle reliably without inducing disease, and these can be used without tetracycline treatment. One such stabilate is being applied in the field and offers considerable advantages over potentially lethal stabilate infections, and savings in the cost of treatment.

1. Stabilate preparation

Infection is established by inoculation of healthy serologically negative cattle with a tick stabilate of *T. parva*, or by application of infected ticks. During the parasitaemic phase of the ensuing disease reaction, clean laboratory-raised nymphs of *Rhipicephalus appendiculatus* are fed on the animals, and the engorged infected ticks are collected. The resultant adult ticks are applied within 3 weeks to 4 months after moulting in ear-bags on healthy rabbits. About 600 ticks are applied to each ear and any unattached ticks are removed after 24 hours. After 4 days, the ticks are removed and counted into batches of approximately 1000. An estimate of the total number of ticks can be obtained by counting and weighing a given number of ticks, and then weighing the total number of ticks. The ticks are washed in a sieve under fast flowing tap water and may be surface disinfected in 1% benzalkonium chloride, or surface sterilised by washing in 70% alcohol, and then again in water. The infection rate is also determined on dissected salivary glands from (usually 60) 4-day fed ticks.

The ticks are placed (~1000) in heavy glass specimen jars or plastic beakers, and 50 ml MEM with Hank's or Earle's salt and 3.5% bovine plasma albumin (BPA), is added. The jars are kept on ice, and the ticks are ground using a tissue grinder homogeniser (for instance Silverson LR2) for 2 minutes using a large aperture disintegrating head, and for 3 minutes using a small aperture head (emulsor screen). The ground-up tick material is usually made up to 50 ml for every 1000 ticks, then centrifuged at 50 ***g*** for 5 minutes, and the supernatant is harvested. An equal volume of cold 15% glycerol in MEM/BPA is added dropwise while the tick material is maintained chilled on ice and stirred by a magnetic stirrer. The final volume will contain sporozoites from the equivalent of ten ticks/ml, but can be adjusted if a different concentration is required because a tick batch was very heavily infected or had a very low infection rate. The final concentration of glycerol in the sporozoite stabilate is 7.5%.

The ground-up tick material is then dispensed into vials by syringe or pipette for small total volumes, or by automatic syringe for larger volumes. Alternatively, artificial insemination equipment for semen dispensation has been used with prelabelled plastic straws. This latter system is ideal for large volume stabilates, and colour coding and labelling provide extra security by identifying each straw. An equilibration time of 30–45 minutes at 4°C should be allowed for small-volume stabilates before they are placed in an ultracold deep freezer (–70°C). For large volumes of stabilate the equilibration time is usually included as part of the dispensing time. Once frozen, the stabilate may be transferred to permanent storage in liquid nitrogen taking care not to allow any significant increase in temperature during transfer.

The infectivity of the stabilate is determined by inoculation of a standard dose of 1.0 ml into susceptible cattle. The stabilate is then titrated, and its infectivity and lethality at different dilutions are established for use in immunisation. The sensitivity to tetracyclines is also determined, essentially to provide a dose of stabilate that is controlled, preferably by a single dose of long-acting tetracycline administered at the same time as inoculation. The immunising dose should induce a very mild or inapparent infection (4), and the animal should develop a serological titre and be immune to lethal homologous challenge. Should a single treatment with tetracycline fail to suppress the infection in all cattle, then either a lower dose of stabilate is examined or two treatments of tetracycline (on days 0 and 4) may be used. An alternative method that has been used involves stabilate infection and treatment with parvaquone at 20 mg/kg on day 8 (depending on the stabilate). This method can be applied where tetracyclines are not reliable, but it requires that the animal be handled more than once. A single treatment with buparvaquone at 2.5 mg/kg at the time of infection has also been shown to be effective with stabilate infections that were not controlled with a single treatment at 20 mg/kg of a long-acting formulation of tetracycline.

Whichever method of immunisation or treatment is adopted, it must be adhered to strictly in the field, or failure or breakdown will occur. It is also important to determine the stabilate and drug/dose regimen in the most susceptible cattle in which it is likely to be used. The method is usually applied using long-acting tetracyline, and it is recommended that the tetracyline be administered before the stabilate, in case an animal escapes.

2. Safety precautions

At a meeting in Malawi in 1988, the following recommendations on safety in the preparation, handling and delivery of *T. parva* infection and treatment vaccines were adopted (4).

a) Field collection of ticks

Consideration should be given to the possible hazard to humans from pathogens present in field-collected ticks. The most important pathogen that has been recognised is Crimean Congo haemorrhagic fever virus, usually associated with ticks of the genus *Hyalomma* and widely prevalent within the geographical distribution of *Rhipicephalus appendiculatus*. Those handling field tick collections should, therefore, be made aware of potential hazards. Ticks of *Hyalomma* species generally should not be removed from hosts; engorged or partially engorged ticks should not be crushed between the fingers. If removed, ticks should be handled with a forceps.

b) Tick-handling facilities

The handling of field-collected ticks in the laboratory must be controlled in order to avoid accidental attachment to personnel. Field-collected ticks should be fed on rabbits and cattle in isolation facilities. Animals on which laboratory-infected or field-collected ticks have fed should be destroyed following transmission and pick-up before leaving the isolation facilities. Following engorgement of field-collected ticks on laboratory animals, aliquots should be homogenised and tested for extraneous human pathogens by inoculation in baby hamster kidney (BHK) and Vero cells. The effects of these inoculations should be studied through three passages. Any unused ticks should be destroyed by chemical means or by incineration.

c) Stabilate preparation

Care should be taken during the preparation of sporozoite stabilates to avoid aerosol infection of personnel with extraneous pathogens when ticks are being ground. Those grinding ticks should be educated in the potential hazards involved; access to areas where ticks are homogenised should be restricted to specified and informed personnel; personnel should wear protective clothing, including gloves and masks; and tick grinding should be carried out under a biohazard hood.

3. Purity of stabilates

Both ticks and experimental mammals are potential sources of contamination of stabilates with extraneous pathogens. In both cases, potential contaminants include *Ehrlichia bovis*, bovine *Borrelia* sp., Orbiviruses, Bunya viruses, and others. Field-collected ticks should therefore not be used for the preparation of bulk stabilates. Well characterised and pathogen-free laboratory colonies of ticks should be used for this purpose. Only healthy cattle and rabbits, free from tick-borne parasites, should be used for tick feeding. The infections to be considered are those transmissible by *R. appendiculatus* and *Hyalomma* ticks. Although conventional laboratory examinations and even advanced techniques do not always detect latent infections in mammals, serological tests and the PCR appear to be the most adequate tests for detecting carriers of silent infections. The tests to be performed depend on the epizootological situation in the area from which animals for breeding ticks are acquired. The most common tick-transmissible infections in bovines are rickettial agents *(Ehrlichia, Coxiella, Anaplasma),* viral agents (Crimean Congo haemmorhagic fever) and protozoan agents (mainly *Theileria* spp.). Stabilates should be prepared as aseptically as possible. Under some conditions, the use of antibiotics at concentrations appropriate for tissue culture may be indicated. Prepared stabilates should be subjected to routine tests for safety by inoculation into BHK and Vero cells, followed by three passages in these systems (as above). Stabilates should be subjected to routine characterisation *in vivo*, which should involve infectivity testing in intact susceptible cattle, sensitivity to tetracyclines and other anti-theilerial drugs, and cross-immunity *in vivo*.

Care must be taken to avoid contamination of the stock being used for preparation of stabilates in the laboratory with other *T. parva* stocks. A set of rules should therefore be established for the handling of infected ticks and the rules should be adhered to rigidly. Tick unit facilities should allow for strict separation of infected and uninfected ticks. Tick unit personnel should use separate overalls for each batch of ticks used in stabilate preparation, and the overalls should be sterilised daily. Simultaneous work on many different stocks should be avoided. Stabilate storage systems should incorporate clear labelling of each stabilate tube or straw.

4. Effect of an immunising stock

The introduction of an immunising stock into an area/country from which it does not originate may result in that parasite, or a component parasite(s) of that stock, becoming established through a carrier state in cattle and transmission by ticks. The long-term effect of the introduction of new (and potentially lethal) parasites on the disease epidemiology should be considered before introduction, and should be monitored carefully following immunisation. This requirement appears to be important mainly for *T. parva* as the attenuated schizonts used for *T. annulata* vaccination do not become a source of infection for ticks.

The characterisation of parasites in target populations should be carried out before immunisation, and at intervals following immunisation. At present, the characterisation of parasite stocks with reference to vaccination relies primarily on immunisation and cross-challenge experiments in cattle. However, a number of methods for characterising parasite stocks *in vitro* have been attempted in laboratories possessing a high degree of expertise. Preliminary studies have shown that parasite stocks that differ in MAb profile may not cross-protect, whereas stocks showing similar profiles give good cross-protection (17). Another method to detect antigenic differences has used T cell clones specific for parasitised cell lines, as T cell responses are believed to be important in mediating immunity against *T. parva* (17). Recently a statistically derived disease reaction index, based on parasitological, clinical and haematological measurements, was proposed for characterising levels of infectivity and virulence of different parasite stocks and assessing the impact of control intervention against theileriosis (28).

5. Vaccination strategy

Unlike *T. annulata*, where a considerable cross-protection is observed among different strains in the field, a very much more complex situation exists for *T. parva*. Two strategies are used to try to overcome this antigenic complexity. A combination of three stocks, which provides a broad spectrum of protection, has been tested in a number of countries. The combination was prepared under strict quality controlled conditions in Malawi in an FAO (Food and Agriculture Organization of the United Nations) project for distribution within the *T. parva*-endemic region. If this combination fails to protect, the breakthrough strain will have to be isolated, characterised and used alone or added to the combination. The other strategy is to prepare national or local stocks for use within defined areas. This latter strategy is more costly in time and resources, but it avoids, to some extent, the introduction of new stocks into an area. The infection and treatment method of immunisation is effective, but the attendant delivery problems and the risk of induction of carrier states and disease transmission, all emphasise the need for the identification of protective antigens for development of subunit vaccines.

REFERENCES

1. ALLSOPP B.A. & ALLSOPP M.T.E.P. (1988). *Theileria parva:* genomic DNA studies reveal non-specific diversity. *Mol. Biochem. Parasitol.,* **28**, 77–84.

2. ALLSOPP B.A., BAYLIS H.A., ALLSOPP M.T.E.P., CAVALIER-SMITH T., BISHOP R.P., CARRINGTON D.M., SOHANPAL B. & SPOONER P. (1993). Discrimination between six species of *Theileria* using oligonucleotide probes which detect small subunit ribosomal RNA sequences. *Parasitology,* **107**, 157–165.

3. ALLSOPP B.A,, CARRINGTON M., BAYLIS H.A., SOHAL S., DOLAN T.T. & IAMS K. (1989). Improved characterization of *Theileria parva* isolates using the polymerase chain reaction and oligonucleotide probes. *Mol. Biochem. Parasitol.*, **35**, 137–148.

4. ANON. (1989). Theileriasis in Eastern, Central and Southern Africa, Dolan T.T., ed. Proceedings of a meeting on East Coast fever immunization held in Malawi, 18–20 September 1988. International Laboratory for Research on Animal Diseases, Nairobi, Kenya, 174–176.

5. BISHOP R.P., ALLSOPP B.A., SPOONER P.R., SOHANPAL B.K., MORZARIA S.P. & GOBRIGHT E.I. (1995). *Theileria:* improved species discrimination using oligonucleotides derived from large subunit ribosomal RNA sequences. *Exp. Parasitol.*, **80**, 107–115.

6. BROWN C.G.D. (1979). Propagation of *Theileria. In:* Practical Tissue Culture Application, Maramorosch K. & Hirumi H., eds. Academic Press, New York, USA, 223–254.

7. BURRIDGE M., BROWN C.G.D. & KIMBER C. (1974). *Theileria annulata*: cross reactions between a cell culture schizont antigen and antigens of East African *Theileria* species in the indirect fluorescent antibody test. *Exp. Parasitol.*, **35**, 374–380.

8. CONRAD P.A., IAMS K., BROWN W.C., SOHANPAL B. & OLE-MOIYOI O.K. (1987). DNA probes detect genomic diversity in *Theileria parva* stocks. *Mol. Biochem. Parasitol.*, **25**, 213–226.

9. DARGHOUTH M.E.A., BOUATTOUR A., BEN-MILED L. & SASSI L. (1996). Diagnosis of *Theileria annulata* – infection of cattle in Tunisia: comparison of serology and blood smears. *Vet. Res.*, **27**, 613–627.

10. DOLAN T.T. (1989). Theileriasis: A comprehensive review. *Rev. sci. tech. Off. int. Epiz.*, **8**, 11–36.

11. D'OLIVEIRA C., VANDERWERDE M., HABELA M., JACQUIET P. & JONGEJAN F. (1995). Detection of *Theileria annulata* in blood samples of carrier cattle by PCR. *J. Clin. Microb.*, **33**, 2665–2669.

12. FOOD AND AGRICULTURE ORGANIZATION OF THE UNITED NATIONS (FAO) (1984). Tick and Tick-borne Disease Control: A Practical Field Manual. FAO, Rome, Italy.

13. FUJISAKI K., KAWAZU S. & KAMIO T. (1994). The taxonomy of the bovine *Theileria* spp. *Parasitology Today,* **10**, 31–33.

14. GODDEERIS B.M., KATENDE J.M., IRVIN A.D. & CHUMO R.S.C. (1982). Indirect fluorescent antibody test for experimental and epidemiological studies on East Coast fever (*Theileria parva* infection of cattle). Evaluation of a cell culture schizont antigen fixed and stored in suspension. *Res. Vet. Sci.*, **33**, 360–365.

15. GRAY M.A., LUCKINS A.G., RAE P.F. & BROWN C.G.D. (1980). Evaluation of an enzyme immunoassay for serodiagnosis of infections with *Theileria parva* and *T. annulata. Res. Vet. Sci.,* **29**, 360–366.

16. HASHEMI-FESHARKI R. (1988). Control of *Theileria annulata* in Iran. *Parasitology Today,* **4**, 36–40.

17. IRVIN A.D. & MORRISON W.I. (1987). Immunopathology, immunology, and immunoprophylaxis of *Theileria* infections. *In:* Immune Responses in Parasitic Infections: Immunology, Immunopathology, and Immunoprophylaxis, Soulsby E.J.L. ed. CRC Press, Boca Raton, Florida, USA, 223–274.

18. KACHANI M., FLACH E.J., WILLIAMSON S., OUHELLI H., EL HASNAOUI M. & SPOONER R.L. (1996). The use of an enzyme-linked immunosorbent assay for tropical theileriosis research in Morocco. *Preventive Vet. Med.* **26**, 329–339.

19. KACHANI M., SPOONER R., RAE P., BELL-SAKYI L. & BROWN D. (1992). Stage-specific responses following infection with *Theileria annulata* as evaluated using ELISA. *Parasitol. Res.*, **78** (1), 43–47.

20. KATENDE J., GODDEERIS B.M., MORZARIA S.P., NKONGE C.K. & MUSOKE A.J. (1990). Identification of *Theileria mutans*-specific antigen for use in an antibody antigen detection ELISA. *Parasitology Immunol.,* **12**, 419–433.

21. MORZARIA S.P., MUSOKE A.J., DOLAN T.T., NENE V., NORVAL R.A.I. & BISHOP R. (1989). Studies on pathogenic *Theileria mutans.* Annual Scientific Report, International Laboratory for Research on Animal Diseases, Nairobi, Kenya, 7–8.

22. MUSOKE A.J., KATENDE J.M., TOYE P.G., SKILTON R.A., IAMS K.P., NENE V. & MORZARIA S.P. (1994). Progress towards development of an antibody detection ELISA for the diagnosis of *Theileria parva. In:* Use of Applicable Biotechnology Methods for Diagnosing Haemoparasites. Proceeding of the Expert Consultation, FAO, Rome, Italy, 174–181.

23. PIPANO E. (1977). Basic principles of *Theileria annulata* control. *In:* Theileriosis, Henson J.B. & Campbell M., eds. International Development Research Centre, Ottawa, Canada, 55–65.

24. PIPANO E. (1989). Bovine theileriosis in Israel. *Rev. sci. tech. Off. int. Epiz.*, **8**, 79–87.

25. PIPANO E. (1989). Vaccination against *Theileria annulata* theileriosis. *In:* Veterinary Protozoan and Hemoparasite Vaccines, Wright I.G., ed. CRC Press, Boca Raton, Florida, USA, 203–234.

26. PIPANO E. (1997). Vaccines against hemoparasitic diseases in Israel with special reference to quality assurance. *Trop. Anim. Health Prod.*, **29**, 86S–90S.

27. RADLEY D.E. (1981). Infection and treatment immunization against theileriosis. *In:* Advances in the Control of Theileriosis, Irvin A.D., Cunningham M.P. & Young A.S., eds. Martinus Nijhoff Publishers, The Hague, The Netherlands, 227–237.

28. ROWLANDS G.J., MUSOKE A.J., MORZARIA S.P., NAGDA S.M., BALLINGALL K.T. & MCKEEVER D.J. (2000). A statistically derived index for classifying East Coast fever reactions in cattle challenged with *Theileria parva* under experimental conditions. *Parasitology,* **120**, 371–381.

29. STEPANOVA N.I. & ZABLOTSKII V.T. (1989). Bovine theileriosis in the USSR. *Rev. sci. tech. Off. int. Epiz.*, **8**, 89–92.

30. WATHANGA J.M., JONES T.W. & BROWN C.G.D. (1986). Cryopreservation of *Theileria* infected lymphoblastoid cells with functional assessment of viability. *Trop. Anim. Health Prod.*, **18**, 191.

*

* *

CHAPTER 2.3.12.

HAEMORRHAGIC SEPTICAEMIA

SUMMARY

Haemorrhagic septicaemia (HS) is an acute, highly fatal septicaemic disease of cattle and buffaloes caused by certain serotypes of Pasteurella multocida. *It is a primary pasteurellosis reproducible in susceptible animals with pure cultures of the causative organism alone.*

The diagnosis of HS depends on the isolation of the causative organism, P. multocida, *from the blood or bone marrow of a dead animal by cultural and biological methods, and the identification of the organism and type by biochemical and serological methods.*

Identification of the agent: *Pure cultures of* P. multocida *can be obtained by streaking material on to artificial media or by the inoculation of suspect infective material into mice, and the subsequent culture of their blood after death in a suitable medium. Identification is made on the basis of the morphological, cultural, and biochemical characteristics of* P. multocida.

The identification of the specific serotype is carried out using one or more serological methods. These include rapid slide agglutination, indirect haemagglutination for 'capsular' typing using sheep red blood cells coated with bacterial extracts, 'somatic' typing by agar gel immunodiffusion tests using heat-treated cell extracts, or agglutination using acid-treated cells.

Serological tests: *Serological tests for detecting specific antibodies are not normally used for diagnostic purposes.*

Requirements for vaccines and diagnostic biologicals: *Vaccines against haemorrhagic septicaemia are simple formalin-killed bacterins, or dense bacterins with adjuvants. The latter enhance the level and prolong the duration of immunity.*

Cultures for the production of vaccines should contain capsulated seed cultures. They are standardised as to their bacterial density on the basis of turbidity tests. Potency tests are most conveniently carried out in mice and/or rabbits.

A. DIAGNOSTIC TECHNIQUES

Haemorrhagic septicaemia (HS) is an acute, highly fatal, septicaemic disease of cattle and buffaloes caused by certain serotypes of *Pasteurella multocida* (2, 7, 9, 10). Presently, two serotypes are recognised – the Asian serotype and the African serotype. Three serotyping methods are available – the 'capsular' typing method using an indirect haemagglutination (IHA) test (4), 'somatic' typing using agglutination, and the agar gel immunodiffusion (AGID) test (11, 15, 16). The Asian strains belong to capsular type B only while the African strains are types B and E (14). Using the somatic typing methods, all strains belong to type 6 by the agglutination tests and type 2 by the AGID test.

A clinical diagnosis can be made on the basis of characteristic signs, gross pathological lesions, herd history, morbidity and mortality patterns, species susceptibility and age group affected. A tentative clinical diagnosis is generally useful in order to initiate control measures.

Laboratory confirmation of diagnosis is by isolation in culture or in mice, followed by identification of the causative agent by biochemical and serological methods as type B or E. Exceptionally, when *in-vitro* culture is not successful, a mouse may be inoculated with the clinical sample. Blood from the mouse is then used for the preparation of blood films on slides and for culture of the organism, which can be used subsequently in rapid slide agglutination tests. Further confirmation is carried out using biochemical and conventional serological tests.

The clinical syndrome of HS consists of an initial phase of temperature elevation (often unnoticed), a phase of respiratory involvement, and a terminal phase of septicaemia and recumbency leading to death. The incubation period is usually 1–3 days, and the course of the disease may range from sudden death, with no observable clinical signs, to a protracted course extending up to 5 days (7, 10).

At post-mortem examination, the first obvious lesion is subcutaneous oedema, particularly in the submandibular and brisket region. Other lesions include petechial to ecchymotic haemorrhages, congestion and/or consolidation of lungs, fibrinous pneumonia, pleurisy and pericarditis (7, 10).

Buffaloes are generally believed to be more susceptible to HS than cattle, and in this species, the disease course is shorter. In endemic areas, most deaths are confined to older calves and young adults. In nonendemic areas, massive epizootics may occur. Case fatality approaches 100% if treatment is not carried out sufficiently early (in the pyrexic stage) (7, 10).

1. Identification of the agent

• Cultural and biochemical methods

The septicaemia in HS occurs at the terminal stage of the disease. Therefore, blood samples taken from sick animals before death may not always contain *P. multocida* organisms. Also, they are not consistently present in the nasal secretions of sick animals.

A blood sample or swab collected from the heart is satisfactory if it is taken within a few hours of death. If the animal has been dead for a long time, a long bone, free of tissue, can be taken. If there is no facility for post-mortem examination, blood can be collected from the jugular vein by incision or aspiration. Blood samples in any standard transport medium should be dispatched on ice and well packed to avoid any leakage.

Blood smears from affected animals are stained with Gram, Leishman's or methylene blue stains. The organisms appear as Gram-negative, bipolar-staining short bacilli. No conclusive diagnosis can be made on the basis of direct microscopic examinations alone.

A suitable medium for the growth of *Pasteurella* is casein/sucrose/yeast (CSY) agar containing 5% blood. The composition of this medium is casein hydrolysate (3 g), sucrose (3 g), yeast extract (5 g), sodium chloride (5 g), anhydrous dipotassium hydrogen orthophosphate (3 g), and distilled water to 1 litre. The pH is adjusted to 7.3–7.4, after which 1.5% agar is added. The medium is autoclaved at 1 bar for 15 minutes. After cooling to 45–50°C, 5% calf blood (antibody-free *P. multocida*) is added (26).

Blood samples, or swabs eluted into 2–3 ml sterile physiological saline, are cultured. Alternatively, the surface of a long bone is swabbed with alcohol, flame sterilised and split open. The marrow is extracted aseptically and cultured. Direct culture is usually satisfactory only if the material is fresh and free from contaminants or post-mortem invaders that would otherwise overgrow any *Pasteurella* present.

For biological examinations, a small volume (0.2 ml) of eluted blood swabs or a portion of bone marrow in saline is inoculated subcutaneously or intramuscularly into mice. The mouse usually serves as a biological 'screen' for extraneous organisms. The mice die in 24–36 hours following inoculation, and a pure growth of *P. multocida* can be seen in blood smears. Pure cultures of *P. multocida* can usually be grown from blood cultures of the mice, even when the original samples come from relatively old carcasses. The organism can be identified by its morphological and cultural characteristics, biochemical reactions and serological tests.

Freshly isolated *P. multocida* forms smooth, greyish glistening translucent colonies, approximately 1 mm in diameter, on blood agar after 24 hours' incubation at 37°C. Colonies grown on CSY agar are larger. Old cultures, particularly those grown on media devoid of blood, may produce smaller colonies. *Pasteurella multocida* does not grow on MacConkey agar. Gram-stained blood or tissue smears show Gram-negative, short, ovoid, bipolar-staining coccoid forms. A degree of pleomorphism will be noted, particularly in old cultures, with longer rods of varying length. The bipolar staining will be more evident with methylene blue or Leishman's stain.

HS organisms produce oxidase, catalase and indole, and will reduce nitrates. They do not produce hydrogen sulphide or urease, and fail to use citrate or liquefy gelatin. Glucose and sucrose are always fermented with the production of acid only. Most strains also ferment sorbitol. Some strains ferment arabinose, xylose and maltose, whereas salicin and lactose are almost invariably not fermented.

One property of HS-causing strains of *P. multocida* is the ability to produce the enzyme hyaluronidase (5). Having identified the genus and species by cultural characteristics and biochemical tests, hyaluronidase production may then be used as a specific test for HS-causing pasteurellae. It should be noted that B serotypes other than B.2 (or 6:B), and type E, are hyaluronidase negative.

A hyaluronic-acid-producing culture is streaked across the centre of a dextrose starch agar plate. The pasteurella culture to be tested for hyaluronidase production is streaked at right angles. The plates are incubated at 37°C for 18 hours. Originally, hyaluronic-acid-producing *Streptococcus equi* were used, but a convenient culture for this purpose is a capsulated mucoid *P. multocida* type A culture. At the point of intersection, the mucoid growth of the hyaluronic acid producer will diminish into a thin line of growth, indicating the production of hyaluronidase by the test culture. Use of freshly prepared plates and a humidified incubator will facilitate hyaluronic acid production and, thereby, the reading of the test.

- **Immunological methods**

Several immunological tests are used for the identification of the HS-causing serotypes of *P. multocida*. These consist of a rapid slide agglutination test (16), an IHA test for capsular typing (4), an agglutination test using hydrochloric-acid-treated cells for somatic typing (17), the AGID test (1, 11, 27), and the counter immunoelectrophoresis test (CIEP) (6).

Hyperimmune antisera for most of these tests are prepared against specific reference strains in rabbits. Cultures in CSY broth (6–8-hours old) are seeded on to CSY blood agar medium. After overnight incubation (18–20 hours) the growth is washed into physiological saline containing 0.3% formalin. The turbidity of the cell suspension is adjusted to that of Brown's tube No. 7. Rabbits are inoculated intravenously at 3–4-day intervals with 0.2, 0.5, 1.0, 1.5 and finally, 2.0 ml of this suspension. The rabbits are inoculated subcutaneously or intramuscularly 1 week after the last injection with 0.5 ml of a similar, but live, suspension. The animals are bled 10 days later. The serum is stored at –20°C, but small quantities for regular use are stored at 4°C with the addition of 1/10,000 merthiolate.

a) Rapid slide agglutination test (capsular typing)

A single colony is mixed with a drop of saline on a slide, a drop of antiserum is added, and the slide is warmed gently. A coarse, floccular agglutination appears within 30 seconds. Old cultures may give a fine, granular agglutination that takes longer to appear.

b) Indirect hemagglutination test (capsular typing)

This was originally performed using antigen-sensitised human type 'O' red blood cells (RBCs) (4), but more recently sheep RBCs have been used (20, 26). The antigen is prepared as follows:

A 6–8-hour broth culture of a reference strain is seeded on to CSY blood agar plates and incubated overnight at 37°C. The growth is harvested in 3 ml physiological saline containing 0.3% formalin. This suspension is then heated at 56°C for 30 minutes, centrifuged at 3000 ***g*** for 15 minutes at 4°C, and the clear supernatant fluid is stored at –20°C. If a refrigerated centrifuge is not available, centrifugation at 1500 ***g*** for 30 minutes gives a supernatant fluid. This is used as the antigen extract. A similar procedure is followed for preparing an antigen extract from an unknown strain that is to be typed.

Sheep blood is collected aseptically into an anticoagulant and centrifuged at 500 ***g*** for 10 minutes. The packed RBCs are washed three times in sterile physiological saline. The antigen extract from an unknown strain prepared by the method described above is used to sensitise the RBCs or absorbed on to the RBCs. This is done by adding 15 volumes of the antigen extract to the RBCs and incubating the mixture for 1 hour at 37°C with frequent shaking. The sensitised RBCs are recovered by centrifugation, washed three times in sterile physiological saline, and made up to a final 1% suspension in physiological saline. The type-specific hyperimmune antiserum (three volumes) is absorbed by the addition of packed RBCs (one volume) for 30 minutes at room temperature, then centrifuged at 500 ***g*** for 10 minutes to pellet the RBCs. The absorbed antiserum is then inactivated by heating at 56°C for 30 minutes.

The test itself can be carried out in tubes or plates, and is performed in two rows. The test described below is for Lucite plates.

i) The capsular extract of the unknown strain is prepared as described above and used to sensitise the sheep RBCs. The known type-specific hyperimmune sera raised in rabbits against types A, B, D and E are diluted as follows:

ii) Using four separate rows of wells the first wells are filled with 0.72 ml saline followed by 0.4 ml in the next six wells or more.

iii) The type-specific hyperimmune sera are each separately diluted in each row by adding 0.08 ml of the serum to the first well and mixing with a pipette. From this well 0.4 ml is transferred to the next well, mixed, and the process carried on until well seven. This constitutes 1/10 dilution in the first well and a doubling dilution thereafter.

iv) All the wells are each filled with 0.4 ml of antigen-adsorbed/sensitised RBCs, shaken slightly and left at room temperature. By the addition of the sensitised blood, the serum dilution in the wells are doubled, i.e. 1/20 in well one, 1/40 in the second, and so on. A positive, negative and saline control are included for each test run.

v) The first reading is taken after 2 hours and a final reading after 18 hours. A course agglutination of the RBCs along the sides of the concave wells is taken as a positive reading, and the formation of a button at the centre of the wells as negative. An arbitrary score of 1–4 is given depending on the size of the agglutination. An unknown strain is identified with the hyperimmune serum that has agglutination. In the absence of agglutination with all sera, the strain is considered to be untypeable.

While IHA can be used for typing unknown strains, the test itself is more efficient when dealing with serotypes B and E and is more reliable as quantitative tests against these strains.

c) Agar gel immunodiffusion tests

AGID tests are used for what is described as 'capsular' as well as 'somatic' typing, depending on the antigens and antisera used. The double diffusion technique is employed. Wells are punched in the solid agar in a circular pattern with one centre well surrounded by six peripheral wells.

i) *Capsular typing:* The gel medium is 1.0% Noble agar, or equivalent product, in 0.2 M phosphate buffer containing merthiolate at a final concentration of 1/10,000 (1, 27). Antigens and antisera are the same as for capsular typing by the IHA method (4). The standard antiserum is placed in the centre well, and the test antigens are placed in the peripheral wells alternately with standard homologous antigen.

ii) *Somatic typing:* The gel medium consists of special Noble agar, or equivalent product, at a concentration of 0.9% in 8.5% sodium chloride solution.

iii) For antigen preparation, the growth from each plate is harvested in 1 ml of 8.5% sodium chloride containing 0.3% formalin. The suspension is heated at 100°C for 1 hour, the cells are sedimented by centrifugation, and the supernatant fluid is used as antigen.

iv) Antisera against 16 somatic types (11) are prepared in chickens. Oil-emulsified bacterin (1 ml) is injected subcutaneously into the mid-portion of the neck of 12–16-week-old male birds. A further injection is made 3 weeks later of 1 ml intramuscularly into the breast, 0.5 ml on each side of the sternum. The birds are bled 1 week later, and the serum is separated and preserved with 0.01% thiomersal and 0.06% phenol. Sera are tested against all somatic types and sera that cross-react are discarded.

v) The test antigen is placed in the centre well and antisera against the different serotypes are placed in the peripheral wells. All haemorrhagic septicaemia serotypes (Asian and African) will react with type 2 antiserum. Cross-reactions may occur with type 5.

d) Counter immunoelectrophoresis

CIEP offers a rapid method for the identification of capsular types B and E cultures.

i) *Preparation of capsular substance:* Capsular substance is prepared in the same manner as described for the IHA test.

ii) *Preparation of hyperimmune antisera:* Antisera are prepared in rabbits as for the IHA test.

iii) *Medium for CIEP:* The medium for the CIEP consists of agarose (2.0 g), barbitone sodium (2.06 g), diethyl barbituric acid (0.37 g), distilled water (180 ml), and 1/1000 merthiolate (20 ml).

iv) *Veronal acetate buffer (barbitone buffer):* The barbitone buffer consists of barbitone sodium (29.24 g), anhydrous sodium acetate (11.70 g), 0.1 N hydrochloric acid (180 ml), and distilled water to 3 litres. The pH should be 8.8.

v) *Preparation of slides:* The electrophoresis plates are prepared by precoating glass slides (57 mm × 70 mm) with 12 ml volumes of the medium. Seven wells, 4 mm in diameter and 7 mm apart, are cut in a row. A parallel set of wells is cut 6 mm (centre to centre) away from the other set of wells.

vi) *Test procedure:* The well on the side of the cathode is loaded with a 20 µl volume of capsular antigen, while an equal volume of type-specific antiserum is loaded on to the well on the side of the anode. Controls included in the test are 0.85% sodium chloride solution against positive antiserum, and capsular extract against negative rabbit serum. The electrophoresis tank is filled with barbitone buffer, pH 8.8. The antigen and antiserum are electrophoresed for 30 minutes at 150 V (25 V/cm). The plates are then examined for precipitation lines.

vii) *Interpretation of the results:* The presence of a distinct line between the antigen and antiserum wells is considered to be a positive result.

e) **Agglutination tests (somatic antigen)**

The somatic 'O' antigen is prepared essentially by a method described previously (15, 17). A 6–8-hour test culture is seeded on to CSY blood agar and incubated overnight. The growth is harvested in 2–3 ml of physiological saline containing 0.3% formalin per plate, and centrifuged at 3000 ***g*** for 15 minutes at 4°C (or 1200–1500 ***g*** for 30–45 minutes at room temperature). The deposited bacteria are resuspended in 25 ml normal HCl saline (0.85% saline in a normal HCl solution) to give an opacity approximately equivalent to Brown's opacity tube No. 6, and incubated overnight. The suspension is again centrifuged, the supernatant fluid is discarded, and the cell residue is washed three times successively in phosphate buffered saline (PBS) at pH 5.0, 6.0 and 7.0, respectively.

Finally, a suspension of the residual cells, equivalent to Brown's opacity tube No. 6, is prepared in PBS at pH 7.0. Any suspensions that autoagglutinate should be discarded.

Antisera are prepared against whole bacterial cell suspensions of the reference strains 6:B (Asian HS), 6:E (African HS) and 11:B (Australian 989, non-HS). Agglutination tests are carried out on a slide and the test antigen is used against the three types of sera. A fine granular agglutination indicates a specific somatic agglutination. Tests carried out against the standard antigens will facilitate reading and interpretation. When nonspecific partial agglutination occurs, the tests carried out with tenfold dilutions of the serum against the test and standard antigens will help to identify somatic antigen.

f) **Serotype designation**

Broadly, two typing systems are adopted. One is 'capsular' typing by Carter's IHA test (4) or by AGID tests (1, 27). The other is 'somatic' typing by the method of Namioka & Murata (15, 17, 18), and by the method of Heddleston, Gallagher & Rebers (11). It is generally agreed that designation of serotypes should be based on a somatic-capsular combination. Two systems commonly in use are the Namioka–Carter and the Carter–Heddleston systems. In the former system, Asian and African HS serotypes are designated 6:B and 6:E, respectively, while in the latter system they are designated B.2 and E.2, respectively.

• **Nucleic acid recognition methods**

Polymerase chain reaction (PCR) amplification of specific DNA sequences allows rapid detection and presumptive identification of organisms directly from either clinical specimens or from small amounts of mixed or pure bacterial cultures. Complex DNA extraction and purification procedures are not required unless blood, urine or faecal specimens are used. PCR-inhibitory compounds present in these materials need to be removed or inactivated prior to amplification.

a) ***Pasteurella-multocida*-specific PCR assay**

PCR technology can be applied for rapid, sensitive and specific detection of *P. multocida* (13, 19, 24). While some disadvantages are evident with each published method, the rapidity and high specificity of the *P.-multocida*-specific PCR assay (24) provides optimal efficiency without the need for additional hybridisation. Although the use of hybridisation can confirm specificity, this approach is usually possible only in specialised laboratories. The *P.-multocida*-specific PCR identifies all subspecies of *P. multocida;* subsp. *multocida*, subsp. *gallicida*, and subsp. *septica* through specific amplification of a ~460 bp DNA fragment within the KMT1 gene. While DNA is also amplified from *Pasteurella canis* biovar 2, these species are readily distinguished by indole fermentation patterns.

A fraction of an isolated colony of the suspect organism is transferred directly into the PCR mixture. Alternatively, template DNA can be obtained from 2 µl of either a mixed or pure broth culture. All currently used methods for the preparation of template DNA produce reproducible results with the KMT1 primers (24), and allow detection of <10 organisms per reaction. The sensitivity and specificity of the *P.-multocida*-specific PCR offer the most compelling argument for the use of PCR technology in laboratory investigation of suspected HS cases. *Pasteurella multocida* can be detected regardless of purity of the specimen, an advantage if the specimen is from an old carcass or from tonsil or nasal swabs. In such cases, the swab should be inoculated in 2 ml CSY broth and incubated on a roller for 2–4 hours; 2 µl of the culture is then added directly to the PCR mixture prior to amplification.

Primer sequences (24):

P.-multocida-specific PCR	KMT1T7	5'-ATC-CGC-TAT-TTA-CCC-AGT-GG-3'
	KMT1SP6	5'-GCT-GTA-AAC-GAA-CTC-GCC-AC-3'

PCR conditions:

Template DNA is added to the PCR mixture (total volume of 25 µl) containing 1 × PCR buffer, 200 µM each deoxynucleotide triphosphate (dNTP), 2 mM $MgCl_2$, 3.2 pmol of each primer and 0.5 u *Taq* DNA polymerase. Cycling parameters are as follows: initial denaturation at 95°C for 5 minutes; 30 cycles of 95°C for 1 minute, 55°C for 1 minute, 72°C for 1 minute; with a final extension at 72°C for 7 minutes. The reaction is held at 4°C until required for electrophoresis; 5 µl of each sample is electrophoresed on a 2% agarose gel in 1 × Tris-acetate running buffer (TAE) at 4 V/cm for 1 hour. The gel is stained with 1% ethidium bromide and DNA fragments are viewed by UV transillumination.

b) HS-causing Type-B-specific PCR assay

Presumptive identification of HS-causing Type B *P. multocida* is also possible by PCR amplification (3, 24). Comparative analysis with the *Haemophilus influenzae* Rd genome indicates that DNA regions amplified in both assays reside in close proximity, yet slight differences in specificity are evident. To date, the HS-causing Type-B-specific PCR (24) remains 100% specific for HS-causing Type B serotypes of isolated *P. multocida*. Type B cultures with the predominant somatic antigen being either type 2 or 5 are identified by the amplification of an ~620 bp fragment with the KTSP61 and KTT72 primers. Reliable identification of Type E *P. multocida* by PCR is not currently available.

Primer sequences (24):

HS-causing Type B specific PCR	KTT72	5'-AGG-CTC-GTT-TGG-ATT-ATG-AAG-3'
	KTSP61	5'-ATC-CGC-TAA-CAC-ACT-CTC-3'

Conditions for HS-causing Type-B-specific PCR are as described for *P.-multocida*-specific PCR.

HS-causing Type-B-specific PCR primers can also be used in a multiplex PCR with the *P.-multocida*-specific primers, dramatically decreasing the time required for *P. multocida* detection and presumptive identification of the HS-serotype. Multiplex PCR conditions are as described above except that 3.2 pmol of each of the four primers and 1 u *Taq* DNA polymerase are used. The use of the multiplex *P.-multocida*-specific/HS-causing Type-B-specific PCR on suspect organisms can confirm the identity and provide a presumptive serotype within 3–4 hours, in comparison with biochemical analysis and conventional serotyping, which can take up to 2 weeks.

c) Genotypic differentiation of isolates

Once presumptive (or definitive) identification has been made, further differentiation of isolates can be achieved by genotypic fingerprinting methods. Restriction endonuclease analysis with the enzyme *Hha*I has proved useful for characterisation of Type B HS-serotypes, with 13 unique fingerprint profiles among 54 isolates resembling the profile of the somatic serotype 2 reference strain (28). In contrast, while a single *Hha*I profile was observed among 13 serogroup E isolates, differentiation of these strains was possible following *Hpa*II digestion. Ribotyping and large DNA separation by pulsed-field gel electrophoresis also provide useful discrimination of serogroup B and E *P. multocida* isolates (22). However, these techniques are largely used for research purposes and require specialised equipment.

PCR fingerprinting is feasible for any laboratory with PCR capability, with several methods previously used for *P. multocida* differentiation. Random amplified polymorphic DNA (RAPD) analysis and arbitrarily primed PCR (AP-PCR), respectively, have been shown to be useful for epidemiological studies of *P. multocida* isolated from rabbits (8) and for differentiating post-vaccination isolates of *P. multocida* obtained from turkeys (12). However, RAPD and AP-PCR analysis of HS-causing *P. multocida* isolates have not been previously described. Repetitive sequence PCR analysis of *P. multocida* has provided useful discrimination of avian and swine isolates, although all HS-causing strains analysed demonstrated similar profiles (23, 25).

2. Serological tests

Serological tests for detecting antibodies are not normally used for diagnosis. The IHA test can be used for this purpose, following a method broadly similar to that described for capsular typing above. High titres detected by the IHA test are indicative of recent exposure to HS. As HS is a disease that occurs mainly in animals reared under unsophisticated husbandry conditions, where disease-reporting systems are also poor, there is often considerable delay in notification of outbreaks. Deaths occur very suddenly and no carcasses are available for examination when notification is made. In such situations, high IHA titres from 1/160 up to 1/1280 or higher among in-contact animals surviving in affected herds, are indicative of recent exposure to HS for the purpose of diagnosis.

B. REQUIREMENTS FOR VACCINES AND DIAGNOSTIC BIOLOGICALS

The three types of vaccines used against HS are bacterins, alum-precipitated vaccine (APV) and oil adjuvant vaccine (OAV). To provide sufficient immunity with bacterins, repeated vaccination is required. Administration of dense bacterins can give rise to shock reactions, which are less frequent with the APV and almost nonexistent with the OAV.

1. Seed management

a) Characteristics of the seed

A local isolate of *P. multocida* representing the prevalent serotype is used. A well capsulated, stable culture that produces large colonies of approximately 2 mm in diameter on CSY blood agar must be maintained. Seed cultures should be stored as semisolid nutrient agar stab cultures at room temperature, or as lyophilised cultures.

b) Method of culture

A calf is infected with the culture, and, within 2–3 hours of its death, blood is collected aseptically from the heart and stored at –20°C in 1 ml aliquots. A fresh aliquot is used for each new batch of vaccine. It is permissible to subculture this aliquot once or twice, provided the colony size does not diminish. A blood aliquot is thawed, plated on to CSY blood agar, and the growth is tested for agglutinability by the appropriate antiserum on a slide. A good culture will give a coarse floccular agglutination in under 30 seconds. A poor culture will yield only a fine granular agglutination.

Seed lots must be shown to be:

i) *Pure:* Free from adventitious agents.
ii) *Safe:* Produce no adverse reaction in the target species when given as recommended.
iii) *Efficacious:* Stimulate effective immunity as indicated by potency tests.

The necessary tests are described in Section 4, below.

2. Method of manufacture

For vaccine production, dense suspensions of bacteria are necessary. They should have a minimum bacterial content of 1.5 g dry weight per litre of suspension. There are two methods of producing dense suspensions. The first is to culture on solid medium in Roux flasks and harvest in formalinised physiological saline, by which means suspensions of any density can be achieved. This is laborious as each flask must be harvested separately and tested for purity. The second and recommended method is the use of a large vessel with aerated cultures in a medium that specifically supports *P. multocida*. A suitable sterilised medium is casein hydrolysate (2 g), sucrose (6 g), yeast extract (6 g), sodium chloride (5 g), anhydrous dipotassium hydrogen orthophosphate (8.6 g), anhydrous potassium dihydrogen orthophosphate (1.36 g), and distilled water to 1 litre. A denser growth is obtained if the casein, sucrose and yeast are prepared as a concentrate, filter-sterilised or autoclaved for 10 minutes at 107°C, and transferred, aseptically, into the tank that has previously been heat-sterilised with the rest of the ingredients.

There are two types of aeration process – by vortexing and sparging. Sterile air is provided by a compressor. In vortex aeration, the culture is stirred by an impeller shaft operating in the air stream, whereas in sparging aeration, the air is dispersed through a sparger. Intermittent aeration seems to produce denser growth (21). The more finely dispersed the air, the better is the bacterial growth. Vessels of 20–40 litres are usually employed, and incubation is at 37°C. In continuous culture systems, once a maximum density has been reached, usually within 15 hours, about 25% of the working volume is harvested and replaced hourly. The harvests of continuous cultures are collected in relatively small volumes into separate vessels, but, after several days, the density diminishes, presumably through loss of capsular antigen. For this reason, batch cultures are preferred. If batch culture vessels are inoculated at a rate of 50 ml/litre of medium, maximum turbidity is obtained within 15–18 hours, when the growth can be terminated by the addition of formalin to a final concentration of 0.5%. This procedure, where a large inoculum is employed and the growth is terminated within a short period, helps to minimise the chances of contamination. The turbidity is standardised against a reference containing the equivalent dry weight/volume of 1.5 g/litre.

Dense cultures are also obtained using fermenters, where heat sterilisation of the tanks and culture can be carried out *in situ*, with automatic temperature, pH and aeration control devices. Liquid sterilisation systems by filtration, for heat-labile components, can also be built into the fermenter. A 100 litre batch fermenter will yield a minimum of 66,000 doses (each of 3 ml) of OAV, and even more doses if the density is high enough for dilution to a reference standard equivalent to 1.5 g/litre, dry weight/volume.

OAV is made by the emulsification of equal volumes of a light mineral oil and the bacterial suspension, with 5% pure anhydrous lanolin as emulsifying agent. The mineral oil and lanolin are first sterilised and, on cooling to 40°C, 0.5% formalin is added to the mixture. The bacterial suspension is added slowly and emulsification is continued for a further 10 minutes. Following overnight storage, the mixture is re-emulsified, bottled and stored at 4°C for 2 weeks prior to use.

APV is prepared by first adjusting the turbidity of the suspension to the reference standard as above, and diluting it with an equal volume of 0.5% formalinised physiological saline. The pH is adjusted to 6.5, and a hot 20% solution of potash alum is added to give a final concentration of 1% alum. After overnight storage with continuous agitation, the vaccine is bottled for use.

3. In-process control

Proper concentration of bacterial growth, the capsulation of the bacteria, purity of culture and efficient inactivation all need to be checked.

4. Batch control

a) Sterility

Tests for sterility and freedom from contamination of biological materials may be found in Chapter I.4.

b) Safety

Two seronegative cattle are vaccinated with twice the recommended dose and observed for 10–14 days for adverse effects.

Five mice are inoculated intramuscularly with 0.2 ml each of the vaccine, and observed for 5 days. The blood of any mouse that dies is cultured for *P. multocida*.

c) Potency

Potency tests can be carried out by any of the following methods:

i) Vaccination of cattle followed by direct challenge or passive mouse protection tests using the bovine sera. This procedure is not very feasible as cattle take a long time to develop adequate immunity after OAV;

ii) Vaccination of rabbits followed by direct challenge or passive mouse protection test using the rabbit sera; or

iii) Potency tests in mice, the most feasible method of the three.

Each of 50 mice are vaccinated intramuscularly with 0.2 ml of vaccine, and again 14 days later. On day 21, the mice are divided into ten groups of five, each group being challenged with respective dilutions of a 6–8-hour broth culture of a field strain in the range 10^{-1}–10^{-10}; 50 unvaccinated controls are similarly challenged, and all mice are observed for 5 days. The median lethal dose (LD_{50}) can then be calculated in order to obtain an indication of the dose that is sufficient to protect cattle: vaccines prepared in the manner described give at least 10^4 units protection in the vaccinated mice.

d) Duration of immunity

A single dose of vaccine administered to young calves 4–6 months of age will protect susceptible animals for 3–4 months when APV is used, and for 6–9 months when OAV is used.

e) Stability

The OAV emulsion should be pure white, and should stick to glass like paint. If the emulsion shows signs of cracking, it should be discarded. Separation of a thin layer of oil on the surface is permissible. It can be stored at 4–8°C for 6 months without any significant loss of potency. It must not be frozen. Increase in the content of lanolin improves stability, but also increases the viscosity – a distinct disadvantage. Use of other emulsifying agents such as 'Arlacel' helps to produce thinner, stable emulsions.

f) Method of use

The vaccine should be administered by deep intramuscular injection. The use of nylon 5 ml volume syringes for a 3 ml dose and a gauge 14–15 needle is advised, and the recommended age for primary vaccination is 4–6 months. For routine, prophylactic vaccination, a single dose of OAV at 4–6 months, a booster 3–6 months later, and annual revaccination thereafter, is recommended. Where husbandry practices are such that reaching individual animals at appropriate times is impracticable, annual vaccination of all animals over 4 months of age, preferably before the season, and vaccination of all calves under 1 year of age, 6 months later, is recommended. In the face of an outbreak in vaccinated animals, one dose of APV, followed by one dose of OAV, is recommended.

g) Precautions (hazards)

Leakage of OAV into subcutaneous tissue can occasionally give rise to fibrous lumps at sites of injection. Rarely, abscesses may develop if sterility conditions are not observed, though most animals are resistant to such infections. APV may occasionally cause shock reactions.

5. Tests on the final product

a) Safety

See Section B.4.b.

b) Potency

See Section B.4.c.

REFERENCES

1. ANON (1981). Simple serological technique recommended for HS diagnosis. *Asian Livestock*, **6**, 41–42.

2. BAIN R.V.S., DE ALWIS M.C.L., CARTER G.R. & GUPTA B.K. (1982). Haemorrhagic Septicaemia. FAO Animal Production and Health Paper No. 33. FAO, Rome, Italy.

3. BRICKELL (1998). Development of a PCR test based on a gene region associated with the pathogenicity of *Pasteurella multocida* serotype B:2, the causal agent of haemorrhagic septicaemia in Asia. *Vet. Microbiol.*, **59**, 295–307.

4. CARTER G.R. (1955). A haemagglutination test for the identification of serological types. *Am. J. Vet. Res.*, **16**, 481–484.

5. CARTER G.R. & CHENGAPPA M.M. (1980). Hyaluronidase production by type B *Pasteurella multocida* from cases of haemorrhagic septicaemia. *J. Clin. Microbiol.*, **11**, 94–96.

6. CARTER G.R. & CHENGAPPA M.M. (1981). Identification of type B and E *Pasteurella multocida* by counterimmuno-electrophoresis. *Vet. Rec.*, **108**, 145–146.

7. CARTER G.R. & DE ALWIS M.C.L. (1989). Haemorrhagic septicaemia. *In: Pasteurella* and Pasteurellosis, Adlam C. & Rutter J.M., eds. Academic Press, London, UK, 131–160.

8. CHASLUS-DANCLA E., LESAGE-DESCAUSES M.C., LEROY-SETRIN S., MARTEL J.L., COUDERT P. & LAFONT J.P. (1996). Validation of random amplified polymorphic DNA assays by ribotyping as tools for epidemiological surveys of *Pasteurella multocida*. *Vet. Microbiol.*, **52**, 91–102.

9. DE ALWIS M.C.L. (1984). Haemorrhagic septicaemia in cattle and buffaloes. *Rev. sci. tech. Off. int. Epiz.*, **3**, 707–730.

10. DE ALWIS M.C.L. (1992). Haemorrhagic septicaemia – a general review. *Br. Vet. J.*, **148**, 99–112.

11. HEDDLESTON K.L, GALLAGHER J.E. & REBERS P.A. (1972). Fowl cholera: gel diffusion precipitin test for serotyping *Pasteurella multocida* from avian species. *Avian Dis.*, **16**, 925–936.

12. HOPKINS B.A., HUANG T.H.M. & OLSON L.D. (1998). Differentiating turkey postvaccination isolants of *Pasteurella multocida* using arbitrarily primed polymerase chain reaction. *Avian Dis.*, **42**, 265–274.

13. KASTEN R.W., CARPENTER T.E., SNIPES K.P. & HIRSH D.C. (1997). Detection of *Pasteurella multocida*-specific DNA in turkey flocks by use of the polymerase chain reaction. *Avian Dis.*, **41**, 676–682.

14. MUSTAFA A.A., GHALIB H.W. & SHIGIDI M.T. (1978). Carrier rate of *Pasteurella multocida* in a cattle herd associated with an outbreak of haemorrhagic septicaemia in the Sudan. *Br. Vet. J.*, **134**, 375–378.

15. NAMIOKA S. (1978). *Pasteurella multocida*. Biochemical characteristics and serotypes. *In:* Methods in Microbiology, 10. Academic Press, London, UK, 272–292.

16. NAMIOKA S. & MURATA M. (1961). Serological studies on *Pasteurella multocida*. I: a simplified method of capsular typing of the organism. *Cornell Vet.*, **51**, 498–507.

17. NAMIOKA S. & MURATA M. (1961). Serological studies on *Pasteurella multocida*. II: characteristics of the somatic (O) antigen of the organism. *Cornell Vet.*, **51**, 507–521.

18. NAMIOKA S. & MURATA M. (1961). Serological studies on *Pasteurella multocida*. III. O antigenic analysis of cultures isolated from various animals. *Cornell Vet.*, **51**, 522–528.

19. NEUMANN S., LEEB T. & BRENIG B. (1998). Vergleich zwischen PCR und kultureller Untersuchung zum Nachweis von Infektionen mit *Pasteurella multocida* beim Hund (Comparison between PCR and multibiological assay for the detection of *Pasteurella multocida* in the dog [in German]). *Kleintierpraxis*, **43**, 69–74.

20. SAWADA T., RIMLER R.B. & RHOADES K.P. (1985). Haemorrhagic septicaemia: naturally acquired antibodies against *Pasteurella multocida* types B and E in calves in the United States. *Am. J. Vet. Res.*, **46**, 1247–1250.

21. THOMAS J. (1968). Studies on haemorrhagic septicaemia oil adjuvant vaccine. I. Methods of production. *Kajian Vet. Malaysia–Singapore*, **1**, 152–158.

22. TOWNSEND K.M., DAWKINS H.J.S. & PAPADIMITRIOU J.M. (1997). Analysis of haemorrhagic septicaemia-causing isolates of *Pasteurella multocida* by ribotyping and field alternation gel electrophoresis (FAGE). *Vet. Microbiol.*, **57**, 383–395.

23. TOWNSEND K.M., DAWKINS H.J.S. & PAPADIMITRIOU J.M. (1997). REP-PCR analysis of *Pasteurella multocida* isolates that cause haemorrhagic septicaemia. *Res. Vet. Sci.*, **63**, 151–155.

24. TOWNSEND K.M., FROST A.J., LEE C.W., PAPADIMITRIOU J.M. & DAWKINS H.J.S. (1998). Development of PCR assays for species- and type-specific identification of *Pasteurella multocida* isolates. *J. Clin. Microbiol.*, **36**, 1096–1100.

25. TOWNSEND K.M., O'BOYLE D., PHAN T.T., HANH T.X., WIJEWARDANA T.G., WILKIE I., TRUNG N.T. & FROST A.J. (1998). Acute septicaemic pasteurellosis in Vietnamese pigs. *Vet. Microbiol.*, **63**, 205–215.

26. WIJEWARDANA T.G., DE ALWIS M.C.L. & BASTIANZ H.L.G. (1986). Cultural, biochemical and pathogenicity studies on strains of *Pasteurella multocida* isolated from carrier animals and outbreaks of haemorrhagic septicaemia. *Sri Lanka Vet. J.*, **34**, 43–57.

27. WIJEWARDENA T.G., DE ALWIS M.C.L. & VIPULASIRI A.A. (1982). An agar gel diffusion test for rapid identification of *Pasteurella multocida* type B (Carter). *Sri Lanka Vet. J.*, **30**, 12–14.

28. WILSON M.A., RIMLER R.B. & HOFFMAN L.J. (1992). Comparison of DNA fingerprints and somatic serotypes of serogroup B and E *Pasteurella multocida* isolates. *J. Clin. Microbiol.*, **30**, 1518–1524.

*

* *

CHAPTER 2.3.13.

BOVINE SPONGIFORM ENCEPHALOPATHY

SUMMARY

Bovine spongiform encephalopathy (BSE) is a fatal neurological disease of adult cattle that was first recognised in Great Britain (GB) in 1986. The pathological changes, the epidemiological pattern, and the transmissibility of the disease indicate that BSE is one of the subacute spongiform encephalopathies caused by unconventional transmissible agents or prions. The archetype for this group of diseases is scrapie of sheep and goats (see Chapter X.9. Scrapie).

The current epizootic of BSE can be explained by oral exposure to a scrapie-like agent in the ruminant-derived protein of meat-and-bone meal included in proprietary concentrates or feed supplements. Initial cases, at least, of BSE in other countries are considered to be the result of exports from GB of infected cattle or contaminated meat-and-bone meal. A ban on the feeding of ruminant-derived protein to ruminants was first implemented in GB in July 1988. Since then, the feeding of mammalian-derived protein to ruminants has, with certain exemptions, been prohibited throughout the European Union and some other countries. From April 1996, this ban, with respect to mammalian meat-and-bone meal, was extended in the UK to all farmed food animals. Experimental transmissibility of BSE to cattle has been demonstrated following parenteral and oral exposure to brain tissue from affected cattle. Epidemiological studies in GB have revealed an increased risk for the offspring of clinical cases of BSE developing the disease themselves, but this enhanced risk will not maintain endemic infection in the national cattle population. As a result of control measures the epizootics in the United Kingdom (UK) and Switzerland are in decline.

The BSE agent is believed also to be the common source of transmissible spongiform encephalopathies (TSEs) in several other species of bovidae and in species of felidae. There is evidence of a causal link between the BSE agent and a new variant form of the human TSE, Creutzfeldt-Jakob disease (CJD).

BSE, as it occurs in GB, has a peak incidence in cattle aged between 4 and 5 years. The clinical course is variable but can extend to several months. Clinical signs are sufficiently distinctive to lead to suspicion of disease, particularly if differential diagnoses are eliminated. In countries with a statutory policy toward the disease, clinically suspect cases must be slaughtered, the brain examined and affected cattle destroyed. Confirmation of the diagnosis is based primarily on histopathological examination of the brain. Lesions have been described only in the central nervous system. Recommendations for safety precautions for handling BSE-infected material now assume that BSE is a zoonosis and a containment category 3 (with derogation) has been ascribed.

***Identification of the agent:** No diagnostic test for the BSE agent in the live animal is presently available. The nature of the agents causing the TSE is unresolved. A disease-specific isoform of a membrane protein PrP (PrP^{Sc}) has a critical importance in the pathogenesis of these diseases and according to the prion hypothesis is the sole component of the infectious agent.*

To confirm the diagnosis of spongiform encephalopathy, histological examination of the brain is necessary. The correlation between the clinical diagnosis and the neurohistological diagnosis in BSE can, with appropriate experience, be greater than 90%. The histopathological examination may also provide a differential diagnosis in clinically suspect cases in which lesions of BSE are not detected. The pathognomonic lesion is spongiform change in grey matter neuropil and neuronal vacuolation of certain brainstem nuclei. This change is usually, but not invariably, bilaterally symmetrical. Detection of accumulations of PrP^{Sc} in the central nervous system of affected cattle by immunochemical methods offers a disease-specific diagnostic approach. PrP^{Sc} can be detected in unfixed brain extracts by immunoblotting and other enzyme immunoassay methods.

Immunohistochemical demonstration of characteristic patterns of accumulation of PrP in formalin-fixed affected brain is now widely used as a confirmatory diagnostic method. Characteristic fibrils, homologous with scrapie-associated fibrils and composed of PrP^{Sc} can be visualised by electron microscopic examination of detergent-treated extracts of unfixed (or formalin-fixed) BSE-affected brains and have also been used to confirm the diagnosis.

BSE can be transmitted from brain tissue of terminally affected cattle to mice by intracerebral/intraperitoneal inoculation or by feeding, but incubation periods of several months precludes bioassay from routine use. This is the only practical method currently available for detection of infectivity.

Serological tests: *Immune responses have not been detected in scrapie or other TSEs.*

Requirements for vaccines and diagnostic biologicals: *There are no biological products available currently.*

A. DIAGNOSTIC TECHNIQUES

A detailed account of bovine spongiform encephalopathy (BSE), its experimental transmissibility (16, 21), occurrence, epidemiology, clinical signs, pathology, diagnosis, prevention, and control has been given previously in English, French and Spanish (30). More recent reviews have provided updated information (13, 14, 35).

BSE is an invariably fatal disease of domestic cattle, cases of which were first recognised in Great Britain (GB) in November 1986 (58). BSE has been shown to belong to that group of disorders known as the transmissible spongiform encephalopathies (TSE) or prion diseases, typified in animal species by scrapie of sheep. These diseases are defined by the pathological accumulation, principally in the central nervous system but also in lympho-reticular tissues, of an abnormal isoform of a host-encoded protein, designated PrP. Retrospective studies have indicated that the first cases of BSE presented around April 1985. The initial epidemiological studies established that the occurrence of BSE was in the form of an extended common source epizootic, due to feedborne infection with a scrapie-like agent in meat-and-bone meal used as a dietary protein supplement.

BSE has occurred in several countries other than the United Kingdom (UK) involving imported and/or indigenous cattle. The origin of such cases is most likely to have resulted directly or indirectly from the export of infected cattle or infected meat-and-bone meal from countries with occurrences of BSE, including historically the UK. It is uncertain whether infection has subsequently been propagated within all countries in which cases have occurred. Cases in indigenous cattle populations outside the UK have been recorded in Belgium, Denmark, France, Ireland, Liechtenstein, Luxembourg, the Netherlands, Portugal and Switzerland.

From July 1988 in GB and from January 1989 in Northern Ireland, the feeding of ruminant-derived protein to ruminants was prohibited. With some exceptions, a ban on the feeding of mammalian-derived protein to ruminant animals has since been introduced elsewhere; in Switzerland (December 1990) (52) and throughout the European Union (June 1994) (35). From April 1996, this ban, at least when protein is presented in the form of meat-and-bone meal, was extended in the UK to all farmed food animals, including horses and fish. Experimentally it has been demonstrated that BSE can be transmitted to cattle following parenteral and oral exposure to brain tissue from affected cattle (16, 56). Epidemiological studies in Britain have revealed an increased risk for the offspring of clinical cases of BSE developing the disease themselves (63). It has not been established if this is due to true maternal transmission. It is considered that this enhanced risk will not maintain endemic infection in the national (UK) cattle population. There is no evidence of horizontal transmission of BSE between cattle. Epidemiological and transmission studies have not revealed evidence of a risk from semen (65) or milk (33, 51). Although experimental studies will not be completed until 2001, there is also no evidence of transmission of BSE through embryos (65). As a result of control measures, the epizootics in the UK and Switzerland are in decline.

The novel occurrence of TSE in several species of captive exotic bovidae and felidae and in domestic cats, during the course of the BSE epizootic is suspected, or, in specific instances, known to have been caused by the BSE agent. Exposure is presumed to have been via feed.

In the past epidemiological studies have found no connection between the exposure of humans to agents causing animal spongiform encephalopathies and the occurrence of the human TSE Creutzfeldt-Jakob disease (CJD). In particular no enhanced occupational or dietary risk from exposure to sheep products has been established, thus suggesting that scrapie agents are not a human health hazard under natural conditions of exposure. However, monitoring of cases of CJD in the UK resulted, in March 1996, in the announcement of the recognition of ten cases of an apparently new variant of sporadic CJD (v-CJD) in the UK (64). As of July 2000, 76 cases of v-CJD have been recorded in the UK. At least one case has been reported in France (12), and another from Ireland. Strain-typing studies of the causal agent of v-CJD in mice (10, 47) have provided strong evidence that the same strain of agent derived from BSE is also found in v-CJD. Studies showing similarities between the Western blot banding and glycosylation patterns of the disease-related isoform of PrP from patients with v-CJD and from certain animal species with naturally acquired or experimentally transmitted BSE, also support this conclusion (15, 25). Therefore, on present evidence, the most likely explanation of cases of v-CJD is exposure to the BSE agent. Because the incubation period of v-CJD is unknown, it is too early to predict the course of the epidemic. The current incidence of the disease must still be viewed with caution. It is therefore now recommended that safety precautions for handling the BSE agent be based on the assumption that BSE is transmissible to humans. Containment category 3 (with derogation) has been assigned (37).

BSE affects adult cattle from approximately 2 years of age, but most cases occur in animals 4–5 years of age. There is no breed predilection, but the incidence of affected herds by functional type is much greater for dairy than beef as, in the UK, it was mainly calves from dairy herds that were fed on concentrate rations containing meat-and-bone meal. Onset of clinical signs is not associated with season or stage of breeding cycle.

BSE has an insidious onset and usually a slowly progressive course (8, 30, 58, 62). Rarely, a case will present with acute signs and then deteriorate rapidly (62). Presenting signs, though variable, usually include behavioural changes, apprehension, and hyper-reactivity. For example, affected cows may be reluctant to enter the milking parlour or may kick vigorously during milking. In dry cows especially, pelvic limb incoordination and weakness can be the first clinical features to be noticed. Neurological signs predominate throughout the clinical course and may include many aspects of altered mental status and behaviour, abnormalities of posture and movement, and aberrant sensation, but the most commonly reported nervous signs are apprehension, pelvic limb ataxia, and hyperaesthesia to touch and sound. The intense pruritus characteristic of some sheep with scrapie is not prominent in cattle with BSE, though in a proportion of cases there is rubbing and scratching activity. Affected cows will sometimes stand with low head carriage, the neck extended and the ears directed caudally (53). Abnormalities of gait include swaying of the pelvic quarters and pelvic limb hypermetria; features that are most readily appreciated when cattle are observed at pasture. Gait ataxia may also involve the pectoral limbs and, with advancing severity of locomotor signs, generalised weakness, resulting in falling and recumbency, can dominate the clinical picture. Reports of reduced rumination (2, 4), also bradycardia and altered heart rhythm (3), though not specific signs, suggest that autonomic disturbance is a feature of BSE. General clinical features of loss of bodily condition, decreasing live weight, and reduction in milk yield often accompany nervous signs as the disease progresses. There has been no change in the clinical picture of BSE over the course of the epizootic in the UK (61). Clinical signs are essentially similar in other countries where BSE has occurred (8). The protracted clinical course, extending usually over a period of weeks or months, would eventually require slaughter on welfare considerations. However, a statutory policy to determine the BSE status of a country requires compulsory notification and diagnostic investigation of clinically suspect cases, their slaughter and the complete destruction of the carcasses of affected cattle (36). Early in the disease course, the signs may be subtle, variable and nonspecific, and thus may prevent clinical diagnosis on an initial examination. Continued observation of such equivocal cases, together with appropriate clinical pathology procedures to eliminate differential diagnoses, especially metabolic disorders, will establish the essential progression of signs. Some early clinical signs of BSE may show similarities with features of nervous ketosis, hypomagnesaemia, encephalitic listeriosis and other encephalitides. Subtle signs may sometimes be exacerbated following stress, such as that caused by transport.

Because of the link recently established between BSE and v-CJD, BSE and related TSE agents are now categorised, in respect to biohazard, with the human TSE (1). Consequently, veterinarians and laboratory workers conducting necropsies on BSE-suspect animals or handling tissues derived from such animals, must conduct the work under appropriate containment conditions (category 3) (37), sometimes with derogations allowed by the nature of the work and the results of local risk assessment. It is important that appropriate protective clothing be worn and that a strict code of practice be followed to prevent exposure to the agent. Laboratories conducting work on BSE must comply with national biocontainment and biosafety regulations. Recommended decontamination procedures may not be completely effective when dealing with high titre material or when the agent is protected within dried organic matter. Recommended physical inactivation is by porous load autoclaving at 134°C–138°C for 18 minutes at 30 lb/in^2. However, temperatures at the higher end of the range may be less effective than those at the lower end and total inactivation may not be achieved under certain conditions, such as when the test material is in the form of a macerate (50). Disinfection is carried out using sodium hypochlorite containing 2% available chlorine, or 2 N sodium hydroxide, applied for more than 1 hour at 20°C for surfaces, or overnight for equipment.

1. Identification of the agent

The nature of the agents causing animal or human TSEs remains unresolved (42). The modified form (PrP^{Sc}) of a host-coded, highly conserved, membrane protein (PrP^{C}) of unknown function, is the only disease-specific macromolecule identified in the scrapie-like diseases. A substantial scientific view is that the agent is composed entirely of the disease-specific isoform of PrP and that the altered form is capable of inducing conversion of the normal form; the protein only or 'prion' hypothesis. The opposing view is that the agent is virus-like and contains nucleic acid. The identification of multiple 'strains' of scrapie agents, with characteristic incubation periods and patterns of neuropathological change when transmitted to mice, is considered to be more in keeping with this latter hypothesis. However, it is difficult to reconcile this view with the extreme resistance of the agent to conventional microbial inactivation procedures, including ultraviolet and ionising irradiation, extremes of temperatures, standard autoclaving and a large range of chemical disinfectants. The molecular basis for strain variation is still unclear.

Characterisation of isolates by transmission of BSE to mice has shown that BSE is caused by a single major strain of agent that differs from characterised strains of the scrapie agent in sheep (9). Uniformity of the pathology among affected cattle has also supported the notion of a single BSE strain and enabled the definition of a particular disease phenotype for BSE (57). This specific pattern of neuropathology in the host species is an important feature of the case definition of BSE.

In the absence of *in-vitro* methods for isolation of the causative agent, the conventional basis of confirmation of the diagnosis in this group of diseases has been the demonstration of the morphological features of spongiform encephalopathy by histopathological examination. This remains necessarily, by definition, the only method by which this characteristic vacuolar pathology can be diagnosed. However, given the essential role of the PrP^{Sc} molecule and increases in technical capabilities in this area, it is now important that diagnostic approaches use one or more methods for the detection of the abnormal form of the protein. The demonstration by electron microscopy on central nervous system extracts of characteristic fibrils, termed scrapie-associated fibrils (SAF), which are composed largely of PrP^{Sc}, is a further morphological diagnostic method. Methods of PrP^{Sc} detection include immunohistochemical demonstration, Western blotting and, most recently, a number of other rapid immunoassays for screening. The use of a particular method will depend on the purpose to which the diagnosis is to be applied in the epidemiological context. This range of purposes will extend from confirmation of the clinical diagnosis in the control of epizootic disease to the screening of healthy populations for evidence of covert or preclinical disease. The pathological case definition adopted will also differ according to whether the method is to be applied for confirmation of a case or for screening of a population. For the former it is important to use approaches that can monitor the pathological phenotype of BSE. Clearly also, the performance of individual methods will be crucial to this process of selection of a single method or a portfolio approach. It must be stressed that the development of methods, particularly rapid screening immunoassays for the detection of PrP^{Sc}, is a rapidly evolving field.

The initial pathological case definition of BSE was based on the histopathological changes in the central nervous system, and this has provided the usual basis for confirmation of the clinical diagnosis of BSE (54, 58). The histopathological examination also allows confirmation of the characteristic neuropathological phenotype of BSE (48, 60). The histopathological changes are neurodegenerative and closely resemble those of scrapie of sheep. The most prominent features are vacuolar and comprise a spongiform change in the neuropil of grey matter and single or multiple vacuoles within neuronal perikarya. The precise appearance of the spongiform change in TSEs, as observed by light microscopy, has been defined previously (31). In BSE, spongiform change is the predominant form of vacuolar change. Both forms of vacuolation are bilaterally distributed and usually symmetrical with a consistent pattern of severity relative to distribution throughout the brain (55, 60). The high frequency of occurrence of neuroparenchymal vacuolation in certain anatomic nuclei of the medulla oblongata at the level of the obex has, in the BSE epizootic in the UK, provided a satisfactory means of establishing a diagnosis on a single section of the medulla (54). However, observation of doubtful lesions in the medulla at this level requires examination of other brain areas to detect cases of BSE with minimal or potentially atypical lesions and, when necessary, to establish pathological differential diagnoses. Neurodegenerative changes other than vacuolation are not prominent in BSE. A gliosis (astrocytosis), as seen in scrapie, is another feature, particularly in sites of vacuolar change. Detection of gliosis is assisted by the use of special stains and immunohistochemistry. For example, astrocytosis can be demonstrated by the immunohistochemical detection of increased glial fibrillary acidic protein (GFAP).

For the preparation of material for diagnostic examination, cattle suspected of having the disease should be killed with an intravenous injection of a concentrated barbiturate solution following sedation, if necessary. The technical procedures concerned with collection, fixation, and histological processing have been described (7, 44) and are revised and summarised below.

In all circumstances of surveillance of neurological disease in adult cattle where the occurrence of BSE within a country or state has not been established or is of low incidence, it is important that a standard neuropathological approach be followed in which representative areas of the whole brain are examined. Departure from this is dependent on local national circumstances, including whether or not a differential diagnosis is required.

Brain tissue should be removed as soon as possible after death. Fresh material for potential use in tests to detect disease-specific PrP should be taken ideally as a complete coronal section (2–4 g) from the medulla, caudal to the obex, specifically avoiding damage to the obex region. The cervical spinal cord and the lateral hemisphere of cerebellum also offer optimal sampling areas that will not encroach on histopathological requirements. This tissue is stored frozen prior to testing. If the remaining whole brain is sampled for the histopathological examination, it should be placed in approximately 4–6 litres of 10% formol saline fixative, which should be changed twice weekly. After fixation for 2 weeks, the brain is cut into coronal slices. The fixation time may be shortened by cutting the fresh brain stem into smaller coronal pieces, leaving intact the diagnostically important areas at the obex, the cerebellar peduncles and the rostral colliculi. Depending on some other factors (temperature, agitation, use of microwave) the fixation time for these small pieces of brainstem may be reduced to 2–5 days. The other formol-fixed parts of the brain may be used for differential diagnosis after completing the standard 2 weeks' fixation. Initially, a single block cut at the obex of the medulla oblongata (Figure 1) should be selected for histological processing by conventional paraffin wax embedding methods for neural tissue. Sections, cut at 5 µm thickness and stained with haematoxylin and eosin, are examined for characteristic spongiform change and neuronal vacuolation. If results are inconclusive because of minimal lesions, or the material is histologically uninterpretable due to autolysis or damage, it is necessary to carry out additional tests, including immunohistochemistry or immunoblotting.

When the occurrence of BSE in a particular country has been established in the indigenous cattle population, and there is evidence that the distribution of lesions is consistent with that seen in the brains of cattle from the UK epizootic, it is adequate for monitoring purposes to remove the hind brain alone (Figure 1). This can be achieved via the *foramen magnum* without removal of the calvarium. This will reduce the amount of fixative required, thereby lowering costs and improving safety, while maintaining representation of the major target areas for histological examination. The diagnosis may be confirmed if completely typical changes are present in the medulla (obex) section. When lesions are not obvious in the medulla (obex), sections of other parts of the brainstem (Figure 1) should be examined. However, given the constant lesion pattern, this is unlikely to contribute additional confirmation in more than 0.5% of cases of BSE where lesions are absent in the medulla (obex) section (54). Clearly this abridged protocol does not allow a full neuropathological examination for differential diagnoses to be established.

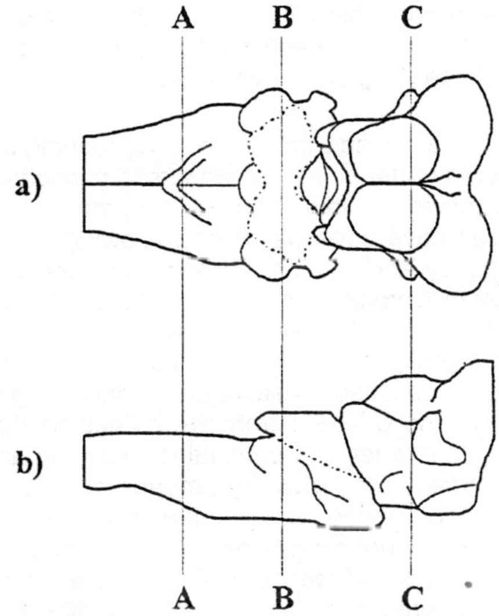

Fig. 1. Brainstem after the removal of the cerebellum, from a) dorsal, and b) lateral aspects.
Recommended levels at which sections should be taken:
A–A = medulla, at the obex;
B–B = medulla through caudal cerebellar peduncles; C–C = midbrain through rostral colliculi.

The interpretation of observed vacuolar changes in the bovine brain must be approached with caution. Vacuoles within the perikarya, indistinguishable from those of BSE, have been reported in neurones of the red and oculomotor nuclei of the midbrain and other brainstem nuclei as an incidental finding in cattle (19, 32, 58). Thus, like the diagnosis of scrapie, which may be confounded by the occurrence of such neuronal vacuolation scattered in the medullae of healthy sheep (see Chapter X.9. Scrapie) (66, 67), histopathological diagnosis of BSE must not rely on the presence of occasional solitary vacuolated neurons. Even relatively numerous vacuolated neurons in the red nucleus must be disregarded. The presence of spongiform change in specific neuroanatomical locations in BSE provides the most confidence of minimising false-positive diagnoses.

As with scrapie of sheep, the possibility of BSE cases occurring in which brain lesions are minimal or undetectable by light microscopy, is a potential problem that can be resolved only by diagnostic criteria independent of histopathology (44, 59).

For routine diagnosis in countries with a high incidence of BSE, histopathological examination confined to the medulla oblongata is the laboratory investigational method used to handle the large number of suspect cases. Demonstration of typical changes provides a definitive diagnosis. Where the result of the histopathological examination is inconclusive or negative or the brain material taken post-mortem was unsuitable for the histological examination because of autolysis or damage, it is important that the disease-specific diagnostic criterion of the detection of abnormal accumulation of PrP be applied. It is also increasingly important to apply such tests in the decaying phase of epizootic occurrence and in surveillance programmes where the most critical monitoring of disease is required. Individual National authorities should apply the use of additional laboratory diagnostic methods such as immunoblotting, immunohistochemistry (IHC) or the detection of scrapie-associated fibrils where their use is considered to be appropriate.

In conjunction with, or even as an alternative to, the histopathological evaluation of medulla sections is the use of IHC to detect PrP^{Sc} accumulation in formalin-fixed, paraffin-embedded material (24, 60). Several different protocols have been applied successfully to the IHC detection of PrP for the diagnosis of BSE (22, 24, 29, 60). Harmonisation toward a fully validated standardised routine diagnostic IHC method is still required. The technique is more sensitive than routine histopathology as it can detect cases in the last months of incubation before the occurrence of vacuolar changes, at least in experimentally induced cases of BSE (56) and possibly also in the natural disease (18). BSE can therefore be diagnosed by IHC in animals with equivocal morphological changes. The technique does not require lengthy tissue fixation and, providing the tissue can be adequately processed histologically, the technique works well in autolysed tissues in which morphological evaluation is no longer possible. IHC is as sensitive as Western blotting for detecting PrP^{Sc} (41). In combination with good histologic preparations IHC allows detection of PrP^{Sc} accumulation and, as PrP^{Sc} accumulation, like the vacuolar pathology, exhibits a typical distribution pattern and appearance, it provides simultaneous evaluation or confirmation of the disease phenotype. In countries with low BSE incidence, IHC is therefore a method of choice for both confirmatory diagnosis and surveillance.

PrP^{Sc} detection by immunohistochemistry is considered to have potential for the preclinical diagnosis of scrapie in sheep using tonsillar (43) or nictitating membrane (38) lymphoid tissue biopsies. Failure to detect infectivity in lymphoid tissues, other than in distal ileum containing Peyer's Patches of experimentally infected cattle, at any time throughout the incubation period and clinical disease course by mouse bioassay (56), suggests that these approaches are currently unlikely to be of use diagnostically in BSE.

Detection of PrP^{Sc} by electrophoretic separation and immunoblotting techniques (20, 26, 49), is carried out on fresh (unfixed) or frozen brain or spinal cord material. Improvements in purification methods for extracting PrP (6, 17) have contributed to increased sensitivity of this method. Automated Western blot and enzyme-linked immunosorbent assay (ELISA) techniques have been developed allowing screening of large numbers of brain samples (34, 41). Such techniques are easy and rapid to perform and are potentially more sensitive than the histopathological evaluation. In a European Commission trial (34) it was demonstrated that one such Western immunoblot method, or either of two specific ELISA methods, when evaluated on brain tissue, were suitable for diagnostic use in specifically targeted populations. This evaluation was restricted to a comparison of the examination of a sample of brains of cattle identified as suspect clinical animals with histopathological changes characteristic of BSE and a sample of brains of cattle from New Zealand that were unexposed to BSE and histopathologically negative. Validation of these tests is continuing, but they do appear to be reliable for large-scale screening and surveillance programmes. They provide a means of initial screening for animals in the late stages (the last few months) of the incubation period, for example in surveys of post-mortem material collected from routinely slaughtered cattle. In countries conducting surveillance for the detection of the novel occurrence of BSE and in those countries in which a means, independent of the system of notification of suspect cases, of assessing the prevalence of BSE, is considered necessary, these recently developed screening tests offer an efficient approach.

The demonstration of characteristic fibrils, the bovine counterpart of SAF (see Chapter X.9. Scrapie), by negative-stain electron microscopy in detergent extracts of fresh or frozen brain or spinal cord tissue (46, 49, 58), has been used as an additional diagnostic method for BSE and may be particularly useful when histopathological approaches are precluded by the occurrence of post-mortem decomposition (45). Recent work on scrapie indicates that, with modification, the method may be applied successfully to formalin-fixed tissue (11). Detection of fibrils has been shown to correlate well with the histopathological diagnosis of BSE (59), but does not offer the specificity or sensitivity available from immunohistochemical or immunoblotting methods.

It must be stressed that the process of full validation of all of these diagnostic methods for BSE has been restrained by the lack of a true gold standard and the consequent need to apply standards of comparison based on relatively small studies. There is therefore a continuing need for the publication of larger scale studies of assay performance. Caution must be exercised in the comparitive interpretation of tests applied to apparently healthy animals as different tests may vary in their sensitivities relative to stage of incubation and pathogenesis of the disease.

BSE infection can be shown by intracerebral/intraperitoneal inoculation (21) or by feeding (5) mice with brain tissue from terminally affected cattle, but bioassay is impractical for routine diagnosis because of the long incubation period (≥292 days). Further development of transgenic mice may offer bioassays with significantly reduced incubation periods for BSE.

2. Serological tests

Similarities with scrapie, in which no immune response in the host has been detected, suggest that there is not likely to be an immune response in BSE.

3. Other tests

There remains the need for a test for BSE that can be applied to the live animal and has a sensitivity capable of detecting PrP^{Sc} at the low levels, such as may occur in the early stages of incubation of the disease. Certain protein markers, notably apolipoprotein E (Apo E), can be detected by two dimensional gel electrophoresis in cerebrospinal fluid of clinically suspected, histopathologically confirmed cases of BSE (28). Apo E is, however, a nonspecific marker for neurodegeneration and has not been shown to be useful for diagnosis of preclinical cases of BSE. Assay of cerebrospinal fluid for the 14-3-3 protein is not of diagnostic use in BSE (40). Similarly, studies of S-100 proteins in cerebrospinal fluid (23) and serum (39) did not give results that would provide diagnostically useful tests for BSE. The electrochemical detection of metabolites in urine (27) has a final performance validation that gave specificity and sensitivity values below that required for it to have a possible independent role in the diagnosis of BSE.

B. REQUIREMENTS FOR VACCINES AND DIAGNOSTIC BIOLOGICALS

There are no biological products available currently.

REFERENCES

1. ADVISORY COMMITTEE ON DANGEROUS PATHOGENS (1998). Transmissible Spongiform Encephalopathy Agents: Safe Working and the Prevention of Infection. Spongiform Encephalopathy Advisory Committee. Her Majesty's Stationery Office, London, UK.

2. AUSTIN A.R, HAWKINS S.A.C., KELAY N.S. & SIMMONS M.M. (1994). New observations on the clinical signs of BSE and scrapie. A Consultation on BSE with the Scientific Veterinary Committee of the Commission of the European Communities held in Brussels, Belgium, 14–15 September 1993. Bradley R. & Marchant B., eds. Document VI/4131/94-EN. European Commission Agriculture, Brussels, Belgium, 347–358.

3. AUSTIN A.R., PAWSON L., MEEK S. & WEBSTER S. (1997). Abnormalities of heart rate and rhythm in bovine spongiform encephalopathy. *Vet. Rec.,* **141**, 352–357.

4. AUSTIN A.R. & SIMMONS M.M. (1993). Reduced rumination in BSE and scrapie. *Vet. Rec.*, **132**, 324–325.

5. BARLOW R.M. & MIDDLETON D.J. (1990). Dietary transmission of bovine spongiform encephalopathy to mice. *Vet. Rec.*, **126**, 111–112.

6. BEEKES M., BALDAUF E., CASENS S., DIRINGER H., KEYES P., SCOTT A.C., WELLS G.A.H., BROWN P., GIBBS C.J. JR & GAJDUSEK D.C. (1995). Western blot mapping of disease-specific amyloid in various animal species and humans with transmissible spongiform encephalopathies using a high-yield purification method. *J. Gen. Virol.*, **76**, 2567–2576.

7. BRADLEY R. & MATTHEWS D. (1992). Subacute, transmissible spongiform encephalopathies: current concepts and future needs. *Rev. sci. tech. Off. int. Epiz.*, **11**, 605–634.

8. BRAUN U., SCHICKER E., PUSTERLA N. & SCHONMANN M. (1998). Kliniche Befunde bei 50 Kuhen mit boviner spongiformer Enzephalopathie (BSE). *Berl. Munch. Tierarztl. Wochenschr.*, **111**, 27–32.

9. BRUCE M.E. (1996). Strain Typing Studies of Scrapie and BSE. *In:* Methods in Molecular Medicine: Prion Diseases, Baker H. & Ridley R.M., eds. Humana Press, Totowa, New Jersey, USA, 223–236.

10. BRUCE M.E., WILL R.G., IRONSIDE J.W., MCCONNELL I., DRUMMOND D., SUTTIE A., MCCARDLE L., CHREE A., HOPE J., BIRKETT C., COUSENS S., FRASER H. & BOSTOCK C.J. (1997). Transmissions to mice indicate that 'new variant' CJD is caused by the BSE agent. *Nature,* **389**, 498–501.

11. CHAPLIN, M.J., ALDRICH, A.D. & STACK, M.J. (1998). Scrapie associated fibril detection from formaldehyde fixed brain tissue in natural cases of ovine scrapie. *Res. Vet. Sci.*, **64**, 41–44.

12. CHAZOT G., BROUSSOLE E., LAPRAS C.I., BLATTLER T., AGUZZI A. & KOPP N. (1996). New variant of Creutzfeldt-Jakob disease in a 26-year-old French man. *Lancet*, **347**, 1181.

13. COLLEE J.G. & BRADLEY R. (1997). BSE: a decade on – part 1. *Lancet,* **349**, 636–641.

14. COLLEE J.G. & BRADLEY R. (1997). BSE: a decade on – part 2. *Lancet,* **349**, 715–721,

15. COLLINGE J., SIDLE K.C.L. MEADS J., IRONSIDE J. & HILL A.F. (1996). Molecular analysis of prion strain variation and the aetiology of 'new variant' CJD. *Nature,* **383**, 685–690.

16. DAWSON M., WELLS G.A.H., PARKER B.N.J., FRANCIS M.E., SCOTT A.C., HAWKINS S.A.C., MARTIN T.C., SIMMONS M.M. & AUSTIN A.R. (1994). Transmission studies of BSE in cattle, pigs and domestic fowl. *In:* A Consultation on BSE with the Scientific Veterinary Committee of the Commission of the European Communities held in Brussels, Belgium, 14–15 September 1993. Bradley R. & Marchant B., eds. Document VI/4131/94-EN. European Commission Agriculture, Brussels, Belgium, 161–167.

17. DIRINGER H., BEEKES M., OZEL M., SIMON D., QUECK I., CARDONE F., POCCHIARI M. & IRONSIDE J.W. (1997). Highly infectious purified preparations of disease-specific amyloid of transmissible spongiform encephalopathies are not devoid of nucleic acids of viral size. *Intervirology,* **40**, 238–246.

18. DOHERR M.G., OESCH B., MOSER M., VANDEVELDE M. & HEIM D. (1999). Targeted surveillance for bovine spongiform encephalopathy. *Vet. Rec.,* **145**, 672.

19. FANKHAUSER R., FATZER R. & FRAUCHIGER E. (1972). Bemerkungen zur spastischen Parese des Rindes. *Schweiz. Arch. Tierheilkd,* **114**, 24–32.

20. FARQUHAR C.F., SOMERVILLE R.A & RITCHIE L.A (1989). Post mortem immunodiagnosis of scrapie and bovine spongiform encephalopathy. *J. Virol. Methods,* **24**, 215–222.

21. FRASER H. & FOSTER J.D. (1994). Transmission to mice, sheep and goats and bioassay of bovine tissues. *In:* A Consultation on BSE with the Scientific Veterinary Committee of the Commission of the European Communities held in Brussels, Belgium, 14–15 September 1993. Bradley R. & Marchant B., eds. Document VI/4131/94-EN. European Commission Agriculture, Brussels, Belgium, 145–159.

22. GRABER H.U., MEYER R.K., FATZER R., VANDEVELDE M. & ZURBRIGGEN A. (1995). *In situ* hybridization and immunohistochemistry for prion protein (PrP) in bovine spongiform encephalopathy (BSE). *J. Vet. Med. Assoc.,* **42**, 453–459.

23. GREEN A.J.E., JACKMAN R., MARSHALL T.A. & THOMPSON E.J. (1999). Increased S-100b in the cerebrospinal fluid of some cattle with bovine spongiform encephalopathy. *Vet. Rec.,* **145**, 107–109.

24. HARITANI M., SPENCER Y.I. & WELLS G.A.H. (1994). Hydrated autoclave pretreatment enhancement of prion protein immunoreactivity in formalin-fixed bovine spongiform encephalopathy-affected brain. *Acta Neuropathol. (Berl.),* **87**, 86–90.

25. HILL A.F., DESBRUSLAIS M., JOINER S., SIDLE K.C.L., GOWLAND I., COLLINGE, J., DOEY L.J. & LANTOS P. (1997). The same prion strain causes vCJD and BSE. *Nature,* **389**, 448–450.

26. HOPE J., REEKIE L.J.D., HUNTEH N., MULTHAUP G., BEYREUTHER K., WHITE H., SCOTT A.C., STACK M.J., DAWSON M. & WELLS G.A.H. (1988). Fibrils from brains of cows with new cattle disease contain scrapie-associated protein. *Nature,* **336**, 390–392.

27. JACKMAN R. & EVEREST S.J., (1994). Further development of the electrochemical analysis of urine from cows with BSE. *In:* Transmissible Spongiform Encephalopathies. A Consultation on BSE with the Scientific Veterinary Committee of the Commission of the European Communities held in Brussels, Belgium, 14–15 September 1993. Bradley R. & Marchant B., eds. Document VI/4131/94-EN. European Commission Agriculture, Brussels, Belgium, 369–376.

28. JONES V., MARTIN T.C, KEYES P. & DAWSON M. (1996). Protein markers in cerebrospinal fluid from BSE-affected cattle. *Vet. Rec.,* **139**, 360–363.

29. KATZ J.B., SHAFER A.L. & MILLER J.M. (1995). Production of antiserum for the diagnosis of scrapie and bovine spongiform encephalopathy using a baculovirus-expressed prion protein. *J. Vet. Diagn. Invest.,* **7**, 245–247.

30. KIMBERLIN R.H. (1992). Bovine spongiform encephalopathy. *Rev. sci. tech. Off. int. Epiz.,* **11**, 347–390 (English), 391–439 (French) and 441–489 (Spanish).

31. MASTERS C.L. & RICHARDSON E.P. JR. (1978). Subacute spongiform encephalopathy (Creutzfeldt-Jakob disease). *Brain,* **101**, 333–334.

32. McGILL I.S. & WELLS G.A.H. (1993). Neuropathological findings in cattle with clinically suspect but histologically unconfirmed bovine spongiform encephalopathy (BSE). *J. Comp. Pathol.*, **108**, 241–260.

33. MINISTRY OF AGRICULTURE, FISHERIES AND FOOD (MAFF) (1999). BSE in GB, A Progress Report, June 1999. MAFF Publications, London, UK.

34. MOYNAGH J. & SCHIMMEL H. (1999). Tests for BSE evaluated. *Nature*, **400**, 105.

35. OFFICE INTERNATIONAL DES EPIZOOTIES (OIE) (1996). Bovine spongiform encephalopathy: an update. *Rev. sci. tech. Off. int. Epiz.*, **15**(3), 1087–1118.

36. OFFICE INTERNATIONAL DES EPIZOOTIES (OIE) (2000). International Animal Health Code: Mammals, Birds and Bees, Ninth Edition. OIE, Paris, France.

37. OFFICE INTERNATIONAL DES EPIZOOTIES (OIE) (2000). Chapter I.5. Human Safety in the Veterinary Microbiology Laboratory. *In:* Manual of Standards for Diagnostic Tests and Vaccines, Fourth Edition, OIE, Paris, France.

38. O'ROURKE K.I., BASZLER T.V., PARISH S.M. & KNOWLES D.P. (1998). Preclinical detection of PrP^{Sc} in nictitating membrane lymphoid tissue of sheep. *Vet. Rec.*, **142**, 489–491.

39. RIOND J.-L., HARTMANN P., JOLLER-JEMELKA H.I. & BRAUN U. (1999). S-100 and bovine spongiform encephalopathy. *Vet. Rec.*, **145**, 114–115.

40. ROBEY W.G., JACKSON R., WALTER R.L., BRACKETT C.A., HARRINGTON C.A. & KILLIAN W.R. (1998). use of cerebrospinal fluid levels of 14-3-3 in predicting neurodegeneration in confirmed BSE symptomatic cattle. *Vet. Rec.*, **143**, 50–51.

41. SCHALLER O., FATZER R., STACK M., CLARK J., COOLEY W., BIFFIGER K., EGLI S., DOHERR M., VANDEVELDE M., HEIM D., OESCH B. & MOSER M. (1999). Validation of a Western immunoblotting procedure for bovine PrP^{Sc} detection and its use as a rapid surveillance method for the diagnosis of bovine spongiform encepahlopathy (BSE). *Acta Neuropathol. (Berl.),* **98**, 437–443.

42. SCHREUDER B.E.C. (1994). BSE agent hypotheses. *Livestock Prod. Sci.*, **38** (Special issue on BSE. EAAP Publication No 1/94), 23–33.

43. SCHREUDER L.J.M., Van KEULEN L.J.M., VROMANS M.E.W., LANGEVELD J.P.M. & SMITS M.A. (1998). Tonsillar biopsy and PrP^{Sc} detection in the preclinical diagnosis of scrapie. *Vet. Rec.,* **142**, 564–568.

44. SCIENTIFIC VETERINARY COMMITTEE (1994). Protocols for the Laboratory Diagnosis and Confirmation of Bovine Spongiform Encephalopathy and Scrapie. A report from the Scientific Veterinary Committee 1994, European Commission, Directorate General for Agriculture, Unit for Veterinary Legislation and Zootechnics. Brussels, Belgium.

45. SCOTT A.C., WELLS G.A.H., CHAPLIN H.J. & DAWSON M. (1991). Bovine spongiform encephalopathy: detection of fibrils in the central nervous system is not affected by autolysis. *Res. Vet. Sci.*, **52**, 332–336.

46. SCOTT A.C., WELLS G.A.H., STACK M.J., WHITE H. & DAWSON M. (1990). Bovine spongiform encephalopathy: detection and quantitation of fibrils, fibril protein (PrP) and vacuolation in brain. *Vet. Microbiol.,* **23**, 295–304.

47. SCOTT M.R., WILL R., IRONSIDE J., NGUYEN H.-O.B., TREMBLAY P., DEARMOND S.J. & PRUSINER S.B. (1999). Compelling transgenetic evidence for transmission of bovine spongiform encephalopathy prions to humans. *Proc. Natl Acad. Sci.* USA, **96**, 15137–15142.

48. SIMMONS M.M., HARRIS P., JEFFREY M., MEEK S.C., BLAMIRE I.W.H. & WELLS G.A.H. (1996). BSE in Great Britain: consistency of the neurohistopathological findings in two random annual samples of clinically suspect cases. *Vet. Rec.*, **138**, 175–177.

49. STACK M.J., KEYES P. & SCOTT A.C. (1996). The diagnosis of bovine spongiform encephalopathy and scrapie by the detection of fibrils and the abnormal protein isoform. *In:* Methods in Molecular Medicine: Prion Diseases, Baker H. & Ridley R.M., eds. Humana Press, Totowa, New Jersey, USA, 85–103.

50. TAYLOR D.M. (1996). Inactivation studies on BSE agent. *Br. Food J.,* **98**, 36–39.

51. TAYLOR D.M., FERGUSON C.E., BOSTOCK C.J. & DAWSON M. (1995). Absence of disease in mice receiving milk from cows with bovine spongiform encephalopathy. *Vet. Rec.*, **136**, 592.

52. VICARI A., HORNLIMANN B. & AUDIGE L. (1997). Risk assessment on the role of meat-and-bone meal in the occurrence of bovine spongiform encephalopathy in Switzerland. *Epidemiol. Sante Anim.*, **31–32,** 06.10.1-06.10.3.

53. WELLS G.A.H. (1989). Bovine spongiform encephalopathy. *In:* Veterinary Annual, 29th Issue, Grunsell C.S.G., Raw M.-E. & Hill F.W.G., eds. Wright, London, UK, 59–63.

54. WELLS G.A.H., HANCOCK R.D., COOLEY W.A., RICHARDS M.S., HIGGINS R.J. & DAVID G.P. (1989). Bovine spongiform encephalopathy: diagnostic significance of vacuolar changes in selected nuclei of the medulla oblongata. *Vet. Rec.*, **125**, 521–524.

55. WELLS G.A.H., HAWKINS S.A.C., CUNNINGHAM A.A., BLAMIRE I.W.H., WILESMITH J.W., SAYERS A.R. & HARRIS P. (1994). Comparative pathology of the new transmissible spongiform encephalopaties. *In:* A Consultation on BSE with the Scientific Veterinary Committee of the Commission of the European Communities held in Brussels, 14–15 September 1993. Bradley R. & Marchant B., eds. Document VI/4131/94-EN. European Commission, Agriculture, Brussels, Belgium.

56. WELLS G.A.H., HAWKINS S.A.C., GREEN R.B., AUSTIN A.R., DEXTER I., SPENCER Y.I., CHAPLIN M.J., STACK M.J. & DAWSON, M. (1998). Preliminary observations on the pathogenesis of experimental bovine spongiform encephalopathy (BSE): an update. *Vet. Rec.*, **142,** 103–106.

57. WELLS G.A.H., HAWKINS S.A.C., HADLOW W.J. & SPENCER Y.I. (1992). The discovery of bovine spongiform encephalopathy and observations on the vacuolar changes. *In*: Prion Disease of Humans and Animals, Prusiner S.B., Collinge J., Powell J. & Anderton B., eds. Ellis-Harwood, Chichester, UK, 256–274.

58. WELLS G.A.H., SCOTT A.C., JOHNSON C.T., GUNNING R.F., HANCOCK R.D., JEFFREY M., DAWSON M. & BRADLEY R. (1987). A novel progressive spongiform encephalopathy in cattle. *Vet. Rec.*, **121**, 419–420.

59. WELLS G.A.H., SCOTT A.C., WILESMITH J.W., SIMMONS M.M. & MATTHEWS D. (1994). Correlation between the results of a histopathological examination and the detection of abnormal brain fibrils in the diagnosis of bovine spongiform encephalopathy. *Res. Vet. Sci.*, **56**, 346–351.

60. WELLS G.A.H. & WILESMITH J.W. (1995). The neuropathology and epidemiology of bovine spongiform encephalopathy. *Brain Pathol.*, **5**, 91–103.

61. WILESMITH J.W., HOINVILLE L.J., RYAN J.B.M. & SAYERS A.R. (1992). Bovine spongiform encephalopathy: aspects of the clinical picture and analyses of possible changes 1986–1990. *Vet. Rec.*, **130**, 197–201.

62. WILESMITH J.W., WELLS G.A.H., CRANWELL M.P. & RYAN J.B.M. (1988). Bovine spongiform encephalopathy: epidemiological studies. *Vet. Rec.*, **123**, 638–644.

63. WILESMITH J.W., WELLS G.A.H., RYAN J.B.M., GAVIER-WIDEN D. & SIMMONS M.M. (1997). A cohort study to examine maternally-associated risk factors for bovine spongiform encephalopathy. *Vet. Rec.*, **141**, 239–243.

64. WILL R.G., IRONSIDE J.W., ZEIDLER M., COUSENS S.N., ESTIBEIRO K., ALPEROVITCH A., POSER S., POCCHIARI M., HOFMAN A. & SMITH P.G. (1996). A new variant of Creutzfeldt-Jakob disease in the UK. *Lancet*, **347**, 921–925.

65. WRATHALL A.E. (1997). Risks of transmitting scrapie and bovine spongiform encephalopathy by semen and embryos. *Rev. sci. tech. Off. int. Epiz.*, **16**, 240–264.

66. ZLOTNIK I. & RENNIE J.C. (1957). The occurrence of vacuolated neurones and vascular lesions in the medullas of apparently healthy sheep. *J. Comp. Pathol.*, **67**, 30–36.

67. ZLOTNIK I. & RENNIE J.C. (1958). A comparative study of the incidence of vacuolated neurones in the medulla from apparently healthy sheep of various breeds. *J. Comp. Pathol.*, **68**, 411–415.

*
* *

SECTION 2.4.

SHEEP AND GOAT DISEASES IN LIST B

CHAPTER 2.4.1.

OVINE EPIDIDYMITIS (*Brucella ovis*)

SUMMARY

Brucella ovis *produces a clinical or subclinical disease in sheep that is characterised by genital lesions in rams, and placentitis in ewes. Accordingly, the main consequences of the disease are reduced fertility in rams, infrequent abortions in ewes, and an increased perinatal mortality. The disease has been reported in Argentina, Australia, Brazil, Canada, Chile, France, Germany, Hungary, Mexico, New Zealand, Peru, Romania, Russia, the Slovak Republic, South Africa, Spain, the United States of America and Uruguay, but probably occurs in most sheep-raising countries.*

Identification of the agent: *The existence of clinical lesions (unilateral or, occasionally, bilateral epididymitis) in rams may be indicative of the existence of infection, but laboratory examinations are necessary to confirm the disease. Laboratory confirmation may be based on direct or indirect methods. Direct diagnosis is made by means of bacteriological isolation of* B. ovis *from semen samples or tissues of rams, or vaginal discharges and milk of ewes, on adequate selective media. Molecular biological methods, such as polymerase chain reaction and pulse-field gel electrophoresis, are being developed. However, indirect diagnosis based on serological tests is preferred for routine diagnosis.*

Serological tests: *Agar gel immunodiffusion (AGID) test, complement fixation (CF) test, and enzyme-linked immunosorbent assay (ELISA) using soluble surface antigens obtained from* B. ovis, *can be used; some ELISAs using recombinant proteins and monoclonal antibodies are being tested in field trials. The sensitivities of the AGID test and ELISA are similar and sometimes the ELISA has higher sensitivity than the CF test. A combination of the AGID test and ELISA seems to give the best results in terms of sensitivity. However, with regard to simplicity and cost, the AGID test is the most practicable test for diagnosis of* B. ovis. *The prescribed test for international trade, however, remains the CF test.*

Requirements for vaccines and diagnostic biologicals: *Seed cultures for antigen or vaccine production should be obtained from internationally recognised laboratories. A single standard dose (10^9 colony-forming units) of the live* B. melitensis *Rev. 1 vaccine, administered subcutaneously or conjunctivally, can be used effectively in rams for the prevention of* B. ovis *infection. This vaccine strain should meet minimal quality standards: adequate concentration, absence of dissociation and adequate residual virulence and immunogenicity (see Chapter 2.4.2. Caprine and ovine brucellosis [excluding* B. ovis *infection]).*

A. DIAGNOSTIC TECHNIQUES

Brucella ovis causes a genital infection of ovine livestock manifested by epididymitis, infrequent abortions, and increased lamb mortality. Passive venereal transmission via the ewe appears to be a frequent route of infection, but ram-to-ram transmission is also common[1] (2). Infected ewes may excrete *B. ovis* in vaginal discharge and milk and, accordingly, ewe-to-ram and lactating ewe-to-lamb transmission could also be determinant mechanisms of infection.

The demonstration of the existence of genital lesions (unilateral or, occasionally, bilateral epididymitis) by palpating the testicles of rams may be indicative of the presence of this infection in a given flock. However, this clinical diagnosis is not sensitive enough because only about 50% of rams infected with *B. ovis* present epididymitis (2). Moreover, the clinical diagnosis is extremely unspecific due to the existence of many other bacteria causing clinical epididymitis. The most frequently reported isolates causing epididymitis in rams include *Actinobacillus seminis*, *A. actinomycetemcomitans*, *Histophilus ovis*, *Haemophilus* spp., *Corynebacterium pseudotuberculosis ovis*, *B. melitensis* and *Chlamydia psittaci* (4, 5, 8, 10, 11, 19, 23, 25). It must be emphasised that many palpable epididymal lesions in rams are sterile, trauma-induced spermatic granulomas.

Although cows, goats and deer have been susceptible to *B. ovis* in artificial transmission experiments, no natural cases have been reported in these species. To date, no human cases have been reported, and *B. ovis* is considered to be nonzoonotic. However, in areas where *B. melitensis* infection coexists with *B. ovis*, special care is required when handling samples, which should be transported to the laboratory in leak-proof containers.

1. Identification of the agent

a) Collection of samples

The most valuable samples for the isolation of *B. ovis* from live animals are semen, vaginal swabs and milk. For the collection of vaginal swabs and milk, see the instructions given in Chapter 2.4.2. Caprine and ovine brucellosis (excluding *B. ovis* infection). Semen (genital fluids) can be collected easily in swabs taken from the preputial cavity after electro-ejaculation. If an electro-ejaculator is not available, swabs can be take' from the vagina of brucellosis-free ewes immediately after natural mating. However, a less contamina sample of semen can be obtained: the penis should be extracted, cleaned and the ejaculate collecte(sterile bottles.

For the isolation of *B. ovis* after necropsy, the preferred organs in terms of probability of isolation are the epididymides, seminal vesicles, and ampullae and inguinal lymph nodes in rams, and the uterus, iliac and supra-mammary lymph nodes in ewes. However, to obtain maximum sensitivity, a complete search that includes other organs and lymph nodes (spleen, cranial, scapular, prefemoral and testicular lymph nodes) should be performed. Dead lambs and placentas should also be examined. The preferred culture sites in aborted or stillborn lambs are abomasal content and lung.

Samples for culture should be refrigerated and transported to the laboratory as soon as possible after collection. The organism remains viable for at least 72 hours at room temperature and survival is enhanced at 4°C or, preferably, by freezing the tissue samples.

b) Staining methods

Semen or vaginal smears can be examined following staining by Stamp's method (1, 7) (see Chapter 2.4.2.), and characteristic coccobacilli should be demonstrated in many infected animals (24). Examination of Stamp-stained smears of suspect tissues (ram genital tract, inguinal lymph nodes, placentas, and abomasal content and lung of fetuses) may also allow a rapid presumptive diagnosis.

However, other bacteria with similar morphology or staining characteristics (*B. melitensis, Coxiella burnetii,* and *Chlamydia* spp.) can also be present in such samples, making the diagnosis difficult for inexperienced personnel. Microscopy results should always be confirmed by culture of the microorganism.

c) Culture

The best direct method of diagnosis is bacteriological isolation on adequate culture media. Semen, vaginal swabs, or milk samples can be smeared directly on to plates with adequate culture media and incubated at 37°C in an atmosphere of 5–10% CO_2. Tissues should be macerated and ground in a small amount of sterile saline or phosphate buffered saline (PBS) with a stomacher or blender, before plating.

[1] Under the semi-extensive production systems (most common in European Mediterranean countries) rams are usually housed together. Direct ram-to-ram transmission during nonbreeding periods is quite frequent and has been suggested to take place by several routes, including the rectal mucosa. Most ram-to-ram infections, however, are produced through the oral route. Housed rams establish hierarchies (head-to-head combats), and it is frequent that 'dominated' rams, after being 'mated' by the dominant rams, lick the prepuce of these dominant rams as an act of submission. If these dominant rams are infected, the probability of having *B. ovis* in the prepuce (excretion in the semen) is very high.

Growth normally appears after 3 days, but cultures should not be discarded as negative until 8–10 days have elapsed. Colonies of *B. ovis* become visible (0.5–2.5 mm) after 3–5 days of incubation, and are rough phase, round, shiny and convex.

Brucella ovis can be isolated in nonselective media, such as blood agar base enriched with 10% sterile ovine or bovine sera, or in blood agar medium with 5–10% sterile ovine blood. However, the inoculum frequently contains other bacteria, which often overgrow *B. ovis*. Accordingly, the use of selective media may be preferred. Various *B. ovis* selective media have been described. The procedure of Brown *et al.* (3), modified as follows (12), is recommended:

The basal ingredients for 1 litre of media are: GC medium base (38 g); haemoglobin (10 g); antibiotics: vancomycin (3 mg); colistin (7.5 mg); nystatin (100,000 International Units [IU] = 17.7 mg); cycloheximide (100 mg); and nitrofurantoin (10 mg). Working solutions are prepared as follows:

Solution A: Add 500 ml of distilled water to the GC medium base, heat the paste carefully while stirring continuously and autoclave at 120°C for 20 minutes.

Solution B: Suspend the haemoglobin in 500 ml of distilled water, adding the water slowly to avoid lumps. Once dissolved, add a magnetic stirrer and autoclave at 120°C for 20 minutes.

Antibiotic solution (prepared daily): Vancomycin, cycloheximide and colistin are suspended in individual tubes containing 1 ml of sterile distilled water; the nystatin is suspended in 1 ml of methanol, and the nitrofurantoin is suspended in 1 ml of a 0.1 M NaOH sterile solution (filtration through 0.22 µm filters). Once autoclaved, stabilise the temperature (45–50°C) of both solutions A and B with continuous stirring. Mix both solutions (adding A to B), avoiding bubble formation. Add the antibiotic solution while stirring continuously and carefully. Dispense into sterile plates.

To avoid contamination, the final concentration of agar (1.2%) may be increased to 2–3%, adding Bacto Agar. Once prepared, the plates should not be stored for long periods, and freshly prepared medium is always recommended. This medium is also suitable for the isolation of *B. melitensis*.

Another suitable, but less effective, antibiotic combination is: Vancomycin (3 mg/litre); colistin (7.5 mg/litre); nystatin (12,500 IU/litre); and nitrofurantoin (10 mg/litre). The antibiotics may be added to 7% sheep blood or 1% (w/v) haemoglobin agar, such as GC medium.

d) Identification and typing

Brucella ovis colonies are not haemolytic. They are circular, convex, have unbroken edges, are always of the nonsmooth type when examined by oblique illumination, and test positive in the acriflavine test (1, 7). *Brucella ovis* lacks urease activity, fails to reduce nitrate to nitrite, is catalase positive and oxidase negative, does not produce H_2S and, although it does not grow in the presence of methyl violet, it usually grows in the presence of standard concentrations of basic fuchsin and thionin. The cultures are not lysed by *Brucella*-phages of the Tb, Wb and Iz groups at the routine test dilution (RTD) or 10^4 RTD, while they are lysed by phage R/C (1, 7). Most laboratories are not equipped for a complete identification, and a practical schedule for presumptive identification is needed. Most *B. ovis* isolates can be correctly identified on the basis of growth characteristics, direct observation using obliquely reflected light, Gram or Stamp's staining, catalase, oxidase, urease and acriflavine tests. However, definitive identification should be carried out by reference laboratories with experience in identification and typing of *Brucella*. Recently, a method using pulse-field gel electrophoresis was developed for *Brucella*. With this method it is possible to differentiate *B. ovis* from other *Brucella* species (15).

2. Serological tests

The most efficient and widely used tests are double agar gel immunodiffusion (AGID), complement fixation (CF), and the indirect enzyme-linked immunosorbent assay (ELISA). Several countries have adopted various standard diagnostic techniques for *B. ovis*, but the only test prescribed by the OIE and the European Union (EU) for international trade is the CF test. However, it has been demonstrated that the AGID test shows similar sensitivity to the CF test, and it is a simpler test to perform. Although standardisation is lacking, numerous independent studies have shown that the ELISA is more sensitive and specific than either the CF or AGID tests. At present there is no internationally standardised test method for the serological diagnosis of *B. ovis*.

- **Antigens**

When rough *Brucella* cells are heat-extracted with saline (hot-saline method, HS), they yield water-soluble antigenic extracts whose major component precipitates with sera to rough *Brucella* (9, 16). For this reason, the HS extracts have been referred to as the 'rough-specific antigen' or, when obtained from *B. ovis*, as the '*B. ovis* specific antigen'. However, the chemical characterisation of the HS extracts from *B. ovis* has shown that they are enriched in rough lipopolysaccharide (R-LPS), group 3 outer membrane proteins and other outer membrane components (17). Thus, HS extracts contain LPS determinants specific for *B. ovis*, but also additional antigenic components, some of them shared with rough and smooth *B. melitensis* and other *Brucella* (20). Such components account for the cross-reactivity that is sometimes observed with the HS method and sera of sheep infected with *B. melitensis* or vaccinated with Rev. 1 (17). The HS extract, due to its water solubility and high content of relevant cell surface epitopes, is the best diagnostic antigen and has been widely used for the serological diagnosis of *B. ovis* infection.

Brucella ovis REO 198, a CO_2-independent strain, is recommended as a source of the HS antigens to be used in serological tests. This strain can be obtained from INRA[2]. Solid media decribed in Section A.1.c. are satisfactory for the growth of *B. ovis* REO 198. Ideally, several biotypes of *B. ovis* should be included in the antigen. HS antigen is prepared as follows:

i) Exponentially grow a suitable, preferably aerobic, strain of *B. ovis*, e.g. REO 198, in one of the following ways: For 48 hours in Trypticase soy broth flasks in an orbital incubator at 37°C and 150 rpm; or in Roux bottles of Trypticase soy agar, or other suitable medium, with 5% serum added; or in a batch-type fermenter as decribed for *B. abortus*, but with the addition of 5% serum to the medium.

ii) Cells are washed twice and then resuspended in 0.85% saline (12 g of dried cells or 30 g of wet packed cells in 150 ml).

iii) The cell suspension is then autoclaved at 120°C for 15–30 minutes.

iv) After cooling, the suspension is centrifuged (15,000 *g*, 4°C, 15 minutes) and the supernatant fluid is filtered and dialysed against distilled water (3 × 100 volumes) at 4°C for at least 2 days.

v) The dialysed fluid is ultracentrifuged (100,000 *g*, 4°C, 6–8 hours), and the sediment is resuspended in a small amount of distilled water and freeze-dried.

HS is then resuspended either in distilled water (for use in the AGID test), veronal buffered saline (for use in the CF test), or carbonate–bicarbonate buffer (for use in the ELISA) and titrated against a set of positive and negative sera.

The resuspended HS is kept at 4°C with 0.5% phenol as preservative (only for use in the AGID test) or freeze-dried. Freezing and thawing should be avoided (9). The CF test antigen should be standardised against the International anti-*B. ovis* Standard Serum[3].

a) Complement fixation test (the prescribed test for international trade)

There is no standardised method for the CF test, but the test is most conveniently carried out using the microtitration method. Some evidence shows that cold fixation is more sensitive than warm fixation (6, 18, 21), but that it is less specific. Anticomplementary reactions, common with sheep serum, are, however, more frequent with cold fixation.

Several methods have been proposed for the CF test using different concentrations of fresh sheep red blood cells (SRBC) (a 2–3% suspension is usually recommended) sensitised with an equal volume of rabbit anti-SRBC serum diluted to contain several times (usually from two to five times) the minimum concentration required to produce 100% lysis of SRBC in the presence of a titrated solution of guinea-pig complement. The latter is independently titrated (in the presence or absence of antigen according to the method) to determine the amount of complement required to produce either 50% or 100% lysis of sensitised SRBC in a unit volume of a standardised suspension; these are defined as the 50% or 100% haemolytic unit of complement ($C'H_{50}$ or $C'H_{100}$), respectively. It is generally recommended to titrate the complement before each set of tests, a macromethod being preferred for an optimal determination of $C'H_{50}$. Usually, 1.25–2 $C'H_{100}$ or 5–6 $C'H_{50}$ are used in the test.

Barbital (veronal) buffered saline (VBS) is the standard diluent for the CF test. This is prepared from tablets available commercially, otherwise it may be prepared according to the formula described elsewhere (see Chapter 2.3.1. Bovine brucellosis). The test sera should be inactivated for 30 minutes in a water bath at 60–63°C, and then diluted (doubling dilutions) in VBS. The stock solution of HS antigen (2.5–20 mg/ml in VBS) is diluted in VBS as previously determined by titration (checkerboard titration). Usually, only one serum dilution is tested (generally 1/10).

2 Institut national de la recherche agronomique (INRA) Laboratoire de Pathologie Infectieuse et Immunologie, 37380 Nouzilly, France.

3 Obtainable from the OIE Reference Laboratory for Brucellosis, VLA Weybridge, Addlestone, Surrey KT15 3NB, United Kingdom.

Using standard 96-well microtitre plates with round (U) bottom, the technique is usually performed as follows:

i) Volumes of 25 µl of diluted inactivated test serum are placed in the well of the first and second rows. Volumes of 25 µl of CF test buffer are added to all wells except those of the first row. Serial doubling dilutions are then made by transferring 25 µl volumes of serum from the second row onwards.

ii) Volumes of 25 µl of antigen, diluted to working strength, and 25 µl of complement, diluted to the number of units required, are added to each well.

iii) Control wells containing diluent only, serum + complement + diluent, antigen + complement + diluent, complement + diluent, are set up to contain 75 µl total volume in each case. A control serum that gives a minimum positive reaction should be tested in each set of tests to verify the sensitivity of test conditions.

iv) The plates are incubated at 37°C for 30 minutes or at 4°C overnight, and a volume (25 or 50 µl according to the techniques) of sensitised SRBC is added to each well. The plates are reincubated at 37°C for 30 minutes.

v) The results are read after the plates have been centrifuged at 1000 ***g*** for 10 minutes at 4°C or left to stand at 4°C for 2–3 hours to allow unlysed cells to settle. The degree of haemolysis is compared with standards corresponding to 0, 25, 50, 75 and 100% lysis. The titre of the serum under test is the highest dilution in which there is 50% or less haemolysis.

- **Standardisation of the results of the complement fixation test**

  There is a unit system that is based on the International Standard for anti-*Brucella ovis* Serum (ISABS, International Standard 1985 [see footnote 2]). This serum contains 1000 IU/ml and gives a titre of 1/100 (50% haemolysis). If this serum is tested in a given method and gives a titre of, for example 200, then the factor for an unknown serum tested by that method can be found from the formula: 1000/200 × titre of test serum = number of ICFTU (International complement fixation test units) of antibody in the test serum per ml. It is recommended that any country using the CF test on a national scale should obtain agreement among the different laboratories performing the test by the same method, to allow the same level of sensitivity to be obtained. Results should always be expressed in international units, calculated in relation to those obtained in a parallel titration with a standard serum, which itself may be calibrated against the ISABS.

vi) *Interpretation of the results:* Generally, sera giving a titre equivalent to 50 ICFTU/ml or more are considered to be positive in the EU.

b) Agar gel immunodiffusion test

The AGID test uses the following reagents: Good grade Noble agar or agarose; sodium chloride (NaCl); borate buffer: boric acid (12.4 g); potassium chloride (14.5 g); and distilled water (1600 ml).

Adjust to pH 8.3 with 0.2 M NaOH solution and complete to 2000 ml with distilled water.

To prepare the gels, dissolve 1 g of agarose (or Noble agar), 10 g of NaCl and 100 ml of borate buffer by boiling while stirring continuously. On a flat surface, cover clean glass slides with the necessary amount of molten gel to form a bed of 2.5 mm depth (3.5 ml approximately for standard microslides). After the gel has solidified (15–20 minutes), holes are cut in the gel using a gel puncher. The holes should be 3 mm in diameter and 3 mm apart, and should be arranged in a hexagonal pattern around a central hole that is also 3 mm in diameter. The test can be adapted to Petri dishes and other patterns.

Sera to be examined are placed in alternate wells separated by a control positive serum (infection proved by bacteriology), with the antigen at its optimum concentration in the central well. The results are read after incubation for 24 and 48 hours at room temperature in a humid chamber. A positive reaction is a clearly defined precipitin line between the central well and the wells of the test sera that gives total or partial identity with that of the positive controls. Precipitin lines not giving total identity may also appear and correspond to minor antigenic components of HS extracts (antibodies to these components can also be common in infections due to *B. melitensis*). These reactions should also be considered to be positive.

The HS (2.5–20 mg/ml) diluted in distilled water and containing 0.5% phenol as a preservative is the antigen used in the AGID test (this preserved antigen can be stored at 4°C for at least 1 month). Dilutions of antigen are tested with a panel of 20–30 sera from *B. ovis* naturally infected rams and with a panel of *Brucella*-free animals. The optimum concentration of antigen is the concentration that gives the clearest line with all the *B. ovis* sera, and is negative with the sera from *Brucella*-free animals.

c) **Enzyme-linked immunosorbent assay**

Several variations of this test have been proposed. The test described here is an indirect ELISA using ABTS (2,2'-Azino-bis-[3-ethylbenzothiazoline-6-sulphonic acid]) as chromogen. Tests are performed on 96-well flat-bottomed ELISA plates. Reagent and serum dilutions are made in PBS, pH 7.2, with the addition of 0.05% Tween 20 (PBST). Antigen dilutions are made in a carbonate–bicarbonate buffer, pH 9.6. Plates are washed after antigen coating and between incubations, where appropriate, usually with PBST. The antigen (HS) and conjugate are checkerboard titrated, and dilutions are selected to give the best ratio between negative and positive standard sera. Secondary (anti-ovine IgG [H+L chains]) antibodies are usually conjugated to horseradish peroxidase, although other enzymes can be used. If a peroxidase conjugate is used, the chromogen, usually ABTS, is diluted in a substrate buffer, pH 4 (composed of citric acid trisodium and citric acid). To this is added the substrate, hydrogen peroxide (H_2O_2), and the plate is incubated for 15–60 minutes at room temperature. The reaction may be stopped with 1 mM sodium azide, and the colour change is read at 405–414 nm (for further details see Chapter 2.3.1.).

The antigen used in the ELISA is the HS in stock solution at 1 mg/ml in coating buffer, titrated in a checkerboard titration, with different dilutions of antigen, conjugate and substrate, against a standard serum or against serial dilutions of a panel of sera that are positive and negative for *B. ovis* to determine the most sensitive dilution (usually 5–10 µg/ml).

- **Test procedure**

i) Microtitre plates are coated by the addition of 100 µl of a predetermined antigen dilution in carbonate buffer, pH 9.6, to each well. Plates are incubated for 2 hours at 37°C or overnight at 4°C. They are then washed four times to remove unbound antigen and dried by tapping firmly upside down on an absorbent paper. The coated plates can be used immediately or dried and stored at 4°C (the stability in these conditions is adequate for at least 1 month).

ii) *Sera:* Dilute test and positive and negative control serum samples 1/200 by the addition of a minimum of 10 µl of serum to 2 ml PBST. Add 100 µl volumes of samples in duplicate to the microtitre plates. The plates are covered, incubated at 37°C for 1 hour, and washed three times with the washing buffer.

iii) *Conjugate:* The titrated conjugate is diluted in PBST, added (100 µl) to the wells, and the plate is covered and incubated for 1 hour at 37°C. After incubation, the plates are washed again three times with PBST.

iv) *Substrate:* The solution of ABTS in substrate buffer is added (100 µl/well) and the plates are incubated 15–60 minutes at room temperature with continuous shaking.

v) *Reading and interpreting the results:* Absorbance is read automatically in a spectrophotometer at 405–414 nm. Absorbance values may be expressed as percentages of the mean absorbance of the positive control or, preferably, transformed into ELISA units calculated either manually or by using a computer and a curve-fitting program from a standard curve constructed with the series of positive control dilution results. The threshold should be calculated by testing a sufficiently large *B.-ovis*-free sheep population, the sensitivity of the test being controlled on *B.-ovis*-infected animals.

Comparative studies have shown that the ELISA has better sensitivity than either the AGID or the CF tests (14, 18, 22, 26, 27). Due to the existence of some ELISA-negative and AGID-positive sera, the combination of the AGID test and ELISA gives optimal sensitivity (14). However, the combination of CF test and ELISA or CF and AGID tests does not improve the sensitivity of ELISA alone (14). Moreover, the CF test has other important disadvantages – such as complexity, obligatory serum inactivation, anticomplementary activity of some sera, the difficulty of performing it with haemolysed sera, and prozone phenomena. Because of its sensitivity, simplicity and easy interpretation, the AGID test is very practicable for routine diagnosis in nonspecialised laboratories.

B. REQUIREMENTS FOR VACCINES AND DIAGNOSTIC BIOLOGICALS

Vaccination is probably the most economical and practical means for medium-term control of *B. ovis* in areas with a high incidence of infection. For long-term control, consideration should be given to the effect of vaccination on serological testing, and *B.-ovis*-free accreditation programmes have to be implemented. The live *B. melitensis* strain Rev. 1 (see Chapter 2.4.2.) is probably the best available vaccine for the prophylaxis of *B. ovis* infection (2). A single standard dose (10^9 colony-forming units) of Rev. 1 administered, subcutaneously (in a 1 ml volume) or conjunctivally (in a 25–30 µl volume), to 3–5-month-old rams confers adequate immunity against *B. ovis*. Conjunctival vaccination has the advantage of minimising the intense and long-lasting serological response evoked by subcutaneous vaccination, thereby improving the specificity of serological tests (2). When used in young animals, the Rev. 1 vaccine is safe enough and side-effects appear to be rare. However, there is limited information concerning the safety of Rev. 1 vaccine when used in adult rams. One study found that the subcutaneous or conjunctival vaccination of 13-month-old rams did not produce undesirable side-effects and protected rams against *B. ovis,* although the number of animals was limited in this study (13). This finding should be reinvestigated using a larger number of adult rams as, in countries with extensive management and high levels of incidence, it would be advisable to vaccinate both young and healthy adult rams.

REFERENCES

1. ALTON G.G., JONES L.M., ANGUS R.D. & VERGER J.M. (1988). Techniques for the Brucellosis Laboratory. INRA, Paris, France.

2. BLASCO J.M. (1990). *Brucella ovis. In:* Animal Brucellosis, Nielsen K. & Duncan J.R., eds. CRC Press, Boca Raton, Florida, USA, 351–378.

3. BROWN G.M., RANGER C.R. & KELLEY D.J. (1971). Selective media for the isolation of *Brucella ovis. Cornell Vet.,* **61**, 265–280.

4. BULGIN M.S. & ANDERSON B.C. (1983). Association of sexual experience with isolation of various bacteria in cases of ovine epididymitis. *J. Am. Vet. Med. Assoc.,* **182**, 372–374.

5. BURGESS G.W. & MCDOWELL J.W. (1981). *Escherichia coli* epididymitis and seminal vesiculitis in a ram. *Aust. Vet. J.,* **57**, 479–480.

6. BURGESS G.W. & NORRIS M.J. (1982). Evaluation of the cold complement fixation test for diagnosis of ovine brucellosis. *Aust. Vet. J.,* **59**, 23–25.

7. CORBEL M.J., GILL K.P.W. & THOMAS E.L. (1978). Methods for the identification of *Brucella.* Ministry of Agriculture, Fisheries and Food, UK, ADAS, RCV 22.

8. DE LONG W.J., WALDHALM D.G. & HALL R.F. (1979). Bacterial isolates associated with epididymitis in rams from Idaho and eastern Oregon flocks. *Am. J. Vet. Res.,* **40,** 101–102.

9. DIAZ R. & BOSSERAY N. (1973). Identification d'un composé antigénique spécifique de la phase rugueuse (R) des *Brucella. Ann. Rech. Vet.,* **4,** 283–292.

10. EKDAHL M.O., MONEY D.F. & MARTIN C.A. (1968). Some aspects of epididymitis of rams in New Zealand. *N. Z. Vet. J.,* **16**, 81–82.

11. LIVINGSTONE C.W. & HARDY W.T. (1964). Isolation of *Actinobacillus seminis* from ovine epididymitis. *Am. J. Vet. Res.,* **25**, 660–663.

12. MARIN C.M., ALABART J.L. & BLASCO J.M. (1996). Effect of antibiotics contained in two *Brucella* selective media on growth of *B. abortus, B. melitensis* and *B. ovis. J. Clin. Microbiol.,* **34**, 426–428.

13. MARIN C.M., BARBERAN M., JIMENEZ DE BAGUES M.P. & BLASCO J.M. (1990). Comparison of subcutaneous and conjunctival routes of Rev. 1 vaccination for the prophylaxis of *Brucella ovis* infection in rams. *Res. Vet. Sci.,* **48**, 209–215.

14. MARIN C.M., JIMENEZ DE BAGUES M.P., BLASCO J.M., GAMAZO C., MORIYON I. & DIAZ R. (1989). Comparison of three serological tests for *Brucella ovis* infection of rams using different antigenic extracts. *Vet. Rec.,* **125**, 504–508.

15. MICHAUX-CHARACHON S., BOURG G., JUMAS-BILAK E., GUIGUE-TALET P., ALLARDET-SERVENT A., O'CALLAHAN D. & RAMUZ M. (1997). Genome structure and phylogeny in genus *Brucella. J. Bacteriol.,* **179**, 3244–3249.

16. MYERS D.M., JONES L.M. & VARELA-DIAZ V. (1972). Studies of antigens for complement fixation and gel diffusion tests in the diagnosis of infections caused by *Brucella ovis* and other *Brucella. Appl. Microbiol.,* **23**, 894–902.

17. RIEZU-BOJ J.I., MORIYON I., BLASCO J.M., MARIN C.M. & DIAZ R. (1986). Comparison of lipopolysaccharide and outer membrane protein-lipopolysaccharide extracts in an enzyme-linked immunosorbent assay for the diagnosis of *Brucella ovis* infection. *J. Clin. Microbiol.,* **23**, 938–942.

18. RIS D.R., HAMEL K.L. & LONG D.L. (1984). Comparison of an enzyme-linked immunospecific assay (ELISA) with the cold complement fixation test for the serodiagnosis of *Brucella ovis* infection. *N. Z. Vet. J.*, **32**, 18–20.

19. RODOLAKIS A. & BERNARD K. (1977). Isolement de *Chlamydia* des organes génitaux de béliers atteints d'épididymite. *Bull. Acad. Vet. Fr.*, **50**, 65–70.

20. SANTOS J.M., VERSTREATE D.R., PERERA V.Y. & WINTER A.J. (1984). Outer membrane proteins from rough strains of four *Brucella* species. *Infect. Immun.*, **46**, 188–194.

21. SEARSON J.E. (1982). Sensitivity and specificity of two microtitre complement fixation tests for the diagnosis of *Brucella ovis* infection in rams. *Aust. Vet. J.*, **58**, 5–7.

22. SPENCER T.L. & BURGESS G.W. (1984). Enzyme-linked immunosorbent assay for *Brucella ovis* specific antibody in ram sera. *Res. Vet. Sci.*, **36**, 194–198.

23. WEBB R.F. (1983). Clinical findings and pathological changes in *Histophilus ovis* infections of sheep. *Res. Vet. Sci.*, **35**, 30–34.

24. WEBB R.F., QUINN C.A., COCKRAM F.A. & HUSBAND A.J. (1980). Evaluation of procedures for the diagnosis of *Brucella ovis* infection in rams. *Aust. Vet. J.*, **56**, 172–175.

25. WILLIAMSON P. & NAIRN M.E. (1980). Lesions caused by *Corynebacterium pseudotuberculosis* in the scrotum of rams. *Aust. Vet. J.*, **56**, 496–498.

26. WORTHINGTON R.W., STEVENSON B.J. & DE LISLE G.W. (1985). Serology and semen culture for the diagnosis of *Brucella ovis* infection in chronically infected rams. *N.Z. Vet. J.*, **33**, 84–86.

27. WORTHINGTON R.W., WEDDELL W. & PENROSE M.E. (1984). A comparison of three serological tests for the diagnosis of *B. ovis* infection in rams. *N.Z. Vet. J.*, **32**, 58–60.

*

* *

CHAPTER 2.4.2.

CAPRINE AND OVINE BRUCELLOSIS (excluding *Brucella ovis* infection)

SUMMARY

Brucella melitensis *(biovars 1, 2 or 3) is the main causative agent of caprine and ovine brucellosis. Sporadic cases caused by* B. abortus *have been observed, but clinical disease is rare.* Brucella melitensis *appears to occur naturally in the Mediterranean region, but infection is widespread world-wide. North America is believed to be free from the agent, as are Northern Europe, South-East Asia, Australia and New Zealand.*

Clinically, the disease is characterised by one or more of the following signs: abortion, retained placenta, orchitis, epididymitis and, rarely, arthritis.

Brucella melitensis *is highly pathogenic for humans, causing one of the most serious zoonoses in the world, and all infected tissues, cultures and potentially contaminated materials should be handled under conditions for a high level of biohazard containment.*

Identification of the agent: *Presumptive evidence of* Brucella *is provided by the demonstration, by modified acid-fast staining of organisms, of* Brucella *morphology in abortion material or vaginal discharge, especially if supported by serological tests. The recently developed polymerase chain reaction methods provide additional means of detection. Whenever possible,* Brucella *spp. should be isolated using plain or selective media by culture from uterine discharges, aborted fetuses, udder secretions or selected tissues, such as lymph nodes, testes or epididymi. Species and biovars should be identified by phage lysis, and by cultural, biochemical and serological criteria.*

Serological and allergic skin tests: *The rose bengal plate agglutination and complement fixation tests are usually recommended for screening flocks and individual animals. The serum agglutination test is not considered to be reliable for use in small ruminants. For pooled samples, there are no useful tests such as the milk ring test in cattle. The brucellin allergic skin test can be used as a screening or complementary test in unvaccinated flocks, provided that a purified, lipopolysaccharide (LPS)-free, standardised antigen preparation is used. Results must then be interpreted in relation to the clinical signs, history, and the results of serological or cultural examination.*

Requirements for vaccines and diagnostic biologicals: Brucella melitensis *strain Rev.1 live vaccine is recommended to immunise sheep and goats at risk of infection from* Brucella melitensis. *Production of* Brucella *antigens or Rev.1 vaccine is based on a seed-lot system. Seed cultures to be used for antigens for serological and allergic skin tests and for vaccines should originate from reference centres. They must conform to minimal standards for viability, smoothness, residual infectivity and immunogenicity, if applicable. Antigens for serological tests should be standardised against reference sera calibrated against the International Standard anti* Brucella abortus *Serum, and the procedures and interpretations should conform to international recommendations. Allergen preparations should be free from LPS to prevent anti-LPS antibody production and local inflammatory reactions.*

A. DIAGNOSTIC TECHNIQUES

Brucella are the causative agents of brucellosis, a zoonosis of world-wide importance, that is also called 'Malta fever', 'Mediterranean fever' *(B. melitensis)* or Bang's disease *(B. abortus)* or 'undulant fever' (either). Brucellosis affects both humans and animals. The main domestic animals that are affected are cattle, sheep, goats, and pigs. A number of wildlife species, such as bison, elk, reindeer and caribou, can also be infected. The principal manifestations of animal brucellosis are reproductive failure, i.e. abortion and birth of unthrifty offspring in females, and orchitis and epididymitis in males. Arthritis is also a rare sign. Brucellosis in humans is usually characterised by an influenza-like clinical disease, which may be severe and may be followed by chronic, intermittent relapses.

Caprine and ovine brucellosis (excluding *B. ovis*) is primarily caused by *B. melitensis*. While sporadic cases caused by *B. abortus* have been observed in sheep and goats, clinical signs are rare. Pathologically and epidemiologically, *B. melitensis* infection in sheep and goats is very similar to *B. abortus* infection in cattle. In most circumstances, the primary route of transmission of *Brucella* is the placenta, fetal fluids and vaginal discharges expelled by infected ewes and goats when they abort or have a full-term parturition. Shedding of *Brucella* is also common in udder secretions and semen, and *Brucella* may be isolated from various tissues, such as lymph nodes from the head and those associated with reproduction, and from arthritic lesions (2).

Brucellae are Gram-negative coccobacilli or short rods with straight or slightly convex sides and rounded ends. They do not ferment carbohydrates in conventional media. The genus *Brucella* is now considered to contain six species: *B. abortus*, *B. melitensis*, *B. suis*, *B. ovis*, *B. canis* and *B. neotomae*. Seven biovars are recognised for *B. abortus*, three for *B. melitensis* and five for *B. suis*. However, the degree of genetic relatedness as shown by DNA hybridisation studies is consistent with the existence of a single species within the genus *Brucella*. *Brucella abortus*, *B. melitensis*, *B. suis* and *B. neotomae* occur normally in the smooth form, while *B. ovis* and *B. canis* are invariably nonsmooth species.

The World Health Organization (WHO) laboratory biosafety manual classifies *Brucella* in Risk group III. Brucellosis is readily transmissible to humans, causing acute febrile illness – undulant fever – which may progress to a more chronic form and can also produce serious complications affecting the musculo-skeletal, cardiovascular, and central nervous systems. Infection is essentially acquired by the oral, respiratory, or conjunctival routes, but ingestion of dairy products constitutes the main risk to the general public. There is an occupational risk to veterinarians and farmers who handle infected animals and aborted fetuses or placentae. Brucellosis is one of the most easily acquired laboratory infections, and strict safety precautions should be observed when handling cultures and heavily infected samples, such as products of abortion. The examination of serum samples presents a minimal hazard and precautions normally required by good laboratory practice are sufficient. The examination of heavily infected material should be carried out in safety cabinets by adequately trained staff. Suitable protective clothing should be worn and facilities for its disinfection and for the safe decontamination of apparatus, discarded cultures, and other hazardous material should be provided. Specific recommendations have been made for the safety precautions to be observed with *Brucella*-infected materials (for further details, see refs 2 and 13).

1. Identification of the agent (2, 3)

Unequivocal diagnosis of *Brucella* infections can be made only by the isolation and identification of *Brucella*, but in situations where bacteriological examination is not practicable, diagnosis must be based on serological methods. There is no single test by which a bacterium can be identified as *Brucella*. A combination of growth characteristics, serological and bacteriological methods is usually needed.

a) Staining methods

Brucella are coccobacilli or short rods measuring from 0.6 to 1.5 µm long and from 0.5 to 0.7 µm wide. They are usually arranged singly, and less frequently in pairs or small groups. The morphology of *Brucella* is fairly constant, except in old cultures where pleomorphic forms may be evident. *Brucella* are nonmotile. They do not form spores, and flagella, pili, or true capsules are not produced. *Brucella* are Gram negative and usually do not show bipolar staining. They are not truly acid-fast, but are resistant to decolorisation by weak acids and thus stain red by the Stamp's modification of the Ziehl–Neelsen method. This is the usual procedure for the examination of smears of organs or biological fluids that have been previously fixed with heat or ethanol, and by this method, *Brucella* organisms stain red against a blue background. However, the method has a low sensitivity in milk and dairy products where *Brucella* are often present in small numbers, and interpretation is frequently impeded by the presence of fat globules. Care must be taken in the interpretation of results because other organisms that cause abortions, *e.g. Chlamydia psittaci* or *Coxiella burnetii*, are difficult to differentiate from *Brucella* organisms. The results, whether positive or negative, should be confirmed by culture.

b) Culture

- **Basal media**

Direct isolation and culture of *Brucella* are usually performed on solid media. This is generally the most satisfactory method as it enables the developing colonies to be isolated and recognised clearly. Such media also limit the establishment of nonsmooth mutants and excessive development of contaminants. However, the use of liquid media may be recommended for voluminous samples or those where *Brucella* are present in small numbers. A wide range of commercial dehydrated basal media is available, e.g. *Brucella* medium base, Trypticase soy or Trypticase soy agar, and Bactotryptose. The addition of 2–5% bovine or equine serum is necessary for the growth of strains such as *B. abortus* biovar 2, and many laboratories systematically add serum to basal media, such as blood agar base (Oxoid) or Columbia agar (BioMérieux), with excellent results. Other satisfactory media, such as serum dextrose agar or glycerol dextrose agar, can be used (2). Serum dextrose agar is usually preferred for observation of colonial morphology. A nonselective, biphasic medium, known as Castañeda's medium, is recommended for the isolation of *Brucella* from blood and other body fluids or milk, where enrichment culture is usually advised. Castañeda's medium is used because brucellae tend to dissociate in broth medium, and this interferes with biotyping by conventional bacteriological techniques.

- **Selective media**

All the basal media mentioned above can be used for the preparation of selective media. Appropriate antibiotics are added in order to suppress the growth of organisms other than *Brucella*. The most widely used selective medium is Farrell's medium, which is prepared by the addition of six antibiotics to a basal medium. The following quantities are added to 1 litre of agar: polymyxin B sulphate (5000 units = 5 mg); bacitracin (25,000 units = 25 mg); cycloheximide (100 mg); nalidixic acid (5 mg); nystatin (100,000 units); vancomycin (20 mg).

A freeze-dried antibiotic supplement is available commercially (Oxoid). However, nalidixic acid and bacitracin, at the concentration used in Farrell's medium, could have inhibitory effects for some *B. melitensis* strains (15). Moreover, Farrell's medium inhibits the growth of *B. ovis*. The sensitivity increases significantly by the simultaneous use of both Farrell's and the modified Thayer–Martin medium. Briefly, the modified Thayer–Martin's medium can be prepared with GC medium base (Difco Laboratories, Detroit, United States of America [USA]) supplemented with 2 g/litre of bacto agar (Difco), haemoglobin (Difco) and colistin methanesulphonate (7.5 mg/litre), vancomycin (3 mg/litre), nitrofurantoin (10 mg/litre), nystatin (100,000 International Units [IU]/litre = 17.7 mg) and cycloheximide (100 mg) (all products from Sigma Chemical, St Louis, United States of America (USA) (15). Contrary to *B. abortus*, growth of *B. melitensis* is not dependent on an atmosphere of 5–10% CO_2.

A selective biphasic medium composed of the basal Castañeda's medium with the addition of the following antibiotics to the liquid phase, is sometimes recommended for isolation of *Brucella* in milk (quantities are per litre of medium): polymyxin B (sulphate) (6000 units = 6 mg); bacitracin (25,000 units = 25 mg); cycloheximide (100 mg); nalidixic acid (5 mg); amphotericin B (1 mg); vancomycin (20 mg); D-cycloserine (100 mg).

On suitable solid media, *Brucella* colonies are visible after a 2-day incubation period. After 4 days' incubation, *Brucella* colonies are round, 1–2 mm in diameter, with smooth margins. They are translucent and a pale honey colour. When plates are viewed in the daylight through a transparent medium. When viewed from above, colonies appear convex and pearly white. Later, colonies become larger and slightly darker.

Smooth (S) *Brucella* cultures have a tendency to undergo variation during growth, especially with subcultures, and to dissociate to rough (R) forms. Colonies are then much less transparent, have a more granular, dull surface, and range in colour from matt white to brown in reflected or transmitted light. Changes in the colonial morphology are generally associated with changes in virulence, serological properties and phage sensitivity.

- **Collection and culture of samples**

For the diagnosis of animal brucellosis by cultural examination, the choice of samples usually depends on the clinical signs observed. The most valuable samples include aborted fetuses (stomach contents, spleen and lung), fetal membranes, vaginal secretions (swabs), milk, semen and arthritis or hygroma fluids. From animal carcasses, the preferred tissues for culture are those of the reticulo-endothelial system (i.e. head, mammary and genital lymph nodes and spleen), the pregnant or early post-parturient uterus, and the udder. Growth normally appears after 2–3 days, but cultures should not be discarded as negative until 8–10 days have elapsed.

Tissues: Samples are removed aseptically with sterile instruments and macerated using a 'Stomacher' or tissue grinder with a small amount of sterile phosphate buffered saline (PBS), before being inoculated on to solid media.

Vaginal discharge: A vaginal swab taken after abortion or parturition is an excellent source for the recovery of *Brucella* in sheep and goats. The swab is then streaked on to solid media.

Milk: Samples of milk must be collected cleanly after washing and drying the whole udder and disinfecting the teats. It is essential that samples should contain milk from all quarters, and 10–20 ml of milk should be taken from each teat. The first streams are discarded and the sample is milked directly into a sterile vessel. Care must be taken to avoid contact between the milk and the milker's hands. The milk is centrifuged at 2000 ***g*** for 15 minutes in sealed tubes (to avoid the risk of aerosol contamination of personnel), and the cream and deposit are spread on solid selective medium, either separately or mixed. If Brucellae are present in bulk milk samples, their numbers are usually low, and isolation from such samples is very unlikely.

Dairy products: Dairy products, such as cheeses, should be cultured on the media described above. As these materials are likely to contain small numbers of organisms, enrichment culture is advised. Samples need to be carefully homogenised before culture, after they have been ground in a tissue grinder or macerated and pounded in a 'Stomacher' or an electric blender with an appropriate volume of sterile PBS. Superficial strata (rind and underlying parts) and the core of the product should be cultured. As Brucellae grow, survive or disappear quite rapidly, their distribution throughout the different parts of the product varies according to the local physico-chemical conditions linked to specific process technologies.

Milk and tissue samples should be cooled immediately after they are taken, and transported to the laboratory in the most rapid way. On arrival at the laboratory, all samples should be frozen if they are not to be cultured immediately.

Use of animals should be avoided unless absolutely necessary but may sometimes provide the only means of detecting the presence of *Brucella*, especially when samples have been shown to be heavily contaminated or likely to contain a low number of *Brucella* organisms. Animal inoculation may be either subcutaneously or through abraided skin in guinea-pigs or, preferably, intravenously in mice. The spleens of mice are cultured 7 days after inoculation and, for guinea-pigs, a serum sample is subjected to specific tests 3 and 6 weeks after inoculation, then the spleens are cultured.

c) Identification and typing

Any colonies of *Brucella* morphology should be checked using a Gram-stained (or a Stamp-stained) smear. As the serological properties, dyes and phage sensitivity are usually altered in the nonsmooth phases, attention to the colonial morphology is essential in the typing tests described below. The recommended methods for observing colonial morphology are Henry's method by obliquely reflected light, the acriflavine test described by Braun & Bonestell, or White & Wilson's crystal violet method of staining colonies (2).

Identification of *Brucella* organisms can be carried out by a combination of the following tests: organism morphology and Gram or Stamp's staining, colonial morphology, growth characteristics, urease, oxidase and catalase tests, and the slide agglutination test with an anti-*Brucella* polyclonal serum. Species and biovar identification requires elaborate tests (such as phage lysis and agglutination with A-, M- or R-specific antisera), the performance of which is left to reference laboratories with expertise in these methods. The simultaneous use of several phages e.g. Tbilissi (Tb), Weybridge (Wb), Izatnagar (Iz) and R/C provides a phage-typing system that, in experienced hands, allows a practical identification of smooth and rough species of *Brucella*. However, several characteristics, for example added CO_2 requirement for growth, production of H_2S (detected by lead acetate papers), and growth in the presence of basic fuchsin and thionin at final concentrations of 20 µg/ml, are revealed by routine tests that can be performed in moderately equipped nonspecialised laboratories.

When sending *Brucella* strains to a reference laboratory for typing, it is essential that smooth colonies be selected. Cultures should be lyophilised and sealed in ampoules packed in screw-capped canisters or subcultured on to appropriate nutrient agar slopes contained in screw-capped bottles. The strains could also be sent suspended in transport media (e.g. Amies), but this could provide an opportunity for the establishment of rough mutants.

Brucella organisms are among the most dangerous bacteria with which to work in terms of the risk of producing laboratory-acquired infections. For transporting *Brucella* cultures through the post, it is recommended that the caps of the bottles or canisters should be screwed tightly down and sealed with PVC tapes. Bottles should be wrapped in absorbent paper or cotton wool, sealed in polyethylene bags and packed into a rigid wooden or metal container. This is then wrapped, addressed and labelled 'infectious substance' and, if necessary, labelled in accordance with the requirements of the International Air Transport Association and any special import regulations (2, 13). Before dispatching samples across national boundaries, prior permission should be obtained from the receiving laboratory.

d) Nucleic acid recognition methods

The recently developed polymerase chain reaction (PCR) provides an additional means of detection and identification of *Brucella* sp. Despite the high degree of DNA homology within the genus *Brucella*, several methods, including PCR-restriction fragment length polymorphism (RFLP) and Southern blot, have been developed that allow, to a certain extent, differentiation between *Brucella* species and some of their biovars. Recently, a method using pulse-field gel electrophoresis was developed for *Brucella*. With this method it is possible to differentiate several *Brucella* species (16). However, none of these methods has been fully evaluated and standardised, and none is widely available (for further details see ref. 11).

2. Serological tests (2, 14)

In situations where bacteriological examination is not practicable, diagnosis of *Brucella* infection must often be based on serological methods. In routine tests, anti-*Brucella* antibodies are detected in serum or milk. The most widely used serum-testing procedures for the diagnosis of *Brucella* infection in sheep and goats are the buffered *Brucella* antigen tests (BBAT), i.e. the card and rose bengal plate agglutination test, which are essentially the same, and the complement fixation (CF) test. The bulk milk ring test, which has great usefulness for locating infected cattle herds, is ineffective in small ruminants. The WHO, the United States Department of Agriculture (USDA), and the European Union (EU), have adopted specific recommendations for standardising the test performance and interpretation of the results for all the different methods mentioned above (2, 13).

In small ruminants, the BBAT and CF test are the most widely used methods (13). While the BBAT is not very specific but appears to be adequate as a screening test for detecting infected flocks or to guarantee the absence of infection in brucellosis-free flocks, discrepancies between the BBAT and CF test results are not rare in infected sheep and goats (5). Thus, the results of the two tests should be considered simultaneously to increase the likelihood of detecting infected individuals and improve the control of the disease in areas where it has not been completely eradicated (1, 3, 5). A few Rev.1 vaccinates, however, may become persistent reactors.

Some success has been achieved in the past few years with enzyme-linked immunosorbent assays (ELISAs) using various antigens, but generally those with a high content of smooth lipopolysaccharide (LPS). A gene (bp26) that expresses a highly immunogenic protein from *B. abortus* (17) and from *B. melitensis* (9) was isolated and the protein used for diagnosis in different host species. Results showed that this antigen could be useful in differentiating S19 and Rev.1 vaccinated from infected bovines and sheep (10, 17). These tests promise increased sensitivity and specificity, but a great deal of work is still required on standardisation of reagents (11).

- **Antigens for the buffered *Brucella* antigen and complement fixation tests**

Brucella abortus biovar 1 strains 99 or 1119-3 are recommended for the preparation of CF test and rose bengal plate agglutination test antigens. These generally consist of inactivated standardised *Brucella* 0.5% phenol saline whole-cell suspensions. Detailed methods for the preparation and standardisation of the antigens are described in Chapter 2.3.1. Bovine brucellosis and in ref. 2.

Brucella abortus strain 99 (Weybridge) or 1119-3 (USDA) original seed should be used[1]. Production of *Brucella* antigens is based on a seed-lot system. Strains should be cultured in a suitable medium. The method of culture should be such as to avoid bacterial dissociation and thereby to maintain the smooth characteristic of the culture. Agar medium should be well dried, and a minimum number of subcultures made before production cultures are seeded. Changes in medium should be avoided. The original seed cultures should be propagated to produce a seed lot that must conform to the properties of the original strains. The bacteria should be suspended in a buffer solution, which may contain a suitable stabiliser, and preserved by lyophilisation or by freezing at liquid nitrogen temperature. All cultures must be pure and must conform to the characteristics of CO_2-independent strains of *B. abortus* biovar 1.

The rose bengal plate agglutination test antigen used in the EU is standardised without reference to the cell concentration, but so that a positive reaction is achieved at a dilution of 1/47.5 of the Second International Standard for anti-*Brucella abortus* Serum (ISABS), and a negative reaction at a dilution of 1/55. However, recent results have shown that the presently accepted international standardisation should be modified to increase the sensitivity of the test in sheep and goats, for example by using an adequate standard serum panel (5). The CF test antigen used in the EU is standardised against the ISABS to give 50% fixation at a dilution of 1/200 of this serum. The antigen is generally issued as a concentrate and is diluted in CF diluent before use in each day's test.

Rose bengal plate agglutination test and other BBAT antigens and CF test antigens are phenol saline *Brucella* whole-cell suspensions. The phenol concentration must not exceed 0.5%.

---

1 Original seed should be obtained from the OIE Reference Laboratory for Brucellosis at VLA Weybridge, New Haw, Addlestone, Surrey KT15 3NB, United Kingdom, or the United States Department of Agriculture (USDA), National Veterinary Services Laboratories (NSVL), 1800 Dayton Avenue, Ames, Iowa 50010, USA.

a) **Buffered *Brucella* antigen test – rose bengal plate agglutination test (a prescribed test for international trade)**

This test is a simple spot agglutination test using antigen stained with rose bengal and buffered to a low pH, usually 3.65±0.05. Note that normally antigen made with *B. abortus* is used to test for *B. melitensis.*

i) Bring the serum samples and antigen to room temperature (22±4°C); only sufficient antigen for the day's tests should be removed from the refrigerator.

ii) Place 25–30 µl of each serum sample on a white tile, enamel or plastic plate, or in a WHO haemagglutination plate.

iii) Shake the antigen bottle well, but gently, and place an equal volume of antigen near each serum spot.

iv) Immediately after the last drop of antigen has been added to the plate, mix the serum and antigen thoroughly (using a clean glass rod for each test) to produce a circular or oval zone approximately 2 cm in diameter.

v) The mixture is agitated gently for 4 minutes at ambient temperature on a rocker or three-directional agitator (if the reaction zone is oval or round, respectively).

vi) Read for agglutination immediately after the 4-minute period is completed. Any visible reaction is considered to be positive. A control serum that gives a minimum positive reaction should be tested before each day's tests are begun to verify the sensitivity of test conditions.

The use of 75 µl of serum and 25 µl of antigen, rather than 25 (to 30) µl of each, increases the sensitivity of the rose bengal plate agglutination test in small ruminants (5).

b) **Complement fixation test (a prescribed test for international trade)**

There is no standardised method for the CF test, but this test is most conveniently done by the microtitration method. Either warm or cold fixation may be used for the reaction between test serum, antigen and complement. In warm fixation, the mixture is held at 37°C for 30 minutes. In cold fixation the mixture is held at 4°C for 14–18 hours. A number of factors affect the choice of the method: anticomplementary activity in serum samples of poor quality is more evident with cold fixation, while fixation at 37°C increases the frequency and intensity of prozones, and a number of dilutions must be tested for each sample.

Several methods have been proposed for the CF test using different concentrations of fresh or preserved sheep red blood cells (SRBCs) (a 2.5% or 3% suspension is usually recommended) sensitised with an equal volume of rabbit anti-SRBC serum diluted to contain several times (usually from two to five times) the minimum concentration required to produce 100% lysis of SRBCs in the presence of a titrated solution of guinea-pig complement. The latter is independently titrated (in the presence or absence of antigen according to the method) to determine the amount of complement required to produce either 50% or 100% lysis of sensitised SRBCs in a unit volume of a standardised suspension; these are defined as the 50% or 100% haemolytic unit of complement ($C'H_{50}$ or $C'H_{100}$), respectively. It is generally recommended to titrate the complement before each set of tests, a macromethod being preferred for an optimal determination of $C'H_{50}$. Usually, 1.25–2 $C'H_{100}$ or 5–6 $C'H_{50}$ are used in the test.

Barbital (veronal) buffered saline is the standard diluent for the CF test. This is prepared from tablets available commercially, otherwise it may be prepared according to the formula described elsewhere (see Chapter 2.3.1. Bovine brucellosis, and refs 2 and 14). The undiluted test sera should be inactivated for 30 minutes in a water bath at 60°C±2°C. Usually, only one serum dilution is tested (generally 1/4 or 1/5 depending on the CF procedure chosen), but serial dilutions could be tested when a serum titration is needed. The minimal temperature for sheep and goats is 58°C, but 60°C is better in order to prevent anticomplementary problems; 62°C is required when testing camel or equine sera.

Using standard 96-well microtitre plates with round (U) bottoms, the technique is usually performed as follows:

i) Volumes of 25 µl of diluted inactivated test serum are placed in the well of the first and second rows. Volumes of 25 µl of CF test buffer are added to all wells except those of the first row. Serial doubling dilutions are then made by transferring 25 µl volumes of serum from the second row onwards.

ii) Volumes of 25 µl of antigen, diluted to working strength, and 25 µl of complement, diluted to the number of units required, are added to each well.

iii) Control wells containing diluent only, serum + complement + diluent, antigen + complement + diluent, complement + diluent, are set up to contain 75 µl total volume in each case. A control serum that gives a minimum positive reaction should be tested in each set of tests to verify the sensitivity of test conditions.

iv) The plates are incubated at 37°C for 30 minutes or at 4°C overnight, and a volume (25 or 50 µl according to the technique) of sensitised SRBCs is added to each well. The plates are reincubated at 37°C for 30 minutes.

v) The results are read after the plates have been centrifuged at 1000 *g* for 10 minutes at 4°C or left to stand at 4°C for 2–3 hours to allow unlysed cells to settle. The degree of haemolysis is compared with standards corresponding to 0, 25, 50, 75 and 100% lysis.

- **Standardisation of results of the complement fixation test**

  There is a unit system that is based on the Second ISABS[2]. This serum contains 1000 IU per ml and gives a titre of 1/100 (50% haemolysis). If this serum is tested in a given method and gives a titre of, for example 200 (50% haemolysis), then the factor for an unknown serum tested by that method can be found from the formula: 1000/200 × titre of test serum = number of ICFTU (International complement fixation test units) of antibody in the test serum per ml. The EU has adopted this as its unit. The EU standard serum[3] contains 1000 EU units/ml, like the ISABS. The ISABS contains specific IgG; national standard sera should also depend on this isotype for their specific complement-fixing activity. Difficulties in standardisation arise because different techniques selectively favour CF by different immunoglobulin isotypes. It is recommended that any country using the CF test on a national scale should obtain agreement among the different laboratories performing the test by the same method, to allow the same level of sensitivity to be obtained. To facilitate comparison between countries, results should always be expressed in IUs, calculated in relation to those obtained in a parallel titration with a standard serum, which in turn may be calibrated against the ISABS.

vi) *Interpretation of the results:* Generally, sera giving a titre equivalent to 20 ICFTU/ml or more are considered to be positive.

3. Dermal hypersensitivity test

Delayed-type hypersensitivity reactions associated with cell-mediated immunity may be induced by either infection or immunisation with living or killed adjuvanted vaccines. Because of this, a number of skin tests have been developed. Antigens that are free of smooth LPS, such as Brucellin-INRA[4] or the commercial Brucellergène OCB[5], are preferable to crude preparations that interfere with serological diagnosis. Reactions are, therefore, specific to the genus *Brucella,* and no reactions are observed in brucellosis-free unvaccinated individuals or flocks that have had no contact with *Brucella* organisms. However, not all infected animals react. The allergic skin test is now more widely used for the surveillance of unvaccinated sheep and goat herds, either as a screening or a complementary test, and has been reported to be very helpful (2, 3, 13).

In sheep and goats, the test is done by injecting intradermally 50 µg of Brucellin-INRA (in 0.1 ml of saline solution) or 0.1 ml of Brucellergène OCB, into the lower eyelid. Reading of the reaction should take place 48 hours after injection, and any visible or palpable reaction of hypersensitivity, such as an oedematous reaction leading to an elevation of the skin or thickening of the eyelid (≥2 mm), should be interpreted as a positive reaction.

B. REQUIREMENTS FOR VACCINES AND DIAGNOSTIC BIOLOGICALS

B1. *Brucella melitensis* strain Rev.1 vaccine

Brucella melitensis Rev.1 vaccine is used as a freeze-dried suspension of live *B. melitensis* Rev.1 strain for the immunisation of sheep and goats. It is normally given to lambs and kids aged between 3 and 6 months as a single subcutaneous injection. The standard dose is between 0.5×10^9 and 4.0×10^9 viable organisms. The use of this vaccine administered by the conjunctival route with a minimum dose of $1–5 \times 10^8$ produces a similar protection without a persistent antibody response. Care must be taken when using this route to avoid the risk of contaminating the environment or causing human infection. In many developing countries, vaccination of adult animals has to be considered as the best option for the control of the disease. However, Rev.1 vaccine is known to often cause abortion and excretion in milk when animals are vaccinated during pregnancy, either with full or

2 Obtainable from the VLA (see footnote 1).

3 Obtainable from Bundesinstitut für gesundheitlichen Verbraucherschutz und Veterinärmedizin, Thielallee 88-92, 14195 Berlin, Postfach 33 00 13, 14191 Berlin, Germany.

4 A national French reference brucellin has been produced by INRA-PII (Nouzilly, France) and is obtainable from the OIE Reference Laboratory for Brucellosis, AFSSA-LERPAZ, BP67, 94703 Maisons-Alfort Cedex, France.

5 Synbiotics Europe, 2 rue Alexander Fleming, 69007 Lyon, France.

reduced dose. These side-effects are considerably reduced when adult animals are vaccinated conjunctivally before mating or during the last month of pregnancy. Therefore, when mass vaccination is the only means of controlling the disease, a vaccination campaign should be recommended using the standard dose of Rev.1 administered by the conjunctival route when the animals are not pregnant or during the lambing season.

The subcutaneous vaccination of young animals at full dose and the vaccination of adult animals, even at reduced doses, may lead to long-term persistence of vaccinal antibodies in a proportion of animals that could create a serious obstacle to the serological diagnosis of brucellosis. Conjunctival vaccination minimises these problems. Therefore, the serological diagnosis of brucellosis should take into account the vaccinal state of the herd and the overall frequency distribution of antibody titres detected in the group of animals tested. Animals from herds with persistent vaccinal antibodies are not suitable for international trade, unless this trade takes place between countries with similar control policies.

1. Seed management

a) Characteristics of the seed

Brucella melitensis strain Rev.1 original seed for vaccine production can be obtained[6]. A European reference Rev.1 strain that possesses the characteristics of the Rev.1 original seed has been recently produced by the European Pharmacopoeia[7].

Production of *Brucella* live vaccines is based on the seed-lot system described above (Section A.2.) for rose bengal plate agglutination test and CF test antigens. Strains should be cultured in a suitable medium. Strain Rev.1 must conform to the characteristics of *B. melitensis* biovar 1, except that it should grow more slowly. Additionally, it should grow on agar containing streptomycin (2.5 µg/ml), and it should be inhibited by the addition to a suitable culture medium of benzylpenicillin sodium (3 µg [5 IU]/ml), thionin (20 µg/ml) or basic fuchsin (20 µg/ml). It must also conform to the characteristics of residual virulence and immunogenicity in mice of the original seed.

b) Method of culture (2, 18)

Serum dextrose agar, and Trypticase soy agar, to which 5% serum or 0.1% yeast extract may be added, are among the solid media that have been found to be satisfactory for propagating the Rev.1 strain. Rev.1 strain does not grow well on potato agar.

For vaccine production, Rev.1 may be grown under conditions similar to those described for strains 99 and 1119-3 (see Chapter 2.3.1. Bovine brucellosis), except that Rev.1 generally needs 3–5 days to grow, the phenol saline is replaced by a freeze-drying stabiliser, and the organisms are not killed but are stored at 4°C while quality control examinations are carried out as described below. Moreover, the specific requirements for Rev.1 vaccine production recommend that each seed lot (i.e. the culture used to inoculate medium for vaccine production) should be no more than three passages removed from an original seed culture and that the harvest of a vaccine lot should be no more than three passages from a seed lot or an original seed. The original seed culture should always be checked for the absence of dissociation before use. The recommended method for preparing seed material is given in ref. 2. The following freeze-drying stabiliser (sterilised by filtration) is of proven value: enzymatic digest of casein (2.5 g); sucrose (5 g); sodium glutamate (1 g); distilled water (100 ml).

c) Validation as a vaccine

Numerous independent studies have confirmed the value of *B. melitensis* strain Rev.1 as a vaccine for protecting sheep and goats from brucellosis. Its virulence is unchanged after passage through pregnant sheep and goats. Abortions may result when the Rev.1 vaccine is inoculated into pregnant ewes or goats. The vaccine-induced abortions are not avoided using reduced doses, and doses as low as 10^6, used either subcutaneously or conjunctivally, have been demonstrated to induce abortions (4).

A Rev.1 vaccine is efficient if it possesses the characteristics of the Rev.1 original strain, i.e. those of *B. melitensis* biovar 1 reference strain 16M (ATCC No. 23456), except those specific for the strain Rev.1 (2, 13), and if it proves to be satisfactory with respect to immunogenicity and residual virulence (7) (see below).

6 Obtainable from Institut National de la Recherche Agronomique (INRA), Laboratoire de Pathologie Infectieuse et Immunologie, 37380 Nouzilly, France.
7 Obtainable from the European Pharmacopoeia, BP 907, 67029 Strasbourg Cedex 1, France.

2. Method of manufacture (2, 18)

For production of *B. melitensis* strain Rev.1 vaccine, the procedures described above for antigens (2) can be used except that the cells are collected in a freeze-drying stabiliser and deposited by centrifugation. The yield from one fermenter run or the pooled cells from a batch of Roux flask cultures inoculated on the same occasion from the same seed lot constitutes a single harvest. More than one single harvest may be pooled to form the final bulk that is used to fill the final containers of a batch of vaccine. Before pooling, each single harvest must be checked for purity, cell concentration, dissociation and identity. The volume of the final bulk is adjusted by adding sufficient stabiliser so that a dose contains an appropriate number of viable organisms. After adjusting the cell concentration of the final bulk, tests for identity, dissociation and absence of contaminating organisms are conducted (see below).

3. In-process control

In-process checks should be made on the growth of Rev.1 vaccine from either solid or liquid medium to verify identity and to ensure purity and freedom from dissociation to rough forms during preparation of seed lots, single harvests, final bulks and the final (filling) lots. At least 99% of cells in seed lots and 95% of cells in final lots should be in the smooth phase.

Cell concentration should be estimated on the bulks and precisely determined on final lots. Immunogenicity and the 50% persistence time or 50% recovery time should also be determined on seed lots and final lots.

4. Batch control

With freeze-dried vaccine, the control tests should be conducted on the vaccine reconstituted in the form in which it will be used.

a) Sterility (or absence of extraneous microorganisms)

The Rev.1 vaccine should be checked for bacterial and fungal contamination as prescribed in Chapter I.4.

b) Safety

The Rev.1 vaccine is a virulent product *per se*, and it should keep a minimal virulence to be efficient (see Section B1.4.c.). A safety test may be performed on sheep and goats when a new manufacturing process is started and when a modification in the innocuousness of the vaccine preparation is expected. This control should be done as follows: The test uses 12 ewe lambs and 12 goat kids, aged 4–6 months. Six young females of each species are injected with one or three recommended doses. Each lot of six young females are kept separately. All animals are observed for 21 days. No significant local or systemic reaction should occur. If, for a given dose and route of administration, this test gives good results on a representative batch of the vaccine, it does not have to be repeated routinely on seed lots or vaccine lots prepared with the same original seed and with the same manufacturing process.

c) Potency

A Rev.1 vaccine is efficient if it possesses the characteristics of the Rev.1 original strain, i.e. if it is satisfactory with respect to identity, smoothness, immunogenicity, and residual virulence (8). Batches should also be checked for the number of viable organisms.

- **Identity**

The reconstituted Rev.1 vaccine should not contain extraneous microorganisms. *Brucella melitensis* present in the vaccine is identified by suitable morphological, serological and biochemical tests and by culture: Rev.1 strain is inhibited by addition to the suitable culture medium of 3 µg (5 IU) per ml of benzyl-penicillin sodium; the strain grows on agar containing 2.5 µg per ml of streptomycin.

- **Smoothness (determination of dissociation phase)**

The Rev.1 vaccine reconstituted in distilled water is streaked across six agar plates (serum dextrose agar or Trypticase soy agar with added serum 5% [v/v] or yeast extract 0.1% [w/v]) in such a manner that the colonies will be close together in certain areas, while semi-separated and separated in others. Slight differences in appearance are more obvious in adjacent than widely separated colonies. Plates are incubated at 37°C for 5 days, and examined by obliquely reflected light (Henry's method) before and after staining (three plates) with crystal violet (White & Wilson's staining method).

Appearance of colonies before staining: S colonies appear round, glistening and blue to blue-green in colour. R colonies have a dry, granular appearance and are dull yellowish-white in colour. Mucoid colonies (M) are transparent and greyish in colour and can be distinguished by their slimy consistency when touched with a loop. Intermediate colonies (I), which are the most difficult to classify, have an appearance intermediate between S and R forms: they are slightly opaque and more granular than S colonies.

Appearance of colonies after staining with crystal violet: S colonies do not take up the dye. Dissociated colonies (I, M, or R) are stained various shades of red and purple and the surface may show radial cracks. Sometimes a stained surface film slips off a dissociated colony and is seen adjacent to it.

The colony phase can be confirmed by the acriflavine agglutination test (2). S colonies remain in suspension, whereas R colonies are agglutinated immediately and, if mucoid, will form threads. Intermediate colonies may remain in suspension or a very fine agglutination may occur.

Sometimes a slight dissociation, difficult to observe, can be seen between small colonies (typical Rev.1, 1–1.2 mm in diameter, according to the medium used, residual moisture in the incubator atmosphere, and to the presence or absence of CO_2) and larger colonies. Dissociation between small and large colonies occurs at a ratio of 1 large to 10^3 small colonies. Both are of the S variety. To avoid an increase in this dissociation along successive passages, it is important to select small colonies for preparation of seed lots.

- **Enumeration of live bacteria**

Inoculate each of at least five plates of Tryptose, serum dextrose or other suitable agar medium with 0.1 ml of adequate dilutions of the vaccine spread with a sterile glass, wire or plastic spreader. Colony-forming units (CFU) per vaccine volume unit are enumerated.

- **Residual virulence (50% persistence time or 50% recovery time) (7, 8)**

i) Inject subcutaneously a suspension containing 10^8 live bacteria of the vaccine to be examined into each of 32 female CD1 mice, aged 5–6 weeks.

ii) Kill the mice by cervical dislocation, in groups of eight selected at random 3, 6, 9 and 12 weeks later.

iii) Remove the spleens and homogenise individually and aseptically with a glass grinder in 10 volumes of PBS, pH 6.8.

iv) Spread the suspension on to plates containing a suitable culture medium, using 0.4 ml per plate and no fewer than three plates per spleen (lower limit of detection: five bacteria per spleen). Carry out, in parallel, a similar test using *B. melitensis* Rev.1 reference strain.

v) Calculate the 50% persistence time or 50% recovery time using the Bonet-Maury probit transformation test (6) (eight mice per point, pooled totals, followed by graphical analysis on log-probit paper, arithmetic time scale). The computerised Probit procedure from the SAS statistical package can also be applied for these calculations with similar efficacy (12). The 50% persistence time or 50% recovery time should not differ significantly from that of the reference strain. For Rev.1 strain, the 50% persistence time or 50% recovery time and confidence limits are usually 7.9±1.2 weeks. A good Rev.1 vaccine should keep enough virulence to be efficient.

If this test has been done with good results on a representative batch of the vaccine, it does not have to be repeated routinely on other vaccine lots prepared from the same seed lot and using the same manufacturing process.

- **Immunogenicity in mice (7, 8)**

This test uses six groups of six female CD1 mice, aged 5–7 weeks, that have been selected at random.

i) Inject subcutaneously a suspension containing 10^5 CFU of live bacteria of the vaccine to be examined into each mouse in four of the six groups (24 mice).

ii) Inject a suspension containing 10^5 CFU of live bacteria of a reference S19 or Rev.1 vaccine into each of six mice of the fifth group. The sixth group will serve as the unvaccinated control group.

The exact number of CFU inoculated should be checked afterwards by spreading 0.2 ml of an appropriate dilution of the vaccine suspension on to four plates containing a suitable culture medium.

iii) All the mice are challenged 30 days after vaccination (and immediately following 16 hours' starvation), intraperitoneally with 2×10^5 CFU of *B. abortus* strain 544 (CO_2-dependent). The challenge dose is controlled by plating 0.2 ml of an appropriate dilution on to four plates containing a suitable culture medium.

iv) Kill the mice by cervical dislocation 15 days later.

v) Each spleen is excised aseptically, the fat is removed, and the spleen is weighed and homogenised. Alternatively, the spleens can be frozen and kept at –20°C for from 24 hours to 7 weeks.

vi) Each spleen is homogenised aseptically with a glass grinder in nine times its weight of PBS, pH 6.8 (19 times when the weight is below 120 mg).

vii) Two fractions (0.2 ml) of this first suspension (spleen diluted 1/10 or 1/20) and of the successive dilutions in PBS (1/10, 1/100, 1/1000) are spread on to plates containing a suitable culture medium, using 0.2 ml per plate, in order to count the organisms. Vaccinal strains may survive in mice longer than 45 days (delay from vaccination to autopsy) and disturb the challenge strain enumeration. To distinguish between them, medium is added either with *i*-erythritol (1 g/litre), which inhibits the growth of strain 19, or benzylpenicillin (3 mg/litre), which inhibits the growth of strain Rev.1.

viii) Colonies of *Brucella* are enumerated on plates showing fewer than 300 CFU. When no colony is seen, the spleen is considered to be infected with five bacteria. Results are first recorded as X, the number of *Brucella* per spleen, and expressed as Y, after the following transformation: Y = log (X/log X). Mean and standard deviation, which are the response of each group of six mice, are then calculated.

ix) Conditions of the control experiment are satisfactory if: the response of unvaccinated mice (mean of Y) is at least 4.5; the response of mice vaccinated with the reference strain 19 or Rev.1 vaccine is lower than 2.5; and the standard deviation calculated on each lot of six mice is lower than 0.8.

x) The vaccine under examination is satisfactory if the response of mice vaccinated with this vaccine calculated on the four groups of mice is lower than 2.5.

If this test has been done with good results on a representative batch of the vaccine, it does not have to be repeated routinely on other vaccine lots prepared from the same seed lot and with the same manufacturing process.

Brucella melitensis strain Rev.1 (original seed) and *B. abortus* strain 19, which have been shown satisfactory with respect to immunogenicity and/or residual virulence, can be obtained from INRA (see footnote 6). A European reference Rev.1 strain that has been shown satisfactory with respect to immunogenicity and 50% persistence time or 50% recovery time has been recently produced by the European Pharmacopoeia (see footnote 7).

d) Duration of immunity

It is accepted that subcutaneous or conjunctival vaccination with standard doses of Rev.1 confers a solid and durable immunity in sheep and goats. However, increasing field evidence shows that the immunity conferred declines with time.

The use of reduced doses produces a less efficient immunity, while side-effects, such as antibody responses or induction of abortion, are not avoided.

e) Stability

Strain Rev.1 vaccine prepared from a satisfactory seed stock from appropriate sources is stable in characteristics, provided that in-process and batch control requirements described above are fulfilled, and shows no tendency to reversion to virulence. The freeze-dried vaccine shows a gradual loss of viable count, but should retain its potency for the recommended shelf life (1 year). However, for good vaccine potency, it is not recommended that the viable count immediately after freeze-drying be well in excess of the maximum requirement.

f) Preservatives

Antimicrobial preservatives must not be used in live Rev.1 vaccine. For preparation of the freeze-dried vaccine, a stabiliser as described in Section B1.1.b. is recommended.

g) Precautions (hazards)

As Rev.1 strain is pathogenic for humans, great care should always be taken in handling cultures, especially in bulk, and precautions should always be taken when inoculating, harvesting, bottling and freeze-drying Rev.1 strain. A hazard warning should be included on the label of the final containers. Specific safety measures are detailed in refs 2 and 13.

5. Tests on the final product

a) Safety

See Section B1.4.b.

b) Potency

For the freeze-dried vaccine, the potency must be determined on the final product. The tests are as described in Section B1.4.c.

B2. Brucellin

Brucellin-INRA is an LPS-free extract from rough *B. melitensis* B115. This preparation does not provoke formation of antibodies reactive in rose bengal plate agglutination and CF tests.

1. Seed management

a) Characteristics of the seed

Production of Brucellin-INRA is based on a seed-lot system as described for antigens and vaccines. *B. melitensis* strain B115 for brucellin production can be obtained from INRA (see footnote 6). The original seed should be propagated to produce a seed lot, which should be preserved by lyophilisation or freezing at liquid nitrogen temperature. It should conform to the properties of a pure culture of a rough strain of *B. melitensis* and must not produce smooth *Brucella* LPS. It should produce reasonable yields of a mixture of protein antigens reactive with antisera to smooth and rough *Brucella* strains.

b) Method of culture (2, 18)

Brucella melitensis strain B115 is best grown in the liquid medium described above for fermenter culture. It may be grown by the batch or continuous method in a fermenter or in flasks agitated on a shaker. Purity checks should be made on each single harvest, and the organisms must be in the rough phase.

c) Validation as an *in-vivo* diagnostic reagent

Laboratory and field studies in France have confirmed that Brucellin-INRA is safe, nontoxic and specific in action. The preparation contains 50–75% proteins, mainly of low molecular weight and 15–30% carbohydrate. It does not contain LPS antigens. Brucellin-INRA does not provoke inflammatory responses in unsensitised animals, and it is not in itself a sensitising agent. It does not provoke antibodies reactive in the standard serological tests for brucellosis. More than 90% of small ruminants infected with *B. melitensis* manifest delayed hypersensitivity to Brucellin-INRA at some stage. The preparation is not recommended as a diagnostic agent for individual animals, but can be useful when used for screening herds. It is given to small ruminants in 100-µg doses by the intradermal route, and provokes a local delayed hypersensitivity reaction visible at 48–72 hours in sensitised animals. Positive reactions can be given by vaccinated as well as by infected animals.

2. Method of manufacture (2)

Brucella melitensis B115 cells are killed after culture by raising the temperature to 70°C for 90 minutes, cooled to 4°C, and harvested by centrifugation at 9000 ***g*** for 15 minutes at 4°C. The cells are washed in cold sterile distilled water and dehydrated by precipitating with three volumes of acetone at –20°C, and then allowed to stand at –20°C for 24–48 hours. After repeated washing in cold acetone, followed by a final rinse in diethyl ether, the cells are dried over calcium chloride and held at 4°C. The dried cells are subjected to a viability check. They are resuspended in sterile 2.5% sodium chloride to a final concentration of 5% (w/v) and agitated for 3 days at 4°C. Bacterial cells are removed by centrifugation as above, and the supernatant is concentrated to one-fourth the volume by ultrafiltration on a Diaflo PM10 membrane (Amicon) and precipitated by addition of three volumes of ice-cold ethanol. The mixture is held at 4°C for 24 hours and the precipitate is recovered by centrifugation, redissolved in sterile water, and dialysed to remove ethanol. After centrifugation at 105,000 ***g*** for 6 hours at 4°C, the supernatant material, comprising the unstandardised brucellin, is subjected to assays for protein and carbohydrate. It may be freeze-dried either as bulk material or after it has been dispensed into its final containers.

3. In-process control

The crude brucellin extract should be checked for sterility after acetone extraction, to ensure killing of *Brucella* cells, and again at the end of the process to check possible contamination. The pH and protein concentration should be determined, and identity tests should be performed on the bulk material before filling the final containers.

4. Batch control

a) Sterility

Allergen preparations should be checked for sterility as described in Chapter I.4.

b) Safety

Samples of brucellin from the final containers should be subjected to the standard sterility test. Brucellin preparations should also be checked for abnormal toxicity. Doses equivalent to 20 sheep and goat doses (2 ml) should be injected intraperitoneally into a pair of normal guinea-pigs that have not been exposed previously to *Brucella* organisms or their antigens. Five normal mice are also inoculated subcutaneously with 0.5 ml of the brucellin to be examined. Animals are observed for 7 days, and there should be no local or generalised reaction to the injection.

Dermo-necrotic capacity is examined by intradermal inoculation of 0.1 ml of the product to be examined into the previously shaved and disinfected flank of three normal albino guinea-pigs that have not been exposed previously to *Brucella* organisms or their antigens. No cutaneous reaction should be observed. Absence of allergic and serological sensitisation is checked by intradermal inoculation of three normal albino guinea-pigs, three times every 5 days, with 0.1 ml of a 1/10 dilution of the preparation to be examined. A fourth similar injection is given, 15 days later, to the same three animals and to a control lot of three guinea-pigs of the same weight but which have not been injected previously. The animals should not become seropositive to the standard tests for brucellosis (rose bengal plate agglutination test, CF test) when sampled 24 hours after the last injection, and should not develop delayed hypersensitivity responses.

c) Potency

The potency of brucellin preparations is determined by intradermal injection of graded doses of brucellin into guinea-pigs that have been sensitised by subcutaneous inoculation of 0.5 ml of reference brucellin (see footnote 4) in Freund's complete adjuvant from 1 to 6 months previously. The erythematous reactions are read and measured at 24 hours and the titre is calculated by comparison with a reference brucellin. This method is only valid for comparing brucellin preparations made according to the same protocol as the sensitising allergen. Initial standardisation of a batch of allergen and the sensitisation and titration in ruminants is described in ref. 2.

d) Duration of sensitivity

Duration of sensitivity is uncertain. Individual animals vary considerably in the degree of hypersensitivity manifested to brucellin. Animals in the very early stages of infection, or with long-standing infection, may not manifest hypersensitivity to intradermal injection.

e) Stability

The freeze-dried preparation retains full potency for several years. The liquid commercial preparation should retain potency for the recommended shelf-life.

f) Preservatives

The use of preservatives is not recommended when the preparation is freeze-dried. In the liquid form, sodium merthiolate (at most 0.1 mg/ml) may be used as a preservative. If freeze-dried, the preparation should not be reconstituted until immediately before use.

g) Precautions (hazards)

Brucellin is not toxic. Nevertheless it may provoke severe hypersensitivity reactions in sensitised individuals who are accidentally exposed to it. Care should be taken to avoid accidental injection or mucosal contamination. Used containers and injection equipment should be carefully decontaminated or disposed of by incineration in a suitable disposable container.

5. Tests on final product

a) Safety

A sterility test should be performed by the recommended method. The *in-vivo* safety tests are as those described for batch control (see Section B2.4.b.). These tests on the batch may be omitted if the full test is performed on the final filling lots.

b) Potency

This is performed by injection of a single dose into guinea-pigs using the procedure described in Section B2.4.c.

REFERENCES

1. ALTON G.G. (1990). *Brucella melitensis. In:* Animal Brucellosis, Nielsen K.H. & Duncan J.R., eds. CRC Press, Boca Raton, Florida, USA, 383–409.

2. ALTON G.G., JONES L.M., ANGUS, R.D. & VERGER J.M. (1988). Techniques for the Brucellosis Laboratory. INRA, Paris, France.

3. BLASCO J.M. (1992). Diagnosis of *Brucella melitensis* infection in small ruminants. *In:* Prevention of Brucellosis in the Mediterranean Countries, Plommet M., ed. Pudoc Scientific, Wageningen, The Netherlands, 272–277.

4. BLASCO J.M. (1997). A review on the use of *B. melitensis* Rev 1 vaccine in adult sheep and goats. *Prev. Vet. Med.*, **31**, 275–283.

5. BLASCO J.M., GARIN-BASTUJI B., MARIN C.M., GERBIER G., FANLO J., JIMENEZ DE BAGUES M.P. & CAU C. (1994). Efficacy of different rose bengal and complement fixation antigens for the diagnosis of *Brucella melitensis* infection in sheep and goats. *Vet. Rec.*, **134**, 415–420.

6. BONET-MAURY P., JUDE A. & SERVANT P. (1954). La mesure statistique de la virulence et l'immunité. Application à l'etude de la virulence du bacille typhique et à la mesure du pouvoir immunisant des vaccins antityphoidiques. *Rev. d'Immun. Th. Antimic.*, **18**, 21–49.

7. BOSSERAY N. (1992). Le vaccin Rev.1: dérive des caractères d'immunogénicité et de virulence indépendante des marqueurs classiques. *In:* Prevention of Brucellosis in the Mediterranean Countries, Plommet M., ed. Pudoc Scientific, Wageningen, The Netherlands, 182–186.

8. BOSSERAY N. (1993). Control methods and thresholds of acceptability for anti-*Brucella* vaccines. *Dev. Biol. Stand.*, **79**, 121–128.

9. CLOECKAERT A., DEBBARH H.S., VIZCAINO N., SAMAN E., DUBRAY G. & ZYGMUNT M.S. (1996). Cloning, nucleotide sequence and expression of the *Brucella melitensis* bp26 gene coding for a protein immunogenic in infected sheep. *FEMS Microbiol. Lett.*, **140**, 139–144.

10. DEBBARH H.S., ZYGMUNT M.S., DUBRAY G. & CLOECKAERT A. (1996). Competitive ELISA using monoclonal antibodies to the *Brucella melitensis* bp26 protein to evaluate antibody response in infected and *B. melitensis* Rev1 vaccinated sheep. *Vet. Microbiol.*, **53**, 325–337.

11. GARIN-BASTUJI B., BLASCO J.M., GRAYON M. & VERGER J.M. (1998). Brucella melitensis infection in sheep: present and future. *Vet. Res.*, **29**, 255–274.

12. GRILLO M.J., BOSSERAY N. & BLASCO J.M. (2000). *In vitro* markers and biological activity in mice of seed lot strains and commercial *Brucella melitensis* Rev.1 and *Brucella abortus* B19 vaccines. *Biologicals*, **28**, 119–127

13. JOINT FOOD AND AGRICULTURE ORGANIZATION OF THE UNITED NATIONS/WORLD HEALTH ORGANIZATION EXPERT COMMITTEE ON BRUCELLOSIS (1986). Technical Report Series 740, Sixth Report. WHO, Geneva, Switzerland.

14. MACMILLAN A. (1990). Conventional serological tests. *In:* Animal Brucellosis, Nielsen K.H. & Duncan J.R., eds. CRC Press, Boca Raton, Florida, USA, 153–197.

15. MARIN C.M., ALABART J.L. & BLASCO J.M. (1996). Effect of antibiotics contained in two *Brucella* selective media on growth of *B. abortus, B. melitensis* and *B. ovis. J. Clin. Microbiol.*, **34**, 426–428.

16. MICHAUX-CHARACHON S., BOURG G., JUMAS-BILAK E., GUIGUE-TALET P., ALLARDET-SERVENT A., O'CALLAHAN D. & RAMUZ M. (1997). Genome structure and phylogeny in genus *Brucella. J. Bacteriol.*, **179**, 3244–3249.

17. ROSSETTI O., ARESE A., BOSCHIROLI L. & CRAVERO S. (1996). Cloning of *Brucella abortus* gene and characterisation of expressed 26 kilodalton periplasmic protein: potential use for diagnosis. *J. Clin. Microbiol.*, **34**, 165–169.

18. WORLD HEALTH ORGANIZATION (1977). Requirements for *Brucella melitensis* strain Rev.1 vaccine (Live – for veterinary use). World Health Organization (WHO) Technical Report Series No. 610, 28th Report, Annex 4. WHO, Geneva, Switzerland, 85–97.

*

* *

CHAPTER 2.4.3.

CONTAGIOUS AGALACTIA

SUMMARY

Contagious agalactia, a disease of sheep and goats that manifests as mastitis, arthritis and keratoconjunctivitis, was originally associated only with Mycoplasma agalactiae. *There are now three other mycoplasmas,* M. capricolum *subsp.* capricolum, M. mycoides *subsp.* mycoides *LC* (MmmLC) *and* M. putrefaciens, *that have been shown to cause similar diseases, at times accompanied by pneumonia.*

Identification of the agent: *Differentiation of the above-mentioned aetiological agents depends on the use of suitable media for isolation, and on carrying out biochemical and serological tests on the isolates.*

Serological tests: *Detection of antibodies in serum by complement fixation, growth inhibition or enzyme-linked immunosorbent assay is useful in diagnosis and in epidemiological studies, but does not replace identification of the causal organism for specific diagnosis.*

Requirements for vaccines and diagnostic biologicals: *Killed vaccines are not considered to be efficacious for the prevention of* M. agalactiae *infection, but show promise for that caused by* MmmLC. *Live vaccines made from attenuated cultures have shown better results than killed vaccines with* M. agalactiae *infection, but are not acceptable in all countries.*

A. DIAGNOSTIC TECHNIQUES

Contagious agalactia is a disease of sheep and goats that manifests itself as mastitis, arthritis and keratoconjunctivitis, which has been known for over 170 years. It occurs mainly in Europe, western Asia and North Africa, and is caused by *Mycoplasma agalactiae* (5). A comprenhensive review of this disease was published in 1997 (4). In recent years, *M. capricolum* subsp. *capricolum (Mcc)* (26) and *M. mycoides* subsp. *mycoides* LC *(MmmLC)* have also been isolated in many countries from sheep and goats with mastitis and arthritis. The clinical signs in these infections were sufficiently similar to those of contagious agalactia to lead Perreau (31) to suggest that these infections could also be considered to be contagious agalactia. For this reason, all three organisms will be included in the present discussion. In addition, cases of mastitis and arthritis in goats associated with *M. putrefaciens* (10) have brought notice to a further condition with characteristics similar to those of contagious agalactia. Whether regulatory authorities will prefer to preserve the name for the disease caused by *M. agalactiae* or whether the conditions caused by these other mycoplasmas will be included under the disease name 'contagious agalactia' remains to be determined. Meanwhile, official reports of contagious agalactia outbreaks should always specify which mycoplasma species is involved.

Clinically, the disease caused by *M. agalactiae* may be recognised by elevated temperature, inappetence, alteration in consistency of the milk in lactating ewes with decline and subsequent failure of milk production, lameness and, in some animals, keratoconjunctivitis (8). Pregnant animals may abort. *Mycoplasma agalactiae* may also be found in vulvovaginitis lesions in goats (37), and in lung lesions, but pneumonia is not a consistent finding. Bacteraemia is common and could account for the isolation of the organism from sites where it is only transiently present.

Mastitis, arthritis, pleurisy, pneumonia, and keratoconjunctivitis may all result from infection with *MmmLC*. This organism is widely distributed – it occurs on all the continents, including some countries to which *M. agalactiae* has not spread or where it occurs rarely (1, 9, 31, 35). With few exceptions, *MmmLC* is confined to goats (30). Cases usually occur sporadically, but the disease may persist and slowly spread within a herd. After parturition, the opportunity for spread in milking animals increases, and kids ingesting infected colostrum and milk become infected. The resulting septicaemia with arthritis and pneumonia gives rise to high mortality in kids (9, 12).

Mcc has occurred in geographically diverse situations (Africa, Australia, Europe and the United States of America), but the frequency of occurrence is low (6, 31). Goats are more commonly affected than sheep, and clinical signs of fever, septicaemia, mastitis, and severe arthritis may be followed rapidly by death (6, 8). Pneumonia may be seen at necropsy. The severe joint lesions seen in experimental infections with this organism are accompanied by intense periarticular subcutaneous oedema affecting tissues to some distance from the joint (8). The genital lesions seen in sheep in the United Kingdom are unusual (21).

There are few records of natural infection with *M. putrefaciens* in goats, and none so far in sheep. Perreau (31) commented that *M. putrefaciens* infection in France was associated with mastitis and agalactia, but not usually with arthritis or ocular lesions. In 1987 in California, a large outbreak of mastitis and agalactia in goats was apparently caused by a pure infection with *M. putrefaciens* (10). There was a high rate of abortion in females, followed by death. Severe arthritis later became a prominent sign in females and progeny, although at no time was pyrexia seen in infected goats (10).

1. Identification of the agents

In the living animal, milk, aspirated joint fluid and nasal exudate are the samples of choice for culture, while at necropsy, udder and associated lymph nodes, joint fluid, and lung lesions are the preferred samples. The organisms may also be isolated from liver, kidney, and spleen. Mycoplasms may be isolated from the blood during the acute stage of the disease when there is mycoplasmaemia. The usual techniques used in the isolation of mycoplasmas apply to all four organisms under discussion. Media containing heart-infusion broth, yeast extract (1–2%), and horse or pig serum (15–20%), with bacterial inhibitors, ampicillin (150 mg/litre) or cycloserine (200 mg/litre), will be adequate to isolate and grow *M. agalactiae, Mcc, MmmLC* and *M. putrefaciens* (8, 26). Thallous acetate has been used in some countries, but it is a highly toxic substance with environmental problems and it inhibits the growth of certain mycoplasmas.

Material obtained aseptically is inoculated into liquid, and plated on solid media. The solid medium is incubated in a humid atmosphere at 37°C in 5% CO_2 or in a candle jar (3% CO_2). Liquid medium is incubated at 37°C and plated on to solid medium either when growth is evident, or at 5–7 days even if growth cannot be seen. All four mycoplasmas grow well producing typical fried-egg colonies, those of *Mcc* and *MmmLC* becoming large (up to 2 mm in diameter) in 3–4 days, depending on growth conditions.

Before proceeding further, the cultures should be purified. From well-separated colonies, single representatives are picked off into liquid medium and incubated. When grown, the culture may be filtered through membranes of 0.22–0.45 µm pore size and the filtrate plated on to solid medium and incubated. This process is repeated twice more (42).

The colony appearance is useful to the experienced eye only, but selected biochemical tests (7, 13) can help with initial screening.

a) Biochemical tests

Growth in liquid medium containing glucose (1%), arginine (0.2%), and phenolphthalein diphosphate (0.01%), on solid medium containing horse serum or egg yolk for the demonstration of film and spots, and on casein agar or coagulated serum agar to test for proteolysis, are among the most useful tests for differentiating among the four mycoplasmas (7).

The characteristics of the four mycoplasmas are:

Organism	Test						
	G	A	F	P	C	S	O
M. agalactiae	–	–	+	+	–	–	–
M. capricolum subsp. *capricolum*	+	+	–	+	+	+	–
M. mycoides subsp. *mycoides* LC	+	–	–	–	+	+	–
M. putrefaciens	+	+	+	+	–	–	+

G = Catabolism of glucose; A = Arginine hydrolysis; F = Production of surface film and spots; P = Presence of phosphatase; C = Digestion of casein; S = Liquefaction of coagulated serum; O = Odour of putrefaction in cultures.

As more strains of each species have undergone testing, variations in some of these results have been found. Some *M. agalactiae* (36) and *M. putrefaciens* strains (Cottew, unpublished data) have failed to produce film and spots. Some strains, otherwise resembling *MmmLC*, have not liquefied coagulated serum (19). *Mcc* strains may be slow to hydrolyse arginine, requiring prolonged incubation (ref. 32, and Cottew, unpublished data) or passages in the medium before hydrolysis is effected. Among the four species, the odour of putrefaction in cultures is peculiar to *M. putrefaciens*. Despite these considerations, the biochemical characteristics can narrow the range of possibilities, but serological tests are required for precise identification. (See also Chapter 2.4.6. Contagious caprine pleuropneumonia, Table 1.)

b) Serological identification

Identification of isolates using specific antisera is usually carried out with the disk growth inhibition test (DGIT) (4), film inhibition test or the indirect fluorescent antibody (IFA) test (13, 27). A comparison with a standard strain is useful.

In the GIT, diluted liquid cultures are seeded on to solid medium and allowed to be absorbed (a streak culture using the 'running drop' method gives good results). Filter paper discs, each saturated with a specific antiserum and allowed to dry, are placed on the agar surface. Stronger reactions are obtained if the antisera are added to wells (4 mm in diameter) made in the agar. Plates are incubated and examined. With suitable homologous antiserum, a zone of up to 7–8 mm in width around the disc or well will be free from growth (complete inhibition). Partial inhibition can occur with weak antisera.

In the IFA test, specific antisera are applied to colonies on growth medium. Homologous antiserum remains attached after washing and is demonstrated by adding fluorescein-conjugated antiglobulin, washing, and viewing the colonies in an epifluorescence microscope (13, 27).

The growth precipitin test is also used (14). This reaction detects antigens that are diffusing from growing culture and is regarded as group-specific rather than species-specific (13).

Antisera for these serological tests have traditionally been prepared against the type strains of the various *Mycoplasma* species, and most field isolates have been readily identified using these antisera. As more strains have been examined, however, some have been found to react poorly with these antisera, while reacting well with antisera to other representative strains of the species. Intraspecific variation in antigenic composition has not been reported for *M. putrefaciens,* but occurs to some degree with *M. agalactiae* (36) and not uncommonly with *Mcc* strains. Thus, diagnosticians may need to have available more than one antiserum to enable all strains of a species to be identified.

Sharing of antigens among species or subspecies can make the allocation of an isolate to a species difficult, as is found in differentiation among strains of *M. capricolum* subsp. *capripneumoniae* (F38), and the bovine Group 7 mycoplasmas (22). The difficulty of placing field isolates into a subspecies of *M. mycoides* is now well known (19). In the diagnostic laboratory, should the suggested use of several representative antisera fail to place an isolate in a species (or subspecies), help from a specialised laboratory could be sought. The identification of first isolates should always be confirmed by a reference laboratory.

c) Nonimmunological identification techniques

In specialised laboratories, work towards speciation of problem strains has made use of nonimmunological techniques, such as the determination of the isoenzyme composition (15) and more complex methods of examining the protein and DNA content of the mycoplasmas, and the use of DNA probes (13), but these techniques are not ready for routine use in a diagnostic laboratory.

Polymerase chain reaction (PCR) assays have been developed and brought into use. The PCR is a relatively stable and robust test for detection of target nucleic acid, and is extremely sensitive. It is used on blood, tissue samples and milk.

Several PCRs specific for *M. agalactiae* have been developed and show similar levels of sensitivity, although based on different gene sequences (11, 38, 39). The PCR has been shown to be more sensitive than culture for detecting *M. agalactiae* in milk samples (40). PCRs have also been reported for *Mmm*LC and *Mcc* (3, 20). To date, no PCRs have been reported for *M. putrifaciens.*

2. Serological tests

a) Complement fixation

Perreau *et al.* (33) reported a standard complement fixation (CF) test that has also been applied to other mycoplasmas involved in the contagious agalactia syndrome. Antigens are prepared from washed organisms, standardised by opacity, and lysed, either ultrasonically or by using sodium lauryl sulphate followed by dialysis. Sera are inactivated at 60°C for 1 hour, and the test is carried out in microtitre plates with overnight fixation in the cold. The haemolytic system is added, and the test is read after complete lysis is shown by the antigen control. A positive result is complete fixation at a serum dilution of 1/40 or greater for the following mycoplasmas: *M. agalactiae, Mcc,* and *MmmLC*. The CF is regarded as a herd test and at least ten sera are tested from each herd, preferably from acute and convalescent cases.

Some sera from healthy flocks react in the CF test using *M. agalactiae* up to a serum dilution of 1/20, but rarely react with the other two antigens. However, in flocks infected with *M. agalactiae*, sera giving a homologous reaction at 1/80 may cross-react at up to 1/40, the positive threshold, with the other two antigens. It is often difficult to perform the CF test with sheep and goat sera, where possible the enzyme-linked immunosorbent assay (ELISA) is to be preferred.

b) Enzyme-linked immunosorbent assay

ELISAs have been reported to be more sensitive than CF tests for the detection of antibody to *M. agalactiae* (4). Problems of nonspecificity have been overcome by the use of monoclonal or protein G conjugates in the ELISA (25). A number of commercial ELISA kits are now available and these are being used for large-scale surveys in France and the United Kingdom. ELISAs are not widely available for the other three causative mycoplasmas.

c) 'Film and spots' inhibition

'Film and spots' production by the standard or field strains growing on solid culture medium is inhibited by serum containing specific anti-*M.-agalactiae* antibodies. The test methodology is similar to that of an antibiogram on solid mycoplasma culture medium: about 20 µl of each serum should be added to a blank paper disc. After 4–6 days of incubation at 37°C, a radial inhibition of the films around the disc wider than 2 mm is regarded as positive (28). The test serum should be free from antibiotics.

Serological testing for *M. putrefaciens* and *M. capricolum* has not been carried out to the same extent as that for the other mycoplasmas under discussion, but the tests mentioned are equally applicable.

B. REQUIREMENTS FOR VACCINES AND DIAGNOSTIC BIOLOGICALS

Vaccines for the prevention of contagious agalactia due to *M. agalactiae* have been used in countries in Europe and western Asia. No single vaccine has been universally adopted, and no standard methods of preparation and evaluation would apply to all vaccines that have been used.

1. Inactivated vaccines for *Mycoplasma agalactiae* infection

In those countries where live vaccines for *M. agalactiae* are not acceptable, research has focused on the use of killed organisms, usually with an adjuvant. In experimental infections, vaccines inactivated with phenol and adjuvanted with saponin gave superior protection, compared with formalin or heat-inactivated vaccines (41). While some inactivated vaccines have given a degree of protection against clinical disease resulting from experimental challenge (16, 17), this type of vaccine is considered to lack efficacy in the field (29). It is possible that in some instances, the apparent lack of protection given by such a vaccine could have resulted from the animals concerned being infected with one of the other three mycoplasmas involved with the syndrome of contagious agalactia.

2. Live attenuated vaccines for *Mycoplasma agalactiae* infection

Live attenuated vaccines prepared from *M. agalactiae* in Turkey produced better protection than dead vaccines in controlled experiments (16, 17); generalised infection and clinical signs were prevented, but transient infection of the udder could occur after challenge. Lambs born to vaccinated ewes were protected. This vaccine has been used successfully in the field in Turkey (Arisoy, personal communication), but it has not been adopted elsewhere in Europe. However, Lambert, working in France, reported that studies on a live attenuated vaccine gave 'considerable but not total, protection' against challenge and also showed no reversion to virulence during or after ten passages in sheep (24).

A thorough review of contagious agalactia by Lambert (23) has summarised important aspects of the application of dead and live vaccines. Live vaccines should not be used in lactating animals, and should be part of a regional plan in which all flocks from which animals are likely to make contact are vaccinated at the same time.

3. *Mycoplasma mycoides* subsp. *mycoides* LC

In Israel, an inactivated vaccine protected kids against infection with *MmmLC* resulting from ingestion of infected milk, and from subcutaneous challenge (2).

4. *Mycoplasma capricolum* subsp. *capricolum* and *M. putrefaciens*

Although infections with *Mcc* and *M. putrefaciens* are severe, their prevalence is relatively low and, as might be expected, little or no work appears to have been carried out on preventive vaccination for these infections.

• General comment

Eventual prevention of contagious agalactia by vaccination may be possible, but it is complex. In sheep, the condition is almost always due to the single mycoplasma, *M. agalactiae,* but in goats any of four mycoplasmas may be involved. Further, should the antigenic variation that occurs with two of these be associated with the protective antigens, then the vaccine may have to contain several representative strains of each species. As has been discussed, effective vaccines have already been described for *M. agalactiae* and *MmmLC,* but the former is a live attenuated culture that may not be acceptable in some countries. The prevalence of these conditions varies among countries, and these differences would affect decisions on whether large-scale, regional or local vaccination should take place. There is much to be done before vaccination will be widely used in prevention of contagious agalactia. Therefore, it is not possible at this stage to establish standard requirements that would be universally acceptable to all concerned.

• Control

It is of value to draw attention to the informative accounts by Gaillard-Perrin & Lenfant (18) and Picavet (34) on control measures and their application in the field in the absence of specific prophylaxis by vaccination.

• Acknowledgement

Parts of this chapter were taken from or based on versions of the chapter in previous editions of this *Manual.*

REFERENCES

1. BAR-MOSHE B. & RAPAPPORT E. (1978). Contagious agalactia-like disease in goats caused by *Mycoplasma mycoides* subsp. *mycoides* (ovine/caprine serogroup 8). *Refu. Vet.*, **35**, 75–77.

2. BAR-MOSHE B., RAPAPPORT E. & BRENNER J. (1984). Vaccination trials against *Mycoplasma mycoides* subsp. *mycoides* (large-colony type) infection in goats. *Israel J. Med. Sci.*, **20**, 972–974.

3. BASHIRUDDIN J.B., TAYLOR T.K. & GOULD A.R. (1994). A PCR-based test for the specific identification of *Mycoplasma mycoides* subsp. *mycoides* SC in clinical material. *J. Vet. Diagn. Invest.*, **6**, 428–434.

4. BERGONIER D., BERTHOLET X. & POUMARAT F. (1997). Contagious agalactia of small ruminants: current knowledge concerning epidemiology, diagnosis and control. *Rev. sci. tech. Off. int. Epiz.*, **16**, 848–873.

5. CLYDE W.A. (1964). Mycoplasma species identification based upon growth inhibition by specific antisera. *J. Immunol.*, **92**, 958–965.

6. CORDY D.R., ADLER H.E. & YAMAMOTO R. (1955). A pathogenic pleuropneumonia-like organism from goats. *Cornell Vet.*, **43**, 50–68.

7. COTTEW G.S. (1983). Recovery and identification of caprine and ovine mycoplasmas. *In:* Methods in Mycoplasmology, Vol. 2. Diagnostic Mycoplasmology, Tully J.G. & Razin S., eds. Academic Press, New York, USA, 91–104.

8. COTTEW G.S. (1985). Infections with Mollicutes in sheep and goats. *In:* Infektionen durch Mycoplasmatales, Gylstorff I., ed. VEB Gustav Fischer Verlag, Jena, Germany, 368–386 (Infektionskrankheiten und ihre Erreger, Bd 21).

9. DA MASSA A.J., BROOKS D.L. & ADLER H.E. (1983). Caprine mycoplasmosis: widespread infection in goats with *Mycoplasma mycoides* subsp. *mycoides* (large-colony type). *Am. J. Vet. Res.*, **44**, 322–325.

10. DA MASSA A.J., BROOKS D.L., HOLMBERG C.A. & MOE A.I. (1987). Caprine mycoplasmosis: an outbreak of mastitis and arthritis requiring the destruction of 700 goats. *Vet. Rec.*, **120**, 409–413.

11. DEDIEU L., MADY V. & LEFEVRE P.-C. (1994). Development of two polymerase chain reaction assays for the identification of contagious agalactia related mycoplasmas. Proceedings of the 10th Congress of the International Organisation on Mycoplasmology, August 1994, Bordeaux, France.

12. EAST N.E., DA MASSA A.J., LOGAN L.L., BROOKS D.L. & MCGOWAN B. (1983). Milkborne outbreak of *Mycoplasma mycoides* subsp. *mycoides* in a commercial goat dairy. *J. Am. Vet. Med. Assoc.*, **182**, 1338–1341.

13. ERNO H. (1987). Mycoplasmas of ruminants: a general introduction. *Rev. sci. tech. Off. int. Epiz.*, **6**, 553–563.

14. ERNO H. & PETERSLUND K. (1983). Growth precipitation test. *In:* Methods in Mycoplasmology, Vol. 1. Mycoplasma Characterization, Razin S. & Tully J.G., eds. Academic Press, New York, USA, 489–492.

15. ERNO H., SIMONSEN K., HARBI M.S.M.A. & SKOVGAARD-SORENSEN K. (1987). Further studies on the presence of certain enzymes as a means of differentiating mycoplasmas within the '*M. mycoides* group'. *Ibid* ref. 36, 99–107.

16. FOGGIE A., ETHERIDGE J.R., ERDAG O. & ARISOY F. (1971). Contagious agalactia of sheep and goats. Studies on live and dead vaccines in lactating sheep. *J. Comp. Pathol.*, **81**, 165–172.

17. FOGGIE A., ETHERIDGE J.R., ERDAG O. & ARISOY F. (1971). Contagious agalactia of sheep and goats. Immunity of lactating ewes vaccinated before mating with live or dead vaccines. *J. Comp. Pathol.*, **81**, 393–400.

18. GAILLARD-PERRIN G. & LENFANT D. (1987). The importance of *Mycoplasma mycoides* subsp. *mycoides* in caprine mammary disease in France. *Ibid* ref. 36, 59–69.

19. GAILLARD-PERRIN G. & LENFANT D. (1987). Difficulties experienced in the isolation and identification of *Mycoplasma mycoides* subsp. *mycoides*. *Ibid* ref. 36, 103–110.

20. HOETZL H., SACHSE K. & PFUTZNER H. (1994). Differentiation of the members of the '*Mycoides* cluster' using PCR. *IOM Lett.*, **3**, 28–35.

21. JONES G.E., RAE A.G., HOLMES R.G., LISTER S.A., JONES J.M.W., GRATER G.S. & RICHARDS N. (1983). Isolation of exotic mycoplasmas from sheep in England. *Vet. Rec.*, **113**, 540.

22. KIBOR-CHINGI A., ERNO H. & WAIYAKI P.G. (1987). Report on serological problems in classification of mycoplasmas from cases of contagious caprine pleuropneumonia in Kenya. *Ibid* ref. 36, 85–89.

23. LAMBERT M. (1987). Agalactie contagieuse des brebis et des chèvres. *Rev. sci. tech. Off. int. Epiz.*, **6**, 681–697.

24. LAMBERT M. (1987). Assessment of a live attenuated vaccine against *Mycoplasma agalactiae*. Contagious Agalactia and other Mycoplasmal Diseases of Small Ruminants. Proceedings of a workshop held in Nice, France, 1985, Jones G.E., ed. Commission of the European Communities, Luxembourg (EUR 10984 EN), 77–83.

25. LAMBERT M., CALAMEL M., DUFOUR P., CABASSE E., VITU C. & PEPIN M. (1998). Detection of false-positive sera in contagious agalactia with a multiantigen ELISA and their elimination with a protein G conjugate. *J. Vet. Diagn. Invest.*, **10**, 326–330.

26. LEACH R.H., ERNO H. & MACOWAN K.J. (1993). Proposals for designation of F38-type caprine mycoplasmas as *Mycoplasma capricolum* subsp. *capripneumonine* subsp. nov. and consequent obligatory relegation of strains currently classified as *M. capricolum* (Tully, Barile, Edward, Theodore and Erno 1974) to an additional new subspecies, *M. capricolum* subsp. *capricolum* subsp. nov. *Int. J. Syst. Bact.*, **43**, 603–605.

27. LEFEVRE P.-C., JONES G.E. & OJO M.O. (1987). Pulmonary mycoplasmosis of small ruminants. *Rev. sci. tech. Off. int. Epiz.*, **6**, 759–799.

28. MACOWAN K.J., BRAND T.F., MCGILLVERAY N. & HUNTER A.R. (1984). Experimental infection of castrated male lambs with *Mycoplasma agalaciae. J. Hyg. (Camb.)*, **93**, 455–463.

29. MIEGE M. (1978). Le foyer d'agalactie contagieuse des chèvres des deux Savoies. *Rev. Med. Vet.*, **129**, 247–259.

30. OKOH A.E. J. & OCHOLI R.A. (1986). Disease associated with *Mycoplasma mycoides* subsp. *mycoides* in sheep in Nigeria. *Vet. Rec.*, **118**, 212.

31. PERREAU P. (1979). Les mycoplasmoses de la chèvre. *Cah. Med. Vet.*, **48**, 71–85.

32. PERREAU P. & BREARD A. (1979). La mycoplasmose caprine à *M. capricolum. Comp. Immunol. Microbiol. Infect. Dis.*, **2**, 87–97.

33. PERREAU P., LE GOFF C. & GIAUFFRET A. (1976). Le diagnostic sérologique de l'agalactie contagieuse des petits ruminants: un test de fixation du complément. *Bull. Acad. Vet. Fr.*, **49**, 185–192.

34. PICAVET D.P. (1984). Evolution de deux foyer d'agalacite contagieuse caprine en Ariège. *Rev. Med. Vet.*, **135**, 517–525.

35. RUHNKE H.L., ROSENDAL S., GOLTZ J. & BLACKWELL T.E. (1983). Isolation of *Mycoplasma mycoides* subsp. *mycoides* from polyarthritis and mastitis of goats in Canada. *Can. Vet. J.*, **24**, 54–56.

36. SARRIS K., ZDRAKAS A., DIMARELI Z., GIAKOUMIS N. & PAPADOPOULOS O. (1987). Intraspecific heterogeneity of *Mycoplasma agalactiae. In:* Contagious Agalactia and other Mycoplasmal Diseases of Small Ruminants. Proceedings of a workshop held in Nice, France, 1985, Jones G.E., ed. Commission of the European Communities, Luxembourg (EUR 10984 EN), 77–83.

37. SINGH N., RAJYA B.S. & MOHANTY G.C. (1974). Granular vulvovaginitis (GVV) in goats associated with *Mycoplasma agalactiae. Cornell Vet.*, **64**, 435–442.

38. SUBRAHAMANIAM S., BERGONIER D., POUMARAT F., CAPUAL S., SCHLATTER Y., NICOLET J. & FREY J. (1998). Species identification of *Mycoplasma bovis* and *Mycoplasma agalactiae* based on the uvrC gene by PCR. *Mol. Cell. Probes*, **12**, 161–169.

39. TOLA S., ANGIOI A., ROCCHIGIANI A.M., IDINI G., MANUNTA D., GALLERI G. & LEORI G. (1997). Detection of *Mycoplasma agalactiae* in sheep milk samples by polymerase chain reaction. *Vet. Microbiol.*, **54**, 17–22.

40. TOLA S., IDINI G., MANUNTA D., GALLERI G., ANGIOI A., ROCCHIGIANI A.M. & LEORI G. (1996). Rapid and specific detection of *Mycoplasma agalactiae* by polymerase chain reaction. *Vet. Microbiol.*, **51**, 77–84.

41. TOLA S., MANUNTA D., ROCCA S., ROCCHIGIANI A.M., IDINI G., ANGIOI A. & LEORI G. (1999). Experimental vaccination against *Mycoplasma agalactiae* using different inactivated vaccines. *Vaccine*, **17**, 2764–2768.

42. TULLY J.G. (1983). Cloning and filtrating techniques for mycoplasmas. *In:* Methods in Mycoplasmology, Vol. 1. Mycoplasma Characterization, Razin S. & Tully J.G., eds. Academic Press, New York, USA, 173–177.

*
* *

CHAPTER 2.4.4/5.

CAPRINE ARTHRITIS/ENCEPHALITIS & MAEDI-VISNA

SUMMARY

Maedi-visna (MV), or ovine progressive pneumonia (OPP), of sheep and caprine arthritis/encephalitis (CAE) of goats are persistent virus infections caused by closely related lentiviruses. Phylogenetic analyses comparing nucleotide sequences of MV virus (MVV) and CAE virus (CAEV) suggest CAEV emerged from related sheep lentiviruses (24). The primary route of transmission of MV/OPP virus to lambs or CAEV to kids is via colostrum or milk during nursing. Ovine lentiviruses have been identified in most of the sheep-rearing countries of the world, with the notable exceptions of Australia and New Zealand. The distribution of CAEV is highest in industrialised countries, and seems to have coincided with the international movement of European breeds of dairy goats. Clinical and subclinical MV and CAE are associated with progressive, mononuclear cell inflammatory lesions in the lungs, joints, udder and central nervous system. Indurative mastitis is common in both species, and its economic significance may be underestimated. Laboured breathing associated with emaciation caused by progressive pneumonitis are the predominant features in clinically affected sheep, whereas polyarthritis is the main disease in goats. However, most lentivirus-infected sheep and goats are largely asymptomatic, but remain persistent carriers of virus and are capable of transmitting infection via colostrum or milk and respiratory secretions. The most practical and reliable approach to confirming a diagnosis of MV or CAE is a combination of serology and clinical evaluation. Although serology represents the most cost-effective method of diagnosing persistently infected, clinically normal animals, it should be understood that testing errors occur, and the frequency of error depends on the performance data for sheep and/or goats of the particular serological assay being used. Serological methods are of greatest value for screening entire populations rather than for the detection of single seropositive animals.

Identification of the agent: *Virus isolation can be attempted from live clinical or subclinical cases by co-cultivating peripheral blood or milk leukocytes with appropriate ovine or caprine cell cultures, such as choroïd plexus (MVV) or synovial membrane (CAEV) cells. However, this is time-consuming and not always successful. Following necropsy, virus isolation is most readily accomplished by establishing explant cultures of affected tissues, e.g. lung, choroïd plexus, synovial membrane or udder. Also, alveolar macrophages may be obtained from the lung at post-mortem and co-cultivated with susceptible cells. The cytopathic effects are characteristic, consisting of the appearance of refractile stellate cells and syncytia. The presence of MVV or CAEV can be confirmed by immunolabelling methods and electron microscopy.*

Nucleic acid recognition methods – polymerase chain reaction, Southern blotting and in situ *hybridisation – can be applied, but such technology is not widely available and details are not included in this chapter. A recent review addresses some of these techniques (14).*

Serological tests: *Most infected sheep and goats possess detectable specific antibodies that can be assayed by a number of different serological tests. The two most commonly used are the agar gel immunodiffusion test and the enzyme-linked immunosorbent assay. Western immunoblotting and immunoprecipitation are also performed, but only in specialised laboratories. A milk antibody assay may be appropriate in dairy goat herds. However, it should be recognised that anti-lentivirus antibody transfers with virus during suckling, and the presence of antibody in the milk of suckling sheep or goats does not aid in preventing transmission. The time required for seroconversion following infection can be relatively prolonged and unpredictable, being measured in months rather* *than in weeks. However, after seroconversion, the antibody response usually persists and antibody-positive sheep and goats are regarded as virus carriers.*

Requirements for vaccines and diagnostic biologicals: *There are no biological products available.*

A. DIAGNOSTIC TECHNIQUES

Maedi-visna (MV), or ovine progressive pneumonia (OPP), of sheep and caprine arthritis/encephalitis (CAE) of goats are persistent virus infections caused by closely related lentiviruses. MV/OPP and CAE are characterised by lifelong persistence of the causal agent in host monocytes and macrophages, and a variable length of time between infection and induction of a serologically detectable antiviral antibody response. Most infected sheep and goats do not exhibit clinical disease, but remain persistently infected and are capable of transmitting virus (2, 3, 4).

Maedi-visna is an Icelandic name that describes two of the clinical syndromes recognised in MVV-infected sheep. 'Maedi' means 'laboured breathing' and describes the disease associated with a progressive interstitial pneumonitis, and 'visna' means 'shrinkage' or 'wasting', the signs associated with a paralysing meningoencephalitis. Whereas progressive lung disease is the primary finding with MVV infection, chronic polyarthritis, with synovitis and bursitis is the primary clinical outcome of CAEV infection. Encephalitis occurs primarily in kids aged between 2 and 6 months following CAEV infection. Indurative mastitis occurs in both syndromes. The lungs of sheep affected by MV do not collapse when removed from the thorax and often retain the impression of the ribs. The lungs and lymph nodes increase in weight (up to 2–3 times the normal weight). The lesions are uniformly distributed throughout the lungs, which are uniformly discoloured or mottled grey-brown in colour and of a firm texture. Udders affected by MV are diffusely indurated and associated lymph nodes may be enlarged.

When MV/OPP or CAE is the suspected cause of clinical disease, confirmation of the diagnosis can be achieved by a combination of clinical evaluation, serology and, when necessary, histological examination of appropriate tissues collected at necropsy. Important tissues to examine include lung for progressive interstitial pneumonitis, brain and spinal cord for meningoencephalitis, udder for indurative mastitis, affected joints and synovium for arthritis, and kidney for vasculitis (5, 7, 8, 17, 18). The nature of the inflammatory reaction in each site is similar, consisting of an interstitial, mononuclear cell reaction, sometimes with large aggregates of lymphoid cells and follicle formation.

1. Identification of the agent

Isolation and characterisation of MVV or CAEV would not normally be attempted for routine diagnostic purposes. Due to the persistent nature of these infections, the establishment of a positive antibody status is sufficient for the identification of virus carriers. However, due to a late seroconversion after infection, negative serology may occur in recently infected animals.

There are two approaches to the isolation of MVV and CAEV: one for use with the live animal, and the second for use with necropsy tissues.

a) Isolation from the live animal

- **Maedi-visna virus**

The MV provirus DNA is carried in circulating monocytes and tissue macrophages. Virus isolation from the live animal therefore requires the establishment of leukocyte preparations, with aseptic precautions, from peripheral blood, or milk during lactation, culturing them together with indicator cells. Sheep choroïd plexus (SCP) cells are commonly used for this purpose. These indicator cells can be prepared as primary explant cultures from fetal or newborn virus-free lambs, and their number can be multiplied over three to four passages for storage in liquid nitrogen. The recovered SCP cells are suitable for co-cultivation for up to 10 or 15 passages. Although the cells continue to grow well thereafter, their susceptibility to MVV may become reduced.

Leukocyte preparations can be made from peripheral blood as buffy coats by the centrifugation at 1000 ***g*** of heparinised ethylene diamine tetra-acetic acid (EDTA) or citrated samples for 15 minutes. The cells are aspirated, suspended in Hanks' balanced salt solution (HBSS), and further purified by centrifugation at 400 ***g*** on to a suitable cushion (e.g. Ficoll Paque [Pharmacia]) for 40 minutes. The interface cells are spin-washed once or twice in HBSS at 100 ***g*** for 10 minutes, and the final cell pellet is resuspended in medium to a concentration of approximately 10^6 cells/ml; 10 ml of this suspension is then added to a washed monolayer of slightly subconfluent SCP cells in a flask with an area of 25 cm^2.

Leukocytes can be similarly deposited from milk by centrifugation, when they are spin-washed, resuspended and finally added to SCP monolayer cultures.

These cultures are maintained at 37°C in a 5% CO_2 atmosphere, changing the medium and passaging as necessary. They are examined for evidence of a cytopathic effect (CPE), which is characterised by the appearance of refractile stellate cells with dendritic processes accompanied by the formation of syncytia. The cultures should be maintained for several weeks before being discarded as uninfected. Once a CPE is suspected, cover-slip cultures should be prepared. These are fixed, and evidence of viral antigen is sought by immunolabelling, usually by means of indirect fluorescent antibody or by the use of indirect immunoperoxidase methods. In addition, the cells of any suspect monolayers are deposited by centrifugation, and preparations are made for the identification of any characteristic lentivirus particles by transmission electron microscopy. Reverse transcriptase in the supernatant of the cell culture is indicative of the presence of retroviruses.

- **Caprine arthritis/encephalitis virus**

The same principles that apply to the isolation of MVV also apply to the isolation of CAEV. CAEV was originally isolated by explantation of synovial membrane from an arthritic goat (5). With live CAEV-infected goats, peripheral blood, milk, and possibly joint fluid aspirate represent the most suitable specimens from which leukocyte preparations can be established. SCP cells (as described above) are suitable indicator cells. Alternatively, co-cultures with other cell types, such as goat synovial membrane, fetal testis or cornea, could also be attempted. If a CPE is suspected, tests for detection of viral antigen should be carried out, as described above.

b) Isolation from necropsy tissues

- **Caprine arthritis/encephalitis virus and Maedi-visna virus**

Samples of suspect tissues, collected as fresh as possible, such as lung, synovial membranes, udder, etc., are collected aseptically into sterile HBSS or cell culture medium and minced finely in a Petri dish using scalpel blades. Individual fragments are collected by Pasteur pipette and transferred to flasks of 25 cm^2, approximately 20–30 fragments per flask, and a drop of growth medium is placed carefully on each. The flasks are then incubated at 37°C in a humid 5% CO_2 atmosphere, and left undisturbed for a few days to allow the individual explants to adhere to the plastic. Fresh medium can be added with care, after which rafts of cells will gradually grow out from the fragments. When there is sufficient cell out-growth, the cultures are trypsin dispersed to allow the development of cell monolayers. These can be examined for CPE, and any suspected virus growth is confirmed in the same way as for the co-cultivations.

Adherent macrophage cultures are easy to establish from lung-rinse material (post-mortem broncho-alveolar lavage) and can be tested for virus production by serology, electron microscopy, or reverse transcriptase assay within 1–2 weeks. Virus isolations can be done by co-cultivation of macrophages and SCP cells as described for leukocytes above.

c) Nucleic acid recognition methods

Most virus disease diagnostic laboratories will be equipped for the basic cell culture procedures described above. However, in more specialised, research-based laboratories, virus identification can be achieved by nucleic acid recognition methods. In the case of MVV and CAEV, these methods, such as the polymerase chain reaction (PCR) followed by Southern blotting and *in situ* hybridisation (13), are all methods that can be applied to the detection and recognition of specific nucleic acid sequences within the proviral DNA of MVV and CAEV. When PCR detection of OPP and CAE viruses becomes routinely available, this detection method could be used in rigorous eradication programmes to determine the infection status of those animals that cannot be definitively diagnosed by serology (14).

2. Serological tests

Ovine and caprine lentivirus infections are persistent, so that antibody detection is a valuable serological tool for identifying virus carriers. MV and OPP viruses are antigenically indistinguishable by methods that employ polyclonal antisera. However, the close antigenic relationship between MVV and CAEV does not extend to identical efficiencies in their use for detection of heterologous antibody (15).

The assays now commonly used are agar gel immunodiffusion (AGID) (6, 10, 23) and the enzyme-linked immunosorbent assay (ELISA) (11, 12, 25). The AGID is specific, reproducible and simple to perform, but experience is required for reading the results. The ELISA is economical, and stages of the process can be automated, thus making it useful for screening large numbers of sera. However, the sensitivity and specificity of the ELISA depends on the quality of the antigen. In the case of MV/OPP and CAE viruses, the production of satisfactory antigen preparations has limited its routine application. Modifications to the MV/OPP and CAE ELISAs are emerging, such as use of recombinant protein antigen (20, 21), double antibody sandwich methods, and monoclonal antibodies (12), which may ultimately result in its wider application. In general, however, AGID remains the most frequently used test.

a) Agar gel immunodiffusion (the prescribed test for international trade)

There are two MV/OPP and CAE viral antigens of major importance in routine serology, a viral envelope glycoprotein commonly referred to as gp135, and a core protein, p28. These are both conserved in an antigen preparation consisting of medium harvested from infected cell cultures and concentrated approximately 50-fold by dialysis against polyethylene glycol. The WLC-1 strain of OPP virus is commonly used[1].

It is important to recognise that the sensitivity of the AGID test for detecting anti-CAEV antibody is dependent on the antigen used (1, 15). It was demonstrated that an AGID test with CAEV gp135 afforded greater sensitivity than an AGID test with CAEV p28 (1). Also, it was shown that when compared with immunoprecipitation, the sensitivity of the AGID test for anti-CAEV antibody was 35% greater with CAEV antigen than OPP virus antigen (15). The most likely explanation for this difference in sensitivity between the CAE and OPP virus antigen for the detection of anti-CAEV antibody is that although the immunoprecipitation assay requires only the binding of a single epitope by antibody to obtain a positive result, precipitation in an agar gel requires multiple epitope–antibody interactions. Although the OPP and CAE viruses are closely related antigenically, the degree of the antigenic relatedness is not known, and it is likely that there are fewer antibody/antigen interactions in the heterologous system. When the appropriate antigen is used, the AGID test performance is high. When compared with immunoprecipitation, the AGID for the detection of anti-CAEV antibody and using CAEV antigen had 92% sensitivity and 100% specificity (15).

In MVV-infected sheep and CAEV-infected goats, the predominant precipitating antibody response detected routinely is directed against the gp135 antigen. An anti-p28 response is usually present at a lower titre than the anti-gp135 response.

In some CAEV-infected goats there is evidence to suggest that an anti-gp135 antibody response is produced, in the absence of an anti-p28 response and vice versa, in a proportion of individuals (9, 21). Hence, for validation of the test, standard sera producing both anti-gp135 and anti-p28 precipitin lines are required.

The gel medium is 0.7–1% agarose in 0.05 M Tris buffer, pH 7.2, with 8.0% NaCl. The test is conveniently performed in plastic Petri dishes, or in 10 cm^2 plastic trays. The pattern and size of the wells will determine the number of sera tested per plate. Various well patterns can be adopted, but a hexagonal arrangement with a central well is usual: for example, a pattern with alternating large (5 mm in diameter) and small (3 mm in diameter) peripheral wells, 2 mm apart and 2 mm from a central antigen well that is 3 mm in diameter. The large peripheral wells are used for test sera and the small ones for standard sera. A weak positive control must be included in each test. The plates are incubated overnight at ambient room temperature in a humid chamber, and then examined for precipitin lines. Plates may be incubated for a further 24 hours if needed.

b) Enzyme-linked immunosorbent assay

Various ELISA protocols have been described. At present, an ELISA using purified whole virus as antigen, appears to be the most practical option for routine diagnosis. Simard & Briscoe (22) reported a simple method with greater sensitivity than the AGID test. Antigen was produced by differential centrifugation and detergent treatment of supernatant from infected cell cultures, and was used to coat microplates. Reagents were added sequentially as follows:

i) test serum,

ii) horseradish peroxidase-conjugated rabbit anti-sheep immunoglobulin,

iii) colour developer,

---

1 This has been distributed by Dr R.C. Cutlip, United States Department of Agriculture, Ames, Iowa, United States of America. Commercially available AGID kits for detection of anti-OPP and CAE antibody are available from: Veterinary Diagnostic Technology, Wheat Ridge, Colorado, USA. Fax: (+1.303) 467.2799; and Veterinary Laboratories Agency, New Haw, Addlestone, Surrey KT15 3NB, United Kingdom. Fax: (+44.1932) 34.70.46.

with specified incubation times, temperatures, and washing procedures between each stage. Positive and negative controls were included, and the test results were measured as absorbance, by photometer (22).

A commercial ELISA kit is available for CAEV antibody detection (25). The ELISA technique is also applicable to milk, but given that lentivirus antibody titres in milk are lower (possibly 10% of those in sera), a much reduced sensitivity would be expected (16). Because the primary route of CAEV transmission is via colostrum and milk, the testing of milk samples for anti-CAEV or anti-MVV antibody would not provide timely information for the prevention of transmission, especially to offspring from the immediate gestation (14).

B. REQUIREMENTS FOR VACCINES AND DIAGNOSTIC BIOLOGICALS

There are no biological products available. Monoclonal antibodies recognising conformational epitopes of the CAEV envelope glycoprotein, gp135 have been described (19).

REFERENCES

1. ADAMS D.S. & GORHAM J.R. (1986). The gp135 of caprine arthritis encephalitis virus affords greater sensitivity than the p28 in immunodiffusion serology. *Res. Vet. Sci.*, **40**, 157–160.

2. ADAMS D.S., KLEVJER-ANDERSON P., CARLSON J.L., MCGUIRE T.C. & GORHAM J.R. (1983). Transmission and control of caprine arthritis-encephalitis virus. *Am. J. Vet. Res.*, **44**, 1670–1675.

3. CORK L.C. (1990). Pathology and epidemiology of lentiviral infection of goats. *In:* Maedi-Visna and Related Diseases, Petursson G. & Hoff-Jørgensen R., eds. Kluwer Academic Press, Dordrecht, The Netherlands, 119–127.

4. CRAWFORD T.B. & ADAMS D.S. (1981). Caprine arthritis-encephalitis: clinical features and presence of antibody in selected goat populations. J. *Am. Vet. Med. Assoc.*, **178**, 713–.719.

5. CRAWFORD T.B., ADAMS D.S., CHEEVERS W.P. & CORK L. C. (1980). Chronic arthritis in goats caused by a retrovirus. *Science*, **207**, 997–999.

6. CUTLIP R.C., JACKSON T.A. & LAIRD O.A. (1977). Immunodiffusion test for ovine progressive pneumonia. *Am. J. Vet. Res.*, **38**, 1081–1084.

7. CUTLIP R.C., LEHMKUHL H.D., BROGDEN K.A. & MCCLURKIN A.W. (1986). Vasculitis associated with ovine progressive pneumonia virus infection in sheep. *Am. J. Vet. Res.*, **46**, 61–64.

8. CUTLIP R.C., LEHMKUHL H.D., WOOD R.L. & BROGDEN K.A. (1985). Arthritis associated with ovine progressive pneumonia. *Am. J. Vet. Res.*, **46**, 65–68.

9. DAWSON M. (1985). The detection of precipitating antibodies to lentivirus antigens in goat sera using two immunodiffusion assays. *In:* Slow Viruses in Sheep, Goats and Cattle, Sharp J.M. & Hoff-Jørgensen R., eds. Commission of the European Communities, EUR 8076, 233–238.

10. DAWSON M., BIRONT P. & HOUWERS D.J. (1982). Comparison of serological tests used in three state veterinary laboratories to identify maedi-visna virus infection. *Vet. Rec.*, **111**, 432–434.

11. HOUWERS D.J., GIELKENS A.L.J. & SCHAAKE J. (1982). An indirect enzyme-linked immunosorbent assay (ELISA) for the detection of antibodies to maedi-visna virus. *Vet. Microbiol.*, **7**, 209

12. HOUWERS D.J. & SCHAAKE J. (1987). An improved ELISA for the detection of antibodies to ovine and caprine lentiviruses, employing monoclonal antibodies in a one-step assay. *J. Immunol. Methods*, **98**, 151–154.

13. JOHNSON L.K., MEYER A.L. & ZINK M.C. (1992). Detection of ovine lentivirus in seronegative sheep by *in situ* hybridization, PCR and cocultivation with susceptible cells. *Clin. Immunol. Immunopathol.*, **65**, 254–260.

14. KNOWLES D.P. (1997). Laboratory diagnostic tests for retrovirus infections of small ruminants. *Vet. Clin. North Am. Food Anim. Pract.*, **13**, 1–11.

15. KNOWLES D.P., EVERMANN J.F., SCHROPSHIRE C., VANDER SCHALIE J., BRADWAY D., GEZON H.M. & CHEEVER W.P. (1994). Evaluation of agar gel immunodiffusion serology using caprine and ovine lentiviral antigens for detection of antibody to caprine-arthritis encephalitis virus. *J. Clin. Microbiol.* **32**, 243–245.

16. MOTHA M.J. & RALSTON J.C. (1994). Evaluation of ELISA for detection of antibodies to CAE in milk. *Vet. Microbiol.*, **38**, 359–367.

17. OLIVER R.E., GORHAM J.R., PARISH S.F., HADLOW W.J. & NARAYAN O. (1981). Ovine progressive pneumonia: pathologic and virologic studies on the naturally occurring disease. *Am. J. Vet. Res.*, **42**, 1554–1559.

18. OLIVER R.E., GORHAM J.R., PERRYMAN L.E. & SPENCER G.R. (1981). Ovine progressive pneumonia: experimental intrathoracic, intracerebral and intra-articular infections. *Am. J. Vet. Res.*, **42**, 1560–1564.

19. OZYORUK F., CHEEVERS W.P., HULLINGER G.A., MCGUIRE T.C., HUTTON M. & KNOWLES D.P. (2001). Monoclonal antibodies to conformational epitopes of the surface glycoprotein of caprine arthritis-encephalitis virus: potential application to competitive-inhibition enzyme-linked immunosorbent assay for detecting antibodies in goat sera. *Clin. Diagn. Lab. Immunol.*, **8**, 44–51.

20. POWER C., RICHARDSON S., BRISCOE M. & PASICK J. (1995). Evaluation of two recombinant Maedi-Visna virus proteins for use in an enzyme-linked immunosorbent assay for the detection of serum antibodies to ovine lentiviruses. *Clin. Diagn. Lab. Immunol.*, **2**, 631–633.

21. RIMSTAD E., EAST N., DEROCK E., HIGGINS J. & PEDERSEN N.C. (1994). Detection of antibodies to caprine arthritis/encephalitis virus using recombinant gag proteins. *Arch. Virol.*, **134**, 345–356.

22. SIMARD C.L. & BRISCOE M.R. (1990). An enzyme-linked immunosorbent assay for detection of antibodies to maedi-visna virus in sheep. A simple technique for production of antigen using sodium dodecyl sulfate treatment. *Can. J. Vet. Res.*, **54**, 446–450.

23. SIMARD C.L. & BRISCOE M.R. (1990). An enzyme-linked immunosorbent assay for detection of antibodies to Maedi-visna virus in sheep. Comparison to conventional agar gel immunodiffusion test. *Can. J. Vet. Res.*, **54**, 451–456.

24. VALAS S., BENOIT C., GUIONAUD C., PERRIN G. & MAMOUN R.Z. (1997). North American and French caprine arthritis-encephalitis viruses emerge from ovine maedi-visna viruses. *Virology*, **237**, 307–318.

25. ZANONI R.G., VOGT H.R., POHL B., BOTTCHER J., BOMMELI W. & PETERHANS E. (1994). An ELISA based on whole virus for the detection of antibodies to small-ruminant lentiviruses. *J. Vet. Med. B*, **41**, 662–669.

*
* *

CHAPTER 2.4.6.

CONTAGIOUS CAPRINE PLEUROPNEUMONIA

SUMMARY

Contagious caprine pleuropneumonia (CCPP) is a severe disease of goats caused by Mycoplasma capricolum *subspecies* capripneumoniae *(Mccp). This organism is closely related to three other mycoplasmas:* M. mycoides *subsp.* mycoides, M. mycoides *subsp.* capri, *and* M. capricolum *subsp.* capricolum. *Unlike true CCPP, which is confined to the thoracic cavity, the disease caused by the latter three mycoplasmas is accompanied by prominent lesions in other organs and/or parts of the body besides the thoracic cavity.*

Typical cases of CCPP are characterised by extreme fever (41–43°C), high morbidity and mortality rates in susceptible herds affecting all ages and both sexes, and abortions in pregnant goats. After approximately 2–3 days of high fever, respiratory signs become apparent: respiration is accelerated and painful, and in some cases is accompanied by a grunt. Coughing is frequent, violent and productive. In the terminal stages, animals are unable to move – they stand with their front legs wide apart, the neck is stiff and extended, and sometimes saliva continuously drips from the mouth. Post-mortem examination reveals fibrinous pleuropneumonia with massive lung hepatisation and pleurisy, accompanied by accumulation of straw-coloured pleural fluid.

Identification of the agent: *Definitive diagnosis requires culture of the causative organism from lung tissue samples and/or pleural fluid taken at post-mortem. After cloning and purification, isolates can be identified by several biochemical, immunological and molecular tests. Recently a polymerase-chain-reaction-based test has been described and shown to be specific, sensitive and applicable to different sample types.*

Serological tests: *Serological tests have not been widely applied for identifying the cause of pleuropneumonia in goats or sheep. Such tests are best used on a herd basis rather than for diagnosis in individual animals. The complement fixation test remains the most widely used serological test for CCPP, except in Kenya where latex agglutination is used. Indirect hemagglutination is also used. A specific competitive enzyme-linked immunosorbent assay has been developed. As with the other serological tests, it does not detect all reactors, but its specificity and suitability for large-scale testing make it an appropriate test for epidemiological investigations.*

Requirements for vaccines and diagnostic biologicals: *Vaccine against CCPP caused by Mccp is available commercially from the Kenya Veterinary Vaccines Production Institute*[1].

A. DIAGNOSTIC TECHNIQUES

Contagious caprine pleuropneumonia (CCPP) is a severe disease of goats occurring in many countries in Africa and Asia where the total goat population is more than 500 million (1). Classical, acute CCPP is caused by *Mycoplasma capricolum* subsp. *capripneumoniae* (Mccp) (17), originally known as the F38 biotype. This organism was first isolated and shown to cause CCPP in Kenya (18–21); it has subsequently been isolated in the Sudan, Tunisia, Oman, Turkey, Chad, Uganda, Ethiopia, Niger, Tanzania and the United Arab Emirates. Disease indistinguishable from naturally occurring CCPP has been experimentally reproduced with Mccp by several groups of workers.

1 Kenya Veterinary Vaccines Production Institute, P.O. Box 53260, Nairobi, Kenya. E-mail: kevevapi@africaonline.co.ke

The diagnosis of outbreaks of respiratory disease in goats, and of CCPP in particular, is complicated, especially where it is endemic. It must be differentiated from other similar clinico-pathological syndromes such as: pestes de petit ruminants, to which sheep are also susceptible; pasteurellosis, which can be differentiated on the basis of distribution of gross lung lesions; and what has been called 'mastitis, arthritis, keratitis, pneumonia and septicaemia syndrome' (36). As the name implies the pneumonia is accompanied by prominent lesions in other organs. The disease caused by Mccp is readily contagious and fatal to susceptible goats of all ages and both sexes, does not affect sheep or cattle, and is characterised histopathologically by an interstitial, intralobular oedema of the lung (14).

1. Identification of the agent

a) Microscopy of lung exudates, impression smears or sections

Mccp shows a branching filamentous morphology *in vivo* that can be observed by dark-field microscopy in exudates or tissue suspensions from lesions or pleural fluid. Alternatively, smears made from cut lung lesions can be stained by the method of May–Grünwald–Giesma and examined by light microscopy. The other caprine mycoplasmas show a short filamentous or coccobacillary morphology. Neither of these techniques provides a definitive diagnosis.

b) Nucleic acid recognition methods

The polymerase chain reaction (PCR) is used to amplify a conserved segment of the 16S rRNA gene of the mycoides cluster. The PCR product is then analysed by restriction enzyme cleavage for the identification of the Mccp amplicon. The test is used directly on clinical materials such as lung tissue and pleural fluid (3). However, isolation of Mccp remains the confirmatory test.

c) Gel precipitin tests to detect antigen in tissue specimens

Mccp releases an antigenic polysaccharide (30) to which a specific monoclonal antibody (MAb) (WM-25) has been produced (31, 32). This MAb specifically immunoprecipitates in agar gel with the polysaccharide produced by Mccp, and is used to identify the causative agent in cases of CCPP, particularly when specimens are no longer suitable for culture because of deterioration during transit.

d) Isolation of mycoplasmas

i) *Selection of samples*

The necropsy samples of choice are lung lesions, particularly from the interface between consolidated and unconsolidated areas, pleural fluid, and mediastinal lymph nodes. If microbiological examination cannot be performed immediately, samples or whole lungs can be stored deep-frozen at –20°C for considerable periods (months) with little apparent loss in mycoplasma viability. During transport, samples should always be kept as cool as possible, as mycoplasma viability diminishes rapidly with increasing temperature. Lung samples can be dispatched to other laboratories in freeze-dried form, but freeze drying reduces the titre of many mycoplasma species, including Mccp.

ii) *Treatment of samples*

Swabs are suspended in 2–3 ml of culture medium. Tissue samples are best minced using scissors, and then shaken vigorously, or pulverised in medium[2] using 1 g of tissue to 9 ml of medium. Tissues should not be ground. The suspension is usually prepared with a mycoplasma medium, but if parallel bacteriological examination is to be carried out, a high quality bacteriological medium, such as nutrient broth, may be used to provide a suspension suitable for both forms of examination. Pleural fluid, or a tissue suspension or swab, is serially diluted through at least three tenfold steps (to a nominal 10^{-4}) in the selected mycoplasma medium. Dilutions should also be plated on to solid medium.

iii) *Mycoplasma media*

The medium used by MacOwan & Minette to culture Mccp organisms (19), is termed 'viande foie goat' (VFG), and includes goat-meat liver broth and goat serum. Alternative suitable media are WJ (13), modified Hayflick's, and modified Newing's tryptose (15)[3]. Media enriched with 0.2% (or up to 0.8%) sodium pyruvate perform considerably better, both for primary isolation and antigen production of

2 For example, with the Stomacher 80, A.J. Seward, London, United Kingdom (UK).
3 A commercial medium called Mycoplasma Experience is also available from Mycoplasma Experience, Reigate, Surrey, UK.

Mccp (23, 24). This forms the basis for Thiaucourt's medium (36, 38) and modified Thiaucourt's medium (3). The formulations of the last two media are as follows:

- *Thiaucourt's medium*

  A. Autoclaved portion (121°C for 15 minutes): Bacto PPLO (pleuropneumonia-like organisms) broth without crystal violet (Difco) (21 g); deionised water (700 ml).

  B. Membrane-filtered portion: Horse (alternatively pig or donkey) serum inactivated at 56°C for 30 minutes (200 ml); fresh yeast extract (100 ml); glucose (sterile solution 0.5 g/ml) (2 ml); and sodium pyruvate (sterile solution 0.5 g/ml) (8 ml).

  Part B is added to A aseptically. Ampicillin (0.1 g/litre) and thallium acetate (250 mg/litre) can be added to prevent contamination in primary isolations. The final pH of the medium should be 7.4–7.6.

- *Modified Thiaucourt's medium*

  A. Autoclaved portion (121°C for 15 minutes): Bacto PPLO broth without crystal violet (Difco) (17.5 g); glass distilled water (650 ml).

  B. Membrane-filtered portion: Horse (pig or donkey) serum inactivated at 56°C for 30 minutes (250 ml); fresh yeast extract (100 ml); 50% glucose (4 ml); 25% sodium pyruvate (8 ml); 5% thallium acetate (4 ml); ampicillin (250 mg); and 0.5% phenol red (4 ml). The pH is adjusted to 7.8 with sodium hydroxide or hydrochloric acid.

  Part B is added to part A aseptically.

  Modified Newing's tryptose broth and agar plates (Gourlay's medium) (11) are routinely used for isolation and maintenance of Mccp at the OIE Reference Laboratory in Kenya (see Table given in Part 4 of this *Manual*).

iv) *Medium production, storage and quality control*

Certain medium components, particularly serum, yeast extract and deionised water, should be regularly monitored for growth-promoting capacity before incorporation into mycoplasma media. Low-passage field isolates should be used for this screening purpose.

Broth media may be stored for at least 6 months at –25°C before use, but penicillin or its analogues should not be added until final dispensing. Broth media are dispensed into bijoux (1.8 ml or 2.7 ml) or screw-capped tubes (4.5 ml), and stored for up to 3 weeks at 4°C. Solid media are best made with agarose (0.9% [w/v]), Noble agar (1.5% [w/v]), or purified agar (0.6% [w/v]). Plates, which are poured to a depth of 6–8 mm, should be as fresh as possible when used, and should be stored for no more than 2 weeks at 4°C before use.

v) *Cultivation*

Cultures are incubated at 37°C. Plates are best incubated in a humid atmosphere of 5% CO_2, 95% air or N_2, or in a candle jar with a moisture source.

Broth cultures are examined daily for evidence of growth – colour change and the appearance of floccular material. Gross turbidity indicates bacterial contamination; cultures showing this should be passed through a 0.45-µm membrane filter before subculture. Broth cultures are subcultured by inoculation of fresh broth medium with one-tenth of their volume, or by streaking agar medium with a loop.

Plate cultures are examined every 1–3 days using a stereo microscope (×5–50 magnification) and transmitted and incident light sources. If negative, the plates are discarded after 14 days. Subculture is carried out by the transfer of excised agar blocks bearing isolated colonies to either agar (on which the blocks are pushed, face down) or broth media. Alternatively, an agar plug bearing one colony is drawn into a Pasteur pipette and discharged into fresh broth medium.

Cloning and purification of isolates is performed by repeated transfer of single colonies representing each morphological type seen. Colony morphology varies with the medium used, the mycoplasma species, its passage level and the age of the culture.

In early passage, many mycoplasma species, including *M. capricolum* subsp. *capricolum* (Mcc), produce colonies of bizarre morphology, often small, centreless, and of irregular shape. This effect is often associated with the use of marginally suitable medium. With passage, such isolates demonstrate conventional 'fried egg' colony morphology, except *M. ovipneumoniae*, which retains centreless colonies. Colonies of *M. mycoides* subsp. *mycoides* Large Colony (MmmLC) and Mcc may be up to 3 mm in diameter.

Filtration of broth cultures through 0.45 µm filters before subculture aids purification by excluding cell aggregates.

Cultures suspected of being L-forms of bacteria should be examined for reversion to bacterial form by three to five passages on solid mycoplasma medium from which antibiotics and thallium acetate have been omitted.

Broth media used for primary isolation and which have shown no indication of growth by 7 days, should be subcultured blind.

Cultures of each sample, including one blind subculture, should be examined for a minimum of 3 weeks before being discarded. Titrations in broths, if performed in full (to 10^{-10}), are also read at 3–4 weeks, and are expressed as colour-changing units per transfer volume. Growth on plates is expressed as colony-forming units (CFU) per ml.

e) Identification of mycoplasmas

i) *Polymerase chain reaction*

Once the organism has been cultured, verification of Mccp can be achieved in 1 day by PCR. The test is based on amplification of a segment of the 16S rRNA gene. The amplified fragment is common to the mycoides cluster. However, when the amplicon is digested with endonuclease *PstI*, a unique cleavage pattern of three fragments for Mccp is observed when the enzyme digests are analysed in agarose gel electrophoresis and stained with ethidium bromide (3).

ii) *Biochemical tests*

Wild strains should be passaged, and preferably cloned, three times before identification is attempted.

Biochemical tests cannot identify an isolate unequivocally, which at present can only be done by serological or genetic means. Intraspecies variation in some biochemical reactions is often considerable, but some tests perform a useful function both as a preliminary screening system and in providing supportive data for serological findings.

The tests most commonly used are glucose breakdown, arginine hydrolysis, 'film and spots' formation, reduction of tetrazolium chloride (aerobically and anaerobically), phosphatase activity, serum digestion and digitonin sensitivity. The first three of these tests are performed routinely in isolation and cultivation procedures. Glucose breakdown is indicated by acid (yellow) change, and arginine hydrolysis by alkaline (red) change in broth media, using phenol red as indicator. Film and spots' describes an apparent wrinkling of the agar surface due to the deposition on it of an iridescent film of lipid, together with the development of black spots within the medium in the vicinity of ageing colonies. This phenomenon, produced by three mycoplasmas of small ruminants, is demonstrated on agar media containing 20% or more serum, preferably of horse or pig origin. Supplementation of the medium with 10% egg yolk emulsion improves the sensitivity of the test.

The remaining biochemical tests require specific media or reagents. The test for tetrazolium reduction provides corroborative evidence of the mycoplasmal nature of *M. agalactiae* isolates, as this organism is neither glycolytic nor arginine-hydrolysing. Serum digestion (8) distinguishes members of ruminant mycoplasmas, and phosphatase production (4) separates Mcc from other members of this cluster. Digitonin sensitivity distinguishes members of the order Mycoplasmatales from those of the order Acholplasmatales (10).

iii) *Serological identification*

Mycoplasmal antigens used in hyperimmune serum production are invariably contaminated with medium constituents. The antibodies stimulated by these contaminants can cause false-positive reactions in serological identification tests. This problem is avoided by absorption of the antiserum with the medium used to produce the antigen (10 mg lyophilised medium per ml of antiserum), or by growing the mycoplasmas to be used as antigens in medium containing homologous animal components, e.g. growth in VFG medium to immunise goats.

Because of the close serological relationships between members of the '*M. mycoides* cluster', isolates from cases of CCPP should, preferably, be identified by at least two of the three tests described below.

- **Growth inhibition test**

The growth inhibition test (GIT) is the simplest and most specific, but the least sensitive, of the tests available. It depends on the direct inhibition of growth on solid medium by specific hyperimmune serum, and detects primarily surface antigens (6).

Mccp appears to be highly homogeneous serologically and wide zones of inhibition free of 'breakthrough' colonies are observed with antiserum to the type strain, regardless of the source of the test strain (13). Mccp cross-reacts with Leach's bovine group 7 (PG50), *M. equigenitalium* and *M. primatum* in the GIT when polyclonal antisera are used, but an MAb specific for Mccp in the GIT has been produced (31). The MAb reagent, WM25, is specific for (Mccp) isolates by the disc growth inhibition method, which will exclude *M. agalactiae*, Mcc and the other members of the '*M. mycoides* cluster' associated with goats, but not bovine group 7 (not found in goats): the latter can be excluded, however, by colony indirect fluorescence tests (2). A small proportion of Mccp isolates also cross-react in the GIT with antiserum to Mcc.

- **Test procedure**

i) Broth culture in mid-to-late logarithmic phase is used at three tenfold dilutions, the selection of which is related to the vigour of growth of the isolate on agar.

ii) Agar plates are dried for 30 minutes at 37°C.

iii) Sterile paper disks of 6–7 mm in diameter are impregnated with a drop (10–20 µl) of undiluted antiserum. Disks may be used wet, in which form they can be stored at –20°C, or they can be lyophilised (6), which allows storage at 4°C.

iv) Using a separate plate for each dilution of culture, 1 ml or 2.5 ml volumes are pipetted on to 5 cm or 10 cm diameter plates, respectively. The inoculum is dispersed evenly over the plate, then the excess is removed.

v) The plates are dried at 20–30°C for 15–20 minutes, preferably under a protective hood, until no visible liquid is present on the surface. Sufficient residual moisture should remain to enable freeze-dried disks to adhere to the agar surface.

vi) Several disks, each impregnated with a different antiserum (selected on the basis of sample source and the biochemical reactions and colony morphology of the isolate), are carefully placed on the agar plates; isolates from CCPP cases should be screened with antisera against Mccp, MmmLC, Mmc, *M. mycoides* subsp. *capri* (Mcc) and *M. ovipneumoniae*. A disk containing 1.5% digitonin should also be included on the plates.

vii) The plates are incubated at 37°C for 2–6 days. Initial overnight incubation at 27°C can increase the sensitivity of the test. Inhibition by digitonin is generally readily apparent; however, inhibition by antiserum may be more difficult to interpret, with suppression rather than total inhibition of growth, depending on the species of mycoplasma, colony density and potency of the antiserum. 'Breakthrough' colonies are commonly observed within zones of inhibition. Circular precipitin bands are occasionally seen around disks. Positive inhibition is regarded as a zone of 2 mm or more.

- **Growth precipitation test**

The growth precipitation test detects soluble cytoplasmic and extramembranous antigens released by growing cultures and allowed to diffuse through solid mycoplasma growth medium towards mycoplasma antiserum during growth (16). As with the gel precipitin test, there are strong cross-reactions within the mycoides cluster. If growth inhibition is performed by using MAb WM25, which is specific for Mccp, both specific inhibition and a growth precipitin line are achieved simultaneously.

- **Indirect fluorescence antibody test**

The direct and indirect fluorescent antibody tests are the most effective of the various serological methods for identifying most mycoplasmas (27). They are simple, rapid, and sensitive, yet economical in the use of antiserum. Several forms have been described, the most commonly used and perhaps best being the indirect fluorescent antibody (IFA) test applied to unfixed colonies on agar. Antiserum against a single strain is sufficient to identify field isolates of that species, and antisera are diluted before use. Cultures do not have to be cloned, but the test is usually applied only after several passages have indicated whether the culture contains more than one species and the growth characteristics of the organism(s) present.

- **Test procedure**

i) Two agar plates are predried at 37°C for 30 minutes. Each one is flooded with a different dilution of test broth culture, the dilutions being selected according to the vigour of growth of the strain on agar medium. Alternatively, a drop of undiluted culture is spread over a single 5 cm plate using an L-shaped glass rod.

ii) The plates are incubated at 37°C until the first evidence of growth is observed. If the IFA test cannot be performed immediately, the plates can be stored at 4°C for up to 4 weeks.

iii) Several blocks of approximately 0.5–1 cm^2 are excised from areas where colonies are numerous, but not confluent. The blocks of each agar culture are cut to the same geometric shape to enable recognition of origin, a different shape being used for each isolate. Several blocks of each isolate are distributed (colony surface facing upwards) on to several different slides, each slide being used for a different mycoplasma antiserum. The colony surface of each block is identified for future reference by undercutting one corner.

iv) Rabbit anti-mycoplasma (ra-m) serum or normal rabbit serum (NRS; as a control on a duplicate block) at a suitable dilution in normal saline or phosphate buffered saline (PBS), pH 7.2, is gently pipetted on to each agar block until the surface area is totally covered. The optimal dilution of ra-m is determined by chequerboard titration against the fluorescein isothiocyanate (FITC)-conjugated anti-rabbit immunoglobulin serum (a-r Ig-FITC) used.

v) The flooded blocks are incubated on their slides at room temperature for 30 minutes in a humid chamber.

vi) All blocks on one slide are tipped into a 10 ml tube containing approximately 7 ml of PBS.

vii) The plugged tubes are rotated at 18–30 rpm for 10 minutes. The PBS is then decanted and replaced with fresh PBS, and the tubes are rotated again for 10 minutes.

viii) The PBS is decanted and the blocks are placed colony surface facing upwards on their respective slides. Excess moisture is blotted off.

ix) All blocks are flooded with a-r Ig-FITC at optimal dilution.

x) The blocks are incubated again for 30 minutes at room temperature in a humid chamber, then tipped into tubes containing fresh PBS, and washed twice by rotating, as before.

xi) The blocks, replaced colony surface facing upwards on their respective slides, are examined by an epi-immunofluorescent microscope using the settings recommended by the manufacturer for FITC.

• *Notes on the indirect fluorescent antibody test*

xii) Working dilutions of ra-m and a-r Ig-FITC should be kept at 4°C, which limits their shelf life to approximately 1 week.

xiii) Isolates from CCPP should be examined using antisera against Mccp, MmmLC, Mmc and Mcc, positive control cultures should comprise their type strains, namely Mccp, Y goat, PG3 and California kid, respectively.

xiv) A negative (NRS-treated) control should always be incorporated for each culture.

xv) Interpretation of the IFA test can be difficult. Autofluorescence is produced by some species, particularly acholeplasmas. Even in pure cultures, a proportion of colonies may not stain positively with the relevant antiserum; this is particularly true of Mcc. Otherwise, poor results are usually ascribable to the use of an agar culture that has been allowed to grow for too long, or to the use of antiserum that has deteriorated with dilution and age.

f) Other identification tests

Metabolism inhibition (35) and tetrazolium reduction inhibition (33) are other tests sometimes used in the identification of caprine mycoplasmas. A gene probe, F38-12, capable of distinguishing Mccp has been developed (34).

2. Serological tests

Serology has not been widely applied to identifying the cause of outbreaks of pleuropneumonia in goats and sheep. Endemic infections with MmmLC and Mmc can produce a background of positive titres to these organisms in a proportion of apparently healthy animals (13), and under experimental conditions seroconversion to *M. mycoides* can occur in goats with no clinical signs of disease. Acute cases caused by Mccp rarely show positive titres to the organism before death (21, 25, 36), perhaps because antibodies are 'eclipsed' by circulating mycoplasma antigens (25). Seroconversion to Mccp in experimentally infected animals is observed by the complement fixation (CF) test and indirect haemagglutination (IHA) test to start 7–9 days after the appearance of clinical signs, to peak between days 22 and 30, and to decline rapidly thereafter (25). These various observations indicate that serology should be applied on a herd, not an individual basis, and that whenever possible, paired serum samples collected 3–8 weeks apart, should be examined.

a) Complement fixation test (the prescribed test for international trade)

The CF test in various forms remains the most widely used serological test for diagnosis of contagious bovine pleuropneumonia (12, 26). In CCPP, the CF test was used for detection of Mccp infection (19) and it has been found to be more specific, though less sensitive, than the IHA test (25). Its main disadvantage is the high level of technical expertise required to perform the test (12).

One method of performing the test is as follows. To prepare the antigen, 2 litres of culture of titre higher than 10^9 CFU/ml is centrifuged at 40,000 ***g*** for 1 hour at 5°C. The deposit is resuspended and washed three times in physiological saline prior to storage in 0.5–1.0 ml volumes at –20°C.

Sterile broth treated as above constitutes sediment antigen, and a freeze-dried broth reconstituted at 200 mg/ml constitutes a second control antigen. Prior to testing, the antigen is diluted 1/60 and ultrasonicated for 3 minutes at low power in a container of iced water. The sonicate is centrifuged at 1250 ***g*** for 30 minutes to remove any debris, and stored at –20°C. If stored for more than 2–3 weeks the antigen should be recentrifuged.

- **Test procedure**

Microtitre plate tests are performed using 0.025 ml volumes, two volumes containing three mean haemolytic doses of complement, and a 1.5% (v/v) final concentration of sheep red blood cells (SRBCs) in U-bottomed microtitre plates as follows:

i) The following are mixed and incubated at 37°C for 45 minutes:

   - 25 µl of doubling dilutions of test serum (heat inactivated at 56°C for 30 minutes) starting with 1/2 dilution;
   - 25 µl of antigen (the dilution of the antigen must be determined in a chequerboard titration using a known positive serum);
   - 25 µl of complement (3 haemolytic units).

ii) 25 µl of sensitised SRBCs, at a final concentration of 1.5% (v/v), is mixed and the plates are incubated at 37°C for 45 minutes.

iii) The plates are incubated at 4°C for 1 hour to allow the unlysed cells to settle.

iv) Reading the results: The titre will be the highest serum dilution that will fix 50% of the complement, i.e. 50% haemolysis.

- **Controls**

In all CF tests a number of controls are required:

i) Indicator systems (RBCs + haemolysin) alone to ensure that RBCs do not lyse spontaneously.

ii) Indicator system with complement only to show that enough complement is present to lyse the cells.

iii) Indicator system with antigen only and no complement to show that antigen alone does not lyse the cells.

iv) Indicator system with serum alone and no complement to show that the serum alone does not lyse the cells.

v) Indicator system with complement and antigen to detect any anticomplementary activity of the antigen.

vi) Indicator system with the complement and serum to detect any anticomplementary activity of the serum.

b) Indirect haemagglutination test

The IHA test (5) has been used for diagnosis of CCPP (25).

The IHA test is most commonly performed with RBCs that are either fresh and tanned, or treated with glutaraldehyde. The former are more sensitive but show greater variability between tests, and require sensitisation of cells with antigen each time the test is performed. Glutaraldehyde treatment of RBCs reduces sensitivity but produces a much more useful diagnostic test, as sensitised RBCs remain effective for 1 year or more if kept refrigerated, and require little further manipulation before use in the test.

The specificity of the IHA test for the '*M. mycoides* cluster' has been evaluated using rabbit hyperimmune sera and glutaraldehyde-treated RBCs sensitised with lightly sonicated mycoplasma cell suspensions (13). MmmLC- and Mccp-sensitised cells cross-reacted with antisera to the other three species, but Mmc- and Mcc-sensitised cells each cross-reacted only with the antiserum to Mccp.

The polysaccharide produced by Mccp has been found to bind to untreated goat RBCs and, as such, was successfully used in an IHA test to identify animals with experimental and natural CCPP (30).

Cells sensitised with the four principal caprine mycoplasmas have been used in field studies in Oman and the Sudan. The conclusions from the two surveys differed. The Oman survey revealed widespread seropositivity to Mmc, whereas Mcc reactors were largely confined to herds in which the Mcc had been shown to occur by cultural means (13). In contrast, more animals with signs of CCPP in the Sudan were seropositive to MmmLC than to any of the mycoplasmas tested, only 7% reacting with Mcc antigen. Seropositivity to two or more antigens was noted in a proportion of animals in both surveys.

c) Latex agglutination test

Latex beads sensitised with the polysaccharide produced by Mccp and present in culture supernatant have been used in a slide agglutination test (28). This test is presently used routinely in Kenya. It is a very useful test in an outbreak because it can be performed at the penside using a drop of whole blood.

Both CF test and IHA test findings emphasise the difficulties inherent in the serological diagnosis of CCPP when using whole cell or membrane preparations as antigen. The use of the more defined antigen, the polysaccharide elaborated by Mccp, provides greater specificity, as there is no cross-reactivity with sera against the other three principal caprine mycoplasmas.

d) Competitive enzyme-linked immusorbent assay (37)

This test is based on the specificity of the MAb for the Mccp epitope and the ability of Mccp-infected goats to make antibodies to this epitope. The two antibodies are made to compete for the Mccp epitope coated on to plates. The test has been described to be specific and to detect antibodies for long periods after infection. However, as with the other serological tests, it does not detect all reactors (it detects between 30% and 60% in an infected herd) (37). The competitive enzyme-linked immunosorbent assay is easier to perform than the CF test, and is suitable for testing many samples at one time. It is therefore a suitable test for epidemiological investigations.

B. REQUIREMENTS FOR VACCINES AND DIAGNOSTIC BIOLOGICALS

The first experimental vaccine against Mccp comprised live Mccp in high passage (22). When inoculated intratracheally, it proved innocuous and protected goats against experimental challenge. More recent work has concentrated, however, on inactivated forms of vaccine. The current form used in Kenya (where inactivated Mccp vaccines have been in use for several years) contains lyophilised Mccp suspended in saponin; this formulation has a shelf life of at least 14 months. The optimal dose of 0.15 mg of mycoplasma provides protection for over 1 year (29).

1. Seed management

a) Characteristics of the seed

The master seed was isolated from the lungs of a sick goat. It is a Yatta isolate and has been confirmed to be Mccp by GIT and PCR, after 15 passages *in vitro*. The master seed should also be pure and free from other contaminants.

b) Method of culture

The master seed is established and stored in a freeze-dried form in 1 ml ampoules. The working seed is prepared by amplifying the master seed in modified Newing's broth to make a bulk of 4 litres. Its growth is arrested at the log phase before filament formation.

This culture is tested for sterility before it is distributed in aliquots of 20 ml volumes and stored frozen at –20°C.

c) Validation as a vaccine

The master seed should be prepared from lung specimens or pleura fluids of a goat that dies of pneumonia, showing all the clinical signs of CCPP. The isolate must be confirmed by GIT or by PCR to be Mccp. It must be checked for sterility, safety, potency and extraneous agents.

2. Method of manufacture

For vaccine production, a working seed is first established by amplifying an aliquot of freeze-dried master seed in modified Newing's broth, to make a bulk of 4 litres of culture. This culture is aliquoted in 20 ml volumes and frozen at –20°C. The vaccine is grown in 5 litre pots containing 4 litres of modified Newing's broth. Each pot is sampled asceptically for sterility testing before 20 ml of working seed is inoculated into each 4 litres of medium.

These pots are incubated at 37°C for 4–6 days depending on how fast the mycoplasma grows. After the filaments sediment, the antigen is harvested by centrifugation at 12,600 ***g*** for 30 minutes from pots that are not contaminated. The pellet is resuspended in sterile normal saline and centrifuged to remove the remnants of the growth medium. The pellet is resuspended again in a small volume of sterile normal saline to make a viscous suspension.

Saponin is added to inactivate the mycoplasma at 3 mg saponin to 1 ml of antigen. It is left agitating overnight at 4°C using a magnetic stirrer.

NOTE: Saponin also acts as an adjuvant. Three samples are taken asceptically from this suspension and tested for sterility, for protein estimation and for the innocuity test.

Protein estimation is done by using the standard opacity tubes and expressed in mg/ml and this determines the total number of doses in the batch of vaccine.

3. In-process control

During production, the following tests are carried out to ensure that the product remains pure and safe. These tests are carried out by quality assurance staff. Each pot is sampled asceptically before inoculation to test for sterility.

After maturity of culture, only pots that have not shown signs of contamination are pooled for centrifugation; the contaminated pots are decontaminated and discarded after autoclaving.

After inactivation with saponin, a sample is taken asceptically for sterility, another one for innocuity and another one for the protein estimation test.

a) Sterility test

This test is aimed at verifying the absence of fungal and bacterial contaminants. Two tubes of thioglycollate are inoculated with 1 ml of the sample each. The tubes contain about 15 ml of broth. These are incubated at 37°C to eliminate aerobics, microaerophilics and anaerobics. The other medium used is soybean casein digest broth. Four tubes are inoculated with 12 ml of sample each.

Two tubes are incubated at 37°C and another two at room temperature (25°C) to eliminate bacterial and fungal contaminants. All media are incubated for 14 days with controls. Absence of any growth shows that the sample is not contaminated.

b) Innocuity test

This test aims to demonstrate the presence of living mycoplasma in the vaccine: 0.3 ml of inactivated antigen is added to 2.7 ml of modified Newing's broth in a tube and tenfold dilutions are made from 10^{-1} to 10^{-9}. A positive control is set up using a viable culture of *M. capripneumonia* and a negative control using three uninoculated tubes of medium. All are incubated at 37°C for 12 days. If there is no growth in the tubes inoculated with test sample, the vaccine passes the test.

c) Protein content estimation

This test uses Brown's opacity tubes. The antigen is dispensed to a similar tube as those containing standards, and its opacity is compared visually with the opacity of each standard opacity tube starting with the lowest. After estimation, the antigen is diluted using sterile normal saline to make 2 mg of protein/ml as the final vaccine.

4. Batch control

a) Sterility

The sterility test on the final batch is carried out as described in B.3.a. except that four bottles from each batch are pooled together and samples of the pool are used.

b) Safety

Every batch of CCPP vaccine must be proven to be safe in laboratory animals. Two guinea-pigs are each inoculated by the intramuscular route in the hind leg and another two guinea-pigs are inoculated by the intraperitoneal route with 0.5 ml containing 5 doses of vaccine.

c) Potency

Research is in progress at the Kenya Agricultural Research Institute, Muguga, Kenya, to develop a test for potency.

The interpretation of results will be a scoring system, whereby a seed lot passes potency in goats if a vaccine prepared from it protects 80% of the vaccinates.

d) Duration of immunity

The vaccine protects goats for 14 months. It is, however, recommended to boost immunity after 1 year.

e) Stability

If stored at 4°C, the vaccine has a shell life of 1 year. Before use the vaccine should be shaken thoroughly, for even distribution of antigen.

f) Preservatives

At present preservatives are not used in the vaccine.

g) Precautions

Side-effects of the CCPP vaccine include development of a swelling at the site of inoculation and fever for 1–2 days following vaccination, accompanied with inappetance. The swelling may last between 1 and 14 days and is due to the saponin adjuvant. Accidental self-injection causes severe irritation.

5. Tests on the final product

a) Safety

Every batch of vaccine should be tested for safety in laboratory animals as described in B.4.b.

b) Potency

Once the potency test has been developed, every batch of vaccine will be required to be tested for potency.

REFERENCES

1. ACHARYA R.M. (1992). Goat production. *In:* Recent advances in goat production. Fifth International Conference on Goats, New Delhi, India, March 1992, 49–94.

2. BELTON D., LEACH R.H., MITCHELMORE D.L. & RURANGIRWA F.R. (1994). Serological specificity of a monoclonal antibody to mycoplasma strain F38, the agent of contagious caprine pleuropneumonia. *Vet. Rec.*, **134**, 643–646.

3. BOLSKE G., MATTSSON J.G., BASCUNANA C.R., BERGSTROM K., WESONGA H. & JOHANSSON K.E. (1996). Diagnosis of contagious caprine pleuropneumonia by detection and identification of *Mycoplasma capricolum* subsp. *capripneumoniae* by PCR and restriction enzyme analysis. *J. Clin. Microbiol.*, **34**, 785–791.

4. BRADBURY J.M. (1983). Phosphate activity. *In:* Methods in Mycoplasmology, Vol. 1, Razin S. & Tully J.G., eds. Academic Press, New York, USA, 363–366.

5. CHO H. J., RUHNKE H.L. & LANGFORD E.V. (1976). The indirect haemagglutination test for detection of antibodies in cattle naturally infected with mycoplasmas. *Can. J. Comp. Med.*, **40**, 20–29.

6. DIGHERO M.W., BRADSTREET C.M.P. & ANDREWS B.E. (1970). Dried paper discs for serological identification of human mycoplasmas. *J. Appl. Bacteriol.*, **33**, 750–757.

7. ERNO H. (1983). Mycoplasmas related to Mycoplasma mycoides subsp. mycoides. *In:* The Diagnosis of Contagious Bovine Pleuropneumonia and Other Infections with *Mycoplasma mycoides* subspecies *mycoides*, Hall S.A., ed. CEC publication EUR 8654, Luxembourg, 33–39.

8. FREUNDT E.A. (1983). Proteolytic activity. *In:* Methods in Mycoplasmology, Vol. 1, Razin S. & Tully J.G., eds. Academic Press, New York, USA, 367–371.

9. FREUNDT E.A. (1983). Culture media for classical mycoplasmas. *In:* Methods in Mycoplasmology, Vol. 1, Razin S. & Tully J.G., eds. Academic Press, New York, USA, 127–135.

10. FREUNDT E.A., ANDREWS B.E., ERNO H., KUNZE M. & BLACK F.T. (1973). The sensitivity of Mycoplasmatales to sodium-polyanethol-sulfonate and digitonin. *Zentralbl. Bant Parasitkde*, (I Abt), **A225**, 104–112.

11. GOURLAY R.N. (1964). Antigenicity of Mycoplasma mycoides. 1. Examination of body fluids from cases of contagious bovine pleuropneumonia. *Res. Vet. Sci.*, **5**, 473–482.

12. GOURLAY R.N. (1983). Serological tests for the diagnosis of contagious bovine pleuropneumonia. *In:* The Diagnosis of Contagious Bovine Pleuropneumonia and Other Infections with *Mycoplasma mycoides* subspecies *mycoides*, Hall S.A., ed. CEC publication EUR 8654, Luxembourg, 27–32.

13. JONES G.E. & WOOD A.R. (1988). Microbiological and serological studies on caprine pneumonia in Oman. *Res. Vet. Sci.*, **44**, 125–131.

14. KALINER G. & MACOWAN K.J. (1976). The pathology of experimental and natural contagious caprine pleuropneumonia in Kenya. *Vet. Med.* [B], **2**, 652–661.

15. KIBOR A.C. & WAIYAKI P.G. (1986). Growth of mycoplasma F38 in medium B (modified Hayflick) and Newings typtose medium. *Bull. Anim. Health Prod. Afr.*, **34**, 157–159.

16. KROGSGAARD-JENSEN A. (1972). Mycoplasma: growth precipitation as a serodiagnostic method. *Appl. Microbiol.*, **23**, 553–558.

17. LEACH R.H., ERNO H. & MACOWAN K.J. (1993). Proposal for designation of F38-type caprine mycoplasmas as *Mycoplasma capricolum* subsp. *capripneumoniae* subsp. nov. and consequent obligatory relegation of strains currently classified as *M. capricolum* (Tully, Garile, Edward, Theodore & Erno, 1974) to an additional new subspecies, *M. capricolum* subsp. *capricolum* subsp. nov. *Int. J. Syst. Bacteriol.*, **43**, 603–605.

18. MACMARTIN D.A., MACOWAN K.J. & SWIFT L.L. (1980). A century of classical contagious caprine pleuropneumonia: from original description to aetiology. *Br. Vet. J.*, **136**, 507–515.

19. MACOWAN K.J. & MINETTE J.E. (1976). A mycoplasma from acute contagious caprine pleuropneumonia in Kenya. *Trop. Anim. Health Prod.*, **8**, 91–95.

20. MACOWAN K.J. & MINETTE J.E. (1977). The role of mycoplasma strain F38 in contagious caprine pleuropneumonia in Kenya. *Vet. Rec.*, **101**, 380–381.

21. MACOWAN K.J. & MINETTE J.E. (1977). Contact transmission of experimental contagious caprine pleuropneumonia (CCPP). *Trop. Anim. Health Prod.*, **9**, 185–188.

22. MACOWAN K.J. & MINETTE J.E. (1978). The effect of high passage mycoplasma strain F38 on the courses of contagious caprine pleuropneumonia (CCPP). *Trop. Anim. Health Prod.*, **10**, 31–35.

23. MILES R.J. & WADHER B.J. (1990). Kinetics and pattern of substrate utilization by *Mycoplasma* spp. *Zentralbl. Bakteriol.* (Suppl.), **20**, 675–676.

24. MOHAN K., MILES R.J. & WADHER B.J. (1990). Growth and biochemical characteristics of mycoplasmas isolated from the lungs of Nigerian goats. *Zentralbl. Bakteriol.* (Suppl.), **20**, 841–843.

25. MUTHOMI E.K. & RURANGIRWA F.R. (1983). Passive haemagglutination and complement fixation as diagnostic tests for contagious caprine pleuropneumonia caused by the F38 strain mycoplasma. *Res. Vet. Sci.*, **35**, 1–4.

26. PERREAU P., LE GOFF C. & GIAUFFREA A. (1976). Le diagnostic serolgique de l'agalaxie contagieuse des petits ruminants: un test de fixation du complement. *Bull. Acad. Vet. Fr.*, **49**, 185–192.

27. ROSENDAL S. & BLACK F.T. (1972). Direct and indirect immunofluorescence of unfixed and fixed mycoplasma colonies. *Acta Pathol. Microbiol. Scand.*, **80**, 615–622.

28. RURANGIRWA F.R., MCGUIRE T.C., KIBOR A. & CHEMA S. (1987). A latex agglutination test for field diagnosis of caprine pleuropneumonia. *Vet. Rec.*, **121**, 191–193.

29. RURANGIRWA F.R., MCGUIRE T.C., KIBOR A. & CHEMA S. (1987). An inactive vaccine for contagious caprine pleuropneumonia. *Vet. Rec.*, **121**, 397–402.

30. RURANGIRWA F.R., MCGUIRE T.C., MAGNUSON N.S., KIBOR A. & CHEMA. S. (1987). Composition of polysaccharide from mycoplasma (F-38) recognized by antibodies from goats with contagious caprine pleuropneumonia. *Res. Vet. Sci.*, **42**, 175–178.

31. RURANGIRWA F.R., MCGUIRE T.C., MUSOKE A.J. & KIBOR A. (1987). Differentiation of F38 mycoplasmas causing contagious caprine pleuropneumonia with a growth-inhibiting monoclonal antibody. *Infect. Immun.*, **55**, 3219–3220.

32. RURANGIRWA F.R., MCGUIRE T.C., WAMBUGU A.N. & KIHARA S.M. (1992). *In:* Ninth International Congress of the International Organization for Mycoplasmology, August 2–7 1992, Ames, Iowa, USA. IOM Letters, Vol. 2 FP5/2, p. 128.

33. SENTERFIT L.B. & JENSEN K.E. (1996). Antimetabolic antibodies to *Mycoplasma pneumonia* measured by tetrazolium reduction inhibition. *Proc. Soc. Exp. Biol. Med.*, **122**, 786–790.

34. TAYLOR T.K., BASHRUDDIN J.B. & GOULD A.R. (1992). Relationship between members of the *Mycoplasma mycoides* cluster as shown by DNA probes and sequence analysis. *Int. J. Syst. Bacteriol.*, **42**, 593–601.

35. TAYLOR-ROBINSON D., PRUCELL R.H., WONG D.C. & CHANOCK R.M. (1966). A colour test for the measurement of antibody to certain mycoplasma species based on the inhibition of acid production. *J. Hyg. (Camb.)*, **64**, 91–104.

36. THIAUCOURT F. & BOLSKE G. (1996). Contagious caprine pleuropneumonia and other pulmonary mycoplasmoses of sheep and goats. *Rev. sci. tech. Off. Int. Epiz.*, **15**, 1397–1414.

37. THIAUCOURT F., BOLSKE G., LIBEAU G., LE GOFF C. & LEFEVRE P.-C. (1994). The use of monoclonal antibodies in the diagnosis of contagious caprine pleuropneumonia (CCPP). *Vet. Microbiol.*, **41**, 191–203.

38. THIAUCOURT F., GUERIN C., MADY V. & LEFEVRE P.-C. (1992). Diagnostic de la pleuropneumonie cantagieuse caprine: ameliorations recentes. *Rev. sci. tech. Off. Int. Epiz.*, **11**, 859–865.

*

* *

CHAPTER 2.4.7.

ENZOOTIC ABORTION OF EWES (ovine chlamydiosis)

SUMMARY

The diagnosis of enzootic abortion, also known as ovine chlamydiosis or chlamydial abortion of ewes, depends on the demonstration or possibly isolation and identification of the causative agent in the products of abortion or vaginal excretions of freshly aborted females. A humoral antibody response may be detected after abortion. Goats as well as sheep and, less commonly, cattle and deer, can be affected. Chlamydiosis of small ruminants is a zoonosis and the organism must be handled with biosafety precautions. Pregnant women are particularly susceptible. Until recently, the causative organism was known as Chlamydia psittaci, *but under a newly introduced nomenclature for the chlamydiae it is now known as* Chlamydophila abortus.

Identification of the agent: *The basis for a positive diagnosis of infection with* C. abortus *depends on a history of abortion in sheep or goats (often in late pregnancy), evidence of necrotic placentitis, and the demonstration of large numbers of the organism in stained smears of affected placentae. The still moist fleece of fetuses or vaginal swabs of females that have freshly aborted are also useful. Care is needed to distinguish cotyledonary damage caused by* Toxoplasma gondii *and, in stained smears, to be aware of the morphological similarities between* C. abortus *and* Coxiella burnetii, *the agent of Q fever.*

Chlamydial antigen can be detected by enzyme-linked immunosorbent assay, or the fluorescent antibody test, whereas chlamydial DNA can be detected by the polymerase chain reaction, the former two being available in kit form.

Chlamydophila abortus *can be isolated only in living cells; thus facilities for growth in chicken embryos or cell cultures, with appropriate biohazard containment, are required.*

Serological tests: *A rise in antibody titre to* C. abortus, *detected by the complement fixation (CF) test, is common after abortion or stillbirth, but this does not occur in every case.* Chlamydophila abortus *shares common antigens with* C. pecorum *and some Gram-negative bacteria, so that the CF test is not wholly specific, nor does it distinguish between responses to vaccination and to infection. Low CF titres need to be interpreted with caution, particularly if these are encountered in individual animals or in flocks with no history of abortion.*

Alternative serological tests have been developed, but none has been sufficiently appraised so far for field use. A delayed hypersensitivity reaction to chlamydial antigen can be elicited in infected sheep, but the procedure is not amenable to routine use.

Requirements for vaccines and diagnostic biologicals: *Inactivated and live vaccines are available that reduce the incidence of abortion, but do not prevent infection. They assist in control of the disease but will not eradicate it. Serological screening during the period after parturition helps to identify infected flocks, to which control measures can then be applied.*

A. DIAGNOSTIC TECHNIQUES

Chlamydophila abortus causes enzootic abortion in sheep and goats and may also impair overall reproductive performance (20). Less frequently, cattle and deer may be affected. The organism has zoonotic potential (7), and therefore must be handled carefully with adequate microbiological precautions and laboratory containment. Sheep also harbour another chlamydial species, *C. pecorum*, distinguishable from *C. abortus* by DNA analysis and specialised serology. There is limited evidence for its pathogenicity (12). Until recently, the causative organism was known as *Chlamydia psittaci* (14), but now a new taxonomic classification of *Chlamydiae* has been adopted (8), in which the family Chlamydiaceae has been divided into two genera and nine species, based on sequence analysis of the 16s and 23s rRNA genes. The two new genera, *Chlamydia* and *Chlamydophila*, correlate with the former species *C. trachomatis* and *C. abortus*. The genus *Chlamydia* includes *C. trachomatis* (human), *C. suis* (swine) and *C. muridarum* (mouse and hamster). The genus *Chlamydophila* includes *C. psittaci* (avian), *C. felis* (cats), *C. abortus* (sheep, goats and cattle), *C. caviae* (guinea-pigs), the former species *C. pecorum* (sheep and cattle) and *C. pneumoniae* (human). The two genera and nine species have merit both on the basis of molecular structure and for the purposes of classification of host range and clinical disease. The species show a high degree of correlation with host range, disease syndrome and virulence, thus assisting in understanding the epidemiology of the various species and serovars affecting mammals and birds. The terms 'chlamydiosis' and 'chlamydia(e)' are used to refer to members of either of the two genera. However, a binomial of the new generic and specific names is used when referring to a particular chlamydial species.

Infected females shed vast numbers of infective *C. abortus* at the time of abortion or parturition, particularly in the placenta and uterine discharges. Human infection may be acquired from these sources or from carelessly handled laboratory cultures of the organism, with effects that range from subclinical infection to acute influenza-like illness. Authenticated cases of human placentitis and abortion caused by *C. abortus* of ovine origin indicate that pregnant women are at special risk and should not be exposed to sources of infection (7).

1. Identification of the agent

a) Smears

Where the clinical history of the flock and the character of lesions in aborted placentae suggest enzootic abortion, a diagnosis can be made by microscopic examination of smears made from affected chorionic villi or adjacent chorion. Several staining procedures are satisfactory, for example, modified Machiavello, Giemsa, *Brucella* differential or modified Ziehl–Neelsen stains (25). In positive cases stained by the latter method and examined under high-power microscopy, large numbers of small (300 nm) coccoid elementary bodies are seen singly or in clumps stained red against the blue background of cellular debris. Under dark-ground illumination, the elementary bodies are pale green. If placental material is not available, smears may be made from vaginal swabs of females that have aborted within the previous 24 hours, or from the moist fleece of a freshly aborted or stillborn lamb that has not been cleaned by its mother. In general, such preparations contain fewer organisms than placental smears.

In morphology and staining characteristics, *C. abortus* resembles the rickettsia *Coxiella burnetii,* which, in some circumstances, may provoke abortion and which, in humans, causes Q fever. Care must be taken to differentiate between these two organisms in cases lacking a good history or evidence of chlamydial-induced placental pathology. Antigenic differences between *C. abortus* and *Coxiella burnetii* can be detected serologically. Fluorescent antibody tests using a specific antiserum or monoclonal antibody may be used for identification of *C. abortus* in smears.

b) Antigen detection

Several chlamydial genus-level antigen detection tests are available commercially. A comparative assessment of several such assays, on nonovine material, indicated that those using enzyme-linked immunosorbent assay (ELISA) methodology were more sensitive than kits employing a fluorescent antibody test (FAT) (31). Under the test conditions used, a kit that detects chlamydial lipopolysaccharide (LPS) was judged to be the most sensitive of the rapid ELISA-based systems investigated. Though occasionally yielding false-positive results, particularly with avian faecal samples, the kit also gave satisfactory results with ovine placental samples (30).

c) DNA

Amplification of chlamydial DNA by polymerase chain reaction (PCR) provides an alternative approach for verifying the presence of chlamydiae in biological samples without resorting to culture. PCR is highly sensitive for this purpose (14, 28), but has the attendant risk of cross-contamination between samples, so appropriate measures must be taken to avoid this. Methods for discriminating between amplified DNA sequences originating from *C. abortus* and *C. pecorum* are emerging (15, 19). At present, these are mainly research techniques, but they are beginning to be introduced into diagnostic laboratories.

d) Tissue sections

Intracellular chlamydial inclusions can be demonstrated by Giemsa staining of thin (≤4 µm) sections taken from target tissues that have been suitably fixed in fluids such as Bouin or Carnoy. More striking results can be obtained by immunological staining procedures. The direct immunoperoxidase method (9) is rapid and simple, while the method with streptavidin–biotin is more complex (1). A commercial FAT (Imagen-Celltech), developed for use in human medicine, gives satisfactory results with ovine placental material (1). Electron microscopy can also be performed using negative contrast, to differentiate chlamydiae from *Coxiella burnetii.*

e) Isolation of the agent

Chlamydophila abortus can be isolated in embryonated chicken eggs or in cell cultures, the latter being the method of choice for isolation of new strains.

Tissue samples, such as diseased cotyledons, placental membranes, fetal lung or liver, or vaginal swabs, that may be subject to any delay before isolation procedures begin, should be maintained in a suitable transport medium in the interim period. The most satisfactory medium is sucrose/phosphate/glutamate medium supplemented with 10% fetal bovine serum, antibiotic (streptomycin and gentamycin are suitable, but not penicillin), and a fungal inhibitor (24). A tissue:medium ratio of 1:10 is commonly employed. Alternatively, approximately 1 g of tissue is ground with sterile sand in 8 ml of transport medium.

Chicken embryos: Test samples are prepared as 10% suspensions in nutrient broth containing streptomycin (not penicillin) (200 µg/ml); 0.2 ml of suspension are inoculated into the yolk sac of 6–8-day old embryos, which are then further incubated at 37°C. Infected embryos die between 4 and 13 days after inoculation. Smears prepared from their vascularised yolk sac membranes reveal large numbers of elementary bodies.

Cell cultures: C. abortus of ovine origin can be isolated in a variety of cell types but McCoy, BGM or baby hamster kidney (BHK) cells are most commonly used. For confirmatory diagnosis, cultured monolayers are suspended in growth medium at a concentration of 2×10^5 cells/ml. Aliquots of 2 ml of the suspension are dispensed into flat-bottomed glass Universal bottles, each containing a single 16 mm cover-slip. Confluent cover-slip monolayers are achieved after incubation for 24 hours at 37°C. The growth medium is removed and replaced by 2 ml of test inoculum, which is then centrifuged at 2500 ***g*** for 30 minutes on to the cover-slip monolayer to promote infection. After further incubation for 2–3 days, the cover-slip monolayers are fixed in methanol and stained with Giemsa or after the method of Gimenez (6, 13). After methanol fixation, infected cultures contain basophilic (Giemsa) or eosinophilic (Gimenez) intracytoplasmic inclusions. Similar procedures are used in culturing *C. abortus* for antigen preparation. Fluorescent antibody techniques can also be used and are equally effective.

Chlamydial activity can be further enhanced by chemical treatment of cultured cells, before or during infection, to favour chlamydial growth. Various substances that have been described for incorporation into the infective inoculum to which cover-slip monolayers are exposed include: cycloheximide (1 µg/ml) in the maintenance medium (16), emetine (1 µg/ml) for 5 minutes before infection (21), and 5-iodo-2-deoxyuridine (2) (80 µg/ml) for 3 days prior to infection. Unless preconditioned cells are available, the latter isolation procedure requires increased time for successful agent isolation.

2. Serological tests

Complement fixation (CF) is the most widely used procedure (26). On a flock basis (ten sera from aborted ewes or goats, 4–8 weeks after abortion or parturition), the CF test will detect evidence of vaccination or infection. Infection is evident principally during active placental infection in the last month of gestation and following the bacteraemia that often accompanies abortion. Consequently, paired sera collected at the time of abortion and again 3 weeks later may reveal a rising CF antibody titre that will provide a basis for a retrospective diagnosis. Antigenic cross-reactivity between *C. abortus* and *C. pecorum,* as well as with some Gram-negative bacteria (e.g. *Acinetobacter*), can give rise to low false-positive CF test results. Thus, titres less than 1/32 in individual animals should be considered to be nonspecific for *C. abortus.*

Antigen is prepared from heavily infected yolk sac membranes obtained from chicken embryos that have been inoculated in the same manner as those used to isolate the organism from field material. Chopped and ground membranes are suspended in phosphate buffer, pH 7.6, at the rate of 2 ml per membrane. After removal of crude debris, the supernatant fluid is centrifuged at 10,000 ***g*** for 1 hour at 4°C, the deposit is resuspended in a small volume of saline, and a smear of this is examined to ensure a high yield of chlamydiae. The suspension is held in a boiling water bath for 20 minutes, or is autoclaved, and sodium azide (0.3%) is added as a preservative. Antigen may also be prepared from cell cultures infected with *C. abortus.* Infected monolayers are suspended in phosphate buffer, pH 7.6, and the cells are disrupted by homogenisation or ultrasonication. Gross debris is removed and subsequent procedures are as for the preparation of antigen from infected yolk sacs. In either case, CF tests with standardised complement and antisera will establish the optimal working dilution for each batch of antigen.

The serological responses to *C. abortus* and *C. pecorum* can be resolved by indirect micro-immunofluorescence (3), but the procedure is too time-consuming for routine diagnostic purposes. ELISAs developed independently by several research groups have not been adapted for general diagnostic work, partly because of difficulties associated with the use of particulate antigens. However, a novel ELISA that incorporates a stable, solubilised antigen has been used to test experimental and field samples, and has given results that, though lacking species specificity, have a higher sensitivity than CF (4, 18). Of note has been the recent application of monoclonal antibody technology in a competitive ELISA to discriminate between antibodies to *C. abortus* and *C. pecorum* (23). Commercial development of the assay is in progress.

B. REQUIREMENTS FOR VACCINES AND DIAGNOSTIC BIOLOGICALS

Inactivated vaccines can be prepared from infected yolk sacs (10) or cell cultures (17, 29), and incorporate whole organisms (5) or fractions of them (27). A recombinant vaccine against *C. abortus* remains a future goal. A chemically induced, temperature-sensitive mutant derived from an ovine abortion strain of *C. abortus* has been tested as live vaccine (22). No adverse effects have been observed in inoculated sheep or goats, and protection against experimental infection is good. Following field trials in Britain, a lyophilised live vaccine was licensed in 1995. Vaccination of naive breeding females afforded substantial protection against challenge and reduced shedding of chlamydiae by vaccinates after infection. Vaccination was less effective in females already carrying infection. The following paragraphs apply to the inactivated vaccine.

1. Seed management

a) Characteristics of the seed

One or more ovine abortion isolates that consistently grow productively in the chosen substrate are suitable, and an early passage of the seed stock can be established. Alternatively, an isolate that has been adapted to the chicken embryo by multiple passage (>100) can be used. This permits more of the embryo to be used for vaccine production (11). Although adaptation to the embryo may diminish the isolate's virulence for sheep, there is no evidence that such change reduces its protective efficacy as an inactivated vaccine (11).

b) Method of culture

For low passage isolates, the procedures described for the preparation of CF antigen are suitably adapted and amplified for bulk production. Once the final harvest suspension is obtained, an aliquot is removed for titration of its infectivity. The bulk is treated with formalin to a final concentration of 0.4%, and stored until sterility tests confirm complete inactivation.

c) Validation as a vaccine

Before inoculation of large numbers of embryos or cell cultures, the viability and freedom from contamination of seed stock should be verified. It may be convenient to collect the total harvest in separate manageable lots. In this case, the infectivity of an aliquot of each lot should be separately titrated to ensure that each matches the requirements (see Section B.2. below). Store under refrigerated conditions.

2. Method of manufacture

The inactivated harvest is centrifuged and resuspended in phosphate buffered saline containing 0.2% formalin to a volume representing a preinactivation infectivity titre of approximately 10^8 infectious units/ml (29). Usually, the aqueous suspension is blended with an oil adjuvant, either directly (29) or after precipitation by potassium alum ($AlK[SO_4]_2.12\ H_2O$) (10). A preservative, such as 0.01% thiomersal, may also be added.

3. In-process control

The main requirements are to ensure adequate growth of *C. abortus*, avoidance of extraneous infection of the culture substrate, completeness of inactivation and biohazard awareness by process workers.

4. Batch control

Each separate batch of manufactured vaccine should be tested for sterility, safety and potency.

a) Sterility

Tests for sterility and freedom from contamination of biological materials may be found in Chapter I.4.

b) **Safety**

Subcutaneous inoculation into two or more seronegative sheep of twice the standard dose (usually 1.0 ml) of manufactured vaccine should elicit no systemic reaction, but oil-adjuvant vaccines can cause a nonharmful swelling at the inoculation site.

c) **Potency**

At present, potency is judged by the occurrence of a serological response in previously unvaccinated sheep given 1 ml of vaccine subcutaneously. Blood samples taken before and 28 days after vaccination are compared. Ultimately, potency has to be judged against experimental challenge or field performance, but no *in vitro* correlation of protective efficacy has yet been established.

d) **Duration of immunity**

No firm data are available, but revaccination is recommended after 1–3 years, according to the exposure risk.

e) **Stability**

Vaccine stored under refrigeration (5±3°C) should remain stable for at least 1 year. Before use it should be held at room temperature for 24 hours, and the container should be shaken vigorously immediately before vaccine is withdrawn.

5. Tests on the final product

a) **Safety**

See Section B.4.b.

b) **Potency**

See Section B.4.c.

REFERENCES

1. AMIN J.D. & WILSMORE A.J. (1994). Detection of *Chlamydia psittaci (ovis)* antigen in tissue sections and McCoy cells using streptavidin–biotin and the Imagen staining method. *Br. Vet. J.*, **150**, 555–560.

2. ANDERSON I.E. (1986). Comparison of five ovine isolates of *Chlamydia psittaci*: an evaluation of three cell culture treatments. *Med. Lab. Sci.*, **43**, 241–248.

3. ANDERSON I.E. (1987). Comparison of some ovine *Chlamydia psittaci* isolates by indirect immunofluorescence. *Vet. Microbiol.*, **13**, 69–74.

4. ANDERSON I.E., HERRING A.J., JONES G.E., LOW J.C. & GREIG A. (1995). Development and evaluation of an indirect ELISA to detect antibodies to abortion strains of *Chlamydia psittaci* in sheep sera. *Vet. Microbiol.*, **43**, 1–12.

5. ANDERSON I.E., TAN T.W., JONES G.E. & HERRING A.J. (1990). Efficacy against ovine enzootic abortion of an experimental vaccine containing purified elementary bodies of *Chlamydia psittaci*. *Vet. Microbiol.*, **24**, 21–27.

6. ARENS M. & WEINGARTEN M. (1981). Vergleichende Untersuchungen an Buffalo Green monkey (BGM) Zellen und Mausen zur Isolierung von *Chlamydia psittaci* aus Kot und Organproben von Vogeln. *Zentralbl. Veterinarmed [B]*, **28**, 301–309.

7. BUXTON D. (1986). Potential danger to pregnant women of *Chlamydia psittaci* from sheep. *Vet. Rec.*, **118**, 510–511.

8. EVERETT K.D.E., BUSH R.M. & ANDERSEN A.A. (1999). Emended description of the order *Chlamydiales,* proposal of *Parachlamydiaceae* fam. nov. and *Simkaniaceae* fam. nov., each containing one monotypic genus of the family *Chlamydiaceae,* including a new genus and five new species, and standards for the identification of organisms. *Int. J. System. Bact.*, **49**, 415–440.

9. FINLAYSON J., BUXTON D., ANDERSON I.E. & DONALD K.M. (1985). Direct immunoperoxidase method for demonstrating *Chlamydia psittaci* in tissue sections. *J. Clin. Pathol.*, **38**, 712–714.

10. FOGGIE A. (1973). Preparation of vaccines against enzootic abortion of ewes. A review of the research work at the Moredun Institute. *Vet. Bull.*, **43**, 587–590.

11. FROST J.W. & WACHENDORFER G. (1986). Ten years' vaccination against chlamydial abortion of ewes. *In:* Chlamydial Diseases of Ruminants, Aitken I.D., ed. Commission of the European Communities, Luxembourg, 67–70.

12. FUKUSHI H. & HIRAI K. (1993). *Chlamydia pecorum* – the fourth species of genus *Chlamydia. Microbiol. Immunol.*, **37**, 515–522.

13. GIMENEZ D.F. (1964). Staining rickettsiae in yolk-sac cultures. *Stain Technol.*, **39**, 135–140.

14. HERRING A.J. (1993). Typing *Chlamydia psittaci* – a review of methods and recent findings. *Br. Vet. J.*, **149**, 455–475.

15. HEWISON R.G., GRIFFITHS P.C., BEVAN B.J., KIRWAN S.E.S., FIELD M.E., WOODWARD M.J. & DAWSON M. (1997). Detection of *Chlamydia psittaci* DNA in avian clincal samples by polymerase chain reaction. *Vet. Microbiol.*, **54**, 155–166.

16. JOHNSON F.W.A., CLARKSON M.J. & SPENCER W.N. (1983). Direct isolation of the agent of enzootic abortion of ewes *(Chlamydia psittaci)* in cell cultures. *Vet. Rec.*, **113**, 413–414.

17. JONES G.E., JONES K.A., MACHELL J., BREBNER J., ANDERSON I.E. & HOW S. (1995). Efficacy trials with tissue-culture grown, inactivated vaccines against chlamydial abortion in sheep. *Vaccine*, **13**, 715–723.

18. JONES G.E., LOW J.C., MACHELL J. & ARMSTRONG K. (1997). Comparison of five tests for the detection of antibodies against chlamydial (enzootic) abortion of ewes. *Vet. Rec.*, **141**, 164–168.

19. KALTENBOECK B., KOUSOULAS K.G. & STORZ J. (1992). Two-step polymerase chain reactions and restriction endonuclease analyses detect and differentiate ompA DNA of *Chlamydia* spp. *J. Clin. Microbiol.*, **30**, 1098–1104.

20. PAPP J.R. & SHEWEN P.E. (1996). Pregnancy failure following vaginal infection of sheep with *Chlamydia psittaci* prior to breeding. *Infect. Immun.*, **64**, 1116–1125.

21. PAUL I.D. (1982). The growth of *Chlamydia* in McCoy cells treated with emetine. *Med. Lab. Sci.*, **39**, 15–32.

22. RODOLAKIS A. (1986). Use of a live temperature-sensitive vaccine in experimental and natural infections. *In:* Chlamydial Diseases of Ruminants, Aitken I.D., ed. Commission of the European Communities, Luxembourg, 71–77.

23. SALTI-MONTESANTO V., TSOLI E., PAPAVASSILIOU P., PSARROU E., MARKEY B.M., JONES G.E. & VRETOU E. (1997). Diagnosis of ovine enzootic abortion, using a competitive ELISA based on monoclonal antibodies against variable segments 1 and 2 of the major outer membrane protein of *Chlamydia psittaci* serotype 1. *Am. J. Vet. Res.*, **58**, 228–235.

24. SPENCER W.N. & JOHNSON F.W.A. (1983). Simple transport medium for the isolation of *Chlamydia psittaci* from clinical material. *Vet. Rec.*, **113**, 535–536.

25. STAMP J.T., MCEWEN A.D., WATT J.A.A. & NISBET D.I. (1950). Enzootic abortion in ewes. I. Transmission of the disease. *Vet. Rec.*, **62**, 251–254.

26. STAMP J.T., WATT J.A.A. & COCKBURN R.B. (1952). Enzootic abortion in ewes. Complement fixation test. *J. Comp. Pathol.*, **62**, 93–101.

27. TAN T.W., HERRING A.J., ANDERSON I.E. & JONES G.E. (1990). Protection of sheep against *Chlamydia psittaci* infection with a subcellular vaccine containing the major outer membrane protein. *Infect. Immun.*, **58**, 3101–3108.

28. THIELE D., WITTENBRINK M.M., FISCHER D. & KRAUSS H. (1992). Evaluation of the polymerase chain reaction (PCR) for detection of *Chlamydia psittaci* in abortion material from ewes. *Zentralbl. Bakteriol.*, **277**, 446–453.

29. WALDHALM D.G., DELONG W.J. & HALL R.F. (1982). Efficacy of bacterin prepared from *Chlamydia psittaci* grown in cell culture for experimental immunisation of ewes. *Vet. Microbiol.*, **7**, 493–498.

30. WILSMORE A.J. & DAVIDSON I. (1991). 'Clearview' rapid test compared with other methods to diagnose chlamydial infection. *Vet. Rec.*, **128**, 503–504.

31. WOOD M.M. & TIMMS P. (1992). Comparison of nine antigen detection kits for diagnosis of urogenital infections due to *Chlamydia psittaci* in koalas. *J. Clin. Microbiol.*, **30**, 3200–3205.

*

* *

SECTION 2.5.

EQUINE DISEASES IN LIST B

CHAPTER 2.5.1.

CONTAGIOUS EQUINE METRITIS

SUMMARY

Contagious equine metritis is an inflammation of the endometrium of mares caused by Taylorella equigenitalis *infection, which usually results in temporary infertility. It is a nonsystemic illness, the effects of which are restricted to the reproductive tract of the mare.*

The chief clinical signs are a copious to slight mucopurulent vaginal discharge and a variable cervicitis and vaginitis. Recovery is uneventful, but prolonged asymptomatic carriage is established in a proportion of infected mares. The infection is most frequently transmitted by sexual contact with carrier stallions, which are always asymptomatic and in which the principal sites of T. equigenitalis *colonisation are the urogenital membranes (urethral fossa, urethra and penile sheath). Inadequate hygiene during the cleansing or examination of the genitalia of horses can also be responsible for the transmission of infection. Carrier mares are colonised on the urogenital membranes, principally in the clitoral sinuses and fossa and very frequently in the uterus. Foals born of carrier mares may also become carriers. The organism can infect equid species other than horses, e.g. donkeys.*

Washing with disinfectants combined with local and systemic antibiotic treatment can eliminate T. equigenitalis, *but vaccination is ineffective.*

The principal means of control is through preventing transmission by the establishment of freedom from infection before breeding commences. Detection of infection depends on the culture of T. equigenitalis *from urogenital swabs of mares and stallions and its accurate identification. Serum antibody to* T. equigenitalis *can be detected in mares for 3–7 weeks after infection and can also be demonstrated in the occasional carrier mare, but not stallion. Serology may therefore be of value in detecting recent, but not chronic, infection in the mare, but the emphasis for control of the disease should be on the detection of carriers by culture.*

Identification of the agent: *Swabs must be transported to the laboratory with precautions to avoid loss of viability. Growth of* T. equigenitalis *is likely to take at least 72 hours and may take up to 13 days, but usually does not take longer than 6 days at 37°C on medium enriched with heated blood and an atmosphere of 5–10% CO_2. A standard incubation time of up to at least 7 days is satisfactory and practical. After 72 hours under appropriate culture conditions colonies may be small – up to 2–3 mm in diameter – watery to opaque and yellowish grey, and are smooth with an entire edge.* Taylorella equigenitalis *is a Gram-negative, small, coccoid rod that is sometimes pleomorphic and exhibits bipolar staining. It produces catalase and phosphatase, and is strongly oxidase positive. It is otherwise unreactive biochemically, and identification is finally dependent on antigenic characterisation of bacteria using specific antibodies.*

Antibody to whole killed T. equigenitalis *and a latex agglutination kit employing these antibodies may be used, but specificity for the organism and evidence for its failure to react with other oxidase positive/catalase positive, Gram-negative bacteria that might be cultured from the urogenital tract of horses is essential. Monoclonal antibodies have been developed that can be used successfully to identify* T. equigenitalis.

***Serological tests:** No serological test described to date will, by itself, reliably detect infection for diagnosis and control. However, serological tests can be used as an adjunct to culture for* T. equigenitalis *in screening mares recently bred with a carrier stallion, but must not be used as a substitute for culture.*

***Requirements for vaccines and diagnostic biologicals:** Effective vaccines that protect against contagious equine metritis or prevent colonisation by* T. equigenitalis *are not yet available.*

A. DIAGNOSTIC TECHNIQUES

Contagious equine metritis was first described in the United Kingdom (UK) in 1977 (9), after which it was diagnosed throughout Europe, North America, Australia and other countries. It was first seen as disease outbreaks characterised by a mucopurulent vaginal discharge originating from inflammation of the endometrium and caused temporary infertility. The fastidious nature and slow growth of the causative bacterium, *Taylorella equigenitalis*, caused difficulties in initial attempts at culture (15), but the disease was reproduced by experimental clitoral challenge with isolated laboratory-grown bacteria (14, 16, 20). Using appropriate culture conditions, *T. equigenitalis* is easily isolated from infective vaginal discharge. Mares may encounter more than one episode of the disease in a short period of time (25). Serum antibody persists for 3–7 weeks after infection, but often it is not detectable shortly after recovery from active disease (11). Most mares recover uneventfully, but some may become carriers of *T. equigenitalis* for many months (14). Colonisation by *T. equigenitalis* is most consistently demonstrated by culture of swabs taken from the recesses of the clitoral fossa and sinuses, but it may be recovered from the cervix and endometrium in more pure culture (14). Carriage does not always affect conception (26), and in such cases pregnancy may proceed so that foals are born, become infected by passage down the birth canal, and thereby also become long-term and asymptomatic carriers (23). Many primary cases of infection with *T. equigenitalis* in the mare are subclinical, and a frequent indicator of infection is a mare returning in early oestrus after being bred to a putative carrier stallion.

Carrier mares and stallions act as reservoirs of infection, but stallions, because they mate with numerous mares, act as the principal means of transmission. The urogenital membranes of stallions become contaminated at coitus, leading to a carrier state that may persist for many months or years (18). Unhygienic examination of mares and insanitary washing of the stallion's penis may also spread infection. Other sites of the horse body are not known to harbour *T. equigenitalis*. Most carrier females are clitoral carriers of *T. equigenitalis*. Long-term persistence of the organism in the uterus has rarely been observed. However, though of rare occurrence, *T. equigenitalis* can cause abortion in the mare.

Prior infection and vaccination are not fully protective (12), and failure of antibody to persist has meant that control of infection has relied on prevention of transmission through the detection of *T. equigenitalis* in swabs of urogenital membranes. In spite of difficulties with the culture of *T. equigenitalis*, screening mares and stallions prior to and while on the stud farm has successfully eliminated the disease from thoroughbred horses in countries using a voluntary code of practice. Many of these are based on the widely adopted UK's Horserace Betting Levy Board's Code of Practice, which is updated annually; the key recommendations of the Code are summarised below.

At the start of the breeding season, swabs are taken from all stallions, including those in their first season, from the urethra, urethral fossa, penile sheath and pre-ejaculatory fluid, on two occasions no fewer than 7 days apart. Mares are classified according to the degree of risk that they represent, and the intensity of sampling is adjusted accordingly. High-risk mares are defined as: (a) those from which *T. equigenitalis* was isolated in the past 7 years; (b) those found to be positive over 7 years ago but not mated since (and hence that have not recently had their fertility tested); (c) any mare mated to a stallion that transmitted infection in the previous year; (d) barren and maiden mares arriving from outside the countries adopting the Code if mated; and (e) mares mated in the previous year to a stallion from outside of these countries. All other mares are considered to be of low risk. A clitoral swab is taken from high-risk mares at home and a negative result should be obtained before the mare is transported to the stallion stud farm. Two further clitoral swabs are taken at the stallion stud farm; one on arrival, and the second during oestrus prior to mating, at which time the endometrium is also swabbed. All swabs should be negative <u>before</u> mating is permitted. In low-risk mares, one clitoral swab (taken at home or at the stallion breeding farm) and one endometrial swab are taken and a result is not required before mating is allowed to proceed.

Results of laboratory tests for *T. equigenitalis* should be entered on a certificate, which is sent to the veterinarians and stallion stud farm managers who are supervising the breeding. The certificate should record the animal's name, the sites and date of swabbing, the name of the veterinarian taking the swab, details of the test laboratory, the date the swabs were received and cultured by the laboratory, and whether the swabs were negative or positive, or whether the culture was overgrown by other bacteria to an extent that the laboratory could not be confident that small numbers of *T. equigenitalis* would be detected and, therefore, requiring another set of swabs to be sent.

Difficulties with the culture of *T. equigenitalis* caused by its fastidious nature necessitate the use of a quality control system that should be passed before a laboratory is permitted to undertake testing for contagious equine metritis and to issue certificates of the results obtained. The task of quality control should be undertaken by a good and impartial microbiology laboratory, authorised for the purpose, which is not involved in routine testing of contagious equine metritis swabs. At 6-month intervals, swabs inoculated into mixed cultures that are designed to test the ability to recover and identify *T. equigenitalis* in the face of contaminants, as well as procedures for reporting results, should be sent to laboratories wishing to participate. A list of those laboratories satisfactorily passing the quality control should be published in a veterinary journal that is widely read by the national veterinarians. The veterinarians and stallion stud farm managers who are supervising the breeding season should accept only certificates provided by laboratories published in the latest list.

Any mares showing abnormal vaginal exudate, or returning to oestrus prematurely, should be investigated and managed as though infected with *T. equigenitalis* until results of laboratory investigations prove otherwise. Other causes of outbreaks of endometritis include *Pseudomonas aeruginosa* and certain capsule types of *Klebsiella pneumoniae*. Swabs should be examined for these bacteria, and an attempt should be made to culture and identify *K. pneumoniae* and *P. aeruginosa* so as to establish a differential diagnosis.

If carriers of *T. equigenitalis* are detected, the organism can be eliminated by treatment with systemic antibiotics combined with disinfectant washing of exposed genital membranes (1). Particular attention should be paid to cleansing of the recesses of the clitoral fossa and sinuses of mares, where colonisation by *T. equigenitalis* is most evident in carriers. A course of treatment may take several weeks and may need to be repeated before intensive swabbing consistently fails to recover *T. equigenitalis* (10). A significant number of carrier mares can be refractive to several courses of treatment. These may require surgery to effect ablation of the clitoral sinuses for permanent elimination of the carrier state in such animals.

Control measures for countries regarded as free from *T. equigenitalis* infection should be based on the screening of animals prior to importation and/or during a post-importation quarantine period using swabbing and testing regimes broadly based on those described above for breeding populations.

1. Identification of the agent (the prescribed test for international trade)

Various bacteria may be present on the urogenital membranes of horses as harmless commensals that interfere with the culture of *T. equigenitalis*. Some may be present in small numbers, but grow in the swab before it is cultured thereby obscuring the presence of *T. equigenitalis*. Swabs must be placed in a transport medium with activated charcoal, such as Amies medium, to absorb inhibitory by-products of bacterial metabolism (21). Numbers of *T. equigenitalis* decline in swabs with time, and this effect is more pronounced at higher temperatures (17). Swabs must be kept cool and transported so that they arrive at the laboratory no later than 24–48 hours after they were taken. Negative culture results from swabs plated out more than 48 hours after they were taken are unreliable. Antibiotic treatment for whatever cause should cease at least 7 days before swabbing. The presence of antibiotics may damage *T. equigenitalis*, which nonetheless persists in the urogenital membranes but will not grow on laboratory media.

Each swab must be inoculated on to two 5% (v/v) heated blood agar plates with a rich peptone agar base containing additional cysteine (0.83 mM), sodium sulphite (1.59 mM) and a fungicide (5 µg/ml amphotericin B). *Taylorella equigenitalis* will grow on blood agar, but it can tolerate less than ideal conditions better when grown on heated blood agar ('chocolate' blood produced by heating at 70–80°C for 12 minutes). Some manufacturers[1] produce a peptone agar base that is quality controlled for its ability to support the growth of *T. equigenitalis*. An important feature of all good *T. equigenitalis* media is the absence of fermentable carbohydrates. These do not enhance the growth of *T. equigenitalis*, but their fermentation by other bacteria inhibits *T. equigenitalis* growth (2, 12). One of the plates should also contain streptomycin sulphate (200 µg/ml). Many isolates of *T. equigenitalis* are resistant to this concentration of antibiotic, which serves to reduce the extent of growth of other bacteria that might otherwise obscure the presence of small numbers of *T. equigenitalis* (21). The plate without streptomycin sulphate is used to isolate a smaller proportion of *T. equigenitalis* strains that are sensitive to this antibiotic. Growth by other bacteria, for example *Proteus mirabilis*, however, may be so extensive on this medium that the laboratory should record that they cannot issue a negative result. In this event, further swabs should be requested in the hope that the problem will not recur.

Occasionally, the urogenital membranes will be persistently colonised by another bacterium that interferes with diagnosis, and it will prove necessary to attempt to eliminate this by washing and antibiotic treatment. Swabbing for *T. equigenitalis* should not recommence until at least 7 days after treatment has stopped. A medium containing trimethoprim (1 µg/ml), clindamycin (5 µg/ml), and amphotericin B (5 µg/ml), to which all *T. equigenitalis* are resistant, has been developed (24) and assessed (2), and is claimed to overcome this

1 For example, Mast Diagnostics, Mast House, Derby Road, Bootle, Merseyside L20 1EA, United Kingdom (UK), and Lab M, Tomley House, Wash Lane, Bury BL9 6AU, UK.

difficulty in most cases. This medium is usefully included routinely in the initial culturing. Additional plates should be inoculated with a culture of *T. equigenitalis* to check that each batch of medium will support growth.

Plates must be incubated at 35–37°C in 5–10% (v/v) CO_2 in air or by use of a candle jar. At least 48 hours is normally required before colonies of *T. equigenitalis* become visible, after which time daily inspection is needed. Visual detection of colonies may take 13 days in rare cases (27). A standard incubation time of up to at least 7 days is satisfactory and practical. Plates should be examined for contaminants after the first 24 hours' incubation. Colonies may be quite small, up to 2–3 mm in diameter, smooth with an entire edge, glossy and yellowish grey.

Taylorella equigenitalis is a Gram-negative, nonmotile, bacillus or cocco-bacillus that is often pleomorphic (up to 6 µm long) and may exhibit bipolar staining. It is catalase positive, phosphatase positive, and strongly oxidase positive (see ref. 3 for methods for examining catalase, phosphatase and oxidase activities). It is otherwise inert in tests for biochemical activity. If a slow-growing organism is isolated that fits the description for cellular morphology and that is strongly oxidase positive, it should be tested for reactivity with *T.-equigenitalis*-specific antiserum.

A variety of serotyping tests have been developed ranging in complexity from slide agglutination to direct or indirect immunofluorescence. Each method has its advantages and disadvantages. The disadvantage of the slide agglutination test is that occasionally autoagglutination of isolates occurs: culturing in bottled CO_2 in air, as opposed to in a candle jar, may reduce autoagglutination (22). It has been suggested that immunofluorescence can be used to identify autoagglutinating isolates, but with this test a degree of cross-reaction with organisms such as *Pasteurella haemolytica* may occur, and it may be necessary to repeat the test using adsorbed antisera (22). The immunofluorescence test can be improved by the use of monoclonal antibodies, which are now becoming available.

Antiserum is produced by vaccinating rabbits with killed *T. equigenitalis*. A number of different immunisation regimes can be employed, ranging from those used for producing *Escherichia-coli*-typing antisera (19), to immunisation together with an adjuvant, such as Freund's incomplete. Monoclonal antibodies are available commercially that provide a highly specific means of identifying *T. equigenitalis*. A standard strain, such as NCTC 11184[2], should be used for immunisation. However, the most important consideration is the specificity of the antiserum produced. It should agglutinate *T. equigenitalis,* but fail to agglutinate other bacteria that might be cultured from horse urogenital membranes, even if rarely. In particular, it should not agglutinate any oxidase-positive and Gram-negative rods, such as *P. haemolytica, Actinobacillus equuli, Bordetella bronchiseptica* (to which *T. equigenitalis* is closely related, see ref. 6), and *Pseudomonas aeruginosa*. Recently a '*Taylorella*-like' bacterium has been isolated from male donkeys in the United States of America. This newly described bacterium does not produce disease but resides in the genital tract of male donkeys and can be passed to other equids during mating. Moreover it has similar, though not identical, colonial appearance and gives identical biochemical test results as those used to confirm the identity of *T. equigenitalis*. There is even serological cross-reactivity between the two organisms. Laboratories should be aware of the existence of the *Taylorella*-like organism and its significance.

A latex agglutination kit for the antigenic identification of *T. equigenitalis* can be purchased[3] that is based on polyclonal antibodies produced using methods similar to those described above. This is widely used by routine testing laboratories for the confirmation of identification of colonies growing on selective medium that give a biochemical reaction consistent with *T. equigenitalis*. As *T. equigenitalis* is antigenically relatively distinct, and small amounts of cross-reactive antibody are easily absorbed during production of the reagent, the test has proved to be highly specific and sensitive.

A polymerase chain reaction (PCR) method has been used for detecting *T. equigenitalis* and was compared with culture methods in the Netherlands (4, 7). In these studies, a much higher rate of detection by PCR was found than by culture, even among horses imported from a source without previous evidence of *T. equigenitalis* infection or clinical disease. The authors proposed that carriage is more widespread than previously believed, and that recently discovered genetic variation among strains (5, 13) may relate to differences in pathogenicity. The PCR has also been used in the UK (8). It was highly specific and was able to detect very small numbers of *T. equigenitalis* in the presence of very large numbers of bacteria arising from the background flora harvested from culture plates inoculated with samples of the equine urogenital tract. The PCR test has not yet proved positive in populations of horses from which *T. equigenitalis* has not been recently cultured (8). This promising technique needs to be more fully and widely evaluated.

---

2 Obtainable from the National Collection of Type Cultures, Colindale, London, UK.

3 Mono Tayl, Obtainable from Bionor, Stromdaljordet 4, Postboks 1868, Gulset, N-3701 Skein, Norway.

2. Serological tests

No serological test described to date will, by itself, reliably detect infection for diagnosis and control. However, serological tests can be used as an adjunct to culture for *T. equigenitalis* in screening mares recently bred with a carrier stallion, but must not be used as a substitute for culture.

B. REQUIREMENTS FOR VACCINES AND DIAGNOSTIC BIOLOGICALS

Effective vaccines that protect against contagious equine metritis or prevent colonisation by *T. equigenitalis* are not yet available.

REFERENCES

1. ANON (1979). Report of an International CEM meeting. *Vet. Rec.*, **105**, 337–338.

2. ATHERTON J.G. (1983). Evaluation of selective supplements used in media for the isolation of the causative organism of contagious equine metritis. *Vet. Rec.*, **113**, 299–300.

3. BARROW G.I. & FELTHAM R.K.A. (1993). Cowan and Steels's Manual for the Identification of Medical Bacteria, Third Edition. Cambridge University Press, Cambridge, UK.

4. BLEUMINK-PLUYM N.M.C., HOUWERS D.J., PARLEVLIET J.M. & COLENBRANDER B. (1993). PCR-based detection of CEM agent. *Vet. Rec.*, **133**, 375–376.

5. BLEUMINK-PLUYM N.M.C., TER LAAK E.A. & VAN DER ZEIJST B.A.M. (1990). Epidemiologic study of *Taylorella equigenitalis* strains by field inversion gel electrophoresis of genomic restriction endonuclease fragments. *J. Clin. Microbiol.*, **28**, 2012–2016.

6. BLEUMINK-PLUYM N.M.C., VAN DIJK L., VAN VLIET A.H., VAN DER GIESSEN J.W. & VAN DER ZEIJST B.A. (1993). Phylogenetic position of *Taylorella equigenitalis* determined by analysis of amplified 16S ribosomal DNA sequences. *Int. J. Syst. Bacteriol.*, **43**, 618–621.

7. BLEUMINK-PLUYM N.M.C., WERDLER M.E.B., HOUWERS D.J., PARLEVLIET J.M., COLENBRANDER B. & VAN DER ZEIJST B.A.M. (1994). Development and evaluation of PCR test for detection of *Taylorella equigenitalis*. *J. Clin. Microbiol.*, **32**, 893–896.

8. CHANTER N., VIGANO F., COLLIN N.C. & MUMFORD J.A. (1998). Use of a PCR assay for *Taylorella equigenitalis* applied to samples from the United Kingdom. *Vet. Rec.*, **143**, 225–227.

9. CROWHURST R.C. (1977). Genital infection in mares. *Vet. Rec.*, **100**, 476.

10. CROWHURST R.C., SIMPSON D.J., GREENWOOD R.E.S. & ELLIS D.R. (1979). Contagious equine metritis. *Vet. Rec.*, **104**, 465.

11. DAWSON F.L.M., BENSEN J.A. & CROXTON-SMITH P. (1978). The course of serum antibody development in two ponies experimentally infected with contagious metritis. *Equine Vet. J.*, **10**, 145–147.

12. FERNIE, BATTY I., WALKER P.D., PLATT H., MACKINTOSH M.E. & SIMPSON D.J. (1980). Observations on vaccine and post-infection immunity in contagious equine metritis. *Res. Vet. Sci.*, **28**, 362–367.

13. LAPAN G., AWAD-MASALMEH M., HARTIG A. & SILBER R. (1991). Investigations on *Taylorella equigenitalis*; cell wall proteins, DNA fingerprints, plasmids, adhesion and cytotoxicity. *J. Vet. Med. [B]*, **38**, 589–598.

14. PLATT H., ATHERTON J.G., DAWSON F.L.M. & DURRANT D.S. (1978). Developments in contagious equine metritis. *Vet. Rec.*, **102**, 19.

15. PLATT H., ATHERTON J.G., SIMPSON D.J., TAYLOR C.E.D., ROSENTHAL R.O., BROWN D.F.J. & WREGHITT T.G. (1977). Genital infection in mares. *Vet. Rec.*, **101**, 20.

16. ROGERSON B.A., CONDRON R.J., BAKER J. & CRAVEN J.A. (1984). Experimental infection of mares with *Haemophilus equigenitalis*. *Aust. Vet. J.*, **61**, 392–395.

17. SAHU S.P., DARDIRI A.H., ROMMEL F.A. & PIERSON R.E. (1979). Survival of contagious equine metritis bacteria in transport media. *Am. J. Vet. Res.*, **40**, 1040–1042.

18. SCHLUTER H., KULLER H., FREIDREICH U., SELBITZ H., MARWITZ T., BEYER C. & ULLRICH E. (1991). Epizootiology and treatment of contagious equine metritis (CEM), with particular reference to the treatment of infected stallions. *Prakt. Tierarzt.*, **72**, 503–511.

19. SOJKA W.J. (1965). *Escherichia coli* in Domestic Animals and Poultry. *Commonwealth Review Series* No.7.

20. SWANEY L.M. & SAHU S.P. (1978). CEM: bacteriological methods. *Vet. Rec.*, **102**, 43.

21. SWERCZEK T.W. (1978). Inhibition of the CEM organism by the normal flora of the reproductive tract. *Vet. Rec.*, **103**, 125.

22. TER LAAK E.A. & WAGENAARS C.M.F. (1990). Autoagglutination and the specificity of the indirect fluorescent antibody test applied to the identification of *Taylorella equigenitalis*. *Res. Vet. Sci.*, **49**, 117–119.

23. TIMONEY P.J. & POWELL D.G. (1982). Isolation of the contagious equine metritis organism from colts and fillies in the United Kingdom and Ireland. *Vet. Rec.*, **111**, 478–482.

24. TIMONEY P.J., SHIN S.J. & JACOBSON R.H. (1982). Improved selective medium for isolation of the contagious equine metritis organism. *Vet. Rec.*, **111**,107–108.

25. TIMONEY P.J., WARD J. & KELLY P. (1977). A contagious genital infection of mares. *Vet. Rec.*, **101**, 103.

26. TIMONEY P.J., WARD J. & MCARDLE J.F. (1978). CEM and the foaling mare. *Vet. Rec.*, **102**, 246–247.

27. WARD J., HOURIGAN M., MCGUIRK J. & GOGARTY A. (1984). Incubation times for primary isolation of contagious equine metritis organism. *Vet. Rec.*, **114**, 298.

*

* *

CHAPTER 2.5.2.

DOURINE

SUMMARY

Dourine is a chronic or acute contagious disease of breeding solipeds that is transmitted directly from animal to animal during coitus. The causal organism is Trypanosoma equiperdum *(Doflein, 1901).*

Dourine is the only trypanosomosis that is not transmitted by an invertebrate vector. Trypanosoma equiperdum *differs from other trypanosomes in that it is primarily a tissue parasite that rarely invades the blood. There is no known natural reservoir of the parasite other than infected equids. It is present in the genital secretions of both infected males and females. The incubation period, severity, and duration of the disease vary considerably; it is often fatal, but spontaneous recoveries do occur. Subclinical infections occur, and donkeys and mules are more resistant than horses and may remain inapparent carriers. Infection is not always transmitted by an infected animal at every copulation. Rats can be infected experimentally, and can be used to maintain strains of the parasite indefinitely.* Trypanosoma equiperdum *strains are best stored in liquid nitrogen.*

The clinical signs are marked by periodic exacerbation and relapse, ending in death or, possibly, recovery. Fever, local oedema of the genitalia and mammary glands, cutaneous eruptions, incoordination, facial paralysis, ocular lesions, anaemia, and emaciation may all be observed. Oedematous cutaneous plaques, 5–8 cm in diameter and 1 cm thick, are pathognomonic.

Identification of the agent: *Definitive diagnosis depends on the recognition of clinical signs and identification of the parasite. As this is rarely possible, diagnosis is usually based on clinical signs, together with serological evidence from complement fixation (CF) tests.*

Serological tests: *Humoral antibodies are present in infected animals whether or not they display clinical signs. The CF test is used to confirm infection in clinical cases or in latent carriers. Noninfected animals, especially donkeys, often yield unclear results. The indirect fluorescent antibody test can be used to confirm infection or resolve inconclusive CF test results. Enzyme-linked immunosorbent assays are also used.*

Requirements for vaccines and diagnostic biologicals: *There are no vaccines available. The only effective control is through the slaughter of infected animals. Good hygiene is essential during assisted matings because infection may be transmitted through contaminated fomites.*

A. DIAGNOSTIC TECHNIQUES

Dourine is a chronic or acute contagious disease of breeding solipeds that is transmitted directly from animal to animal during coitus. The causal organism is *Trypanosoma equiperdum* (Doflein, 1901). Dourine is also known under other names: mal de coït, el dourin, morbo coitale maligno, Beschälseuche, slapsiekte, sluchnaya bolyezn, and covering disease (1, 6).

Although the disease has been known since ancient times, its nature was established only in 1896 when Rouget discovered trypanosomes in infected Algerian horses. Dourine is the only trypanosomosis that is not transmitted by an invertebrate vector. *Trypanosoma equiperdum* differs from other trypanosomes in that it is primarily a tissue parasite that is rarely detected in the blood. There is no known natural reservoir of the parasite other than infected equids.

Infection is transmitted during copulation, more commonly from stallion to mare, but also from mare to stallion, due to the presence of the parasite in the seminal fluid and mucous exudate of the penis and sheath of the infected male, and in the vaginal mucus of the infected female. Initially, parasites are found free on the surface of the mucosa or between the epithelial cells of a newly infected animal. Invasion of the tissues takes place, and oedematous patches appear in the genital tract. Parasites then may pass into the blood, where they are carried to other parts of the body. In typical cases, this metastatic invasion gives rise to characteristic cutaneous plaques.

The incubation period, severity and duration of the disease vary considerably. In South Africa, the disease is typically chronic, usually mild, and may persist for several years (4). In other areas, such as northern Africa and South America, the disease tends to be more acute, often lasting only 1–2 months or, exceptionally, 1 week. Although dourine is a fatal disease with an average mortality of 50% (especially in stallions), spontaneous recovery can occur. Subclinical infections are recognised. Donkeys and mules are more resistant than horses.

As trypanosomes are not continually present in the genital tract throughout the course of the disease, transmission of the infection does not necessarily take place at every copulation involving an infected animal. Transmission of infection from mare to foal can occur via the mucosa, such as the conjunctiva. Mares' milk has been shown to be infectious. Animals other than equids can be infected experimentally. Rat-adapted strains can be maintained indefinitely; infected rat blood can be satisfactorily cryopreserved. Antigens for serological tests are commonly produced from infected laboratory rats.

The disease is marked by stages of exacerbation, tolerance or relapse, which vary in duration and which may occur once or several times before death or recovery. The signs most frequently noted are: pyrexia, tumefaction and local oedema of the genitalia and mammary glands, oedematous cutaneous eruptions, knuckling of the joints, incoordination, facial paralysis, ocular lesions, anaemia, and emaciation. A pathognomonic sign is the oedematous plaque consisting of an elevated lesion in the skin, up to 5–8 cm in diameter and 1 cm thick. The plaques usually appear over the ribs, although they may occur anywhere on the body, and usually persist for between 3 and 7 days. They are not a constant feature.

Generally, the oedema disappears and returns at irregular intervals. During each recess, an increasing extent of permanently thickened and indurated tissue can be seen. The vaginal mucosa may show raised and thickened semitransparent patches. Folds of swollen membrane may protrude through the vulva. It is not uncommon to find oedema of the mammary glands and adjacent tissues. Depigmentation of the genital area, perineum, and udder may occur. In the stallion, the first clinical sign is a variable swelling involving the glans penis and prepuce. The oedema extends posteriorly to the scrotum, inguinal lymph nodes, and perineum, with an anterior extension along the inferior abdomen. In stallions of heavy breeds, the oedema may extend over the whole floor of the abdomen.

Pyrexia is intermittent; nervous signs include incoordination, mainly of the hind limbs, lips, nostrils, ears, and throat. Facial paralysis is usually unilateral. In fatal cases, the disease is usually slow and progressive, with increasing anaemia and emaciation, although the appetite remains good almost throughout.

At post-mortem examination, gelatinous exudates are present under the skin. In the stallion, the scrotum, sheath, and testicular tunica are thickened and infiltrated. In some cases the testes are embedded in a tough mass of sclerotic tissue and may be unrecognisable. In the mare, the vulva, vaginal mucosa, uterus, bladder, and mammary glands may be thickened with gelatinous infiltration. The lymph nodes, particularly in the abdominal cavity, are hypertrophied, softened and, in some cases, haemorrhagic. The spinal cord of animals with paraplegia is often soft, pulpy and discoloured, particularly in the lumbar and sacral regions.

1. Identification of the agent

A definitive diagnosis depends on the recognition of the clinical signs and the demonstration of the parasite. This is rarely possible because: (a) although the clinical signs and gross lesions in the developed disease may be pathognomonic, they cannot always be identified with certainty, especially in the early stages or in latent cases; they can be confused with other conditions, such as coital exanthema (moreover, in some countries [e.g. in South America], *T. evansi* infections give rise to similar clinical signs); (b) the trypanosomes are only sparsely present and are extremely difficult to find, even in oedematous areas; and (c) the trypanosomes are only fleetingly present in the blood, and in small numbers that defy detection.

In practice, diagnosis is based on clinical evidence supported by serology.

In infected animals, trypanosomes are present, in low numbers only, in lymph and oedematous fluids of the external genitalia, in the vaginal mucus, and fluid contents of plaques. They are usually undetectable in the blood, but may be found in the urethral or vaginal mucus collected from preputial or vaginal washings or scrapings 4–5 days after infection.

Later, parasites may be found in the fluid contents of oedemas and plaques, especially shortly after their eruption. The skin of the area over the plaque should be washed, shaved and dried, and the fluid contents aspirated by syringe. Blood vessels should be avoided. The fresh aspirate is examined microscopically for motile trypanosomes. These are present for a few days only, so that lesions should be examined at intervals. The parasite is rarely found in thick blood films, but is sometimes detectable after centrifuging blood and examining the recentrifuged plasma.

As dourine is the only trypanosome to affect horses in temperate climates, the observation of trypanosomes in thick blood films is sufficient for a positive diagnosis. In countries where nagana or surra occur, it is difficult to distinguish *T. equiperdum* microscopically (morphology, motility) from other members of the subgenus Trypanozoon *(T. evansi, T. brucei)*. In particular, *T. equiperdum* and *T. evansi* cannot be differentiated on the basis of morphological criteria. Both are monomorphic, slender trypomastigotes with a free flagellum, although pleomorphic, stumpy, proteonuclear forms are recognised.

Typical strains of the parasite range in length from 15.6 to 31.3 µm.

2. Serological tests

Humoral antibodies are present in infected animals, whether they display clinical signs or not. The complement fixation (CF) test (9) is used to confirm clinical evidence and to detect latent infections. Uninfected equids, particularly donkeys and mules, often give inconsistent or nonspecific reactions because of the anticomplementary effects of their sera. In the case of anticomplementary sera, the indirect fluorescent antibody (IFA) test is of advantage. There is no internationally adopted protocol. Cross-reactions are possible due to the presence in some countries of other trypanosomes, for example, *T. cruzi* and *T. evansi.* Enzyme-linked immunosorbent assays (ELISAs) are also used.

a) Complement fixation test (the prescribed test for international trade)

Standard or microtitre techniques may be used (5). Guinea-pig serum (available commercially) is used as a source of complement. Other reagents are sheep red blood cells (RBCs) washed in veronal buffer, and rabbit haemolytic serum (commercial).

- **Antigen production**

i) A rat is inoculated with *T. equiperdum* cryopreserved stock. It must be free from *T. lewisi*, which can be achieved by injection with neoarsphenamine. At maximum parasitaemia, blood is collected into an anticoagulant, such as heparin.

ii) Twenty large rats are inoculated intraperitoneally with 0.3 ml of this stock culture. All rats are to have a heavy infection concurrently. Rats usually die within 3–5 days; prior to this, blood is taken from the tail for thick smears and examined microscopically. When parasitaemia is maximal, the rats are bled into citrated saline. If parasitaemia is not synchronous, rats can be bled and their blood held in acid-citrate-dextrose saline at 4°C until they have all been bled.

iii) The blood is filtered through muslin gauze and centrifuged at 800 ***g*** for 4 minutes. The RBCs are mostly deposited while the trypanosomes remain in suspension.

iv) The supernatant fluid is transferred to a fresh tube, the upper layer of RBCs is mixed with trypanosomes to a second tube, and the next layer to a third. Citrate saline is added to tubes 2 and 3 to prevent clotting of cells. All tubes are mixed and centrifuged at 1500 ***g*** for 5 minutes.

v) The supernatant fluid is discarded and the upper white layer of trypanosomes is transferred from all tubes into a clean tube. The next pink layer is transferred into a second tube, and the lower layer to a third tube.

vi) Physiological saline is added and mixed and the tubes are centrifuged again at 1500 ***g*** for 5 minutes to separate the trypanosomes. The washing step is repeated until all the trypanosomes are collected as a pure white mass. Ten rats should produce 3–5 g of antigen. This procedure of purification can also be carried out using a column of DEAE (diethylaminoethyl) cellulose in a solution of phosphate buffered saline (PBS) containing glucose, pH 8.0 (8).

vii) The concentrated trypanosomes are diluted with two volumes of veronal buffer and 5% polyvinylpyrrolidone as a cryopreservative. Before use in CF tests, the antigen must be dispersed to a fine suspension with a Griffiths tube (11). This antigen may be divided into aliquots and lyophilised.

The antigen is standardised by titration against a 1/5 dilution of a standard low-titre antiserum.

Sera: Positive and negative sera should be inactivated at 58°C for 30 minutes before being used in the tests. Mule and donkey sera are normally inactivated at 62°C for 30 minutes. Dilutions of sera that are positive in the screening test are titrated against two units of antigen. Test sera are screened at a dilution of 1/5. Sera showing more than 50% fixation at this dilution are usually deemed to be positive.

Anticomplementary sera: If the anticomplementary control shows only a trace, this may be ignored. For all other anticomplementary sera, the activity must be titrated. A duplicate series of dilutions is made and the sample is retested using *T. equiperdum* antigen in the first row and veronal buffer only in the second. The second row gives the titre of the anticomplementary reaction. Provided the first row shows an end-point that is at least three dilutions greater than the second, the anticomplementary effect may be ignored and the sample rated as positive. If the results are any closer, a fresh sample of serum must be requested. Dilution of the serum 1/2 and heat inactivation at 60–63°C for 30 minutes may result in reduction or removal of the anticomplementary effect.

Buffers and reagents: 0.15 M veronal buffered saline, pH 7.4, is used for diluting reagents and for washing sheep RBCs. Antigen is pretested by checkerboard titration, and two units are used in the test. Guinea-pig complement (C) is tested for its haemolytic activity, and diluted to provide two units for the test. Sheep RBCs in Alsever's solution are washed three times. A 3% solution is used for the haemolytic system. Titrated rabbit-anti-sheep RBCs – the rabbit haemolytic serum – is taken at double the concentration of its haemolytic titre (two units). All test sera, including positive and negative control sera, are inactivated at a 1/5 dilution before testing.

- **Primary dilutions**

i) 100 µl of test serum is diluted with 400 µl of veronal buffer (1/5).

ii) 100 µl of both positive and negative control sera is diluted with 400 µl of veronal buffer (1/5).

iii) The solutions are incubated in a water bath at 58°C for 30 minutes to inactivate complement and destroy anticomplementary factors.

- **Screening test procedure**

i) 25 µl of inactivated test serum is placed in each of three wells.

ii) 25 µl of inactivated control serum is placed in each of three wells.

iii) 25 µl of *T. equiperdum* antigen diluted to contain two units is placed in the first well only for each serum.

iv) 25 µl of complement diluted to contain two units is added to the first two wells only for each serum.

v) 25 µl veronal buffer, pH 7.4, is added to the second well for each serum (anticomplementary well).

vi) 50 µl veronal buffer, pH 7.4, is added to the third well for each serum (lysis activity well).

vii) The complement control is prepared.

viii) The plate is shaken on a microshaker sufficiently to mix the reagents.

ix) The plate is incubated for 1 hour in a water bath at 37°C.

x) The haemolytic system is prepared. After the first 50 minutes of incubation, the sheep RBCs are sensitised by mixing equal volumes of rabbit haemolytic serum, diluted to contain two units per 50 µl, and a 3% suspension of washed RBCs; the solution is mixed well and incubated for 10 minutes at 37°C.

xi) After incubation, 50 µl of haemolytic system is added to each well.

xii) The plate is shaken on a microshaker sufficiently to mix the reagents.

xiii) The plate is incubated for 30 minutes at 37°C.

xiv) *Reading the results:* the plate is viewed from above with a light source beneath it. The fixation in every well is assessed by estimating the proportion of cells not lysed. The degree of fixation is expressed as 0, 1+, 2+, 3+, 4+ (0%, 25%, 50%, 75% or 100% cells not lysed). Reactions are interpreted as follows: 4+, 3+, 2+ = positive, 1+ = suspicious, trace = negative, complete haemolysis = negative.

xv) *End-point titration:* All sera with positive reactions at 1/5 are serially double diluted and tested according to the above procedure for end-point titration.

b) Indirect fluorescent antibody test

An IFA test for dourine can also be used (9) as a confirmatory test or to resolve inconclusive results obtained by the CF test. The test is performed as follows:

Antigen: (For method, see preparation of CF test antigen above). Blood is collected into heparinised vacutainers or into a solution of acid–citrate–dextrose from an animal in which the number of trypanosomes is still increasing (about ten parasites per low power microscope field should be present).

i) The blood is centrifuged for 10 minutes at 800 ***g***.

ii) One to two volumes of PBS is added to the packed RBCs, the mixture is agitated, and smears are made that evenly cover the whole slide.

iii) The smears are air-dried and then wrapped in bundles of four, with paper separating each slide. The bundles of slides are wrapped in aluminium foil, sealed in an airtight container over silica gel, and stored at –20°C or –76°C.

iv) Slides stored at –20°C should retain their activity for about 1 year, at –76°C they should remain useable for longer.

Acid/citrate/dextrose solution: Use 15 ml per 100 ml of blood.

Conjugate: Fluorescein-labelled sheep anti-horse immunoglobulins.

- **Test procedure**

i) The antigen slides are allowed to reach room temperature in a desiccator.

ii) The slides are marked out.

iii) Separate spots of test sera diluted in PBS are applied, and the slides are incubated in a humid chamber in a water bath at 37°C for 30 minutes.

iv) The slides are washed in PBS, pH 7.2, three times for 5 minutes each, and air-dried.

v) Fluorescein-labelled conjugate is added at the correct dilution. Individual batches of antigen and conjugate should be titrated against each other using control sera to optimise the conjugate dilution. The slides are incubated in a humid chamber in a water bath at 37°C for 30 minutes.

vi) The slides are washed in PBS, three times for 5 minutes each, and air-dried.

vii) The slides are mounted in a 50% solution of gylcerol in PBS.

viii) The slides are then examined under UV illumination. Incident light illumination is used with barrier filter K 530 and exciter filter BG 12. Slides may be stored at 4°C for 4–5 days. Sera diluted at 1/80 and above showing strong fluorescence of the parasites are usually considered to be positive. Estimating the intensity of fluorescence demands experience on the part of the observer.

Standard positive and negative control sera should be included in each batch of tests, and due consideration should be given to the pattern of fluorescence in these controls when assessing the results of test sera.

c) Enzyme-linked immunosorbent assay

The ELISA has been developed and compared with other serological tests for dourine (10, 12).

Carbonate buffer, pH 9.6, for antigen coating on to microtitre plates: Na_2CO_3 (1.59 g); $NaHCO_3$ (2.93g); and distilled water (1 litre).

Blocking buffer: Carbonate buffer + 3% fetal calf serum (FCS).

PBS, pH 7.4, with Tween 20 (PBST) for washing: KH_2PO_4 (0.2 g); $Na_2HPO_4 \times 12\ H_2O$ (2.94 g); NaCl (8.0 g); KCl (0.2 g in 1 litre distilled water), and Tween 20 (0.5 ml).

Sample and conjugate buffer: PBST + 6% FCS.

Citric phosphate buffer: Citric acid monohydrate (4.2 g in 200 ml distilled water); $Na_2HPO_4 \times 12\ H_2O$ (in 200 ml distilled water). Both components are mixed at equal volumes.

Substrate indicator system: ABTS (2,2'-Azino-bis-[3-ethylbenzothiazoline-6-sulphonic acid]) (40 mg) is dissolved in citric phosphate buffer (100 ml), and stored at 4°C in the dark. Just before use, 100 µl of 1/40 H_2O_2 is added to 10 ml of ABTS.

Conjugate: Rabbit anti-horse IgG (H+L) PO or IgY anti-horse Ig-PO.

Antigen: Lyophilised *T. equiperdum* antigen (0.5 ml) is reconstituted with coating buffer (5 ml), sonicated twice for 10 seconds each at 12 µm peak to peak, and centrifuged at 10,000 ***g*** for 4 minutes. The supernatant is further diluted to a pretested working dilution (e.g. 1/500).

- **Test procedure**

i) Wells in columns 2, 4, 6, etc., are charged with 50 µl of antigen, columns 1, 3, 5, etc., are charged with the same amount of carbonate buffer. The plate is incubated for 40 minutes at 37°C in a humid chamber, washed in tap water, and 50 µl of blocking buffer is added to each well. The plate is incubated for 20 minutes, washed in tap water followed by three wash cycles with PBST, with soaking times of 3 minutes/cycle.

ii) 50 µl of test samples and equine control sera prediluted 1/100 in sample/conjugate buffer is added in parallel to wells with and without antigen. The plate is incubated for 30 minutes, washed in tap water, followed by three wash cycles with PBST.

iii) Properly diluted conjugate in sample/conjugate buffer is added in volumes of 50 µl to all wells. The plate is incubated for 30 minutes with subsequent washing as above.

iv) 100 µl of substrate indicator system is added to all wells.

v) The reaction is stopped after 15 minutes at room temperature by the addition of 25 µl of 37 mM NaCN. Alternatively, commercially available detergents can be used after pretesting. The results are read photometrically at a wavelength of 405 nm.

vi) Calculation of results: absorbance (with antigen) minus absorbance (without antigen) = net extinction. A reaction exceeding a net extinction of 0.3 is regarded as a positive result.

d) Other serological tests

Other serological tests have been used, including radioimmunoassay, counter immunoelectrophoresis and agar gel immunodiffusion (AGID) tests (2, 3). The AGID has been used to confirm positive tests and to test anticomplementary sera. A seven-well pattern in 0.8% agarose in Tris buffer is used, with the CF test antigen in the centre well and positive control sera and unknown sera in alternate peripheral wells. Recently, a method has been published for diagnosing equine piroplasmosis, glanders and dourine at the same time, using immunoblotting (7).

B. REQUIREMENTS FOR VACCINES AND DIAGNOSTIC BIOLOGICALS

There are no biological products available. Control of the disease depends on compulsory notification and slaughter of infected animals. Good hygiene at assisted matings is also essential.

REFERENCES

1. Barner R.D. (1963). Protozoal diseases. *In:* Equine Medicine and Surgery, Bone J.F. *et al.*, eds. American Veterinary Publications, Santa Barbara, California, USA, 205–210.

2. Caporale V.P., Biancifiori F., Di Matteo A., Nannini D. & Urbani G. (1981). Comparison of various tests for the serological diagnosis of *Trypanosoma equiperdum* infection in the horse. *Comp. Immunol. Microbiol. Infect. Dis.*, **4**, 243–246.

3. Hagebock J.M., Chieves L., Frerichs W.M. & Miller C.D. (1993). Evaluation of agar gel immunodiffusion and indirect fluorescent antibody assays as supplemental tests for dourine in equids. *Am. J. Vet. Res.*, **54**, 1201–1208.

4. Henning M.W. (1955). Animal Diseases in South Africa, Third Edition. Central News Agency, South Africa.

5. Herr S., Huchzermayer H.F.K.A., Te Brugge L.A., Williamson C.C., Roos J.A. & Schiele G.J. (1985). The use of a single complement fixation technique in bovine brucellosis, Johne's disease, dourine, equine piroplasmosis and Q fever serology. *Onderstepoort J. Vet. Res.*, **52**, 279–282.

6. Hoare C.A. (1972). The Trypanosomes of Mammals. A Zoological Monograph. Blackwell Scientific Publications, Oxford & Edinburgh, UK.

7. KATZ J.B., CHIEVES L.P., HENNAGER S.G., NICHOLSON J.M., FISHER T.A. & BYERS P.E. (1999). Serodiagnosis of equine piroplasmosis, dourine and glanders using an arrayed immunoblotting method. *J. Vet. Diagn. Invest.*, 11, 292–294.

8. LANHAM S.M. & GODFREY D.G. (1970). Isolation of salivarian trypanosomes from man and other mammals using DEAE-cellulose. *Exp. Parasitol.*, **28**, 521–534.

9. MINISTRY OF AGRICULTURE, FISHERIES AND FOOD (1986). A Manual of Veterinary Parasitological Laboratory Techniques, Third Edition. Her Majesty's Stationery Office, London, UK.

10. WASSALL D.A., GREGORY R.J.F. & PHIPPS L.P. (1991). Comparative evaluation of enzyme-linked immunosorbent assay (ELISA) for the serodiagnosis of dourine. *Vet. Parasitol.*, **39**, 233–239.

11. WATSON A.E. (1920). Dourine in Canada 1904–1920. History, Research and Suppression. Dominion of Canada Department of Agriculture, Health of Animals Branch, Ottawa, Canada.

12. WORKING PROTOCOLS, BGVV: ELISA ON DOURINE (1995). Bundesinstitut f. gesundheitlichen Verbraucherschutz u. Veterinärmedizin (BgVV). PO Box 33 00 13, D-14191 Berlin, Germany.

*

* *

CHAPTER 2.5.3.

EQUINE ENCEPHALOMYELITIS (Eastern and Western)

SUMMARY

Eastern and Western equine encephalomyelitis viruses belong to the genus Alphavirus of the family Togaviridae. These viruses cycle between birds and mosquitoes. The disease occurs sporadically in horses and humans from mid-summer to late autumn. Horses and humans are tangential dead-end hosts. The disease in horses is characterised by fever, anorexia, and severe depression. Eastern equine encephalomyelitis (EEE) virus infection in horses is often fatal, while Western equine encephalomyelitis (WEE) virus can cause a subclinical or mild disease with less than 30% mortality. EEE and WEE have been reported to cause disease in poultry, game birds and ratites.

EEE and WEE viruses cause disease in humans, and severe infections and death in laboratory workers have been reported. Work with these viruses should be performed only by immunised personnel using certified biosafety cabinets in a biocontainment facility.

***Identification of the agent:** A presumptive diagnosis of EEE or WEE can be made when susceptible horses display the characteristic somnolence and other signs of neurological disease in areas where haematophagous insects are active. There are no characteristic gross lesions. Histopathological lesions can provide a presumptive diagnosis. EEE virus can usually be isolated from the brain and sometimes other tissues of dead horses; however, WEE virus is rarely isolated. EEE and WEE viruses can be isolated from field specimens by inoculating newborn mice, embryonating chicken eggs, cell cultures, or newly hatched chickens. The virus is identified by complement fixation (CF), immunofluorescence, or plaque reduction neutralisation (PRN) tests.*

***Serological tests:** Antibody can be identified by PRN, haemagglutination inhibition, CF tests, or IgM capture enzyme-linked immunosorbent assay.*

***Requirements for vaccines and diagnostic biologicals:** EEE and WEE vaccines are safe and immunogenic. They are produced in cell culture and inactivated with formalin.*

A. DIAGNOSTIC TECHNIQUES

Eastern equine encephalomyelitis (EEE) and Western equine encephalomyelitis (WEE) viruses are members of the genus Alphavirus of the family Togaviridae. The viruses cycle between birds and mosquitoes; from mid-summer to late autumn, clinical disease may be observed in humans and horses, both of which are dead-end hosts for these agents. EEE is usually a fatal disease of horses and has been diagnosed in Quebec and Ontario in Canada, Texas and the states east of the Mississippi River in the United States of America (USA), the Caribbean Islands, Mexico, and Central and South America. WEE can be subclinical, and the mortality in horses with clinical disease is less than 30%. Disease caused by the WEE virus has been reported in the western USA and Canada, Mexico, and Central and South America (6, 8, 14). Highlands J virus, antigenically related to WEE virus, has been isolated in eastern USA. Although it is generally believed not to cause disease in mammals, it has been isolated from the brain of a horse dying of encephalitis in Florida (3).

Even though the mortality is lower for WEE, the clinical signs of EEE and WEE can be identical. Following an incubation period of 5–14 days, clinical signs include fever, anorexia, and depression. In severe cases, the disease in horses progresses to hyperexcitability, blindness, ataxia, severe mental depression, recumbency, convulsions, and death. A presumptive diagnosis of EEE or WEE virus infection in unvaccinated horses can be made if the characteristic somnolence is observed during the summer in temperate climates or the wet season in tropical and subtropical climates, when the mosquito vector is plentiful. However, a number of other diseases, such as West Nile virus, produce similar clinical signs and the diagnosis must be confirmed by the described diagnostic test methods. WEE virus infection in horses is often observed over a wide geographical area, e.g. sporadic cases over 1000 square miles. EEE virus infections are usually observed in limited geographical areas. WEE and EEE virus infections have been reported to cause high mortality in captive-raised game birds, primarily pheasants, chukars and quail. Most encephalomyelitis infections in domestic fowl are caused by EEE virus and occur on the east coast states of the USA. The virus is introduced by mosquitoes, but transmission within the flocks is primarily by feather picking and cannibalism. Both EEE and WEE viruses have caused a fatal disease in ratites. Haemorrhagic enteritis has been observed in emus infected with EEE and WEE viruses, and morbidity and mortality rates may be greater than 85%. Recently, Highlands J and EEE viruses have been found to produce depression, somnolence, decreased egg production, and increased mortality in turkeys (2). EEE virus has been reported to cause disease in swine (1).

EEE virus causes severe disease in humans with a mortality rate of approximately 65% and a high frequency of permanent sequelae in patients who survive. WEE is usually mild in adult humans, but can be a severe disease in children. The fatality rate is between 3 and 14%. Severe infection and death caused by EEE and WEE viruses have been reported in laboratory workers; therefore, any work with these viruses must be performed in a biosafety level 3 laboratory using biological safety cabinets, or biosafety level 2 when personnel have been immunised against EEE and WEE viruses (12). Precautions should also be taken to prevent human infection when performing post-mortem examinations on horses suspected of being infected with the equine encephalomyelitis viruses.

Gross pathological lesions are rarely observed in horses and, if present, consist only of the congestion of the brain and meninges. Ecchymotic haemorrhages of traumatic origin may be observed. Microscopic lesions are usually found throughout the central nervous system and can be diagnostic. There is widespread evidence of a severe inflammatory response involving the grey matter. Neuronal degeneration with infiltration by polymorphonuclear leukocytes, diffuse and focal gliosis, and perivascular cuffing with lymphocytes and neutrophils are seen. Also observed are neuronophagia, and liquefaction of the neuropil. The extent of the lesions depends on the severity of the infection and the duration of the neurological involvement (14). Immunohistochemical procedures for diagnosis of EEE have been described (7).

Brain lesions caused by WEE virus infection are focal and have lymphocytic infiltrations. Brain lesions caused by EEE virus infection are more severe and are found throughout the grey matter. They are characterised by a larger number of neutrophils among the inflammatory cells.

1. Identification of the agent

The most definitive method for diagnosis of EEE or WEE is the isolation of the viruses. EEE virus can usually be isolated from the brains of horses, unless more than 5 days have elapsed between the appearance of clinical signs and the death of the horse. EEE virus can frequently be isolated from brain tissue even in the presence of a high serum-antibody titre. WEE virus is rarely isolated from tissues of infected horses. Brain is the tissue of choice for virus isolation, but the virus has been isolated from other tissues, such as the liver and spleen. It is recommended that a complete set of these tissues be collected in duplicate, one set for virus isolation and the other set in formalin for histopathological examination. Specimens for virus isolation should be sent refrigerated if they can be received in the laboratory within 48 hours of collection; otherwise, they should be frozen and sent with dry ice. A complete set of tissues will allow the performance of diagnostic techniques for other diseases. For isolation, a 10% suspension of tissue is prepared in phosphate buffered saline (PBS), pH 7.8, containing bovine serum albumin (BSA) (fraction V; 0.75%), penicillin (100 units/ml), and streptomycin (100 µg/ml). The suspension is clarified by centrifugation at 1500 ***g*** for 30 minutes.

The newborn mouse is considered to be a sensitive host system. Inoculate intracranially one or two litters of 1–4-day-old mice with 0.02 ml of inoculum using a 26-gauge 3/8 inch (9.3 mm) needle attached to a 1 ml tuberculin syringe. The inoculation site is just lateral to the midline into the midportion of one lateral hemisphere. Mice are observed for 10 days; dead mice are collected daily and frozen at –70°C. Mouse brains are harvested for virus identification by aspiration using a 20-gauge 1 inch (2.5 cm) needle attached to a 1 ml tuberculin syringe. A second passage is made only if virus cannot be identified from mice that die following inoculation.

The chicken embryo is considered to be less sensitive than newborn mice when used for primary isolation of EEE and WEE viruses. Tissue suspensions can be inoculated by the yolk-sac route into 6–8-day-old embryonating chicken eggs. There are no diagnostic signs or lesions in the embryos infected with these viruses. Inoculated embryos should be incubated for 7 days, but deaths usually occur between 2 and 4 days post-inoculation. Usually only one passage is made, unless there are dead embryos from which virus cannot be isolated. Newly hatched chickens are susceptible and have been used for virus isolation. If this method is used, precautions must be taken to prevent aerosol exposure of laboratory personnel, as infected birds can shed highly infectious virus.

EEE and WEE viruses can also be isolated in a number of cell culture systems. The most commonly used cell cultures are primary chicken or duck embryo fibroblasts, continuous cell lines of African green monkey kidney

(Vero), rabbit kidney (RK-13), or baby hamster kidney (BHK-21). Isolation is usually attempted in 25 cm^2 cell culture flasks. Confluent cells are inoculated with 1.0 ml of tissue suspension.

Following a 1–2-hour absorption period, maintenance medium is added. Cultures are incubated for 7 days, and one blind passage is made. EEE and WEE viruses will produce a cytopathic change in cell culture. Cultures that appear to be infected are frozen. The fluid from the thawed cultures is used for virus identification.

When the complement fixation (CF) test is used, EEE or WEE viruses can be identified in infected mouse or chicken brains, cell culture fluid, or amnionic-allantoic fluid. A 10% brain suspension is prepared in veronal (barbitone) buffer; egg and cell culture fluids are used undiluted or diluted 1/10 in veronal buffer. The fluid or suspension is centrifuged at 9000 ***g*** for 30 minutes, and the supernatant fluid is tested against hyperimmune serum or mouse ascitic fluid prepared against EEE and WEE viruses using a standard CF procedure (11). The CF test requires the overnight incubation at 4°C of serum-antigen with 7 units of complement. Virus can be identified in cell culture by direct immunofluorescent staining. The less commonly used method of virus identification is the neutralisation test, as outlined below.

EEE virus nucleic acid in mosquitoes and tissues has been identified by the polymerase chain reaction (PCR) using primers selected from the capsid gene (13). RNA is extracted using guanidium iso-thiocyanate-acid phenol. Forty repetitions of the three-step amplification cycle of nucleic acid denaturisation, primer annealing and primer extension are used. Temperature and duration of each step are optimised for the specific primer pair, reagents and thermal cycler used in the PCR cycles. Reaction products or their fragments are analysed on 2.0–2.6% agarose gels that have been stained with 1 µg/ml of ethidium bromide. An alternate identification procedure is by hybridisation with an oligonucleotide probe. An alternative reverse-transcription PCR has been described (5).

2. Serological tests

Serological confirmation of EEE or WEE virus infection requires a four-fold or greater increase or decrease in antibody titre in paired serum samples collected 10–14 days apart. Most horses infected with EEE and WEE virus have a high antibody titre when clinical disease is observed. Horses infected with EEE or WEE virus usually have antibody titres in the acute stage of the disease. Consequently, a presumptive diagnosis can be made if an unvaccinated horse with appropriate clinical signs has antibody against only EEE or WEE virus. The detection of IgM antibody by the enzyme-linked immunosorbent assay (ELISA) can also provide a presumptive diagnosis of acute infection (9). The plaque reduction neutralisation (PRN) test or, preferably, a combination of PRN and haemagglutination inhibition (HI) tests are the procedures most commonly used for the detection of antibody against EEE and WEE viruses. There are cross-reactions between antibody against EEE and WEE virus in the CF and HI tests. CF antibody against both EEE and WEE viruses appears later and does not persist; consequently, it is less useful for the serological diagnosis of disease.

a) Complement fixation

The CF test is frequently used for the demonstration of antibodies, although the antibodies detected by the CF test may not persist for as long as those detected by the HI or PRN tests. A sucrose/acetone mouse brain extract is commonly used as antigen. The positive antigen is inactivated by treatment with 0.1% beta-propiolactone.

In the absence of an international standard serum, the antigen should be titrated against a locally prepared positive control serum. The normal antigen, or control antigen, is normal mouse brain similarly extracted and diluted.

Sera are diluted 1/4 in veronal buffered saline containing 1% gelatin (VBSG), and inactivated at 56°C for 30 minutes. Titrations of positive sera may be performed using additional twofold dilutions. The CF antigens and control antigen (normal mouse brain) are diluted in VBSG to their optimal amount of fixation as determined by titration against the positive sera; guinea-pig complement is diluted in VBSG to contain 5 complement haemolytic units-50% (CH_{50}). Sera, antigen, and complement are reacted in 96-well round-bottom microtitre plates at 4°C for 18 hours. The sheep red blood cells (SRBCs) are standardised to 2.8% concentration. Haemolysin is titrated to determine the optimal dilution for the lot of complement used. Haemolysin is used to sensitise 2.8% SRBCs and the sensitised cells are added to all wells on the microtitre plate. The test is incubated for 30 minutes at 37°C. The plates are then centrifuged (200 ***g***), and the wells are scored for the presence of haemolysis. The following controls are used: (a) serum and control serum each with 5 CH_{50} and 2.5 CH_{50} of complement; (b) CF antigen and control antigen each with 5 CH_{50}, and 2.5 CH_{50} of complement; (c) complement dilutions of 5 CH_{50}, 2.5 CH_{50}, and 1.25 CH_{50}; and (d) cell control wells with only SRBCs and VBSG diluent. These controls test for anticomplementary antigen, anticomplementary serum, activity of complement used in the test, and integrity of the SRBC indicator system in the absence of complement, respectively.

To avoid anticomplementary effects, sera should be separated from the blood as soon as possible. Positive and negative control sera should be used in the test.

b) **Haemagglutination inhibition**

The antigen for the HI test is the same as described above for the CF test. The antigen is diluted so that the amount used in each haemagglutinating unit (HAU) is from four to eight times that which agglutinates 50% of the RBCs in the test system. The haemagglutination titre and optimum pH for each antigen are determined with goose RBCs diluted in pH solutions ranging from pH 5.8 to pH 6.6, at 0.2 intervals.

Sera are diluted 1/10 in borate saline, pH 9.0, and then inactivated at 56°C for 30 minutes. Kaolin treatment is used to remove nonspecific serum inhibitors. Sera should be absorbed before use by incubation with a 0.05 ml volume of washed packed goose RBCs for 20 minutes at 4°C.

Following heat inactivation, kaolin treatment and absorption, twofold dilutions of the treated serum are prepared in borate saline, pH 9.0 with 0.4% bovalbumin. Serum dilutions (0.025 ml/well) are prepared in a 96-well round-bottom microtitre plate in twofold dilutions in borate saline, pH 9.0, with 0.4% bovalbumin. Antigen (0.025 ml/well) is added to the serum. Plates are incubated at 4°C overnight. RBCs are derived from normal white male geese[1] and washed three times in dextrose/gelatin/veronal (DGV), and a 7.0% suspension is prepared in DGV. The 7.0% suspension is then diluted 1/24 in the appropriate pH solution, and 0.05 ml per well is added immediately to the plates. Plates are incubated for 30 minutes at 37°C. Positive and negative control sera are incorporated into each test. A test is considered to be valid only if the control sera give the expected results. Titres of 1/10 and 1/20 are suspect, and titres of 1/40 and above are positive.

c) **Enzyme-linked immunosorbent assay**

The ELISA is performed by coating flat-bottomed plates with anti-equine IgM capture antibody (9). The antibody is diluted 1/400 in 0.5 M carbonate buffer, pH 9.6, and 50 µl is added to each well. The plates are incubated at 37°C for 1 hour, and then at 4°C overnight. Prior to use, the coated plates are washed twice with 200 µl/well of 0.01 M PBS containing 0.05% Tween 20 with 3% BSA. After the second wash, 200 µl/well of PBS/Tween/BSA is added and the plates are incubated at 37°C for 2 hours. Following incubation, the plates are washed again three times with PBS/Tween/BSA. Test and control sera are diluted 1/100 and 1/1000 in 0.01 M PBS, pH 7.2, containing 0.05% Tween 20, and 50 µl is added to each well. The plates are incubated at 37°C for 2 hours and then washed three times. Next, 50 µl of viral antigen diluted 1/20 in PBS with Tween 20 is added to all wells. The plates are incubated for 75 minutes at 37°C, and washed three times. Then, 50 µl of horseradish-peroxidase-conjugated monoclonal antibody (MAb) to encephalitis virus[2] is added. The plates are incubated for 60 minutes at 37°C and then washed three times. Finally, 50 µl of freshly prepared ABTS (2,2'-Azino-bis-[3-ethylbenzo-thiazoline-6-sulphonic acid]) substrate + hydrogen peroxidase is added, and the plates are incubated at room temperature for 15–40 minutes The absorbance of the test serum is measured at 405 nm. A test serum is considered to be positive if the absorbance of the test serum is twice the mean absorbance of the negative control sera.

d) **Plaque reduction neutralisation**

The PRN test is very specific and can be used to differentiate between EEE and WEE virus infections. The PRN test is performed in duck embryo fibroblast, Vero, or BHK-21 cell cultures. The sera can be screened at a 1/10 and 1/100 final dilution. Endpoints can be established using the PRN or HI test. Serum used in the PRN assay is tested against 100 plaque-forming units of virus. The virus/serum mixture is incubated at 37°C for 75 minutes before inoculation on to confluent cell culture monolayers in 25 cm^2 flasks. The inoculum is adsorbed for 1 hour, followed by the addition of 6 ml of overlay medium. The overlay medium consists of two solutions that are prepared separately. Solution I contains 2 × Earle's Basic Salts Solution without phenol red, 6.6% yeast extract lactalbumin hydrolysate, 4% fetal bovine serum, 800 units/ml penicillin, 400 µg/ml streptomycin, 200 µg/ml nystatin, 6% of a 7.5% solution of sodium bicarbonate, and 3.3% of a 1/1500 dilution of neutral red (1/8000). Solution II consists of 2% Noble agar that is sterilised and maintained at 47°C. Equal volumes of solutions I and II are adjusted to 47°C and mixed together just before use. The test is incubated for 48–72 hours, and endpoints are based on a 90% reduction in the number of plaques compared with the virus control flasks, which should have about 100 plaques.

1 RBCs from adult domestic white male geese are preferred, but RBCs from other male geese can be used. If cells from female geese are used, there may be more test variability. It has been reported that rooster RBCs cause a decrease in the sensitivity of the test.

2 Available from: Centers for Disease Control and Prevention, Biological Reference Reagents, 1600 Clifton Road NE, Mail Stop C21, Atlanta, Georgia 30333, United States of America.

B. REQUIREMENTS FOR VACCINES AND DIAGNOSTIC BIOLOGICALS

Inactivated vaccines against EEE and WEE viruses are available commercially. Attenuated EEE and WEE virus vaccines have not proven satisfactory. The vaccines licensed for use in the USA are prepared using the following combinations: EEE and WEE; EEE, WEE, and Venezuelan equine encephalomyelitis (VEE); and EEE and VEE. In addition, tetanus toxoid and inactivated influenza virus have been combined with EEE and WEE or EEE, WEE, and VEE.

Early vaccines were produced from virus propagated in embryonating chicken eggs and inactivated with formalin. Current vaccines are prepared from virus propagated in cell culture, and inactivated with formalin (4) or monoethylamine.

1. Seed management

a) Characteristics of the seed

Standard strains of EEE and WEE viruses that were isolated over 20 years ago have been used for vaccine production and have been proven to produce good immunity. Strains of EEE virus that differ antigenically and in molecular structure have been identified from different geographical regions. However, the North American and Caribbean isolates appear to be similar (15). Strains of WEE virus isolated from different countries have been found to be similar both by MAb testing and RNA oligonucleotide fingerprinting analysis (8). A recent well-characterised isolate from the country where the vaccine is to be used would be advantageous. Viruses that are selected must be immunogenic and replicate to high titres in cell culture.

b) Method of culture

Primary chicken embryo fibroblasts and Vero cells have been used for propagation of viruses used for vaccine production. The fibroblasts should be prepared from specific pathogen free embryos. Other susceptible cell lines could also be used.

c) Validation as a vaccine

If a cell line is used, the master cell stock is tested to confirm the identity of the cell line, species of origin, and freedom from extraneous agents. If primary cell cultures are used, a monolayer from each batch of each subculture should be tested for extraneous agents including bacteria, fungi, mycoplasma, and viruses. The master seed virus should also be tested to ensure freedom from bacteria, fungi, mycoplasma, and extraneous viruses.

The vaccines are administered by the intramuscular (in most cases) or intradermal route in the cervical region in two doses given 2–4 weeks apart. Annual revaccination is recommended. All foals vaccinated before 1 year of age should be revaccinated before the next vector season.

2. Method of manufacture

Details of the manufacture of vaccines currently on the market are not available. Consequently, the information provided here is intended only as background reference material on the vaccines and not as a method of manufacture. The virus and cell culture system should be selected so that a high virus titre, $\geq 10^6$ $TCID_{50}$ (50% tissue culture infective dose) per ml, is obtained in under 48 hours. Virus for vaccine production can be prepared from the supernatant fluid from infected cell cultures. The fluid is harvested when 70–100% of the monolayers have the characteristic cytopathic changes. The virus titre is determined by titration in cell culture or mice. The fluid is clarified by low speed centrifugation and filtered through gauze. The virus is inactivated by adding formalin to a final concentration of 1/2000 (0.05%) and holding at 37°C for 24 hours. Residual formaldehyde is neutralised by sodium bisulphite (4). The residual free formalin content in the inactivated vaccine should not exceed 0.2% formaldehyde.

3. In-process control

Cultures should be examined daily for virus-induced cytopathic effect. The harvested virus should be tested for microbial contamination. The efficacy of the inactivation process should be checked by testing for viable virus.

4. Batch control

a) Sterility

Tests for sterility and freedom from contamination of biological materials may be found in Chapter I.4.

b) Safety

The inactivated vaccine is safety tested by inoculating subcutaneously at least ten 6–12-hour-old chickens with 0.5 ml of the vaccine. The chickens are observed each day for 10 days for unfavourable reactions that are attributable to the vaccine (10). Safety testing can also be carried out by inoculating intracerebrally at least eight 1–4-day-old mice with 0.02 ml of the vaccine, and observing for 7 days. It is critical that safety tests be conducted on each lot of vaccine to insure that there is no residual virulent virus present.

c) Potency

Potency testing is performed by inoculating each of ten guinea-pigs with either EEE or WEE virus, using one-half the horse dose on two occasions, 14–21 days apart, by the route recommended for the horse. Serum samples from each vaccinate and each control are tested 14–21 days after the second dose using the PRN test. The EEE titres should be ≥1/40, and the WEE titres should be ≥1/40 (10), using Vero cells. If duck embryo fibroblasts are used in the PRN test, the titres will be lower. An alternative potency test is to use intracerebral challenge, 14–21 days after the second vaccination. Each guinea-pig is inoculated with 0.1 ml of virus containing 100 LD_{50} (50% lethal dose). Simultaneous titration is carried out. In order for the vaccine to be approved, 80% of the guinea-pigs must survive both viruses.

d) Duration of immunity

Comprehensive studies on duration of immunity are not available. An annual revaccination is recommended. Foals that are vaccinated before 1 year of age should be revaccinated before the next vector season.

e) Stability

The lyophilised vaccine is stable and immunogenic for 3 years if kept refrigerated at 2–7°C. After 3 years, vaccine should be discarded. The vaccines should be used immediately after reconstitution.

f) Preservatives

The preservatives used are thimerosal at a 1/10,000 dilution and antibiotics (neomycin, polymyxin amphotercin B and gentamicin).

g) Precautions (hazards)

Severe infection and death caused by EEE and WEE viruses have been reported in laboratory workers; therefore, any work with these viruses must be carried out at least in a biosafety level 2 laboratory using biological safety cabinets, and personnel should be immunised against EEE and WEE viruses (12).

Pregnant mares and foals under 2 weeks old should not be vaccinated.

5. Tests on the final product

a) Safety

See Section B.4.b.

b) Potency

See Section B.4.c.

REFERENCES

1. ELVINGER F., BALDWIN C.A., LIGGETT A.D., TANK K.N., & STALLKNECHT D.E. (1996). Prevalence of exposure to eastern equine encephalomyelitis virus in domestic and feral swine in Georgia. *J. Vet. Diagn. Invest.*, **8**, 481–484.

2. GUY J.S. (1997). Arbovirus Infections. *In:* Diseases of Poultry, Calnek B.W., Barnes H.J., Beard C.W., McDougald L.R., & Saif Y.M., ed. Iowa State University Press, Ames, Iowa, USA, 765–772.

3. KARABATSOS N., LEWIS A.L., CALISHER C.H., HUNT A.R. & ROEHRIG J.T. (1988). Identification of Highland J virus from a Florida horse. *Am. J. Trop. Med. Hyg.*, **39**, 603–606.

4. MAIRE L.F. III, MCKINNEY R.W. & COLE F.E. Jr (1970). An inactivated eastern equine encephalomyelitis vaccine propagated in chick-embryo cell culture. I. Production and testing. *Am. J. Trop. Med. Hyg.*, **19**, 119–122.

5. MONROY A.M., SCOTT T.W. & WEBB B.A. (1996). Evaluation of reverse transcriptase polymerase chain reaction for the detection of eastern equine encephalomyelitis virus during vector surveillance. *J. Med. Entomol.*, **33**, 449–457.

6. MORRIS C.D. (1989). Eastern equine encephalomyelitis. *In:* The Arboviruses: Epidemiology and Ecology, Vol. 3, Monath T.P., ed. CRC Press, Boca Raton, Florida, USA, 1–12.

7. PATTERSON J.S., MAES R.K., MULLANEY T.P., & BENSON C.L. (1996). Immunohistochemical Diagnosis of Eastern Equine Encephalomyelitis. *J. Vet. Diagn. Invest.*, **8**, 156–160.

8. REISEN W.K. & MONATH T.P. (1989). Western equine encephalomyelitis. *In:* The Arboviruses: Epidemiology and Ecology, Vol. 5, Monath T.P., ed. CRC Press, Boca Raton, Florida, USA, 89–137.

9. SAHU S.P., ALSTAD A.D., PEDERSEN D.D. & PEARSON J.E. (1994). Diagnosis of eastern equine encephalomyelitis virus infection in horses by immunoglobulin M and G capture enzyme-linked immunosorbent assay. *J. Vet. Diagn. Invest.*, **6**, 34–38.

10. UNITED STATES CODE OF FEDERAL REGULATIONS (2000). Encephalomyelitis vaccine: Eastern and Western killed virus. Title 9, Part 113, Section 113.207. US Government Printing Office, Washington DC, USA, 601–602.

11. UNITED STATES DEPARTMENT OF HEALTH, EDUCATION AND WELFARE (1974). A Guide to the Performance of the Standardised Complement Fixation Method and Adaptation to Micro Test. Centers for Disease Control, Atlanta, Georgia, USA.

12. UNITED STATES DEPARTMENT OF HEALTH AND HUMAN SERVICES (1999). Biosafety in Microbiological and Biomedical Laboratories. US Government Printing Office, Washington DC, USA, 183–184.

13. VODKIN M.H., MCLAUGHLIN G.L., DAY J.F., SHOPE R.E. & NOVAK R.J. (1993). A rapid diagnostic assay for eastern equine encephalomyelitis viral RNA. *Am. J. Trop. Med. Hyg.*, **49**, 772–776.

14. WALTON T.E. (1981). Venezuelan, eastern, and western encephalomyelitis. *In:* Virus Diseases of Food Animals. A World Geography of Epidemiology and Control. Disease Monographs, Vol. 2, Gibbs E.P.J., ed. Academic Press, New York, USA, 587–625.

15. WEAVER S.C., HAGENBAUGH A., BELLEW L.A., GOUSSET L., MALLAMPALLI V., HOLLAND J.J. & SCOTT T.W. (1994). Evolution of Alphaviruses in the eastern equine encephalomyelitis complex. *J. Virol.*, **68**, 158–169.

*

* *

CHAPTER 2.5.4.

EQUINE INFECTIOUS ANAEMIA

SUMMARY

Equine infectious anaemia (EIA) is caused by a lentivirus. It can be diagnosed on the basis of clinical signs, pathological lesions and serology. Infected horses can remain viraemic carriers for life and will yield a positive serological result. Antibody response usually persists and antibody-positive animals, older than 6 months, are identified as virus carriers (below 6 months of age, serological reactions can be due to maternal antibodies). They can potentially transmit the infection to other horses.

Identification of the agent: *Virus from a horse can be isolated by inoculating suspect blood into a susceptible horse or on to leukocyte cultures prepared from susceptible horses. Recognition of infection in horses that have been inoculated experimentally may be made on the basis of clinical signs, haematological changes and a positive antibody response determined by an immunodiffusion test or enzyme-linked immunosorbent assay (ELISA). A successful virus isolation in horse leukocyte cultures is confirmed by the detection of specific EIA antigen, by immunofluorescence assay, polymerase chain reaction, reverse-transcriptase assay, or by the inoculation of culture fluids into susceptible horses. Virus isolation is rarely attempted because of the time, difficulty and expense involved.*

Serological tests: *Agar gel immunodiffusion (AGID) tests and ELISAs are simple, reliable tests for the demonstration of EIA virus infection. When ELISAs are positive they should be confirmed using the AGID test. The precipitating antigen can be prepared from infected tissue cultures or by using recombinant technology.*

Requirements for vaccines and diagnostic biologicals: *There are no biological products currently available.*

A. DIAGNOSTIC TECHNIQUES

Equine infectious anaemia (EIA) occurs world-wide. The disease is characterised by recurrent febrile episodes, thrombocytopaenia, anaemia, rapid loss of weight and oedema of the lower parts of the body; it tends to become an inapparent infection if death does not result from one of the acute clinical attacks. The incubation period is normally 1–3 weeks, but may be as long as 3 months. In acute cases, lymph nodes, spleen and liver are hyperaemic and enlarged. Histologically these organs are infiltrated with nests of immature lymphocytes and plasma cells. Kupffer cells in the liver often contain haemosiderin or erythrocytes. The enlarged spleen may be felt on rectal examination.

Once a horse is infected with EIA virus, its blood is likely to remain infectious for the remainder of its life. This means that the horse is a viraemic carrier and can potentially transmit the infection to other horses (3). Transmission occurs by transfer of blood from an infected horse. In nature, spread of the virus is most likely via interrupted feeding of bloodsucking horseflies on a clinically ill horse and then on susceptible horses, or from the use of contaminated needles. However, *in utero* infection of the fetus does occur (8).

Agar gel immunodiffusion (AGID) tests (6) and enzyme-linked immunosorbent assays (ELISAs) (14) are accurate, reliable tests for the detection of EIA in horses, except for animals in the early stages of infection and foals of infected dams. In other rare circumstances, misleading results may occur when the level of virus circulating in the blood during an acute episode of the disease is sufficient to bind available antibody, and if initial antibody levels never rise high enough to be detectable (15). Although the ELISA will detect antibodies somewhat earlier and at lower concentrations than the AGID test, positive ELISAs are confirmed using the AGID test. This is because false-positive results have been noted with the ELISA. The AGID test also has the advantage of distinguishing between EIA and non-EIA antigen–antibody reactions by lines of identity.

The EIA virus is a lentivirus, a subfamily of the Retroviridae, which also includes maedi-visna virus, caprine arthritis/encephalitis, bovine immunodeficiency and the human immunodeficiency viruses. Nucleic acid sequence comparisons have demonstrated a marked relatedness.

1. Identification of the agent

Virus isolation is usually not necessary to make a diagnosis.

Isolation of virus from suspect horses may be made by inoculating their blood on to leukocyte cultures prepared from horses free of infection. Any virus produced in cultures can be confirmed by detection of specific EIA antigen by ELISA (14), by immunofluorescence assay (16), or by subinoculation into susceptible horses. Virus isolation is rarely attempted because of the difficulty of growing horse leukocyte cultures.

When the exact status of infection of a horse cannot be ascertained, the inoculation of a susceptible horse with suspect blood should be employed. In this case, a horse that has previously been tested for antibody and shown to be negative is given an immediate blood transfusion from the suspect horse, and its antibody status and clinical condition are monitored for at least 45 days. Usually, 1–25 ml of whole blood given intravenously is sufficient to demonstrate infection, but in rare cases it may be necessary to use a larger volume of blood (250 ml) or washed leukocytes from such a volume (4).

2. Serological tests

a) Agar gel immunodiffusion test (the prescribed test for international trade)

Precipitating antibody is rapidly produced as a result of EIA infection, and can be detected by the AGID test. Specific reactions are indicated by precipitin lines between the EIA antigen and the test serum and confirmed by their identity with the reaction between the antigen and the positive standard serum. Horses in the first 2–3 weeks after infection will usually give negative serological reactions.

- **Preparation of antigen**

Specific EIA antigen may be prepared from the spleen of acutely infected horses (5), from infected equine tissue culture (10), from a persistently infected canine thymus cell line (2), or from proteins expressed in bacteria or baculovirus using the recombinant DNA technique (1, 9). Preparation from infected cultures gives a more uniform result than the use of spleen cells and allows for better standardisation of reagents.

To obtain a satisfactory antigen from spleen, a horse must be infected with a highly virulent strain of EIA virus. The resulting incubation period should be 5–7 days, and the spleen should be collected 9 days after inoculation, when the virus titre is at its peak and before any detectable amount of precipitating antibody is produced. Undiluted spleen pulp is used in the immunodiffusion test as antigen (5). Extraction of antigen from the spleen with a saline solution and concentration with ammonium sulphate does not give as satisfactory an antigen as selection of a spleen with a very high titre of EIA antigen.

Alternatively, equine fetal kidney or dermal cells or canine thymus cells are infected with a strain of EIA virus adapted to grow in tissue culture (American Type Culture Collection). Virus is collected from cultures by precipitation with 8% polyethylene glycol or by pelleting by ultracentrifugation. The diagnostic antigen p26 is released from the virus by treatment with detergent or ether (10). EIA virus core proteins, expressed in bacteria or baculovirus, are commercially available and find practical use as high quality antigens for serological diagnosis.

The p26 is an internal structural protein of the virus that is coded for by the *gag* gene. This gene is stable and no variation has been found between strains (11).

- **Preparation of standard antiserum**

A known positive antiserum may be collected from a horse previously infected with EIA virus. This serum should yield a single dense precipitation line that is specific for EIA, as demonstrated by a reaction of identity with a known standard serum. It is essential to match the antigen and antibody concentrations in order to ensure the optimal sensitivity of the test. Reagent concentrations should be adjusted to form a narrow precipitation line approximately equidistant between the two wells containing antigen and serum.

- **Test procedure (5, 12)**

i) Immunodiffusion reactions are carried out in a layer of agar in Petri dishes. For Petri dishes that are 100 mm in diameter, 15 ml of 1% Noble agar is used. Six wells are punched out of the agar surrounding a central well of the same diameter. The wells are 5.3 mm in diameter and 2.4 mm apart. Each well must contain the same volume of reagent.

ii) The antigen is placed in the central well and the standard antiserum is placed in alternate exterior wells. Serum samples for testing are placed in the remaining three wells.

iii) The dishes are maintained at room temperature in a humid environment.

iv) After 24–48 hours the precipitation reactions are examined over a narrow beam of intense, oblique light and against a black background. The reference lines should be clearly visible at 24 hours, and at that time any test sera that are strongly positive may also have formed lines of identity with those between the standard reagents. A weakly positive reaction may take 48 hours to form and is indicated by a slight bending of the standard serum precipitation line between the antigen well and the test serum well. Sera with high precipitating antibody titres may form broader precipitin bands that tend to be diffuse and to fade with time. These are not difficult to recognise because they will dissolve the reference line about half-way across its normal position. Such reactions can be confirmed as specific for EIA by dilution at 1/2 or 1/4 prior to retesting; these then give a more distinct line of identity. Sera devoid of EIA antibody will not form precipitation lines and will have no effect on the reaction lines of the standard reagents.

v) *Interpretation of the results:* Horses that are in the early stages of an infection may not give a positive serological reaction in an AGID test. Such animals should be bled again after 1–2 weeks. In order to make a diagnosis in a young foal, it may be necessary to determine the antibody status of the dam. If the mare possesses any EIA antibody, then a period of about 6 months or longer after birth must be allowed for the maternal antibody to wane; the foal is then retested to determine whether an initial positive reaction was due to maternal antibody or infection.

b) Enzyme-linked immunosorbent assay

There are two ELISAs that have been approved by the United States Department of Agriculture for the diagnosis of equine infectious anaemia: a competitive ELISA and a synthetic antigen ELISA. The competitive ELISA detects antibody against the same p26 core protein antigen as used in the AGID test (an example of the protocol is given below). The synthetic antigen ELISA test detects antibody against the gp45 (viral transmembrane protein) antigen. Typical ELISA protocols are used in both tests. The ELISA using p26 as an antigen is useful in detecting antibody because of its high sensitivity and rapidity compared with the AGID test (13).

- **Preparation of antigen**

EIA virus p-337-EFD strain is grown in equine fetal dermal (EFD) cell line. The virus is concentrated by ultrafiltration and ultracentrifugation for 90 minutes at 51,000 ***g***, and then subjected to ultracentrifugation on a 45% sucrose cushion for 2 hours at 75,000 ***g***. Virus is collected, diluted in TNE buffer and pelleted by ultracentrifugation. The resulting pellet is disrupted by treatment with ether. This antigen consists mainly of p26 protein.

- **Selection of standard weak positive serum**

Serum that gives a weak precipitation line in AGID tests is selected as the standard weak positive serum. The ELISA is adjusted so that the standard serum gives absorbance values of from 0.3 to 0.7.

- **Test procedure**

i) 50 µg/well of p26 antigen is added to wells of the ELISA plates, which are then freeze-dried overnight.

ii) The ELISA plates are coated with 1% gelatin for 1 hour.

iii) 50 µl each of test sera and standard positive and negative sera diluted 1/800 are added to wells of the ELISA plates, which are then incubated for 40 minutes at 37°C.

iv) 50 µl of horseradish-peroxidase-labelled anti-horse IgG is added to each well, and the plates are incubated for 20 minutes at 37°C.

v) 50 µl of thymol blue solution is added to each well, and the plates are incubated for 10 minutes at room temperature.

vi) The reaction is stopped by adding 50 µl 0.5 M sulphuric acid.

vii) Absorbance values are read at 450 nm wavelength. Serum that gives a higher value than that of the standard positive serum is judged to be positive. With this procedure, the rate of false-positive reactions is lower than 0.3%.

Reagents for EIA serological tests such as AGID and competitive and synthetic antigen ELISA are available commercially from several companies. A positive test result by ELISA should be retested using the AGID test to confirm the diagnosis because some false-positive results have been noted with the ELISA. The results can also be confirmed by the immunoblot technique. A standard antiserum for immunodiffusion, which contains the minimum amount of antibody that should be detected by laboratories, is available from the OIE Reference

Laboratories (see Table given in Part 4 of this *Manual*). Uniform methods for EIA control have been published (7).

B. REQUIREMENTS FOR VACCINES AND DIAGNOSTIC BIOLOGICALS

No biological products are available currently.

REFERENCES

1. ARCHAMBAULT D., WANG Z., LACAL J.C., GAZIT A., YANIV A., DAHLBERG J.E. & TRONICK S.R. (1989). Development of an enzyme-linked immunosorbent assay for equine infectious anaemia virus detection using recombinant Pr55gag. *J. Clin. Microbiol.*, **27**, 1167–1173.

2. BOUILLANT A.M.P., NELSON K., RUCKERBAUER C.M., SAMAGH B.S. & HARE W.C.D. (1986). The persistent infection of a canine thymus cell line by equine infectious anaemia virus and preliminary data on the production of viral antigens. *J. Virol. Methods*, **13**, 309–321.

3. CHEEVERS W.M. & MCGUIRE T.C. (1985). Equine infectious anaemia virus; immunopathogenesis and persistence. *Rev. Infect. Dis.*, **7**, 83–88.

4. COGGINS L. & KEMEN M.J. (1976). Inapparent carriers of equine infectious anaemia (EIA) virus. *In:* Proceedings of the IVth International Conference on Equine Infectious Diseases. University of Kentucky, Lexington, Kentucky, USA, 14–22.

5. COGGINS L., NORCROSS N.L. & KEMEN M.J. (1973). The technique and application of the immunodiffusion test for equine infectious anaemia. *Equine Infect. Dis.*, **III**, 177–186.

6. COGGINS L., NORCROSS N.L. & NUSBAUM S.R. (1972). Diagnosis of equine infectious anaemia by immunodiffusion test. *Am. J. Vet. Res.*, **33**, 11–18.

7. COMMITTEE ON INFECTIOUS DISEASES OF HORSES (1997). *Proc. U.S. Anim. Health Assoc.*, **101**, 236–246.

8. KEMEN M.J. & COGGINS L. (1972). Equine infectious anaemia: transmission from infected mares to foals. *J. Am. Vet. Med. Assoc.*, **161**, 496–499.

9. KONG X. K., PANG H., SUGIURA T., SENTSUI H., ONODERA T., MATSUMOTO Y. & AKASHI H. (1997). Application of equine infectious anaemia virus core proteins produced in a Baculovirus expression system, to serological diagnosis. *Microbiol. Immunol.*, **41**, 975–980.

10. MALMQUIST W.A., BARNETT D. & BECVAR C.S. (1973). Production of equine infectious anaemia antigen in a persistently infected cell line. *Arch. Gesamte Virusforsch.*, **42**, 361–370.

11. MONTELARO R.C., PAREKH B., ORREGO A. & ISSEL C.J. (1984). Antigenic variation during persistent infection by equine infectious anaemia, a retrovirus. *J. Biol. Chem.*, **16**, 10539–10544.

12. PEARSON J.E. & COGGINS L. (1979). Protocol for the immunodiffusion (Coggins) test for equine infectious anaemia. *Proc. Am. Assoc. Vet. Lab. Diagnosticians*, **22**, 449–462.

13. SHANE B.S., ISSEL C.J. & MONTELARO R.C. (1984). Enzyme-linked immunosorbent assay for detection of equine infectious anemia virus p26 antigen and antibody. *J. Clin. Microbiol.*, **19**, 351–355.

14. SUZUKI T., UEDA S. & SAMEJINA T. (1982). Enzyme-linked immunosorbent assay for diagnosis of equine infectious anaemia. *Vet. Microbiol.*, **7**, 307–316.

15. TOMA B. (1980). Réponse sérologique négative persistante chez une jument infectée. *Rec. Med. Vet.*, **156**, 55–63.

16. WEILAND F., MATHEKA H.D. & BOHM H.O. (1982). Equine infectious anaemia: detection of antibodies using an immunofluorescence test. *Res. Vet. Sci.*, **33**, 347–350.

*

* *

CHAPTER 2.5.5.

EQUINE INFLUENZA

SUMMARY

Equine influenza is an acute, contagious respiratory disease caused by two distinct subtypes (subtype 1: H7N7 and subtype 2: H3N8) of influenza A viruses within the genus Influenzavirus A, B, of the family Orthomyxoviridae. In fully susceptible Equidae, clinical signs include pyrexia, and a harsh dry cough followed by a mucopurulent nasal discharge. In partially immune vaccinated animals, one or more of these signs may be absent. Characteristically, influenza spreads rapidly in a susceptible population. Diagnosis of influenzavirus infections is based on virus isolation from horses with acute respiratory illness, or on the demonstration of increased antibody titres in paired sera taken in the acute and convalescent stages of the disease. Ideally, both methods are used. Infection may also be demonstrated by detection of viral antigen in respiratory secretions using an enzyme-linked immunosorbent assay. Spread of infection and severity of disease may be reduced by the use of potent equine influenza vaccines containing epidemiologically relevant virus strains.

Identification of the agent: *Embryonated chicken eggs or cell cultures can be used for virus isolation from nasopharyngeal swabs or nasal and tracheal washes. Eggs are preferred for virus isolation because they are more permissive to equine influenza and less likely to select variant viruses.*

Viral growth is monitored by haemagglutination (HA) or, in cell cultures, by haemadsorption (HAD) using chicken or guinea-pig red blood cells. If HA or HAD are positive, isolates can be typed by haemagglutination inhibition (HI) using strain-specific antisera. Isolates should always be sent immediately to International Reference Laboratories (OIE and World Health Organization) for typing and strain collection. Samples that yield negative results (i.e. show no HA or HAD after one passage) should be repassaged. Up to five passages may be necessary to isolate viruses from vaccinated horses.

Serological tests: *Diagnosis of influenzavirus infections can usually only be accomplished by tests on paired sera; the first sample should be taken as soon as possible after the onset of clinical signs, and the second approximately 2 weeks later. Both serum samples should be tested at the same time, due to potential test variability, even within the same laboratory. Sera are heat-inactivated and pretreated to reduce nonspecific reactions. Antibody titres are determined by HI or single radial haemolysis (SRH). For SRH, pretreatment and serial dilution of sera are usually not required. HI and SRH give comparable results, but SRH may be more sensitive for infections in vaccinated horses.*

Requirements for vaccines and diagnostic biologicals: *Inactivated equine influenza virus vaccines contain strains of subtypes 1 and 2 that are propagated in embryonated chicken eggs or tissue culture, concentrated, and purified before inactivation with agents such as formalin or beta-propiolactone. Vaccines provide protection by inducing humoral antibody to HA. Responses are generally short-lived and multiple doses are required to maintain protective levels of antibody. An adjuvant is usually required to stimulate durable protective levels of antibody. A modified live equine A2 influenza vaccine for intranasal administration has recently become available commercially in some countries.*

Influenza vaccines are widely available and are routinely used in competition horses in Europe, the Americas, and Asia. In some countries, vaccination is mandatory for sport horses that are competing under rules of equestrian organisations. Vaccines are not widely used on the Indian subcontinent, China or Australia, the latter region, along with New Zealand, having remained free from infection. Vaccination should not occur before 9 months of age. Following a primary course of three doses at 0, 1 and 6 months, an annual booster is the minimum requirement. In some regions, repeated vaccinations are given every 3–6 months.

Vaccines have been highly successful in preventing infection with A/equine/1 viruses, but frequent reports of vaccine breakdown occur during outbreaks of A/equine/2 infections. This has been attributed to inadequate vaccine potency, inappropriate vaccination schedules, and outdated vaccine viruses that have become irrelevant as a result of antigenic drift. Some biologicals companies are now marketing vaccines that contain recent isolates to counter the effects of antigenic drift. An improved in-vitro *potency test (single radial diffusion) has been developed that can be used for in-process testing of the product before addition of an adjuvant. Levels of antibody required for protection of horses have been identified. A surveillance programme is underway to monitor antigenic drift among equine influenza viruses and to provide information on strain selection for vaccines.*

A. DIAGNOSTIC TECHNIQUES

Equine influenza is caused by two subtypes: subtype 1 (H7N7) and subtype 2 (H3N8) of influenza A viruses of the genus *Influenzavirus* A, B, of the family Orthomyxoviridae. Although these are not genuine human pathogens, humans can become infected with equine influenza virus subtypes. Such infections are unusual and subclinical, but may represent a potential biohazard to laboratory personnel.

All influenza viruses are highly contagious for susceptible hosts, including embryonated chicken eggs and cell cultures. Care must therefore be taken during the handling of infected eggs or cultures to avoid accidental cross-contamination (17). Standard strains should not be propagated in the diagnostic laboratory, at least never at the same time or in the same place where diagnostic samples are being processed. All working areas must be efficiently disinfected before and after virus manipulations, which should preferably be conducted within biohazard containment.

It is important to obtain samples as soon as possible after the onset of clinical signs. These samples include nasopharyngeal swabs or nasal and tracheal washings, the latter taken by endoscopy. Swabs consist of absorbent cotton wool sponge/gauze on wire, or similar, and should be passed via the ventral meatus into the nasopharynx and held there for approximately 10 seconds to absorb respiratory secretions. Swabs should be transferred to a vial containing transport medium immediately after use. This medium consists of phosphate buffered saline (PBS) containing 40% glycerol, or PBS containing 2% tryptose phosphate broth, 2% antibiotic solution (penicillin [10,000 units], streptomycin [10,000 units] in sterile distilled water [100 ml]), and 2% fungizone (250 mg/ml stock). If the samples are to be inoculated within 1–2 days, they may be held at 4°C but, if kept for longer, they should be stored at –60°C or below. Preferably, samples should also be transported on ice.

Only one sample is processed at a time. The liquid is expelled from the swab, which is then disposed of suitably. Further antibiotics may be added if samples appear to be heavily contaminated. The remainder of the fluid is stored at –60°C. Samples treated with antibiotics are allowed to stand on ice for 30 minutes, then centrifuged at 1500 ***g*** for 15 minutes to remove bacteria and debris; the supernatant fluids are used for inoculation. Filtration of samples is not advised as influenza virus may adsorb on to the filter and be lost from the sample.

1. Identification of the agent

Isolation of infectious virus may be carried out in embryonated eggs or cell cultures. Comparison of A/equine/2 viruses isolated in eggs and Madin–Darby canine kidney (MDCK) cells indicates that MDCK cells are capable of selecting variant viruses that are not representative of the predominant virus in clinical specimens. For this reason, eggs are preferred for isolation, particularly if viruses are to be used as vaccine strains (6).). However, in recent years some viruses have been isolated in MDCK cells and not eggs and for this reason both substrates should be used.

a) Embryonated chicken eggs

Fertile eggs are set in a humid incubator at (37–38°C) and turned twice daily; after 10–11 days, they are examined by candling. Only live embryonated eggs are selected for use. The area above the air sac is cleansed with alcohol and a small hole is drilled through the shell. Three eggs/sample are inoculated (0.1 ml) into the amniotic cavity. The syringe is withdrawn approximately 1 cm and a further 0.1 ml is inoculated into the allantoic cavity. Alternatively, the sample may be inoculated into the allantoic cavity alone. The hole is sealed with wax or Sellotape™, and the eggs are incubated at (34–35°C) for 3 days.

The eggs are then transferred to 4°C for 4 hours or overnight to kill the embryos and to reduce bleeding at harvest. The shells are disinfected, and the allantoic and amniotic fluid is harvested by pipette, each harvest being kept separate. These are tested for haemagglutination (HA) activity using a 1% suspension of chicken red blood cells (RBCs) or 0.4% guinea-pig RBCs in PBS. Nonagglutinated RBCs form a 'stream' when the tube or plate is tilted. If there is no HA activity, aliquots of each harvest are pooled and repassaged into further eggs. All HA positive samples are divided into aliquots and stored at –70°C; one aliquot is titrated for HA immediately and, if it has a titre of 1/16 or more, the isolate is typed using antisera against subtype 1 and subtype 2 viruses. If titres are low, positive samples should be passaged. Care should be taken to avoid generation of defective interfering particles by prediluting the inoculum 1/10, 1/100, 1/1000. Positive samples arising from the highest dilution should be selected as stocks for storage. It may be necessary to undertake as many as five passages to isolate the virus, particularly from vaccinated horses. If virus has not been recovered by the fifth passage, further passages are unlikely to be successful.

b) Cell cultures

Cultures of the MDCK cell line (MDCK, ATCC CCL34) may be used to isolate equine influenza viruses if eggs are unavailable. The cells are grown to confluence in tubes and then infected in triplicate with 0.25–0.5 ml of each sample, processed as described above. The cultures are maintained with serum-free medium containing 0.5–2 µg/ml trypsin (TPCK-treated [L-1-tosylamide-2-phenylethyl chloromethyl ketone] to remove chymotrypsin – available pretreated, for example from Sigma), and examined daily for evidence of cytopathic effect (CPE). If positive, or after 7 days in any case, the supernatant fluids are tested for HA. Fluids with titres of >1/16 are typed immediately. Negative fluids and those with titres <1/16 are repassaged.

Alternatively, the cells are screened for evidence of haemadsorption (HAD). This procedure detects expression of viral antigens at the cell surface. The medium is removed from the cultures and the tubes are washed with PBS. One or two drops of a 50% suspension of chicken or guinea-pig RBCs are added, the tubes are rotated carefully, and kept at 22°C (±2°C) for 30 minutes. Unbound RBCs are washed off with PBS, and the cultures are examined microscopically for evidence of HAD.

c) Haemagglutinin

Typing of new isolates of equine influenza viruses is best done by haemagglutination inhibition (HI) using specific antisera. The species in which antibodies are raised will influence the cross-reactivity of the antiserum, with ferrets providing the most strain-specific antibody (10). Isolates may first be treated with Tween 80/ether, which destroys viral infectivity and reduces the risk of cross-contamination. In the case of A/equine/2 viruses particularly, this treatment enhances the HA activity (7).

For HI, both macro- and microtests may be used. The antigens are prepared to final HA dilutions of 1/4 or 1/8 per well. Antisera, treated with potassium periodate to reduce nonspecific haemagglutinins (for details see Section A.2.a. Pretreatment of sera, below), are serially diluted in PBS, antigen is added, and the mixtures are left to react for 30 minutes at 22°C (±2°C). The RBCs (1% chicken or 0.4% guinea-pig) are added, gently mixed and allowed to stand at 22°C (±2°C) for 30 minutes. The volumes of the microtest are 0.025 ml for PBS, sera and antigen, respectively, followed by 0.05 ml for the RBC suspension. In the macrotest, 0.5 ml volumes are used throughout. The HI titres are read as the highest dilution of serum giving complete inhibition of agglutination, i.e. the RBCs form a 'stream' when the plates are tilted. Incomplete inhibition is always scored as agglutination. All isolates should be sent immediately to the International Reference Laboratories designated by the OIE and the World Health Organization (WHO) (see Table given in Part 4 of this *Manual*) for inclusion in the strain surveillance programme to monitor antigenic drift and emergence of new viruses.

Standard antigens must be titrated in parallel with tests to identify viruses and should include: subtype 1 (e.g. A/equine/Prague/56 and A/equine/Newmarket/77) and subtype 2 (e.g. A/equine/Miami/63, A/equine/-Fontainebleau/79, A/equine/2/Newmarket/2/93, and A/equine/Kentucky/94). Additionally, recent isolates from the same geographical area should be included if available. The standard antigens should be treated with Tween 80/ether to avoid cross-contamination. Test antigens and standard antigens are always back-titrated to confirm their antigen content.

d) Neuraminidase

Typing of neuraminidase requires specific antisera and no routine technique is available. Such typing is best done, therefore, in reference laboratories.

e) Detection of viral antigen by enzyme-linked immunosorbent assay

In situations where laboratory facilities for virus isolation are unavailable, influenza virus antigen in nasal secretions may be detected directly by an antigen-capture enzyme-linked immunosorbent assay (ELISA) employing a monoclonal antibody (MAb) against the nucleoprotein (1, 2, 8). (Commercial self-contained kits are available.)

This approach provides a rapid result on which management decisions may be based. It should not be used in preference to virus isolation, as it is essential that new viruses be isolated and sent to reference laboratories for typing as part of the surveillance programme to monitor antigenic drift and emergence of new viruses. Positive ELISA results are useful in the selection of samples for virus isolation attempts if resources are limited.

- **Test procedure**

i) Dispense 100 µl aliquots of nasal swab extract into microstrips coated with polyclonal rabbit anti-H3N8, and incubate for 90 minutes at 22°C (±2°C). Wash the microstrips three times with PBS containing 0.05% Tween 20 (PBST).

ii) Add 100 µl of MAb-horseradish-peroxidase conjugate diluted 1/150 in dilution buffer, then incubate for 1 hour at 37°C. Wash the microstrips six times with PBST.

iii) Add 100 µl aliquots of tetramethyl benzidine and incubate for 10 minutes at 22°C (±2°C). Stop the reaction by adding 100 µl of 0.18 M sulphuric acid, and measure the absorbance at 450 nm.

Reagents may be obtained from the OIE Reference Laboratory, Newmarket (see Table given in Part 4 of this *Manual*).

2. Serological tests

Infections are detected by performing serological tests on paired sera to show a rise in antibody titre. These tests should be carried out whether virus isolation has been attempted or not. Two simple methods exist, HI and single radial haemolysis (SRH), each equally efficient and widely used. The complement fixation (CF) test can also be applied, but is not standardised or in general use. Both of the paired serum samples should be tested together at the same time, to minimise test variability.

a) Haemagglutination inhibition test

The standard antigens are described above. If available, isolates from recent cases should be included. The antigen is first treated with Tween 80/ether in order to increase the sensitivity of the test, particularly for A/equine/2 viruses. Lyophilised-treated antigens for equine influenza viruses are available from the European Pharmacopoeia. Freeze-dried post-infection antisera to recent A/equine/2 viruses are available from the OIE Reference Laboratory (Newmarket). The test is best done in microtitre plates using the appropriate dilution equipment. Sera are pretreated to remove nonspecific haemagglutinins, and are inactivated by heating at 56°C for 30 minutes. Pretreatments include the use of one of the following: (a) kaolin and RBC absorption, (b) potassium periodate (details given below), or (c) *Vibrio cholerae* receptor-destroying enzyme. All three procedures yield similar results. The treated sera are diluted in PBS, antigen with a titre of 1/4 is added, and these are kept at 22°C (±2°C) for 30 minutes after gentle mixing. RBCs are added and the test is read 30 minutes later. The HI titres are the highest dilutions of serum that completely inhibit HA. Titre increases of four-fold or more between paired sera indicate recent infections (17).

- **Microtitre method for haemagglutination inhibition tests**

Chicken RBCs in Alsever's solution (1% [v/v] packed cells); V-bottomed or U-bottomed microtitre plates; PBS; influenza antigen (whole virus or Tween 80/ether-treated); potassium periodate (KIO_4); and glycerol.

- **Tween 80/ether treatment of the virus**

i) To 40 ml of infective allantoic fluid, add 0.5 ml of a 10% (v/v) suspension of Tween 80 in PBS to give a 0.125% (v/v) concentration of Tween 80.

ii) After mixing gently at room temperature for 5 minutes, add 20 ml of diethyl ether to give a final concentration of 33.3% by volume, and mix the suspension well at 4°C for 15 minutes.

iii) After allowing the layers to separate by standing, remove the aqueous layer containing the disrupted virus particles to a glass bottle with a loose lid and allow the excess ether to evaporate off overnight (7).

- **Titration of haemagglutination**

i) Add 25 µl of PBS to all wells in a row.

ii) Add 25 µl of virus to the first well (dilution = 1/2) and titrate through leaving the last well as a control.

iii) Add an extra 25 µl of PBS to all wells.

iv) Add 50 µl of 1% RBCs to all wells. Leave at 22°C (±2°C) for 30 minutes. The HA titre is taken as the last virus dilution giving 50% HA.

- **Pretreatment of sera**

i) Mix one volume (150 µl) of serum with two volumes (300 µl) of freshly prepared 0.016 M potassium periodate (0.38 g in 100 ml PBS), and leave at 22°C (±2°C) for 15 minutes.

ii) Add a further volume of 3% glycerol in PBS to neutralise any excess periodate solution, mix and leave at 22°C (±2°C) for 15 minutes.

iii) Heat inactivate in a 56°C water bath for 30 minutes.

- **Test procedure**

i) Dispense 25 µl of PBS to all wells of the microtitre plate.

ii) Add sera (25 µl) to the first row of 12, and titrate leaving the last well as a control (1/8 to 1/512).

iii) Dilute the antigen to give a dose of 4 HA units (4 × minimum agglutinating dose, i.e. titre/4).

iv) Add 25 µl to each well, and incubate at 22°C (±2°C) for 30 minutes.

v) Add 50 µl of 1% RBCs to each well. Leave at 22°C (±2°C) for 30 minutes.

vi) Read the results by tilting the plate to 70°, no agglutination is recorded as a positive result.

b) Single radial haemolysis

In this test, viral antigens are coupled to fixed RBCs that are suspended in agarose containing guinea-pig complement (C'). Wells are punched in the agarose and filled with test sera. Influenza antibodies and C' lyse the antigen-coated RBCs, resulting in a clear, haemolytic zone around the well; the size of this zone can be measured (9, 15, 16).

Special immunodiffusion plates (Hyland; Miles Scientific) may be used for the assay, but simple Petri dishes are also suitable. Sheep RBCs are collected into Alsever's solution and washed three times. The C' can be obtained commercially, or normal guinea-pig serum can be used. The antigens are allantoic fluids or purified preparations; the strains used are the same as for the HI tests. The viruses are coupled to RBCs by potassium periodate or by chromic chloride. The coupled antigen/RBC preparations are mixed with C', together with a 1% solution of agarose (low melting grade) in PBS. Care must be taken to ensure that the temperature is not allowed to rise above 42°C at any time. The mixture is poured into plates and left overnight at 4°C. Wells of 3 mm in diameter and 12 mm apart are punched in the solidified agarose, 6 mm from the edge of the plates. Such plates may be stored at 4°C for 1–2 weeks. Plates are prepared for each antigen and pretested with known positive and negative antisera.

Sera are heat inactivated at 56°C for 30 minutes, but no further treatment is necessary. Paired sera should be assayed in duplicate on the same plate; all sera are tested in a control plate containing all components except virus. Alternatively, an irrelevant virus, such as an H1N1 virus, may be used in the control plate. Sera that show haemolytic activity for sheep RBCs must be pre-absorbed with sheep RBCs. Zones of lysis should be clear, and not hazy or translucent. All clear zones should be measured and the area of haemolysis calculated.

- **Materials**

NaCl; KCl; HEPES (N-2-hydroxyethy-piperazine, N-2-ethanesulphonic acid); virus antigen; BSA (bovine serum albumin); Na_2HPO_4; KH_2PO_4; agarose; control antiserum; NaOH; chromium chloride; guinea-pig serum for complement; 3 mm hole punch; plastic boxes; zone measuring apparatus; perspex immunoplates (6 × 11 cm); template for hole punching; water bath; incubator; and sodium azide.

- **Preparation of reagents**

i) *Saline/HEPES:* 0.85% NaCl (4.25 g/500 ml); 0.05 M HEPES (5.95 g/500 ml); and 0.02% sodium azide. Make to pH 6.5 with NaOH.

ii) *Saline/HEPES/BSA:* as saline/HEPES with 0.2% (w/v) BSA.

iii) *$CrCl_3$ stock solution (2.25 M) 6 g/10 ml:* For use make fresh 1/400 dilution in 0.85% NaCl.

iv) *PBS (London)/PBS 'A':* NaCl (10.00 g); KCl (0.25 g); Na_2PO_4 (1.45 g); KH_2PO_4 (0.25 g); and Na azide (0.20 g). Make up to 1 litre with distilled H_2O.

v) *Agarose in PBS:* Place flask containing 1 litre PBS 'A' on a stirrer. Slowly add 10 g agarose to the stirring solution. Liquefy in a pressure cooker. Dispense into glass bottles for storage at 22°C (±2°C).

vi) *Virus antigen:* Allantoic fluid containing infectious virus is harvested and stored at –70°C. A short titration curve determines the optimum volume of allantoic fluid to be used when preparing sensitised sheep RBCs. The H7N7 influenza strains always produce clear zones; the H3N8 strains sometimes produce hazy zones, in which case it is necessary to concentrate the virus by ultracentrifugation.

vii) *Sheep blood:* Collect blood into an equal volume of Alsever's solution and store at 4°C. It may be necessary to test bleed several sheep, as characteristics of RBCs from individual sheep vary. Keep the blood for 2 days before use, it may then be usable for up to 3 weeks, providing sterility is maintained.

viii) *Complement:* Collect serum from young guinea-pigs of 300–350 g and store in small volumes at –70°C. For use, thaw in cold H_2O and hold at 4°C prior to mixing.

ix) *Treatment of sera:* Use undiluted sera. Heat inactivate at 56°C for 30 minutes. Avoid repeated freeze–thawing.

- **Test procedure**

i) Wash sheep RBCs at least three times in saline/HEPES.

ii) Prepare an appropriate volume of 8% RBCs (v/v packed cells) in saline/HEPES, having first calculated the number of plates required and allowing 1 ml per plate and 1–2 ml extra.

iii) Add a predetermined volume of clarified allantoic fluid to the 8% RBCs solution. Hold the mixture at 4°C for 10 minutes. Haemagglutination may be observed.

iv) SLOWLY add $CrCl_3$ (1/400 of stock solution in 0.85% NaCl) at half the total volume of virus/RBC suspension. Hold at 22°C (±2°C) for 5 minutes with occasional mixing.

v) Sediment the sensitised RBCs by centrifugation at 1500 ***g*** for 5 minutes.

vi) Gently resuspend in saline/HEPES/BSA and centrifuge at 1500 ***g*** for 5 minutes.

vii) Resuspend RBCs to an 8% suspension in PBS 'A'.

During the sensitisation process, melt the agarose in a pressure cooker. Shortly before use, pipette 7.8 ml volumes to Universal bottles and retain at 42°C. Check that the agar has cooled to 42°C before use.

- **Preparation of plates**

i) Add 0.9 ml of virus-sensitised sheep RBCs to 7.8 ml of agarose (42°C). Mix quickly, but gently.

ii) Add 0.3 ml of undiluted guinea-pig serum. Mix again and pour into immunoplates on a levelling table. Allow to set and air dry without a lid for 5 minutes.

iii) Place lids on plates and store at 4°C in a humid box until used.

iv) Prepare control plates with unsensitised cells to check for nonspecific lysis. Alternatively, control cells can be prepared by sensitising with a nonrelated influenza virus (e.g. a human H1N1 virus). Batches of prepared plates can be stored for several weeks.

v) Punch 3 mm holes in the set gels to a prepared template – allow for 16 test sera and a positive control serum. On antigen control plates, prepare five rows of eight wells.

vi) Pipette 10 µl of heat-inactivated (56°C for 30 minutes) test sera and a positive control serum to appropriate wells. Incubate at 34°C for 20 hours in a humid box.

vii) Measure zone diameters, and calculate areas of haemolysis after the area of the well has been deducted.

Table 1. *Example of titration of antigen*

Red blood cells	Virus	$CrCl_3$	Final volume in PBS
2 ml	0.6 ml (0.3/litre)	1.3 ml	2 ml
2 ml	1.2 ml (0.6/ litre)	1.6 ml	2 ml
2 ml	1.8 ml (0.9/ litre)	1.9 ml	2 ml

Optimum volume of antigen is that which results in the largest and most obvious zone.

Control sera: Subtype-specific antisera should be included in one well on each plate.

- **Interpretation of the results**

For results to be valid, positive and negative control sera should give results consistent with those expected on the basis of prior experience. Areas of haemolysis for the control sera should be clear and vary no more than 10% from the designated value for the control serum. Results may be expressed as mm^2 or as a ratio of the control serum value. Sera giving positive results in the control plate should be adsorbed with sheep RBCs. For diagnostic purposes, acute and convalescent sera should be tested in duplicate on the same plate. Increases in zone areas produced by convalescent sera compared with acute sera are evidence of infection. The increase in area deemed to be significant depends on the reproducibility of the test within the laboratory, but should be equivalent to a twofold or more increase in antibody concentration. This area can be calculated from a standard curve generated from a dilution series of a standard antiserum.

B. REQUIREMENTS FOR VACCINES AND DIAGNOSTIC BIOLOGICALS

Equine influenza virus vaccines usually consist of inactivated whole virus subtypes 1 and 2, or their subunits, with or without adjuvant. However, the Expert Surveillance Panel of OIE and WHO Reference Laboratories has now recommended that the A/equine-1 component should be omitted as no infections with that subtype have been substantiated during the past 20 years. A modified live equine A2 influenza vaccine for intranasal administration has recently become available commercially in some countries. Requirements for such a vaccine may be anticipated to differ in some particulars from the following, which are appropriate to inactivated vaccines.

1. Seed management

a) Characteristics of the seed

An ongoing surveillance programme by OIE and WHO Reference Laboratories aimed at providing information on suitable vaccine strains is being coordinated by the OIE Reference Laboratory (Newmarket) (13). Recommendation on vaccine strains will be published annually in the *OIE Bulletin*.

The vaccine should contain representatives of subtype 2 viruses and should only contain subtype 1 viruses if there is evidence of field infection.

Subtype 1: A subtype 1 strain, such as A/equine/Prague/1/56, or a more recent subtype 1 strain may be used (5).

Subtype 2: Antigenic variants of subtype 2 viruses co-circulate (3). It is important to include recent isolates that are epidemiologically relevant to the region in which the vaccine is to be used. Typical European isolates include A/equine/Suffolk/89, A/equine/Borlange/91, and A/equine/Newmarket/2/93. Typical American isolates are represented by A/equine/Kentucky/94. American-like viruses appear on a regular basis and European viruses occasionally affect horses in America. Therefore it is recommended that vaccines contain representatives of both subfamilies, particularly where equine populations from several continents mix. Some vaccines also contain the original prototype strain A/equine/Miami/63. Vaccines containing Miami/63-like virus will not provide adequate protection against viruses currently circulating and the original prototype strain should be removed from vaccines.

b) Method of culture

Virus strains may be obtained from OIE Reference Laboratories (see Table given in Part 4 of this *Manual*). Viruses selected as vaccine strains should be described in terms of origin and passage history. The strains are propagated in the allantoic cavity of 10-day-old embryonated chicken eggs or cell cultures, such as MDCK. All manipulations must be conducted separately for each strain. Viral growth is monitored by HA tests. Passaged virus is identified by serological tests, such as HI or SRH. If vaccine virus is grown in cell culture, antigenic studies with ferret sera and MAbs should be undertaken to ensure that variant viruses have not been selected during passage to prepare master and working seed viruses. Master and working seed viruses are divided into aliquots and stored in freeze-dried form at –20°C or at –70°C following testing for extraneous agents. Records of storage conditions should be maintained.

The master seed lot of each vaccine strain selected should be processed at one time to assure a uniform composition, tested for extraneous agents, and fully characterised. Antisera, or MAbs for characterisation in HI tests, may be obtained from OIE and WHO reference laboratories.

Working seed lots are derived from a master seed lot and should be of uniform composition, free of extraneous agents, and fully characterised. Aliquots of the working seed are used for production of vaccine.

Master and working seed lots must be prepared in SPF (specific pathogen free) eggs and, as a minimum, in eggs derived from a healthy flock.

If MDCK cells are used to propagate vaccine virus, master cell lines should be established and stored in liquid N_2, and should test free from extraneous agents according to National Control Authority Guidelines.

Examination of seed viruses for extraneous agents including mycoplasmas and other equine viruses should be performed by appropriate techniques, including inoculation of susceptible tissue cultures and examination for CPE or application of fluorescent antibodies for antigen detection.

The presence of other common equine respiratory pathogens, e.g. equine herpesviruses 1, 4, 2, equine picornaviruses, equine viral arteritis, and equine adenoviruses, should be specifically excluded.

Absence of bacteria should be confirmed by standard sterility tests and toxicity tests in small animals.

c) Validation as a vaccine

For each vaccine strain, a prototype batch should be prepared to establish its suitability as a vaccine strain, i.e. purity and safety should be confirmed by standard techniques. The ability of seed-lot viruses to grow to high titre and generate sufficient antigenic mass to stimulate adequate antibody responses in the target species, should be confirmed.

Additionally, vaccine virus derived in MDCK cells should be fully characterised to ensure that antigenic variants have not arisen during the culture process, such that the vaccine virus is no longer representative of the original isolate.

2. Method of manufacture

Production is based on a seed-lot system that has been validated with respect to the characteristics of the vaccine strains. Each strain of virus is inoculated separately into the allantoic cavity of 9–11-day-old embryonating chicken eggs from a healthy flock. The eggs are incubated at a suitable temperature for 2–3 days, and the allantoic fluid is collected. The viral suspensions of each strain are collected separately and inactivated. If necessary, they may be purified. Suitable adjuvants and antimicrobial preservatives may be added.

Monovalent virus pools should be inactivated as soon as possible after their preparation, by a method approved by the National Control Authority. If formalin (40% formaldehyde) or beta-propiolactone (2-oxetanone) is used, the concentration by volume should not exceed 0.1%. Ideally, pools should be held at 4°C and should be inactivated within 5 days of harvest. The virus must be shown to have been inactivated. A suitable method consists of inoculating 0.2 ml of undiluted monovalent pool and 1/10 and 1/100 dilutions of the monovalent pool into the allantoic cavities of groups of fertile eggs (ten eggs in each group), and incubating the eggs at 33–37°C for 3 days. At least eight of the ten eggs should survive at each dosage level. A volume of 0.5 ml of allantoic fluid is harvested from each surviving egg. The fluid harvested from each group is pooled, and 0.2 ml of each of the three pools are inoculated, undiluted, into a further group of ten fertile eggs. Haemagglutinin activity should not be detected in these new groups of eggs. In some countries, the requirement that 80% of the eggs should survive during incubation may be impossible to satisfy. The National Control Authority should then specify the requirement to be satisfied. Before inactivation, samples should be collected for bacterial and fungal sterility tests.

Monovalent material may be concentrated and purified by high-speed centrifugation or other suitable methods approved by the National Control Authority, either before or after the inactivation procedure. It is important to concentrate and purify the virus under optimum conditions, e.g. temperatures that preserve its antigenic properties.

3. In-process control

Relevant in-process controls should be applied before and after inactivation and before and after concentration and purification.

In-process controls include: (a) identity of virus strains (tested by HI); (b) sterility; (c) virus titre; (d) haemagglutinin content (tested by chicken RBC agglutinating units – CCA); and (e) immunologically active HA (tested by single radial diffusion – SRD).

- **Single radial diffusion test**

SRD is a reliable method for measuring immunologically active HA in terms of µg HA, and is used routinely for potency testing human influenza vaccines (20).

The potency of inactivated equine influenza vaccine depends on the concentration of immunologically active haemagglutinin (14, 18, 19).

Assessment of the antigenic content of the vaccine by CCA alone may be misleading, as the sensitivity of this assay is a reflection of the ability of virus strains to agglutinate RBCs. Disruption of virus may lead to an apparent increase in HA as measured by CCA. CCAs do not provide a measure of the antigenic properties of the HA (HA may retain its properties to bind to RBCs while losing its ability to stimulate antibody).

The composition of some equine influenza vaccines is unusual in that products may contain more than one variant of the A/equine/2 (H3N8) subtype. In this situation, it is not possible to judge the potency of individual A/equine/2 components from serological tests performed on sera collected from horses or small animals vaccinated with the final product, because of cross-reactivity between the two isolates of the same subtype. Thus, it is important that a reliable method, such as SRD, be used to measure the potency of individual components, before and after inactivation and prior to mixing and adjuvanting.

In the SRD test, virus preparations are compared with a calibrated reference preparation of known HA content. Antigens are allowed to diffuse through a gel containing an antiserum specific for a particular haemagglutinin. The distance diffused by the antigen before precipitation by the antibody incorporated in the gel is directly related to the concentration of haemagglutinin in the antigen preparations (11).

Standard reagents for SRD testing are available from the WHO International Laboratory for Biological Standards[1]. At present, reagents for A/equine/1, Prague/56 (H7N7), A/equine/2/Miami/63, A/equine/2/ Kentucky/81 (H3N8), A/equine/2/Newmarket/1/93 (American-like), and A/equine/2/Newmarket/2/95 (European-like) viruses are available.

4. Batch control

a) Sterility

Tests for sterility and freedom from contamination of biological materials may be found in Chapter I.4.

b) Safety

i) Using no fewer than two horses, each horse is inoculated intramuscularly at two different sites with the dose of vaccine specified by the manufacturer; these inoculations are repeated 4 weeks later. The animals are kept under observation for 10 days after the second set of injections. No abnormal local or systemic reactions should ensue.

ii) If vaccine is to be used in mares, safety should be demonstrated by giving two doses of vaccine to no fewer than two pregnant mares at the prescribed interval within the trimester for which the vaccine is recommended.

c) Potency

Following mixing of viral antigens and adjuvants, aliquots should be potency tested *in vivo* using horses and guinea-pigs. Adjuvants cause interference in quantitative *in-vitro* tests, such as CCA and SRD, although SRD may be used on the final product as a qualitative assay to demonstrate the presence of antigen for each vaccine strain. For repeated batch tests, only guinea-pigs are used, subject to agreement of the National Control Authority.

i) *Serological responses in horses*

For a valid *in-vivo* potency test, naive seronegative horses must be selected for vaccination and serological tests to measure the antibody response to haemagglutinin must be standardised.

Young horses or ponies should be screened for the presence of antibody using recently isolated viruses relevant to the area from which the horses have been collected. If HI tests are used for screening, A/equine/2 viruses should be treated with Tween 80/ether to maximise the sensitivity of the test. Alternatively, SRH may be used to establish seronegative status of animals to A/equine/1 and A/equine/2 viruses.

To test a vaccine for efficacy in horses, a volume of the vaccine under test corresponding to one vaccine dose is injected by the recommended route into each of five susceptible seronegative horses.

1 National Institute for Biological Standards and Control, Blanche Lane, South Mimms, Potters Bar, Hertfordshire EN6 3QG, UK.

After a period of time recommended between the first and second doses, as stated on the label, a volume of vaccine corresponding to the second dose of vaccine is injected into each horse.

Three blood samples are collected from each animal, the first at the time of vaccination, the second 1 week after the first vaccination, and the third 2 weeks after the second vaccination.

The sera are tested by the HI or SRH test for antibodies to the A/equine/1 and A/equine/2 viruses contained in the vaccines (see Sections A.2.a. and A.2.b.).

The antibody titre of each serum, taken after the second vaccination in each test, should not be less than 1/64 (calculated for the original serum, taking into account the predilution of 1/8). If the titre found for any horse after the first vaccination indicated that there has been an anamnestic response, that result is not taken into account. A supplementary test is carried out, as described above, replacing the horses that showed an anamnestic response with an equal number of new animals. Alternatively, antibody may be measured by SRH, in which case the antibody titre should not be less than 150 mm^2. This is higher than the titre required in the European Pharmacopoeia Monograph for inactivated equine influenza vaccines (85 mm^2) as it is not considered to be protective.

HI tests, and to a lesser extent, SRH tests, vary in sensitivity between laboratories. Standard sera should be tested in parallel with the test sera to ensure that the test is valid with respect to sensitivity. Standard sera may be obtained from the OIE Reference Laboratories. Alternatively, the antibody levels stimulated by the vaccine under test should be shown to be at least equal to the antibody levels stimulated by a standard vaccine tested in parallel that has been shown previously to protect horses against challenge infection.

ii) *Challenge studies in horses*

It may be desirable in certain cases to undertake challenge studies in horses to demonstrate potency, particularly if vaccines are being assessed for their ability to protect against antigenically dissimilar viruses. Challenge studies may be carried out by exposing six vaccinated horses/ponies to an aerosol of virulent influenza virus no fewer than 2 weeks after the second dose of vaccine. Comparisons of clinical signs, virus excretion and serological responses are made with a group of six unvaccinated control animals challenged at the same time (11, 12). The timing of the challenge procedure will reflect the claims to be made on the data sheet regarding duration of immunity.

If tests for potency in horses have been carried out with satisfactory results on a representative batch of vaccine, these tests may be omitted as a routine control on other batches of vaccine prepared using the same seed-lot system, subject to agreement by the National Control Authority.

iii) *Serological responses of guinea-pigs*

In each of ten guinea-pigs free from specific antibodies, inject the dose stated on the label. Collect blood samples 21 days later, and separate the serum. Inactivate each serum by heating at 56°C for 30 minutes, and treat the sera as described above for horse sera.

Perform the tests of each serum using, respectively, the antigen(s) prepared from the strain(s) used in the production of the vaccine. Using each diluted serum, prepare a series of twofold dilutions. To 0.025 ml of each dilution, add 0.025 ml of a suspension of each antigen treated with ether or Tween 80/ether, respectively, and containing 4 HA units. Allow the mixtures to stand at 22°C (±2°C) for 30 minutes, and add 0.5 ml of a 0.5% suspension of chicken RBCs. Allow to stand at 22°C (±2°C) for 1 hour and note the last serum dilution that still completely inhibits HA. The antibody titre of each serum in each test should not be less than the titre stimulated by a standard vaccine that has been shown to stimulate protective levels of antibody in horses.

d) Duration of immunity

Where claims for duration of immunity are made on the data sheet, these should be supported with data on the duration of protective levels of antibody maintained in horses vaccinated according to the recommended schedule. Antibody levels quoted as protective should be validated in challenge studies (see Section B.4.c.ii.) or by comparison with published reports.

e) Stability

Vaccines should be stored at 5±3°C and protected from light. The shelf life quoted on the data sheet should be demonstrated by testing the potency of aliquots over time using the guinea-pig potency test (see Section B.4.c.iii.).

f) Preservatives

Preservatives are not normally included.

g) Precautions (hazards)

The contents of each opened vial should be used within 1 hour of opening. Aseptic precautions should be observed during administration, and only healthy horses should be vaccinated. Occasionally, transient local and/or general reactions may occur, and rest may be advisable for 24–48 hours after vaccination.

5. Tests on the final product

a) Safety

Tests are performed as described in Section B.4.b.i. Once safety has been demonstrated on a prototype batch, safety testing in pregnant mares may be omitted for routine testing of subsequent batches.

b) Potency

See Section B.4.c.iii. As a minimum, serological testing in guinea-pigs should be performed on each batch.

c) Maintaining epidemiologically relevant strains in vaccines

To enable vaccine manufacturers to respond quickly to recommendations from the Expert Surveillance Panel to update vaccine strains, the Committee for Veterinary Medicinal Products for the European Agency for the Evaluation of Medicinal Products has developed a fast-track licensing system when vaccine strains are updated (4).

REFERENCES

1. Chambers T.M., Shortridge K.F., Li P.H., Powell D.G. & Watkins K.L. (1994). Rapid diagnosis of equine influenza by the Directigen FLU-A enzyme immunoassay. *Vet. Rec.*, **135**, 275–279.

2. Cook R.F., Sinclair R. & Mumford J.A. (1988). Detection of influenza nucleoprotein antigen in nasal secretions from horses infected with A/equine influenza (H3N8) viruses. *J. Virol. Methods.*, **20**, 1–12.

3. Daly J.M., Lai A.C.K., Binns M.M., Chambers T.M., Barrandeguy M. & Mumford J.A. (1996). Antigenic and genetic evolution of equine H3N8 influenza A viruses. *J. Gen. Virol.*, **77**, 661–671.

4. European Agency for the Evaluation of Medicinal Products (EMEA), Committee for Veterinary Medicinal Products (CVMP) (1998). Note for Guidance: Harmonisation of Requirements for Equine Influenza Vaccines Specific Requirements for Substitution or Addition of a Strain or Strains. Document EMEA/CVMP/112/98-FINAL, EMEA, London, UK.

5. Gibson C.A., Daniels C.A., Oxford J.S. & McCauley J.W. (1992). Sequence analysis of the equine H7 influenza virus haemagglutinatinin gene. *Virus Res.*, **22**, 93–106.

6. Ilobi C.P., Henfrey R., Robertson J.S., Mumford J.A., Erasmus B.J. & Wood J.M. (1994). Antigenic and molecular characterisation of host-cell mediated variants of equine H3N8 influenza viruses. *J. Gen. Virol.*, **75**, 669–673.

7. John T.J. & Fulginiti V.A. (1966). Parainfluenza 2 virus: increase in haemagglutinin titre on treatment with Tween-80 and ether. *Proc. Soc. Exp. Biol. Med.*, **121**, 109–111.

8. Livesay G.J., O'Neill T., Hannant D, Yadav M.P. & Mumford J.A. (1993). The outbreak of equine influenza (H3N8) in the United Kingdom in 1989; diagnostic use of an antigen capture ELISA. *Vet. Rec.*, **133**, 515–519.

9. Morley P.S., Bogdan J.R., Townsend H.G.G. & Haines D.M. (1995). The effect of changing single radial haemolysis assay method when quantifying influenza A antibodies in serum. *Vet. Microbiol.*, **44**, 101–110.

10. Mumford J.A. (1992). Progress in the control of equine influenza. *In:* Equine Infectious Disease VI: Proceedings of the Sixth International Conference, Plowright W., Rossdale P.D. & Wade J.F., eds. Newmarket, R & W Publications, UK, 207–217.

11. MUMFORD J.A., HANNANT D. & JESSETT D.M. (1990). Experimental infection of ponies with equine influenza (H3N8) viruses by intranasal inoculation or exposure to aerosols. *Equine Vet. J.*, **22**, 93–98.

12. MUMFORD J.A. & WOOD J. (1993). Establishing an acceptability threshold for equine influenza vaccines. *Dev. Biol. Stand.*, **79**, 137–146.

13. MUMFORD J.A. & WOOD J. (1993). WHO/OIE Meeting: Consultation on Newly Emerging Strains of Equine Influenza. *Vaccine*, **11**, 1172–1175.

14. MUMFORD J., WOOD J.M., SCOTT A.M., FOLKERS C. & SCHILD G.C. (1983). Studies with inactivated equine influenza vaccine 2. Protection against experimental infection with influenza virus A/equine/Newmarket/79 (H3N8). *J. Hyg. (Camb.)*, **90**, 385–395.

15. PLATEAU E. & CRUCIERE C. (1983). Study on radial haemolysis method for the detection of anti influenza equiantibodies in equine sera: reliability and expression of the results. *Zentralbl. Veterinarmed [B]*, **30**, 512–520.

16. SCHILD G.C., PEREIRA, M.S. & CHAKRAVERTY P. (1975). Single radial haemolysis: a new method for the assay of antibody to influenza haemagglutinin. *Bull. WHO*, **52**, 43–50.

17. UNITED STATES DEPARTMENT OF HEALTH AND HUMAN SERVICES (1982). Concepts and Procedures for Laboratory-Based Influenza Surveillance. Centers for Disease Control, Atlanta, Georgia, USA, 81–835.

18. WOOD J.M., MUMFORD J., FOLKERS C., SCOTT A.M. & SCHILD G.C. (1983). Studies with inactivated equine influenza vaccine 1. Serological responses of ponies to graded doses of vaccine. *J. Hyg. (Camb.)*, **90**, 371–84.

19. WOOD J.M., SCHILD G.C., FOLKERS C., MUMFORD J. & NEWMAN R.W. (1983). The standardisation of inactivated equine influenza vaccines by single-radial immunodiffusion. *J. Biol. Stand.*, **11**, 133–136.

20. WOOD J.M., SCHILD G.C., NEWMAN R.W. & SEAGROATT V. (1977). An improved single-radial-immunodiffusion technique for the assay of influenza haemagglutinin antigen. Application for potency determinations of inactivated whole virus and subunit vaccines. *J. Biol. Stand.*, **5**, 237–247.

*

* *

CHAPTER 2.5.6.

EQUINE PIROPLASMOSIS

SUMMARY

Equine piroplasmosis or babesiosis is a tick-borne protozoal disease of horses, mules, donkeys and zebra. The aetiological agents are blood parasites named Babesia equi *(which has recently been described as* Theileria equi*) and* B. caballi. *Infected animals may remain carriers of these parasites for long periods and act as sources of infection for ticks, which act as vectors.*

Parasites occur in the blood of infected animals. The introduction of carrier animals into areas where tick vectors are prevalent can lead to an epizootic spread of the disease.

Identification of the agent: *Infected horses can be identified by demonstrating the parasites in stained blood or organ smears. Romanovsky-type staining methods, such as Giemsa, give the best results. In carrier animals low parasitaemias make it extremely difficult to detect parasites, especially in the case of* Babesia caballi *infections, although they may sometimes be demonstrated by using a thick blood smear technique.*

Paired merozoites joined at their posterior ends are a diagnostic feature of B. caballi *infection. The merozoites of* B. equi *are less than 2–3 µm long, and are round or amoeboid. A characteristic of* B. equi *is the arrangement of four parasites in a tetrad or 'Maltese cross'.*

When equivocal results are encountered in serological tests, the subinoculation of a large quantity of whole blood transfused into a susceptible splenectomised horse will assist diagnosis. The recipient horse is observed for clinical signs of disease and its red blood cells are examined for parasites. Alternatively, a specific tick vector is fed on a suspect animal and Babesia *may then be identified either in the vector or through transmission by the vector to another susceptible animal.*

Serological tests: *Infections in carrier animals are best demonstrated by testing their sera for the presence of specific antibodies.*

Currently, the complement fixation (CF) test is the primary test used for qualifying horses for importation. Other serological techniques are the indirect fluorescent antibody (IFA) test and enzyme-linked immunosorbent assay (ELISA). The IFA test can be used to distinguish between B. equi *and* B. caballi *infections. ELISA may be used to detect antibodies to both species in infected horses, although cross-reactions between* B. equi *and* B. caballi *occur, so that this cannot yet be recommended as a differential diagnostic test. However, recent advances using recombinant* B. equi *and* B. caballi *merozoite proteins and monoclonal antibodies to these proteins in competitive inhibition ELISAs appear to be very promising. The competitive ELISA may be superior to CF tests, at least for* B. equi, *especially for detecting long-term infected animals in which the CF titre has waned but which remain IFA seropositive.*

Requirements for vaccines and diagnostic biologicals: *There are no biological products available.*

A. DIAGNOSTIC TECHNIQUES

Equine piroplasmosis or babesiosis is a tick-borne protozoal disease of horses, mules, donkeys and zebra. The aetiological agents of equine piroplasmosis are *Babesia equi* and *B. caballi.* Twelve species of ixodid ticks in the genera *Dermacentor, Rhipicephalus* and *Hyalomma* have been identified as trans-stadial vectors of *B. caballi* and *B. equi*, while eight of these species were also able to transmit *B. caballi* infections transovarially (3, 24, 29, 30). Infected animals may remain carriers of these blood parasites for long periods and will act as sources of infection for vector ticks.

The parasites occur in southern Europe, Asia, countries of the former Union of Soviet Socialist Republics, Africa, Cuba, South and Central America, and certain parts of the southern United States of America. *Babesia equi* has also been reported from Australia (but, apparently never established itself in this region), and is now believed to have a wider general distribution than *B. caballi*.

1. Identification of the agent

Horses that are already infected may be identified by demonstrating the parasites in stained blood or organ smears. For this, Romanowsky-type staining methods, such as the Giemsa method, usually give the best results (28).

The low parasitaemias of carrier animals make it extremely difficult to detect the parasites in smears, especially in the case of infections with *B. caballi*. When the parasites occur at such low levels, experienced workers can sometimes detect them by the use of a thick blood smear technique (19). Thick films are made by placing a small drop (approximately 50 µl) of blood on to a clean glass slide. This droplet is then air-dried, heat fixed at 80°C for 5 minutes, and stained in 5% Giemsa for 20–30 minutes.

An accurate identification of the species of the parasite is sometimes desirable, as mixed infections of *B. equi* and *B. caballi* probably occur frequently.

a) Clinical signs

The clinical signs of equine piroplasmosis are often nonspecific, and the disease can easily be confused with other conditions.

Piroplasmosis can occur in peracute, acute and chronic forms. The acute cases are more common, and are characterised by a fever that usually exceeds 40°C, reduced appetite and malaise, elevated respiratory and pulse rates, congestion of mucous membranes, and smaller and drier than normal faecal balls.

Clinical signs in subacute cases are similar. In addition, affected animals show loss of weight, and the fever is sometimes intermittent. The mucous membranes vary from pale pink to pink, or pale yellow to bright yellow. Petechiae and/or ecchymoses may also be visible on the mucous membranes. Normal bowel movements may be slightly depressed and the animals may show signs of mild colic. Mild oedematous swelling of the distal part of the limbs sometimes occurs.

Chronic cases usually present nonspecific clinical signs such as mild inappetence, poor performance and a drop in body mass. The spleen is usually found to be enlarged on rectal examination.

A rare peracute form where horses are found either dead or moribund, has been reported (17).

b) The parasites

During the life cycle of *Babesia*, the merozoites invade red blood cells (RBCs) where they transform into trophozoites (6, 26). In this situation the trophozoites grow and divide into two round, oval or pear-shaped merozoites. The mature merozoites are now capable of infecting new RBCs and the division process is then repeated.

Babesia caballi: the merozoites in the RBCs are pear-shaped, 2–5 µm long and 1.3–3.0 µm in diameter (16). The paired merozoites joined at their posterior ends are considered to be a diagnostic feature of *B. caballi* infection (20).

Babesia equi (which has recently been described as *Theileria equi* [21]): the merozoites of this organism are relatively small, less than 2–3 µm long (16), and are round or amoeboid. Often four parasites are to be found together in the form of a tetrad or so-called 'Maltese cross' arrangement. This is a characteristic feature of *B. equi* (9).

It has been shown that sporozoites inoculated into horses via a tick bite invade the lymphocytes (27). The sporozoites undergo development in the cytoplasm of these lymphocytes and eventually form *Theileria*-like schizonts. Apparently, merozoites released from these schizonts enter other RBCs. The taxonomic position of *B. equi* appears to be uncertain at present. Further support for the close relation between *B. equi* and *Theileria* spp. has recently come from the homology found between 30 and 34 kDa *B. equi* surface proteins and similar sized proteins of various *Theileria* spp. (12, 14). However, comparison of the small subunit ribosomal RNA genes of various *Babesia*, *Theileria* and *Cytauxzoon* parasites indicates that *B. equi* falls into a distinct group different from both the *Babesia* and *Theileria* groups (1).

2. Serological tests

It is extremely difficult to diagnose the organisms in carrier animals by means of the microscopic examination of blood smears. Furthermore, it is by no means practical on a large scale. The serological testing of animals is therefore recommended as a preferred method of diagnosis, especially when horses are destined to be imported into countries where the disease does not occur, but the vector is present.

Sera should be collected and dispatched to diagnostic laboratories in accordance with the specifications of that laboratory. Horses for export that have been subjected to serological tests and shown to be free from infection, should be kept free of ticks to prevent accidental infections.

A number of serological techniques have been used in the diagnosis of babesiosis, such as the complement fixation (CF) test, the indirect fluorescent antibody (IFA) test, and the enzyme-linked immunosorbent assay (ELISA).

a) Complement fixation (a prescribed test for international trade)

The CF test is the primary test used by some countries to qualify horses for importation (31). A detailed description of antigen production and test protocol has been given, for example by the United States Department of Agriculture (USDA) (2, 5, 33). Because the CF test may not identify all infected animals, especially those that have been treated, and because of the anticomplementary reactions produced by some sera, the IFA test has also been accepted for use as a prescribed test for international trade. An example of a CF protocol is given below.

- **Solutions**

Alsever's solution: prepare the volume of Alsever's solution required by using the following amounts of ingredients per litre: 20.5 g glucose; 8.0 g sodium citrate; 4.2 g sodium chloride; sufficient distilled water to dissolve, and make up to 1 litre with distilled water. Adjust to pH 6.1 using citric acid. Sterilise by filtration.

Stock veronal buffer (5X): dissolve the following in 1 litre distilled water: 85.0 g sodium chloride; 3.75 g sodium 5.5 diethyl barbiturate; 1.68 g magnesium chloride ($MgCl_2.6H_2O$); 0.28 g calcium chloride. Dissolve 5.75 g of 5.5 diethyl barbituric acid in 500 ml hot (near boiling) distilled water. Cool this acid solution and add to the salt solution. Make up to 2000 ml with distilled water and store at 4°C. To prepare a working dilution, add one part stock solution to four parts distilled water. Final pH should be from 7.4 to 7.6.

- **Antigen production**

Blood is collected, in an equal volume of Alsever's solution as an anticoagulant, from horses at the height of the reaction (3–7% parasitaemia for *B. caballi* and 60–85% for *B. equi*). The plasma/Alsever's supernatant and buffy coat is removed when the RBCs have settled to the bottom of the flask. The RBCs are washed several times with cold veronal buffer and then disrupted. The antigen is recovered from the lysate by centrifugation at 30,900 *g* for 30 minutes.

The recovered antigen is washed several times in cold veronal buffer by centrifugation at 20,000 *g* for 15 minutes. Polyvinyl pyrrolidone 40,000 (1–5%[w/v]) is added as a stabiliser and the preparation is mixed on a magnetic stirrer for 30 minutes, strained through two thicknesses of sterile gauze, dispensed into 2 ml volumes and freeze-dried. The antigen can then be stored at below –50°C for several years.

- **Test procedure**

i) The specificity and potency of each batch of antigen should be checked against standard antisera of known specificity and potency. Optimal antigen dilutions are also determined in a preliminary checkerboard titration.

ii) Test sera are inactivated for 35 minutes at 58°C (donkey and mule sera are inactivated at 62.5°C for 35 minutes) and tested in dilutions of 1/5 to 1/5120. Veronal buffer is used for all dilutions.

iii) Complement is prepared and titrated spectrophotometrically to determine the 50% haemolytic dose ($C'H_{50}$) (30). In the test 5.0 $C'H_{50}$ are used. The haemolytic system consists of equal parts of a 2% sheep (RBCs) suspension and veronal buffer with 5 minimum haemolytic doses (MHDs) of haemolysin (amboceptor) (33). Some laboratories use twice the 100% haemolytic dose, which gives equivalent sensitivity.

iv) The test has been adapted to microtitration plates (8). The total volume of the test is 0.125 ml, made up of equal portions (0.025 ml) of antigen, complement (5.0 $C'H_{50}$) and diluted serum. Incubation is performed for 1 hour at 37°C.

v) A double portion (0.05 ml) of the haemolytic system is added and the plates are incubated for a further 45 minutes at 37°C with shaking after 20 minutes.

vi) The plates are centrifuged for 1 minute at 200 ***g*** before being read over a mirror.

vii) A lysis of 50% is recorded as positive, with the titre being the greatest serum dilution giving 50% lysis. A titre of 1/5 is regarded as positive. A full set of controls (positive and negative sera) must be included in each test as well as control antigen prepared from normal (uninfected) horse RBCs.

Anticomplementary samples are examined by the IFA test. Donkey sera are frequently anticomplementary.

b) Indirect fluorescent antibody test (a prescribed test for international trade)

The IFA test has been successfully applied to the differential diagnosis of *B. equi* and *B. caballi* infections (18). The recognition of a strong positive reaction is relatively simple, but any differentiation between weak positive and negative reactions requires considerable experience in interpretation. A detailed description of the protocol of the IFA test has been given (18, 23). An example of an IFA protocol is given below.

- **Antigen production**

Blood for antigen is obtained from horses with a rising parasitaemia, ideally 2–5%. Carrier animals are not suitable for antigen production as they have already produced antibodies. Blood (about 15 ml) is collected into 235 ml of phosphate buffered saline (PBS), pH 7.2. The RBCs are washed three times in cold PBS (1000 ***g*** for 10 minutes at 4°C). The supernatant fluid and the white cell layer are removed after each wash. After the last wash, the packed RBCs are reconstituted to normal volume with 4% bovine serum albumin fraction V made up in PBS, i.e. the original packed cell volume = 30%, so that one-third consists of RBCs. If the original RBC volume is 15 ml, then 5 ml of packed RBCs + 10 ml of 4% bovine albumin in PBS constitutes the antigen. After thorough mixing, the antigen is placed in prepared wells on a glass slide using a template or a syringe (23). Alternatively, the cells can be spread smoothly on to microscope slides, covering the entire slide with an even, moderately thick film. These slides are allowed to dry, wrapped in soft paper and sealed in plastic bags or wrapped in aluminium foil, and stored at –20°C for up to 1 year.

- **Test procedure**

i) Each sample of serum is tested against an antigen of *B. caballi* and of *B. equi*.

ii) Prior to use, the antigen smears are removed from storage at –20°C and incubated at 37°C for 10 minutes.

iii) The antigen slides are then removed from their protective covering and fixed in cold dry acetone (–20°C) for 1 minute.

iv) If smears were prepared, squares (14–21 in number, i.e. 2–3 rows of 7 each) are formed on the antigen slides with nail varnish.

v) Test, positive and negative control sera are diluted from 1/80 to 1/1280 in PBS. Negative and positive control sera are included in each test.

vi) Sera are applied (10 µl each) at appropriate dilutions to the different wells or squares on the antigen slide, incubated at 37°C for 30 minutes, and washed several times in PBS and once in water.

vii) An anti-horse immunoglobulin prepared in rabbits is conjugated with fluorescein isothiocyanate and applied to the slide, which is then incubated and washed as before.

viii) After the final wash, two drops of a solution containing equal parts of glycerin and PBS are placed on each slide and mounted with a cover-slip.

ix) The slides are then examined for the fluorescing parasites. Sera diluted 1/80 or more that show strong fluorescence are usually considered to be positive, although due consideration is also given to the patterns of fluorescence of the positive and negative controls.

c) Enzyme-linked immunosorbent assay

The ELISA has also been used to detect antibodies to both species of the parasite in experimentally infected horses (7, 22). It is apparent that cross-reactions between *B. equi* and *B. caballi* occur (7, 22, 34). It appears, therefore, that more studies are required before the ELISA can be recommended as a diagnostic method to differentiate between species of *Babesia*.

Recent advances in this field have shown that a recombinant *B. equi* merozoite protein and a specific monoclonal antibody (MAb), which defines this merozoite surface protein epitope, can be used successfully in a competitive inhibition ELISA (C-ELISA) (13). This C-ELISA overcomes the problem of antigen purity, as the specificity of this test depends only on the MAb used. A 94% correlation was shown between the C-ELISA and CF test in detecting antibodies to *B. equi.* Sera that gave discrepant results were evaluated for their ability to immunoprecipitate ^{35}S-methionine-labelled *in-vitro* translated products of *B. equi* merozoite mRNA. Samples that were C-ELISA (+) CF (–) clearly precipitated multiple *B. equi* proteins. However, immunoprecipitation results with serum samples that were C-ELISA (–) CF (+) were inconclusive (15). Limited data at this stage would suggest that the C-ELISA is specific for *B. equi* (15). Recombinant antigens produced in *Escherichia coli* have the obvious advantage of removing the need to infect horses for antigen production, and provide a consistent source of antigen for international distribution and standardisation.

d) DNA probes

Sensitive and specific DNA probes have been isolated for both *B. equi* and *B. caballi* (25). In this test, parasite DNA is extracted from a blood sample, spotted on to a nylon membrane, and then examined with the relevant radiolabelled DNA probe. These probes have been shown to detect parasites in some carrier animals and could provide a possible solution to the problems experienced with serological tests, where horses are destined for the export market and need to be free of the parasites. However, these tests need further refinement and the sensitivity must be increased before they can be used to certify horses to be free from either *B. equi* or *B. caballi.*

3. Biological tests

• Subinoculation of blood

False-negative or false-positive reactions may be encountered in the course of serological tests (4, 5, 32). In such cases the passage of whole blood, although a cumbersome and expensive exercise, is a very useful technique to determine the true position. Large quantities of whole blood (500 ml) are transfused into a susceptible, preferably splenectomised, horse. This animal is then kept under close observation for clinical signs of disease. Diagnosis is confirmed by the presence of parasites in its RBCs.

In an additional technique, a specific clean vector tick is fed on a suspect animal, and the organism can then either be identified in the tick itself, or through the transmission of the organism by the vector tick to another susceptible animal.

• *In-vitro* cultivation

Success in the establishment of long-term *in-vitro* cultures of *B. equi* and *B. caballi* may be one alternative to supplement the methods described above, in order to identify carriers of the parasites (10, 11, 35, 36). *Babesia caballi* parasites were successfully cultured from the blood of two horses that tested negative by the CF test (11). Similarly, *B. equi* could be cultured from horses that did not show any patent parasitaemias at the time of the initiation of the cultures (34, 35).

B. REQUIREMENTS FOR VACCINES AND DIAGNOSTIC BIOLOGICALS

No biological products are available currently.

REFERENCES

1. ALLSOPP M.T.E.P., CAVALIER-SMITH T., DE WAAL D.T. & ALLSOPP B.A. (1994). Phylogeny and evolution of the piroplasms. *Parasitol.*, **108**, 147–152.

2. BROWN G.M. (1979). Equine piroplasmosis complement fixation test antigen production. USDA, APHIS, National Veterinary Services Laboratories. Diagnostic Reagents Laboratory, Ames, Iowa. USA NVSL Diagnostic Production Guide No. R–72/73/74.

3. DE WAAL D.T. & POTGIETER F.T. (1987). The transstadial transmission of *Babesia caballi* by *Rhipicephalus evertsi evertsi. Onderstepoort J. Vet. Res.*, **54**, 655–656.

4. DONNELLY J., JOYNER L.P., GRAHAM-JONES O. & ELLIS C.P. (1980). A comparison of the complement fixation and immunofluorescent antibody titres in a survey of the prevalence of *Babesia equi* and *Babesia caballi* in horses in the Sultanate of Oman. *Trop. Anim. Health Prod.*, **12**, 50–60.

5. FRERICHS W.M., HOLBROOK A.A. & JOHNSON A.J. (1969). Equine piroplasmosis: Complement-fixation titres of horses infected with *Babesia caballi*. *Aust. J. Vet. Res.*, **30**, 697–702.

6. FRIEDHOFF K. (1970). Studies on the fine structure of *Babesia bigemina, B. divergens* and *B. ovis*. Proceedings of the Second International Congress of Parasitology. *J. Parasitol.*, **56**, Section 2 (1), 110.

7. GOTZ F. (1982). Untersuchungen über die Brauchbarkeit von ELISA, IFAT, IHA, und KBR zum Nachweis von *Babesia equi* Infectionen. Vet. Med. Diss., Munich. Germany.

8. HERR S., HUCHZERMEYER H.F.K.A., TE BRUGGE L.A., WILLIAMSON C.C., ROOS J.A. & SCHIELE G.J. (1985). The use of a single complement fixation test technique in bovine brucellosis, Johne's disease, dourine, equine piroplasmosis and Q fever serology. *Onderstepoort J. Vet. Res.*, **52**, 279–282.

9. HOLBROOK A.A., JOHNSON A.J. & MADDEN B.S. (1968). Equine piroplasmosis: Intraerythrocytic development of *Babesia caballi* (Nuttall) and *Babesia equi* (Laveran). *Am. J. Vet. Res.*, **29**, 297–303.

10. HOLMAN P.J., CHIEVES L., FRERICHS W.M., OLSON D. & WAGNER G.G. (1994). *Babesia equi* erythrocytic stage continuously cultured in an enriched medium. *J. Parasitol.*, **80**, 232–236

11. HOLMAN P.J., FRERICHS W.M., CHIEVES L. & WAGNER G.G. (1993). Culture confirmation of the carrier status of *Babesia caballi*-infected horses. *J. Clin. Microbiol.*, **31**, 698–701.

12. KAPPMEYER L.S., PERRYMAN L.E. & KNOWLES D.P (1993). A *Babesia equi* gene encodes a surface protein with homology to *Theileria* species. *Mol. Biochem. Parasitol.*, **62**, 121–124.

13. KNOWLES D.P., KAPPMEYER L.S. & PERRYMAN L.E. (1997). Genetic and biochemical analysis of erythrocyte-stage surface antigens belonging to a family of highly conserved proteins of *Babesia equi* and *Theileria* species. *Mol. Biochem. Parasitol.*, **90**, 69–79.

14. KNOWLES D.P., KAPPMEYER L.S., STILLER D., HENNAGER S.G. & PERRYMAN L.E. (1992). Antibody to a recombinant merozoite protein epitope identifies horses infected with *Babesia equi*. *J. Clin. Microbiol.*, **30**, 3122–3126.

15. KNOWLES D.P., PERRYMAN L.E. & KAPPMEYER L.S. (1991). Detection of equine antibody to *Babesia equi* merozoite proteins by a monoclonal antibody-based competitive inhibition enzyme-linked immunosorbent assay. *J. Clin. Microbiol.*, **29**, 2056–2058.

16. LEVINE N.D. (1985). Veterinary Protozoology. Iowa State University Press, Ames, Iowa, USA.

17. LITTLEJOHN A. (1963). *In:* Babesiosis, Bone J.F., Catcott E.J., Gabel A.A., Johnson L.E. & Riley W.F., eds. Equine Medicine and Surgery. American Veterinary Publications, California, USA, 211–220.

18. MADDEN P.A. & HOLBROOK A.A. (1968). Equine piroplasmosis: Indirect fluorescent antibody test for *Babesia caballi*. *Am. J. Vet. Res.*, **29**, 117–123.

19. MAHONEY D.F. & SAAL J.R. (1961). Bovine babesiosis: Thick blood films for the detection of parasitaemia. *Aust. Vet. J.*, **37**, 44–47.

20. MEHLHORN H. & SCHEIN E. (1984). The piroplasms: Life cycle and sexual stages. *Adv. Parasitol.*, **23**, 37–103.

21. MEHLHORN H. & SCHEIN E. (1998). Redescription of *Babesia equi* Laveran, 1901 as *Theileria equi*. *Parasitol. Res.*, **84**, 467–475.

22. MERKLE F.J. (1983). Untersuchungen über die Brauchbarkeit von KBR, IFAT, und ELISA zum Nachweis der *Babesia caballi*-Infectionen des Pferdes. Vet. Med. Diss., Munich, Germany.

23. MORZARIA S.P., BROCKLESBY D.W. & HARRADINE D.L. (1977). Evaluation of the indirect fluorescent antibody test for *Babesia major* and *Theileria mutans* in Britain. *Vet. Rec.*, **100**, 484–487.

24. NEITZ W.O. (1956). Classification, transmission and biology of piroplasms of domestic animals. *Ann. N.Y. Acad. Sci.*, **64**, 56–111.

25. POSNETT E.S. & AMBROSIO R.E. (1989). Repetitive DNA probes for the detection of *Babesia equi*. *Mol. Biochem. Parasitol.*, **34**, 75–78.

26. POTGIETER F.T. & ELS H.J. (1977). The fine structure of intra-erythrocytic stages of *Babesia bigemina*. *Onderstepoort J. Vet. Res.*, **44**, 157–168.

27. SCHEIN E., REHBEIN G., VOIGT W.P. & ZWEYGARTH E. (1981). *Babesia equi* (Leveran, 1901). 1. Development in horses and in lymphocyte culture. *Tropenmed. Parasitol.*, **32**, 223–227.

28. SHUTE P.G. (1966). The staining of malaria parasites. *Trans. R. Soc. Trop. Med. Hyg.*, **60** , 412–416.

29. STILLER D. & FRERICHS W.M. (1979). Experimental transmission of *Babesia caballi* to equids by different stages of the tropical horse tick, *Anocentor nitens*. *Recent Adv. Acarol.*, **2**, 262–268.

30. STILLER D., FRERICHS W.M., LEATCH G. & KUTTLER K.L. (1980). Transmission of equine babesiosis and bovine anaplasmosis by *Dermacentor albipictus* (Packard) (Acari: Ixodidae). *J. N.Y. Ent. Soc.*, **88**, 75–76.

31. TAYLOR W.M., BRYANT J.E., ANDERSON J.B. & WILLERS K.H. (1969). Equine piroplasmosis in the United States – A review. *J. Am. Vet. Med. Assoc.*, **155**, 915–919.

32. TENTER A.M. & FRIEDHOFF K.T. (1986). Serodiagnosis of experimental and natural *Babesia equi* and *B. caballi* infections. *Vet. Parasitol.*, **20**, 49–61.

33. UNITED STATES DEPARTMENT OF AGRICULTURE (USDA) ANIMAL AND PLANT HEALTH INSPECTION SERVICE, VETERINARY SERVICES (1997). Complement fixation test for the detection of antibodies to *Babesia caballi* and *Babesia equi* – microtitration test. USDA, National Veterinary Services Laboratories, Ames, Iowa, USA.

34. WEILAND G. (1986). Species-specific serodiagnosis of equine piroplasma infections by means of complement fixation test (CFT), immunofluorescence (IFF), and enzyme-linked immunosorbent assay (ELISA). *Vet. Parasitol.*, **20**, 43–48.

35. ZWEYGARTH E., JUST M.C. & DE WAAL D.T. (1995). Continuous *in vitro* cultivation of erythrocytic stages of *Babesia equi*. *Parasitol. Res.*, **81**, 355–358.

36. ZWEYGARTH E., JUST M.C. & DE WAAL D.T. (1997). *In vitro* cultivation of *Babesia equi:* detection of carrier animals and isolation of parasites. *Onderstepoort J. Vet Res.*, **64**, 51–56.

*

* *

CHAPTER 2.5.7.

EQUINE RHINOPNEUMONITIS

SUMMARY

Equine rhinopneumonitis (ER) is a collective term for any one of several highly contagious, clinical disease entities of equids that may occur as a result of infection by either of two closely related herpesviruses, equid herpesvirus-1 and -4 (EHV-1 and EHV-4). Both EHV-1 and EHV-4 are world-wide in distribution and constitute an extremely prevalent health risk for domestic horses of all ages and categories, as well as for other members of the Equidae family.

Infection by either EHV-1 or EHV-4 is characterised by a primary respiratory tract disease of varying severity that is related to age and immunological status of the infected animal. Infections by EHV-1 in particular are capable of progression beyond the respiratory mucosa to cause the more serious disease manifestations of abortion, perinatal foal death, or neurological dysfunction. In most cases, primary EHV-1 or EHV-4 infection is followed by virus latency. In response to naturally encountered stresses (weaning, transport, social disruption, etc.), the viruses may be reactivated in latently infected animals and transmitted to other susceptible horses.

***Identification of the agent:** The standard method of identification of the herpesviral agents of ER continues to be laboratory isolation of the virus from appropriate clinical or necropsy material followed by seroconfirmation of their identity. The viruses can be readily isolated in equine cell culture from nasopharyngeal samples taken from horses during the febrile stage of respiratory tract infection, from liver, lung, spleen, or thymus of aborted fetuses, and from the leukocyte fraction of the blood of animals with acute EHV-1 disease. Positive identification of viral isolates as EHV-1 or EHV-4 can be achieved by immunofluorescence with type-specific monoclonal antibodies.*

A rapid presumptive diagnosis of rhinopneumonitis abortion can be achieved by direct immunofluorescent detection of viral antigen in cryostat sections of tissues from aborted fetuses, using conjugated polyclonal antiserum.

Sensitive and reliable methods for EHV-1/4 detection by polymerase chain reaction or immunoperoxidase staining have been developed recently and are useful adjuncts to standard virus cultivation techniques for diagnosis of ER.

Post-mortem demonstration of the characteristic histopathological lesions of EHV-1 in tissues from aborted fetuses or in the central nervous system of neurologically affected animals complements the laboratory diagnosis of ER.

***Serological tests:** Because most horses will possess some level of antibody to EHV-1/4, the demonstration of specific antibody in the serum collected from a single blood sample is not sufficient for a positive diagnosis of recent, active ER. Paired, acute and convalescent sera from animals suspected of being infected with EHV-1 or EHV-4 can be tested for a significant rise in virus-specific antibody titre by either complement fixation (CF), virus neutralisation, or enzyme linked immunosorbent assay. If a single convalescent serum is the only sample available, the CF test is the most informative serological test to perform.*

***Requirements for vaccines and diagnostic biologicals:** Both live attenuated and inactivated viral vaccines of varying composition are commercially available for use in assisting in the control of ER. While vaccination is helpful in reducing the incidence of abortion in mares, and in ameliorating the severity of clinical signs of respiratory infection in young horses, it should not be considered to be a substitute for strict adherence to the well-established tenets of sound management practices known to reduce the risk of rhinopneumonitis. Revaccination at frequent* *intervals is recommended with each of the products, as the duration of vaccine-induced immunity is relatively short.*

Standards for production and licensing of both attenuated and inactivated EHV vaccines are established by appropriate veterinary regulatory agencies in the countries of vaccine manufacture and use. A single set of internationally recognised standards for ER vaccines is not available. In each case, however, vaccine production is based on the system of a detailed outline of production employing a well-characterised cell line and a master seed lot of vaccine virus that has been validated with respect to virus identity, safety, virological purity, immunogenicity, and the absence of extraneous microbial agents.

A. DIAGNOSTIC TECHNIQUES

Equine rhinopneumonitis (ER) is a historically derived term that describes a constellation of several disease entities of horses that may include respiratory disease, abortion, neonatal foal pneumonitis, or myeloencephalopathy (1, 6, 8). The disease has been recognised for over 60 years as a threat to the international horse industry, and is caused by either of two members of the Herpesviridae family, equid herpesvirus-1 and -4 (EHV-1 and EHV-4). EHV-1 and EHV-4 are closely related alphaherpesviruses of the horse with nucleotide sequence identity within individual homologous genes ranging from 55% to 84%, and amino acid sequence identity from 55% to 96% (23, 24). The two herpesviruses are enzootic in all countries in which large populations of horses are maintained as part of the cultural tradition or agricultural economy. Herpesviruses closely related to EHV-1/4 have been isolated from several equid species other than the domestic horse, e.g. zebras, onagers, and donkeys. In rare instances, EHV-1 infection has been documented in some nonequid animal species, e.g. domestic cattle (abortion), llamas and alpacas (optic nerve neuropathy and blindness), and captive gazelle (encephalitis). There is no recorded evidence that the two herpesviruses of ER pose any health risks to humans working with the agents.

ER is highly contagious among susceptible horses, with viral transmission to cohort animals occurring by inhalation of aerosols of virus-laden respiratory secretions. Extensive use of vaccines has not eliminated EHV infections, and the world-wide annual financial burden from these equine pathogens is immense. Development of bioengineered mutants and vector-delivered subunit constructs of EHV-1 is in progress and may show some promise in the development of future vaccines, including marker vaccines.

In horses under 3 years of age, clinical ER usually takes the form of an acute, febrile respiratory illness that spreads rapidly through the group of animals. The viruses infect and multiply in epithelial cells of the respiratory mucosa. Signs of infection become apparent 2–8 days after exposure to virus, and are characterised by fever, inappetence, depression, and nasal discharge. The severity of respiratory disease varies with the age of the horse and the level of immunity resulting from previous vaccination or natural exposure. Subclinical infections with EHV-1/4 are common, even in young animals. Although mortality from uncomplicated ER is rare and complete recovery within 1–2 weeks is the normal pattern, the respiratory infection is a frequent and significant cause of interrupted schedules among horses assembled for training, racing, or competitive equestrian events. Fully protective immunity resulting from infection is of short duration, and convalescent animals are susceptible to reinfection by EHV-1/4 after several months. Although reinfections by the two herpesviruses cause less severe or clinically inapparent respiratory disease, the risks for subsequent abortion and/or central nervous system (CNS) disease are not eliminated.

Though respiratory disease is, in economic terms, the most costly result of EHV-1/4 infections, by far the greatest clinical threats to individual breeding, racing, or pleasure horse operations posed by ER are the potential abortigenic and neurological sequelae of EHV-1 respiratory infection. A fortuitous combination of several unique biological properties possessed by this member of the equine herpesvirus pair accounts for its capacity for systemic spread beyond the local environment of the horse's respiratory tract to cause abortion and/or paralytic disease: (a) its propensity for systemic dissemination within virus-infected, circulating leukocytes; (b) its capacity for direct spread from an infected leukocyte to contiguous cells without a required extracellular phase; and (c) its tropism for vascular endothelial cells. The end pathogenetic result of these specialised properties of EHV-1 is infection of endothelial cells by virus-infected leukocytes as they circulate through the vasculature of the gravid mare's endometrium, or the CNS of any category of horse (2). The former may result in abortion with or, more rarely, without infection of the fetus, and the latter may result in EHV-1-related neurological disorders. In contrast, EHV-4 is infrequently associated with sporadic abortions in mares.

Herpesvirus abortion in mares is a disease of the final 4 months of gestation. The preceding EHV-1 respiratory tract infection, which may occur from 7 to 80 days before the abortion event, is in most cases clinically unnoticeable in mares of breeding age. Each abortion occurs as a sudden event without warning signs in the mare. The proportion of at-risk mares that abort cannot be predicted and may be as low as a single animal or as high as 70% of those exposed to the virus. Mares infected very late in gestation with EHV-1 may give birth to infected, live foals with severe interstitial viral pneumonitis complicated by secondary bacterial pneumonia. Such foals invariably die within a few days after birth from overwhelming respiratory tract pathology.

EHV-1 and EHV-4 neurological disease may affect any age or gender of horse, including mares within a group in which abortion is occurring. Although the range and severity of neurological signs associated with EHV-1 infection are broad, some form of hindlimb incoordination and weakness is common to most cases. More severely affected animals may exhibit further progression to either hindlimb or quadripedal paralysis, accompanied by sternal or lateral recumbency. Both morbidity and mortality rates in horses with EHV-1 neurological disease are highly variable from outbreak to outbreak. Following recovery from ER, horses usually remain latently infected with the virus for life. Such latently infected carrier animals provide a large, clinically inapparent reservoir for the two herpesviruses that serves as a source for initiation of new outbreaks of infection and disease. Natural reactivation of latent equine herpesviruses is associated with management activities that produce stress – weaning, transport, castration, climatic extremes, and the introduction of new animals into established social groups. Strict adherence to farm or stable management practices designed to minimise the occurrence of such environmental stress factors is important, therefore, for reducing the risk of rhinopneumonitis.

1. Identification of the agent (3, 26)

Because ER is a highly contagious disease with the potential for occurring as explosive outbreaks with high mortality from abortigenic or neurological sequelae, rapid diagnostic methods are important. Although several rapid and innovative diagnostic techniques based on enzyme-linked immunosorbent assay (ELISA), polymerase chain reaction (PCR), immunohistochemical staining with peroxidase, or nucleic acid hybridisation probes have been recently described, their use is often restricted to specialised reference laboratories, and thus the method of choice for diagnosis of ER by diagnostic virology laboratories handling many routine samples continues to be the traditional methodology of cell culture isolation followed by sero-identification of the isolated viruses. Successful laboratory isolation of EHV-1/4 depends on strict adherence to proper methods for both sample collection and laboratory processing.

a) Collection of samples

Samples of nasopharyngeal exudate for virus isolation are best obtained from horses during the very early, febrile stages of the respiratory disease, and are collected via the nares by swabbing the nasopharyngeal area with a 5 × 5 cm gauze sponge attached to the end of a 50 cm length of flexible, stainless steel wire encased in latex rubber tubing. After collection, the swab should be removed from the wire and transported immediately to the virology laboratory in 3 ml of cold (not frozen) fluid transport medium (serum-free MEM [minimal essential medium] with antibiotics). Virus infectivity can be prolonged by the addition of appropriate concentrations of bovine serum albumin or gelatin.

Virological examination of fetal tissues from suspect cases of EHV-1 abortion is most successful when performed on aseptically collected samples of liver, lung, thymus, and spleen. The tissue samples should be transported to the laboratory and held at 4°C until inoculated into tissue culture. Samples that cannot be processed within a few hours should be stored at –70°C. In ante-mortem cases of EHV-1 neurological disease, the virus can often be isolated from the leukocyte fraction of the blood of acutely infected horses or, less often, from the nasopharynx of the affected animal or cohort animals. For attempts at virus isolation from blood leukocytes, a 15–20 ml sample of sterile blood, collected in citrate, EDTA (ethylene diamine tetra-acetic acid), or heparin anticoagulant, should be transported without delay to the laboratory on ice, but not frozen. Although the virus has, on occasion, been isolated from post-mortem cases of EHV-1 neurological disease by culture of samples of brain and spinal cord, such attempts to isolate virus are often unsuccessful.

b) Virus isolation

For efficient primary isolation of EHV-4 from horses with respiratory disease, equine-derived cell cultures must be used. Both EHV-1 and EHV-4 may be isolated from nasopharyngeal samples using primary equine fetal kidney cells or cell strains of equine fibroblasts derived from dermal (E-Derm) or lung tissue. The nasopharyngeal swab along with its accompanying 3 ml of transport medium are transferred into the barrel of a sterile 10 ml syringe. Using the syringe plunger, the fluid is squeezed from the swab into a sterile tube. A portion of the expressed fluid is then filtered through a sterile, 0.45 µm membrane syringe filter unit into a second sterile tube. Recently prepared cell monolayers in 25 cm² tissue culture flasks are inoculated with 0.5 ml of the filtered, as well as the nonfiltered, nasopharyngeal swab extract. Multiwell plates may also be used. Virus is allowed to attach by incubating the inoculated monolayers at 37°C on a platform rocker for 1.5–2 hours. Monolayers of uninoculated control cells should be incubated in parallel with sterile transport medium only.

At the end of the attachment period, the inocula are removed and the monolayers are rinsed twice with phosphate buffered saline (PBS) to remove virus-neutralising antibody that may be present in the nasopharyngeal secretions. After addition of 5 ml of supplemented maintenance medium (MEM containing 2% fetal calf serum [FCS] and twice the standard concentrations of antibiotics [penicillin, streptomycin, gentamicin, and amphotericin B]), the flasks are incubated at 37°C. The use of positive control virus samples to validate the isolation procedure carries the risk that this may lead to eventual contamination of diagnostic specimens. This risk can be minimised by using routine precautions and good laboratory technique, including the use of biosafety cabinets, inoculating positive controls after the diagnostic specimens, decontaminating the surfaces in the hood while the inoculum is asorbing and using a positive control of relatively low titre. Inoculated flasks should be inspected daily by microscopy for the appearance of characteristic herpesvirus cytopathic effect (CPE) (focal rounding, increase in refractility, and detachment of cells). Cultures exhibiting no evidence of viral CPE after 1 week of incubation may be blind-passaged into freshly prepared monolayers of cells, using small aliquots of both media and cells as the inoculum. Blind passage is usually not productive.

A number of cell types may be used for isolation of EHV-1 from the tissues of aborted fetuses or from post-mortem cases of neurological disease (e.g. rabbit kidney [RK-13], baby hamster kidney [BHK-21], Madin–Darby bovine kidney [MDBK], etc.), but equine-derived cell cultures are most sensitive and must be used if the infrequent cases of EHV-4 abortion are to be detected. Around 10% (w/v) pooled tissue homogenates of liver, lung, thymus, and spleen (from aborted fetuses) or of CNS tissue (from cases of neurological disease) are used for virus isolation. These are prepared by first mincing small samples of tissue into 1 mm cubes in a sterile Petri dish with dissecting scissors, followed by macerating the tissue cubes further in serum-free culture medium with antibiotics using a mechanical tissue grinder (e.g. Ten-Broeck or Stomacher). After centrifugation at 1200 ***g*** for 10 minutes, the supernatant is removed and 0.5 ml is inoculated into duplicate cell monolayers in 25 cm^2 flasks. Following incubation of the inoculated cells at 37°C for 1.5–2 hours, the inocula are removed and the monolayers are rinsed twice with PBS. After addition of 5 ml of supplemented maintenance medium, the flasks are incubated at 37°C for up to 1 week or until viral CPE is observed.

Culture of peripheral blood leukocytes for the presence of EHV-1 is frequently successful in horses during the early stages of the paralytic disease. On receipt by the diagnostic laboratory, the tube of chilled blood, containing citrate or heparin as anticoagulant, is mixed by inversion and allowed to stand for 1 hour at room temperature. The top layer of leukocyte-rich plasma is removed and centrifuged at 640 ***g*** for 15 minutes. After decanting the supernatant, the leukocyte pellet is resuspended in the small volume of residual supernatant by brief vortexing of the tube. The resuspended cells are then rinsed twice with 10 ml of sterile PBS by centrifugation (300 ***g*** for 10 minutes) and resuspension. After the last centrifugation, the leukocyte pellet is resuspended in 1 ml of MEM containing 2% FCS and the resulting cell suspension is used for inoculating duplicate monolayers of equine fibroblast or RK-13 cell cultures. Then 0.5 ml of the rinsed leukocyte suspension harvested from each tube of blood is added to each of two 25 cm^2 flasks of cells containing 8–10 ml of freshly added maintenance medium. The flasks are incubated at 37°C for 7 days; the inoculum is not removed. Because CPE may be difficult to detect in the presence of the massive inoculum of leukocytes, each flask of cells is freeze–thawed after 7 days of incubation. Finally, 0.5 ml of the cell-free culture medium from each flask is transferred to freshly made cell monolayers. These are incubated and observed for viral CPE for at least 5–6 days before discarding as negative.

c) Seroconfirmation of virus identity

The basis for identification of any herpesvirus isolate recovered from specimens submitted from suspected cases of ER is its immunoreactivity with specific antisera. Specific identification of an isolate as EHV-1 or EHV-4 can be quickly and simply accomplished by immunofluorescent detection of viral antigen in the infected cell culture using type-specific monoclonal antibodies (MAbs). The test, which is type-specific and accurate, can be performed on a small aliquot of infected cells from the same container inoculated with clinical or post-mortem material. An isolate made in a laboratory that lacks MAbs can be confirmed as EHV-1/4 using a polyclonal antiserum.

Cell monolayers infected with the isolate are removed by scraping from the flask when at least 75% CPE is evident. The cells are pelleted from the culture medium and resuspended in 0.5 ml of PBS. 50 µl of the cell suspension are placed into two wells of a multiwell microscope slide, air-dried, and fixed for 10 minutes with 100% acetone. Control cell suspensions (uninfected, EHV-1 infected, or EHV-4 infected) are also spotted into each of two wells of the same slide. Control cells may be prepared in advance and stored frozen in small aliquots. A drop of an appropriate dilution of MAb specific for EHV-1 is added to one well of each cell pair, and a drop of MAb specific for EHV-4 is added to each of the other wells. After 30 minutes' incubation at 37°C in a humid chamber, unreacted antibody is removed by two 10-minute washes with PBS. MAbs bound to viral antigen can be detected with goat anti-mouse IgG conjugated with fluorescein isothiocyanate (FITC). A drop of diluted conjugate is added to each well and, after 30 minutes at 37°C, the wells are again washed twice with PBS. Cells are examined with a fluorescence microscope, and positive fluorescence with the antibody of appropriate specificity indicates the virus type.

d) Virus detection by direct immunofluorescence

Direct immunofluorescent detection of EHV-1 antigens in samples of post-mortem tissues collected from aborted equine fetuses provides an indispensable method to the veterinary diagnostic laboratory for making a rapid preliminary diagnosis of herpesvirus abortion (10). Side-by-side comparisons of the immunofluorescent and cell culture isolation techniques on more than 100 cases of equine abortion have provided evidence that the diagnostic reliability of direct immunofluorescent staining of fetal tissues obtained at necropsy approaches that of virus isolation attempts from the same tissues. In the United States of America (USA), specific and potent polyclonal antiserum to EHV-1, prepared in swine and conjugated with FITC, is provided to veterinary diagnostic laboratories for this purpose by the National Veterinary Services Laboratory of the United States Department of Agriculture (USDA). The antiserum cross-reacts with EHV-4 and hence is not useful for serotyping. Freshly dissected samples (5 × 5 mm pieces) of fetal tissue (lung, liver, thymus, and spleen) are frozen, sectioned on a cryostat at –20°C, mounted on to microscope slides, and fixed with 100% acetone. After air-drying, the sections are incubated at 37°C in a humid atmosphere for 30 minutes with an appropriate dilution of the conjugated swine antibody to EHV-1. Unreacted antibody is removed by two washes in PBS, and the tissue sections are then covered with aqueous mounting media and a cover-slip, and examined for fluorescent cells indicating the presence of EHV-1 antigen. Each test should include a positive and negative control consisting of sections from known EHV-1 infected and uninfected fetal tissue.

Cytocentrifuge preparations of peripheral blood mononuclear cells (PBMC) collected from suspect ante-mortem cases of EHV-1 myeloencephalopathy may also be examined for viral antigen by immunofluorescence after incubation, as described above, with virus-specific, FITC-conjugated antiserum. The sensitivity of the latter test for EHV-1 antigen is greatly enhanced if performed on leukocyte preparations cultured *in vitro* for 2–4 days in the presence of a T cell mitogen (e.g. pokeweed mitogen), which amplifies the frequency of virus-infected cells (20, 22).

e) Virus detection by immunoperoxidase staining

Enzyme immunohistochemical (IH) staining methods (e.g. immunoperoxidase) have been developed recently as procedures for detecting EHV-1 antigen in paraffin-embedded tissues of aborted equine fetuses or neurologically affected horses (19, 29). Such ancillary IH techniques for antigen detection may facilitate identification of the virus in archival tissue samples or in clinical cases in which traditional laboratory methods for EHV-1 detection have been unsuccessful. Immunoenzymatic staining for EHV-1 is particularly useful for the simultaneous evaluation of morphological lesions and the identification of the infectious agent. Adequate controls must be included with each immunoperoxidase test run for evaluation of both the method specificity and antibody specificity (11).

f) Virus detection by polymerase chain reaction

The PCR can be used for rapid amplification and diagnostic detection of nucleic acids of EHV-1 and -4 in clinical specimens, paraffin-embedded archival tissue, or inoculated cell cultures (4, 5, 12–18, 21, 27, 28). A variety of type-specific PCR primers have been designed to distinguish between the presence of EHV-1 and EHV-4. The correlation between PCR and virus-isolation techniques for diagnosis of EHV-1 or EHV-4 is of the order of 85% (4, 13, 17, 21, 27). Diagnosis of ER by PCR is rapid, sensitive, and does not depend on the presence of infectious virus in the clinical sample. It now forms an integral part of a range of diagnostic tests currently available for ER, each with its own advantages and limitations.

For diagnosis of active infection by EHV, PCR methods are most reliable with samples from aborted fetuses or from nasopharyngeal swabs of foals and yearlings; they are most useful in explosive epizootics of abortion or respiratory tract disease in which a rapid identification of the virus is critical for guiding management strategies. The interpretation of the amplification by PCR of genomic fragments of EHV-1 or EHV-4 in tissues (lymph nodes, peripheral blood leukocytes, or CNS) from adult horses is complicated by the high prevalence of latent EHV-1 and EHV-4 DNA in circulating lymphocytes and the trigeminal ganglia of such animals (28).

g) Histopathology

Histopathological examination of sections of formalin-fixed, paraffin-embedded tissues from aborted fetuses or from neurologically affected horses is an essential part of the laboratory diagnosis of these two clinical manifestations of ER. In aborted fetuses, typical herpetic intranuclear inclusion bodies present within bronchiolar epithelium or in cells at the periphery of areas of hepatic necrosis are pathognomonic lesions for EHV-1. The characteristic, but not pathognomonic, microscopic lesion associated with EHV-1 neuropathy is a degenerative thrombotic vasculitis of small blood vessels in the brain or spinal cord (perivascular cuffing and infiltration by inflammatory cells, endothelial proliferation and necrosis, and thrombus formation).

2. Serological tests

Because of the ubiquity of the viral agents of ER and the high seroprevalence among horses in most parts of the world, the demonstration of a negative antibody titre to EHV-1/4 by serological testing of horses designated for export is not part of present veterinary regulations that seek to prevent international spread of infectious diseases of horses. Serological testing can, however, be a useful adjunct procedure for assisting in the diagnosis of ER in horses. Serodiagnosis of ER is based on the demonstration of significant increases in antibody titres in paired sera taken during the acute and convalescent stages of the disease. The results of tests performed on sera from a single collection date are, in most cases, impossible to interpret with any degree of confidence. The initial (acute phase) serum sample should be taken as soon as possible after the onset of clinical signs, and the second (convalescent phase) serum sample should be taken 3–4 weeks later. Samples of cerebrospinal fluid may also be of value in serodiagnosis of EHV-1 neurological disease. 'Acute phase' sera from mares after abortion or from horses with EHV-1 neurological disease may already contain maximal titres of EHV-1 antibody, with no increase in titres detectable in sera collected at later dates. In such cases, serological testing of paired serum samples from clinically unaffected cohort members of the herd for rising antibody titres against EHV-1/4 may provide information useful for retrospective diagnosis of ER within the herd. Finally, the serological detection of antibodies to EHV-1 in heart or cord blood or other fluids of equine fetuses can be of diagnostic value in rare cases of virologically negative fetuses aborted as a result of EHV-1 infection.

Serum antibody levels to EHV-1/4 may be determined by ELISA (9), virus neutralisation (VN) (25), or complement fixation (CF) tests (25). Because CF antibody titres to EHV-1/4 become negative within a few months following recovery from infection, the CF test is most useful in diagnosing recent infection by the herpesviruses if a convalescent serum is the only sample available for testing. The CF test performed on sera collected from horses with the paralytic form of EHV-1 infection is also useful for making the rapid diagnosis necessary for initiating appropriate measures for control of the spread of this contagious disease. Because there are no internationally recognised reagents or standardised techniques for performing any of the serological tests for detection of EHV-1/4 antibody, antibody titre determinations on the same serum may differ from one laboratory to another. Furthermore, all of the serological tests mentioned detect antibodies that are cross-reactive between EHV-1 and EHV-4. Nonetheless, the demonstration, by any of the tests, of a four-fold or greater rise in antibody titre to EHV-1 or EHV-4 during the course of a clinical illness provides serological confirmation of recent infection with one of the viruses. The ELISA and CF test have the advantage that they are quicker to provide results and do not require cell culture facilities. Recently, a type-specific ELISA that can distinguish between antibodies to EHV-1 and EHV-4 was developed and is made commercially available (7). The microneutralisation test is a widely used and sensitive serological assay for detecting EHV-1/4 antibody and will thus be described here.

a) Virus neutralisation test

This serological test is most commonly performed in flat-bottom 96-well microtitre plates (tissue culture grade) using a constant dose of virus and doubling dilutions of equine test sera. At least two replicate wells for each serum dilution are required. Serum-free MEM is used throughout as a diluent. Virus stocks of known titre are diluted just before use to contain 100 $TCID_{50}$ (50% tissue culture infective dose) in 25 µl. Monolayers of E-Derm or RK-13 cells are monodispersed with ethylene diamine tetra-acetic acid/trypsin and resuspended at a concentration of 5×10^5/ml. Note that RK-13 cells can be used with EHV-1 but do not give clear CPE with EHV-4. Antibody positive and negative control equine sera and controls for cell viability, virus infectivity, and test serum cytotoxicity, must be included in each assay. End-point VN titres of antibody are calculated by determining the reciprocal of the highest serum dilution that protects 100% of the cell monolayer from virus destruction in both of the replicate wells.

A suitable test procedure is as follows:

i) Inactivate test and control sera for 30 minutes in a water bath at 56°C.

ii) Add 25 µl of serum-free MEM to all wells of the microtitre assay plates.

iii) Pipette 25 µl of each test serum into duplicate wells of both rows A and B of the plate. The first row serves as the serum toxicity control and the second row as the first dilution of the test. Make doubling dilutions of each serum starting with row B and proceeding to the bottom of the plate by sequential mixing and transfer of 25 µl to each subsequent row of wells. Six sera can be assayed in each plate.

iv) Add 25 µl of the appropriately diluted EHV-1 or EHV-4 virus stock to each well (100 $TCID_{50}$/well) except those of row A, which are the serum control wells for monitoring serum toxicity for the indicator cells. Note that the final serum dilutions, after addition of virus, run from 1/4 to 1/256.

v) A separate control plate should include titration of both a negative and positive horse serum of known titre, cell control (no virus), virus control (no serum), and a virus titration to calculate the actual amount of virus used in the test.

vi) Incubate the plates for 1 hour at 37°C in 5% CO_2 atmosphere.

vii) Add 50 µl of the prepared E-Derm or RK-13 cell suspension (5 × 10^5 cells/ml) in MEM–10% FCS to each well.

viii) Incubate the plates for 4–5 days at 37°C in an atmosphere of 5% CO_2 in air.

ix) Examine the plates microscopically for CPE and record the results on a worksheet. Alternatively, the cell monolayers can be scored for CPE after fixing and staining as follows: after removal of the culture fluid, immerse the plates for 15 minutes in a solution containing 2 mg/ml crystal violet, 10% formalin, 45% methanol, and 45% water. Then, rinse the plates vigorously under a stream of running tap water.

x) Wells containing intact cell monolayers stain blue, while monolayers destroyed by virus do not stain. Verify that the cell control, positive serum control, and serum cytotoxicity control wells stain blue, that the virus control and negative serum control wells are not stained, and that the actual amount of virus added to each well is between $10^{1.5}$ and $10^{2.5}$ $TCID_{50}$. Wells are scored as positive for neutralisation of virus if 100% of the cell monolayer remains intact. The highest dilution of serum resulting in complete neutralisation of virus (no CPE) in both duplicate wells is the end-point titre for that serum.

xi) Calculate the neutralisation titre for each test serum, and compare acute and convalescent phase serum titres from each animal for a four-fold or greater increase.

B. REQUIREMENTS FOR VACCINES AND DIAGNOSTIC BIOLOGICALS

Both live attenuated and inactivated vaccines are available as licensed, commercially prepared products for use as prophylactic aids in reducing the burden of disease in horses caused by EHV-1/4 infection. Clinical experience has demonstrated that none of the vaccine preparations should be relied on to provide an absolute degree of protection from ER. Multiple doses, repeated annually, of each of the currently marketed ER vaccines are recommended by their respective manufacturers, with vaccination schedules that vary with the particular vaccine.

In the USA, eight vaccine products for ER, each containing different permutations of EHV-1, EHV-4, and the two subtypes of equine influenza virus, are currently marketed by four veterinary biologicals manufacturers. Four of the ER vaccines contain equine herpesviruses only; these vaccines contain prototypic and B-variant strains of EHV-1, or a single strain of EHV-1, or both EHV-1 and EHV-4. The only live virus ER vaccine currently licensed for use in the USA consists of a strain of EHV-1 attenuated by multiple serial passages in porcine and rabbit cell cultures. This vaccine is available either as EHV-1 alone or as a combination of live EHV-1 and inactivated equine influenza subtypes 1 and 2.

The clinical indications stated on the product label for use of the several available vaccines for ER are either herpesvirus-associated respiratory disease, abortion, or both. Of the eight vaccines manufactured for ER in the USA, only two have met the United States Department of Agriculture (USDA) regulatory requirements for claiming efficacy in providing protection from herpesvirus abortion as a result of successful vaccination and challenge experiments in pregnant mares. None of the vaccine products has been tested for their ability to prevent the occurrence of neurological disease sometimes associated with EHV-1 infection.

Each of the four manufacturers of vaccines for ER in the USA also markets a combination vaccine product containing a mixture of equine herpesvirus and both subtypes of inactivated equine influenza virus. The herpesvirus component of the combined vaccines may be either inactivated EHV-4, inactivated EHV-1 and EHV-4, or live attenuated EHV-1.

Additional ER vaccine preparations, both live-attenuated and inactivated, are manufactured in Europe under guidelines set forth in the European Pharmacopoeia. Several other vaccine manufacturers are presently at some stage in development of their own lines of vaccine for ER. These include bioengineered vector constructs expressing EHV-1 antigens, as well as EHV-1 mutants lacking one or more genes required for full virulence in the horse. The latter are intended for testing as live-attenuated virus vaccine candidates.

1. Seed management

a) Characteristics and culture

The master seed virus (MSV) for ER vaccines must be prepared from strains of EHV-1 and/or EHV-4 that have been positively and unequivocally identified by both serological and genetic tests. Seed virus must be propagated in a cell line approved for equine vaccine production by the appropriate regulatory agency. A complete record of original source, passage history, medium used for propagation, etc., shall be kept for the master seed preparations of both the virus(es) and cell stock(s) intended for use in vaccine production. Permanently stored stocks of both MSV and master cell stock (MCS) used for vaccine production must be demonstrated to be pure, safe and, in the case of MSV, also immunogenic. Generally, the fifth passage from the MSV and the twentieth passage from the MCS are the highest allowed for vaccine production. Results of all quality control tests on master seeds must be recorded and made a part of the licensee's permanent records.

b) Validation as a vaccine

i) *Purity*

Tests for master seed purity include prescribed procedures that demonstrate the virus and cell seed stocks to be free from bacteria, fungi, mycoplasmas, and extraneous viruses. Special tests must be performed to confirm the absence of equine arteritis virus, equine infectious anaemia virus, equine influenza virus, equine herpesvirus-2, -3, and -5, equine rhinovirus, the alphaviruses of equine encephalomyelitis, bovine viral diarrhoea virus (BVDV – common contaminant of bovine serum), and porcine parvovirus (PPV – potential contaminant of porcine trypsin). The purity check should also include the exclusion of the presence of EHV-1 from EHV-4 MSV and vice versa.

ii) *Safety*

Samples of each lot of MSV to be used for preparation of live attenuated ER vaccines must be tested for safety in horses determined to be susceptible to the virulent wild-type virus, including pregnant mares in the last 4 months of gestation.

Vaccine safety must be demonstrated in a 'safety field trial' in horses of various ages from three different geographical areas. The safety trial should be conducted by independent veterinarians using a prelicensing batch of vaccine. EHV-1 vaccines making a claim for efficacy in controlling abortion must be tested for safety in a significant number of late gestation pregnant mares, using the vaccination schedule that will be recommended by the manufacturer for the final vaccine product.

iii) *Immunogenicity*

Tests for immunogenicity of the EHV-1/4 MSV stocks should be performed in horses on an experimental test vaccine prepared from the highest passage level of the MSV allowed for use in vaccine production. The prescribed test for MSV immunogenicity consists of vaccination of horses with low antibody titres to EHV-1/4, with doses of the test vaccine that will be recommended on the final product label. Second serum samples should be obtained and tested for significant increases in neutralising antibody titre against the virus, 21 days after the final dose.

iv) *Efficacy*

An important part of the validation process is the capacity of a prelicensing lot of the ER vaccine to provide a significant level of clinical protection in horses from the particular disease manifestation of EHV-1/4 infection for which the vaccine is offered, when used under the conditions recommended by the manufacturer's product label. Serological data are not acceptable for establishing the efficacy of vaccines for ER. Efficacy studies must be designed to ensure appropriate randomisation of test animals to treatment groups, blinding of the recording of clinical observations, and the use of sufficient numbers of animals to permit statistical evaluation for effectiveness in prevention or reduction of the specified clinical disease. The studies should be performed on fully formulated experimental vaccine products (a) produced in accordance with, (b) at or below the minimum antigenic potency specified in, and, (c) produced with the highest passage of MSV and MCS allowed by the approved 'Outline of Production' (see section B.2.). Vaccine efficacy is demonstrated by vaccinating a minimum of 20 EHV-1/4-susceptible horses possessing low serum neutralising antibody titres, followed by challenge of the vaccinates and 10 nonvaccinated control horses with virulent virus. A significant difference in the clinical signs of ER must be demonstrated between vaccinates and nonvaccinated control horses. The vaccination and challenge study must be performed on an identical number of pregnant mares and scored for abortion if the vaccine product will make a label usage claim 'for prevention of' or 'as an aid in the prevention of' abortion caused by EHV-1.

2. Method of manufacture

A detailed protocol of the methods of manufacture to be followed in the preparation of vaccines for ER must be compiled, approved, and filed as an Outline of Production with the appropriate licensing agency. Specifics of the methods of manufacture for ER vaccines will differ with the type (live or inactivated) and composition (EHV-1 only, EHV-1 and EHV-4, EHV-4 and equine influenza viruses, etc.) of each individual product, and also with the manufacturer.

3. In-process control

Cells, virus, culture medium, and medium supplements of animal origin that are used for preparation of production lots of vaccine must be derived from bulk stocks that have passed the prescribed tests for bacterial, fungal, and mycoplasma sterility; nontumorigenicity; and absence of extraneous viral agents.

4. Batch control

Each bulk production lot of ER vaccine must pass tests for sterility, safety, and immunogenic potency.

a) Sterility

Samples taken from each batch of completed vaccine are tested for bacteria, fungi, and mycoplasma contamination. Procedures to establish that the vaccine is free from extraneous viruses are also required; such tests should include inoculation of cell cultures that allow detection of the common equine viruses, as well as techniques for the detection of BVDV and PPV in ingredients of animal origin used in the production of the batch of vaccine.

b) Safety

Tests to assure safety of each production batch of ER vaccine must demonstrate complete inactivation of virus (for inactivated vaccines) as well as a level of residual virus-killing agent that does not exceed the maximal allowable limit (e.g. 0.2% for formaldehyde). Safety testing in laboratory animals is also required.

c) Potency

Batch control of antigenic potency for EHV-1 vaccines may be tested by measuring the ability of dilutions of the vaccine to protect hamsters from challenge with a lethal dose of hamster-adapted EHV-1 virus. Although potency testing on production batches of ER vaccine may also be performed by vaccination of susceptible horses followed by either viral challenge or assay for seroconversion, the recent availability of virus type-specific MAbs has permitted development of less costly and more rapid *in-vitro* immunoassays for antigenic potency. The basis for such *in-vitro* assays for ER vaccine potency is the determination, by use of the specific MAb, of the presence of at least the minimal amount of viral antigen within each batch of vaccine that correlates with the required level of protection (or seroconversion rate) in a standard animal test for potency.

d) Duration of immunity

Tests to establish the duration of immunity to EHV-1/4 achieved by immunisation with each batch of vaccine are not required. The results of many reported observations indicate that vaccination-induced immunity to EHV-1/4 is not more than a few months in duration; these observations are reflected in the frequency of revaccination recommended on ER vaccine product labels.

e) Stability

At least three production batches of vaccine should be tested for shelf life before reaching a conclusion on the vaccine's stability. When stored at 4°C, inactivated vaccine products generally maintain their original antigenic potency for at least 1 year. Lyophilised preparations of the live virus vaccine are also stable during storage for 1 year at 4°C. Following reconstitution, live virus vaccine is unstable and cannot be stored without loss of potency.

5. Tests on the final product

Before release for labelling, packaging, and commercial distribution, randomly selected filled vials of the final vaccine product must be tested by prescribed methods for freedom from contamination and safety in laboratory test animals.

a) Safety

See Section B.4.b.

b) Potency

See Section B.4.c.

REFERENCES

1. ALLEN G.P. & BRYANS J.T. (1986). Molecular epidemiology, pathogenesis and prophylaxis of equine herpesvirus-1 infections. *In:* Progress in Veterinary Microbiology and Immunology, Vol. 2, Pandey R., ed. Karger, Basel, Switzerland & New York, USA, 78–144.

2. ALLEN G.P., KYDD J.H., SLATER J.D. & SMITH K.C. (1999). Recent advances in understanding the pathogenesis, epidemiology, and immunological control of equid herpesvirus-1 (EHV-1) abortion. *Equine Infect. Dis.*, **8**, 129–146.

3. ALLEN G.P., KYDD J.H., SLATER J.D. & SMITH K.C. (2000). Equid herpesvirus-1 (EHV-1) and -4 (EHV-4) infections. *In:* Infectious Diseases of Livestock, Coetzer J.A.W., Thomson G.R. & Tustin R.C., eds. Oxford University Press, Cape Town, South Africa (in press).

4. BALLAGI-PORDANY A., KLINGEBORN B., FLENSBURG J. & BELAK S. (1990). Equine herpesvirus type 1: detection of viral DNA sequences in aborted fetuses with the polymerase chain reaction. *Vet. Microbiol.*, **22**, 373–381.

5. BORCHERS K. & SLATER J. (1993). A nested PCR for the detection and differentiation of EHV-1 and EHV-4. *J. Virol. Methods*, **45**, 331–336.

6. BRYANS J.T. & ALLEN G.P. (1988). Herpesviral diseases of the horse. *In:* Herpesvirus Diseases of Animals, Wittman G., ed. Kluwer, Boston, USA, 176–229.

7. CRABB B.S. , MACPHERSON C.M., REUBEL G.H., BROWNING G.F., STUDDERT M.J. & DRUMMER H.E. (1995). A type-specific serological test to distinguish antibodies to equine herpesviruses 4 and 1. *Arch. Virol.*, **140**, 245–258.

8. CRABB B.S. & STUDDERT M.J. (1995). Equine herpesvirus 4 (equine rhinopneumonitis virus) and 1 (equine abortion virus). *Adv. Virus Res.*, **45**, 153–190.

9. DUTTA S.K., TALBOT N.C. & MYRUP A.C. (1983). Detection of equine herpesvirus-1 antigen and the specific antibody by enzyme-linked immunosorbent assay. *Am. J. Vet. Res.*, **44**, 1930–1934.

10. GUNN H.M. (1992). A direct fluorescent antibody technique to diagnose abortion caused by equine herpesvirus. *Irish Vet. J.*, **44**, 37–40.

11. HAINES D.M. & CHELACK B.J. (1991). Technical considerations for developing enzyme immunohistochemical staining procedures on formalin-fixed paraffin-embedded tissues for diagnostic pathology. *J. Vet. Diagn. Invest.*, **3**, 101–112.

12. KIRASAWA R., ENDO A., IWAI H. & KAWAKAMI Y. (1993). Detection and identification of equine herpesvirus-1 and -4 by polymerase chain reaction. *Vet. Microbiol.*, **36**, 57–67.

13. LAWRENCE G.L., GILKERSON J., LOVE D.N., SABINE M. & WHALLEY J.M. (1994). Rapid, single-step differentiation of equid herpesvirus 1 and 4 from clinical material using the polymerase chain reaction and virus-specific primers. *J. Virol. Methods*, **47**, 59–72.

14. MACKIE J.T., MACLEOD G.A., TEUBEL G.H. & STUDDERT M.J. (1996). Diagnosis of equine herpesvirus 1 abortion using polymerase chain reaction. *Aust. Vet. J.*, **74**, 390–391.

15. O'KEEFE J.S., JULIAN A., MORIARTY K., MURRAY A. & WILKS C.R. (1994). A comparison of the polymerase chain reaction with standard laboratory methods for the detection of EHV-1 and EHV-4 in archival tissue samples. *N. Z. Vet. J.*, **42**, 93–96.

16. O'KEEFE J.S., MURRAY A., WILKS C.R. & MORIARTY K.M. (1991). Amplification and differentiation of the DNA of an abortigenic (type 1) and a respiratory (type 4) strain of equine herpesvirus by the polymerase chain reaction. *Res. Vet. Sci.*, **50**, 349–351.

17. RIMSTAD E. & EVENSEN O. (1993). The identification of equid herpesvirus 1 in paraffin-embedded tissues from aborted fetuses by polymerase chain reaction and immunohistochemistry. *J. Vet. Diagn. Invest.*, **5**, 174–183.

18. RIMSTAD E. & HYLLSETH B. (1994). Equine herpesviruses 1 and 4: amplification and differentiation by polymerase chain reaction. *Acta Vet. Scand.*, **35**, 303–306.

19. SCHULTHEISS P.C., COLLINS J.K. & CARMAN J. (1993). Use of an immunoperoxidase technique to detect equine herpesvirus-1 antigen in formalin-fixed paraffin-embedded equine fetal tissues. *J. Vet. Diagn. Invest.*, **5**, 12–15.

20. SCOTT J.C., DUTTA S.K. & MYRUP A.C. (1983). *In vivo* harboring of equine herpes virus 1 in leukocyte populations and subpopulations and their quantitations from experimentally infected ponies. *Am. J. Vet. Res.*, **44**, 1344–1348.

21. SHARMA P.C., CULLINANE A.A., ONIONS D.E. & NICOLSON L. (1992). Diagnosis of equid herpesviruses -1 and -4 by polymerase chain reaction. *Equine Vet. J.*, **24**, 20–25.

22. SMITH D.J., IQBAL J., PUREWAL A., HAMBLIN A.S. & EDINGTON N. (1998). *In vitro* reactivation of latent equid herpesvirus-1 from CD5+/CD8+ leukocytes indirectly by IL-2 or chorionic gonadotrophin. *J Gen. Virol.*, **79**, 2997–3004.

23. TELFORD E.A.R., WATSON M.S., MCBRIDE K. & DAVISON A.J. (1992). The DNA sequence of equine herpesvirus-1. *Virology*, **189**, 304–316.

24. TELFORD E.A.R., WATSON M.S., PERRY J., CULLINANE A.A. & DAVISON A.J. (1998). The DNA sequence of equine herpesvirus 4. *J. Gen. Virol.*, **79**, 1197–1203.

25. THOMSON G.R., MUMFORD J.A., CAMPBELL J., GRIFFITHS L. & CLAPHAM P. (1976). Serological detection of equid herpesvirus 1 infections of the respiratory tract. *Equine Vet. J.*, **8**, 58–65.

26. TIMONEY P.J. (1992). Rhinopneumonitis and viral abortion. *In:* Veterinary Diagnostic Virology: A Practitioner's Guide, Castro A. & Heuschele W., eds. Mosby Year Book Publishers, USA, 173–177.

27. WAGNER W.N., BOGDAN J., HAINES D., TOWNSEND H.G.G. & MISRA V. (1992). Detection of equine herpesvirus and differentiation of equine herpesvirus type 1 from type 4 by the polymerase chain reaction. *Can. J. Microbiol.*, **38**, 1193–1196.

28. WELCH H.M., BRIDGES C.G., LYON A.M., GRIFFITHS L. & EDINGTON N. (1992). Latent equid herpesviruses 1 and 4: detection and distinction using the polymerase chain reaction and cocultivation from lymphoid tissues. *J. Gen. Virol.*, **73**, 261–268.

29. WHITWELL K.E., GOWER S.M. & SMITH K.C. (1992). An immunoperosidase method applied to the diagnosis of equine herpesvirus abortion, using conventional and rapid microwave techniques. *Equine Vet. J.*, **24**, 10–12.

*

* *

CHAPTER 2.5.8.

GLANDERS

SUMMARY

Glanders is a contagious and fatal disease of horses, donkeys, and mules, and is caused by infection with the bacterium Burkholderia mallei *(the name recently changed from* Pseudomonas mallei *and was previously classified variously as* Pfeifferella, Loefflerella, Malleomyces *or* Actinobacillus*). The disease causes nodules and ulcerations in the upper respiratory tract and lungs. A skin form also occurs, known as 'farcy'. Control of glanders requires testing of suspect clinical cases, screening of apparently normal equids, and elimination of positive reactors. It is easily transmitted to humans, in whom 95% of cases are fatal. All infected or potentially infected material must be handled in the laboratory under conditions of strict biocontainment.*

Identification of the agent: *Smears from fresh material may reveal Gram-negative nonsporulating, nonencapsulated rods. The bacteria grow aerobically and prefer media that contains glycerol. Unlike the* Pseudomonas *species,* Burkholderia mallei *is nonmotile. Guinea-pigs are highly susceptible, and males are used for testing of potentially infected material. Intraperitoneal injections are given to attempt to elicit the Strauss reaction (orchitis).*

Mallein and serological tests: *The mallein test is a sensitive and specific clinical test for glanders. Mallein, a protein fraction of the organism, is injected intradermo-palpebrally or given by eyedrop. In infected animals, the eyelid swells markedly in 1–2 days. A complement fixation test and an enzyme-linked immunosorbent assay are the most accurate and reliable serological tests for diagnostic use.*

Requirements for vaccines and diagnostic biologicals: *There are no vaccines. Mallein purified protein derivative is currently available commercially from institutes in The Netherlands and Romania (see footnote 1).*

A. DIAGNOSTIC TECHNIQUES

Glanders is a bacterial disease of solipeds with zoonotic potential that has been known since ancient times, and that is caused by infection with the bacterium *Burkholderia mallei* (the name recently changed from *Pseudomonas mallei* and was previously classified variously as *Pfeifferella, Loefflerella, Malleomyces* or *Actinobacillus*). Carnivores may become infected by eating infected meat, but cattle, sheep and pigs are resistant (12). Glanders in the acute form occurs most frequently in donkeys and mules, which run a high fever and exhibit respiratory signs (swollen nostrils, dyspnoea, and pneumonia): death occurs within a few days. In horses, glanders generally runs a more chronic course and they may survive for several years. Chronic and subclinical 'occult' cases are dangerous sources of infection.

In horses, inflammatory nodules and ulcers develop in the nasal passages and give rise to a sticky yellow discharge, accompanied by enlarged firm submaxillary lymph nodes. Stellate scarring follows healing of the ulcers. The formation of nodular abscesses in the lungs is accompanied by progressive debility, febrile episodes, coughing and dyspnoea. Diarrhoea and polyuria can also occur. In the skin form ('farcy'), the lymphatics are enlarged and nodular abscesses ('buds') of 0.5–2.5 cm develop, which ulcerate and discharge yellow oily pus. Discharges from the respiratory tract and skin are infective, and transmission between animals, which is facilitated by close contact, is by inhalation, ingestion of contaminated material (e.g. from infected feed and water troughs), or by inoculation (e.g. via a harness). The incubation period is from a few days to many months (13).

Glanders is transmissible to humans by direct contact with sick animals or infected materials. In the untreated acute disease, there is 95% mortality within 3 weeks. A chronic form with abscessation also occurs. When handling suspect or known infected animals or fomites, stringent precautions should be taken to prevent self-infection or transmission of the bacterium to other equids. Laboratory samples should be securely packaged, kept cool and labelled 'Glanders suspect'. In the laboratory, all manipulations with potentially infected material must be performed in conditions of biohazard containment.

Glanders has been eradicated from many countries by statutory testing, elimination of infected animals, and import restrictions. It persists in some Eastern European, Asian, and African countries.

1. Identification of the agent

Cases for specific glanders investigation should be differentiated on clinical grounds from other chronic infections of the nasal mucosae or sinuses, and from strangles (*Streptococcus equi* infection), ulcerative lymphangitis (*Corynebacterium pseudotuberculosis)* and sporotrichosis (*Sporotrichium* spp.). Glanders should be excluded positively from suspected cases of epizootic lymphangitis (caused by *Histoplasma farciminosum*), with which it has many clinical similarities. In humans in particular, glanders should be distinguished from melioidosis (*P. pseudomallei* infection), which is caused by an organism with close similarities to *B. mallei* (12).

a) Morphology of *Burkholderia mallei*

The organisms are fairly numerous in smears from fresh lesions, but in older lesions they are scanty (16). They should be stained by methylene blue or Gram stain. The organisms are mainly extracellular, fairly straight Gram-negative rods with rounded ends, 2–5 µm long and 0.5 µm wide, often stain irregularly and do not have capsules or form spores. Unlike other organisms in the *Pseudomonas* group, *Burkholderia mallei* have no flagellae and are therefore nonmotile (8). The organisms are difficult to demonstrate in tissue sections, where they may have a beaded appearance (11). In culture media, they vary in appearance depending on the age of the culture and type of medium. In older cultures, there is much pleomorphism. Branching filaments form on the surface of broth cultures.

b) Cultural characteristics

It is preferable to attempt isolation from unopened uncontaminated lesions (11). The organism is aerobic and facultatively anaerobic only in the presence of nitrate (5, 8), growing optimally at 37°C (10). It grows well, but slowly, on ordinary culture media; glycerol enrichment is particularly useful. After a few days on glycerol agar, there is a confluent slightly cream coloured growth that is smooth, moist, and viscid. With continued incubation, the growth thickens and becomes dark brown and tough. It also grows well on glycerol potato agar and in glycerol broth, on which a slimy pellicle forms. On plain nutrient agar, the growth is much less luxuriant, and growth is poor on gelatin (14).

Alterations to characteristics may occur *in vitro*, so fresh isolates should be used for identification reactions. Litmus milk is slightly acidified by *B. mallei*, and coagulation may occur after long incubation. The organism reduces nitrates. Although some workers have claimed that glucose is the only carbohydrate that is fermented (slowly and inconstantly), other workers have shown that if an appropriate medium and indicator are used, glucose and other carbohydrates, such as arabinose, fructose, galactose and mannose, are consistently fermented by *B. mallei* (4). Indole is not produced, horse blood is not haemolysed and no diffusible pigments are produced in cultures (8). A commercial laboratory test kit (e.g. API [Analytical Profile Index] system: Analytab Products or BioMerieux) can be used for easy confirmation that an organism belongs to the *Pseudomonas* group. Lack of motility is then of special relevance.

In contaminated samples, supplementation of media with substances that inhibit the growth of Gram-positive organisms (e.g. crystal violet, proflavine) has proved useful, as has pretreatment with penicillin (1000 units/ml for 3 hours at 37°C) (16). A selective medium has been developed (17) composed of polymyxin E (1000 units), bacitracin (250 units), and actidione (0.25 mg) incorporated into nutrient agar (100 ml) containing glycerine (4%), donkey or horse serum (10%), and ovine haemoglobin or trypton agar (0.1%).

Outside the body, the organism has little resistance to drying, heat, light or chemicals, so that survival beyond 2 weeks is unlikely. Under favourable conditions, however, it can probably survive a few months. *Burkholderia mallei* can remain viable in tap water for at least 1 month (14). For disinfection, benzalkonium chloride or 'roccal' (1/2000), sodium hypochlorite (500 ppm available chlorine), iodine, mercuric chloride in alcohol, and potassium permanganate have been shown to be highly effective against *B. mallei* (10). Phenolic disinfectants are less effective.

c) Laboratory animal inoculation

Guinea-pigs, hamsters and cats have been used for diagnosis when necessary. If isolation in a laboratory animal is considered unavoidable, suspected material is inoculated intraperitoneally into a male guinea-pig. Positive material will cause a severe localised peritonitis and orchitis (the Strauss reaction). The number of organisms and their virulence determines the severity of the lesions. Additional steps are used when the test material is heavily contaminated (6). The Strauss reaction is not specific for glanders, and other organisms can elicit it. Bacteriological examination of infected testes should confirm the specificity of the response obtained.

d) Other methods

There have been recent advances in the application of molecular biological techniques to the detection of glanders. A polymerase chain reaction for the specific detection of *B. mallei* DNA has been developed (2) that allows differentiation between *B. mallei* and *B. pseudomallei*. An immunoblotting method has been developed (7) that shows promise, especially for testing sera that give anticomplementary or other spurious reactions in the complement fixation (CF) test. As neither of these techniques have yet been fully validated or gained wide acceptance, details are not given here.

2. Mallein and serological tests

a) The mallein test (a prescribed test for international trade)

The mallein purified protein derivative (PPD), which is available commercially, is a solution of water-soluble protein fractions of heat-treated *B. mallei*. The test depends on infected horses being hypersensitive to mallein. Advanced clinical cases in horses and acute cases in donkeys and mules may give inconclusive results requiring additional methods of diagnosis to be employed (1).

- **The intradermo-palpebral test**

This is the most sensitive, reliable and specific test for detecting infected solipeds, and has largely displaced the ophthalmic and subcutaneous tests (3); 0.1 ml of concentrated mallein PPD is injected intradermally into the lower eyelid and the test is read at 24 and 48 hours. A positive reaction is characterised by marked oedematous swelling of the eyelid, and there may be a purulent discharge from the inner canthus or conjunctiva. This is usually accompanied by a rise in temperature. With a negative response, there is usually no reaction or only a little swelling of the lower lid.

- **The ophthalmic test**

This is less reliable than the intradermo-palpebral test. A few drops of mallein are instilled into the eye at the canthus. In an infected animal, the eyelids, and sometimes the side of the face, become swollen and there may be a little discharge from the eye. The reaction may also occur to a lesser extent in the opposite eye.

- **The subcutaneous test**

This test interferes with subsequent serological diagnosis and so the other two mallein tests are preferred. The test may also not be acceptable in some countries. The horse's temperature has to be under 102°F (38.8°C) on the day before the test, at the time of the injection, and at 9, 12 and 15 hours after the injection. A 10 cm square skin patch in the middle of the neck is clipped and disinfected; 2.5 ml of dilute mallein are injected subcutaneously into the centre of the patch. With a positive test, the horse develops a pyrexia of 104°F (40.0°C) or over during the first 15 hours, and a firm painful swelling with raised edges develops within 24 hours at the injection site. In nonglandered horses, there is no, or minimal, transient local swelling. Doubtful reactors may be retested after 14 days using a double dose of mallein.

b) Complement fixation test (a prescribed test for international trade)

Although not as sensitive as the mallein test, the CF test is an accurate serological test that has been used for glanders diagnosis for many years (3). It is reported to be 90–95% accurate, serum being positive within 1 week of infection and remaining positive for a long time in chronic cases (14). The antigen for the CF test has been prepared from young cultures by growing the organism on glycerol–agar slopes for 12 hours, and washing off with normal saline. The suspension is then heated for 1 hour at 65°C.

Serum is diluted 1/5 in veronal (barbiturate) buffered saline containing 0.1% gelatin (VBSG) or CFD (complement fixation diluent – available as tablets) without gelatin, and inactivated for 30 minutes at 56°C. Serum of equidae other than horses should be inactivated at 63°C for 30 minutes. Twofold dilutions of the sera are prepared in 96-well round-bottom microtitre plates. Guinea-pig complement is diluted in the chosen buffer and 5 (or optionally 4) complement haemolytic units-50% (CH_{50}) are used. Sera, complement and antigen are reacted in the plates and incubated for 1 hour at 37°C. (Some laboratories prefer to use overnight incubation at 4°C.) A 2% suspension of sensitised washed sheep red blood cells is added, and the plates are incubated for 45 minutes at 37°C, then centrifuged for 5 minutes at 600 *g*.

A sample that produces 100% haemolysis at the 1/5 dilution is negative, 25–75% haemolysis is suspicious, and no haemolysis (100% fixation) is positive. Unfortunately false-positive results can occur as some strains cross-react with *P. pseudomallei* (3), and healthy horses can have a CF titre for a variable period following a mallein test.

c) Avidin–biotin dot enzyme-linked immunosorbent assay

The avidin–biotin dot enzyme-linked immunosorbent assay (dot ELISA) is a promising test that has not yet been widely validated. The antigen is prepared from a 5-day growth on glycerine dextrose agar, suspended in sterile distilled water to give a thick suspension, and inactivated by heat at 100°C for 1 hour. The sample is centrifuged at 20,000 ***g*** for 1 hour, and the volume of water is adjusted to give a 20% packed cell volume. Phenyl methyl sulphonyl fluoride, at 2 mM concentration, is added to inhibit protease, and the sample is freeze–thawed six times in liquid nitrogen. It is then centrifuged at 20,000 ***g*** for 1 hour, and the supernatant is filtered through a 0.23 µm membrane filter. Protein is estimated (9) and the antigen is stored at –20°C with merthiolate (1/10,000). The antigen is used at a concentration of 0.6 mg protein/ml.

- **Test procedure**

i) Dot approximately 1 µl of optimally diluted antigen on to the centre of a nitrocellulose dipstick (East Panjab Manufacturing, India) with a micropipette, and allow to dry at 37°C for 15 minutes.

ii) Unbound nitrocellulose sites are blocked by incubating the dipsticks in 3% skimmed milk in phosphate buffered saline (PBS) at 37°C for 30 minutes.

iii) After rinsing in PBS, incubate the dipsticks in an appropriate dilution of equine serum for 30 minutes at 37°C, and then wash them in three changes of 0.05% PBS/Tween 20 (PBST) with a minimum of five shakings in each wash.

iv) Further incubation is carried out in optimally diluted biotinylated anti-horse IgG in PBS (Vector Laboratories, United States of America) at 37°C for 20 minutes.

v) Wash the dipsticks again as before, and immerse in optimally diluted horseradish peroxidase–avidin D (Vector Laboratories) in 0.5% gelatin–PBS for 8 minutes at room temperature.

vi) After washing as before, the enzyme reaction is developed with a substrate solution containing 0.3 mg/ml of diamino-benzidine and 1 µl/ml of H_2O_2 solution (30%) in PBS.

vii) The reaction is developed for 5 minutes and stopped by washing the dipsticks in tap water.

viii) A positive reaction is indicated by the appearance of a clearly visible brown dot in the antigen-coated area.

Using antigen dotted, preblocked dipsticks, the test can be completed in approximately 1 hour. Serum or whole blood can be used for the test, and partial haemolysis does not impart any background colour to the antigen-coated area on the nitrocellulose.

Low antibody levels, 1/100 or less, can be demonstrated in the normal equine population. Naturally infected and sensitised horses have dot ELISA titres ranging from 1/400 to 1/25,600. With the limited data available from infected horses at this stage, a 1/200 dilution of the serum is recommended as a positive threshold (15). Positive dot ELISA titres may be seen on day 4 post-infection, but are present from day 6 and persist for 7 weeks, although some animals may still be positive at 11 weeks. Test results are unreliable for up to 6 weeks after a mallein test.

d) Agglutination and precipitin tests

The accuracy of these tests is unsatisfactory for use in control programmes. Horses with chronic glanders and those in a debilitated condition give negative or inconclusive results.

B. REQUIREMENTS FOR VACCINES AND DIAGNOSTIC BIOLOGICALS

No vaccines are available.

Mallein PPD for use in performing the intradermo-palpebral and ophthalmic tests is produced commercially by two institutes[1].

The ID-Lelystad has provided the following information on requirements for mallein PPD.

1. Seed management

Three strains of *Burkholderia mallei* are employed for production of mallein PPD, namely strain Bogor (originating from Indonesia), strain Mukteswar (India) and strain Zagreb (Yugoslavia). The seed material is kept as a stock of freeze-dried cultures. The strains are subcultured on to glycerol agar at 37°C for 1–2 days. For maintaining virulence and antigenicity, the strains may be passaged through guinea-pigs.

2. Method of manufacture

For production of mallein PPD, Dorset–Henley medium, enriched by the addition of trace elements, is used. The liquid medium is inoculated with a thick saline suspension of *B. mallei*, grown on glycerol agar. The production medium is incubated at 37°C for about 10 weeks. The bacteria are then killed by steaming for 3 hours in a Koch's steriliser. The fluid is then passed through a layer of cotton wool to remove coarse bacterial clumps. The resulting turbid fluid is cleared by membrane filtration, and one part trichloroacetic acid 40% is immediately added to nine parts culture filtrate. The mixture is allowed to stand overnight and a light brownish to greyish precipitate settles.

The supernatant fluid is pipetted off and discarded. The precipitate is centrifuged for 15 minutes at 2500 ***g*** and the layer of precipitate is washed three or more times in a solution of 5% NaCl, pH 3, until the pH is 2.7. The washed precipitate is dissolved by stirring with a minimum of an alkaline solvent. The fluid is dark brown and a pH of 6.7 will be obtained. This mallein concentrate has to be centrifuged thoroughly and the supernatant is diluted with an equal amount of a glucose buffer solution. The protein content of this product is estimated by the Kjeldahl method and freeze-dried after it has been dispensed into ampoules.

3. In-process control

During the period of incubation, the flasks are inspected frequently for any signs of contamination, and suspect flasks are discarded. A typical growth of the *B. mallei* cultures comprises turbidity, sedimentation, some surface growth with a tendency towards sinking, and the formation of a conspicuous slightly orange-coloured ring along the margin of the surface of the medium.

4. Batch control

Each batch of mallein PPD is tested for sterility, safety, preservatives, protein content and potency.

Sterility testing is performed according to the European Pharmacopoeia guidelines.

The examination for safety is conducted on from five to ten normal healthy horses by carrying out the intradermo-palpebral test. The resulting swelling should be, at most, barely detectable and transient, without any signs of conjunctival discharge.

Preparations containing phenol as a preservative should not contain more than 0.5% (w/v) phenol. The protein content should be not less than 0.95 mg/ml and not more than 1.05 mg/ml.

Potency testing is performed in guinea-pigs and horses. The animals are sensitised by subcutaneous inoculation with a concentrated suspension of heat-killed *B. mallei* in paraffin oil or incomplete Freund's adjuvant. Cattle can also be used instead of horses. The production batch is bioassayed against a standard mallein PPD by intradermal injection in 0.1 ml doses in such a way that complete randomisation is obtained.

In guinea-pigs, the different areas of erythema are measured after 24 hours, and in horses the increase in skin thickness is measured by calipers. The results are statistically evaluated, using standard statistical methods for parallel-line assays.

1 Institute for Animal Science and Health (ID-Lelystad), Edelhertweg 15, 8219 PH, Lelystad, The Netherlands, and Min Agr Si Industr. Institut Die Cercertari Si Biopreparate 'Pasteur', R-7000 - Bucuresti, 77.826 SOS Giulesti Nr 333, Romania.

REFERENCES

1. ALLEN H. (1929). The diagnosis of glanders. *J. R. Army Vet. Corps,* **1**, 241–245.

2. BAUERNFEIND A., ROLLER C., MEYER D., JUNGWIRTH R. & SCHNEIDER I. (1998). Molecular procedure for rapid detection of *Burkholderia mallei* and *Burkholderia pseudomallei. J. Clin. Microbiol.,* **36**, 2737–2741.

3. BLOOD D.C. & RADOSTITS O.M. (1989). Diseases caused by bacteria. *In:* Veterinary Medicine, Seventh Edition. Balliere Tindall, London, UK, 733–735.

4. EVANS D. (1966). Utilization of carbohydrates by *Actinobacillus mallei. Can. J. Microbiol.,* **12**, 625–639.

5. GILARDI G.L. (1985). Pseudomonas. *In:* Manual of Clinical Microbiology, Fourth Edition, Lenette E.H., Bulawo A., Hausler W.J. & Shadomy H.J., eds. American Society for Microbiology, Washington DC, USA, 350–372.

6. GOULD J.C. (1950). *In:* Mackie and McCartney's Handbook of Bacteriology, Eighth Edition, Cruickshank R., ed. E. & S. Livingstone, Edinburgh, UK, 391–394.

7. KATZ J.B., CHIEVES., HENNAGER S.G., NICHOLSON J.M., FISHER T.A. & BYERS P.E. (1999). Serodiagnosis of equine piroplasmosis, dourine and glanders using an arrayed immunoblotting method. *J. Vet. Diagn. Invest.*, **11**, 292–294.

8. KRIEG N.R. & HOLT J.G., eds. (1984). Gram-negative aerobic rods and cocci. *In:* Bergey's Manual of Systematic Bacteriology Vol. 1. Williams & Wilkins, Baltimore, USA & London, UK, 174–175.

9. LOWRY O.H., ROSEBROUGH N.J., FARR A.L. & RANDALL R.J. (1951). Protein measurement with the Folin phenol reagent. *J. Biol. Chem.,* **193**, 265–275.

10. MAHADERAN S., DRAVIDAMANI S. & DARE B.J. (1987). Glanders in horse. *Centaurus,* **III**, 135-138.

11. MILLER W., PANNEL L., CRAVITZ L., TANNER A. & INGALLS M. (1948). Studies on certain biological characteristics of *Malleomyces mallei* and *Malleomyces pseudomallei* I. Morphology, cultivation, viability, and isolation from contaminated specimens. *J. Bacteriol.,* **55**, 115-126.

12. MINETT F.C. (1959). Glanders (and melioidosis). *In:* Infectious Diseases of Animals. Vol. 1. Diseases due to Bacteria, Stableforth A.W. & Galloway I.A., eds. Butterworths Scientific Publications, London, UK, 296–309.

13. MONLUX W.S. (1984). Diseases affecting food and working animals. *In:* Foreign Animal Diseases. United States Department of Agriculture, US Government Printing Office, Washington DC, USA, 178–185.

14. STEELE J.H. (1980). Bacterial, rickettsial and mycotic diseases. *In:* CRC Handbook Series in Zoonoses, Section A, Vol. I, Steele J.H., ed. CRC Press, Boca Raton, USA, 339–351.

15. VERMA R.D., SHARMA J.K., VENKATESWARAN K.S. & BATRA H.V. (1990). Development of an avidin-biotin dot enzyme-linked immunosorbent assay and its comparison with other serological tests for diagnosis of glanders in equines. *Vet. Microbiol.,* **25**, 77–85.

16. WILSON G.S. & MILES A.A. (1964). Glanders and melioidosis. *In:* Topley and Wilson's Principles of Bacteriology and Immunity. E. Arnold, London, UK, 1714–1717.

17. XIE X., XU F., XU B., DUAN X. & GONG R. (1980). A New Selective Medium for Isolation of Glanders Bacilli. Collected papers of veterinary research. Control Institute of Veterinary Biologics, Ministry of Agriculture, Peking, China, **6**, 83–90.

*

* *

CHAPTER 2.5.10.

EQUINE VIRAL ARTERITIS

SUMMARY

Equine viral arteritis (EVA) is a contagious viral disease of equids caused by equine arteritis virus (EAV), an RNA virus that is classified in the family Arteriviridae. The virus is found in horse populations in many countries world-wide. EVA cannot be differentiated clinically from a number of other respiratory and systemic equine diseases. While laboratory-confirmed outbreaks of EVA have been infrequently reported in the past, the incidence of the disease appears to be on the increase.

Although many cases of EAV infection are subclinical, certain virus strains can cause disease of varying severity characterised principally by fever, depression, anorexia, dependent oedema, especially of the limbs, scrotum and prepuce in the stallion, conjunctivitis, an urticarial-type skin reaction, abortion and, rarely, a fulminating pneumonia or pneumo-enteritis in young foals. Apart from mortality in young foals, the case-fatality rate in outbreaks of EVA is very low. Affected horses almost invariably make complete clinical recoveries. A long-term carrier state can occur in a high percentage of infected stallions, but not in mares or nonbreeding horses.

***Identification of the agent:** Diagnosis of EAV infection is based on virus isolation, detection of viral antigen or nucleic acid, or demonstration of a specific antibody response. Virus isolation should be attempted from nasopharyngeal and conjunctival swabs, unclotted blood samples, and semen from possible carrier stallions. In suspect cases of EVA-related mortality or abortion, isolation can be attempted from a wide range of tissues, especially lung, spleen and other lymphoreticular tissues, and from placental and fetal fluids and tissues. Isolation of EAV from clinical or post-mortem specimens should be attempted in rabbit, equine, or monkey kidney cell culture. The identity of isolates of EAV should be confirmed by neutralisation test or by immunocytochemical methods, namely indirect immunofluorescence or avidin–biotin–peroxidase techniques.*

Detection and identification of EAV in clinical or post-mortem specimens can also be attempted using the reverse-transcription polymerase chain reaction assay and appropriate viral RNA primers.

Where mortality is associated with a suspected outbreak of EVA, a wide range of tissues should be examined for histological evidence of panvasculitis that is especially pronounced in the small arteries throughout the body. The characteristic vascular lesions present in the mature animal are not a notable feature in EVA-related abortions.

***Serological tests:** A variety of serological tests, including neutralisation, complement fixation (CF), indirect fluorescent antibody, agar gel immunodiffusion and the enzyme-linked immunosorbent assay (ELISA), have been used for the detection of antibody to EAV. The test currently in widest use is a complement-enhanced microneutralisation test. It is a sensitive and highly specific assay of proven value in diagnosing acute infection and in seroprevalence studies. The CF test is less sensitive but can be used for diagnosing recent infection. Several ELISAs have been developed, some of which appear to offer comparable specificity and sensitivity to the neutralisation test.*

***Requirements for vaccines and diagnostic biologicals:** Two commercial tissue culture vaccines have been produced against EVA. One is a modified live virus (MLV) vaccine prepared from virus that has been attenuated for horses by multiple serial transfers in equine and rabbit cell cultures. It has been shown to be safe and protective for stallions and nonpregnant mares. Vaccination of foals under 6 weeks of age and of pregnant mares in the final 2 months of gestation is contraindicated. The second vaccine is an inactivated, adjuvanted product prepared from virus* *grown in equine cell culture that can be used in nonbreeding and breeding horses. In the absence of appropriate safety data, the vaccine is not currently recommended for use in pregnant mares.*

A. DIAGNOSTIC TECHNIQUES

Equine viral arteritis (EVA) is a contagious viral disease of equids caused by equine arteritis virus (EAV), a positive-sense, single-stranded RNA virus, which is the prototype member of the genus Arterivirus, family Arteriviridae, order Nidovirales (6). Epizootic lymphangitis pinkeye, fievre typhoide and rotlaufseuche are some of the descriptive terms used in the past to refer to a disease that was very probably EVA. The natural host range of EAV would appear to be restricted to equids and the virus does not present a human health hazard (46, 52). EAV is present in the horse population of many countries world-wide. Although relatively few outbreaks of EVA have been confirmed in the past, there has been an apparent increase in the incidence of the disease in recent years (52).

While the majority of cases of acute infection with EAV are subclinical, certain strains of the virus can cause disease of varying severity (52). Typical cases of EVA can present with any combination of the following clinical signs: fever, depression, anorexia, leukopenia, dependent oedema, especially of the limbs, scrotum and prepuce of the stallion, conjunctivitis, ocular discharge, supra or periorbital oedema, rhinitis, nasal discharge, a local or generalised urticarial skin reaction, abortion and, rarely, a fulminating pneumonia or pneumo-enteritis in young foals. Regardless of the severity of clinical signs, affected horses almost invariably make complete recoveries. The case-fatality rate in outbreaks of EVA is very low; mortality is usually only seen in very young foals, especially those congenitally infected with the virus (34, 52).

EAV replicates and is shed in large quantities from the respiratory tract of acutely infected animals (38). It is also shed in the semen of acutely infected stallions, a variable percentage of which become long-term carriers in the reproductive tract and constant semen shedders of the virus (52, 53). The carrier state has only been found in the stallion, not in the mare, gelding or sexually immature colt (52).

1. Identification of the agent

a) Virus isolation

In the case of a suspected outbreak of EVA or when attempting to confirm subclinical EAV infection, virus isolation should be attempted from nasopharyngeal and conjunctival swabs, unclotted blood samples, and semen from stallions considered to be possible carriers of the virus (52). To optimise the chances of virus isolation, the relevant specimens should be obtained as soon as possible after the onset of fever in affected horses. Heparin is contraindicated as an anticoagulant when attempting virus isolation from blood as there is evidence that it inhibits the growth of EAV in RK 13 cells (1). Where EVA is suspected in cases of mortality in young foals or older animals, isolation of EAV can be attempted from a variety of tissues, especially the lymphatic glands associated with the alimentary tract and related organs, also the lungs, liver and spleen (38). In outbreaks involving abortion, placental and fetal fluids and a wide range of placental, lymphoreticular and other fetal tissues can be productive sources of virus (52).

Although not always successful in natural cases of EAV infection (22, 39, 55), virus isolation should be attempted from clinical specimens or necropsied tissues using rabbit, equine or monkey kidney cell culture (38, 52). Selected cell lines, e.g. RK-13 (ATCC CCL-37), LLC-MK_2 (ATCC CCL-7), and African green monkey kidney (Vero) (ATCC CCL81) cells or primary horse or rabbit kidney cell culture can be used, with early passage RK-13 cells being the cell system of choice. There is evidence that higher passage levels of RK-13 cells can be less permissive for the primary isolation of EAV, especially from semen. Several other factors have been shown to have an influence on the primary isolation of EAV from semen in RK-13 cells (45). Higher isolation rates have been obtained using 3–5-day-old monolayers, a large inoculum size in relation to the cell surface area in the inoculated flasks or multiwell plates, and the incorporation of carboxymethyl cellulose in the overlay medium. It should be noted that most RK-13 cells, including ATCC CCL-37, are contaminated with bovine viral diarrhoea virus, the presence of which appears to enhance sensitivity of this cell system for the primary isolation of EAV.

Inoculated cultures are examined daily for the appearance of viral cytopathic effect (CPE), which is usually evident within 2–6 days. In the absence of visible CPE, culture supernatants should be subinoculated on to fresh cell monolayers after 5–7 days. The majority of isolations of EAV are made in the first or second passage in cell culture (53). The identity of isolates of EAV can be confirmed in a one-way neutralisation test or by an immunocytochemical method, namely indirect immunofluorescence (12, 56) or the avidin–biotin–peroxidase (ABC) technique (33, 43). A polyclonal rabbit antiserum has been used to identify EAV in infected cell cultures (28). Mouse monoclonal antibodies (MAbs) to the nucleocapsid (N) protein and envelope G_L protein of EAV (3, 13, 24) and a monospecific polyclonal rabbit antiserum to the envelope (M) protein have also been developed and these can detect various strains of the virus in RK-13 cells as early as 12–24 hours after infection (2, 33). Viral antigen has been detected in the tissues of infected horses by immunofluorescence using conjugated equine antiserum to EAV (12) or by the ABC technique using mouse MAbs to the N or G_L proteins of the virus (34, 43, 56).

Virus isolation from semen (a prescribed test for international trade)

There is considerable evidence that short- and long-term carrier stallions shed EAV constantly in the semen but not in respiratory secretions or urine; nor has it been demonstrated in the buffy coat of the blood of such animals (53). Stallions should first be tested using the virus neutralisation (VN) test on serum. Virus isolation should be attempted from the semen of stallions that are positive for antibodies to EAV and that do not have a satisfactory history of vaccination against EVA. Virus isolation is also indicated in the case of shipped semen where a blood sample from the donor stallion is not available. It is recommended that virus isolation from semen be attempted from two samples, which can be collected on the same day, on consecutive days or after an interval of several days or weeks. There is no evidence that the outcome of attempted virus isolation from particular stallions is influenced by the interval between collections or time of the year. Isolation of EAV should be carried out preferably on a portion of an entire ejaculate collected using an artificial vagina or a condom and a teaser or phantom mare. When it is not possible to obtain semen by this means, a less preferable alternative is to collect a dismount sample at the time of breeding. Care should be taken to ensure that no antiseptics/disinfectants are used in the cleansing of the external genitalia of the stallion prior to collection. Samples should contain the sperm-rich fraction of the ejaculate with which EAV is associated. The virus is not present in the pre-sperm fraction of semen (53). Immediately following collection, the semen should be refrigerated on crushed ice or on freezer packs for transport to the laboratory with a minimum of delay. Where there is likely to be a delay in submitting a specimen for testing, the semen can be frozen at or below –20°C for a varying period of days or weeks before being dispatched to the laboratory. Freezing a sample has not been found to militate against isolation of EAV from the semen of a carrier stallion.

- **Test procedure**

i) Semen samples are pretreated before inoculation into cell culture by short-term sonication (for three 15-second cycles) followed by centrifugation at 1000 ***g*** for 10 minutes at 4°C to sediment the spermatozoa.

ii) After removal of culture medium, 3–5-day-old confluent monolayer cultures of RK-13 cells, either in 25 cm^2 tissue culture flasks or multiwell plates, are inoculated with serial decimal dilutions (10^{-1}–10^{-3}) of seminal plasma in tissue culture maintenance medium containing 2% fetal bovine serum and antibiotics. An inoculum of 1 ml per 25 cm^2 flask is used and no fewer than two flasks per dilution of seminal plasma are inoculated. Inoculum size and number of wells inoculated per dilution of a specimen should be pro-rated where multiwell plates are used. Appropriate dilutions of a virus positive control semen sample or virus control of known titre diluted in culture medium should be included in each test.

iii) The flasks or cover plates are closed and gently rotated to disperse the inoculum over the cell monolayers.

iv) Inoculated cultures are then incubated for 1 hour at 37°C either in an aerobic incubator or an incubator containing a humidified atmosphere of 5% CO_2 in air, depending on whether flasks or multiwell plates are used.

v) Without removing any of the inoculum or washing the cell monolayers, the latter are overlaid with 0.75% carboxymethyl cellulose containing medium with antibiotics.

vi) The flasks or plates are reincubated at 37°C and checked microscopically for viral CPE, which is usually evident within 2–6 days.

vii) In the absence of visible CPE, culture supernatants are subinoculated on to fresh cell monolayers after 5–7 days. After removal of the overlay medium, monolayers are stained with 0.1% formalin-buffered crystal violet solution.

The identity of any virus isolates should be confirmed by using immunolabelling, a fluorescent antibody method or virus neutralisation with monospecific antisera or MAbs as indicated above.

In the one-way neutralisation test, serial decimal dilutions of the virus isolate are tested against an MAb or monospecific antiserum prepared against the prototype Bucyrus strain of EAV (ATCC VR 796) and also a serum negative for neutralising antibodies to the virus. Corresponding titrations of the prototype Bucyrus virus with the same reference antibody reagents are included as test controls. The test is performed in either 25 cm^2 tissue culture flasks or multiwell plates. Appropriate quantities of the known EAV positive and negative antibody reagents are inactivated for 30 minutes in a water bath at 56°C and diluted 1/4 in phosphate buffered saline, pH 7.2; then 0.3 ml of diluted antibody reagent is dispensed into five tubes for each virus isolate to be tested. Serial decimal dilutions (10^{-1}–10^{-5}) of each virus are made in Eagles Minimal Essential Medium containing 10% fetal bovine serum, antibiotics and 10% freshly diluted guinea-pig complement. Then, 0.3 ml of each virus dilution is added to the tubes containing positive and negative antibody reagents. The tubes are shaken and the virus/antibody mixtures are incubated for 1 hour at 37°C. The mixtures are then inoculated on to 3–5-day-old confluent monolayer cultures of RK-13 cells, either in 25 cm^2 flasks or multiwell plates, using two flasks or wells per virus dilution. Each flask is inoculated with 0.25 ml of virus/antibody mixture; the inoculum size is pro-rated where multiwell plates are used. Inoculated flasks or plates are incubated for 2 hours at 37°C, gently rocking after 1 hour to disperse the inoculum over the cell monolayers. Without removing any of the inoculum or washing the cell monolayers, the latter are overlaid with 0.75% carboxymethyl cellulose containing medium and incubated for 4–5 days at 37°C, either in an aerobic incubator or an incubator containing a humidified atmosphere of 5% CO_2 in air. After removal of the medium, monolayers are stained with 0.1% formalin-buffered crystal violet solution. Plaques are counted and the virus infectivity titre determined both in the presence and absence of EAV antibodies using the Spearman–Kärber method. Identification of a virus isolate is based on the extent of plaque reduction compared with that of the prototype Bucyrus strain of EAV.

Most EAV isolates from carrier stallions are made in the first passage in cell culture using the described test procedure. The occurrence of nonviral cytotoxicity or bacterial contamination of specimens are not significant problems when attempting isolation of this virus from stallion semen. Nonviral cytotoxicity, if observed, usually affects monolayers inoculated with the 10^{-1} and, much less frequently, the 10^{-2} dilution of seminal plasma. Treatment of seminal plasma with polyethylene glycol (Mol. wt 6000) prior to inoculation has been used with some success in overcoming this problem (21). The method described involves the addition of polyethylene glycol to the 10^{-1}–10^{-3} dilutions of seminal plasma to give a final concentration of 10% in each dilution. The mixtures are held overnight at 4°C with gentle stirring, after which they are centrifuged at 2000 ***g*** for 30 minutes and the supernatants are discarded. The precipitates are suspended in cell culture maintenance medium to one-tenth the volume of the original dilutions and the mixtures are homogenised. They are then centrifuged at 2000 ***g*** for 30 minutes and the supernatants are taken off and used for inoculation. There is no evidence to indicate that pretreatment of seminal plasma in this manner reduces sensitivity of the virus isolation procedure.

The presence of anti-EAV antibody in the seminal plasma of certain virus-shedding stallions has not been found to prevent detection of the carrier state in these animals.

b) Nucleic acid detection

The reverse-transcription polymerase chain reaction (RT-PCR) assay is an additional method (to virus isolation in cell culture) for EAV detection. Single and nested RT-PCR assays have been developed and evaluated for detection of various strains of the virus in cell culture (5, 8, 23, 48, 50). Single-step extraction of RNA followed by reverse transcription and amplification have been described (5, 23, 48). Detection of amplified products can be performed either by agarose gel electrophoresis or by enzyme-linked immunosorbent assay (ELISA)–PCR assay using commercial reagents. The RT-PCR assay provides a means of identifying virus-specific RNA in clinical specimens, namely nasopharyngeal swab filtrates, buffy coats, semen and urine and in post-mortem tissue samples (2, 5, 8, 23, 48, 50). Comparable results to virus isolation have been obtained with a nested RT-PCR assay that takes only 2 days to complete (2, 5, 23). The assay has the advantage of not requiring viable virus for performance of the test. Because of the high sensitivity of the procedure, however, there is the potential for cross-contamination of a sample in the laboratory giving rise to a false-positive result. To minimise the risk of this occurring, considerable care needs to be taken, especially during the steps of RNA extraction and amplification, and relevant EAV positive and negative controls and, where appropriate, RNA extracted from the tissue culture fluid of uninfected cells need to be included in each PCR assay.

Primer selection is critical to the sensitivity of the RT-PCR assay with primers preferably designed from the most conserved regions of the viral genome. Sequences chosen from the viral polymerase, nucleocapsid (N) or envelope (M) protein genes are reportedly effective in a single or nested RT-PCR assay (5, 8, 23, 48, 50). Until such time as a complete consensus or universal primer set for EAV has been identified, however, it is advisable to use the RT-PCR assay in conjunction with and not as an alternative to virus isolation to maximise detection of EAV in clinical or post-mortem specimens.

It should be emphasised that as the RT-PCR assay will not distinguish between infectious and noninfectious or incomplete virus, the assay cannot determine the current infectivity status of a particular animal or sample of semen, a factor of considerable importance with respect to the international trade in horses and equine semen.

Strains of EAV isolated from different regions of the world have been classified into different phylogenetic groups by sequence analysis of the envelope (G_L, G_S, M) protein genes and the nucleocapsid (N) protein gene (4, 9, 49, 51). The relationships between strains demonstrated by nucleotide sequencing is a useful molecular epidemiological tool for tracing the origin of outbreaks of EVA (2).

c) Histopathological examination

Where mortality is associated with a suspected outbreak of EVA, a wide range of tissues should be examined for histological evidence of panvasculitis that is especially pronounced in the small arteries throughout the body, particularly in the caecum, colon, spleen, associated lymphatic glands and adrenal cortex (12, 30). The presence of a disseminated necrotising arteritis involving endothelial and medial cells of affected vessels is considered to be pathognomonic of EVA. The characteristic vascular lesions present in the mature animal are not, however, as prominent a feature in EAV-related abortions (29).

EAV antigen can be identified in various tissues of EVA-affected animals either in the presence or absence of lesions (12). It can be detected within the cytoplasm of infected cells using equine polyclonal or murine MAbs on fresh or fixed tissues (32).

2. Serological tests

A variety of serological tests including neutralisation (microneutralisation [47] and plaque reduction [36]), complement fixation (18), indirect fluorescent antibody test (12), agar gel immunodiffusion (12), and ELISA (7, 10, 26, 27, 31, 32) have been used to detect antibody to EAV.

The test currently in widest use to diagnose infection, carry out seroprevalence studies, and test horses for export, is a microneutralisation (VN) test in the presence of complement. Besides the VN assay, the complement fixation test, although less sensitive, has also been used for diagnosing recent infections because complement-fixing antibody titres are relatively short lived (18). In contrast, neutralising antibody titres to EAV can persist for several years after natural infection (52). Although the ELISA has been used for diagnosis and seroprevalence studies (7, 10, 31, 32, 46), it is not yet widely accepted as having equivalent sensitivity and specificity to the VN test (7, 26, 27, 46). Unlike the VN test, a positive reaction in the ELISA is not necessarily reflective of protective immunity against EVA as both non-neutralising and neutralising antibodies are involved.

Antiserum to unpurified EAV has been prepared in horses and in rabbits using conventional immunisation protocols. Also, mouse monoclonal and monospecific rabbit polyclonal antibodies have been developed to the nucleocapsid (N) protein (13, 14) envelope (G_L) protein (3, 13, 14, 24), envelope (M and G_S) proteins (42) and other proteins of EAV (13).

OIE Standard Sera for EAV are available[1] and these can facilitate international standardisation of the microneutralisation test and ELISA.

Only one major serotype of EAV has been recognised so far (35, 52). This is represented by the prototype Bucyrus strain (ATCC VR 796), from which the reference virus used in all EAV serological assays has been derived. Virus stock is grown in the RK-13 cell line, clarified of cellular debris by low speed centrifugation and stored in aliquots at –70°C. Several frozen aliquots are thawed and the infectivity of the stock virus is determined by titration in RK-13 cells.

a) Virus neutralisation (a prescribed test for international trade)

The VN test is used to screen stallions for evicence of EAV infection and determine whether there is a need to attempt virus isolation from semen. It can also be used for diagnostic purposes to confirm infection in suspect cases of EVA. The VN test procedure in current widest use is that developed by the National Veterinary Service Laboratories of the United States Department of Agriculture (47). It is recommended that the test be carried out in RK-13 cells using the approved CVL-Bucyrus (Weybridge) strain of EAV as reference virus[2]. Originally derived from the prototype Bucyrus virus, the passage history of the CVL (Weybridge) strain is not fully documented. The sensitivity of the VN test for detection of antibodies to EAV can be significantly influenced by several factors, especially the source and passage history of the strain of virus used (16, 17). The CVL-Bucyrus strain and the highly attenuated vaccine strain of EAV are of comparable sensitivity for detecting low-titred positive sera, especially from EVA-vaccinated horses. For this test, it is important to obtain a sterile blood sample as contamination of serum can interfere with the result. Efforts continue to establish uniformity of the testing protocol and consistency of serological results among laboratories providing the VN test.

---

1 Dr P.J. Timoney, Director, Maxwell H. Gluck Equine Research Center, Dept of Veterinary Science, University of Kentucky, Lexington, Kentucky 40546-0099, United States of America.

2 Dr D.J. Paton, Veterinary Laboratories Agency, Weybridge, New Haw, Addlestone KT15 3NB, United Kingdom.

- **Test procedure**

i) Sera are inactivated for 30 minutes in a water bath at 56°C (control sera, only once).

ii) Serial twofold dilutions of the inactivated test sera in cell culture medium (25 µl volumes) are made in a 96-well, flat-bottomed, cell-culture grade microtitre plate starting at a 1/2 serum dilution and using duplicate rows of wells for each serum to be tested. Most sera are screened initially at a 1/4 and 1/8 serum dilution (i.e. final serum dilution after addition of an equal volume of the appropriate dilution of stock virus to each well). Positive samples at the 1/8 dilution can, if desired, should be retested and titrated out for end-point determination. Individual serum controls, together with negative and known low- and high-titred positive control sera are also included in each test.

iii) A dilution of stock virus to contain from 100 to 300 $TCID_{50}$ (50% tissue culture infective dose) per 25 µl is prepared using as diluent cell culture medium containing antibiotics and fresh guinea-pig complement at a final concentration of 10%.

iv) 25 µl of the appropriate dilution of stock virus is added to every well containing 25 µl of each serum dilution, except the test serum control wells.

v) A virus back titration of the working dilution of stock virus is included, using four wells per tenfold dilution, to confirm the validity of the test results.

vi) The plates are covered and shaken gently to facilitate mixing of the serum/virus mixtures.

vii) The plates are incubated for 1 hour at 37°C in a humid atmosphere of 5% CO_2 in air.

viii) A suspension of cells from 3–5-day-old cultures of RK-13 cells are prepared using a concentration that will result in confluent monolayers in the microtitre plate wells within 18–24 hours after seeding.

ix) 100 µl of cell suspension is added to every well, the plates are covered with plate lids or sealed with tape and shaken gently.

x) The plates are incubated at 37°C in a humid atmosphere of 5% CO_2 in air.

xi) The plates are read microscopically for viral CPE after 48–72 hours' incubation. The validity of the test is confirmed by establishing that the working dilution of stock virus contained 30–300 $TCID_{50}$ virus and that the titres of the positive serum controls are within 0.3 $\log_{10}$ units of their predetermined titres.

A serum dilution is considered to be positive if there is an estimated 75% or perferably 100% reduction in the amount of viral CPE in the serum test wells compared with that present in the wells of the lowest virus control dilution. End-points are then calculated using the Spearman–Kärber method. A titre of 1/4 or greater is considered to be positive. A negative serum should only have a trace (less than 25%) or no virus neutralisation at the lowest dilution tested. Antibody titres may, on occasion, be difficult to define as partial neutralisation may be observed over a range of several serum dilutions. Infrequently, sera will be encountered that cause toxic changes in the lower dilutions tested. In such cases it may not be possible to establish whether the sample is negative or a low-titred positive. Testing another serum sample from the animal in question may resolve the problem.

b) Enzyme-linked immunosorbent assay

A number of direct or indirect ELISAs have been developed for the detection of antibodies to EAV (7, 10, 26, 27, 31, 32). These have been based on the use of purified virus or recombinant-derived viral antigens. The usefulness of earlier assays was compromised by the frequency of false-positive reactions (11, 32). These latter were associated with the presence of antibodies to various tissue culture antigens in the sera of horses that had been vaccinated with tissue-culture-derived antigens (11). Identification of the importance of the viral G_L protein in stimulation of the humoral antibody response to EAV led to the development of several ELISAs that employ a portion of, or the entire recombinant protein produced in a bacterial or baculovirus expression system (3, 10, 13, 24, 26). Some of these assays appear to offer comparable sensitivity and specificity to the VN test and may detect EAV-specific antibodies prior to a positive reaction being obtainable in the VN test (7). False-negative reactions can occur, however, even with some of these assays. An ELISA based on the use of a combination of the G_L, M or N structural proteins of EAV expressed from recombinant baculoviruses successfully detected viral antibody in naturally or experimentally infected horses but not in EVA-vaccinated animals (26). Of major importance with respect to any G_L protein-based ELISA for EAV is the fact that test sensitivity will vary depending on the ectodomain sequence(s) of this viral protein used in the assay. Considerable amino acid sequence variation within this domain has been found between isolates of EAV (4, 24). Therefore, to maximise sensitivity of a G_L-based ELISA, it may be necessary to include multiple ectodomain sequences representative of known phylogenetically different isolates of EAV rather than depend on a single ectodomain sequence. A more recently developed blocking ELISA involving MAb produced against the G_L protein has been reported to have a sensitivity of 99.4% and a specificity of 97.7% compared with the VN test (10). Screening a random peptide-phage library with polyclonal sera from EAV-infected horses has led to the identification of ligands, which have been purified and used as antigen in an ELISA for EAV (27). No correlation has been found, however, between absorbency values obtained with this assay and neutralising antibody titres, indicating that the antibodies being detected are largely against nonsurface epitopes of the virus. It is expected that an ELISA will be available soon that can provide equivalent sensitivity and specificity to the VN test.

B. REQUIREMENTS FOR VACCINES AND DIAGNOSTIC BIOLOGICALS

Two tissue culture vaccines have been commercially developed against EVA. The first is a modified live virus (MLV) vaccine prepared from virus that has been attenuated for horses by multiple serial transfers in equine and rabbit cell cultures. This vaccine is licensed for use in stallions, nonpregnant mares and in nonbreeding horses. Whereas nonbreeding horses can be vaccinated at any time, stallions and mares should be vaccinated not less than 3 weeks prior to breeding. The vaccine is not recommended for use in pregnant mares, especially in the last 2 months of gestation, nor in foals under 6 weeks of age unless in the face of significant risk of exposure to natural infection. The vaccine is commercially available in the USA and Canada.

The second commercial vaccine developed against EVA is an inactivated product prepared from virus grown in equine cell culture, which is filtered, chemically inactivated and then combined with a metabolisable adjuvant. This vaccine is licensed for use in nonbreeding and breeding horses. In the absence of appropriate safety data, the vaccine is currently not recommended for use in pregnant mares. The initial vaccination regimen involves two doses of vaccine administered intramuscularly 3–6 weeks apart. Booster vaccination is recommended at 6-month intervals. The inactivated vaccine is licensed for commercial use in certain European countries, including Denmark, Ireland and the United Kingdom.

An additional inactivated vaccine against EVA has been developed in Japan for use should an outbreak of EVA occur in that country (20). It is an aqueous formalin-inactivated vaccine that has been shown to be safe and effective for use in nonbreeding and breeding horses. For optimal immunisation with this vaccine, horses require a primary course of two injections given at an interval of 4 weeks, with a booster dose administered every 6–12 months. As it is currently not commercially available, no details will be provided on the production of this vaccine.

1. Seed management

a) Characteristics of the seed

Both MLV and inactivated commercial vaccines are derived from the prototype Bucyrus strain of EAV (ATCC VR 796). Available evidence points to the existence of only one major serotype of the virus, and strain variation is not considered to be of significance in relation to vaccine efficacy (35, 52).

In the case of the MLV vaccine, the prototype virus was attenuated by serial passage in primary cultures of horse kidney (HK-131), rabbit kidney (RK-111), and a diploid equine dermal cell line, ATCC CCL57 (ECID-24) (15, 25, 35). The indications from the use of this vaccine are that the virus is safe and immunogenic between its 80th and 111th passage in primary rabbit kidney (15, 25, 35, 37, 40, 41, 54).

The inactivated adjuvanted vaccine is prepared from the unattenuated prototype Bucyrus strain of EAV (ATCC VR 796) that has been plaque purified and in its fourth serial passage in the diploid equine dermal cell line (ECID-4). After growth in cell culture, the virus is then purified by filtration before being chemically inactivated and adjuvanted.

Suitable lots of master seed virus for each vaccine should be maintained in liquid nitrogen or its equivalent.

b) Method of culture

The virus for both MLV and inactivated vaccines should be grown in a stable cell culture system, such as equine dermal cells, using an appropriate medium supplemented with sterile bovine serum or bovine serum albumin as replacement for bovine serum in the growth medium. Cell monolayers should be washed prior to virus inoculation to remove traces of bovine serum. Extensive virus growth as evidenced by the appearance of cytopathic changes in 80–100% of the cells should be obtained within 2–3 days.

c) Validation as a vaccine

In the case of both MLV and inactivated vaccines, the respective virus strains should be grown in an appropriate cell culture system that has been officially approved for vaccine production and confirmed to be free from extraneous bacteria, fungi, mycoplasmas and viruses (44). The identity of the vaccine virus in the master seed should be confirmed by neutralisation with homologous anti-EAV serum. Incomplete neutralisation of EAV by homologous horse or rabbit antisera has been scientifically documented (47) and is a problem when screening master seed virus for extraneous viruses and when attempting to confirm the identity of the vaccine virus. The problem has been circumvented by reducing the infectivity titre of the master seed virus below that required for seed virus production before conducting a neutralisation test on the diluted virus. Virus/serum mixtures are tested for residual live virus by serial passage in cell culture. No evidence of cytopathic viruses, haemadsorbing viruses, or noncytopathic strains of bovine virus diarrhoea virus should be found, based on attempted virus isolation in cell culture. If cells of equine origin are used, they should be confirmed to be free from equine infectious anaemia virus. The newer technologies of PCR and antigen-capture ELISA may be used in the future as adjuncts to virus isolation in screening for adventitious agents.

The MLV vaccine has been shown to be both safe and effective for use in stallions and nonpregnant mares (40, 41, 54). Vaccination confers a high level of protective immunity that persists for at least several years (25, 35). Based on experimental studies and extensive field use of the vaccine for over 14 years, there is no evidence of back reversion to virulence of the vaccine virus, nor of recombination of the vaccine virus with naturally occurring strains of EAV. Furthermore, there are ample data to confirm that the attenuated strain of EAV in the current vaccine is not shed in the semen of stallions after vaccination nor does it localise and set up the carrier state in the reproductive tract of the stallion (41, 52, 54).

The commercial inactivated vaccine has been shown to be nonreactive and safe for use in healthy nonbreeding and breeding horses. Limited field studies of this vaccine indicate that it is immunogenic, stimulating a satisfactory degree of immunity, the duration of which has yet to be reported.

Although there are no published reports on the efficacy of either commercial vaccine in preventing establishment of the carrier state in the stallion, an aqueous formalin inactivated vaccine against EVA has been shown to prevent virus persistence in the reproductive tract of vaccinated stallions following subsequent experimental challenge with EAV (19).

2. Method of manufacture

Both the MLV and inactivated vaccines are produced by cultivation of the respective seed viruses in an equine dermal cell system. Cell monolayers should be washed prior to inoculation with seed virus to remove traces of bovine serum in the growth medium. Inoculated cultures should be maintained on an appropriate maintenance medium. Harvesting of infected cultures should take place when almost the entire cell sheet shows the characteristic CPE. Supernatant fluid and cells are harvested and clarified of cellular debris and unwanted material by filtration. In the case of the inactivated vaccine, the purified virus is then chemically inactivated and adjuvanted with a metabolisable adjuvant.

3. In-process control

The MLV and inactivated vaccines should be produced in a stable cell line that has been tested for identity and confirmed to be free from contamination by bacteria, fungi, mycoplasmas or other adventitious agents. In addition to the preproduction testing of the master seed virus for each vaccine and the cell line for adventitious contaminants, the cell cultures infected with the respective vaccine viruses should be examined macroscopically for evidence of microbial growth or other extraneous contamination during the incubation period. If growth in a culture vessel cannot be reliably determined by visual examination, subculture, microscopic examination, or both should be carried out.

4. Batch control

a) Sterility

Tests for sterility and freedom from contamination of biological materials may be found in Chapter I.4.

b) Safety

In the case of both MLV and inactivated vaccines, each production lot of vaccine should be checked for extraneous bacterial, fungal and mycoplasmal contaminants. The vaccine should be safety tested by the intramuscular inoculation of at least two horses seronegative for neutralising antibodies to EAV with one vaccine dose of lyophilised virus each (44). None of the inoculated horses should develop any clinical signs of disease other than mild pyrexia during the ensuing 2-week observation period. In addition, nasopharyngeal swabs should be collected daily from each horse for attempted virus isolation; white blood cell counts and body temperatures should also be determined on a daily basis. No significant febrile or haematological changes should supervene following vaccination (41, 52, 54). Limited shedding of vaccine virus by the respiratory route for at most 7 days may be demonstrated in the occasional vaccinated horse (54). There is no evidence of virus shedding in the semen of stallions following vaccination (41, 54).

To ensure complete inactivation of the vaccine virus, each serial lot of the inactivated vaccine should be checked for viable virus by three serial passages in equine dermal cells and by direct fluorescent antibody staining with specific EAV conjugate before being combined with adjuvant. This should be followed by a safety test in guinea-pigs and mice.

c) **Potency**

Potency of the vaccine in the final containers is determined by plaque infectivity assay in monolayer cultures of equine dermal cells and by a vaccination challenge test in horses (44). The vaccine must be tested in triplicate in cell culture, the mean infectivity titre calculated and the dose rate determined on the basis that each dose of vaccine shall contain not less than 3×10^4 plaque-forming units of attenuated EAV. The *in-vivo* potency of the MLV and inactivated vaccines is evaluated in a single vaccination challenge test using 17–20 vaccinated and 5–7 control horses or in two tests each comprising ten vaccinates and five controls.

The viral antigen concentration in the inactivated vaccine is over one-thousand times the concentration of viral antigen present in the MLV vaccine.

d) **Duration of immunity**

Detectable neutralising antibody titres to EAV should develop in the majority of horses within 3 weeks of vaccination with the MLV vaccine (37, 40, 41, 52, 54). Responses to primary vaccination are characterised by a rapid fall in antibody titres with a significant number of animals reverting to seronegativity 1–3 months after vaccination (54). Revaccination with this vaccine results in an excellent anamnestic response, however, with the development of high antibody titres that remain relatively undiminished for 12 months or longer (52).

Experimental studies have shown that most horses vaccinated with the inactivated vaccine develop low to moderate neutralising antibody titres to EAV by day 14 after the second vaccination. There is no published information on the duration of immunity conferred by this vaccine.

e) **Stability**

The lyophilised MLV vaccine can be stored for at least 3–4 years at 2–7°C without loss in infectivity, provided it is kept in the dark (25). Infectivity should be preserved for much longer periods if vaccine is frozen at –20°C or below. Once rehydrated, however, the vaccine should be used within 1 hour or else destroyed. The inactivated vaccine is stored as a liquid suspension at 2–8°C, with no loss of potency for at least 1 year, provided it is protected from light.

f) **Preservatives**

The preservatives added to the MLV and inactivated vaccines are neomycin, polymyxin B and amphotericin B, and those added to the inactivated vaccine are neomycin, polymyxin B, amphotericin B and thiomersal.

g) **Precautions (hazards)**

Pregnant mares should not be vaccinated with the MLV vaccine during the last 2 months of gestation, as there is a risk, albeit minimal, of fetal invasion by the vaccine virus. The possibility of a vaccinally induced anaphylactic reaction, though very rare, could result from the administration of either the MLV or inactivated vaccine. In the absence of appropriate safety data, the inactivated vaccine is currently not recommended for use in pregnant mares.

5. Tests on the final product

a) **Safety**

With the exception of the inactivated vaccine, which needs to be sterility tested a second time to ensure freedom from contamination, no further safety tests are required on the inactivated or MLV vaccines.

b) **Potency**

No potency tests additional to those conducted on each production lot of the MLV or inactivated vaccines are required on either final product.

REFERENCES

1. ASAGOE T., INABA Y., JUSA E.R., KOUNO M., UWATOKO K. & FUKUNAGA Y. (1997). Effect of heparin on infection of cells by equine arteritis virus. *J. Vet. Med. Sci.*, **59**, 727–728.

2. BALASURIYA U.B.R., EVERMANN J.F., HEDGES J.F., MCKEIRNAN A.J., MITTEN J.Q., BEYER J.C., MCCOLLUM W.H., TIMONEY P.J. & MACLACHLAN N.J. (1998). Serologic and molecular characterization of an abortigenic strain of equine arteritis virus isolated from infective frozen semen and an aborted equine fetus. *J. Am. Vet. Med. Assoc.*, **213**, 1586–1589.

3. BALASURIYA U.B.R., MACLACHLAN N.J., DE VRIES A.A.F., ROSSITTO P.V. & ROTTIER P.J.M. (1995). Identification of a neutralisation site in the major envelope glycoprotein (G_L) of equine arteritis virus. *Virology*, **207**, 518–527.

4. BALASURIYA U.B.R., TIMONEY P.J., MCCOLLUM W.H. & MACLACHLAN N.J. (1995). Phylogenetic analysis of open reading frame 5 of field isolates of equine arteritis virus and identification of conserved and nonconserved regions in the G_L envelope glycoprotein. *Virology*, **214**, 690–697.

5. BELAK S., BALLAGI-PORDANY A., TIMONEY P., MCCOLLUM W.H, LITTLE T.V., HYLLSETH B. & KLINGEBORN B. (1995). Evaluation of a nested PCR assay for the detection of equine arteritis virus infection. Proceedings of the 7th International Conference on Equine Infectious Diseases, Tokyo, Japan, 1994, 33–38.

6. CAVANAGH D. (1997). Nidovirales: A new order comprising Coronaviridae and Arteriviridae. *Arch. Virol.*, **142**, 629–633.

7. CHIRNSIDE E.D., FRANCIS P.M., DE VRIES A.A.F., SINCLAIR R. & MUMFORD J.A. (1995). Development and evaluation of an ELISA using recombinant fusion protein to detect the presence of host antibody to equine arteritis virus (EAV). *J. Virol. Methods*, **54**, 1–13.

8. CHIRNSIDE E.D. & SPAAN W.J.M. (1990). Reverse transcription and cDNA amplification by the polymerase chain reaction of equine arteritis virus (EAV). *J. Virol. Methods*, **30**, 133–140.

9. CHIRNSIDE E.D., WEARING C.M., BINNS M.M. & MUMFORD J.A. (1994). Comparison of M and N gene sequences distinguishes variation amongst equine arteritis virus isolates. *J. Gen. Virol.*, **75**, 1491–1497.

10. CHO H.J., ENTZ S.C., DEREGT D., JORDAN L.T., TIMONEY P.J. & MCCOLLUM W.H. (2000). Detection of antibodies to equine arteritis virus by a monoclonal antibody-based blocking ELISA. *Can. J. Vet. Res.*, **64**, 38–43.

11. COOK R.F., GANN S.J. & MUMFORD J.A. (1989). The effects of vaccination with tissue culture-derived viral vaccines on detection of antibodies to equine arteritis virus by enzyme-linked immunosorbent assay (ELISA). *Vet. Microbiol.*, **20**, 181–189.

12. CRAWFORD T.B. & HENSON J.B. (1973). Immunofluorescent, light microscopic and immunologic studies of equine viral arteritis. Proceedings of the Third International Conference on Equine Infectious Diseases, Paris, 1972. Karger, Basel, Switzerland, 282–302.

13. DEREGT D., DE VRIES A.A.F., RAAMSMAN M.J.B., ELMGREN L.D. & ROTTIER P.J.M. (1994). Monoclonal antibodies to equine arteritis virus identify the G_L protein as a target for virus neutralization. *J. Gen. Virol.*, **75**, 2439–2444.

14. DE VRIES A.A.F., CHIRNSIDE E.D., HORZINEK M.C. & ROTTIER P.J.M. (1992). Structural proteins of equine arteritis virus. *J. Virol.*, **66**, 6294–6303.

15. DOLL E.R., BRYANS J.T., WILSON J.C. & MCCOLLUM W.H. (1968). Immunisation against equine viral arteritis using modified live virus propagated in cell cultures of rabbit kidney. *Cornell Vet.*, **48**, 497–524.

16. EDWARDS S., CASTILLO-OLIVARES J., CULLINANE A., LABLE J., LENIHAN P., MUMFORD J.A., PATON D.J., PEARSON J.E., SINCLAIR R., WESTCOTT D.G.F., WOOD J.L.N., ZIENTARA S. & NELLY M. (1999). International harmonisation of laboratory diagnostic tests for equine viral arteritis. Proceedings of the Eighth International Conference on Equine Infectious Diseases, Dubai, UAE, 1998, 359–362.

17. FUKUNAGA Y., MATSUMURA T., SUGIURA T., WADA R., IMAGAWA H., KANEMARU T. & KAMADA M. (1994). Use of the serum neutralisation test for equine viral arteritis with different virus strains. *Vet. Rec.*, **136**, 574–576

18. FUKUNAGA Y. & MCCOLLUM W.H. (1977). Complement fixation reactions in equine viral arteritis. *Am. J. Vet. Res.*, **38**, 2043–2046.

19. FUKUNAGA Y., WADA R., MATSUMURA T., ANZAI T., IMAGAWA H., SUGIURA T., KUMANOMIDO T., KANEMARU T. & KAMADA M. (1992). An attempt to protect against persistent infection of equine viral arteritis in the reproductive tract of stallions using formalin inactivated-virus vaccine. Proceedings of the Sixth International Conference on Equine Infectious Diseases, Cambridge, UK, 1991, 239–244.

20. FUKUNAGA Y., WADA R., MATSUMURA T., SUGIURA T. & IMAGAWA H. (1990). Induction of immune response and protection from equine viral arteritis (EVA) by formalin inactivated-virus vaccine for EVA in horses. *J. Vet. Med. (B)*, **37**, 135–141.

21. FUKUNAGA Y., WADA R., SUGITA S., FUJITA Y., NAMBO Y., IMAGAWA H., KANEMARU T., KAMADA M., KOMATSU N. & AKASHI H. (2000). *In vitro* detection of equine arteritis virus from seminal plasma for identification of carrier stallions. *J. Vet. Med. Sci.*, **62**, 643–646.

22. GERBER H., STECK F., HOFER B., WALTHER L. & FRIEDLI U. (1978). Serological investigations on equine viral arteritis. Proceedings of the Fourth International Conference on Equine Infectious Diseases, Princeton, New Jersey, USA, 1976, Veterinary Publications, 461–465.

23. GILBERT S.A., TIMONEY P.J., MCCOLLUM W.H. & DEREGT D. (1997). Detection of equine arteritis virus in the semen of carrier stallions using a sensitive nested PCR assay. *J. Clin. Microbiol.*, **35**, 2181–2183.

24. GLASER A.L., DE VRIES A.A.F. & DUBOVI E.J. (1995). Comparison of equine arteritis virus isolates using neutralizing monoclonal antibodies and identification of sequence changes in G_L associated with neutralization resistance. *J. Gen. Virol.*, **76**, 2223–2233.

25. HARRY T.O. & MCCOLLUM W.H. (1981). Stability of viability and immunising potency of lyophilised, modified equine arteritis live-virus vaccine. *Am. J. Vet. Res.*, **42**, 1501–1505.

26. HEDGES J.F., BALASURIYA U.B.R., SHABBIR A., TIMONEY P.J., MCCOLLUM W.H., YILMA T. & MACLACHLAN N.J. (1998). Detection of antibodies to equine arteritis virus by enzyme linked immunosorbant assays utilizing G_L, M and N proteins expressed from recombinant baculoviruses. *J. Virol. Methods*, **76**,127–137.

27. INIGUEZ P., ZIENTARA S., MARAULT M., MACHIN I. B., HANNANT D. & CRUCIERE C. (1998). Screening of horse polyclonal antibodies with a random peptide library displayed on phage: identification of ligands used as antigens in an ELISA test to detect the presence of antibodies to equine arteritis virus. *J. Virol. Methods*, **73**, 175–183.

28. INOUE T., YANAGAWA R., SHINAGAWA M. & AKIYAMA Y. (1975). Immunofluorescent studies on the multiplication of equine arteritis virus in Vero and E. Derm (NBL-6) cells. *Jpn J. Vet. Sci. (Nippon Juigaku Zasshi)*, **37**, 569–575.

29. JOHNSON B., BALDWIN C., TIMONEY P. & ELY R. (1991). Arteritis in equine fetuses aborted due to equine viral arteritis. *Vet. Pathol.*, **28**, 248–250.

30. JONES T.C., DOLL E.R. & BRYANS J.T. (1957). The lesions of equine viral arteritis. *Cornell Vet.*, **47**, 52–68.

31. KONDO T., FUKUNAGA Y., SEKIGUCHI K., SUGIURA T. & IMAGAWA H. (1998). Enzyme-linked immunosorbent assay for serological survey of equine arteritis virus in racehorses. *J. Vet. Med. Sci.*, **60**, 1043–1045.

32. LANG G. & MITCHELL W.R. (1984). A serosurvey by ELISA for antibodies to equine arteritis virus in Ontario racehorses. *J. Equine Vet. Sci* **4**, 153–157.

33. LITTLE T.V., DEREGT D., MCCOLLUM W.H., & TIMONEY P.J. (1995). Evaluation of an immunocytochemical method for rapid detection and identification of equine arteritis virus in natural cases of infection. Proceedings of the Seventh International Conference on Equine Infectious Diseases, Tokyo, Japan, 1994, 27–31.

34. LOPEZ J.W., DEL PIERO F., GLASER A. & FINAZZI M. (1996). Immunoperoxidase histochemistry as a diagnostic tool for detection of equine arteritis virus antigen in formalin fixed tissues. *Equine Vet. J.*, **28**, 77–79.

35. MCCOLLUM W.H. (1969). Development of a modified virus strain and vaccine for equine viral arteritis. *J. Am. Vet. Med. Assoc.*, **155**, 318–322.

36. MCCOLLUM W.H. (1970). Vaccination for equine viral arteritis. Proceedings of the Second International Conference on Equine Infectious Diseases, Paris, 1969, Karger, Basle, Switzerland, 143–151.

37. MCCOLLUM W.H. (1986). Responses of horses vaccinated with avirulent modified-live equine arteritis virus propagated in the E. Derm (NBL-6) cell line to nasal inoculation with virulent virus. *Am. J. Vet. Res.*, **47**, 1931–1934.

38. MCCOLLUM W.H., PRICKETT M.E. & BRYANS J.T. (1971). Temporal distribution of equine arteritis virus in respiratory mucosa, tissues and body fluids of horses infected by inhalation. *Res. Vet. Sci.*, **2**, 459–464.

39. MCCOLLUM W.H. & SWERCZEK T.W. (1978). Studies of an epizootic of equine viral arteritis in racehorses. *J. Equine Med. Surg.*, **2**, 293–299.

40. MCCOLLUM W.H. TIMONEY P.J., ROBERTS A.W., WILLARD J.E. & CARSWELL G.D. (1988). Response of vaccinated and non-vaccinated mares to artificial insemination with semen from stallions persistently infected with equine arteritis virus. Proceedings of the Fifth International Conference on Equine Infectious Diseases, Lexington, 1987, University Press of Kentucky, Lexington, Kentucky, USA, 13–18.

41. MCKINNON A.O., COLBERN G.C., COLLINS J.K., BOWEN R.A., VOSS J.L. & UMPHENOUR N.W. (1986). Vaccination of stallions with modified live equine viral arteritis virus. *J. Equine Vet. Sci.*, **6**, 66–69.

42. MACLACHLAN N.J., BALASURIYA U.B.R., HEDGES J.F., SCHWEIDLER T.M., MCCOLLUM W.H., TIMONEY P.J., HULLINGER P.J. & PATTON J.F. (1998). Serologic response of horses to the structural proteins of equine arteritis virus. *J. Vet. Diagn. Invest.*, **10**, 229–236.

43. MACLACHLAN N.J., BALASURIYA U.B.R., ROSITTO P.V., HULLINGER P.A., PATTON J.F. & WILSON W.D. (1996). Fatal experimental equine arteritis virus infection of a pregnant mare: immunohistochemical staining of viral antigens. *J. Diagn. Invest.*, **8**, 367–374.

44. MOORE B.O. (1986). Development and evaluation of three equine vaccines. *Irish Vet. J.*, **40**, 105–107.

45. OSTLUND E.N., PETERS J.C, STOKER A.M, MCCOLLUM, W.H & TIMONEY P.J. (1997). Enhancement of cell culture growth of two arteriviruses by carboxymethyl cellulose overlay. Abstract. Proceedings of the Annual Meeting of the American Association of Veterinary Laboratory Diagnosticians, Louisville, Kentucky, USA, p. 33.

46. PAWESKA J.T., BINNS M.M., WOODS P.S.A. & CHIRNSIDE E.D. (1997). A survey for antibodies to equine arteritis virus in donkeys, mules and zebra using virus neutralisation (VN) and enzyme linked immunosorbent assay (ELISA). *Equine Vet. J.*, **29**, 40–43.

47. SENNE D.A., PEARSON J.E. & CABREY E.A. (1985). Equine viral arteritis: A standard procedure for the virus neutralisation test and comparison of results of a proficiency test performed at five laboratories. *Proc. U.S. Anim. Health Assoc.*, **89**, 29–34.

48. ST-LAURENT G., MORIN G. & ARCHAMBAULT D. (1994). Detection of equine arteritis virus following amplification of structural and nonstructural viral genes by reverse transcription-PCR. *J. Clin. Microbiol.*, **32**, 658–665.

49. STADEJEK T., BJORKLUND H., BASCUNANA C.R., CIABATTI I.M., SCICLUNA M.T., AMADDEO D., MCCOLLUM W.H., AUTORINO G.L., TIMONEY P.J., PATON D.J., KLINGEBORN B. & BELAK S. (1999). Genetic diversity of equine arteritis virus. *J. Gen. Virol.*, **80**, 691–699.

50. SUGITA S., IMAGAWA H., WADA R. & FUKUNAGA Y. (1997). RT-PCR detection of equine arteritis virus from various samples of an experimentally infected pregnant mare. *J. Equine Sci.*, **8**, 29–33.

51. SUGITA S., KONDO T., SEKIGUCHI K., YAMAGUCHI S., KAMADA M., NEROME K. & FUKUNAGA Y. (1994). Molecular evolution of the M gene of equine arteritis virus. Proceedings of the Seventh International Conference on Equine Infectious Diseases, Tokyo, Japan, 1994, 39–43.

52. TIMONEY P.J. & MCCOLLUM W.H. (1993). Equine viral arteritis. *Vet. Clin. North Am. Equine Pract.*, 9, 295–309.

53. TIMONEY P.J., MCCOLLUM W.J., MURPHY T.W., ROBERTS A.W., WILLARD J.G. & CARSWELL G.D. (1987). The carrier state in equine arteritis virus infection in the stallion with specific emphasis on the venereal mode of virus transmission. *J. Reprod. Fertil.* (Suppl.), **35**, 95–102.

54. TIMONEY P.J., UMPHENOUR N.W. & MCCOLLUM W.H. (1988). Safety evaluation of a commercial modified live equine arteritis virus vaccine for use in stallions. Proceedings of the Fifth International Conference on Equine Infectious Diseases, Lexington, 1987, University Press of Kentucky, Lexington, Kentucky, USA, 19–27.

55. TRAUB-DARGATZ J., RALSTON S., BENNETT D. & COLLINS J. (1985). Outbreak of EVA at CSU-VTH. *J. Equine Vet. Sci.*, 5,168.

56. WADA R., KONDO T., FUKUNAGA Y. & KANEMARU T. (1995). Histopathological and immunofluorescent studies on the uterus of aborted mares experimentally infected with equine arteritis virus. *J. Equine Sci.*, **5**, 41–43.

*

* *

CHAPTER 2.5.12.

VENEZUELAN EQUINE ENCEPHALOMYELITIS

SUMMARY

Venezuelan equine encephalomyelitis (VEE) viruses, of the genus Alphavirus of the family Togaviridae, cause disease ranging from mild febrile reactions to fatal encephalitic zoonoses in Equidae and humans. They are transmitted by haematophagous insects.

High infection rates in humans have been documented following exposure to aerosols from infected laboratory animals or from laboratory accidents. Severe clinical disease or death can occur in humans. Neither infective VEE viruses nor their antigens prepared from infected tissues or cell cultures must ever be handled by personnel who do not possess demonstrable immunity in the form of neutralising antibody. All laboratory manipulations must be carried out within certified biological safety cabinets with facilities for efficient biocontainment and an adequately filtered air exhaust system.

VEE viruses are divided into six antigenic subtypes (I–VI). Within subtype I there are five antigenic variants (variants AB–F). Antigenic variants I-AB and I-C are associated with epizootic activity in equids. The other three variants of subtype I (I-D, I-E, I-F) and the other five subtypes of VEE have been associated with natural enzootic cycles. These variants and subtypes have been considered to be nonpathogenic for equids, although they can cause clinical disease in humans. These are known as enzootic VEE viruses; they cycle between rodents, mosquitoes, and birds. During 1993 and 1996; however, an outbreak of encephalitis in horses in Mexico was shown to be caused by enzootic VEE viruses of subtype I-E.

***Identification of the agent:** Diagnosis of VEE virus infection can be confirmed by the isolation, identification, and antigenic classification of the isolated virus.*

A presumptive diagnosis of equine encephalomyelitis can be made when susceptible animals in tropical or subtropical areas display clinical signs of encephalomyelitis where haematophagous insects are active. VEE virus can be isolated in cell cultures or in laboratory animals using the blood or serum of febrile animals that have been exposed to clinical cases of encephalitis by the bites of infected mosquitoes. It is recovered less frequently from the blood or brains of encephalitic animals.

VEE virus can be identified by complement fixation, haemagglutination inhibition, plaque reduction neutralisation (PRN), or immunofluorescence tests using VEE-specific antibodies. Specific identification of epizootic VEE variants can be made by the indirect fluorescent antibody test, or a differential PRN test using subtype- or variant-specific monoclonal antibody, or by nucleic acid sequencing.

***Serological tests:** Specific antibodies may be demonstrated by PRN tests against epizootic VEE virus variants or by IgM capture enzyme-linked immunosorbent assay.*

Any diagnosis of VEE in an individual that is based on seroconversion in the absence of an epizootic should be made with care. Although enzootic subtypes and variants are normally of low pathogenicity for equids, subclinical infection will stimulate antibody production to epizootic VEE virus variants.

Infections of equids with enzootic VEE viruses will usually produce a low level viraemia accompanied by antibody development, but without clinical disease in most cases.

***Requirements for vaccines and diagnostic biologicals:** The only acceptable vaccines against VEE are an attenuated virus vaccine, made with strain TC-83, or inactivated virus preparations* *also made from this strain. Attenuated virus is immunogenic when given by intramuscular injection, but sometimes causes adverse reactions in the recipient.*

Formalin-inactivated virulent VEE virus preparations should never be used in equids, as residual virulent virus can remain after formalin treatment, and thereby cause severe illness in both animals and humans. Epizootics of VEE have occurred from the use of such formalin-treated viruses.

A. DIAGNOSTIC TECHNIQUES

The Venezuelan equine encephalomyelitis (VEE) complex of viruses, of the genus Alphavirus of the family Togaviridae, are mosquito-transmitted, zoonotic pathogens that produce from mild to severe febrile, occasionally fatal, encephalitic diseases in equines and humans. Infections by aerosols have originated from the cage debris of infected laboratory rodents and from laboratory accidents. Those who handle infectious VEE viruses or their antigens prepared from infected tissues or cell cultures should be vaccinated and shown to have demonstrable immunity in the form of VEE virus-specific neutralising antibody (1, 4). All procedures producing aerosols from VEE virus materials should be conducted in biosafety cabinets with biocontainment and efficient filtration of the exhaust air from the laboratory (6, 7).

The VEE virus complex is composed of six subtypes (I–VI). Within subtype I, there are five antigenic variants (AB–F) (2–4, 8, 10). Originally, subtypes I-A and I-B were considered to be distinct variants, but they are now considered to be identical (I-AB). Within subtype III, there are three antigenic variants (A–C). Antigenic variants I-AB and I-C have been associated with epizootic VEE in equids and concurrent epidemics in humans (3, 4, 8–10). These equine pathogens are known as epizootic variants; they have been isolated from equids, humans, and haematophagous insects (primarily mosquitoes) only during equine epizootics. Subtype I-C was isolated in Venezuela in 1993 and Venezuela and Colombia in 1995. Subtype I-D was isolated from Peru in 1994 and 1995. The recent epizootic isolates appear to have evolved from enzootic I-D subtype (5).

The variants of subtype I (I-D, I-E, and I-F) and the other five subtypes (II–VI) have been associated with naturally occurring cycles. Normally, enzootic VEE viruses do not produce clinical encephalomyelitis in the equine species (9), but in 1993 and 1996 in Mexico, an enzootic subtype caused a limited epizootic in horses. These enzootic variants and subtypes can produce clinical disease in humans (3, 4, 8, 10). Infections with both epizootic and enzootic variants and subtypes have been acquired by laboratory workers (6).

Historically, epizootic VEE was limited to northern and western South America (Venezuela, Colombia, Ecuador, Peru and Trinidad) (4). From 1969 to 1972, however, epizootic activity occurred in Guatemala, El Salvador, Nicaragua, Honduras, Costa Rica, Belize, Mexico, and the United States of America (USA) (Texas). Epizootics of VEE caused by I-AB or I-C virus have not occurred in North America and Mexico since 1972. The only recent isolation of epizootic VEE virus variants was I-C from horses and humans in Venezuela in 1993 and 1996, and Venezuela and Colombia in 1995. In addition, an enzootic variant (I-E) caused disease in horses in Mexico in 1993. In contrast, enzootic VEE variants and subtypes exist continuously in enzootic foci in the tropical and subtropical Americas including the Florida Everglades (subtype II), Mexico (variant I-E), the Central American countries (variant I-E), Panama (variants I-D and I-E), Venezuela (variant I-D), Colombia (variant I-D), Peru (variant III-C), French Guiana (variant III-B and subtype V), Ecuador (variant I-D), Suriname (variant III-A), Trinidad (variant III-A), Brazil (variants I-F and III-A and subtype IV), and Argentina (subtype VI). In an atypical ecological niche, variant III-B has been isolated in the USA (Colorado and South Dakota) in an unusual association with birds (3, 4, 8, 10).

The foci of enzootic variants and subtypes are found in areas classified as tropical wet forest, i.e. those areas with a high water table or open swampy areas with meandering sunlit streams. These are the areas of the Americas where rainfall is distributed throughout the year or areas permanently supplied with water. Enzootic viruses cycle among rodents, and perhaps birds, by the feeding of mosquitoes (3, 4, 8, 10).

A tentative diagnosis of viral encephalomyelitis in equids can be based on the occurrence of acute neurological disease during the summer in temperate climates or in the wet season in tropical or subtropical climates. These are the seasons of haematophagous insect activity. Virus infection will result in clinical disease in many equids concurrently rather than in isolated cases. Epizootic activity can move vast distances through susceptible populations in a short time (3, 4, 8, 10).

1. Identification of the agent

A confirmatory diagnosis of VEE is based on the isolation and identification of the virus or on the demonstration of seroconversion. The period of viraemia coincides with the onset of pyrexia within 12–24 hours of infection. Viraemia terminates 5–6 days after infection, and coincides with the production of neutralising antibodies and the appearance of clinical neurological signs. Frequently, VEE viruses cannot be isolated from the brains of infected equids. Blood samples for virus isolation should be collected from febrile animals that are closely associated with clinical encephalitic cases.

Virus may be isolated from the blood or sera of infected animals by inoculating 1–4-day-old mice or hamsters intracerebrally or by the inoculation of other laboratory animals, such as guinea-pigs and weaned mice. It may also be isolated by the inoculation of various cell cultures including African green monkey kidney (Vero), rabbit kidney (RK-13), baby hamster kidney (BHK-21), or duck or chicken embryo fibroblasts, or by inoculation of embryonated chicken eggs. Details of virus identification techniques are described in Chapter 2.5.3. Equine encephalomyelitis (Eastern and Western).

Isolates can be identified as VEE virus by complement fixation (CF), haemagglutination inhibition (HI), or plaque reduction neutralisation (PRN) tests, or by immunofluorescence. The VEE virus isolates can be characterised by the indirect fluorescent antibody test or PRN using monoclonal antibody or by nucleic acid sequencing. The VEE virus characterisation should be carried out in a reference laboratory (see Table given in Part 4 of this *Manual*).

2. Serological tests

Diagnosis of VEE virus infection in equids requires the demonstration of specific antibodies in paired serum samples collected in the acute and convalescent phases. After infection, PRN antibodies appear within 5–7 days, CF antibodies within 6–9 days, and HI antibodies within 6–7 days. The second convalescent phase serum sample should be collected 4–7 days after the collection of the first acute phase sample or at the time of death. The serological procedures are described in detail in Chapter 2.5.3.

Any diagnosis of VEE in an individual that is based on seroconversion in the absence of an epizootic should be made with care. Although enzootic subtypes and variants are nonpathogenic for equids, infection will stimulate antibody production to epizootic VEE virus variants.

B. REQUIREMENTS FOR VACCINES AND DIAGNOSTIC BIOLOGICALS

The acceptable vaccines against VEE infection are an attenuated virus vaccine, strain TC-83, and an inactivated virus preparation made from that strain (3, 4, 8, 10). The inactivated vaccine is now the most widely used, and is marketed in EEE/VEE and EEE/WEE/VEE combinations.

Inactivated vaccine should be administered in two doses with an interval of 2–4 weeks between doses. Annual revaccination is recommended.

Attenuated vaccine should be reconstituted with physiological saline and used immediately. Multidose vials are kept on ice while the vaccine is being used. Any vaccine not used within 4 hours of reconstitution should be safely discarded. Foals under 2 weeks of age and pregnant mares should not be vaccinated. Animals are vaccinated subcutaneously in the cervical region with a single dose. Revaccination is not recommended.

NOTE: Formalin-treated preparations of virulent epizootic VEE virus should never be used in equids. Residual virulent virus can remain after formalin treatment, and result in severe illness. Epizootics of VEE have occurred in Central and Southern America from the use of such preparations (8, 11).

1. Seed management[1]

a) Characteristics of the seed

Attenuated VEE virus vaccine, strain TC-83, originated from the Trinidad donkey strain (a variant of I-AB) of epizootic VEE virus isolated in 1944. This strain was derived by serial passage of the Trinidad donkey strain in fetal guinea-pig heart cells. It is safe and immunogenic at the established passage levels, and induces protective immunity in vaccinated equids, although adverse reactions can sometimes occur. The vaccine was originally developed for use in personnel involved in high-risk VEE virus research. Suitable seed lots should be maintained at –70°C in a lyophilised state.

1 Sections on Seed management, Manufacture, In-process control, and Batch control are taken from the Biotechnology, Biologics, and Environmental Protection Division of the United States Department of Agriculture's Animal and Plant Health Inspection Service (APHIS).

b) Method of culture

The virus is grown in fetal guinea-pig heart cell cultures in a suitable medium.

c) Validation as a vaccine

The cells used for vaccine production must be free from bacterial, fungal, mycoplasmal, and viral contamination. VEE virus is identified in batches of vaccine by PRN tests against hyperimmune serum. For inactivated vaccines of cell culture origin, strain TC-83 virus is treated with formaldehyde.

2. Method of manufacture[1]

Vaccine is produced by harvesting supernatant fluid from fetal guinea-pig heart monolayers in which the replication of attenuated VEE virus has occurred. The monolayers are maintained at approximately 37°C. The time of harvesting is determined by the occurrence of characteristic cytopathic changes when approximately 70–100% of the cell sheet is affected, that is 1–3 days after infection. The supernatant fluid is clarified by low speed centrifugation and suitable stabilisers are added to protect the virus during freezing and lyophilisation.

3. In-process control[1]

Cultures should be examined daily for cytopathic changes. After harvesting, the virus suspension should be tested for the presence of microbial contaminants.

Inactivated vaccines derived from attenuated strain TC-83 virus should be checked to exclude the presence of viable virus after formalin treatment.

4. Batch control[1]

a) Sterility

Tests for sterility and freedom from contamination of biological materials may be found in Chapter I.4.

b) Safety

Safety tests of the inactivated vaccine are described in Chapter 2.5.3.

Safety tests of the attenuated vaccine are conducted in mice. A 0.5 ml dose is injected intraperitoneally or subcutaneously into each of eight mice, and the animals are kept under observation for 7 days. If adverse reactions attributable to the product occur during this period, the product is considered to be unsatisfactory.

c) Potency

Potency tests of the inactivated vaccine are described in Chapter 2.5.3. except that antibody titre in inoculated guinea-pigs will be ≥1/4.

Potency of the attenuated vaccine can be determined by testing in horses. Each of 20 susceptible horses is inoculated subcutaneously with 1 ml of lyophilised vaccine that has a reconstituted virus titre of at least 2.5 $\log_{10}$ $TCID_{50}$ (50% tissue culture infective dose) per ml. For a valid test, at least 19 of 20 vaccinated horses must have HI antibody titres of at least 1/20 or serum neutralising antibody titres of at least 1/40 within 21–28 days of vaccination.

When tested at any time within the expiration period following lyophilisation, the product must have a virus titre of 0.7 $\log_{10}$ greater than that used to test horses as described above, but no less than 2.5 $\log_{10}$ $TCID_{50}$/dose.

The final product must be free from bacterial, fungal, mycoplasmal, or extraneous viral contaminants.

d) Duration of immunity

Comprehensive studies on duration of immunity are not available. An annual revaccination is recommended for the inactivated vaccine. Foals that are vaccinated at under 1 year of age should be revaccinated before the next vector season. Revaccination with the attenuated vaccine is not recommended.

e) Stability

The lyophilised vaccine is stable and immunogenic for 3 years if kept refrigerated at 2–7°C. After 3 years, vaccine should be discarded. The vaccines should be used immediately after reconstitution. Multidose vials of the attenuated vaccine should be kept on ice while being used. All unused vaccine should be safely discarded 4 hours after reconstitution.

f) Preservatives

The preservatives used are thimerosal at a 1/1000 dilution and antibiotics (neomycin, polymyxin, amphotercin B, and gentamicin).

g) Precautions (hazards)

Pregnant mares and foals under 2 weeks of age should not be vaccinated.

All personnel handling infectious VEE viruses or their antigens prepared from infected tissues or cell cultures should be vaccinated and shown to have demonstrable immunity in the form of VEE virus-specific neutralising antibody. All procedures producing aerosols from VEE virus materials should be conducted in biosafety cabinets with biocontainment and efficient filtration of the exhaust air from the laboratory (6, 7).

5. Tests on the final product

a) Safety and potency

Safety and potency tests are as outlined above under Batch control (Sections B.4.b. and B.4.c.). The attenuated vaccine must have a virus titre of no less than 2.5 $\log_{10}$ $TCID_{50}$/dose.

REFERENCES

1. BERGE T.O., BANKS I.S. & TIGERTT W.D. (1961). Attenuation of Venezuelan equine encephalomyelitis virus by *in vitro* cultivation in guinea pig heart cells. *Am. J. Hyg.*, **73**, 209–218.

2. CALISHER C.H., SHOPE R.E., BRANDT W., CASALS J., KARABATSOS N., MURPHY F.A., TESH R.B. & WIEBE M.F. (1980). Proposed antigenic classification of registered arboviruses. I. *Togavirus Alphavirus. Intervirology*, **14**, 229–232.

3. MONATH T.P. & TRENT D.W. (1981). Togaviral diseases of domestic animals. *Comp. Diagn. Vir. Dis.*, **4**, 331–440.

4. PAN AMERICAN HEALTH ORGANIZATION (1972). Venezuelan encephalitis. *In:* Proceedings of a Workshop/ Symposium on Venezuelan Encephalitis Virus. Sci. Publ. No. 243, Washington DC, USA, 416 pp.

5. POWERS A.M., OBERSTE M.S., BRAULT A.C., RICO-HESSE R., SCHMURA S.M., SMITH J.F., KANG W, SWEENEY W.P. & WEAVER S.C. (1997). Repeated emergence of epidemic/epizootic Venezuelan equine encephalitis from a single genotype of enzootic subtype ID virus. *J. Virol.*, **71**, 6697–6705.

6. SUBCOMMITTEE ON ARBOVIRUS LABORATORY SAFETY OF THE AMERICAN COMMITTEE ON ARTHROPOD-BORNE VIRUSES (1980). Laboratory safety for arboviruses and certain viruses of vertebrates. *Am. J. Trop. Med. Hyg.*, **29**, 1359–1381.

7. UNITED STATES DEPARTMENT OF HEALTH AND HUMAN SERVICES (1999). Biosafety in Microbiological and Biomedical Laboratories. US Government Printing Office, Washington DC, USA, 190–196.

8. WALTON T.E. (1981). Chapter 24. Equine encephalomyelitis. *In:* Virus Diseases of Food Animals. A World Geography of Epidemiology and Control. Disease Monographs, Vol. 2, Gibbs E.P.J., ed. Academic Press, New York, USA, 587–625.

9. WALTON T.E., ALVAREZ O. Jr, BUCKWALTER R.M. & JOHNSON K.M. (1973). Experimental infection of horses with enzootic and epizootic strains of Venezuelan equine encephalomyelitis virus. *J. Infect. Dis.*, **128**, 271–282.

10. WALTON T.E. & GRAYSON M.A. (1989). Chapter 46. Venezuelan equine encephalomyelitis. *In:* The Arboviruses: Epidemiology and Ecology, Vol. 4, Monath T.P., ed. CRC Press, Boca Raton, Florida, USA, 203–231.

11. WEAVER S.C., PFEFFER M., MARRIOTT K., KANG W. & KINNEY R.M. (1999) Genetic evidence for the origins of Venezuelan equine encephalitis virus subtype IAB outbreaks. *Am. J. Trop. Med. Hyg.*, **60**, 441–448.

*

* *

CHAPTER 2.5.13.

EPIZOOTIC LYMPHANGITIS

SUMMARY

Epizootic lymphangitis is a contagious, chronic disease of horses and other Equidae characterised clinically by a spreading, suppurative, ulcerating pyogranulomatous dermatitis and lymphangitis. This is seen particularly in the neck, legs and chest. It can also present as an ulcerating conjunctivitis, or multifocal pneumonia. Transmission is by contact with traumatised skin, biting flies, or inhalation. The causative agent, Histoplasma capsulatum *var.* farciminosum, *is a dimorphic fungal soil saprophyte. Differential diagnoses include glanders (farcy), caused by* Burkholderia mallei, *ulcerative lymphangitis due to* Corynebacterium pseudotuberculosis, *sporotrichosis caused by* Sporothrix schenckii, *and the skin lesions of histoplasmosis caused by* Histoplasma capsulatum *var.* capsulatum. *Amphotericin B is the drug of choice for the treatment of clinical cases of epizootic lymphangitis.*

Identification of the agent: *Identification of the agent is made by its appearance in smears of the exudate or in histological sections of the lesion material. The yeast form of the organism is present in large numbers in well established lesions, and appears as pleomorphic ovoid to globose structures, approximately 2–5 µm in diameter, located both extracellularly and intracellularly in macrophages and giant cells. Organisms are usually surrounded by a 'halo' when stained with Gram stain, haematoxylin and eosin, Periodic acid–Schiff reaction or Gomori methenamine–silver stain. The mycelial form of the organism grows slowly under aerobic conditions at 25–30°C on a variety of media, including Mycobiotic agar, Sabouraud's dextrose agar, brain–heart infusion agar, and pleuropneumonia-like organism nutrient agar.*

Serological and other tests: *Antibodies to* H. capsulatum *var.* farciminosum *develop at or before the onset of clinical signs. Assays reported for detection of antibody include fluorescent antibody, enzyme-linked immunosorbent assay, and passive haemagglutination tests. In addition, a skin hypersensitivity test has been described.*

Requirements for vaccines and diagnostic biologicals: *Killed and live vaccines have been used on a limited scale in endemic areas, but they are not readily available.*

A. DIAGNOSTIC TECHNIQUES

Epizootic lymphangitis is a contagious, chronic disease of horses and other Equidae. The disease is characterised clinically by a suppurative, ulcerating, and spreading pyogranulomatous, multifocal dermatitic and lymphangitis. It is seen most commonly in the extremities, chest wall and the neck, but it can also be present as an ulcerating conjunctivitis of the palpebral conjunctiva, or as a multifocal pneumonia. It has also been called pseudofarcy or pseudoglanders. Another synonym is equine histoplasmosis, which may be a more accurate name for the disease, as not all clinical cases present obvious lymphangitis. The form that the disease takes seems to depend primarily on the route of entry (14). The skin form of the disease occurs when contaminated soil contacts traumatised skin. The conjunctival form of the disease is believed to be spread by biting flies of the *Musca* or *Stomoxys* genera. The pulmonary form of the disease is infrequent and is presumed to occur after inhalation of the organism. In all cases, the lesions are nodular and granulomatous in character, and the organism, once established, spreads locally by invasion and then via the lymphatics. There is often thickening, or 'cording', of lymphatics, with the formation of purulent nodules. Regional lymph nodes may by enlarged and inflamed. The causative agent, *Histoplasma capsulatum* var. *farciminosum*, is a dimorphic fungus. The mycelial form is present in soil; the yeast form is most commonly found in lesions. *Histoplasma farciminosum* was formerly described as an independent species, but this assessment has been changed and it is now considered to be a variety of *H. capsulatum* due to the close morphological similarities of both the mycelial and yeast forms (19). Antigenically, *H. capsulatum* var. *farciminosum* and *H. capsulatum* var. *capsulatum* are indistinguishable (10).

The cutaneous form of the disease could be confused with glanders, which is caused by *Burkholderia mallei*, with ulcerative lymphangitis, which is caused by *Corynebacterium pseudotuberculosis*, sporotrichosis caused by *Sporothrix schenckii*, and histoplasmosis caused by *H. capsulatum* var. *capsulatum* (9, 11).

The disease is endemic in parts of Africa, the Middle East, and Asia. It is most frequently reported from North Africa, but has also been described in other parts of Africa. The disease has been well documented in India. Reports from other parts of the world are sporadic and need to be carefully examined before the existence of the disease elsewhere can be validated. The incidence of the disease increases with assembling of animals; it was much more common, historically, when large numbers of horses were stabled together for cavalry and other transportation needs. Mainly, it is horses, mules, and donkeys that are affected by the disease, although infection may occur in camels and cattle. Experimentally, other animals are refractory to infection subsequent to inoculation, with the exception of certain laboratory animal species such as mice and rabbits (14). Infection in humans has also been reported (2, 3, 8). Amphotericin B is the drug of choice for the treatment of clinical cases of epizootic lymphangitis.

As the clinical signs of epizootic lymphangitis can be confused with those of other diseases in the field, definitive diagnosis rests on laboratory confirmation.

1. Identification of the agent

Material should be collected directly from the suppurative and nodular lesions. For microbiological isolation, the material should be placed in a liquid nutrient medium with antibacterials and kept refrigerated until culturing, which should be attempted as soon as possible. For direct examination, swabs of lesion material can be smeared on glass slides and fixed immediately. For histopathology, sections of lesion material, including both viable and nonviable tissue, should be placed in 10% neutral buffered formalin. Confirmation of the disease is dependent on the demonstration of *H. capsulatum* var. *farciminosum*.

a) Direct microscopic examination

- **Gram-stained smears**

Smears can be stained directly with Gram stain and examined for the typical yeast form of the organism, which will appear as Gram-positive, pleomorphic, ovoid to globose structures, approximately 2–5 µm in diameter (2). They may occur singly or in groups, and may be found within macrophages or extracellularly. A halo around the organisms (unstained capsule) is frequently observed.

- **Histopathology**

In haematoxylin and eosin (H&E)-stained histological sections, the appearance of the lesion is quite characteristic and consists of pyogranulomatous inflammation with fibroplasia. Langhans giant cells are common. The presence of numerous organisms, both intra- and extracellularly in tissue sections stained with H&E, Periodic acid–Schiff reaction and Gomori methenamine–silver stain is of diagnostic value (12). There is some indication that the number of organisms increases with chronicity. The organisms are pleomorphic, often described as slightly lemon-shaped basophilic masses, varying from 2 to 5 µm in diameter. Budding is often seen intracellularly within macrophages or giant cells.

- **Electron microscopy**

Electron microscopy has been applied to skin biopsy samples of 1.5–2.0 mm immediately prefixed in phosphate buffered 2% glutaraldehyde solution at 4°C and post-fixed in 1% osmium tetroxide. Ultra-thin sections were cut and stained with uranyl acetate and lead citrate. Examination demonstrated the fine internal structure of the organism, *H. capsulatum* var. *farminosum,* including the cell envelope, plasma membrane, cell wall, capsule and inner cell structures (1).

- **Polymerase chain reaction**

DNA sequences of four protein-coding genes have been analysed to elucidate the evolutionary relationships of *H. capsulatum* varieties. This indicated that *H. capsulatum* var. *farciminosum* is deeply buried in the branch of SAm Hcc group A, (H60 to -64, -67, -71, -74 and -76), looking as if it were an isolate of South American *H. capsulatum* var. *capsulatum* (10).

b) Culture

The mycelial form of *H. capsulatum* var. *farciminosum* grows slowly on laboratory media (2–8 weeks at 26°C). The recommended medium is Mycobiotic agar (2). Other media include Sabouraud's dextrose agar medium enriched with 2.5% glycerol, brain–heart infusion agar supplemented with 10% horse blood, and pleuropneumonia-like organism (PPLO) nutrient agar enriched with 2% dextrose and 2.5% glycerol, pH 7.8 (8, 13). Addition of antibiotics to the media is recommended: cycloheximide (0.5 g/litre) and chloramphenicol (0.5 g/litre). Colonies appear in 3–8 weeks as dry, yellow to dark brown, granular, wrinkled mycelia. Aerial forms occur, but are rare. Microscopically, hyphae from cultured colonies are hyaline, septate, branched, pleomorphic (1–4 µm in diameter), and variable with Gram stain.

As a confirmatory test the yeast form of *H. capsulatum* var. *farciminosum* can be induced by subculturing some of the mycelium into brain–heart infusion agar containing 5% horse blood or by using Pine's medium alone at 35–37°C. Yeast colonies are flat, raised, wrinkled, white to greyish brown, and pasty in consistency (13). On culture, *H. capsulatum* var. *farciminosum* should be distinguished from *H. capsulatum* var. *capsulatum* (11).

c.) Animal inoculation

Experimental transmission of *H. capsulatum* var. *farciminosum* has been attempted in mice, guinea-pigs and rabbits. Immunosuppressed mice are highly susceptible to experimental infection and can be used for diagnostic purposes (1).

2. Serological tests

There are published reports of various tests to detect antibodies as well as a skin hypersensitivity test for detection of cell-mediated immunity.

a) Fluorescent antibody tests

- **Indirect fluorescent antibody test**

The following procedure is as described by Fawi (4).

i) Antigen slides are made by smearing the lesion contents on to a glass slide or by emulsifying the cultured yeast phase of the organism in a saline solution and creating a thin film on a glass slide.

ii) The slides are heat-fixed by passing the slide through a flame.

iii) The slides are then washed in phosphate buffered saline (PBS) for 1 minute.

iv) Undiluted test sera are placed on the slides, which are then incubated for 30 minutes at 37°C.

v) The slides are washed in PBS three times for 10 minutes each.

vi) Fluorescein isothiocyanate (FITC)-conjugated anti-horse antibody at an appropriate dilution is flooded over the slides, which are then incubated for 30 minutes at 37°C.

vii) Washing in PBS is repeated three times for 10 minutes each.

viii) The slides are examined using fluorescence microscopy.

- **Direct fluorescent antibody test**

The following procedure is as described by Gabal *et al.* (5).

i) The globulin fraction of the test serum is precipitated, and then resuspended to its original serum volume in saline. The serum is then conjugated to FITC.

ii) Small colony particles of the cultured mycelial form of the organism are suspended in 1–2 drops of saline on a glass slide. With a second slide, the colony particles are crushed and the solution is dragged across the slide to create a thin film.

iii) The smears are heat-fixed.

iv) The slides are washed in PBS.

v) The slides are incubated with dilutions of conjugated serum for 60 minutes at 37°C.

vi) The slides are washed in PBS three times for 5 minutes each.

vii) The slides are examined using fluorescence microscopy.

b) Enzyme-linked immunosorbent assay

The following procedure is as described by Gabal & Mohammed (7).

i) The mycelial form of the organism is produced on Sabouraud's dextrose agar in tubes 20 × 125 mm, and incubated for 4 weeks at 26°C. Three colonies are ground in 50 ml of sterile PBS. The suspension is diluted 1/100 and the microtitre plates are coated with 100 µl/well.

ii) The plates are incubated at 4°C overnight.

iii) The plates are washed with PBS containing Tween 20 (0.5 ml/litre) three times for 3 minutes each.

iv) The plates are incubated with 5% bovine serum albumin, 100 µl/well, at 23–25°C for 30 minutes, with shaking.

v) The plates are washed with PBS containing Tween 20 (0.5 ml/litre) three times for 3 minutes each.

vi) Peroxidase-labelled goat anti-horse IgG is diluted 1/800 and used at 100 µl/well, with incubation for 30 minutes at 23–25°C, with shaking.

vii) The plates are washed with PBS containing Tween 20 (0.5 ml/litre) three times for 3 minutes each.

viii) Finally, 100 µl/well of hydrogen peroxide and ABTS (2,2'-Azino-bis-[3-ethylbenzothiazoline-6-sulphonic acid]) in a citric acid buffer, pH 4, is added.

ix) The plates are read at 60 minutes in a spectrophotometer at wavelength 405 nm.

x) The absorbance values are obtained twice from each serum dilution and the standard deviation and average percentage of the absorbance values of the different serum samples are considered in the interpretation of the results.

c) Passive haemagglutination test

The following procedure is as described by Gabal & Khalifa (6).

i) The organism is propagated for 8 weeks on Sabouraud's dextrose agar. Five colonies are scraped, ground, suspended in 200 ml of saline, and sonicated for 20 minutes. The remaining mycelial elements are filtered out, and the filtrate is diluted 1/160.

ii) Normal sheep red blood cells (RBCs) are washed, treated with tannic acid, washed, and resuspended as a 1% cell suspension.

iii) Different dilutions of the antigen preparation are mixed with the tanned RBCs and incubated in a water bath at 37°C for 1 hour. The RBCs are collected by centrifugation, washed three times in buffered saline and resuspended to make a 1% cell suspension.

iv) Test sera are inactivated by heating at 56°C for 30 minutes and then absorbed with an equal volume of washed RBCs.

v) Dilutions of serum (0.5 ml) are placed in test tubes with 0.05 ml of antigen-coated tanned RBCs.

vi) Agglutination is recorded at 2 and 12 hours.

vii) Agglutination is detected when the RBCs form a uniform mat on the bottom of the tube. A negative test is indicated by the formation of a 'button' of RBCs at the bottom of the tube.

d) Skin hypersensitivity tests

Two skin hypersensitivity tests for the diagnosis of epizootic lymphangitis have been described. The first test was described by Gabal & Khalifa (6).

i) The organism is propagated for 8 weeks on Sabouraud's dextrose agar. Five colonies are scraped, ground, suspended in 200 ml of saline, and sonicated for 20 minutes. The remaining mycelial elements are filtered out and the filtrate is diluted 1/100. Sterility of the preparation is verified by incubating an aliquot on Sabouraud's dextrose agar at 26°C for 4 weeks.

ii) Animals are inoculated intradermally with 0.2 ml in the neck.

iii) The inoculation site is examined for the presence of a local indurated and elevated area at 48–72 hours post-injection.

Alternatively, a 'histofarcin' test has been described by Soliman *et al.* (17).

i) The mycelial form of the organism is grown on polystyrene discs floating on 250 ml of PPLO media containing 2% glucose and 2.5% glycerine at 23–25°C for 4 months.

ii) The fungus-free culture filtrate is mixed with acetone (2/1) and held at 4°C for 48 hours.

iii) The supernatant is decanted and the acetone is allowed to evaporate.

iv) Precipitate is suspended to 1/10 original volume in distilled water.

v) Animals are inoculated intradermally with 0.1 ml of antigen in the neck.

vi) The inoculation site is examined for the presence of a local indurated and elevated area at 24, 48 and 72 hours post-injection.

B. REQUIREMENTS FOR VACCINES AND DIAGNOSTIC BIOLOGICALS

Control of the disease is usually through elimination of the infection. This is achieved by culling infected horses and application of strict hygiene practices to prevent spread of the organism. There are published reports on the use of killed (2) and live attenuated vaccines (19) in areas where epizootic lymphangitis is endemic, apparently with relatively good results. The antigen used for skin hypersensitivity testing is described in the previous section.

REFERENCES

1. AL-ANI F.K. (1999). Epizootic lymphangitis in horses: a review of the literature. *Rev. sci. tech. Off. int. Epiz.*, **18**, 691–699.

2. AL-ANI F.K., ALI A.H. & BANNA H.B. (1998). *Histoplasma farciminosum* infection of horses in Iraq. *Veterinarski Arhiv.*, **68**, 101–107.

3. CHANDLER F.W., KAPLAN W. & AJELLO L. (1980). Histopathology of Mycotic Diseases. Year Book Medical Publishers, Chicago, USA, 70–72 and 216–217.

4. FAWI M.T. (1969). Fluorescent antibody test for the serodiagnosis of *Histoplasma farciminosum* infections in Equidae. *Br. Vet. J.*, **125,** 231–234.

5. GABAL M.A., BANA A.A. & GENDI M.E. (1983). The fluorescent antibody technique for diagnosis of equine histoplasmosis (epizootic lymphangitis). *Zentralbl. Veterinarmed. [B]*, **30,** 283–287.

6. GABAL M.A. & KHALIFA K. (1983). Study on the immune response and serological diagnosis of equine histoplasmosis (epizootic lymphangitis). *Zentralbl. Veterinarmed. [B]*, **30,** 317–321.

7. GABAL M.A. & MOHAMMED K.A. (1985). Use of enzyme-linked immunosorbent assay for the diagnosis of equine *Histoplasma farciminosi* (epizootic lymphangitis). *Mycopathologia*, **91,** 35–37.

8. GUERIN C., ABEBE S. & TOUATI F. (1992). Epizootic lymphangitis in horses in Ethiopia. *J. Mycol. Med.*, **2**, 1–5.

9. JUNGERMAN P.F. & SCHWARTZMAN R.M. (1972). Veterinary Medical Mycology. Lea & Febiger. Philadelphia, USA.

10. KASUGA T., TAYLOR T.W. & WHITE T.J. (1999). Phylogenetic relationships of varieties and geographical groups of the human pathogenic fungus *Histoplasma capsulatum* darling. *J. Clin. Microbiol.*, **37**, 653–663.

11. LEHMANN P.F. HOWARD D.H. & MILLER J.D. (1996). Veterinary Mycology. Springer-Verlag, Berlin, Germany, **96**, 251–263.

12. ROBINSON W.F. & MAXIE M.G. (1993). The cardiovascular system. *In:* Pathology of Domestic Animals, Vol. 3. Academic Press, New York, USA, 82–84.

13. SELIM S.A., SOLIMAN R., OSMAN K., PADHYE A.A. & AJELLO L. (1985). Studies on histoplasmosis farciminosi (epizootic lymphangitis) in Egypt. Isolation of *Histoplasma farciminosum* from cases of histoplasmosis farciminosi in horses and its morphological characteristics. *Eur. J. Epidemiol.*, **1,** 84–89.

14. SINGH T. (1965). Studies on epizootic lymphangitis. I. Modes of infection and transmission of equine histoplasmosis (epizootic lymphangitis). *Indian J. Vet. Sci.*, **35,** 102–110.

15. SINGH T. (1967). Studies on epizootic lymphangitis. Study of clinical cases and experimental transmission. *Indian J. Vet. Sci.*, **36,** 45–47.

16. SINGH T & VARMANI B.M.L. (1966). Studies on epizootic lymphangitis: A note on pathogenecity of *Histoplasma farciminosum (rivolta)* for laboratory animals. *Indian J. Vet. Sci.*, **36,** 164–167.

17. SOLIMAN R., SAAD M.A. & REFAI M. (1985). Studies on histoplasmosis farciminosii (epizootic lymphangitis) in Egypt. III. Application of a skin test ('histofarcin') in the diagnosis of epizootic lymphangitis in horses. *Mykosen,* **28,** 457–461.

18. STANDARD P.G. & KAUFMAN L. (1976). Specific immunological test for the rapid identification of members of the genus *Histoplasma. J. Clin. Microbiol.*, **3**, 191–199.

19. WEEKS R.J., PADHYE A.A. & AJELLO L. (1985). *Histoplasma capsulatum* variety *farciminosum:* a new combination for *Histoplasma farciminosum. Mycologia*, **77**, 964–970.

*
* *

CHAPTER 2.5.14.

JAPANESE ENCEPHALITIS

SUMMARY

Japanese encephalitis virus is a mosquito-borne flavivirus that causes encephalitis, principally in horses. It also infects humans, and causes abortions in pigs. Pigs act as amplifiers of the virus, and birds can also be involved in its spread.

A definitive diagnosis of Japanese encephalitis in horses depends on the isolation of virus from affected or dead animals. As the isolation rate of virus is usually very low, clinical, serological and pathological findings are useful in diagnosis.

***Identification of the agent:** For virus isolation, brain material is collected from affected or dead horses that showed the clinical signs of encephalitis. Isolation procedures include the inoculation of unweaned mice and cell cultures. A suspension of brain material in buffered saline containing calf serum (or bovine serum albumin) and antibiotics is inoculated intracerebrally into 2–4-day-old mice. If the mice show neurological signs followed by death within 14 days, then virus identification can be carried out by cell culture. The virus is also isolated in cell cultures made from chicken embryos, in porcine or hamster kidney cells, African green monkey kidney (Vero) cells, the MD-BK cell line, and mosquito cell lines.*

A cytopathic effect appears in some cell cultures, but it is usually unclear. Identification of the virus in mice or in tissue cultures is confirmed by serological methods.

***Serological tests:** Antibody assay is a useful technique for determining the prevalence of infection in a horse population, and also for diagnosing Japanese encephalitis in diseased individuals. The assay methods include virus neutralisation (VN), haemagglutination inhibition, and complement fixation tests. The VN test is the most specific because of its ability to differentiate Japanese encephalitis virus infection from other flavivirus infections. It is best performed as a plaque reduction test.*

***Requirements for vaccines and diagnostic biologicals:** There is an inactivated vaccine prepared from a virus suspension derived from infected mouse brains or infected cell cultures.*

A. DIAGNOSTIC TECHNIQUES

Japanese encephalitis is a disease of horses caused by a mosquito-borne flavivirus that elicits clinical signs of encephalitis in infected animals, and can be fatal (3, 4). It also infects humans, and causes abortions in pigs. Pigs act as amplifiers of the virus, and birds can also be involved in its spread. Only a single serotype has been identified among Japanese encephalitis virus isolates, although strain variation was recognised by serological and molecular studies. Haemagglutination inhibition and neutralisation tests combined with antigen absorption procedures could distinguish at least two subtypes, Nakayama and JaGAr-01, among Japanese encephalitis virus (5).

The definitive diagnosis of Japanese encephalitis in horses depends on the isolation of the causal virus. The isolation rate of virus from diseased or dead horses is usually very low, which may be due to the instability of the virus under certain environmental conditions, and also to the presence of antibody in infected animals. Clinical, serological and pathological findings are of assistance in diagnosis. Diagnosis is also possible by the detection of specific IgM and IgG antibodies in cerebrospinal fluid by enzyme immunoassay methods (1).

The materials required for virus isolation are obtained from a portion of the corpus striatum, cortex or thalamus of the brains of affected horses. Blood and spinal cord samples are also used for isolation. All materials should be kept cool immediately after they are collected, and frozen to –80°C if virus is to be isolated at a later date. Any potentially infected materials must be handled under biocontainment conditions, to prevent the risk of human infection. Humans may be infected by a scratch from an infected and develop encephalitis.

1. Identification of the agent

Samples of brain and spinal cord are homogenised in a 10% suspension in buffered saline, pH 7.4, containing calf serum (2%) or bovine serum albumin (0.75%), streptomycin (100 µg/ml) and penicillin (100 units/ml). The calf serum should be free from Japanese encephalitis antibodies. The suspension is centrifuged at 1500 ***g*** for 15 minutes, and the supernatant fluid is removed for inoculation: 0.02 ml is inoculated intracerebrally into 2–4-day-old mice. The inoculated mice are kept under clinical observation for 14 days. No clear clinical signs may develop, but anorexia becomes evident by the disappearance of the white milk spot on the abdomen. The skin then changes colour from pinkish to dark red, and convulsions develop immediately before the mice die. Brains of dead or moribund mice are collected and stored at –80°C for a further passage.

To identify the virus, sucrose/acetone-extracted antigen is prepared from the infected mouse brains of a second passage in mice. This antigen is checked for its ability to agglutinate the red blood cells (RBCs) of 1-day-old chickens or of geese at different pH levels between pH 6.0 and 7.0, at intervals of pH 0.2, according to the method described (2). Briefly, RBC suspensions of 1/24 dilution are prepared in the diluent with different pH values. In a 96-well plate with a U-shaped bottom, the extracted antigen is diluted serially with 25 µl volumes. Then, 25 µl of the diluted RBCs is added to each well. The plate is incubated at 37°C for 1 hour, and the haemagglutination result is read. If the antigen is able to haemagglutinate, it is used in a haemagglutination inhibition (HI) test using a Japanese encephalitis antiserum.

Primary cultures of chicken embryo or hamster kidney cells, or a mosquito cell line C6/36 (a cloned cell line from *Aedes albopictus*) may be used for virus isolation. The specimens, such as brain and blood taken from animals suspected of being infected, and the brain suspension from mice after inoculation, are inoculated into the cultures; monoclonal antibodies specific to flavivirus and Japanese encephalitis virus may be used to identify the virus by the indirect fluorescent antibody test (6).

2. Serological tests

Serological tests are useful to determine the prevalence of infection in an animal population, the geographical distribution of the virus, and the degree of antibody production in vaccinated horses. To apply the tests to diagnosis in individual horses, it should be remembered that horses in an endemic area may have been inapparently infected with the virus for some time or may have been immunised with a vaccine. Valid data depend on a significant rise in antibody titre within paired sera collected in the acute and convalescent phases. The specificity of each serological test should also be considered.

In some regions of the world, there is a need to perform additional tests on related viruses before an unequivocal diagnosis of Japanese encephalitis can be made. For example, in Australia and Papua New Guinea, the antigenically closely related virus of Murray Valley encephalitis occurs.

a) Virus neutralisation

The plaque reduction test using chicken embryo primary cultures, African green monkey kidney (Vero) cells or baby hamster kidney (BHK) cells is sensitive and reliable.

Japanese encephalitis virus (Nakayama strain or JaGAr-01 strain) is propagated by intracerebral inoculation in 1-day-old mice. Moribund or dead mice are obtained, from which brain contents are collected and made into a 10% suspension in phosphate buffered saline (PBS), pH 7.2, containing 10% fetal calf serum. The suspension is centrifuged at 5000 ***g*** for 20 minutes at 4°C. The supernatant is stored in aliquots at –80°C.

- **Test procedure**

i) Inactivate sera for 30 minutes in a water bath at 56°C.

ii) Make serial dilutions of the sera in cell culture medium from 1/10 to 1/160 using a 24-well (17 mm in diameter) flat-bottomed microplate (or test tubes).

iii) Dilute stock virus to make 100 plaque-forming units (PFU)/0.2 ml in cell culture medium.

iv) Mix one volume of each diluted serum with an equal volume of diluted virus. Include virus control with culture medium, negative serum control and positive serum control in each plate.

v) Incubate for 90 minutes at 37°C.

vi) Add 200 µl of the virus/serum mixture to wells of BHK-21 cell monolayer formed on 24-well culture plates.

vii) Incubate the plates in a CO_2 atmosphere for 90 minutes at 37°C.

viii) Remove the inoculum and add 1 ml of overlay medium (1.5% carboxymethyl cellulose, 1% fetal calf serum in Eagle's medium).

ix) Incubate the plates in a CO_2 atmosphere for 4 days at 37°C.

x) After removing the culture fluid, fix the plates in a solution containing 2.5% potassium dichromate, 5% glacial acetic acid and 5% formalin for 30 minutes at room temperature. Wear rubber gloves when handling the fixing solution.

xi) Stain the plate in 0.1% crystal violet solution for 30 minutes at room temperature.

xii) Discard the stain and rinse the cells with tap water.

xiii) Air dry the cells and count the plaques.

xiv) Estimate the serum dilution that reduces the number of plaques by 50% or more of the control without serum.

b) Haemagglutination inhibition

The HI test is widely used for the diagnosis of Japanese encephalitis, but has cross-reactivity with other flaviviruses. For this test, the sera must first be treated with acetone or kaolin, and then absorbed with homotypic RBCs to remove any nonspecific haemagglutinins. The RBCs of geese or of 1-day-old chickens are used at the optimum pH (6.6–7.0). The test should be conducted with the treated sera and 8 units of standard antigen; this is commercially available in some countries.

- **Haemagglutination (HA)**

- **Preparation of virus antigen**

1. *Sucrose–acetone extraction of antigen from infected suckling mouse brains (SMB)*

   i) Homogenise infected SMB with 4 volumes of 8.5% sucrose.

   ii) Add the homogenate drop-wise to 20 times its volume of cold acetone.

   iii) Centrifuge (500 ***g*** for 5 minutes), then remove the supernatant.

   iv) Resuspend the sediment with the same volume as above of cold acetone, and keep in an ice bath for 1 hour.

   v) Centrifuge (500 ***g*** for 5 minutes), then remove the supernatant.

   vi) Pool the sediment with cold acetone in a single tube.

   vii) Centrifuge (500 ***g*** for 5 minutes), then remove the supernatant.

   viii) Spread the sediment inside the tube and vacuum dry for 1–2 hours.

   ix) Dissolve the dry sediment with saline: 0.4 volume of original homogenate.

   x) Centrifuge (8000 ***g*** for 1 hour, 4°C). The supernatant is ready for use.

2. *Infected fluid of* Aedes albopictus, *clone C6/36, cells*

   i) Harvest the infected fluid 1 week after incubation at 28°C.

   ii) Centrifuge (1000 ***g*** for 15 minutes). The supernatant is ready for use.

- **Preparation of goose red blood cells**

1. *Solutions*

   Acid-citrate-dextrose (ACD): 11.26 g sodium citrate ($Na_3C_6H_5O_7.2H_2O$); 4.0 g citric acid ($H_3C_6H_5O_7.H_2O$); 11.0 g dextrose ($C_6H_{12}O_6$); distilled water to a final volume of 500 ml. Autoclave at 10 lb (1.7 unit pressure) for 10 minutes.

   Dextrose-gelatine-veronal (DGV): 0.58 g veronal (Barbital); 0.60 g gelatine; 0.38 g sodium veronal (sodium barbital); 0.02 g (0.026 g) $CaCl_2$ (for $CaCl_2.2H_2O$); 0.12 g $MgSO_4.7H_2O$; 8.50 g NaCl; 10.0 g dextrose; distilled water to a final volume of 1000 ml. Autoclave at 10 lb (1.7 unit pressure) for 10 minutes (five times stock volume is easier to prepare).

2. *Bleeding*

   1.5 ml of ACD + 8.5 ml of blood (0.5 ml of ACD + 2.8 ml of blood).

3. *Washing (sterile)*

   i) Total blood + 2.5 volume of DGV. Centrifuge (500 ***g*** for 15 minutes), then remove the supernatant.

   ii) Resuspend the sedimented RBCs in three volumes (total blood) of DGV.

   iii) Centrifuge (500 ***g*** for 15 minutes), then remove the supernatant. Repeat steps 2 and 3 twice more (total four spin cycles).

   iv) Transfer the final RBC suspension to a flask with aluminium foil cover.

4. *Adjusting the RBC concentration*

   i) 0.2 ml of the RBC suspension + 7.8 ml of 0.9% NaCl (1/40 dilution).

   ii) Read the optical density $(OD)_{490}$ in a spectophotometer with 10 mm tube.

   iii) Adjust the RBC stock so that 1/40 dilution gives 0.450 of OD_{490}. (Final volume = Initial volume × absorbance $OD_{490}/0.450$.)

   iv) Store the RBC stock in a refrigerator for up to 3 weeks.

   v) Before use, resuspend the RBCs gently and dilute 1/24 in VAD.

- **Antigen dilution**

1. Stock solutions (should be kept at 4°C): *1.5 M NaCl:* 87.7 g NaCl and distilled water to a final volume of 1000 ml; *0.5 M boric acid:* 30.92 g H_3BO_3 and hot distilled water to a final volume of 700 ml (dissolve boric acid and cool down); *1 N NaOH:* 40.0 g NaOH and distilled water to a final volume of 1000 ml; *borate saline (BS), pH 9.0:* 80 ml 1.5 M NaCl, 100 ml 0.5 M H_3BO_3, 24 ml 1.0 N NaOH, and distilled water to a final volume of 1000 ml; *4% bovine albumin:* 4 g bovine albumin fraction V (Armour), 90 ml BS, pH 9.0, adjust pH to 9.0 with 1 N NaOH, and BS, pH 9.0, to make a final volume of 1000 ml.

2. *Antigen diluent:* 0.4% bovine albumin/borate saline (BABS): 10 ml 4% bovine albumin, pH 9.0, and 90 ml BS, pH 9.0.

3. Twofold serial dilution of antigen with BABS on microtitre (U-shaped microtray).

- **Addition of goose red blood cells**

1. *Stock solutions:*

   1.5 M NaCl

   0.5 M Na_2HPO_4: 70.99 g Na_2HPO_4 (for Na_2HPO_4, 12 H_2O: 179.08 g), and distilled water to a final volume of 1000 ml.

   1.0 M NaH_2PO_4: 138.01 g $NaH_2PO_4.H_2O$ (for Na_2PO_4, $2H_2O$: 156.01 g), and distilled water to a final volume of 1000 ml.

2. *Working solution: virus adjusting diluent (VAD)*

VAD	1.5 M NaCl	0.5 M Na_2HPO_4	1.0 M NaH_2PO_4	
6.0	100	32	184	
6.2	100	62	160	and distilled
6.4	100	112	144	water to a
6.6	100	160	120	final volume of
6.8	100	192	104	1000 ml
7.0	100	240	80	

Values of VADs are not the pH of each VAD, but the pH after each VAD is mixed with an equal volume of BABS, pH 9.0.

3. *Procedures*

   i) 1 volume of stock goose RBCs + 23 volumes of VAD (1/24 dilution).

   ii) Add 25 µl of diluted RBCs to each well on microtitre tray containing diluted antigen (25 µl/well).

   iii) Incubate at 37°C for 1 hour, then read the result.

   ++ Complete agglutination (uniformly thin pellicle of RBCs following the curvature of the well bottom)

   + Partial agglutination (a ring associated with a rough or thinner pellicle)

   ± Minimal agglutination (a button on a thin or scattered pellicle)

   – Negative agglutination (clearly defined button with no RBC film)

   End point is the last dilution (highest dilution) in which ++ or + is observed.

   Titre: the reciprocal of the end point dilution.

- **Haemagglutination inhibition**

- **Preparation of test sera**

1. *Bleeding and separation of the sera*

   i) Incubate blood specimen at 37°C for 1 hour and then at 4°C overnight.

   ii) Centrifuge (2000 ***g*** for 15 minutes) to separate the serum from the clot.

   iii) Heat inactivate at 56°C for 30 minutes.

   iv) Store at –20°C if not processed immediately.

2. *2-mercaptoethanol treatment*

   i) Place 50 µl of the sera into two small test tubes.

   ii) Add 150 µl of 0.13 M 2-mercaptoethanol in PBS into one test tube, and 15 µl PBS into another tube.

   iii) Incubate at 37°C for 1 hour, then cool in an ice bath.

3. *Acetone extraction*

   i) Place 2.5 ml of cold acetone into each tube. Apply rubber stoppers and extract for 5 minutes in an ice bath.

   ii) Centrifuge cold (1500 ***g*** for 5 minutes), then remove the supernatant.

   iii) Repeat steps i and ii once more.

   iv) Spread the sediment inside tubes and vacuum dry at room temperature for 1 hour.

   v) Add 0.5 ml of BS, pH 9.0, to each tube. Apply rubber stoppers. Dissolve the sediment overnight at 4°C to make 1/10 dilution of the sera.

4. *Kaolin extraction as an alternative to acetone extraction*

   i) 25% acid-washed kaolin (Fischer) in BS, pH 9.0.

   ii) 1 volume of sera + 4 volumes of BS + 5 volumes of 25 % kaolin.

   iii) Extract at room temperature for 20 minutes with occasional shaking.

   iv) Centrifuge (1000 ***g*** for 30 minutes). The supernatant is 1/10 dilution of the sera.

5. *Absorption with goose RBCs*

   i) To each treated serum add 1/50 volume of packed goose RBCs.

   ii) Absorb for 20 minutes in an ice bath.

   iii) Centrifuge (800 ***g*** for 10 minutes). The supernatant is ready for the HI test (1/10 dilution).

- **Haemagglutination inhibition test**

1. *Primary haemagglutination titration of antigen*

   Dilute the antigen to make 4–8 units/0.05 ml.

2. *Serial twofold dilution of test sera on microtray*

   Serum–antigen reaction

   Add 25 µl of diluted antigen into each well containing diluted test sera. Place the remainder of the antigen in empty wells and incubate at 4°C overnight.

3. *Secondary haemagglutination titration of the antigen*

   i) Collect antigen distributed in empty wells and HA test by serial twofold dilution in 25 µl system.

   ii) Add 25 µl of BABS to each well to make 50 µl/well.

4. *Addition of goose RBCs*

   i) Dilute RBC stock (1/24) in VAD.

   ii) Distribute 50 µl into each well containing 50 µl of serum antigen mixture or secondary titration of antigen.

   iii) Incubate at 37°C for 1 hour then read the result.

   Serum HI titre: the reciprocal of the highest dilution of the test sera showing complete inhibition of HA.

5. *Interpretation of the results*

   Four-fold difference between the titre in the acute and convalescent sera is considered to be a significant rise or fall and is diagnostic of infection with a virus antigenically related to that used in the test.

c) Complement fixation

Complement fixation (CF) is sometimes used for serological diagnosis. The antigen for this test is extracted with acetone/ether from the brains of inoculated mice.

- **Antigen preparation**

i) Extract and weigh the brains of the inoculated dead mice.

ii) Add to the brains, 20 volumes of cold acetone, kept at –20°C, and homogenise.

iii) Centrifuge the suspension at 5000 ***g*** for 5 minutes at 4°C, and remove the supernatant.

iv) Add to the pellet the same volume of cold acetone as used in step ii above, and mix well.

v) Extract with acetone by keeping the pellet at –20°C for 20 minutes, and repeat the centrifugation described in step iii above.

vi) Repeat steps iv and v.

vii) Repeat steps iv and v, but this time use cold acetone/ether (equal volume mixture).

viii) Repeat steps iv and v twice using cold ether.

ix) Remove the supernatant by aspirator and spread the pellet over the centrifuge tube.

x) Vacuum dry for 1–2 hours.

xi) Dissolve the pellet in cold saline (2 ml/g of brain) and keep at 4°C overnight.

xii) Centrifuge at 5000 ***g*** for 1 hour. The supernatant is the antigen.

- **Test procedure**

i) Heat-inactivate the test sera at 1/4 dilution in gelatin–veronal buffer.

ii) Serially dilute the sera twofold in a 96-well microtray (25 µl).

iii) Add 25 µl of 4 units of antigen and mix by vibration.

iv) Add 50 µl of 2 units of complement (pooled fresh guinea-pig serum).

v) Mix by vibration and incubate at 4°C for 18 hours.

vi) Leave the microtray at room temperature for 15 minutes.

vii) Add 25 µl of sensitised sheep RBCs to each well.

viii) Mix by vibration and incubate at 37°C for 30 minutes, then read the result.

ix) The highest dilution of test sera showing no haemolysis is the titre of the sera by CF test. A rise or drop of four-fold or more in the titre is considered to be significant.

B. REQUIREMENTS FOR VACCINES AND DIAGNOSTIC BIOLOGICALS

The vaccine for Japanese encephalitis in horses is prepared by the inactivation of a virus suspension derived from infected mouse brains or cell cultures.

1. Seed management

a) Characteristics of the seed

The Beijing-1 strain of Japanese encephalitis virus is used for vaccine production in Japan. The strain must be lethal for mice when inoculated intracerebrally, and must be able to grow in a primary culture of porcine kidney. This strain has the capacity to haemagglutinate the RBCs of geese, 1-day-old chickens or pigeons. The virus must be able to be neutralised by a standard antiserum to Japanese encephalitis virus.

b) Method of culture

The original and seed viruses should be grown in mouse brains or cell cultures. The passage levels should not exceed three times that of the original virus and twice that of the seed virus.

c) Validation as a vaccine

The vaccine product from this strain provides immunity to encephalitis in equines and prevents stillbirths in pregnant sows.

It is recommended that the original and seed viruses be maintained below –70°C, or below 5°C after lyophilisation.

2. Method of manufacture

The virus is grown in the brains of mice aged 3–4 weeks or in a monolayer culture. Uninoculated control cultures should not show any cytopathic effects caused by any other virus. Seed virus is inoculated intracerebrally into mice. The brains of those mice that show severe clinical signs of encephalitis are collected. These brains are homogenised in PBS, centrifuged at 1500 ***g*** for 30 minutes, and the supernatant fluid is processed as the virus suspension.

Seed virus is inoculated into cell cultures and the fluids are later harvested separately from each batch when virus replication is at its maximum. This fluid is filtered, or centrifuged at 1500 ***g*** for 30 minutes, and the supernatant fluid is processed as the virus suspension.

Formalin (0.5%) is added to the suspension to inactivate any live virus; this is considered to be the 'undiluted virus suspension'. Adjuvant may be added to enhance its immunogenicity.

3. In-process control

The virus suspension should be examined for bacterial contamination by culture techniques and for virus infectivity by intracerebral mouse inoculation or inoculation into cell cultures. The inactivated undiluted virus suspension should be re-examined for contamination by culture and by microscopy after staining, and should be checked by intracerebral mouse inoculation to ensure complete inactivation by the formalin.

4. Batch control

a) Sterility

Tests for sterility and freedom from contamination of biological materials may be found in Chapter I.4.

b) Safety

Ten 3-day-old mice are inoculated intracerebrally with 0.02 ml of the final product, and observed for 14 days to ensure (by the absence of any deaths) the complete inactivation of live virus.

5. Tests on the final product

a) Sterility

Tests for sterility and freedom from contamination of biological materials may be found in Chapter I.4.

b) Safety

See Section B.4.b.

c) Formalin determination

The formalin concentration should be less than 0.2% (v/v) by general quantification procedures.

d) Potency

The final product must be checked for immunogenicity by mouse protection tests. The product is diluted one part to ten parts of PBS; 30 mice aged 2–3 weeks are inoculated intraperitoneally with 0.1 ml of the diluted product twice at 3-day intervals. There should be an equivalent uninoculated control group. All mice are challenged intraperitonally with graded doses of live virus 8 days following the first inoculation, and observed for 14 days. The survival rate should be more than 40% in the immunised group and the mortality rate in the control group should be more than 90%. The titre of challenge virus should be not less than 10^3 LD_{50} (50% lethal dose) per 0.2 ml.

d) Stability

The final product must be shown to be fully effective for 12 months when stored at 4°C.

REFERENCES

1. Burke D.S., Hisalak A. & Ussery M.A. (1982). Japanese encephalitis. *In:* Proceedings of International Seminar on Viral Diseases in SE Asia and the Western Pacific, Mackenzie J.S., ed. Academic Press, Sydney, Australia, 537-540.

2. Clarke D.H. & Casals I. (1958). Techniques for haemagglutination with arthropod-borne viruses. *Am. J. Trop. Med. Hyg.*, **7**, 561–573.

3. Fenner F.J., Gibbs E.P.J., Murphy F.A., Rott R., Studdert M.J. & White D.O. (1992). Flaviviridae. *In:* Veterinary Virology, Second Edition. Academic Press, New York, USA, 441–455.

4. Hoke C.H. Jr & Gingrich J.B. (1994). Japanese encephalitis. *In:* Handbook of Zoonoses, Second Edition, Beran G.W., ed. CRC Press, Boca Raton, Florida, USA, 59–69.

5. Igarashi A. (1994). Japanese encephalitis virus. *In:* Encyclopedia of Virology, Webster R.G. & Granoff A., eds. Academic Press, New York, USA, 746–751.

6. Kimura-Kuroda J. & Yasui K. (1986). Antigenic comparison of envelop protein E between Japanese encephalitis virus and some other flaviviruses using monoclonal antibodies. *J. Gen. Virol.*, **67**, 2663–2672.

SECTION 2.6.

SWINE DISEASES IN LIST B

CHAPTER 2.6.1.

ATROPHIC RHINITIS OF SWINE

SUMMARY

Atrophic rhinitis, a severe progressive form of rhinitis, is an infectious disease of swine generally characterised by purulent nasal discharge combined with shortening or twisting of the snout, atrophy of the turbinate (conchal) bones and reduced productivity.

It is caused by infection with toxigenic strains of Pasteurella multocida *alone or in combination with* Bordetella bronchiseptica *and perhaps other components of the nasal flora. Infections with* B. bronchiseptica *alone can cause a less severe form, with mild or moderate, nonprogressive turbinate bone atrophy, generally with moderate snout changes.*

Virtually all apparently normal pig herds are infected with B. bronchiseptica *and possibly nontoxigenic* P. multocida, *some with evidence of a degree of turbinate atrophy. Infection with toxigenic* P. multocida *often results in clinical evidence of severe atrophic rhinitis. This may occur enzootically, or more sporadically, depending on a variety of factors including the herd immunity. Turbinate bone atrophy may only be obvious at slaughter, or may be detected in the live animal, for example by radiography.*

Identification of the agent: *The diagnosis of atrophic rhinitis of swine depends on clinical and post-mortem observations assisted by the recovery and characterisation of* P. multocida *and* B. bronchiseptica *in affected swine. The isolation of* P. multocida *is often complicated by the more profuse growth of other organisms. This may be overcome by preservation of the nasal or tonsillar swab at 4–8°C and by using a selective culture medium, usually blood agar containing antibiotics.* Pasteurella multocida *can be identified by biochemical tests; toxigenicity of isolates can be demonstrated by testing for cytotoxicity in cultured cells. A commercially available enzyme-linked immunosorbent assay is now widely used to differentiate toxigenic from nontoxigenic isolates, as well as to detect toxin production by bacteria from primary culture plates without the need for prior isolation and identification of individual colonies. This test is increasingly used as the preferred test for control of the progressive form of the disease.*

Isolates can be characterised by their capsular and somatic antigens. Capsular types A and D are usually isolated from swine; toxigenic strains belong to type A or type D, but severe progressive atrophic rhinitis is usually associated with type D. Capsular antigens may be distinguished serologically by indirect haemagglutination or immunofluorescence tests, chemically by flocculation in acriflavine, or by susceptibility to hyaluronidase. Somatic antigens are detected by precipitation or agglutination tests.

Bordetella bronchiseptica *is isolated by the use of selective culture media. It forms characteristic colonies and can be identified antigenically by slide agglutination tests.*

Serological tests: *Detection of antibodies to* P. multocida *and* B. bronchiseptica *is of no value for identifying diseased or carrier animals, as nontoxigenic strains of* P. multocida *share cross-reactive antigens with toxigenic strains, and* B. bronchiseptica *can be isolated from swine of most herds. A serological test based on detection of antibodies to the* P. multocida *toxin has been described and is commercially available. Its usefulness is limited by the fact that some infected swine do not* *develop antibodies to the toxin, or only develop them late, and also by widespread vaccination with* P. multocida *toxoid, which induces antibodies of vaccinal origin.*

Requirements for vaccines and diagnostic biologicals: *Several vaccines are available commercially that contain bacterins of* B. bronchiseptica *and a mixture of toxigenic and/or nontoxigenic strains of* P. multocida *or a toxoid derived from* P. multocida *or from a recombinant* Escherichia coli.

A. DIAGNOSTIC TECHNIQUES

Atrophic rhinitis is an infectious disease of swine characterised by shortening or twisting of the snout, turbinate (conchal bone) atrophy and reduced productivity. Two forms of the disease have been recognised:

a) A severe progressive form caused by toxigenic isolates of *Pasteurella multocida* alone or in combination with *Bordetella bronchiseptica* and perhaps other components of the nasal flora.

b) A less severe form with mild to moderate turbinate atrophy, usually without significant snout changes, associated with infections with toxigenic *B. bronchiseptica,* alone or perhaps in combination with other components of the nasal flora (10, 26). Herds have been recognised in the United Kingdom in which some swine at slaughter have snout damage consistent with the progressive form of the disease, but from which repeated efforts to isolate toxigenic *P. multocida* (17) or detect them by enzyme-linked immunosorbent assay (ELISA) have failed. Repeated exposure to *B. bronchiseptica* may cause severe damage to turbinate bones (20) and atmospheric ammonia alone may cause moderate turbinate damage.

Increased severity of these infections is associated with intensive production, overstocking, and poor management, housing and environment. Elevated concentrations of atmospheric ammonia, often found in weaner and fattening houses, experimentally reproduced moderate turbinate damage. Reduced productivity has generally been associated with the severe progressive form of atrophic rhinitis and therefore by implication with toxigenic *P. multocida*. However, the precise relationship between infection with these bacteria and reduced weight gains has not been adequately elucidated. Some experts believe that the major factors influencing the severity of the disease in a herd are managemental and environmental rather than microbiological. Toxigenic *P. multocida* spp. *multocida, P. multocida* ssp. *septica, P. avium* and *P. canis*, and closely related bacteria have been recovered from pig workers (13), rabbits (25), goats (2) and cattle (19). The role of these in atrophic rhinitis of swine, if any, is not yet clear.

As many pig herds are infected with *B. bronchiseptica* and nontoxigenic *P. multocida*, the presence of some degree of turbinate atrophy can be expected in most apparently normal herds. However, infection with toxigenic *P. multocida* appears to occur in herds with clinical evidence or a history of the more severe form of atrophic rhinitis. This may occur either as a herd problem or sporadically in a few slaughtered swine; such herds are important because of the risk of transferring infection to other herds previously free from toxigenic *P. multocida* and the risk of progression to the severe form of the disease.

The diagnosis of atrophic rhinitis of swine depends on clinical, pathological and microbiological investigations. The latter are particularly important for herds capable of spreading the disease that may be subclinically infected with toxigenic *P. multocida.* It is now generally accepted that a progressive atrophic rhinitis herd is one in which toxigenic *P. multocida* is present whether or not the herd has shown signs of the disease (23). Control in many countries has, therefore, centred on detection of infection, even in asymptomatic animals that are considered to be potential carriers.

Clinical signs include sneezing, nasal discharge, shortening or twisting of the snout, accompanied by atrophy of the nasal turbinate bones, a reduced growth rate and, in severe cases, difficulty in eating. Turbinate atrophy may only be seen at slaughter when snout sections at the level of the second premolar tooth are examined, but radiography as well as endoscopy have also been used to detect this change in live animals (11, 30). Several scoring systems for these gross changes are in use and are particularly useful for monitoring disease.

Diagnosis is assisted by histopathological examination of any turbinate atrophy, and the isolation and characterisation of *P. multocida* and *B. bronchiseptica.* The histopathological changes include fibrous replacement of the bony plates of the ventral conchae, sometimes with varying degrees of inflammatory and reparative changes (12). Demonstration of toxigenic *P. multocida* either by culture or by detection of its toxin can confirm the diagnosis of progressive atrophic rhinitis (7, 16), or may indicate subclinically infected swine.

1. Identification of the agent

Nasal or tonsillar swab samples are collected from swine aged 8–10 weeks with clinical signs of atrophic rhinitis or from swine whose carrier status is being investigated. These should be placed in charcoal transport medium (1) or isotonic saline if there is to be any delay before further investigation.

Cultures are made on selective medium. The cultures should produce individual colonies of *B. bronchiseptica* on Bordet–Gengou agar that contains furaltadone, penicillin, and streptomycin (29). Other agars used for the isolation of *B. bronchiseptica* include: MacConkey agar with added glucose (14); trypticase-soya and/or blood agar (blood agar containing cephalexin [4 mg in 1 ml water]; add 5 ml sheep blood and 1 ml of cephalexin solution to 100 ml of basic agar). Another effective alternative is Smith–Baskerville medium (31), which is very selective against the interfering bacterial flora of the nasal cavity. A 5% horse blood agar with added neomycin (1 mg/ml), bacitracin (1 mg/ml) is used for *P. multocida* (28, 30). Isolation of *P. multocida* has been improved beyond that achieved in mice by preservation of swabs during transit below 8°C for periods of up to 24 hours before they reach the laboratory for culture on selective medium (5).

Isolates of *P. multocida* are identifiable by their colony morphology. Gram staining reveals Gram-negative bipolar pleomorphic rods; these fail to grow on MacConkey agar, but yield a positive oxidase reaction and produce indole. Isolates producing the type D capsule form a heavy flocculate in 1/1000 aqueous acriflavine, and the growth of *P. multocida* with the type A capsule appears to be inhibited in the presence of hyaluronidase, which digests the capsule (27). *Bordetella bronchiseptica* is identified by its characteristic colony morphology on Bordet–Gengou medium and by a slide agglutination test using hyperimmune rabbit serum (25).

Toxigenic isolates of *P. multocida* can be differentiated from nontoxigenic strains by the toxicity of the supernatant fractions of broth cultures for embryonic bovine lung (EBL) cells (27) or African green monkey kidney (Vero) cells (24). The bacteria are grown in brain heart infusion broth incubated at 37°C for 24 hours. These are centrifuged and the supernatant fractions are sterilised by filtration, and titrated in EBL monolayer cultures in microtitre plates. These are incubated for 2–3 days, after which the cells are stained with crystal violet and examined microscopically to detect cytopathic effects. Difficulty with the general availability of cell culture facilities has meant that this test has not been adopted widely.

A rapid cell culture test may be used in which colonies resembling *P. multocida* can be selected from the medium used for primary isolation and subcultured on an agar overlay of EBL cells. After 18 hours' incubation, toxigenic isolates produce sufficient toxin to diffuse through the agar and cause the cells to separate from each other (7). This method has the advantage that isolates do not need to be identified unless they are toxigenic, and that many isolates per sample with a suitable colony morphology may be tested.

An ELISA that is based on monoclonal antibodies can detect toxin (16) in mixtures of bacteria recovered from primary isolation media. This test was made commercially available[1] approximately 8 years ago and has been widely adopted as an aid to identifying carriers and preventing transmission. The test is standardised, highly reproducible, more sensitive than cell culture methods and does not require specialised facilities. The improved sensitivity comes, in part, from the potential ability of the test to detect toxin production by just one toxigenic colony from among many colonies that may be nontoxigenic. To obtain a positive result from a sample such as this by the rapid cell culture method would require testing of each colony on primary isolation medium; this kind of extensive testing is not usually practicable. The test is not prone to false-positive results, but a positive result without previous history of disease or suspicious signs should be thoroughly investigated to recover toxigenic isolates. The ELISA should be repeated until it can be established that the original result was due to the presence of the organism in the animal from which it came.

Gene probes based on fragments of the *P. multocida* toxin gene have been described (18). Diagnostic tests, based on detection of DNA fragments have also been described (21) and in future could offer great advantages in detecting toxigenic *P. multocida* in samples where bacterial culture is not possible.

2. Serological tests

At present there are no satisfactory serological tests that can be relied on to detect those animals infected with toxigenic *P. multocida* and capable of developing or spreading the disease. Detection of antibodies to *P. multocida* is not helpful, as nontoxigenic strains share many cross-reacting antigens with toxigenic strains. A serological test based on detection of antibodies to the *P. multocida* toxin has been described (15) and is available (see footnote 1). However, many animals infected with toxigenic *P. multocida* fail to produce antibodies to the toxin, and widespread use of toxoid-containing vaccines will limit its diagnostic value to herds with no history of vaccination or to detection of vaccine response in vaccinated herds.

1 Available from Dako A/S, Produktionsvej 42, DK-2600 Glostrup, Denmark.

Infection with *B. bronchiseptica* can be detected serologically by agglutination tests (26), but as most pig herds are infected, antibodies to this organism will usually be present.

B. REQUIREMENTS FOR VACCINES AND DIAGNOSTIC BIOLOGICALS

There are several commercially available vaccines that contain bacterins of *B. bronchiseptica* and a mixture of toxigenic and nontoxigenic strains of *P. multocida*, or a *P. multocida* toxoid. Vaccines based on a *P. multocida* toxoid, which became available approximately 10 years ago, seemed likely from experimental work (6, 15) to offer specific protection against the action of the toxin, which by itself can be used to reproduce all of the major signs of this disease. It has also been shown that stimulating antibody to the toxin in pregnant sows would reduce colonisation by toxigenic *P. multocida* in piglets as well as protect against disease (6, 22). Observations of natural disease since the introduction of the toxoid-based vaccines has fulfilled these expectations, particularly with respect to clinical and histopathological signs of the progressive disease; prevalence of toxigenic *P. multocida* carriage has also been reduced, but the organism can nonetheless be detected by extensive swabbing in some herds that were originally affected by atrophic rhinitis, in which disease has been prevented by use of the vaccine.

Precise details of standards for the production of effective commercial vaccines are not available, but they are known to contain 10^{10} cells of formalin-killed *B. bronchiseptica* and 10 µg of *P. multocida* toxoid per dose. It is also clear that purified toxoid (inactivated by formaldehyde) is more immunogenic than crude toxoid (3, 6), and that the immunogenicity of the inactivated form is not affected by mixture with a *B. bronchiseptica* bacterin. A recently released vaccine (4) contains only the purified toxoid produced from a recombinant *Escherichia coli*. This would be expected to be effective where toxigenic *P. multocida* are the major infective component of the disease. The toxin in this recombinant has been inactivated by deletion of a portion of the gene that does not compromise protective immunogenicity. All commercially available vaccines contain either an oil adjuvant or aluminium hydroxide gel.

Bordetella bronchiseptica used for vaccine production should be phase I virulent cultures, and the *P. multocida* isolates should be toxigenic. Seeds of *B. bronchiseptica* and toxigenic *P. multocida* of established identity and passage history should be stored by conventional means. A defined number of passages should be used to give the production culture. *Bordetella bronchiseptica* should be inactivated by formaldehyde. As the toxin of *P. multocida* has an intracellular location and is released on cell lysis during the stationary phase, the culture supernatant should be harvested approximately 48 hours after the end of the exponential phase of growth.

1. Seed management

a) Characteristics of the seed

The seed-lot system should be employed for the bacterial strains used to prepare whole cell bacterins, as well as for the strains from which purified antigens are derived.

In the case of whole cell bacterins, the origin and history of both the *P. multocida* and *B. bronchiseptica* strains should be described and the full characterisation of the master seeds should be laid down in a master seed batch protocol.

Working seeds used for vaccine production should be derived from the master seed and checked for all relevant properties as described in the master seed batch protocol.

b) Method of culture

All bacterial strains should be grown in suitable media that support the growth and the expression of relevant antigens efficiently.

c) Validation as a vaccine

i) *Purity*

Both the master seed and the working seed must be pure cultures, free from bacterial, mycotic, mycoplasmal and viral contamination.

Identity of the bacterial species and the production of relevant antigens should be confirmed.

ii) *Safety*

Although inactivation of the bacterial cultures by a validated method is a standard procedure, both bacterial species produce dermonecrotic toxins; detoxification of these toxins should be confirmed when toxoids are used as vaccine components. Standard safety tests for inactivated vaccines should be carried out (8, 9).

iii) *Efficacy*

The efficacy of a trial vaccine should be measured by vaccinating groups of pregnant sows. Their progeny should be challenged by virulent cultures of *B. bronchiseptica* and toxin-producing *P. multocida*. Significant protection should be obtained against the clinical signs of the progressive form of atrophic rhinitis, i.e. tubinate atrophy. The clinical signs induced in the controls and vaccinates may be compared according to the scoring system of Done (11).

2. Method of manufacture

Both *B. bronchiseptica* and *P. multocida* cultures should be propagated in media that supports their growth efficiently and allows optimal expression of the antigens that are relevant for the induction of protective antibodies. *Bordetella bronchiseptica* should be confirmed to be a phase I culture, and for *P. multocida,* it should be confirmed that the culture contains sufficient levels of toxin.

Bordetella bronchiseptica cells and either *P. multocida* cells and/or toxin are inactivated, detoxified and formulated with an adjuvant. Commonly used adjuvants are aluminum salts or oil emulsions.

3. In-process control

During the manufacturing process, the following in-process controls are carried out.

a) Purity and identity of the seed cultures

Cultures are inoculated on to blood agar plates and incubated. No nonspecific colonies should grow on these plates.

b) Purity and identity of the production cultures

Cultures are inoculated on to blood agar plates and incubated. No nonspecific colonies should grow on these plates.

c) Inactivation of cultures before further processing

Cultures are inactivated with formaldehyde. Tests are performed to check the effectiveness of the inactivation process and to test for residual formaldehyde.

d) Quantification of antigens

This is carried out by performing a total cell count using a bacterial counting chamber for enumerating whole cells or an antigenic mass determination for defined antigens, e.g. *P. multocida* toxin, by quantitative enzyme-immunoassay.

4. Batch control

a) Sterility

Every batch of vaccine should be tested for sterility according to standard methods (see Chapter I.4.) described in the European Pharmacopoeia or the US Code of Federal Regulations.

b) Safety

Every batch of vaccine should be tested for safety in the target animal, by giving a double dose by the recommended route of vaccination, and a second, single dose 2 weeks later. No abnormal local or systemic reactions should occur.

c) Potency

Every batch of vaccine should be tested for potency using a validated serological test that correlates with the protection obtained in the efficacy experiment, as described under Section B.1.c.iii. The potency test is not necessarily carried out in the target animal – mice or rabbits can be used. In that case, correlation has to be shown with protective antibody levels in the target animal.

d) Duration of immunity

Normally, the vaccine is applied during the late stage of pregnancy, so that progeny will be protected by the uptake of colostral antibodies.

When the vaccine may be applied irrespective of the stage of pregnancy, duration of immunity should be at least 6 months, so that booster vaccinations twice a year should maintain effective antibody levels.

e) Stability

Every batch of vaccine should be subjected to an accelerated shelf-life test, which has been correlated with real-time shelf-life testing.

f) Preservatives

When a preservative is used, the concentration should be measured for each batch. It must not exceed the maximum permitted level.

g) Precautions

When an oil emulsion is used as the adjuvant, accidental injection of the operator can cause a severe local reaction. Medical attention should be sought immediately, treating the wound as a grease-gun injury.

5. Tests on the final product

a) Safety

Every batch of vaccine should be tested for safety, as described in Section B.4.b.

b) Potency

Every batch of vaccine should be tested for potency, as described in Section B.4.c.

REFERENCES

1. AMIES C.R. (1967). A modified formula for the preparation of Stuart's transport medium. *Can. J. Public Health*, **58**, 296–300.

2. BAALSRAD K.J (1987). Atrophic rhinitis in goats in Norway. *Am. J. Vet. Res.*, **47**, 730–737.

3. BORDING A. & FOGED N.T. (1991). Characterisation of the immunogenicity of formaldehyde detoxified *Pasteurella multocida* toxin. *Vet. Microbiol.*, **29**, 267–280.

4. BORDING A., NYMORK K. & SMIDT E. (1994). Field trials with a new genetically engineered vaccine for protection against progressive atrophic rhinitis in pigs. *Acta Vet. Scand.*, **35**, 155–163.

5. CHANTER N, GOODWIN R.F.W. & RUTTER J.M. (1989). Comparison of methods for the sampling and isolation of toxigenic *Pasteurella multocida* from the nasal cavity of pigs. *Res. Vet. Sci.*, **47**, 355–358.

6. CHANTER N. & RUTTER J.M. (1990). Colonisation by *Pasteurella multocida* in atrophic rhinitis of pigs and immunity to the osteolytic toxin. *Vet. Microbiol.*, **25**, 253–265.

7. CHANTER N., RUTTER J.M. & LUTHER P.D. (1986). Rapid detection of toxigenic *Pasteurella multocida* by an overlay technique. *Vet. Rec.*, **119**, 629–630.

8. COMMISSION EUROPEAN COMMUNITIES (1992). Commission Directive 92/18/EEC of the 20th March 1992 modifying the annex to Council Directive 81/852/EEC on the approximation of the laws of member states relating to analytical, pharmotoxicological and clinical standards and protocols in respect of the testing of veterinary medical products. *Off. J. European Communities.*

9. COMMISSION OF THE EUROPEAN COMMUNITIES (1994). CVMP Working Party on the Efficacy of Veterinary Medicines. Note for Guidance. Rue de la Loi 200, B-1049, Brussels, Belgium.

10. DE JONG M.K. (1993). *In:* Diseases of Swine, Seventh Edition, Leman A.D., Straw B.E., Mengeling W.L., d'Allaire S. & Taylor D.J., eds. Iowa State University Press, Ames, Iowa, USA, 414–435.

11. DONE J.T. (1976). Porcine atrophic rhinitis: snout radiography as an aid to diagnosis and detection of the disease. *Vet. Rec.*, **98**, 23–28.

12. DONE J.T. (1983). Atrophic rhinitis: Pathomorphological diagnosis. *In:* Atrophic Rhinitis of Pigs, Pedersen K.B. & Nielsen N.C., eds. Commission of the European Communities, Eur 8643 En, Luxembourg, 3–12.

13. DONNIO P.Y., AVRIL J.L., ANDRE P.M & VAUCEL J. (1991). Dermonecrotoxic toxin production by strains of *Pasteurella multocida* isolated from man. *J. Med. Microbiol.*, **34**, 333–337.

14. FARRINGTON D.O. & SWITZER W.P. (1977). Evaluation of nasal culturing procedures for the control of atrophic rhinitis caused by *Bordetella bronchiseptica* in swine. *J. Am. Vet. Med. Assoc.*, **170**, 34–36.

15. FOGED N.T., NIELSEN J.P. & JORSAL S.E. (1989). Protection against progressive atrophic rhinitis by vaccination with *Pasteurella multocida* toxin purified by monoclonal antibodies. *Vet. Rec.*, **125**, 7–11.

16. FOGED N.T., NIELSEN J.P. & PEDERSEN K.B. (1988). Differentiation of toxigenic from non-toxigenic isolates of *Pasteurella multocida* by enzyme-linked immunosorbent assay. *J. Clin. Microbiol.*, **26**, 1419–1420.

17. GOODWIN R.F.W., CHANTER N. & RUTTER J.M. (1990). Screening pig herds for toxigenic *Pasteurella multocida* and turbinate damage in a health scheme for atrophic rhinitis. *Vet. Rec.*, **127**, 83–86.

18. KAMPS A.M.I.E., BUGS W.E.C.M., KAMP E.M. & SMITS M.A. (1990). Specificity of DNA probes for the detection of toxigenic *Pasteurella multocida* subsp. *multocida* strains. *J. Clin. Microbiol.*, **28**, 1858–1861.

19. KEMP E.M., TER LAAK E.A. & DE JONG M.F. (1990). Atypical pasteurella strains producing a toxin similar to the dermonecrotoxic toxin of *Pasteurella multocida* subspecies *multocida*. *Vet. Rec.*, **126**, 434–437.

20. KOBISCH M. & NOVOTNY P. (1990). Identification of a 68 kilodalton outer membrane protein as the major protective antigen of *Bordetella bronchiseptica* by using specific pathogen free piglets. *Infect. Immun.*, **58**, 352–357.

21. NAGAI S., SOMENO S. & YAGIHASHI T. (1994). Differentiation of toxigenic from nontoxigenic isolates of *Pasteurella multocida* by PCR. *J. Clin. Microbiol.*, **32**, 1004–1010.

22. NIELSEN J.P., FOGED N.T., SORENSEN V., BARFOD K, BORDING A. & PETERSEN S.K. (1991). Vaccination against progressive atrophic rhinitis with a recombinant *Pasteurella multocida* toxin derivative. *Can. J. Vet. Res.*, **55**, 128–138.

23. PEDERSEN K.B., NIELSEN J.P, FOGED N.T., ELLING F., NIELSEN N.C. & WILLEBERG P. (1988). Atrophic rhinitis in pigs. Proposal for a revised definition. *Vet. Rec.*, **122**, 190–191.

24. PENNINGS A.M.M.A. & STORM P.K. (1984). A test in VERO cell monolayers for toxin production by strains of *Pasteurella multocida* isolated from pigs suspected of having atrophic rhinitis. *Vet. Microbiol.*, **9**, 503–508.

25. RIMLER R.B & BROGDEN K.A. (1986). *Pasteurella multocida* isolated from rabbits and swine: serologic types and toxin production. *Vet. Rec.*, **121**, 350–353.

26. RUTTER J.M. (1981). Quantitative observations on *Bordetella bronchiseptica* infection in atrophic rhinitis of pigs. *Vet. Rec.*, **108**, 451–454.

27. RUTTER J.M. (1985). Atrophic rhinitis in swine. *Adv. Vet. Sci. Comp. Med.*, **29**, 240–275.

28. RUTTER J.M. & LUTHER P.D. (1984). Cell culture assay for toxigenic *Pasteurella multocida* from atrophic rhinitis of pigs. *Vet. Rec.*, **114**, 393–396.

29. RUTTER J.M., TAYLOR R.J., CRIGHTON W.G., ROBERTSON I.B. & BENSON J.A. (1984). Epidemiological study of *Pasteurella multocida* and *Bordetella bronchiseptica* in atrophic rhinitis. *Vet. Rec.*, **115**, 615–619.

30. SCHOSS P. (1983). Clinical diagnosis of atrophic rhinitis. *In:* Atrophic Rhinitis of Pigs. Pedersen K.B. & Nielsen N.C., eds. Commission European Communities, Eur 8643 En, Luxembourg, 13–21.

31. SMITH I.M. & BASKERVILLE A.J. (1979). A selective medium facilitating the isolation and recognition of *Bordetella bronchiseptica* in pigs. *Res. Vet. Sci.*, 27, 187–192.

*

* *

CHAPTER 2.6.2.

PORCINE BRUCELLOSIS

SUMMARY

Brucellosis in pigs is caused by Brucella suis, *a bacterial infection that, after an initial bacteraemia, causes chronic inflammatory lesions localised in the reproductive organs of both sexes, and in the bones.* Brucella suis *species consists of five biovars, but the infection in pigs is caused by* B. suis *biovars 1, 2 or 3. The disease caused by biovars 1 and 3 is similar, while that caused by biovar 2 differs from 1 and 3 in its host range, its limited geographical distribution and its pathology. Biovar 2 is rarely pathogenic for humans, whereas biovars 1 and 3 are highly pathogenic causing severe disease. Porcine brucellosis is of widespread occurrence; generally, however, the prevalence is low, with the exception of South America and South-East Asia where the prevalence is higher. In some areas,* B. suis *infection has become established in wild or feral pigs – diagnostic methods recommended for wild and feral pigs are the same as for domestic pigs. Various biovars of* B. suis *cause infections in animals other than pigs, such as reindeer, caribou, hares and various murine species and occasionally in cattle and dogs.* Brucella suis *infections in animals other than pigs are dealt with in an appendix at the end of this chapter.*

Signs of disease in sows include abortion at any stage of gestation, and birth of dead or weak piglets. In boars, the most prominent sign is orchitis, and the secondary sex organs may be affected. Brucella suis *may be present in the semen, sometimes in the absence of clinical signs. Transmission during copulation is more common than is the case with brucellosis in ruminants. In both sexes, bones and especially joints and tendon sheaths may be affected, causing lameness and sometimes paralysis. Pigs are susceptible to artificial infection with* B. abortus *and* B. melitensis, *but reports of natural disease in pigs being caused by either of these organisms are rare. In humans, the infection is usually confined to those who are occupationally exposed to pigs, and to laboratory workers. However,* B. suis *is capable of colonising the bovine udder, causing serious human epidemics.*

Identification of the agent: Brucella suis *is readily isolated from live pigs by culture of birth products, and from carcasses by culture of lymph nodes and organs. Selective media are available for culture of contaminated samples. In nature,* B. suis *occurs invariably in the smooth phase – the appearance on solid medium is typical of smooth brucellae. Biovars of porcine origin agglutinate with monospecific anti-A serum, and not with anti-M serum. Definite identification of species and biovars may be effected by phage typing and biochemical tests, preferably carried out in specialised laboratories.*

Serological tests: *To date, none of the conventional serological tests has been shown to be entirely reliable in routine diagnosis in individual pigs and they are rather used for the identification of infected herds. The buffered* Brucella *antigen tests (BBATs), i.e. the buffered plate agglutination test (BPAT) and the rose bengal test (RBT), are more reliable in practice than other conventional tests. The indirect enzyme-linked immunosorbent assay (ELISA) and competitive ELISA have recently been developed, showing improved sensitivity and specificity values. A fluorescence polarisation assay has also been developed. The procedures for the BBATs are the same as those described in Chapter 2.3.1. Bovine brucellosis. The allergic skin test is also useful for identifying infected herds.*

Requirements for vaccines and diagnostic biologicals: Brucella suis *strain 2 vaccine has been used for immunising pigs in the People's Republic of China. Confirmation of the results obtained in China is required before strain 2 vaccine can be recommended for general use. In other countries, experimental work has shown that* B. mellitensis *Rev 1 vaccine is superior to* B. suis *strain 2.* Brucella abortus *RB51 vaccine has also been shown to be effective in swine. In practice, no* *product has yet found general acceptance. Preparation, testing and use of an established allergen, brucellysate (or brucellin fraction F) are described.*

A. DIAGNOSTIC TECHNIQUES

Porcine brucellosis is an infection caused by biovar 1, 2 or 3 of *Brucella suis*. It occurs in almost every country where pigs are raised. Generally, the prevalence is low, but in some areas, such as South America and South-East Asia, the prevalence is much higher. Porcine brucellosis may be a serious, but presently unrecognised, problem in some countries. *Brucella suis* biovar 1 infections have been reported from feral pigs in some of the southern States of the United States of America, and in Queensland, Australia. In Queensland, a number of human infections have been reported from people who hunt and handle material taken from feral pigs (11).

The disease is generally transmitted by consumption of feed contaminated by birth and/or abortion products and uterine discharges. Pigs will readily eat aborted fetuses and membranes. Transmission during copulation also occurs frequently, and this has implications for those practising artificial insemination.

In pigs, as in ruminants, after the initial bacteraemia, *B. suis* colonises cells of the reproductive tract of either sex. In females, placentas and fetuses are invaded, while in males, invasion occurs in one or more of the following: testis, epididymis, seminal vesicles, and/or bulbo-urethral glands. In males, the lesions, which are most often unilateral, start with a hyperplasia that may progress to abscess formation; the final stage is characterised by sclerosis and atrophy. Arthritis may occur in various joints, and sometimes spondylitis occurs.

The most common manifestation of brucellosis in female pigs is abortion, occurring very early or at any time during gestation. Vaginal discharge is not often evident, and the problem may appear to be infertility rather than abortion. In males, brucellosis is more likely to be persistent, with lesions in the genital tract often leading to interference with sexual activity, which can be temporary or permanent. The boar may excrete brucellae in the semen without any apparent abnormality in the sex organs or interference with sexual activity.

In both sexes, there may be swollen joints and tendon sheaths, lameness and, occasionally, posterior paralysis. A significant proportion of both male and female pigs will recover from the infection, often within 6 months, but many will remain permanently infected.

Brucellosis caused by *B. suis* biovar 2 differs from infection caused by biovars 1 and 3 in its host range – in addition to domestic and wild pigs, biovar 2 affects the European hare *(Lepus capensis)*; in its limited geographical range – the infection is restricted to Scandinavia, most of Europe and the Balkan Peninsula; and in its pathology – in pigs, persistent purulent lesions are more common, with miliary lesions in the wall of both the gravid and nongravid uterus. To date, biovar 2 has only once been reported as the cause of human brucellosis. An extensive outbreak caused by biovar 2 in pigs in Denmark has been meticulously recorded (14).

The common biovars of *B. suis* (1 and 3) are serious human pathogens and precautions are needed when handling and disposing of potentially infective material. This is especially so in the laboratory after culture has greatly increased the number of organisms present. Laboratory manipulation of the cultures or contaminated material from infected animals must be done under strict biosecurity conditions to safely handle this dangerous zoonotic agent. Biosecurity containment level 3 is recommended.

1. Identification of the agent

In porcine brucellosis, culture methods are at least as sensitive as serology (2). As the produce of almost all pig-raising enterprises passes through abattoirs, surveillance methods (serology and culture) can be applied effectively at this point. Samples for culture should be transported to the laboratory on ice as soon as possible after collection.

Suitable samples for culture from live animals include fetuses, placentas, vaginal swabs, semen, exudate from joints, and abscesses. From carcasses, a limited number of lymph nodes, such as mandibular, retropharyngeal and iliac, in addition to material from any suspicious lesion, can be expected to yield *B. suis* from most infected animals. Routine culture of semen in artificial insemination centres is important in endemic areas, especially in view of the unreliability of conventional serological tests.

In many areas, traditional village pig breeding is now accompanied by the development of larger commercial units, thereby increasing the use of artificial insemination. Whereas artificial insemination using brucellosis-free boars can be a valuable aid in the control of porcine brucellosis, the inadvertent use of infected semen could, obviously, cause incalculable damage.

Media used for other species of brucellae are suitable for *B. suis*. The addition of serum is not essential, but basal medium containing 5% serum is a satisfactory medium, both for isolation, maintenance of cultures and typing. The addition of CO_2 to the atmosphere is not required.

For the culture of materials that may be contaminated with extraneous organisms, selective media can be prepared. For most purposes, the following procedure is adequate: natamycin (50 mg), bacitracin (25,000 units), and polymyxin B sulphate (6000 units) are added per litre of medium that has been melted and cooled to 56°C. The medium is then poured into Petri plates. Where a greater degree of selectivity is required, vancomycin (20 mg), nalidixic acid (5 mg), and nystatin (100,000 units) may be added to each litre of the above selective medium. Both agar and broth are used as media. Agar plates are kept for at least 7 days at 37°C in a conventional incubator and checked daily for the presence of visible growth. *Brucella* broth (10 ml in tubes) is incubated in a conventional environment for 20 days. Every 4 days a sample of 0.1 ml of broth is removed for direct plating on to agar as previously described.

In nature, *B. suis* invariably occurs in the smooth form and colonies are indistinguishable from other smooth brucellae, described in Chapter 2.3.1. Bovine brucellosis.

Biovars 1, 2 and 3 of *B. suis* are all A surface antigen dominant, and growth may be presumptively identified by slide agglutination with monospecific A serum. Confirmatory identification of species and biovar should be performed in a specialised reference laboratory. The OIE Reference Laboratories for brucellosis are listed in the the Table given in Part 4 of this *Manual.*

Confirmation of species and biovar depends on phage tests, production of H_2S (only biovar 1 produces H_2S), and growth in the presence of dyes. Some strains of *B. suis* biovar 1 are atypical in that they grow on media containing 20 µg/ml of basic fuchsin. Most strains of *B. suis* are inhibited by safranin O at a concentration of 1/10,000, whereas *B. suis* reacts more rapidly in the urease test than either *B. abortus* or *B. melitensis.* Oxidative metabolic tests are particularly useful in distinguishing *B. suis* from other smooth species, especially their ready use of amino acids of the urea cycle, e.g. arginine.

The possibilities for applying molecular genetic methodology to the study of taxonomy and to detection of brucellae in samples apply equally to *B. suis* as to *B. abortus.* (see Chapter 2.3.1).

2. Serological tests

None of the conventional serological tests used for the diagnosis of porcine brucellosis are reliable for diagnosis in individual pigs. A significant problem is the fact that weaners up to 2–3 months of age are susceptible to infection with *B. suis,* but their agglutinating antibody response to the infection is very limited.

These conventional tests use antigens that are dependent on smooth lipopolysaccharide (LPS) for their activity. Due to the sharing of an 'O' chain polysaccharide, such antigens react equally with the LPS of *Yersinia enterocolitica* serotype 0.9 and are not, therefore, able to distinguish between antibodies to these two infections. *Yersinia enterocolitica* infection in pigs is not uncommon in some areas (15). Use of the fluorescence polarisation assay (8) eliminates the cross-reactivity with *Y. enterocolitica.* Swine serum may sometimes also contain nonspecific antibody, thought to be IgM, further reducing the specificity of conventional serology, especially the serum agglutination test (SAT). Also, swine complement interacts with guinea-pig complement to produce a pro-complementary activity that reduces the sensitivity of the complement fixation (CF) test. Sensitivity levels as low as 38% (9) and 49% (12) have been reported for the CF test; therefore this test cannot be recommended for the diagnosis of brucellosis in individual pigs. For international and other trade, e.g. purchasing boars, the disease status of the herd and of the area in which the herd is situated are of more importance than tests on individual animals. In spite of this, the European Union and some other countries still insist that only pigs whose serum shows an agglutination titre <30 International Units (IU) per ml and a CF test of less than 20 ICFTU (international CF test units) should be allowed to cross international boundaries.

a) Enzyme-linked immunosorbent assay

- **Indirect ELISA**

Indirect and competitive enzyme-linked immunosorbent assays (ELISAs) have been developed for the diagnosis of brucellosis in individual pigs and for screening large numbers of sera. These techniques promise to be more efficient than any of the tests mentioned above, and the competitive ELISA appears to be better at distinguishing antibody reactions due to *Y. enterocolitica* serotype 0.9 from those due to *Brucella.* The method for the indirect ELISA is described in detail in Chapter 2.3.1, however, monoclonal antibody specific for porcine IgG conjugated with horseradish peroxidase (HRPO) can be used.

- **Competitive ELISA**

Competitive ELISA procedures for detection of porcine antibody to *Brucella* sp. (8) are identical to the procedures used for bovine antibody to *B. abortus* described in Chapter 2.3.1. This assay is capable of eliminating most reactions due to *Y. enterocolitica* serotype 0.9 and other cross-reacting antibody, such as IgM, will not compete well. The cELISA is recommended as a confirmatory test as its sensitivity and specificity exceeds those of the agglutination tests.

b) Fluorescence polarisation assay

The fluorescence polarisation assay (FPA) for detection of porcine antibody to *Brucella* sp. is essentially the same as that described for cattle (for more details see Chapter 2.3.1); an example serum dilution used is 1/25 for the tube test and 1/10 for the plate test (8). It is a simple technique for measuring antigen/antibody interaction and may be performed in the laboratory or in the field. The analytes are mixed in one tube and the result is read 2 minutes later. This assay may assist in eliminating much of the reactivity resulting from exposure to *Y. enterocolitica* serotype 0.9 and other cross-reacting antibody. Lyophilised porcine sera tend to increase background activity in this assay. The FPA may be used as a screening and/or confirmatory test.

- **Test procedure**

i) 1 ml of PBSAL buffer (0.1 M phosphate buffer, pH 7.2, containing 0.15 M sodium chloride, 0.1% sodium azide and 0.05% lithium dodecyl sulphate) is added to a 10 × 75 mm borosilicate glass tube. 10 µl of swine serum or 20 µl of EDTA-treated blood is added to the tube and mixed well. A reading is obtained on the fluorescence polarisation meter (FPM) to determine light scatter (FPM reading in millipolarisation units, mP).

ii) A volume of antigen that results in a total fluorescence intensity of $250–300 \times 10^3$ is added to the tube and mixed well. This volume will vary from batch to batch, but is generally in the range of about 10 µl. A second reading is obtained on the FPM after incubation at ambient temperature for approximately 2 minutes.

iii) A reading above the predetermined threshold is indicative of a positive reaction.

iv) The following are included in each batch of tests: a strong positive, a weak positive, a negative working standard serum (calibrated against the OIE ELISA Standard Sera).

Controls should be tested before the test sera and after the testing has been completed or with each 100 samples tested.

c) Buffered *Brucella* antigen tests (prescribed tests for international trade)

For screening purposes or complete herd tests, the buffered *Brucella* antigen tests (BBAT), i.e. the card test, the rose bengal plate agglutination test (RBT) or the buffered plate agglutination test (BPAT), are recommended. The preparation and standardisation of BBAT antigens and the methods of performing the tests are described in Chapter 2.3.1. Bovine brucellosis. All biovars of *B. suis* affecting pigs have the same immunodominant A antigen as do most of the *B. abortus* biovars, which makes the *B. abortus* antigens appropriate for testing swine sera.

3. Allergic (hypersensitivity) tests

Allergic tests have been widely used in Eastern Europe, the former Union of Soviet Socialist Republics (USSR), and in the People's Republic of China for the diagnosis of brucellosis in herds of pigs. The specificity is very high. However, the sensitivity of the allergic test is similar to that of the serological tests (BBATs) and is not reliable for diagnosis in individual pigs. Some infected animals that are negative serologically, react positively to the skin test, and vice versa. Thus, where practicable, it is useful to perform both tests. As the active principle of the allergic test is protein, there should be no cross-reaction with *Y. enterocolitica* serotype 0.9, at least in theory. The authors are not aware of any demonstration of this attribute.

Many different allergens have been used for diagnosis, but one that is simple to prepare, that has been used effectively as a herd test in pigs, and that is still in use in some countries is an acid hydrolysate, sometimes called brucellysate or brucellin fraction F. Despite containing some polysaccharide, this preparation does not stimulate agglutinins or complement-fixing antibodies, nor does it sensitise animals (5). A method of preparation is given in Section B.

More recently, Brucellin-INRA has been developed for use in ruminants; the authors are not aware of it having been used in pigs. A rough strain is used in its preparation, thereby avoiding the presence of smooth LPS. The preparation, testing, and use of Brucellin-INRA is described in detail in Chapter 2.4.2. Caprine and ovine brucellosis (excluding *B. ovis* infection).

B. REQUIREMENTS FOR VACCINES AND DIAGNOSTIC BIOLOGICALS

Numerous attempts have been made to develop a vaccine to immunise pigs against *B. suis*. Only one product has found any acceptance for field use – *B. suis* strain 2 (S2) vaccine used extensively in south China (People's Republic). To date, it does not appear to have been used elsewhere in pigs, probably because it has been shown to confer less protection that the Rev. 1 vaccine. The *B. abortus* RB51 vaccine has also been shown to be effective in swine (7).

B1. *Brucella suis* strain 2 vaccine

S2 is a smooth, stable, naturally attenuated strain of *B. suis* biovar 1. Extensive studies have failed to detect any characteristic to distinguish S2 from field strains of biovar 1, except the level of virulence, which, as judged by its persistence in mice and guinea-pigs, is much lower than that of the average field strain. The low level of virulence and its stability has been demonstrated by passage in pregnant sows and boars (16).

The S2 vaccine may be given orally, for example in China it is often mixed in food, although it is warned that fermented food rapidly inactivates the vaccine. Oral vaccination could be an attractive possibility for the control of brucellosis in feral pigs. Challenge experiments in both sexes have shown appreciably lower levels of infection in the vaccinated compared with unvaccinated control animals, even in sows challenged with infected semen. For oral vaccination, doses of around 2×10^{10} are required, and usually two doses are given at an interval of approximately 2 months. Antibody produced in response to oral vaccination is said to disappear by 6 months after vaccination. Liang Xingxian (6) reports that in Guangdong Province in south China, porcine brucellosis has been controlled by a combination of annual serological testing of breeding stock with elimination of serologically positive animals and vaccination of serologically negative animals. In 1985, the reactor rate was 10%; in 1987 it had fallen to 1.2%, and no reactive boars had been found in the 4 years to 1991. Before the S2 vaccine is accepted for use in countries outside China, its safety and immunogenicity should be thoroughly investigated under the conditions pertaining in each country.

1. Seed management

Freeze-dried seed cultures for the experimental production and use of S2 vaccines are available from recognised institutions[1]. This freeze-dried material may be propagated by culture on nutrient agar or Trypticase soy agar for 2–3 days to produce seed lots that should not be more than three subcultures away from the material received.

Any country interested in introducing this vaccine should organise adequate challenge experiments and field trials in pigs.

2. Method of manufacture

The S2 vaccine is produced in fermenters using the same procedures and media as described for *B. abortus* Strain 19 (see Chapter 2.3.1. Bovine bruellosis). However, for the propagation of S2 vaccine on solid medium, either nutrient agar or trypticase soy agar is preferred to potato agar.

3. In-process control and further testing

In-process control, batch control and tests on the final product are all the same as for *B. abortus* strain 19. As regards the length of immunity, annual revaccination is recommended.

B2. Brucellysate (brucellin fraction F)

a) Preparation

i) Grow a smooth culture of *Brucella* (e.g. *B. suis*) on agar medium or in a fermenter.

ii) Harvest cells grown on solid medium in normal saline (0.15 M NaCl).

iii) Deposit by centrifugation and resuspend to 50–100 × 10^9 cells/ml in normal saline.

Iv) Add 1 N hydrochloric acid and adjust the pH to 1.2–2.0. Incubate at room temperature for 90 minutes.

v) Autoclave at 120°C for 25 minutes and leave overnight in the autoclave.

vi) Separate the cells by centrifugation.

vii) Adjust the pH of the supernatant hydrolysate to 6.8–7.0. Warm in a water bath at 80°C for 30 minutes.

viii) Pass through a sterilising filter.

ix) Estimate the nitrogen content of the concentrated hydrolysate. Adjust the protein nitrogen content to 25–30 mg/100 ml.

---

1 Obtainable from the National Institute for the Control of Veterinary Products and Pharmaceuticals, Ministry of Agriculture, 30 Baishiqiao Road, Beijing 100081, People's Republic of China, or from VLA Weybridge, Surrey KT15 3NB, United Kingdom. Supply from Weybridge laboratory needs the prior permission of the World Health Organization.

x) Check for sterility. Check for lack of toxicity by injecting 0.5 ml into each of from three to five mice.

Potency may be tested in sensitised guinea-pigs in comparison with a product of known potency. Guinea-pigs may be sensitised by repeated injections of killed *B. suis* in Freund's incomplete adjuvant (1).

b) Field use

As a diagnostic agent in pigs, 0.2 ml of the allergen is injected intradermally into the skin at the base of the ear. The reaction is read after 48 hours. A positive reaction shows erythema on nonpigmented skin and an oedematous swelling. In severe reactions there may also be some necrosis.

APPENDIX: *BRUCELLA SUIS* INFECTIONS IN ANIMALS OTHER THAN PIGS

1. Rangiferine brucellosis

Brucella suis biovar 4 causes serious disease in reindeer or caribou (*Rangifer tarandus* and its various subspecies) throughout the Arctic region, Siberia, Canada and Alaska (10). Some of these animals are domesticated, others are wild and migratory. *Rangifer tarandus* is very susceptible to *B. suis* infection, which causes fever, depression and various local signs, such as abortion, retained placentas, metritis, sometimes with blood-stained discharge, mastitis, bursitis and orchitits. In the Arctic region, *B. suis* biovar 4 constitutes a serious zoonosis (3). Transmission to humans may be by direct contact or through consumption of milk and other inadequately heated products from reindeer. Bone marrow, which is considered to be a special delicacy in this region, is a source of human infection.

The methods already described for isolating and identifying *B. suis* in samples taken from pigs are equally applicable to *B. suis* biovar 4 in samples taken from reindeer. Biovar 4 grows well on all the usual media used for the culture of *Brucella*. It reacts positively with both A and M monospecific sera. For serology, the tube agglutination test has been reported to be satisfactory, with titres from 1/20 being considered to be diagnostic. The CF test has also been used but the clinical interpretation of these tests in reindeer has not been established.

Vaccination of reindeer with *B. abortus* strain 19 vaccine, or alternatively with *B. abortus* 45/20 adjuvant vaccine, has been tried experimentally without any clear-cut result. In the case of strain 19, the reaction to vaccination was rather severe and immunity in the vaccinated animals could only be demonstrated against challenge with very small doses of *B. suis* biovar 4.

2. *Brucella suis* infection in other nonporcine species

There are two different types of epidemiological situation with regard to *B. suis* infection in other nonporcine species. In the first case, *B. suis* infection occurs in animals that are not the natural host of the particular infection through the ingestion of contaminated materials or by co-habitation with infected natural hosts. For example, Arctic foxes and wolves may contract *B. suis* biovar 4 from reindeer; dogs and rodents, such as rats and mice, may acquire other *B. suis* biovars by cohabitation with infected hosts. Cattle may become infected by cohabitation with infected feral swine. The infecting bacteria are invariably the well defined biovars of the natural host species.

In the second case, wildlife species that are natural hosts for *B. suis* or *B.-suis*-like infections become infected. One example is the so-called murine brucellosis of the former USSR, where small rodents are infected with *B. suis* biovar 5. Other similar situations have been reported from Queensland, Australia and from Kenya. In all three cases, *B. suis* strains with different characteristics were involved, and at least one of them was difficult to classify.

Brucellosis caused by *B. suis* biovar 2 is perhaps a special case. The reservoir of infection is in the European hare *(Lepus capensis)* (13), or in wild pigs *(Sus scrofa)* living in the same area (4), or in both. Biovar 2 infection appears to be confined to the area inhabited by the European hare, and within this area is more prevalent in hares and wild pigs than in domestic pigs. However, having invaded domestic pig herds, biovar 2 is likely to spread as rapidly as biovars 1 and 3. The disease in hares is characterised by the formation of nodules, varying in size from that of a millet seed to a cherry or even larger; these often become purulent. Such nodules may occur in almost any location, sometimes subcutaneosly or intramuscularly, in the spleen, liver or lung and in the reproductive organs of either sex. The bodily condition of the hare may be surprisingly unaffected.

Serological investigations in nonporcine species are usually carried out for screening purposes. In these particular circumstances, specificity is more important than sensitivity. Here the CF test is recommended, although the buffered *Brucella* plate agglutination test may be useful because of its simplicity. In many previous investigations, the tube agglutination test was used, apparently with satisfaction. However, in nonporcine species the interpretation of serological results may be problematic. Where supposedly positive samples are encountered, serological screening should be followed by bacteriological investigation.

For bacteriological investigations in situations such as these, where the infecting organisms may have unusual characteristics, it is advisable to duplicate the culture on selective media by culture on plain medium supplemented with 5% serum, and to broaden the investigation by incubating the cultures in an atmosphere containing 10% CO_2. Colonies resembling *Brucella* can be tentatively identified by Gram staining, by slide agglutination tests with monospecific A and M serum, and by anti-rough *Brucella* serum. *Brucela suis* biovar 5 is unusual in that it reacts with monospecific M serum, and not with monospecific A serum. Further identification as outlined in Section A.1. is best carried out in a specialised laboratory.

REFERENCES

1. ALTON G.G., JONES L.M., ANGUS R.D. & VERGER J.M. (1988). Techniques for the Brucellosis Laboratory. INRA, Paris, France.

2. FERRIS R.A., SCHOENBAUM M.A. & CRAWFORD R.P. (1995). Comparison of serologic tests and bacteriologic culture for detection of brucellosis in swine from naturally infected herds. *J. Am. Vet. Med. Assoc.*, **207**, 1332–1333.

3. FORBES L.B. (1991). Isolates of *B. suis* biotype 4 from animals and humans in Canada, 1982–1990. *Can. Vet. J.*, **32**, 686–688.

4. GODFROID J., MICHEL P., UYTTERHAIEGEN L., DE SMEDT C., RASSENEUR F., BOELAERT F., SAEGERMAN C. & PATIGNY X. (1994). Brucellose enzootique a *Brucella suis* biotype 2 chez le sanglier *(Sus scrofa)* en Belgique. *Ann. Med. Vet.*, **138**, 263–268.

5. JOINT FOOD AND AGRICULTURE ORGANIZATION OF THE UNITED NATIONS (FAO)/WORLD HEALTH ORGANIZATION (WHO) EXPERT COMMITTEE ON BRUCELLOSIS (1986). Sixth Report. Technical Report Series 740. WHO, Geneva, Switzerland.

6. LIANG XINGXIAN (1991). The prevalence, prevention and control of swine brucellosis in Guangdong Province, China. Document AGU/BRU/92/21 Food and Agriculture Organization of the United Nations (FAO), Rome, Italy.

7. LORD V.R., CHERWONOGRODZKY J.W., SCHURIG G.G., LORD R.D., MARCANO M.J. & MELENDEZ G.E. (1998). Venezuelan field trials of vaccines against brucellosis in swine. *Am. J. Vet. Res.*, **59**, 546–551.

8. NIELSEN K., GALL D., SMITH P., VIGLIOCCO A., PERREZ B., SAMARTINO L., DAJER A., ELZER P. & ENRIGHT F. (1999). Validation of the fluorescence polarization assay as a serological test for the presumptive diagnosis of porcine brucellosis. *Vet. Microbiol.*, **68**, 245–253.

9. PRIADI A., CHASANAH U., HIRST R.G., EMMINS J.J., VAN DER GIESSEN J. & SEOROSO M. (1995). Development of an enzyme-linked immunosorbant assay (ELISA) for detecting antibody to *Brucella* suis in porcine sera. *Penyakit Hewan.*, **17**, 66–70 (*Vet. Bull.*, **56**, abstract 7528).

10. ORLOW E.S. (1963). Brucellosis in reindeer. Proceedings of the 17th World Veterinary Congress, Hanover, Germany, 1, 585–588.

11. ROBSON J.M., HARRISON M.W., WOOD R.N., TILSE M.H., MCKAY A.B. & BRODRIBB T.R. (1993). Brucellosis: reemergence and changing epidemiology in Queensland. *Med. J. Aust.*, **159**, 153–158.

12. ROGERS R.J., COOK D.R., KETTERER P.J., BALDRODCK, F.C., BLACKALL P.J. & STEWART R.W. (1989). An evaluation of three serological tests for antibody to *Brucella suis* in pigs. *Aust. Vet. J.*, **66**, 77–80.

13. SZULOWSKI K., IWANIAK W., PILASZEK J., TRUSZCZYNSKI M. & CHROBOCINSKA M. (1999). The ELISA for the examination of hare sera for anti-Brucella antibodies. *Comp. Immunol. Microbiol. Infect. Dis.*, **22**, 33–40.

14. THOMSEN A. (1935). *Brucella* infection in swine. *Acta Path. Microbiol. Scand.* Supplement xxi.

15. WRATHALL A.E., BROUGHTON E.S., GILL K.P.W. & GOLDSMITH G.P. (1983). Serological reactions to *Brucella* species in British pigs. *Vet. Rec.*, **132**, 449–454.

16. XIE XIN (1986). Orally administrable brucellosis vaccine: *Brucella suis* strain 2 vaccine. *Vaccine*, **4**, 212–216.

*
* *

CHAPTER 2.6.3.

ENTEROVIRUS ENCEPHALOMYELITIS (previously Teschen/Talfan diseases)

SUMMARY

Enterovirus encephalomyelitis was first described as a particularly virulent, highly fatal, nonsuppurative encephalomyelitis of pigs, known as Teschen disease. It was caused by strains of porcine enterovirus serotype 1 (PEV-1) of the Picornaviridae family. Less severe forms of the disease were first recognised in the United Kingdom (Talfan disease) and in Denmark (poliomyelitis suum). The viruses involved in these conditions also belong to the genus Enterovirus. *In addition to PEV-1 strains, the milder form of the disease was caused by other types of PEV, including PEV-2–6, 8, and 12–13.*

The disease was first described in Czechoslovakia in 1929. During the 1940s and 1950s it caused serious losses in European countries. The clinical disease is now rare in Europe, although serological evidence indicates that virus variants of low pathogenicity may circulate in pig populations in some countries.

It is not possible to differentiate between encephalomyelitis due to porcine enterovirus and other viral encephalomyelitides based only on clinical signs and gross pathology. The most suitable methods for diagnosis are demonstration of characteristic microscopic lesions in the central nervous system of affected pigs, isolation and subsequent identification of PEV, and demonstration of specific antibodies. At post-mortem, microscopic lesions, which are characterised by inflammatory lesions with perivascular lymphocyte infiltration, occur in the grey matter of the brain and in the spinal cord. The later stages of the disease are characterised by a degeneration of neurons and their replacement by glial connective tissue.

***Identification of the agent:** Tissue suspensions of brain and spinal cord from affected pigs are inoculated into tissue culture derived from porcine kidney. If PEV is present, it gives rise to specific cytopathic effects characterised by round refractile cells. For PEV identification and serotyping, suitable tests are employed using specific antisera or monoclonal antibodies against standard strains of PEV. Virus neutralisation tests and indirect fluorescent antibody tests are preferred.*

***Serological tests:** Because the seroprevalence of PEV-1 may exceed 60% in healthy pig populations in some countries of Central Europe, and identical clinical signs may be caused by other viruses – including other serotypes of PEV – a single serological test for PEV-1 giving positive results does not indicate that neurological signs observed are actually caused by PEV-1. A four-fold rise in titre together with typical signs should be considered to be an indication of a PEV-1 infection having caused clinical disease. For screening for specific antibodies in pig populations, it is usual to use the virus neutralisation test in microtitre plates or the enzyme-linked immunosorbent assay.*

***Requirements for vaccines and diagnostic biologicals:** Vaccines are available. Inactivated vaccine produced from virus propagated on tissue cultures from porcine kidney is recommended for active immunisation. The virus is usually inactivated by formaldehyde or other suitable inactivants having a linear rate of inactivation, and adsorbed on to aluminium hydroxide or mixed with oil adjuvant. The vaccine is injected subcutaneously, if adjuvanted, or intramuscularly.*

A. DIAGNOSTIC TECHNIQUES

Enterovirus encephalomyelitis (previously Teschen/Talfan diseases) is an acute condition of pigs characterised by central nervous system (CNS) disorders. Teschen is the name of the town in Czechoslovakia where the disease was first recognised in 1929 (4). The causal agents were porcine enteroviruses of serotype I (PEV-1) (2, 5). However, sporadic outbreaks of encephalomyelitis in later years were additionally caused by porcine enteroviruses of other serotypes, including PEV-2, PEV-3, PEV-4, PEV-5, PEV-6, PEV-8, PEV-12 and PEV-13 (15). All these viruses belong to the genus *Enterovirus* in the Picornaviridae family (12). The porcine encephalomyelitis observed in Canada during the 1960s was caused by a coronavirus and is not discussed in this chapter.

Three groups of PEV can be distinguished by serological cross-reactivity, type of cytopathic effect (CPE) in pig kidney cells, physico–chemical properties and genomic conformity (group I: PEV-1–7, 11–13; group II: PEV-8; group III: PEV-9–10). PEV may be identified and serotypes may be differentiated by using a virus neutralisation (VN) test, complement fixation test (1, 6) or indirect fluorescent antibody (IFA) test. In the course of enterovirus encephalomyelitis, the virus propagates in the CNS, causing a nonsuppurative encephalomyelitis with associated degeneration of motor ganglion cells. The disease is most commonly seen in suckling or weaner pigs, in which it causes fever, anorexia, ataxia, leg paralysis and convulsions. Morbidity and mortality rates vary considerably, but can be high. Small amounts of virus are present in faeces for a long time after clinical recovery, so that convalescent animals become an continuing source of infection. The pathological lesions caused by the virus are nonpurulent encephalitis and myelitis associated with degeneration of motor ganglion cells.

Laboratory diagnosis of the disease is based on histological examination of brain and spinal cord, on identification of the agent in the CNS of affected pigs, and on the detection of specific antibodies in the blood of convalescent animals.

For histological diagnosis, samples of cerebrum, cerebellum, diencephalon, medulla oblongata and cervical and lumbar spinal cord are collected. The samples are fixed in formaldehyde and sections are stained using conventional histological methods. Microscopic examination reveals nonsuppurative perivascular lymphocyte infiltrations (4). The infiltrations are confined to the grey matter with occasional involvement of the white matter. Changes are observed in the ventral horns of the spinal cord, in the diencephalon and cerebellum, and to a lesser extent in the cerebral hemispheres. Degeneration of neurons and their replacement by glial connective tissue develops in the late stage of the disease. Electron microscopic studies indicate that the target organelle in the infected neuron appears to be the endoplasmic reticulum, which undergoes vesiculation leading to irreversible degeneration. Nonpurulent leptomeningitis, especially in the cerebellum, is often seen.

The virus enters the organism via the oral or nasal cavity. The incubation period is, on average, about 14 days. The main signs of the prodromal stage are fever up to 41.5°C, lassitude, anorexia and locomotor disturbances. This stage is followed by hypersensitivity: touching the skin provokes painful squeals and gritting of the teeth. Tremors, clonic spasms of the legs, opisthotonos and nystagmus are also observed. The final clinical stage is paralysis proceeding from the hind part through the loins to the fore part of the body. Paralysis of the thermoregulatory centre results in hypothermy. When respiratory muscles are paralysed, the animal dies of suffocation.

No pathological lesions are seen at necropsy; congestion of cerebrospinal meninges and nasal mucosa may occur.

1. Identification of the agent

Samples of brain and spinal cord are collected from pigs slaughtered at an early clinical stage of the disease. When not processed immediately, the samples should be placed in a solution prepared from equal parts of phosphate buffered isotonic saline (PBS), pH 7.4, and glycerol.

Pieces of tissues are minced to prepare a 10% (w/v) suspension in PBS solution. The suspension is centrifuged lightly and the supernatant fluid is used for inoculation of tissue cultures. Monolayer cultures of primary porcine kidney or testes cells or established cell lines derived from porcine kidney, for example PK-15, or testes are suitable for isolation of PEV.

Ten monolayers of confluent cells are used. Each tube is opened to discard the growth medium, and then inoculated with 0.1 ml of suspect tissue homogenate, closed and placed on a roller drum. After 1 hour, the inoculum is discarded and each tube is washed three times with PBS. Finally, each tube is replenished with 1 ml of maintenance medium without calf serum. The tubes are then returned to the roller drum and incubated at 37°C. Microscopic examination should be performed daily. If the sample contains live PEV, development of the characteristic CPE will be seen after 3–4 days. The CPE is characterised by small foci of rounded refractile cells. With further incubation, the CPE generalises and all cells detach from the glass. After several passages the virus grows better and produces complete CPE after 24–48 hours. The identity of PEV can be confirmed by the use of specific antiserum or monoclonal antibodies. VN and IFA tests are best suited to this purpose. Once an isolate has been identified serologically as PEV, piglet inoculation is the only certain means of determining that the given isolate is pathogenic.

Standard antisera have been prepared by hyperimmunisation of guinea-pigs, rabbits or colostrum-deprived piglets with the standard strain of PEV serotypes 1–13.

a) Virus neutralisation test for porcine enterovirus identification

The virus harvested from cell cultures is diluted in tissue culture maintenance medium over the range 10^{-1} to 10^{-6} in tenfold steps. For enterovirus serotyping, 14 rows of each dilution are prepared, equal volumes of standard antisera to PEV-1–13 diluted 1/10 are added to the rows 1–13 and an equal volume of negative serum to the last row. Mixtures are incubated overnight at 4°C or for 1 hour at 37°C and thereafter inoculated into roller tube cultures or into wells of microtitration plates. Assessment is carried out 72 hours later and every following day up to day 10, depending on when the CPE is seen. The identification of a PEV serotype is confirmed if the titre of the isolated virus in the presence of that antiserum is at least 10^3 lower than that virus incubated with negative serum.

b) Indirect fluorescent antibody test for the confirmation of porcine enterovirus antigen in cells

The IFA test is based on the reaction of the antigens in infected cells with specific antibodies in positive serum (13). The reaction is visualised by a fluorescein isothiocyanate (FITC)-conjugated antiglobulin, using a microscope with a UV or a blue light source. The antigen is detectable in cells 12 hours after the infection with PEV, i.e. before the development of CPE. Polyclonal antisera often show cross-reactivity with different PEV types, which can confuse the interpretation of results.

- **Test procedure**

i) Monolayers of porcine kidney cells on cover-slips are inoculated with the suspected material. Positive and negative controls should be processed in parallel with the test specimens.

ii) After incubation for 12–16 hours, the cover-slips are removed, washed twice in PBS, air-dried and fixed in cold acetone for 5–15 minutes.

iii) The cover-slips are placed into a wet box and flooded with rabbit or pig hyperimmune anti-PEV serum optimally diluted 1/10 with PBS or with PEV-specific monoclonal antibody at working dilution.

iv) The wet box is closed and incubated at 37°C for 60 minutes.

v) The cover-slips are removed and washed three times in PBS, then flooded with FITC-conjugated anti-rabbit or anti-pig goat serum, at a previously assessed working dilution, and incubated at 37°C for 30 minutes.

vi) The cover-slips are then washed three times with PBS, air-dried and mounted in 0.1 M Tris-buffered glycerol, pH 8.6.

After processing, the cover-slips are examined microscopically. The control slides are examined first to confirm that the fluorescence observed is specific. The fluorescence is apple green in colour and occurs in the cell cytoplasm and at the periphery of the nucleus. Instead of cover-slips, multispot slides or multiwell plates can also be used.

2. Serological tests

Because the seroprevalence of PEV-1 may exceed 60% in healthy pig populations in some countries of Central Europe, and identical clinical signs may be caused by other viruses – including other serotypes of PEV – a single serological test for PEV-1 giving positive results does not indicate that neurological signs observed are actually caused by PEV-1. A four-fold rise in titre together with typical signs should be considered to be an indication of a PEV-1 infection having caused clinical disease. For screening for specific antibodies in pig populations, it is usual to use the VN test in microtitre plates or the enzyme-linked immunosorbent assay (ELISA).

Pigs that have recovered from disease, or those with inapparent disease, produce specific antibodies. Several serological methods are available for their detection, of which the VN test is the most useful. Originally the test was carried out in tubes using porcine kidney cell cultures as the indicator system for infectivity. Later, the microtitre modification was introduced, in the interests of economy (10). More recently, an ELISA has been developed that is more sensitive and rapid, but which requires special equipment and considerable laboratory experience (3).

For serological diagnosis it is necessary to have standard strains of PEV serotypes propagated in cell cultures and hyperimmune serum monospecific for PEV types.

- **Standard strain of porcine enterviruses**

Characteristics: Following long experience, the strain 'Zabreh', isolated in Czechoslovakia during the period of peak incidence of the disease, was selected as the standard strain to generate the severe form of enterovirus encephalomyelitis. The pathogenicity of the strain is maintained by intracerebral passages in healthy, colostrum-deprived piglets. The virus produces typical signs of enterovirus encephalomyelitis after an incubation period of 5–7 days. For serological diagnosis, the following strains of PEV serotypes should be used as standard strains: Type 1 – Talfan, type 2 – T80, type 3 – O2b, type 4 – PS36, type 5 – F26, type 6 – PS37, type 7 – F43, type 8 – V13, type 9 – UKG/410/73, type 10 – LP54/Eng/75, type 11 – UKG/173/74, type 12 – 2899/84, type 13 – 460/88.

Stock virus: Standard strains are propagated on monolayers of tissue culture either from primary porcine kidney or testes or from an established cell line, for example PK-15. A 10% suspension in PBS, pH 7.4, is prepared from the brain and spinal cord of piglets infected experimentally with PEV. Some types are isolated from faeces. The suspension is centrifuged and the supernatant is used for the inoculation of cell cultures. The procedure for the cultivation of PEV in cell cultures is as follows:

The growth medium is removed from the cell culture and after rinsing with buffered saline, cells are inoculated with the virus suspension at 37°C. The size of the inoculum should be equal to 10% of the growth medium. After 1 hour of incubation at 37°C, the fluid is decanted, the cultivation vessel is rinsed with buffered saline, and the cells are overlayed with serum-free Earle's medium with antibiotics. CPE is apparent within 48 hours, and the monolayer disintegrates more or less completely during the next 48–72 hours. In the subsequent three to five passages in cell culture, the development of the CPE accelerates and the concentration of virions increases. Titration of the virus is performed in tube cultures or on microtitre plates. A cell-adapted strain usually reaches $TCID_{50}$ (50% tissue culture infective dose) titres of 10^6–10^7 per ml.

The fluid harvest is checked for specificity using known specific hyperimmune antiserum. Treatment with 5% chloroform and cultivation in human and bovine cell cultures and chicken embryos, is used to exclude contamination with other viruses. PEV is chloroform resistant and multiplies only in cultures of swine origin. Immunofluorescent antibody staining is useful to detect possible contaminants that are also chloroform resistant and propagate on cells of swine origin (e.g. parvovirus), or that are noncytopathogenic. The stock virus should be divided into small aliquots and preserved at –60°C. Frozen virus retains its properties for several years. For stock virus that is to be used in the neutralisation test, a constant dose of 100 $TCID_{50}$ is recommended.

- **Specific hyperimmune serum**

Specific hyperimmune serum is obtained by repeated immunisation of guinea pigs, rabbits or colostrum-deprived piglets with PEV. The standard strains should be used. Rabbits are immunised either intravenously, using virus suspension alone, or subcutaneously or intraperitoneally, using the virus suspension with 10% oil adjuvant. Good results may be obtained by administering three doses of 2 ml of virus suspension + 0.2 ml oil adjuvant, at intervals of 2 weeks. The rabbits are bled 10 days after the last immunisation. Piglets are immunised in the same way. The harvested sera are clarified by centrifugation and stored in small aliquots at –20°C. The sera are titrated using a neutralisation test and constant antigen. Only sera with an antibody titre of at least 1/256 can be used for the identification of the virus.

a) Virus neutralisation test in microtitre plates

The test is performed in flat-bottomed tissue culture microtitre plates, using low passage porcine kidney or testes cells or cell lines derived from porcine tissue. Stock virus is grown in cell monolayers. The virus harvested from cell cultures is clarified by centrifugation and stored in aliquots at –20°C. Culture medium, such as Eagle's complete medium LYH (Hanks balanced salt solution with yeast extract, lactalbumin and antibiotics), is used as diluent.

- **Test procedure**

i) Inactivate swine sera for 30 minutes in a water bath at 56°C.

ii) The sera to be tested are diluted in cell culture medium in twofold steps from 1/2 to 1/64, four wells per dilution and 50 µl volumes per well.

iii) Controls include positive and negative sera, cells and medium control.

iv) Add to each well 50 µl of virus stock previously diluted in culture medium to provide 100 $TCID_{50}$.

v) Incubate for 1 hour at 37°C with plates covered. The residual virus stock is also incubated.

vi) Make back titrations of the residual virus stock in four tenfold dilution steps using 50 µl per well and four wells per dilution.

vii) Add 50 µl of porcine kidney cell suspension at 5×10^5 cells per cm^3.

viii) After further shaking, the plates are sealed and incubated at 37°C in a CO_2 atmosphere for 2–3 days or longer, to a maximum of 8 days.

ix) Read the plates microscopically for CPE. The test should be validated by checking the back titration of virus and titration of controlled positive serum. Virus should give a value of 100 $TCID_{50}$ with a permissible range of 30–300. The standard positive serum should give a titre within 0.3 log_{10} units from its predetermined mean. A negative serum should give no neutralisation at the lowest dilution tested, i.e. 1/2.

x) The VN results are determined by the Spearman–Kärber method as the dilution of serum that neutralised the virus in 50% of the wells.

xi) Virus neutralisation titres are regarded as positive if the corresponding serum neutralises the virus at an initial serum dilution of 1/8 or higher.

b) **Enzyme-linked immunosorbent assay**

An alternative method for the detection and titration of specific antibodies against PEV is the ELISA technique (3). The test is performed in microtitre plates using PEV grown on tissue cultures as antigen. The technique can be carried out using the following steps.

- **Antigen preparation**

i) The stock virus is multiplied in established cell lines as described in Section B below.

ii) The harvested virus is clarified by centrifugation at 200 ***g*** for 15 minutes, and then precipitated with a final 50% saturated $(NH_4)_2SO_4$ for 120 minutes at 4°C.

iii) After centrifugation at 2000 ***g***, the resulting precipitate is suspended in TEN buffer (Tris-hydroxymethyl-methylamine [0.01 M], ethylene diamine tetra-acetic acid [1 mM] and NaCl [0.15 M]), pH 7.4, to 1/100 of the initial volume.

iv) The concentrated viral suspension is extracted by shaking with freon 3/1 for 10 minutes at 4°C.

v) Following further centrifugation, the supernatant is divided into two separate phases. The upper aqueous phase, containing the viral antigen, is desalinated by passage through a 2.5 × 40 cm cylinder packed with sephadex G 25.

vi) The viral solution is finally concentrated by ultracentrifugation at 160,000 ***g*** for 3 hours.

vii) The pellet is suspended in TEN buffer, pH 7.4, in approximately 1000th the initial volume of virus.

viii) Insoluble proteins are separated by light centrifugation, and the supernatant is used as the positive antigen in the ELISA.

- **Test procedure**

i) Plates are sensitised with prediluted antigen in phosphate buffered saline (PBS), pH 7.2, by adding 100 µl to each well. The absorption of antigen to the surface of the plate takes place overnight at 4°C. Parallel rows of the plate should be treated with negative antigen.

ii) The plate is washed five times in PBS to remove excess antigen.

iii) Test sera are diluted 1/20 with PBST (PBS solution containing 0.05% Tween 20). 50 µl of the diluted sera is placed into each of two wells with positive antigen and into two wells with negative antigen. The plate is incubated for 1 hour at 37°C.

iv) The plates are washed five times with PBST.

v) A predetermined dilution of horseradish peroxidase conjugated with anti-swine immunoglobulin prepared in rabbits is added in 50 µl quantities to each well. The plates are incubated for a further 1 hour at room temperature.

vi) The plates are washed five times in PBS.

vii) Substrate solution (0.1% orthophenyl-endiamine with 0.03% hydrogen peroxide in PBS, pH 6.0) is added in 100 µl quantities to each well.

viii) After the addition of substrate, positive samples change colour to dark brown. When a sufficient degree of colour reaction is seen in the wells of known positive sera, the reaction is stopped by addition of 50 µl of 2 M sulphuric acid to each well. The absorbance of the wells is measured at a wavelength of 492 nm, preferably using an automatic multichannel spectrophotometer with print-out mechanism. Positive and negative sera and noninfected cells should be processed as controls in parallel with the test specimens.

ix) The absorbance of a serum is the mean reading of two wells with positive antigen minus the mean reading of two wells with negative antigen. Absorbance readings of test sera that exceed by more than twofold the mean reading of standard negative sera are regarded as positive.

B. REQUIREMENTS FOR VACCINES AND DIAGNOSTIC BIOLOGICALS

• Vaccines against enterovirus encephalomyelitis

During the period of highest incidence of the disease in central Europe and Madagascar, active immunoprophylaxis was an important means for the control of this infection (14). Initially, the brains and spinal cords of experimentally infected piglets were used as antigen for vaccine manufacture. After establishing the cultivation of PEV virus on monolayers of porcine kidney cells (11), the virus propagated *in vitro* is used to prepare vaccine. The following two types of vaccines have been developed:

i) Killed vaccines prepared from virus inactivated as described in Section B.2., and adsorbed on to aluminium hydroxide or mixed with oil adjuvant for parenteral administration (7, 9).

ii) Live attenuated virus vaccines obtained by serial passages in porcine kidney cultures. This type of vaccine has been successful when administered intranasally or periorally (7, 8), but is not commercially available.

1. Seed management

a) Characteristics of the seed

Local strains of PEV isolated from natural outbreaks of enterovirus encephalomyelitis are recommended as antigen for inactivated vaccine production.

b) Method of culture

The virus is propagated on tissue cultures and specificity is confirmed by neutralisation tests as described in Section A.2.a. Viruses shown to be identical to the standard strain are tested for freedom from contamination, and the virus content is estimated by titration on monolayer cultures of porcine kidney cells. The master seed is distributed in small aliquots and stored at –60°C. It is recommended that at least three such strains of PEV are maintained.

2. Method of manufacture

The viruses from master seeds are propagated on tissue culture to a sufficient volume for the production of one batch of vaccine. The best facility for virus production is a roller drum apparatus turning at approximately eight revolutions per hour. The harvested virus is checked for specificity, sterility and virus content. The virus has to be neutralised by standard hyperimmune serum and be free from any microbiological contamination. The virus should contain 10^6 $TCID_{50}$ per ml when titrated on porcine kidney cell cultures. The batch of virus is inactivated using formaldehyde or other suitable chemicals, such as binary ethylenimine. Where formaldehyde is used, this can be done by using formalin at a final concentration of formaldehyde 1/2500 at 37°C for 48 hours. The virus must be tested to show complete inactivation before it is adsorbed on to aluminium hydroxide or mixed with mineral oil emulsion adjuvant. It is administered by subcutaneous injection.

3. In-process control

The porcine kidney cells, growth media and harvested virus have to be free from bacteria, mycoplasmas and fungi. Tests for sterility and freedom from contamination of biological materials may be found in Chapter I.4.

The harvested virus is further checked for specifity and virus content. Methods are fully described in Section A.1.

4. Batch control

a) Sterility

Tests for sterility and freedom from contamination of biological materials can be found in Chapter I.4.

b) Safety

The safety test is carried out by inoculation of from two to four piglets at 2 months of age with double the field dose of the final product vaccine. The animals are observed for 21 days, during which time they must remain healthy, without any signs of disease that could be attributable to the vaccine.

c) Potency

The potency test is performed on five piglets, at 2 months of age, inoculated with the minimum recommended dose as determined by previous assays. After 21 days the vaccinated piglets, together with two unvaccinated controls, are challenged intranasally with 10 LD_{50} (50% lethal dose) of a virulent field strain of PEV. The potency of the vaccine is satisfactory if 60% of the vaccinated animals survive with no signs of disease but the two controls fall ill within 14 days. Potency may also be estimated by measuring the increase in specific antibodies as described in Sections A.2.a. and A.2.b. A serum-neutralising titre of at least 1/32 is required. For subsequent batches it is sufficient to carry out the VN only.

d) Duration of immunity

The killed vaccine protects swine for up to 6 months. Pigs vaccinated before parturition transfer colostral immunity, which lasts 6–8 weeks, to piglets.

e) Stability

The shelf life for this vaccine was experimentally determined as 1 year.

f) Preservatives

The vaccine may be stored at 2–8°C. It should be protected from light and frost.

g) Precautions (hazards)

The vaccine contains inactivated virus and the aluminium hydroxide adjuvant is not usually associated with harmful reactions. If the vaccine is an oil-emulsion vaccine, care should be taken to avoid accidental self-injection as this will cause a painful local reaction.

5. Tests on the final product

a) Safety

As in Section B.4.b.

b) Potency

As in Section B.4.c.

REFERENCES

1. AUERBACH J., PRAGER D., NEUHAUS S., LOSS U. & WITTE K.H. (1994). Grouping of porcine enteroviruses by indirect immunofluorescence and description of new serotypes. *J. Vet. Med. [B]*, 41, 277–282.

2. BETTS A.O. (1960). Studies on enteroviruses of the pig. VI. The relationship of the T 80 strain of a swine polioencephalomyelitis virus to some other viruses as shown by neutralization tests in tissue cultures. *Res. Vet. Sci.*, 1, 296–300.

3. HUBSCHLE O.J.B., RAJOANARISON J., KOKO M., RAKOTONDRAMARY E. & RASOLFOMANANA P. (1983). ELISA for detection of Teschen virus antibodies in swine serum samples. *Dtsch Tierarztl. Wochenschr.*, **90**, 86–88.

4. KLOBOUK A. (1931). Encephalomyelitis enzootica suum. *Zverolekarsky obzor*, **24**, 436–480.

5. KLOBOUK A. (1933). Aetiology of the so-called Teschen disease – Encephalomyelitis enzootica suum. *Zverolekarske rozpravy*, **8**, 85–96.

6. KNOWLES N.J. & BUCKLEY L.S. (1980). Differentiation of porcine enterovirus sertoypes by complement fixation. *Res. Vet. Sci.*, **29**, 113–115.

7. MADR V. (1959). Propagation of the Teschen disease virus in cell cultures. *Veterinarstvi*, **IX**, 298–301.

8. MAYR A. (1958). Attenuation of pathogenicity of the Teschen disease virus by passaging in cell cultures. *Monatsh. Tierheilkd*, **10**, 186–191.

9. MAYR A. (1958). A tissue culture vaccine against Teschen disease 1. Communication. Preparation of vaccine. *Zentralbl. Bakteriol. [I. Orig.]*, **172**, 465–480.

10. MAYR A. & BIBRACK B. (1971). Demonstration of Teschen Talfan infection using a micromodification of neutralization test. *Zentralbl. Veterinarmed. [B]*, **18**, 657–664.

11. MAYR A. & SCHWOEBEL W. (1957). Propagation of the Teschen disease virus in porcine kidney cell cultures and properties of the cultured virus. 1.2.3. part. *Zentralbl. Bakteriol. [I. Orig.]*, **168**, 329–359.

12. MINOR P.D., BROWN F., DOMINGO E., HOEY E., KING A., KNOWLES N., LEMON S., PALMENBERG A., RUECKERT R.R., STANWAY G., WIMMER E. & YIN-MURPHY S.H. (1995). Family Picornaviridae. *In:* Virus Taxonomy. Classification and Nomenclature of Viruses, Murphey F.A., Fauquet C.M., Bishop H.D.L., Ghabrial S.H., Jarvis A.W., Martelli G.P., Mayo M.A. & Summers M.D., eds. Sixth Report of the International Committee on Taxonomy of Viruses. *Arch. Virol., (Suppl.)* ,**10**, 329–336.

13. ROMANENKO V.F., PRUSS O.G., BELYI YU.A. & KUPNOVSKAYA L.V. (1982). Immunofluorescent diagnosis of porcine encephalomyelitis. *Veterinariia*, **4**, 69–72.

14. THAUB E. (1942). Active immunization against Teschen disease using vaccines adsorbed on aluminium hydroxide. *Arch. Tierheilkd*, **77**, 52–66.

15. WITTE VON K.H., AUERBACH J., LOSS K.U., NEUHAUS S. & PRAGER D. (1994). Typisierung von 17 porzinen Enterovirusisolaten aus Polioenzephalomyelitisfällen der Jahre 1983–1991. *DTW Dtsch. Tierarztl. Wochenschr.*, **101**, 453–492.

*

* *

CHAPTER 2.6.4.

TRANSMISSIBLE GASTROENTERITIS

SUMMARY

Transmissible gastroenteritis (TGE) is an enteric disease of pigs caused by TGE virus (TGEV), a member of the Coronaviridae. Since 1984, a distinct respiratory variant (porcine respiratory coronavirus or PRCV) has spread throughout many parts of the world. This virus is probably a deletion mutant of TGEV. PRCV does not appear to be an important primary pathogen, but it has greatly complicated the diagnosis of TGE, particularly by serological means.

Laboratory diagnosis is made by demonstrating the presence of virus, viral antigens or viral nucleic acid in material from suspected cases, or by demonstrating virus-specific humoral antibodies.

***Identification of the agent:** Virus may be identified by virus isolation in tissue culture, electron microscopy, various immunodiagnostic assays, and more recently by specific detection of viral RNA. The most commonly employed rapid assays are probably the immunodiagnostic ones, particularly enzyme-linked immunosorbent assays (ELISAs) on faeces and fluorescent antibody tests on cryostat sections of intestine. Detection of virus by reversed passive haemagglutination has also been described. Another enteric disease, porcine epidemic diarrhoea, is caused by a serologically distinct coronavirus that nevertheless has an identical appearance under the electron microscope. Diagnostically, immune electron microscopy circumvents this problem.*

***Serological tests:** The most widely used methods are virus neutralisation tests and ELISAs. Only in the latter case is differentiation from PRCV possible, as TGEV and PRCV antibodies show complete cross-neutralisation. Passive haemagglutination and haemagglutination inhibition tests have also been developed for TGE serology.*

***Requirements for vaccines and diagnostic biologicals:** There are no commercial biological products available internationally. However, several countries practise vaccination, and in the United States of America licences have been issued authorising the production and distribution of monovalent and combined vaccines.*

A. DIAGNOSTIC TECHNIQUES

Transmissible gastroenteritis (TGE) is an enteric disease of pigs caused by TGE virus (TGEV), a member of the Coronaviridae. Since 1984, a distinct respiratory variant (porcine respiratory coronavirus or PRCV) has spread throughout many parts of the world. TGEV multiplies in and damages the enterocyte lining of the small intestine, producing villous atrophy and enteritis. Diarrhoea and vomiting occur in pigs of all ages; mortality is highest in neonates. Extra-intestinal sites of virus multiplication include the respiratory tract and mammary tissues (18), but the virus is most readily isolated from the intestinal tract and from faeces. By contrast, porcine respiratory coronavirus (PRCV) is most readily isolated from the upper respiratory tract, the tonsils or the lungs, and little if any enteric multiplication of virus occurs (10, 24, 30). PRCV is probably a deletion mutant of TGEV (32).

As TGE is a contagious disease that can occur as explosive epizootics, rapid diagnostic methods for its confirmation are particularly important. The disease can also take the form of a low-level endemic problem of post-weaning diarrhoea, which is more difficult to diagnose.

1. Identification of the agent

Virus may be identified by virus isolation in tissue culture (12), electron microscopy, various immunodiagnostic assays, and more recently by specific detection of viral RNA (2, 3, 28, 40, 43, 51). An alternative diagnostic method that has been recommended for laboratories lacking facilities for specialised tests is the oral dosing of susceptible piglets with suspect intestinal contents. However, laboratory tests are still required to confirm susceptibility of the inoculated pigs and to show that any illness induced in these animals is due to TGE. The most commonly employed rapid assays are probably the immunodiagnostic ones, particularly enzyme-linked immunosorbent assays (ELISAs) on faeces (5, 20, 48) and fluorescent antibody tests (FAT) on cryostat sections of intestine (31). Detection of virus by reversed passive haemagglutination has also been described (1). Another enteric disease, porcine epidemic diarrhoea, is caused by a serologically distinct coronavirus that nevertheless has an identical appearance under the electron microscope. Diagnostically, immune electron microscopy circumvents this problem (35, 47).

a) Virus isolation in tissue culture

Apart from the inoculation of live piglets (12), this is the most definitive method of diagnosis. However, for routine use it is slow and laborious.

Isolation is usually attempted from faeces or from carcass material, particularly the small intestine. Loops of affected small intestine, ligated at each end to retain the contents, are the preferred specimens. As the virus is heat labile, all samples should be fresh or chilled.

Sample material is homogenised in cell culture medium or phosphate buffered saline (PBS), pH 7.2, containing antibiotics, e.g. penicillin (1000 U/ml), dihydrosteptomycin (1000 µg/ml), and mycostatin (20 U/ml), to produce a 10% suspension. This is allowed to stand out of direct sunlight for 30 minutes at room temperature. The suspension is then sonicated and clarified by low speed centrifugation. The supernatant fluid may be mixed with an equal volume of heat-inactivated bovine serum in order to reduce the cytotoxic effect of the material and it is then used to inoculate susceptible tissue cultures, such as 3–4-day-old primary or secondary pig kidney monolayers. Other low passage porcine cultures (such as thyroid or testis) and some cell lines (15, 21) may also be used for primary virus isolation. After incubation at 37°C for 1 hour, the cell sheets are overlaid with a medium, such as Earle's yeast lactalbumin (EYL) balanced salt solution, containing sodium bicarbonate and antibiotics, e.g. penicillin (100 U/ml), dihydrostreptomycin (100 µg/ml), mycostatin (20 U/ml), and 1% fetal calf serum. Incorporation of trypsin into the culture medium may enhance primary viral recovery (6, 15). Uninoculated control cultures are established concurrently and all cultures are incubated at 37°C.

Viral cytopathic effect (CPE) may be observed after 3–7 days, characterised by cell rounding, enlarging, forming syncytia and detaching into the medium. Plaque formation is sometimes more reliable and easier to recognise. A suitable plaquing overlay is 1.6% noble agar in 2 × minimal essential medium with 1% $NaCO_3$, antibiotics (as above), 0.7% neutral red and 1% DEAE (diethylaminoethyl) (100 µg/ml). Wild-type TGEV does not grow readily in tissue culture, so several subpassages may be necessary before these distinctive changes become apparent. Cytopathic isolates must be confirmed as TGEV by immunostaining or by *in-vitro* neutralisation tests using appropriate TGEV-specific antisera (6). If suitable monoclonal antibodies (MAbs) are available they can be used to distinguish between TGEV and PRCV by immunostaining methods (13, 42). Differentiation of TGEV from PRCV can also be accomplished by TGEV-specific cDNA probes (2) or by discriminatory reverse-transcription polymerase chain reaction (RT-PCR) (49).

b) Fluorescent antibody test for viral antigens

This is a rapid, sensitive and specific means of identifying TGE viral antigens in cryostat sections of intestine. A freshly dead pig is required, and the ideal animal should be under 4 weeks of age (preferably less than 1 week) and just starting to show clinical signs of the disease (that is, within 24–28 hours of infection). Within 30 minutes of death, 2 cm lengths from four different regions of the posterior part of the small intestine should be removed. Lengths of 5–10 mm are cut from these for snap freezing with solid CO_2. Correct orientation of the material is important to ensure that subsequent cutting by cryostat yields true transverse sections. Sections are cut 6 µm thick, mounted on cover-slips, air-dried and fixed in acetone. Fixed positive and negative control sections are stored at –20°C for staining in parallel. After washing with Tris buffer, pH 8.7, or PBS, the sections are stained with a diluted solution of fluorescein isothiocyanate (FITC)-conjugated TGEV antibody, and placed in a humid incubator at 37°C for 30 minutes. Any unbound stain is removed by washing in Tris buffer. If desired, the sections are counterstained with a 10^{-5} dilution of Evans blue in Tris buffer and mounted in glycerol.

Stained sections should be examined by ultraviolet light microscopy as soon as possible. The quality of the staining is assessed by reference to the controls. An accurate interpretation depends on the preservation of the villous architecture, the epithelial cells of which are examined for intracytoplasmic fluorescence.

A peroxidase–antiperoxidase method for the demonstration of TGEV has been developed recently for detection of TGEV and PRCV in both frozen and formalin-fixed, and paraffin-embedded tissues (17, 41).

c) Enzyme-linked immunosorbent assay detection of faecal virus antigens

A double antibody sandwich system may be used, for instance with a capture MAb and a polyclonal enzyme-linked detector antibody. The anti-TGEV MAb is directed towards a conserved epitope on the viral nucleoprotein, and is in the form of clarified ascitic fluid. It is applied to 96-well microplates in a bicarbonate buffer, pH 9.6, and incubated overnight at 4°C. Faecal samples are prepared in McIlvaine's buffer[1], pH 6.0, and then diluted in PBS, pH 7.2, containing 0.05% Tween 20, 1% gelatin, 1% Nonidet and a proprietary dried-milk product. Plates are washed twice with washing buffer (PBS containing 0.05% Tween 20) before adding the prepared faecal samples. The plates are incubated at 37°C for 2 hours. After a further wash, a peroxidase-linked, porcine, polyclonal TGEV antiserum is added in a buffer of PBS containing 0.05% Tween 20, 1% gelatin and 5% normal pig serum; this mixture is incubated at 37°C for 2 hours. The plates are washed six times before adding the enzyme substrate, which is tetramethyl benzidine (0.1 mg/ml) in 0.1 M acetate buffer, pH 6.0, with 0.00225% hydrogen peroxide. The reaction is stopped after 5 minutes by the addition of 2.0 M sulphuric acid, and the absorbance of the well contents are assessed. A control negative and a control weak positive antigen well are included on each plate.

d) Nucleic acid recognition methods

In situ hybridisation (ISH) and RT-PCR methods have been described for the direct detection of TGEV in clinical samples, with differentiation from PRCV (28, 43). A second round of nested PCR may significantly enhance the sensitivity (27). Differentiation between TGE viruses may be achieved by analysing PCR products with restriction endonuclease enzymes (51) or by sequencing (29).

2. Serological tests

Serology may be diagnostic if a rising titre of antibody can be demonstrated. In addition, a single seropositive result has diagnostic value if collected from a population previously known to be seronegative. As the possibility of acquiring carrier virus status among pigs can be reduced by accepting only seronegative animals, serological testing is also a common precondition for importation.

Following infection with TGEV or PRCV, viral antibodies can be detected in serum from 6 or 7 days post-infection, and such antibodies persist at least for many months. Although PRCV and TGEV antibodies show complete neutralisation of either virus, there are differences in the specificities of some of the non-neutralising antibodies (8, 13, 42), as PRCV lacks certain epitopes present on the TGEV. MAbs to such regions can be incorporated into competitive ELISAs to detect serum antibody that is entirely TGEV specific. While such tests are reliable in that they do not produce false-positive results with PRCV antisera, false negatives may occur because of a reduced sensitivity compared with neutralisation tests, and because of strain variation among TGE viruses, such that no single TGEV-specific MAb will recognise all strains (7, 42). The problem of insensitivity can be reduced by using the test on a group or herd basis.

a) Transmissible gastroenteritis virus/porcine respiratory coronavirus tests

These tests detect antibody to both TGEV and PRCV, and include virus neutralisation (VN) tests, indirect ELISAs (14, 16, 22, 33) and competitive ELISAs based on TGEV/PRCV group-specific MAbs (26).

VN tests can be performed with a variety of cell types and viral strains. Commonly used cell lines include swine testes (21) or primary or continuous porcine kidney cells. Such tests have been very widely used for many years and are commonly regarded as standards against which to assess new assays. A modification of the method of Witte (50) uses flat-bottomed tissue-culture grade microtitre plates, a cell line of A72 cells derived from a dog rectal tumour, and a field strain of virus adapted to grow in such cells: 100 $TCID_{50}$ (50% tissue culture infective dose) of virus is incubated with heat-inactivated test sera, and neutralisation is indicated by absence of CPE after further incubation with A72 cells in Leibovitz 15 medium (Sigma, United Kingdom) with added antibiotics, 10% fetal calf serum and 1% L-glutamine. The total volume of reagents in all wells should be 150 µl.

- **Virus neutralisation: test procedure**

i) Sera are inactivated for 30 minutes in a water bath at 56°C.

ii) Doubling dilutions of test sera are made in cell culture medium beginning with undiluted serum (this gives a neutralisation stage dilution of 1/2 when mixed with an equal volume of virus). The dilutions are prepared in a 96-well flat-bottomed cell-culture grade microtitre plate using, optimally, three wells per dilution and 25 µl volumes per well. Positive and negative control sera are also included in the test. No

---

1 McIlvaine's buffer A: citric acid (8.4 g), distilled water (400 ml). McIlvaine's buffer B: Na_2HPO_4 (18.45 g), distilled water (650 ml). McIlvaine's buffer: buffer A (368.5 ml) + buffer B (631.5 ml). Adjust to pH 6.0; can be stored for 2 months in a refrigerator.

standard sera are available, but internal positive standards should be prepared and titrated in an appropriate range.

iii) 25 µl TGEV stock is added to each well at a dilution in culture medium calculated to provide 100 $TCID_{50}$ per well. Virus should be added to two out of the three wells containing serum at each dilution. The third well serves as a serum-only control and should receive 25 µl per well of culture medium instead of virus.

iv) The residual virus is back titrated in four tenfold steps using 25 µl per well and at least four wells per dilution; 25 µl of culture medium is added to each of the back-titration wells to compensate for the absence of a test serum.

v) The plates are agitated briefly and then incubated for 1 hour in a CO_2 atmosphere at 37°C.

vi) 100 µl of, for example, A72 cell suspension at 2×10^5 cells per ml is added to each well.

vii) The plates are incubated for 3–7 days in a CO_2 atmosphere at 37°C.

viii) The plates are read microscopically for CPE. The test is validated by checking the back titration of virus (which should give a value of 100 $TCID_{50}$ with a permissible range of 50–200 $TCID_{50}$) and the control sera. The standard positive serum should give a value within 0.3 $\log_{10}$ units either side of its predetermined mean. Readings of each test serum dilution should be made with reference to the appropriate serum-only control to distinguish viral CPE from serum-induced cytotoxicity or contamination.

ix) The test serum results are determined by the Spearman–Kärber method as the dilution of serum that neutralised the virus in 50% of wells.

x) A negative serum should give no neutralisation at the lowest dilution tested (i.e. undiluted serum, equivalent to a dilution of 1/2 at the neutralisation stage).

b) Transmissible-gastroenteritis-virus-specific tests

These are ELISAs employing an MAb that recognises TGEV but not PRCV (7, 9, 42, 46). Test sera from pigs previously infected with a strain of TGEV recognised by the MAb will contain antibodies of the same specificity that can compete with it for binding to TGEV-antigen-coated ELISA plates. ELISA antigens may be prepared from cell lysates of kidney cell lines that were either inoculated with tissue-culture-adapted strains of TGEV, or uninfected. Alternatively TGEV-infected or uninfected swine testes cells fixed in 80% acetone have been used as an antigen source (42). Positive and negative antigens are coated to alternate rows of microtitre plates using bicarbonate buffer, pH 9.6. Diluted test sera, including positive and negative controls, are added to appropriate wells and incubated overnight before further addition of diluted MAb to all wells. Bound MAb is detected by a peroxidase-conjugated anti-mouse antibody that induces a colour reaction in the presence of an appropriate substrate. The colour changes are measured by spectrophotometer and for each test sample the net result is the difference in absorbance between the positive and negative antigen wells, expressed as a percentage of the result obtained with the negative control serum. The negative–positive cut-off value for the test must be determined by previous testing of known negative and positive populations.

Haemagglutination-based tests described to date (19, 23, 39) were validated before the appearance of PRCV. However, they may be TGEV specific as TGEV, but not PRCV, is haemagglutinating (38).

B. REQUIREMENTS FOR VACCINES AND DIAGNOSTIC BIOLOGICALS

Vaccination against TGE is carried out in several countries.

Information on experimental work or field trials of TGEV vaccines licensed for use in the United States of America (USA) has been reviewed, including possible limitations in their field efficacy and concepts related to the design of optimal TGEV vaccines (34, 36, 37). Eight manufacturers are licensed to produce TGEV vaccines in the USA: the vaccines include six modified live and two inactivated vaccines. The modified live vaccines are used for oral administration to pregnant sows (to induce passive immunity) or have also been licensed for oral administration to nursing or weaned pigs (to induce active immunity). Inactivated TGEV vaccines are licensed for parenteral inoculation of pregnant sows by the intramuscular route or for intraperitoneal administration to nursing or weaned pigs. In general, these vaccines induced marginal passive protection against TGEV challenge of nursing piglets when evaluated under controlled experimental conditions or in the field. Although they fail to adequately protect against epizootic TGE, data suggest that these vaccines may provide some efficacy against enzootic TGEV by stimulating an anamnestic antibody response to TGEV in serum and milk (36, 37).

The main reason proposed for TGEV vaccine failures was their inability to stimulate high levels of secretory IgA (SIgA) antibodies in milk analogous to the SIgA antibody responses found in the milk of sows naturally infected with TGEV (36, 37). Furthermore, these vaccines did not adequately protect the sow against TGE, such that illness in the sow often resulted in anorexia, agalatica and failure to passively protect her piglets. Thus the modified live vaccines may fail to replicate to the extent required to induce protective immunity in the intestine, or if given to seronegative neonatal animals, concerns exist regarding their possible reversion to virulence. Killed vaccines given parenterally do not induce SIgA antibodies; cell-mediated immune responses are often poor and the duration of immunity may be short-lived. Although use of PRCV strains as vaccine candidates for TGE has been proposed, experimental studies regarding their efficacy against TGEV have shown a lack of efficacy (25) or only partial cross-protection (4, 11, 45). However, the widespread prevalence of PRCV infections in the swine population in Europe appears to have dramatically reduced the incidence of epizootic TGE in Europe (30). Newer recombinant DNA strategies for the development of TGEV vaccines include the possible use of an S protein subunit vaccine (contingent upon the development of mucosal delivery systems and adjuvants) or the use of live recombinant viral or bacterial vectors that express TGEV genes important for the induction of immunity (34, 36).

There are a number of general requirements (e.g. produced in a licensed facility, label rules, tracking capability, etc.) that apply to all biological products including vaccines. A set of regulations exist (called standard requirements, or SRs) that describe testing to be done on the vaccine and parent materials. Detailed information on SRs for vaccines in the USA are contained in the Code of Federal Regulations (CFR) Title 9, Volume 1, Part 113 (abbreviated below as 9 CFR, 113) (44). The European Pharmacopoeia also contains information. Unfortunately, there is no specific standard requirement for TGEV vaccines.

1. Seed management

a) Characteristics of the seed

The seed virus must be tested for purity and identity. The purity includes freedom from bacteria and fungi (9 CFR 113:27), mycoplasmas (9 CFR 113:28), and extraneous viruses (9 CFR 113:55) (44). The demonstration of identity is usually accomplished by VN or FAT. Genetically engineered vaccines or naturally selected vaccines with claims of antigen-coding gene deletion/inactivation are required to provide evidence (genotypic and/or phenotypic) of that identity.

b) Method of culture

Culture must be carried out on proven uncontaminated (approved) cells, and the number of cell culture passages is limited (usually to five). It is not required that the species of origin of the cell line be that of the target species.

c) Validation as a vaccine

Vaccine validation takes two forms. The master seed is considered to be immunogenic if a vaccine made at the highest passage, and according to the outline of production, is shown to be protective. The lowest antigenic level (modified live virus titre or inactivated antigen mass) shown to be protective becomes the baseline for all future serials (lots) of the product. In the case of live products, factors for titration variation and the death curve over time would be added. These trial vaccines should be tested for purity, safety, and efficacy by the manufacturer. Protection must be shown against the natural disease, with the virulent challenge virus. Virulent challenge virus is defined as the dose that causes disease in ≥95% of the susceptible controls. Three prelicense serials must subsequently be made and tested by the manufacturer and by the licensing authority, for potency, sterility and safety.

2. Method of manufacture

This is proprietary information for each manufacturer and hence not available.

3. In-process control

This is largely proprietary. Some in-process controls refer directly to production (e.g. O_2 concentration in the fermenter). Another category, however, includes tests similar to the final container potency test. For all vaccines, the simpler the final batch or container potency test, the more likely it is that it may be used as a monitoring/blending test: for example, virus titration on sub-batches may be used to predict final blended batch titre. Ingredients of animal origin must be sterilised or shown to be free from contamination.

4. Batch control

Batches must be blended to the final specifications and bottling specifications (e.g. fermentation runs may be pooled, or one run may be split and pooled with each of three others, etc.). In some countries, bulk and process control define the product and are the subject of intense regulation and scrutiny. The emphasis in the USA is on the final product. Batch control techniques must be detailed in the outline of production and must be meaningful, trackable, and the manufacturer must discard product that fails to meet specifications. If a batch is to be exported to another country for bottling or blending, then it is subjected to all the testing as though it were final product.

a) **Sterility**

All products must be tested for sterility. The manufacturer may also run sterility tests on batches for monitoring. Tests are similar to those described in Section B.1.a.

b) **Safety**

Safety tests are done before the licence is granted, and then on the final container (Sections B.5.a. and B.5.b.).

c) **Potency**

Potency would normally only be done if the potency test were a simple test (e.g. ELISA) to confirm the blending calculations before bottling.

d) **Duration of immunity**

Duration of immunity is tested in the prelicence (efficacy) serial test, not the batch control. New products are required to support label claims for revaccination schedules with efficacy trials (challenge) at the specified time after vaccination.

e) **Stability**

Stability is established before the licence is granted. Usually accelerated ageing (37°C) is used to estimate the lifetime so that the products do not have to be kept at storage temperature (4°C) for the real time period. This can be adjusted with real-time data later. The manufacturer is not required to do stability testing. Manufacturers are required to state the amount of antigenic material that will be in their product throughout the shelf life. Samples of product are selected (usually live) and tested within 30 days of expiration to see if, for example, the titre is at the level stated in the manufacturer's outline. Stability is also affected by moisture. Moisture left in a desiccated product can shorten its life, so this has to be tested in the final product or In-process.

f) **Preservatives**

There are restrictions on the maximum amounts of antibiotics that can be in a product. Restrictions on some vaccine components are related to their safety and to whether the stated withdrawal period is long enough for the component to have cleared before the animal is slaughtered. Preservatives used are proprietary.

g) **Precautions (hazards)**

Any risks to vaccinates need to be clearly stated on the label. This usually applies to pregnancy warnings for abortogenic live viruses, and the general anaphylaxis warning, but may also attempt to warn the user about soreness or swelling at the injection site, or transient fever or inappetence in some cases. No unusual label precautions apply to the TGE vaccines currently licensed.

5. Tests on the final product

a) **Safety**

Usually this will be a mouse and/or a guinea-pig or swine safety test (9 CFR 113:33, and ref. 50). Sterility tests are also carried out on the final product.

b) **Potency**

There is no single test for release potency. Whatever test is used must be correlated to protection in the host animal (the efficacy tests). The potency of live TGEV vaccines can be evaluated by *in-vitro* titration of the viral infectious dose in cell culture (34). This titre must be correlated with the minimum viral titre required to induce protective immunity against experimental challenge, and also against natural challenge under field conditions. The potency of killed vaccines is evaluated by vaccination and challenge tests using different doses of the vaccine. Titres of neutralising antibodies induced by inoculation of laboratory animals with the vaccine may be accepted if there is an established correlation with development of protective immunity.

Particular viral antigens associated with the induction of neutralising antibodies and protection against challenge can be quantified in killed vaccines using specific MAbs in ELISA, such as neutralising MAbs to the S protein of TGEV (34).

REFERENCES

1. ASAGI M., OGAWA T., MINETOMA T., SATO K. & INABA Y. (1986). Detection of transmissible gastroenteritis virus in feces from pigs by reversed passive haemagglutination. *Am. J. Vet. Res.*, **47**, 2161–2164.

2. BAE I., JACKWOOD D.J., BENFIELD D.A., SAIF L.J., WESLEY R.D. & HILL H. (1991). Differentiation of transmissible gastroenteritis virus from porcine respiratory coronavirus and other antigenically related coronaviruses by using cDNA probes specific for the 5' region of the S glycoprotein gene. *J. Clin. Microbiol.*, **29**, 215–218.

3. BENFIELD D.A., JACKWOOD D.J., BAE I., SAIF L.J. & WESLEY R.D. (1991). Detection of transmissible gastroenteritis virus using cDNA probes. *Arch. Virol.*, **116**, 91–106.

4. BERNARD S., BOTTREAU E., AYNAUD, J.M., HAVE P. & SZYMANSKY J. (1989). Natural infection with the porcine respiratory coronavirus induces protective lactogenic immunity against transmissible gastroenteritis virus. *Vet. Microbiol.*, **21**, 1–8.

5. BERNARD S., LANTIER I., LAUDE H. & AYNAUD J.M. (1986). Detection of transmissible gastroenteritis coronavirus antigens by a sandwich enzyme-linked immunosorbent assay technique. *Am. J. Vet. Res.*, **47**, 2441–2444.

6. BOHL E.H. (1979). Diagnosis of diarrhea in pigs due to transmissible gastroenteritis or rotavirus. *In:* Viral Enteritis in Humans and Animals, Bricout F. & Scherrer R., eds. INSERM, Paris, France, **90**, 341–343.

7. BROWN I.H. & PATON D.J. (1991). Serological studies of transmissible gastroenteritis in Great Britain, using a competitive ELISA. *Vet. Rec.*, **128**, 500–503.

8. CALLEBAUT P., CORREA I., PENSAERT M., JIMENEZ G. & ENJUANES L. (1988). Antigenic differentiation between transmissible gastroenteritis virus of swine and a related porcine respiratory coronavirus. *J. Gen. Virol.*, **69**, 1725–1730.

9. CALLEBAUT P., PENSAERT M.B. & HOOYBERGHS J. (1989). A competitive inhibition ELISA for the differentiation of serum antibodies from pigs infected with transmissible gastroenteritis virus (TGEV) or with the TGEV-related porcine respiratory coronavirus. *Vet. Microbiol.*, **20**, 9–19.

10. COX E., HOOYBERGHS J. & PENSAERT M.B. (1990). Sites of replication of a porcine respiratory coronavirus related to transmissible gastroenteritis virus. *Res. Vet. Sci.*, **48**, 165–169.

11. COX E., PENSAERT M.B. & CALLEBAUT P. (1993). Intestinal protection against challenge with transmissible gastroenteritis virus of pigs after infection with the porcine respiratory coronavirus. *Vaccine*, **11**, 267–272.

12. DULAC G.C., RUCKERBAUER G.M. & BOULANGER P. (1977). Transmissible gastroenteritis: demonstration of the virus from field specimens by means of cell culture and pig inoculation. *Can. J. Comp. Med.*, **41**, 357–363.

13. GARWES D.J., STEWART F., CARTWRIGHT S.F. & BROWN I. (1988). Differentiation of porcine respiratory coronavirus from transmissible gastroenteritis virus. *Vet. Rec.*, **122**, 86–87.

14. HOHDATSU T., EIGUCHI Y., IDE S., BABA H. & YAMAGISHI H. (1987). Evaluation of an enzyme-linked immunosorbent assay for the detection of transmissible gastroenteritis virus antibodies. *Vet. Microbiol.*, **13**, 93–97.

15. HONDA E., TAKAHASHI H., OKAZAKI K., MINETOMA T. & KUMAGAI T. (1990). The multiplication of transmissible gastroenteritis viruses in several cell lines originated from porcine kidney and effects of trypsin on the growth of the viruses. *Jpn J. Vet. Sci.*, **52**, 217–224.

16. HUANG C-C., JONG M.H. & LAI S.Y. (1988). Preparation of an enzyme-linked immunosorbent assay (ELISA) kit and its application in diagnosis of transmissible gastroenteritis. *Taiwan J. Vet. Med. Anim. Husbandry,* **51**, 57–63.

17. JEAN Y.H., KANG M.I., HWANG E.K., KWON Y.B., CHUNG U.I. & LEE J.B. (1987). Detection of transmissible gastroenteritis virus in tissue by peroxidase–antiperoxidase method. Research Reports Rural Development Administration (Livestock & Veterinary), Korea, **29**, 48–53.

18. KEMENY L.J., WILTSEY V.L. & RILEY J.L. (1975). Upper respiratory infection of lactating sows with transmissible gastroenteritis virus following contact exposure to infected piglets. *Cornell Vet.,* **65**, 352–362.

19. LABADIE J.P., AYNAUD J.M., VAISAIRE J. & RENAULT L. (1977). Porcine transmissible gastroenteritis. Antibody detection by passive haemagglutination test: applications to diagnosis and epidemiology. *Rec. Med. Vet.,* **153**, 931–936.

20. LANZA I., SHOUP D.I. & SAIF L.J. (1995). Lactogenic immunity and milk antibody isotypes to transmissible gastroenteritis virus in sows exposed to porcine respiratory coronavirus during pregnancy. *Am. J. Vet. Res.,* **56**, 739–748.

21. MCCLURKIN A.W. & NORMAN J.O. (1966). Studies on transmissible gastroenteritis of swine. II. Selected characteristics of a cytopathogenic virus common to five isolates from transmissible gastroenteritis. *Can. J. Comp. Med.,* **30**, 190–198.

22. NELSON L.D. & KEHLING C.L. (1984). Enzyme-linked immunosorbent assay for detection of transmissible gastroenteritis virus antibody in swine sera. *Am. J. Vet. Res.,* **45**, 1645–1657.

23. NODA M., YAMASHITA H., ICOIDE F., KODOI K., ORNON T., ASAGI M. & INABA Y. (1987). Haemagglutination with transmissible gastroenteritis. *Arch. Virol.,* **96**, 109–115.

24. O'TOOLE D., BROWN I.H., BRIDGES A. & CARTWRIGHT S.F. (1989). Pathogenicity of experimental infection with 'pneumotropic' porcine coronavirus. *Res. Vet. Sci.,* **47**, 23–29.

25. PATON D.J. & BROWN I.H. (1990). Sows infected in pregnancy with porcine respiratory coronavirus show no evidence of protecting their suckling piglets against transmissible gastroenteritis. *Vet. Res. Commun.,* **14**, 329.

26. PATON D.J., BROWN I.H. & VAZ E.K. (1991). An ELISA for the detection of serum antibodies to both transmissible gastroenteritis virus and porcine respiratory coronavirus. *Br. Vet. J.,* **147**, 370–372.

27. PATON D.J., IBATA G., MCGOLDRICK A., JONES T.O. & PRITCHARD G.C. (1998). Attempted isolation and characterisation of recent British isolates of transmissible gastroenteritis. Proceedings of the 15th IPVS Congress, Birmingham, UK, 5–9 July 1998.

28. PATON D., IBATA G., SANDS J. & MCGOLDRICK A. (1997). Detection of transmissible gastroenteritis virus by RT-PCR and differentiation from porcine respiratory coronavirus. *J. Virol. Methods,* **66**, 303–309.

29. PATON D. & LOWINGS P. (1997). Discrimination between transmissible gastroenteritis virus isolates. *Arch. Virol.,* **142**, 1703–1711.

30. PENSAERT M., CALLEBAUT P. & VERGOTE J. (1986). Isolation of a porcine respiratory, non-enteric coronavirus related to transmissible gastroenteritis. *Vet. Q.,* **8**, 257–261.

31. PENSAERT M.B., HALTERMAN E.O. & BERNSTEIN T. (1968). Diagnosis of transmissible gastroenteritis in pigs by means of immunofluorescence. *Can. J. Comp. Med.,* **32**, 555–561.

32. RASSCHAERT D., DUARTE M. & LAUDE H. (1990). Porcine respiratory coronavirus differs from transmissible gastroenteritis virus by a few genomic deletions. *J. Gen. Virol.,* **71**, 2599–2607.

33. RUKHADZE G.G., ALIPER T.I. & SERGEEV V.A. (1989). Isolation of peplomer glycoprotein E2 of transmissible gastroenteritis virus and application in enzyme-linked immunosorbent assay. *J. Clin. Microbiol.,* **27**, 1754–1758.

34. SAIF L.J. (1993). Coronavirus immunogens. *Vet. Microbiol.,* **37**, 285–297.

35. SAIF L.J., BOHL E.H., KOHLER E.M. & HUGHES J.H. (1977). Immune electron microscopy of transmissible gastroenteritis virus and rotavirus (reovirus-like agent) of swine. *Am. J. Vet. Res.*, **38**, 13–20.

36. SAIF L.J. & JACKWOOD D.J. (1990). Enteric virus vaccines: Theoretical considerations, current status and future approaches. *In:* Viral Diarrheas of Man and Animals, Saif L.J. & Theil K.W., eds. CRC Press, Boca Raton, Florida, USA, 313–329.

37. SAIF L.J. & WESLEY R. (1992). Transmissible gastroenteritis virus. *In:* Diseases of Swine, Seventh Edition, Leman A.D. *et al.*, eds. Iowa State University Press, Ames, Iowa, USA, 362–386.

38. SCHULTZE B., KREMPL C., BALLESTEROS M.L., SHAW L., SCHAUER R., ENJUANES L. & HERRLER G. (1996). Transmissible gastroenteritis coronavirus, but the related porcine respiratory coronavirus, has a sialic acid (N-glycolylneuramic acid) binding activity. *J. Virol.*, **70**, 5634–5637.

39. SHIMIZU M. & SHIMIZU Y. (1977). Micro-indirect haemagglutination test for detection of antibody against transmissible gastroenteritis virus of pigs. *J. Clin. Microbiol.*, **6**, 91–95.

40. SHOCKLEY L.J., KAPKE P.A., LAPPS W., BRIAN D., POTGIETER L.N.D. & WOODS R. (1987). Diagnosis of porcine and bovine enteric coronavirus infections using cloned cDNA probes. *J. Clin. Microbiol.*, **25**, 1591–1596.

41. SHOUP D.I., SWAYNE D.E., JACKWOOD D.J. & SAIF L.J. (1996). Immunohistochemistry of transmissible gastroenteritis virus antigens in fixed paraffin-embedded tissues. *J. Vet. Diagn Invest.*, **8**, 161–167.

42. SIMKINS R.A., WEILNAU P.A., BIAS J. & SAIF L.J. (l992). Antigenic variation among transmissible gastroenteritis virus (TGEV) and porcine respiratory coronavirus strains detected with monoclonal antibodies to the S protein of TGEV. *Am. J. Vet Res.*, **53**, 1253–1258.

43. SIRINARUMITR T., PAUL P.S., KLUGE J.P. & HALBUR P.G. (1996). *In situ* hybridization technique for the detection of swine enteric and respiratory coronaviruses, transmissible gastroenteritis virus (TGEV) and porcine respiratory coronavirus (PRCV), in formalin-fixed paraffin-embedded tissues. *J. Virol. Methods*, **56**, 149–160.

44. UNITED STATES DEPARTMENT OF AGRICULTURE (USDA) (1995). Code Of Federal Regulations, Title 9, Parts 1–199. US Government Printing Office, Washington D.C., USA.

45. VAN COTT J., BRIM T., LUNNEY J. & SAIF L.J. (1994). Contribution of antibody secreting cells induced in mucosal lymphoid tissues of pigs inoculated with respiratory or enteric strains of coronavirus to immunity against enteric coronavirus challenge. *J. Immunol.*, **152**, 3980–3990.

46. VAN NIEUWSTADT A.P. & BOONSTRA J. (1991). A competitive ELISA to distinguish TGEV- from PRCV-infected pigs. International Pig Veterinary Society Proceedings 1990, 265.

47. VAN NIEUWSTADT A.P., CORNELISSEN J.B. & VREESWIJK J. (1988). Solid phase immune electron microscopy for diagnosis of transmissible gastroenteritis in pigs. *Res. Vet. Sci.*, **44**, 286–294.

48 VAN NIEUWSTADT A.P., CORNELISSEN J.B. & ZETSTRA T. (1988). Comparison of two methods for detection of transmissible gastroenteritis virus in feces of pigs with experimentally induced infection. *Am. J. Vet. Res.*, **49**, 1836–1843.

49. VAUGHN E.M., HALBUR P.G. & PAUL P.S. (1994). Three new isolates of porcine respiratory coronavirus with various pathogenicities and spike (S) gene deletions . *J. Clin. Microbiol.*, **32**, 1809–1812.

50. WITTE K.H. (1971). Micro-colour test for assay of transmissible gastroenteritis virus neutralizing antibodies. *Arch. Gesamte Virusforsch.*, **33**, 171–176.

51. WOODS R.D. (1997). Development of PCR-based techniques to identify porcine transmissible gastroenteritis coronavirus isolates. *Can. J. Vet. Res.*, **61**, 167–172.

*
* *

SECTION 2.7.

AVIAN DISEASES IN LIST B

CHAPTER 2.7.1.

INFECTIOUS BURSAL DISEASE (Gumboro disease)

SUMMARY

Infectious bursal disease (IBD) is caused by a virus that is now classified as a member of the genus Avibirnavirus of the family Birnaviridae. Although turkeys, ducks, guinea fowl and ostriches may be infected, clinical disease occurs solely in chickens. Only young birds are clinically affected. Severe acute disease of 3–6-week-old birds is associated with high mortality, but a less acute or subclinical disease is common in 0–3-week-old birds. This can cause secondary problems due to the effect of the virus on the bursa of Fabricius. IBD virus (IBDV) causes lymphoid depletion of the bursa, and if this occurs in the first 2 weeks of life, significant depression of the humoral antibody response may result. Two serotypes of IBDV are recognised. These are designated serotypes 1 and 2. Both serotypes can be differentiated by cross-neutralisation assays. Clinical disease has been associated with and vaccines prepared against serotype 1 only. Serological variants of IBD serotype 1 occur and these may require special vaccines for maximum protection. Very virulent strains of classical serotype 1 are now common and are causing serious disease in many countries.

Clinical disease due to infection with the IBDV, also known as Gumboro disease, can usually be diagnosed by a combination of characteristic signs and post-mortem lesions. Laboratory confirmation, or detection of subclinical disease, can be carried out by demonstration of a humoral immune response in unvaccinated chickens or by detecting the presence of viral antigen in tissues. In the absence of such tests, histological examination of bursae may be helpful.

***Identification of the agent:** Isolation of IBDV is not usually carried out as a routine diagnostic procedure. Specific antibody-negative chickens may be used for this purpose as may cell cultures or embryonating eggs from specific antibody-negative sources. However, some difficulty may be experienced if using the latter two systems as the virus does not readily adapt to them. If successful, the identity of the virus can be confirmed by the virus neutralisation (VN) test.*

The agar gel immunodiffusion (AGID) test can be used to detect viral antigen in the bursa of Fabricius. A portion of the bursa is removed, homogenised, and used as antigen in a test against known positive antiserum. This is particularly useful in the early stages of the infection, before the development of an antibody response. An immunofluorescence test using IBD-virus-specific chicken antiserum can also be used to detect antigen in bursal tissue. The reverse-transcription polymerase chain reaction with specific primers may be used to detect viral genomic RNA in the bursa of Fabricius.

***Serological tests:** An AGID, VN or enzyme-linked immunosorbent assay may be carried out on serum samples. The infection usually spreads rapidly within a flock of birds. Because of this, only a small percentage of the flock needs to be tested to detect the presence of antibodies. If positive reactions are found in unvaccinated birds then the whole flock must be regarded as infected.*

***Requirements for vaccines and diagnostic biologicals:** Both live attenuated and inactivated (killed) vaccines are available to control the disease. It is important that live vaccines be stable, with no tendency to revert to virulence on passage. To be effective, the inactivated vaccines need to have a high antigen content.*

Live vaccines are used to produce an active immunity in young chickens. An alternative to this is to provide chickens with passive protection by vaccinating the parents using a combination of live and killed vaccines. Effective vaccination of breeding stock is therefore of great importance.

Live vaccines: *Attenuated strains of IBD viruses are used. These are referred to as either mild, intermediate, or 'intermediate plus' ('hot') vaccines. The mild vaccines cause no bursal damage, while the intermediate and intermediate plus vaccines cause some lymphocytic depletion in the bursa of Fabricius. None of the vaccine types causes immunosuppression when used in birds over 14 days old.*

Mild vaccines are rarely used in broilers, but are used widely to prime broiler parents prior to inoculation with inactivated vaccine. Intermediate and 'hot' vaccines are more capable of overcoming low levels of maternally derived antibodies (MDA). They may be administered by intramuscular injection, spray or in drinking water. In the absence of MDA, mild vaccines are given at 1-day old. When MDA are present at 1 day of age, vaccination should be delayed until MDA in most of the flock has waned. The best schedule can be determined by serological testing of the birds to detect the time at which MDA has fallen to a low level. More recently, vaccines have been developed that can be administered in ovo *at 18 days of incubation.*

Killed vaccines: *These are used to stimulate high and uniform levels of antibody in parent chickens so that the progeny will have high and uniform levels of MDA. The killed vaccines are manufactured in oil emulsion adjuvant and given by injection. They must be used in birds already sensitised by primary exposure, either to live vaccine or to field virus. This can be checked serologically. High levels of MDA can be obtained in breeder birds by giving, for example, live vaccine at approximately 8 weeks of age, followed by inactivated vaccine at approximately 18 weeks of age.*

A. DIAGNOSTIC TECHNIQUES

Two distinct serotypes of infectious bursal disease virus (IBDV) are known to exist. Type 1 virus causes clinical disease in chickens younger than 10 weeks. Older chickens usually show no clinical signs. Antibodies are sometimes found in other avian species, but no signs of infection are seen. Type 2 antibodies are very widespread in turkeys and are sometimes found in chickens and ducks. There are no reports of clinical disease caused by infection with Type 2 virus (6).

Isolation and identification of the agent provide the most certain diagnosis, but are not usually attempted for routine diagnostic purposes (7). In practice, laboratory diagnosis of IBD depends on detection of specific antibodies to the virus, or on detection of the virus in tissues, using immunological methods.

1. Identification of the agent

Clinical IBD has clearly characteristic signs and post-mortem lesions. A flock will show very high morbidity with severe depression in most birds lasting for 5–7 days. Mortality rises sharply for 2 days then declines rapidly over the next 2–3 days. Usually between 5% and 10% of birds die, but mortality can reach 30–40%. The main clinical signs are watery diarrhoea, ruffled feathers, reluctance to move, anorexia, trembling and prostration. Post-mortem lesions include dehydration of the muscles with numerous ecchymotic haemorrhages, enlargement and orange discoloration of the kidneys with urates in the tubules. The bursae of Fabricius shows the main diagnostic lesions. In birds that die at the peak of the disease outbreak, the bursa is enlarged and turgid with a pale yellow discoloration. Intrafollicular haemorrhages may be present and in some cases, the bursa may be completely haemorragic giving the appearance of a black cherry. Peribursal straw-coloured oedema with be present in many bursa. Confirmation of clinical disease or detection of subclinical disease is best done by using immunological methods as the IBDV is difficult to isolate. For virus isolation, the methods described below should be followed. Differentiation between serotypes 1 and 2 or between serotype 1 subtypes should be undertaken by a specialised laboratory (e.g. the OIE Reference Laboratories for Infectious Bursal Disease [see Table given in Part 4 of this *Manual*]).

a) Sample preparation

Remove the bursae of Fabricius aseptically from approximately five affected chickens in the early stages of the disease. Chop the bursae using two scalpels, add a small amount of peptone broth containing penicillin and streptomycin (1000 µg/ml each), and homogenise in a tissue blender. Centrifuge the homogenate at 3000 ***g*** for 10 minutes. Harvest the supernatant fluid for use for the following investigations. Filtration through a 0.22 µ filter may prove necessary to further control bacterial contamination although this may cause a reduction in virus titre.

b) Isolation of virus in cell culture

Inoculate 0.5 ml of sample into each of four freshly confluent chicken embryo fibroblast cultures (from a specific pathogen free [SPF] source) in 25 cm^2 flasks. Adsorb at 37°C for 30 minutes, wash twice with Earle's balanced salt solution and add maintenance medium to each flask. Incubate the cultures at 37°C, observing daily for evidence of cytopathic effect (CPE). This is characterised by small round refractive cells. If no CPE is observed after 6 days, discard the medium, then freeze and thaw the cultures and inoculate the resulting lysate into fresh cultures. This procedure may need to be repeated at least three times. If CPE is observed, the virus should be tested against IBD antiserum in a tissue culture virus neutralisation (VN) test (see below).

c) Isolation of virus in embryos

Inoculate 0.2 ml of sample into the yolk sac of five 6–8-day-old specific antibody negative (SAN) chicken embryos and on to the chorioallantoic membrane of five 9–11-day-old SAN chicken embryos. Candle daily and discard dead embryos up to 48 hours post-inoculation. SAN embryos are derived from flocks shown to be serologically negative to IBDV. Embryos that die after this time are examined for lesions. Type 1 IBD produces dwarfing of the embryo, subcutaneous oedema, congestion and haemorrhages. The liver is usually swollen, with patchy congestion producing a mottled effect. In later deaths, the liver may be swollen and greenish, with areas of necrosis. The spleen is enlarged and the kidneys are swollen and congested, with a mottled effect.

IBDV usually causes death in at least some of the embryos on primary isolation.

d) Isolation of virus in chickens

Inoculate, by eyedrop, five susceptible and five IBD-immune chickens (3–7 weeks of age) with 0.05 ml of sample. Kill the chickens 72–80 hours after inoculation, and examine their bursae of Fabricius. The bursae of IBDV-infected chickens appear yellowish (sometimes haemorrhagic) and turgid, with prominent striations. Peribursal oedema is sometimes present, and plugs of caseous material are occasionally found. The plicae are petechiated.

The presence of lesions in the bursae of susceptible chickens along with the absence of lesions in immune chickens is diagnostic for IBD. The bursae from both groups may be used as antigen in an agar gel immunodiffusion (AGID) test against known positive IBD antiserum.

e) Identification by immunofluorescence

Sections of bursa are prepared using a microtome cryostat, dried at room temperature and then fixed in cold acetone. Fluorescent-labelled IBDV-specific antisera are applied to the sections, which are then incubated at 37°C for 1 hour in a humid atmosphere. At the end of the incubation period, they are washed for 30 minutes using PBS, pH 7.2, then rinsed in distilled water. The sections are mounted using buffered glycerol, pH 7.6, and examined by UV microscopy for IBDV-specific fluorescence (9).

f) Identification by molecular techniques

Molecular virological techniques are being developed that allow IBDV to be identified more quickly than by virus isolation. An example is the use of the reverse-transcription polymerase chain reaction. This method could detect IBDV, which is unable to grow in cell culture, because it is not necessary to grow the virus before amplification. However, these methods will require more research and development before they are suitable for general use.

2. Serological tests

a) Agar gel immunodiffusion test

The AGID test is the most useful of the serological tests for the detection of specific antibodies in serum, or for detecting viral antigen or antibodies in bursal tissue.

Blood samples should be taken early in the course of the disease, and repeat samples should be taken 3 weeks later. Because the virus spreads rapidly, only a small proportion of the flock needs to be sampled.

Usually 20 blood samples are enough. For detection of antigen in the bursa of Fabricius, the bursae should be removed aseptically from about ten chickens at the acute stage of infection. The bursae are minced using two scalpels in scissor movement, then small pieces are placed in the wells of the AGID plate against known positive serum.

- **Preparation of positive control antigen**

Inoculate 3–5-week-old susceptible chickens, by eyedrop, with a clarified 10% (w/v) bursal homogenate known to contain viable IBDV[1]. Kill the birds 3 days post-inoculation, and harvest the bursae aseptically. Discard haemorrhagic bursae and pool the remainder, weigh and add an equivalent volume of cold distilled water and an equivalent volume of undiluted methylene chloride. Thoroughly homogenise the mixture in a tissue blender and centrifuge at 2000 ***g*** for 30 minutes. Harvest the supernatant fluid and dispense into aliquots for storage at –40°C. The antigen contains live virus and should be handled only in suitable containment facilities such as a class II safety cabinet.

- **Preparation of positive control antiserum**

Inoculate 4–5-week-old susceptible chickens, by eyedrop, with 0.05 ml of a clarified 10% (w/v) bursal homogenate known to contain viable IBDV[1]. Exsanguinate 28 days post-inoculation. Pool and store serum in aliquots at –20°C.

- **Preparation of agar**

Dissolve sodium chloride (80 g) and phenol (5 g) in distilled water (1 litre). Add agar (12.5 g) and steam until the agar has dissolved. While the mixture is still very hot, filter it through a pad of cellulose wadding covered with a few layers of muslin. Dispense the medium in 20 ml volumes into glass bottles and store at 4°C until required for use.

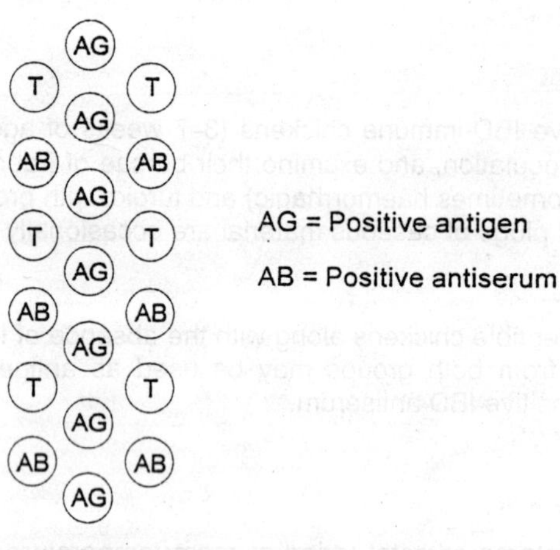

Fig. 1. Protocol for tests for antibody.

T = test sera

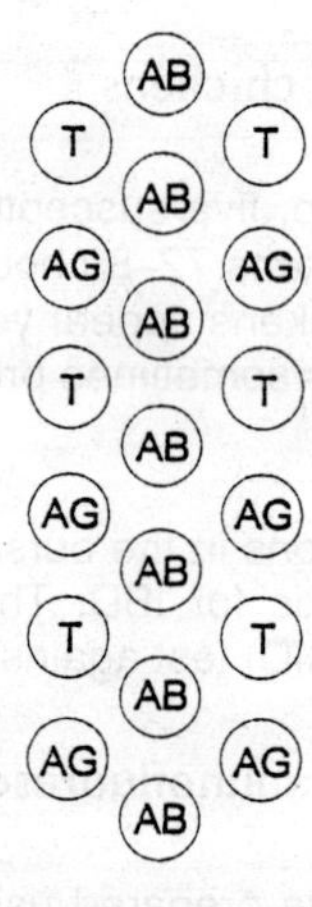

Fig. 2. Protocol for tests for antigen.

T = test tissues

Notes:

1. The linear pattern of wells is preferred although a hexagonal pattern may be used. Each test serum or bursa should be placed adjacent to a positive control antibody (AB) or antigen (AG), respectively.
2. Wells, 3 mm deep, 6 mm in diameter, and 3 mm apart, are used.

- **Test procedure**

i) Prepare plates from 24 hours to 7 days before use. Dissolve the agar by placing in a steamer or boiling water bath. Take care to prevent water entering the bottles.

ii) Pour the contents of one bottle into each of the required number of 9 cm plastic Petri dishes laid on a level surface. (Some laboratories prefer to pour the gel on 25 × 75 mm glass slides, 3 mm deep.)

iii) Cover the plates and allow the agar to set, and then store the plates at 4°C. Poured plates may be stored for up to 7 days at 4°C. (If the plates are to be used the same day that they are poured, dry them by placing them opened but inverted at 37°C for from 30 minutes to 1 hour.)

1 A suitable strain of IBDV (type 1) is the strain 52/70, obtainable from VLA Weybridge, New Haw, Addlestone, Surrey KT15 3NB, United Kingdom (UK).

iv) Cut three vertical rows of wells 6 mm in diameter and 3 mm apart, using a template and tubular cutter.

v) Remove the agar from the wells using a pen and nib, taking care not to damage the walls of the wells.

vi) Using a pipette, dispense 50 µl of the test sera into the wells as shown in Figure 1.

OR

Dispense small pieces of finely minced test bursae by means of curved fine pointed forceps into the wells, as shown in Figure 2, to just fill the wells.

vii) Dispense 50 µl of the positive and negative control reagents into the relevant wells.

viii) Incubate the plates at between 22°C and 37°C for up to 48 hours in a humid chamber to avoid drying the agar.

ix) Examine the plates against a dark background with an oblique light source after 24 and 48 hours.

- **Quantitative agar gel immunodiffusion tests**

The AGID test can also be used to measure antibody levels, by using dilutions of serum in the test wells, and taking the titre as the highest dilution to produce a precipitin line (2). This can be very useful for measuring maternal or vaccinal antibodies and for deciding on the best time for vaccination.

b) Virus neutralisation tests

VN tests are carried out in cell culture. The test is more laborious and expensive than the AGID test, but is more sensitive in detecting antibody. This sensitivity is not required for routine diagnostic purposes, but may be useful for evaluating vaccine responses or to differentiate between IBDV 1 and 2 serotypes.

First, 0.05 ml of virus diluted in tissue culture medium to contain 100 $TCID_{50}$ (50% tissue culture infective doses) per 0.05 ml is placed in each well of a tissue-culture grade microtitre plate (Spearman–Kärber [1] or the Reed & Muench [11]). The test sera are heat-inactivated at 56°C for 30 minutes. Serial doubling dilutions of the sera are made in the diluted virus. After 30 minutes at room temperature, 0.2 ml of SPF chicken embryo fibroblast cell suspension is dispensed into each well. Plates are sealed and incubated at 37°C for 4–5 days, after which the monolayers are observed microscopically for typical CPE. The end-point (serum titre) is expressed as the reciprocal of the highest serum dilution that did not show CPE. To reduce test-to-test and operator-to-operator variation, a European Pharmacopoeia Standard Reference Serum may be included with each batch of tests. The results are then expressed as Ph. Eur. units/ml[2].

c) Enzyme-linked immunosorbent assay

ELISAs are in use for the detection of antibodies to IBD. Coating the plates requires a purified, or at least semipurified, preparation of virus, necessitating specialist skills and techniques. Methods for preparation of reagents and application of the assay were described by Marquardt *et al.* in 1980 (8). Commercial kits are available.

The test sera are diluted according to the established protocol or kit instructions and each is dispensed into the requisite number of wells. After incubation under the appropriate conditions, the sera are discarded from the plates, and the wells are washed thoroughly. Anti-chicken immunoglobulins conjugated to an enzyme are dispensed into the wells, and the plates are again incubated as appropriate. The plates are emptied and rewashed before substrate containing a chromogen that gives a colour change in the presence of the enzyme used is added to the plate. After a final incubation step, the substrate/chromogen reaction is stopped by addition of a suitable stopping solution and the colour reactions are quantified by measuring the optical density of each well. The Sample to Positive (S/P) ratio for each test sample is calculated.

d) Interpretation of results

The AGID test is surprisingly sensitive, though not as sensitive as the VN test; the latter will often give a titre when the AGID test is negative. Positive reactions indicate infection in unvaccinated birds without maternal antibodies. As a guide, a positive AGID reaction in a vaccinated bird or young bird with maternal antibody indicates a protective level of antibody. ELISA gives more rapid results than VN or AGID and is less costly in terms of labour, although the reagents are more expensive. VN and AGID titres correlate well, but as VN is more sensitive, AGID titres are proportionally lower. Correlation between ELISA and VN and between ELISA and AGID is more variable depending on the source of the ELISA reagents. A formula has been

---

2 The Ph. Eur. Standard Reference Serum together with instructions for use and calculation of untis/ml, is obtainable from VLA Weybridge (see footnote 1).

devised that allows ELISA titres to be used to calculate the optimal age for vaccination (5), which will vary depending on the vaccine used. Nonspecific positive reactions may occur with most ELISAs because they are usually designed for monitoring vaccine responses, in which case sensitivity is regarded as more important than specificity. This should be taken into account when the ELISA is used for diagnosis.

B. REQUIREMENTS FOR VACCINES AND DIAGNOSTIC BIOLOGICALS

Two types of vaccine are available for the control of IBD. These are live attenuated vaccines or inactivated oil-emulsion adjuvanted vaccines (15).

To date, IBD vaccines have been made from type 1 IBDV only, although a type 2 virus has been detected in poultry. The type 2 virus has not been seen to be associated with disease, but its presence will stimulate antibodies. Type 2 antibodies do not confer protection against type 1 infection, neither do they interfere with the response to type 1 vaccine. There have been numerous descriptions of serological variants of type 1 virus (12). Cross-protection studies have shown that inactivated vaccines prepared from 'classical' type 1 virus require a high antigenic content to provide good protection against some of these variants. IBD vaccines that contain both classical and variant IBD type 1 viruses are now licensed.

- **Live vaccines: methods of use**

Live IBD vaccines are produced from fully or partially attenuated strains of virus, known as 'mild', 'intermediate', or 'intermediate plus' ('hot'), respectively.

Mild or intermediate vaccines are used in parent chickens to produce a primary response prior to vaccination near to point-of-lay using inactivated vaccine. They are susceptible to the effect of maternally derived antibody (MDA) so should be administered only after all MDA has waned. Application is by means of intramuscular injection, spray or in the drinking water, usually at 8 weeks of age (13).

Intermediate vaccines are used to protect broiler chickens and commercial layer replacements. They are also used in young parent chickens if there is a high risk of natural infection with virulent IBD. Intermediate vaccines are susceptible to the presence of MDA, but are sometimes administered at 1-day old, as a coarse spray, to protect any chickens in the flock that may have no or only minimal levels of MDA. This also establishes a reservoir of vaccine virus within the flock that allows lateral transmission to other chickens when their MDA decays. Second and third applications are usually administered, especially when there is a high risk of exposure to virulent forms of the disease. The timing of these will depend on the antibody titres of the parent birds at the time the eggs were laid. As a guide, the second dose is usually given at 10–14 days of age when about 10% of the flock is susceptible to IBD, and the third dose 7–10 days later. The route of administration is by means of spray or in the drinking water. Intramuscular injection is used rarely. If the vaccine is given in the drinking water, clean water must be used free from smell or taste of chlorine or metals. Skimmed milk powder may be added at a rate of 2 g per litre. Care must be taken to ensure that all birds receive their dose of vaccine. To this end, all water should be removed (cut off) for 2–3 hours before the medicated water is made available. It is preferable to divide the medicated water into two parts, giving the second part 30 minutes after the first.

Recently, technology has been developed to deliver live vaccine into eggs during the incubation period. Live vaccine virus is blended with IBD antibody and the complex is injected *in ovo* at 18 days of incubation. The eggs go on to hatch and the vaccine virus is released when the chicks are about 7 days of age. In this way, the problem of maternally derived IBD antibody is overcome and the chicks are effectively immunised (4).

Live IBD vaccines are generally regarded as compatible with other avian vaccines. However, IBD vaccines that cause bursal damage could interfere with the response to other vaccines. Only healthy birds should be vaccinated. Vaccine should be kept at temperatures between 2°C and 8°C up to the time of use.

- **Inactivated vaccines: method of use**

Inactivated IBD vaccines are used to produce high, long-lasting and uniform levels of antibodies in breeding hens that have previously been primed by live vaccine or by natural exposure to field virus during rearing (3). The usual programme is to administer the live vaccine at about 8 weeks of age. This is followed by the inactivated vaccine at 16–20 weeks of age. The inactivated vaccine is manufactured as a water-in-oil emulsion, and has to be injected into each bird. The preferred route is intramuscular into the leg muscle, avoiding proximity to joints, tendons or major blood vessels. A multidose syringe may be used. All equipment should be cleaned and sterilised between flocks, and vaccination teams should exercise strict hygiene when going from one flock to another. Vaccine should be stored at between 4°C and 8°C. It should not be frozen or exposed to bright light or high temperature.

Only healthy birds, known to be sensitised by previous exposure to IBDV, should be vaccinated. Used in this way the vaccine should produce such a good antibody response that chickens hatched from those parents will have passive protection against IBD for up to about 30 days of age (16). This covers the period of greatest susceptibility to the disease and prevents bursal damage at the time when this could cause immunosuppression. It has been shown that bursal damage occurring after about 15 days of age has little effect on immunocompetence as by that time the immunocompetent cells have migrated into the peripheral lymphoid tissues. However, if there is a threat of exposure to infection with very virulent IBDV, live vaccines should be applied as described above. The precise level and duration of immunity conferred by inactivated IBD vaccines will depend mainly on the concentration of antigen present per dose. The manufacturing objective should be to obtain a high antigen concentration and hence a highly potent vaccine.

1. Seed Management

a) Characteristics of the seed

- **Live vaccine**

The seed virus must be shown to be free from extraneous viruses, bacteria, mycoplasma and fungi, particularly avian pathogens. This includes freedom from contamination with other strains of IBDV. For vaccine strains that claim to be attenuated and nonimmunosuppressive, the seed virus must be shown to be stable, with no tendency to revert to virulence. This can be confirmed by carrying out at least six consecutive chicken-to-chicken passages at 3–4 day intervals using bursal suspension as inoculum in 3–6-week-old SPF chickens. It must be shown that the virus was transmitted. A histological comparison is then made to show that there is no difference between bursae from birds inoculated with the initial and the final passage material. Bursal scoring (10) and imaging techniques have been developed. Some live vaccine strains in the 'intermediate' or 'intermediate plus' categories cannot be expected to pass such a test.

Test for immunosuppression: An important characteristic is that the virus should not produce such damage to the bursa of Fabricius that it causes immunosuppression in susceptible birds. (Live vaccines of the 'intermediate' type may be licensed even though they may be capable of causing immunosuppression.) The vaccine is administered by injection or eyedrop, one field dose per bird, to each of 20 SPF chickens, at 1-day old. A further group of birds of the same age and source are housed separately as controls. At 2 weeks of age, each bird in both groups is given one field dose of live Newcastle disease vaccine by eyedrop. The haemagglutination inhibition (HI) response of each bird to Newcastle disease vaccine is measured 2 weeks later, and the protection is measured against challenge with $10^{6.5}$ ELD_{50} (50% embryo lethal doses) Herts 33/56 strain (or similar) of Newcastle disease virus. The IBD vaccine fails the test if the HI response and protection afforded by Newcastle disease vaccine is significantly less (<0.01) in the group given IBD vaccine than in the control group. In countries where Newcastle disease virus is exotic, an alternative is to use sheep erythrocytes or *Brucella abortus* killed antigen as the test antigen, measuring the response with haemagglutination or serum agglutination test, respectively. However, another live vaccine is a preferable test system because it also evaluates cell-mediated immunity.

- **Killed vaccine**

For killed vaccines the most important characteristics are high yield and good antigenicity. Both virulent and attenuated strains have been used. The seed virus must be shown to be free from extraneous viruses, bacteria, mycoplasma and fungi, particularly avian pathogens (14).

b) Method of culture

Seed virus may be propagated in various culture systems, such as SPF chicken embryo fibroblasts, or chicken embryos. In some cases, propagation in the bursa may be used. The bulk is distributed in aliquots and freeze-dried in sealed containers.

c) Validation as a vaccine

Data on efficacy should be obtained before bulk manufacture of vaccine begins. The vaccine should be administered to birds in the way in which it will be used in the field. Live vaccine can be given to young birds and the response measured serologically and by resistance to experimental challenge. In the case of killed vaccines, a test must be carried out in older birds that go on to lay, using the recommended vaccination schedule, so that their progeny can be challenged to determine resistance due to MDA at the beginning and end of lay.

- **Live vaccine**

Efficacy test: Administer one field dose of the minimum recommended titre to each of 20 SPF chickens of the minimum age of vaccination. Inoculate separate groups for each of the recommended routes of application. Leave 20 chickens from the same hatch as uninoculated controls. After 14 days, challenge each of the chickens by eyedrop with approximately 100 CID_{50} (50% chicken infective dose) of a virulent strain of IBDV such as CVL 52/70 (see footnote 1). Observe the chickens for 10 days. The vaccine fails the test unless at least 90% of the vaccinated chickens survive without showing either clinical signs or severe lesions in the bursae of Fabricius. If more than half the controls do not show severe lesions of the bursa of Fabricius, the test is invalid. Lesions are considered to be severe if at least 90% of follicles show greater than 75% depletion of lymphocytes. Providing results are satisfactory, this test need be carried out on only one batch of all those batches prepared from the same seed lot.

- **Killed vaccine**

Efficacy test: At least 20 unprimed SPF birds are given one dose of vaccine at the recommended age (near to point-of-lay) by one of the recommended routes, and the antibody response is measured by serum neutralisation with reference to a standard antiserum[3] between 4 and 6 weeks after vaccination. The vaccine must induce mean antibody levels of at least 10,000 Ph. Eur. units per ml.

Eggs are collected for hatching 5–7 weeks after vaccination, and 25 progeny chickens are then challenged at 3 weeks of age by eyedrop with approximately 100 CID_{50} of a recognised virulent strain of IBDV, such as strain CVL 52/70 (see footnote 1). Ten control chickens of the same breed but from unvaccinated parents are also challenged. Protection is assessed 3–4 days after challenge by removing the bursa of Fabricius from each bird; each bursa is then subjected to histological examination or tested for the presence of IBD antigen by the agar gel precipitin test. Not more than three of the chickens from vaccinated parents should show evidence of IBD infection, whereas all those from unvaccinated parents should be affected.

These procedures should be repeated towards the end of the period of lay, but, on this occasion challenge the progeny should be undertaken when they are 15 days old. The test needs to be performed once only using a typical batch of vaccine.

2. Method of manufacture

The vaccine must be manufactured in suitable clean and secure accommodation, well separated from diagnostic facilities or commercial poultry.

Production of the vaccine should be on a seed-lot system using a suitable strain of virus of known origin and passage history. SPF eggs must be used for all materials employed in propagation and testing of the vaccine. Live vaccines are made by growth in eggs or cell cultures. Inactivated IBD vaccines may be made using virulent virus grown in the bursae of young birds, or using attenuated, laboratory-adapted strains of IBDV grown in cell culture or embryonated eggs. A high virus concentration is required. These vaccines are made as water-in-oil emulsions. A typical formulation is to use 80% mineral oil to 20% suspension of bursal material in water, with suitable emulsifying agents.

3. In-process control

Antigen content: Having grown the virus to high concentration, its titre should be assayed by use of cell cultures, embryos or chickens as appropriate to the strain of virus being used. The antigen content required to produce satisfactory batches of vaccine should be based on determinations made on test vaccine that has been shown to be effective in laboratory and field trials.

Inactivation of killed vaccines: This is often done with either beta-propiolactone or formalin. The inactivating agent and the inactivation procedure must be shown under the conditions of vaccine manufacture to inactivate the vaccine virus and any potential contaminants, e.g. bacteria, that may arise from the starting materials.

Prior to inactivation, care should be taken to ensure a homogeneous suspension free from particles that may not be penetrated by the inactivating agent. A test for inactivation of the vaccine should be carried out on each batch of both the bulk harvest after inactivation and the final product. The test selected should be appropriate to the vaccine virus being used and should consist of at least two passages in susceptible cell cultures, embryos or chickens, with ten replicates per passage. No evidence of the presence of any live virus or microorganism should be observed.

Sterility of killed vaccines: Oil used in the vaccine must be sterilised by heating at 160°C for 1 hour, or by filtration, and the procedure must be shown to be effective. Tests appropriate to oil-emulsion vaccines are carried out on each batch of final vaccine as described, for example, in the European Pharmacopoeia.

---

3 For quantitative agar gel immunodiffusion tests, the British Standard serum is available from VLA Weybridge (see footnote 1).

4. Batch control

a) Sterility

Tests for sterility and freedom from contamination of biological materials may be found in Chapter I.4.

b) Safety

- **Live vaccine safety test**

Ten field doses of vaccine are administered by eyedrop to each of 15 SPF chickens of the minimum age recommended for vaccination. The chickens are observed for 21 days. If more than two chickens die, the test must be repeated. The vaccine fails the test if any chickens die or show signs of disease attributable to the vaccine or if, 21 days after inoculation, more than moderate bursal lesions are present. This test is performed on each batch of final vaccine.

- **Killed vaccine safety test**

Ten SPF birds, 14–28 days of age, are inoculated by the recommended routes with twice the field dose. The birds are observed for 3 weeks. No abnormal local or systemic reaction should develop. The test is performed on each batch of final vaccine.

c) Potency

- **Live vaccine potency test**

The method described in Section B.1.c. Live vaccine (efficacy test) may be used. The test need be carried out on only one batch of all the batches prepared from the same seed lot. Alternatively, a potency test in eggs or cell cultures may be carried out on each serial (batch) of vaccine produced.

- **Killed vaccine potency test**

Ten SPF chickens, approximately 4 weeks of age, are each vaccinated with one dose of vaccine given by the recommended route. An additional ten control birds of the same source and age are housed together with the vaccinates. The antibody response of each bird is determined with reference to a standard antiserum 4–6 weeks after vaccination. The mean antibody level of the vaccinated birds should not be significantly less than the level recorded in the test for protection. No antibody should be detected in the control birds. This test must be carried out on each batch of final vaccine.

d) Duration of immunity (killed vaccine)

Evidence should be provided to show that progeny hatched from eggs taken at the end of the laying cycle are as adequately protected as those taken soon after vaccination. Information should be provided on the duration of antibody levels in the breeders throughout the laying cycle. The test may be performed on primed birds vaccinated by the recommended schedule, but the final dose of vaccine is given at the earliest recommended age and the final observations of progeny protection and antibody levels are made when the vaccinated birds are at least 60 weeks of age. Chickens are hatched from fertile eggs collected at the end of lay, and reared to 3 weeks of age. These are then tested for protection against challenge as described for the killed vaccine efficacy test (see Section B.1.c.).

e) Stability

Evidence should be provided on three batches of vaccine to show that the vaccine passes the batch potency test at 3 months beyond the requested shelf life.

f) Preservatives

A preservative is normally required for vaccine in multidose containers. The concentration of the preservative in the final vaccine and its persistence throughout shelf life should be checked. A suitable preservative already established for such purposes should be used.

g) Precautions (hazards)

Oil-emulsion vaccines cause serious injury to the vaccinator if accidentally injected into the hand or other tissues. In the event of such an accident the person should go at once to a hospital, taking the vaccine package with them. Each vaccine bottle and package should be clearly marked with a warning of the serious consequences of accidental self-injury. Such wounds should be treated by the casualty doctor as a 'grease gun injury'.

5. Tests on the final product

a) Safety

See Section B.4.b.

b) Potency

See Section B.4.c.

REFERENCES

1. AMERICAN ASSOCIATION OF AVIAN PATHOLOGY (1989). Chapter 43. *In:* Laboratory Manual for the Isolation and Identification of Avian Pathogens, Third Edition. Kendall/Hunt Publishing, Dubuque, Iowa, USA.
2. CULLEN G.A. & WYETH P.J. (1975). Quantitation of antibodies to infectious bursal disease. *Vet. Rec.*, **97**, 315.
3. CULLEN G.A. & WYETH P.J. (1976). Response of growing chickens to an inactivated IBD antigen in oil emulsion. *Vet Rec.*, **99**, 418.
4. HADDAD E.E., WHITFILL C.E., AVAKIAN A.P., RICKS C.A., ANDREWS P.D., THOMA J.A. & WAKENELL P.S. (1997). Efficacy of a novel infectious bursal disease virus immune complex vaccine in broiler chickens. *Avian Dis.*, **41**, 882–889.
5. KOUWENHOVEN B. & VAN DER BOS J. (1993). Control of very virulent infectious bursal disease (Gumboro disease) in the Netherlands with so called 'hot' vaccines. Proceedings of the 42nd Western Poultry Disease Conference, Sacramento, California, USA, 37–39.
6. LASHER H.N. & SHANE S.M. (1994). Infectious bursal disease. *World's Poult. Sci.*, **50**, 133–166.
7. LUKERT P.D. & SAIF Y.M. (1997). Infectious bursal disease. *In:* Diseases of Poultry, Tenth Edition, Calnek B.W., ed. Iowa State University Press, Ames, Iowa, USA, 721–738.
8. MARQUARDT W.W., JOHNSON R.B., ODENWALD W.F. & SCHLOTTHOKEN B.A. (1980). An indirect enzyme-linked immunosorbent assay (ELISA) for measuring antibodies in chickens infected with infectious bursal disease virus. *Avian Dis.*, **24**, 375–385.
9. MEULEMANS G., ANTOINE O. & HALEN P. (1977). Application de l'immunofluorescence au diagnostic de la Maladie de Gumboro. *Bull. OIE*, **88**, 225–229.
10. MUSKETT J.C., HOPKINS I.G., EDWARDS K.R. & THORNTON D.H. (1979). Comparison of two infectious bursal disease vaccine strains: Efficacy and potential hazards in susceptible and maternally immune birds. *Vet. Rec.*, **104**, 332–334.
11. REED L.J. & MUENCH H. (1938). A simple method of estimating fifty percent end points. *Am. J. Hyg.*, **27**, 493–497.
12. ROSENBERGER J.K. & CLOUD S.S (1986). Isolation and characterization of variant infectious bursal disease viruses. *J. Am. Vet. Med. Assoc.*, **189**, 357.
13. SKEELES J.K., LUKERT P.D., FLETCHER O.J. & LEONARD J.D. (1979) Immunisation studies with a cell-culture adapted infectious bursal virus. *Avian Dis.*, **23**, 456–465.
14. THORNTON D.H. & MUSKETT J.C. (1982). Quality control methods for inactivated infectious bursal disease vaccines. *Dev. Biol. Stand.*, **51**, 235–241.
15. THORNTON D.H. & PATTISON M. (1975). Comparison of vaccines against infectious bursal disease. *J. Comp. Pathol.*, **85**, 597–610.
16. WYETH P.J. & CULLEN G.A. (1979). The use of an inactivated infectious bursal disease oil emulsion vaccine in commercial broiler parent chickens. *Vet. Rec.*, **104**, 188–193.

*

* *

CHAPTER 2.7.2.

MAREK'S DISEASE

SUMMARY

Marek's disease (MD) is a lymphomatous and neuropathic disease of domestic fowl caused by a herpesvirus.

Diagnosis is made on clinical signs and gross or microscopic lesions. Chickens may become persistently infected with MD virus without developing clinical disease. Infection by MD virus is detected by virus isolation and demonstration of viral antigen or antibodies.

MD is prevented by vaccination with monovalent or multivalent live virus vaccines of various types. The vaccine is injected in ovo *or at hatch.*

In chickens, MD occurs at 3–4 weeks of age or older and is most common between 12 and 30 weeks of age. Paralysis of the legs and wings, with enlargement of peripheral nerves, is pathognomonic, but nerve involvement is sometimes not seen, especially in adult birds. Depending on the strain of MD virus, lymphomatosis can occur, especially in the ovary, liver, spleen, kidneys, lungs, heart, proventriculus and skin. As opposed to the uniform cell population that comprises the tumours caused by lymphoid leukosis, the nerve infiltration and lymphomas caused by MD virus consist of lymphoid cells of various types. Differentiation of MD from lymphoid leukosis is important. Lesions caused by reticuloendotheliosis virus can also be confused with those of MD.

Identification of the agent: *Under field conditions, most chickens become infected with MD virus during the first few weeks of life and then carry the infection throughout their lives, often without developing overt disease. The infection is usually detected by inoculating live buffy coat cells into monolayer cultures of chicken kidney cells or duck embryo fibroblasts, in which characteristic viral plaques develop within a few days. Two serotypes of MD virus are recognised – 1 and 2 – and a third serotype is represented by the related herpesvirus of turkeys (HVT). MD viral antigen can be detected in the feather tips of infected birds using a radial precipitin test.*

Serological tests: *Antibodies to MD virus develop within 1–2 weeks of infection and are commonly recognised by the agar gel immunodiffusion test, the indirect fluorescent antibody test, and sometimes by other serological tests such as enzyme-linked immunosorbent assay.*

Requirements for vaccines and diagnostic biologicals: *MD is prevented by vaccinating chickens* in ovo *or at 1 day of age. Live viral vaccines are used. HVT, in either a cell-free (lyophilised) form, or a cell-associated ('wet') form, is most commonly used. Attenuated variants of serotype 1 strains of MD virus are also used as vaccines, and serotype 2 strains may also be used, particularly in bivalent vaccines, together with HVT (serotype 3). Serotype 1 and 2 vaccines are only available in the cell-associated form. Bivalent vaccines consisting of serotypes 1 and 3 or trivalent vaccines consisting of serotypes 1, 2, and 3 are also used. The bivalent and trivalent vaccines have been introduced to combat the very virulent strains of MD virus that are not well controlled by the usual monovalent vaccines containing HVT alone.*

Vaccination greatly reduces clinical disease, but not persistent infection by MD virus. The vaccine viruses are also carried throughout the life of the fowl.

A. DIAGNOSTIC TECHNIQUES

Marek's disease (MD) (5, 17, 19) is a disease of domestic fowl (chickens) caused by a herpesvirus. It occurs at 3–4 weeks of age or older and is most common between 12 and 30 weeks of age. In the classical form of the disease, characterised by mainly neural involvement, mortality rarely exceeds 10–15% and can occur over a few weeks or many months. In the acute form, in which there is usually lymphoma formation in the viscera, a disease incidence of 10–30% of the flock is not uncommon and outbreaks involving up to 70% can occur. Mortality may increase rapidly over a few weeks and then cease, or can continue at a steady or slowly falling rate for several months. Currently, the acute form of the disease with extensive visceral lymphomas is most prevalent. In its classical form, the most common clinical sign of MD is partial or complete paralysis of the legs and wings. In the acute form, birds are often severely depressed and some may die without showing preceding signs.

In the classical form, the characteristic finding is enlargement of one or more peripheral nerves. Those most commonly affected and easily seen at post-mortem are the brachial and sciatic plexuses, coeliac plexus, abdominal vagus and intercostal nerves. Affected nerves are often two or three times their normal thickness, the normal cross-striated and glistening appearance is absent, and the nerve may appear greyish or yellowish, and sometimes oedematous. Lymphomas are sometimes present in the classical form of MD, most frequently as small, soft, grey tumours in the ovary, and sometimes also in the lungs, kidneys, heart, liver and other tissues.

In the acute form, the typical finding is widespread, diffuse lymphomatous involvement of the liver, gonads, spleen, kidneys, lungs, proventriculus and heart. Sometimes lymphomas also arise in the skin around the feather follicles and in the skeletal muscles. Affected birds usually have enlarged peripheral nerves, as in the classical form. In younger birds, liver enlargement is usually moderate in extent, but in adult birds the liver may be greatly enlarged and the gross appearance identical to that seen in lymphoid leukosis, from which the disease must be differentiated. Nerve lesions are often absent in adult birds with MD.

In both the classical and acute forms of MD, the disease starts as a proliferation of lymphoid cells, which is progressive in some cases and regressive in others. The peripheral nerves may be affected by proliferative, inflammatory or minor infiltrative changes, which are termed type A, B, and C lesions, respectively. The A-type lesions consist of infiltration by proliferating lymphoblasts, large, medium and small lymphocytes, and macrophages, and appears to be neoplastic in nature. The B-type lesion is characterised by interneuritic oedema, infiltration by mainly small lymphocytes and plasma cells, and Schwann cell proliferation, and appears to be inflammatory. The C-type lesion consists of a light scattering of mainly small lymphocytes, and is often seen in birds that show no gross lesions or clinical signs. It is thought to be a regressive, inflammatory lesion. Demyelination frequently occurs in nerves affected by the A- and B-type lesions, and is responsible for the clinical paralysis.

Lymphomas in the visceral organs and other tissues are similar cytologically to the lymphoproliferations in the A-type lesions in nerves. Usually the lymphoid cells are of mixed types, often with a preponderance of small and medium lymphocytes, but sometimes, particularly in acute MD in adult birds, large lymphocytes and lymphoblasts may predominate.

The heterogeneous population of lymphoid cells in MD lymphomas, as seen in haematoxylin-and-eosin-stained sections, or in impression smears of lymphomas stained by May–Grünwald–Giemsa, is an important feature in differentiating the disease from lymphoid leukosis, in which the lymphomatous infiltrations are composed of uniform lymphoblasts. Another important difference is that, in lymphoid leukosis, gross lymphomas occur in the bursa of Fabricius, and the tumour has an intrafollicular origin and pattern of proliferation. In MD, although the bursa is sometimes involved in the lymphoproliferation, the tumour is less apparent, diffuse and interfollicular in location. Peripheral nerve lesions are not a feature of lymphoid leukosis as they are in MD. The greatest difficulty comes in distinguishing between lymphoid leukosis and forms of MD sometimes seen in adult birds in which the tumour is lymphoblastic with marked liver enlargement and absence of nerve lesions. Here it may be necessary to resort to specialised techniques, such as detection by immunofluorescence of T-cell antigens of MD tumour-associated surface antigen (MATSA) on MD tumour cells, or of B-cell antigens or IgM on the tumour cells of lymphoid leukosis. However, a diagnosis can usually be made on gross lesions and histopathology if several affected birds are examined at post-mortem.

Nerve lesions and lymphomatous proliferations induced by certain strains of reticuloendotheliosis virus are similar, both grossly and microscopically, to those present in MD. Although reticuloendotheliosis virus is not common in chicken flocks, it should be borne in mind as a possible cause of lymphoid tumours; its recognition depends on virological and serological tests on the flock. Reticuloendotheliosis virus can also cause neoplastic disease in turkeys, ducks, quail and other species. Another retrovirus also causes lymphoproliferative disease in turkeys. Although chicken flocks may be seropositive for reticuloendotheliosis virus, neoplastic disease is rare. The main features in the differential diagnosis of MD, lymphoid leukosis and reticuloendotheliosis are shown in Table 1.

There are no recognised health risks to humans working with MD virus or the related herpesvirus of turkeys (HVT).

1. Identification of the agent

Infection by MD virus in a flock may be detected by isolating the virus from the tissues of infected chickens. Commonly used sources are buffy coat cells from heparinised blood samples, or suspensions of lymphoma cells or spleen cells. As MD virus is highly cell associated, it is essential that these cell suspensions contain viable cells. The cell suspensions are inoculated into monolayer cultures of chicken kidney cells or duck embryo fibroblasts (chicken embryo fibroblasts are less sensitive for primary virus isolation). Serotype 2 and 3 viruses (see Section B.1.a.) are more easily isolated in chicken embryo fibroblasts than in chicken kidney cells. Usually a 0.2 ml suspension containing from 10^6 to 10^7 live cells is inoculated into duplicate monolayers grown in plastic cell culture dishes (60 mm in diameter). Inoculated and uninoculated control cultures are incubated at 38.5°C in a humid incubator containing 5% CO_2. Alternatively, closed culture vessels may be used. Culture medium is replaced at 2-day intervals. Areas of cytopathic effects, termed plaques, appear within 3–5 days and can be enumerated at about 7–10 days.

***Table 1.** Features useful in differentiating Marek's disease from lymphoid leukosis and reticuloendotheliosis*

Feature	Marek's disease	Lymphoid leukosis	Reticuloendotheliosis*
Age	Any age. Usually 6 weeks or older	Not under 16 weeks	Not under 16 weeks
Signs	Frequently paralysis	Nonspecific	Nonspecific
Incidence	Frequently above 5% in unvaccinated flocks. Rare in vaccinated flocks	Rarely above 5%	Rare
Macroscopic lesions			
Neural involvement	Frequent	Absent	Infrequent
Bursa of Fabricius	Diffuse enlargement or atrophy	Nodular tumours	Nodular tumours
Tumours in skin, muscle and proventriculus	May be present	Usually absent	Absent
Microscopic lesions			
Neural involvement	Yes	No	Infrequent
Liver tumours	Often perivascular	Focal or diffuse	Focal
Spleen	Diffuse	Often focal	Focal or diffuse
Bursa of Fabricius	Interfollicular tumour and/or atrophy of follicles	Intrafollicular tumour	Intrafollicular tumour
Central nervous system	Yes	No	No
Lymphoid proliferation in skin and feather follicles	Yes	No	No
Cytology of tumours	Pleomorphic lymphoid cells, including lymphoblasts, small, medium and large lymphocytes and reticulum cells. Rarely can be only lymphoblasts	Lymphoblasts	Lymphoblasts
Category of neoplastic lymphoid cell	T cell	B cell	B cell

* Reticuloendotheliosis virus may cause several different syndromes. The bursal lymphoma syndrome is most likely to occur in the field and is described here.

Another, less commonly used source of MD virus for diagnostic purposes is feather tips, from which cell-free MD virus can be extracted. Tips about 5 mm long, or minced tracts of skin containing feather tips, are suspended in an SPGA/EDTA (sucrose, phosphate, glutamate and albumin/ethylene diamine tetra-acetic acid) buffer for extraction and titration of cell-free MD virus (4). The buffer is made as follows: 0.2180 M sucrose (7.462 g); 0.0038 M monopotassium phosphate (0.052 g); 0.0072 M dipotassium phosphate (0.125 g); 0.0049 M L-monosodium glutamate (0.083 g); 1.0% bovine albumin powder (1.000 g); 0.2% EDTA (0.200 g); and distilled water (100 ml). The buffer is sterilised by filtration and should be at approximately pH 6.5.

This suspension is ultrasonicated and then filtered through a 0.45 µm membrane filter for inoculation into 24-hour-old drained chicken kidney cell monolayers. After absorption for 40 minutes, the medium is added and cultures are incubated as above for 7–10 days.

Using these methods, MD virus of serotypes 1 and 2 may be isolated, together with the HVT (serotype 3), if it is present as a result of vaccination. With experience, plaques caused by the different virus serotypes can be differentiated fairly accurately on the basis of time of appearance, rate of development, and plaque morphology. HVT plaques appear earlier and are larger than serotype 1 plaques, whereas serotype 2 plaques appear later and are smaller than serotype 1 plaques.

MD virus and HVT plaques may be identified as such using specific fluorescent antibodies raised in chickens. Monoclonal antibodies may be used to differentiate serotypes (12, 22).

- **Polymerase chain reaction**

Polymerase chain reaction (PCR) tests have been described that allow differentiation of some oncogenic and nononcogenic strains of serotype 1 MD virus, and of MD virus vaccine strains of serotypes 2 and 3 (1, 21, 27). PCR may also be used to quantify the MDV genome in cells (2).

2. Serological tests

The presence of antibodies to MD virus in nonvaccinated chickens from about 4 weeks of age is an indication of infection. Before that age, such antibodies may represent maternal transmission of antibody via the yolk and are not evidence of active infection.

Viruses, antigens and antisera are usually available from OIE Reference Laboratories for Marek's Disease (see Table given in Part 4 of this *Manual*), but international standard reagents have not yet been produced.

a) Agar gel immunodiffusion

There is no prescribed test for trade, but the agar gel immunodiffusion (AGID) test is employed most commonly to detect antibody. The test is conducted using glass slides coated with 1% agar in phosphate buffered saline containing 8% sodium chloride. Adjacent wells are filled with antigen or serum and these are incubated in a humid atmosphere at 37°C for 24 hours for diffusion to take place; positive sera show reactions of identity with known positive serum and antigen. The antigen used in this test is either disrupted MD virus-infected tissue culture cells or an extract of feather tips, or skin containing feather tracts obtained from MD virus-infected chickens. The cell culture antigen is prepared by propagating MDV in chicken kidney cells or chicken embryo fibroblast cells. When cytopathic effect is confluent, the cells are detached from the culture vessel and suspended in culture medium or phosphate buffered saline without tryptose phosphate broth (presence of tryptose phosphate broth may produce nonspecific precipitin lines) at a concentration of about 1×10^7 cells/ml. This suspension is then freeze–thawed three times and used as antigen.

- **Test procedure**

i) Make a 1% solution of Difco Bactoagar in 8% sodium chloride by standing the mixture in a boiling water bath.

ii) Pipette 4 ml of the agar solution on to a 7.5 cm × 2.5 cm microscope slide and allow to set.

iii) Cut holes in the agar using a template and No. 1 cork borer. The diameter of wells should be 5 mm, and the wells should be 2 mm apart. Remove agar plugs with a swab stick or pen nib.

iv) Pipette test sera into the top and bottom rows of wells, and standard positive serum and antigen alternately along the centre row.

v) Incubate the slide for 24 hours at 37°C in a humid container and read the results over a lamp in a darkened room.

A variation of the AGID test may be used to detect MD virus antigen in feather tips as an indication of infection by MD virus. Glass slides are prepared with a coating of 0.7% agarose (e.g. A37) in 8% sodium chloride, containing MD virus antiserum. Tips of small feathers are taken from the birds to be examined and are inserted vertically into the agar, and the slides are maintained as described above. The development of radial zones of precipitation around the feather tips denotes the presence in the feather of MD virus antigen and hence of infection in the bird.

b) Other tests

Other tests for MD virus antibody include the direct and indirect fluorescent antibody test. These demonstrate the ability of a test serum to stain MD virus plaques in cell cultures (12, 23). These tests are group specific and more sensitive than the AGID test. A virus neutralisation test for the ability of a serum to neutralise the plaque-forming property of cell-free MD virus can also be employed (3). However, this test is more suitable for research purposes than for routine diagnostic use. An enzyme-linked immunosorbent assay for detecting MD virus antibodies is available (6, 10). To prepare antigen for the enzyme-linked immunosorbent assay, wells of a 96-well microtitre plate are coated with MDV-infected chicken embryo fibroblast cells. The details of the procedure have been published (6, 19).

B. REQUIREMENTS FOR VACCINES AND DIAGNOSTIC BIOLOGICALS

Commercial biological products used in the control of MD are the cell-associated or cell-free (lyophilised) live virus or HVT, respectively. Although genetically engineered recombinant vaccines have been developed (15, 18) they are currently not in commercial use. Marek's disease vaccines are injected *in ovo* at the 17th or 18th day of embryonation (20) or subcutaneously at hatch. The requirements for producing vaccines are outlined below, but other sources should be consulted for further information on the procedures (7–9, 11, 13, 14, 16, 24, 26). Protocols are given in the British Pharmacopoeia Monograph 589, and the US Code of Federal Regulations, Volume 9, part 113 (25).

1. Seed management

a) Characteristics of the seed

Viruses of the MD virus group are classified under three serotypes – 1, 2 and 3 – on the basis of their antigenic relatedness.

Serotype 1: This includes all the pathogenic strains of the virus, ranging from strains that are very virulent plus (e.g. 648A), very virulent (e.g. Md/5, Md/11, Ala-8, RB-1B), virulent (e.g. HPRS-16, JM, GA), mildly virulent (e.g. HPRS-B14, Conn A) and finally to weakly virulent (e.g. CU-2, CVI-988). These strains may be attenuated by passage in tissue culture, with loss of pathogenic properties but retention of immunogenicity, to provide strains that have been used as vaccines. Those that have been used commercially include attenuated HPRS-16 and CVI-988 (Rispens) strains. Attenuated variants of the very virulent stains have been used in experimental vaccines to protect against the variant form of acute MD caused by the very virulent stains, and the R2/23 vaccine strain derived from Md/5 is licensed in the United States of America. Serotype 1 vaccines are prepared in a cell-associated ('wet') form that must be stored in liquid nitrogen.

Serotype 2: This includes naturally avirulent strains of MD virus (e.g. SB-1, HPRS-24, 301B/1, HN-1), and several of these have been shown to provide protection against virulent strains. The SB-1 and 301B/1 strains have been developed commercially and used, particularly with HVT, in bivalent vaccines for protection against the very virulent strains. Serotype 2 vaccines exist only in the cell-associated form.

Serotype 3: This contains the strains of naturally avirulent HVT (e.g. FC126, PB1), which are widely used as a monovalent vaccine, and also in combination with serotype 1 and 2 strains in bivalent or trivalent vaccines against the very virulent strains of MD virus. HVT may be prepared in a cell-free form as a freeze-dried (lyophilised) vaccine or in a cell-associated ('wet') form.

b) Method of culture

The substrates used for commercial vaccine production are primary chicken embryo fibroblasts (CEF) derived from specific pathogen free (SPF) flocks or duck embryo fibroblasts. CEF from SPF flocks are preferred to duck cells because more is known about chicken-embryo-transmitted pathogens and methods for their detection.

c) Validation as a vaccine

Methods for testing SPF flocks for freedom from infection are available (14, 24). SPF chicken flocks should be free from avian adenoviruses, including egg-drop syndrome 76 virus, avian encephalomyelitis virus, avian leukosis virus (subgroups A, B and J), avian nephritis virus, avian reoviruses, avian rotaviruses, chicken anaemia virus, fowl pox virus, infectious bronchitis virus, infectious bursal disease virus, infectious laryngotracheitis virus, influenza type A virus, MD virus, *Mycoplasma gallisepticum, Mycoplasma synoviae,* Newcastle disease virus, reticuloendotheliosis virus, *Salmonella* spp., and turkey rhinotracheitis virus.

SPF duck flocks should be free from avian adenoviruses, avian reoviruses, *Chlamydia,* duck virus enteritis, duck virus hepatitis types I and II, influenza type A virus, Newcastle disease virus, *Pasteurella* (now *Riemerella*) *anatipestifer,* reticuloendoetheliosis virus, and *Salmonella* infections.

Freedom from other infections may also be required as they become recognised.

The master seed virus should be shown to be nonpathogenic for chickens by inoculating ten times the field dose into 1-day-old SPF chickens of a strain susceptible to MD, to ensure that it does not cause gross lesions or significant microscopic lesions of MD by 120 days of age. It should be noted that some vaccine strains of MD virus and HVT may produce minor and transient microscopic nerve lesions under these circumstances.

No increase in virulence should occur during six serial passages of the vaccine strain in 1-day-old SPF MD-susceptible chickens. Ten times the field dose of vaccine is inoculated initially and then passaged by inoculation of heparinised blood at 5–7-day intervals, and tests for viraemia are run to check that virus is transferred at each passage. The birds receiving the final passage are kept for 120 days and should be free from MD lesions. However, some strains, such as Rispens, may cause some mild MD lesions. The important observation is that the virulence should not change. This is a difficult test because the genetic resistance of the chickens fundamentally affects the apparent virulence of the virus, so does the type of inoculum. After successful completion of laboratory safety tests, the safety of the strain should be confirmed in extensive field trials.

Seed virus must be free from the agents listed for SPF flocks and from other contaminants that may be acquired in the laboratory. A vaccine strain derived from turkeys must also be free from lymphoproliferative disease virus and haemorrhagic enteritis virus.

The ability of the master seed virus – and derived virus at the limit of the passage range used to produce vaccinal virus (usually not more than five tissue culture passages) – to protect against MD must be determined. Standardised protection tests are published. They involve vaccination of MD-susceptible SPF chickens at 1 day of age and challenge with sufficient virulent MD virus 8 days later to cause at least a 70% incidence of MD in unvaccinated chickens. Two types of tests are used. In the protection index test, a single field dose (1000 PFU) (plaque-forming units) of vaccine is given and the incidence of MD in vaccinated birds is compared with that in unvaccinated birds. Protective indices should be greater than 80, i.e. vaccinated birds should show at least 80% reduction in the incidence of gross MD, compared with unvaccinated controls.

A PD_{50} (50% protective dose) test is also used, involving the inoculation of five four-fold serial dilutions of vaccine virus selected to provide protection above and below the 50% level, followed by challenge 8 days later to determine the PD_{50} value. The assays are conducted using a standard reference vaccine for comparison. The PD_{50} may be as low as 4 PFU, but higher values can be obtained depending on the vaccine strain, whether cell-free or cell-associated and the presence or absence of maternal antibodies in the test chickens. On the basis of the PD_{50} test, it has been suggested that the minimum vaccine field dose should be the greater of two values: 10^3 PFU or 100 PD_{50}.

Extensive field trials of a new vaccine strain in the presence of field challenge should be conducted using different breeds of birds of varying MD virus maternal antibody status, to ensure efficacy and persistence of immunity. Experience suggests that vaccinal immunity, once acquired, is lifelong.

2. Method of manufacture

Substrate cells are seeded into flat-bottomed vessels for stationary incubation, or into cylindrical vessels for rolled incubation. Media commonly used are Eagle's minimal essential medium, or 199 medium, buffered with sodium bicarbonate and supplemented with 5% calf serum. Incubation is at 38–39°C for 48 hours.

For cell-associated vaccine, cultures are infected with production HVT or MD virus seed virus stock, in cell-associated form, which is usually two passages beyond the master seed stock. Cultures are incubated for

48 hours then the infected cells are harvested by treating the washed cell sheet with an EDTA/trypsin solution to allow the cells to begin to detach. The flasks are then returned to the incubator (38.5°C) to allow complete detachment. The cells are subjected to low speed centrifugation, and then resuspended in the freezing mixture consisting of cell growth medium containing 7.5–15% dimethyl sulphoxide, and held at 4°C or dispensed immediately into the final vaccine containers, usually glass ampoules, which are flame-sealed and frozen in liquid nitrogen.

Cell-free lyophilised vaccine may be prepared from HVT, but not from MD virus strains. For the production of this form of vaccine, HVT-infected cultures are incubated for 72 hours, infected cells are detached from the vessel as described above, or scraped from the walls of the vessel. The cells are suspended in a small volume of growth medium, centrifuged, and resuspended in a buffered stabiliser solution containing 8% sucrose, but free from protein to prevent frothing. The cell suspension is sonicated to release virus, the cell debris is removed, the suspension is diluted with a complete stabiliser – such as SPGA – filled into the final containers, and lyophilised.

The dilution rate for both cell-associated and cell-free vaccines is based on previous experience, as is the number of doses required per container, because the virus content of the harvested material cannot be assayed prior to filling the final containers. The virus content of the finished product can subsequently be added to the label.

3. In-process control

For optimal results in preparing cell-associated vaccine, a slow rate of freezing (1–5°C per minute) and rapid thawing are essential. The infectivity titre of the infected cells, and hence the number of doses per ampoule, are determined after filling the ampoules. Similarly for cell-free vaccine, the virus content of the final suspension, and hence the number of doses per container, is determined after filling.

4. Batch control

a) Identity

Using monospecific neutralising serum, checks should be carried out to show that the product is of the same specificity as the seed virus. This is best done using monoclonal antibodies.

b) Safety and sterility

Extensive testing is required of the materials used to produce the vaccine, and of the final product. Substrate cells should come from an SPF flock and, in particular, be free from vertically transmitted agents. Substances of animal origin used in the preparation of vaccines such as serum, trypsin, and bovine serum albumin, must be free from extraneous agents.

Batches of the final vaccine produced should be tested for freedom from contaminating bacteria, fungi, mycoplasma and the viruses listed for SPF flocks: tests for purity of the diluent should also be conducted. Suitable tests for the detection of extraneous agents at all stages of vaccine production are recommended by several official bodies (14, 16, 24) and in Chapter I.4.

Ten doses of vaccine or a quantity of diluent equivalent to two doses of vaccine should be inoculated into separate groups of ten 1-day-old SPF chickens. No adverse reactions should occur during a 21-day observation period.

c) Potency

The standard dose of each type of vaccine is 1000 PFU per chicken or egg. Virus content assays are conducted on batches of vaccine to ensure that the correct dose per bird will be achieved.

d) Duration of immunity

A test for duration of immunity is carried out on the seed virus only. Such immunity is apparently lifelong.

e) Stability

Tests for stability are carried out on six representative batches of vaccine to show that titre is maintained during the stated shelf life of the vaccine. These tests should be conducted under the conditions of storage of the vaccine. The lyophilised product should have a shelf life of 12 months when stored at 2–8°C.

Manufacturers may double the virus content of the vaccine to compensate for some loss of titre during storage. Appropriate diluting fluids are provided for use with cell-associated and freeze-dried vaccines. The stability of reconstituted vaccine over a 2-hour period should be tested.

f) Preservatives

Preservatives are not included in the vaccine or diluent.

g) Precautions (hazards)

With cell-associated vaccine, care is necessary to avoid injury from ampoules that may explode when they are removed from liquid nitrogen. Eye protection must be worn. During use, reconstituted vaccine must be kept cool and cell-associated vaccine should be agitated to keep cells in suspension.

5. Tests on the final product

a) Safety

See Section B.4.b

b) Potency

See Section B.4.c.

REFERENCES

1. BECKER Y., ASHER Y., TABOR E., DAVIDSON I., MALKINSON M. & WEISMAN Y. (1992). Polymerase chain reaction for differentiation between pathogenic and non-pathogenic serotype 1 Marek's disease virus (MDV) and vaccine viruses of MDV-serotypes 2 and 3. *J. Virol. Methods*, **40**, 307– 322.

2. BUMSTEAD N., SILLIBOURNE J., RENNIE M., ROSS N. & DAVISON F. (1997). Quantification of Marek's disease virus in chicken lymphocytes using the polymerase chain reaction with fluorescence detection. *J Virol. Methods*, **65**, 75–81.

3. CALNEK B.W. & ADLDINGER H.K. (1971). Some characteristics of cell-free preparation of Marek's disease virus. *Avian Dis.*, **15**, 508–517.

4. CALNEK B.W., HITCHNER S.B. & ADLDINGER H.K. (1970). Lyophilization of cell-free Marek's disease herpesvirus and a herpesvirus from turkeys. *Appl. Microbiol.*, **20**, 723–726.

5. CALNEK B.W. & WITTER R.L. (1997). Marek's disease. *In:* Diseases of Poultry, Tenth Edition, Calnek B.W., Barnes H.J. Beard C.W., McDougald L.R. & Saif Y.M., eds Iowa State University Press, Ames Iowa, USA, 369–413.

6. CHENG Y.-Q., LEE L.F., SMITH E.J. & WITTER R.L. (1984). An enzyme-linked immunosorbent assay for the detection of antibodies to Marek's disease virus. *Avian Dis.*, **28**, 900–911.

7. CHURCHILL A.E. (1985). Production of vaccines. *In:* Marek's Disease, Payne L.N. ed. Martinus Nijhoff, Boston, USA, 251–265.

8. COUNCIL OF EUROPE (1997). Marek's Disease Vaccines (Live). *In:* European Pharmacopoeia, Third Edition. Editions of the Council of Europe, Strasbourg, France, 1814–1818. ISBN 92-871-2990-8.

9. COUNCIL OF EUROPE (1997). Vaccines for Veterinary Use. Chapter 5.2.2. Chicken flocks free from specified pathogens for the production and quality control of vaccines. *In:* European Pharmacopoeia, Third Edition. Editions of the Council of Europe, Strasbourg, France, 301–304. ISBN 92-871-2990-8.

10. DAVIDSON I., MALKINSON M., STRENGER C. & BECKER Y. (1988). An improved ELISA method, using a streptavidin–biotin complex, for detecting Marek's disease virus antigens in feather-tips of infected chickens. *J. Virol. Methods*, **14**, 237–241.

11. INTERNATIONAL ASSOCIATION OF BIOLOGICAL STANDARDIZATION (1979). Report of the Avian Products Standardisation Committee.

12. LEE L.F., LIU X. & WITTER R.L. (1983). Monoclonal antibodies with specificity for three different serotypes of Marek's disease virus in chickens. *J. Immunol.*, **130**, 1003–1006.

13. MERIEUX C., HULSE E.C., GAUDRY D., ALLAN W.H., REGAMEY R.H., eds (1974). International Symposium on Requirements for Poultry Virus Vaccines. Proceedings of the 42nd Symposium, organised by the International Association of Biological Standardization, Lyon, France, August 1973. *Dev. Biol. Stand.*, **25**, 423.

14. MINISTRY OF AGRICULTURE, FISHERIES AND FOOD (1990). Guidelines for the Production and Control of Avian Virus Vaccine. MAL 74. HMSO, London, UK.

15. NAZERIAN K., LEE LF., YANAGIDA N. & OGAWA R. (1992). Protection against Marek's disease by a fowlpox virus recombinant expressing the glycoprotein B of Marek's disease virus. *J. Virol.*, **66**, 1409–13.

16. OFFICE OF FEDERAL REGULATIONS (1989). Animals and Animal Products. Code of Federal Regulations, Vol. 9. National Archives of the United States, USA.

17. PAYNE L.N., ed. (1985). Marek's Disease. Martinus Nijhoff, Boston, USA, pp. 359.

18. REDDY S.K., SHARMA J.M., AHMAD J., REDDY D.N., MCMILLEN J.K., COOK S.M., WILD M.A. & SCHWARTZ R.D. (1996). Protective efficacy of a recombinant herpesvirus of turkeys as an *in ovo* vaccine against Newcastle and Marek's diseases in specific-pathogen-free chickens. *Vaccine,* **14**, 469–77.

19. SHARMA J.M. (1998). Marek's disease. *In:* A Laboratory Manual for the Isolation and Identification of Avian Pathogens, Fourth Edition, Swayne D.E. *et al.*, eds. American Association of Avian Pathologists, 116–124.

20. SHARMA J.M. (1999). Introduction to poultry vaccines and immunity. *Adv. Vet. Med.*, **41**, 481–494.

21. SILVA R.F. (1992). Differentiation of pathogenic and non-pathogenic serotype 1 Marek's disease viruses (MDVs) by the polymerase chain reaction amplification of the tandem direct repeats within the MDV genome. *Avian Dis.*, **36**, 521–528.

22. SILVA R.F., CALVERT J.G. & LEE L.F. (1997). A simple immunoperoxidase plaque assay to detect and quantitate Marek's disease virus plaques. *Avian Dis.,* **41**, 528–34.

23. SPENCER J.L. & CALNEK B.W. (1970). Marek's desease: application of immuofluorescence for detection of antigen and antibody. *Am. J. Vet. Res.*, **31**, 345–358.

24. THORNTON D.H. (1985). Quality control and standardisation of vaccines. *In:* L.N. Payne, ed. *Op. cit.*, 267–291.

25. UNITED STATES DEPARTMENT OF AGRICULTURE (USDA) (1995). Code Of Federal Regulations, Title 9, Parts 1–199. US Government Printing Office, Washington D.C., USA

26. WITTER R.L. (1985). Principles of vaccination. *In:* L.N. Payne, ed. *Op. cit.*, 203–250.

27. ZHU G.-S., OJIMA T., HIRONAKA T., IHARA T., MIZUKOSHI N., KATO A., UEDA S. & HIRAI K. (1992). Differentiation of oncogenic and non-oncogenic strains of Marek's disease virus type 1 by using polymerase chain reaction DNA amplification. *Avian Dis.*, **36**, 637–645.

*

* *

CHAPTER 2.7.3.

AVIAN MYCOPLASMOSIS
(Mycoplasma gallisepticum)

SUMMARY

Mycoplasma gallisepticum *(MG) can cause significant economic loss in chickens and turkeys due to chronic respiratory disease, downgrading of carcasses in meat-type birds and loss of production in layers. Infection is diagnosed by demonstration of the organism or its DNA or by the detection of specific humoral antibodies. Other pathogenic mycoplasmas infecting poultry are* M. synoviae *in the chicken and turkey, and* M. meleagridis *and* M. iowae *in the turkey.*

Identification of the agent: *MG can be detected in two ways. It can be identified by immunological tests after isolation in mycoplasma media or the presence of its DNA can be demonstrated in field samples or cultures.*

Samples for isolation consist of swabs of organs or tissues, exudates or diluted tissue homogenates. Culture may also be attempted from aspirates from the infraorbital sinuses or joint cavities and from yolk or embryos. The sample selected will be influenced by the clinical signs and by any lesions present. Broth and agar are used for isolation, but it is normally necessary to obtain mycoplasma colonies on agar before attempting identification. If there is difficulty, an initial passage of the material through mycoplasma-free chicken embryos or mycoplasma-free chickens may be helpful.

Although some basic biochemical tests can be helpful in preliminary classification of mycoplasma isolates, final identification must be by serological tests. The most satisfactory of these are the indirect fluorescent antibody test and the immunoperoxidase test.

DNA detection methods, mainly based on the polymerase chain reaction, have come into use in specialised laboratories. A commercial kit has been marketed in several countries and can be used to detect field strains and to distinguish them from the vaccine F strain.

Serological tests: *Several serological tests have been used to detect MG antibodies, but specificity and sensitivity have been lacking to some degree in all of them. They are more satisfactory for flock screening than for testing individual birds.*

The most commonly used are the rapid serum agglutination (RSA) test, the enzyme-linked immunosorbent assay (ELISA) and the haemagglutination inhibition (HI) test. In the RSA test, sera from individual birds are tested for agglutination using commercially produced stained MG antigen. Chicken or turkey sera that yield agglutination reactions with the antigen within 2 minutes should be heated at 56°C for 30 minutes and retested. Sera that still react, especially when diluted, are considered to be positive. These may then be confirmed by an ELISA or a HI test. Doubtful results should be checked by performing RSA tests with M. synoviae *antigen, as infection with this organism sometimes causes cross-reactions. Several commercial MG antibody ELISA kits are available, including a blocking ELISA that uses a monoclonal antibody.*

Requirements for vaccines and diagnostic biologicals: *Although the preferred method of control is maintenance of MG-free flocks, both live and inactivated vaccines have been used. Vaccination should be considered only on multi-age sites where it is inevitable that flocks will become infected. The usual use of vaccination is to prevent egg production losses in commercial layers, although vaccines may also be used to reduce the level of egg transmission in breeding stock or as a tool for MG eradication on multi-age production sites. It is important for either live or killed vaccine to be administered before the flock is exposed to field infection with MG.*

Available live vaccines are generally produced from the F strain of MG, and, more recently, strains ts-11 and 6/85, which are apathogenic strains with improved safety characteristics. Administration of the F strain by the intranasal or eyedrop route is preferred, but aerosol or drinking water administration may be used. The eyedrop method is recommended for ts-11, while a fine spray is recommended for 6/85. Pullets are generally vaccinated between 12 and 16 weeks of age. A single dose is sufficient and vaccinated birds remain permanent carriers. Long-term use of the F strain on a multi-age site results in displacement of the field strain with the vaccine strain. F strain displaces virulent wild-type MG strains more efficiently than 6/85 or ts-11, but ts-11 has been successfully used to eradicate F strain MG in multi-age commercial layers. Multi-age production sites are also known to test serologically negative for MG after long-term use of 6/85. The F strain is fully virulent for turkeys.

Bacterins consist of a concentrated suspension of MG organisms in an oil emulsion. These are ordinarily administered to growing pullets at 12–16 weeks of age. They are administered parenterally, usually subcutaneously in the neck. Although two doses are desirable, a single dose is usually given because of cost and labour considerations. Bacterins are effective in preventing egg-production losses and respiratory disease, but they do not prevent infection with wild-type MG.

A. DIAGNOSTIC TECHNIQUES

Mycoplasma gallisepticum (MG) belongs to the class Mollicutes, order Mycoplasmatales, family Mycoplasmataceae. MG is particularly important in chickens and turkeys as a cause of respiratory disease and decreased production (13, 20) and can also cause upper respiratory disease in game birds (10). More recently it has been recognised as a cause of conjunctivitis in house finches in North America (18, 21). Under certain circumstances, MG may be associated with acute respiratory disease in chickens and turkeys, especially in young birds, with the turkey being more susceptible. The severity of the disease is greatly affected by the degree of secondary infection with viruses such as Newcastle disease and infectious bronchitis, and/or bacteria such as *Escherichia coli*. A more chronic form of the disease may occur and can cause reduced egg production in breeders and layers. The infection is spread vertically through infected eggs and horizontally by close contact. Other methods of spread are less well documented. It should be noted that *M. synoviae*, *M. meleagridis* and *M. iowae* can also cause disease in poultry.

The presence of MG can be confirmed by isolating the organism in a cell-free medium or by detecting its DNA directly in infected tissues or swab samples. When results are equivocal, chicken embryos or chickens may be inoculated with suspect material. Serological tests are also widely used for diagnosis.

1. Identification of the agent

- **Culture**

Samples are taken from live birds, fresh carcasses or the carcasses of birds that have been frozen when fresh. Samples may also be collected from dead-in-shell embryos or chickens or poults that have broken the shell but failed to hatch. From live birds, swabs may be taken from the choanal cleft, oropharynx, oesophagus, trachea, cloaca and phallus. In the case of dead birds, samples may be taken from the nasal cavity, infraorbital sinus, trachea, or air sacs. Exudates can be aspirated from the infraorbital sinuses and joint cavities.

Samples can be taken from embryonated eggs, e.g. from the inner surface of the vitelline membrane, and from the oropharynx and air sacs.

All samples should be examined as soon as possible after collection. If transportation is necessary, small pieces of tissue should be placed in mycoplasma broth, or swabs should be agitated in 1–2 ml of mycoplasma broth and then discarded. Alternatively, the swabs can be dipped in mycoplasma broth before the specimens are taken (31) and then replaced in the swab holders for transportation. An ice pack or some other means of chilling should be included. Serial dilutions of specimens may be of value as the presence of specific antibodies or antibiotics or inhibitory substances in tissues may inhibit mycoplasma growth unless they are diluted out.

Several suitable culture media have been formulated (9, 12). They generally contain a protein digest and a meat-infusion base supplemented with serum or a serum fraction, yeast factors, glucose and bacterial inhibitors. It is important that each new batch of medium be tested with recently isolated MG cultures of low *in-vitro* passage because some components, especially the yeast extract and the serum, may vary in their ability to support growth (25).

For the growth of MG the following broth and agar media are satisfactory:

- Part A: Pleuropneumonia-like organism (PPLO) broth base without crystal violet (Difco) (14.7 g); distilled or deionised water (700 ml).

- Part B: Pig serum (heated at 56°C for 30 minutes) (150 ml): 25% (w/v) fresh yeast extract (100 ml); 10% (w/v) glucose solution (10 ml); 5% (w/v) thallous acetate (10 ml); 200,000 International Units (IU)/ml penicillin G (5 ml); and 0.1% (w/v) phenol red solution (20 ml). The pH is adjusted to 7.8. The pig serum may be replaced by horse serum, but it is important to ascertain that it supports the growth of MG.

Part A is autoclaved at 121°C, at 1 atmosphere for 15 minutes and, after cooling, is added to Part B, which has been previously sterilised by filtration.

For the corresponding solid medium, 10 g of purified agar, known to support the growth of MG, is added to part A above. The mixture is autoclaved as before and kept in a water bath at 56°C. The constituents of part B, omitting the phenol red, are mixed separately and then incubated at 56°C. Parts A and B are mixed carefully to avoid the production of air bubbles, and are dispensed into 50 mm dishes using 7–9 ml/dish. Excess surface moisture can be removed by a short incubation at 37°C. Plates are stored in an airtight container at approximately 4°C for up to 2 weeks.

Fresh yeast extract is available commercially, although it is preferable to prepare it 'in-house' by taking active dry baker's yeast (250 g) and suspending it in distilled water (1 litre). This is heated to boiling point, cooled and then centrifuged for 20 minutes at 3000 *g*. The supernatant fluid is decanted and adjusted to pH 8.0 with 0.1 M NaOH. This is clarified by centrifugation or by filtration, and then sterilised by filtration. The extract is stored at –20°C. Reagent grade glucose (10 g) is dissolved in distilled or deionised water (100 ml) and adjusted to pH 7.8–8.0 with 0.1 M NaOH. It is sterilised by filtration and stored at 4°C. Reagent grade thallous acetate is dissolved (5 g) in distilled or deionised water (100 ml), filter-sterilised and stored at –20°C. Penicillin solution (10^6 IU benzyl penicillin in 5 ml distilled water) is stored at 4°C, and has a shelf life of 1 week. Phenol red (0.1g) is ground in 0.1 M NaOH (2.8 ml), and then made up to 100 ml in sterile distilled water and autoclaved at 115°C and at 1 atmosphere for 30 minutes. It is stored at 4°C. (Note: Thallous acetate is highly toxic and ampicillin and colistin may be used to replace this and penicillin.)

Specimens are inoculated on to mycoplasma agar and into broth. Solid medium may help detection of slow-growing mycoplasma colonies, which can be overgrown by saprophytes in broth. It may be necessary to make serial dilutions up to 10^{-3} for successful isolation. Inoculated plates are incubated at 37°C in sealed containers. Increased humidity and CO_2 tension in the atmosphere have been reported to enhance growth; these conditions may be obtained by the inclusion of damp paper or cotton wool, and by flushing the container with 5–10% CO_2 in nitrogen, by placing a lighted candle in the container, or by using a CO_2 incubator.

The caps of liquid medium containers should be tightly sealed before incubation at 37°C to avoid spurious changes in pH. For the first few days, the plates are examined daily for colonies with a stereoscopic microscope; after that they are examined less frequently. Cultures from field material should not be discarded as negative for at least 20 days.

Broth medium should be examined daily for acidity, indicated by a change from red to orange or yellow in the indicator. Any observable growth is subcultured on to solid medium immediately. Even if no colour change occurs, subculture on to solid medium should be made after 7–10 days or earlier as the presence of an arginine-hydrolysing (alkali-producing) mycoplasma species may mask the acid colour change produced by MG.

Mycoplasma colonies on solid medium can usually be recognised, although they may not have the typical 'fried egg' appearance. Bacterial colonies may appear on the first passage, but they are often more pigmented and fail to passage on mycoplasma media.

Biochemical reactions (e.g. fermentation of glucose and failure to hydrolyse arginine) can assist in identification, but they are not specific for MG and necessitate purification of the culture by cloning. Immunological and DNA methods are used to identify mycoplasma isolates, although the former are still more commonly employed. They include: the indirect fluorescent antibody (IFA) and immunoperoxidase (IP) tests, both of which are simple, sensitive, specific and rapid to perform; growth inhibition (GI); and metabolism inhibition (MI). Purified (cloned) cultures are required for the GI and MI tests, but not for the IFA or IP test. IFA and IP can detect the presence of more than one species of mycoplasma, as the colonies specific for the antiserum will react while the others will not. However, *M. imitans*, a mycoplasma species that is serologically related to MG and that presents the same biochemical properties (2) has been isolated from ducks, geese and sometimes from other nondomestic bird species in some countries. It may be distinguished from MG by use of a PCR–RFLP (polymerase chain reaction –restriction fragment length polymorphism), as described by Kempf (14). Alternatively, colonies of the isolate can be examined by immunofluorescence using serial dilutions of antisera to MG and *M. imitans* in parallel. The homologous antiserum should have a considerably higher titre.

DNA detection methods for identifying MG directly in tissues or for identifying laboratory isolates are discussed below and are usually based on the PCR.

In certain circumstances where results of the above methods are not conclusive, inoculation of chicken embryos or bioassays in live chickens may be appropriate. The specimens required for inoculation of chicken embryos are the same as those used for the inoculation of artificial media. They are prepared in broth from which thallous acetate is omitted, incubated for 30–60 minutes at 37°C, and then a 0.05–0.1 ml aliquot is inoculated into the yolk sac of several 6–8-day-old chicken embryos derived from MG-free flocks. The eggs are candled daily and embryos that die within 24 hours of inoculation are discarded. Any further dead embryos are kept refrigerated until cultured and those surviving after 5 days are placed at 4°C for 4 hours to kill them and to reduce haemorrhages on opening. The yolk is subcultured into broth and on to agar. Yolk lipid tends to obscure colonies so it is essential to streak the yolk thinly or, preferably, to dilute it first in mycoplasma broth.

Bioassays may be performed by the inoculation of a homogenate of suspect material into at least four 8–16 week-old susceptible mycoplasma-free chickens. Diagnosis is confirmed by the recovery of MG from these birds and/or the demonstration of specific antibodies (22). Such procedures should rarely be necessary. When required, a suitable procedure is as follows:

Samples such as nasal turbinate, infraorbital sinus, trachea, lungs, air sacs, oviduct, or joint fluid are homogenised in from 5 to 10 volumes of broth, and immediately inoculated into at least four test birds intranasally, supra-conjunctivally, intratracheally, into the infraorbital sinus and the air sacs. The birds are kept in isolation. Two additional control birds are inoculated by the same routes with broth only and kept separately in isolation.

At 14, 21, 28 and 35 days after inoculation, the sera of all birds are tested for MG antibodies by the rapid serum agglutination (RSA) test. After the final bleed, all birds are killed and examined for gross and microscopic lesions. Tissues, especially those showing gross lesions, are cultured for mycoplasma. The original samples are considered to be positive for MG if the organism is recovered from the birds inoculated with the homogenate, or if they develop an RSA titre of 1/4 or more. Titres less than this are interpreted as being doubtful. An enzyme-linked immunosorbent assay (ELISA) or a haemagglutination inhibition (HI) test should be performed. The organism should not be recovered from the control birds, nor should they develop any RSA titres. There should be no RSA reaction to *M. synoviae* in either group of birds.

- **Immunological methods**

Immunofluorescence and IP procedures for diagnosis are generally applied to suspect laboratory isolates rather than directly to infected exudates or tissues. This is because the organisms are too small to recognise conclusively under the light microscope and because the corresponding negative and positive control exudate/tissue is unlikely to be readily available.

a) Indirect fluorescent antibody test

The recommended technique for the IFA test (24) requires an agar culture of the unknown isolate, consisting of numerous small discrete colonies, a known MG culture as a positive control, and a culture of a further mycoplasma species, such as *M. synoviae* or *M. gallinarum,* as a negative control. Also required are rabbit anti-MG serum, a normal rabbit serum and an anti-rabbit immunoglobulin fluorochrome-conjugated serum. Sera may be prepared in species other than rabbits. Suitable working dilutions in sterile phosphate buffered saline (PBS; 0.01 M, pH 7.1) of the anti-MG serum and the conjugate are first determined by cross-titration, and are selected for use at two-to-four-fold dilutions less than the actual end-points. These are applied to the colonies of mycoplasmas to be identified that have been previously grown on agar plates as indicated below.

Blocks of about 1.0 × 0.5 cm are cut from the plates and placed, with the colonies uppermost, on to microscope slides. To make subsequent orientation possible, the lower right-hand corner of the block is cut off. A block with the unknown isolate, a block with the known MG culture, and a block with a different but known mycoplasma culture are placed on one slide. A block of the unknown isolate is placed on another slide. A drop of suitably diluted MG antiserum is added to each block of the first slide and the normal rabbit serum is added to the single block on the second slide. All blocks are incubated for 30 minutes at room temperature in a humid atmosphere. Each block is placed in a labelled tube containing PBS, pH 7.2, washed for 10 minutes in a rotary mixer, then similarly rewashed, and finally returned to the original microscope slides. Excess moisture is blotted from the sides of the blocks. One drop of the diluted conjugate is placed on each block, which are then incubated and washed as before. Finally, the blocks are returned to their original slides, and the colonies are examined by incident light using fluorescence microscopy.

Interpretation of the results is subjective and requires some expertise; comparisons with the controls are essential, and they must give the correct reactions.

Some laboratories use fluorescein-conjugated antiserum in a direct immunofluorescence test (direct IMF). A widely used technique for direct IMF is performed by applying the reagents successively within stainless steel rings placed on the original mycoplasma agar plate. Although this is quick and easy to perform, the results obtained are less specific than using the indirect method, which is therefore preferred.

b) Indirect immunoperoxidase test

This involves a similar principle to the IFA test except that the binding of specific antibodies to colonies *in situ* is detected by adding an anti-rabbit immunoglobulin that has been conjugated to the enzyme peroxidase. A positive reaction is then developed by adding an appropriate substrate which, on oxidation, produces coloured colonies. An immunobinding procedure can also be used in which the test colonies are blotted on to nitrocellulose (16) and then reacted in a similar manner. The advantage of the IP test over immunofluorescence is that the former does not require an expensive fluorescence microscope.

c) Growth inhibition test

In the GI test, the growth of mycoplasmas is inhibited by specific antiserum, enabling species to be identified. It is relatively insensitive and sera must be high-titred, monospecific and prepared in mammalian hosts as poultry sera do not inhibit mycoplasma growth efficiently. The organism under test must be in pure culture (cloned) and several dilutions should be tested; a concentration of 10^4 colony-forming units (CFU/ml) is optimal. The rate of growth of the organism may influence growth inhibition, and it is helpful to retard growth initially by incubating at 27°C for 24 hours, followed by incubation at 37°C thereafter. Details of the test and its interpretation are published elsewhere (6).

d) Nucleic acid recognition methods

An alternative to conventional culture and identification is the use of specific DNA-detection methods. MG may be detected by hybridisation with DNA probes, but now it is much more common to use the PCR to amplify specific portions of DNA in the test material. One commercial MG DNA test kit uses a PCR directly on material extracted from swabs, and the amplified product, if present, is detected by a nonradiolabelled probe. Two versions are available; one that detects field strains of MG and one that identifies the vaccine F strain. Several 'in-house' PCR-based tests have also been published for MG. Several are cited by Kempf (14) and, in addition, a manual published in 1998 contains a well validated PCR assay for MG and other avian mycoplasmas (17). A multiplex PCR, which is designed to detect all four avian mycoplasma pathogens, has been described recently (27), but has not yet been validated with clinical samples.

At present these tests tend to be carried out by specialist laboratories and should probably be regarded as useful adjuncts to the present diagnostic methods until their validity has been firmly established. Great care needs to be taken to avoid contamination of samples with MG DNA from nearby culture laboratories or from positive amplificates from previous PCR runs. However the commercial kit referred to above is now licensed by the United States Department of Agriculture (USDA) as a diagnostic method and approved for use in the National Poultry Improvement Plan (NPIP).

Molecular methods are also available for differentiation of MG strains (14), but their usage also tends to be restricted at present to specialist laboratories.

2. Serological tests

The serological tests in common use may lack specificity and/or sensitivity; their use is advised for monitoring flocks rather than for testing individual birds.

The most commonly used tests are RSA, ELISA and HI, although several others have been described such as radioimmunoassay, microimmunofluorescence and indirect IP assay. Poultry companies using ELISA technology for screening large numbers of sera for virus antibodies may also find this type of assay convenient for mycoplasma testing (3, 5). The ELISA technology will not be described here because several MG kits are available commercially. Instead, the details of the HI test are provided as the reagents needed for this test are not commercially available.

a) Rapid serum agglutination test

Sera are collected from a sample of the flock and, if not tested immediately, stored at 4°C and not frozen. The number of sera to be tested depends on the level of detection and confidence limits required. The test should be carried out at room temperature within 72 hours of sera collection. Prior centrifugation will reduce nonspecific reactions. One volume (approximately 0.02 ml) of serum is dropped on to a white tile followed by one volume of stained MG antigen. The tile is rotated to ensure mixing. Agglutination is indicated by clumping within 2 minutes. Known positive and negative controls should be incorporated in the test. The antigens are available commercially but may vary in specificity and sensitivity from different manufacturers and from batch to batch. Any sera that agglutinate should be heated at 56°C for 30 minutes and retested. If they still react strongly, they are considered to be positive, especially if they do so on dilution (1/4 or more). A high proportion of positive sera in a flock (10% or more) indicates MG infection, especially if confirmed by HI test or ELISA. For further confirmation, the flock should be retested within a month. Inconclusive results make it necessary to attempt to isolate the organism. Doubtful results should be checked by performing tests with *M. synoviae* antigen as infection with this organism sometimes causes cross-reactions.

Tests can be conducted on yolk as well as sera although the yolk must first be diluted or extracted.

b) Haemagglutination inhibition test

MG is capable of haemagglutinating avian red blood cells (RBCs), and specific antibodies in sera cause inhibition. A strain should be selected that grows well and haemagglutinates reliably. The HI test requires a satisfactory haemagglutinating MG antigen, washed fresh chicken or turkey RBCs, and the test sera. The antigen can be either a fresh broth culture or a concentrated washed suspension of MG in PBS. It may be difficult to sustain a supply of high titred broth culture antigen; however, the use of concentrated antigen (usually containing 25–50% glycerol and stored at –70°C), increases the likelihood of nonspecific reactions.

The HI test follows well known procedures (1). The haemagglutination (HA) titre of the antigen is first determined in doubling dilutions, the HA unit being defined as the least amount of antigen giving complete HA in the test system employed. The HI test should be performed using 4 HA units by the following method or a method having equivalent sensitivity as determined by tests with known positive sera.

- **Test procedure**

All HA titrations and HI tests are best performed in multiwell plastic plates with V-shaped wells and using constant volumes of 50 µl. A positive and negative control serum are incorporated into each test. One row of eight wells is required for each serum under test. To the first well in each row, add 50 µl of PBS. To the second well in each row, add 8 HA units of antigen in 50 µl volumes, and to each of wells 3 to 8, add 50 µl of 4 HA units of antigen. A 1/5 dilution of serum under test, that has already been prepared, is added in a volume of 50 µl to the first well, mixed, and 50 µl are transferred to the second well, and so on, with 50 µl being discarded from the last well. The first well is the serum control well.

For the antigen control, six wells are required. To wells 2 to 6, inclusive, add 50 µl of PBS, and to wells 1 and 2, add 50 µl of the 8 HA unit antigen. Mix the contents of well 2 and transfer 50 µl to well 3, mix and repeat up to well 6, and discard 50 µl. For the RBC control, two wells are required, into each of which 50 µl of PBS is added. To all wells, add 50 µl of a 0.5% suspension of RBCs (chicken cells for chicken serum and turkey for turkey serum).

The plate is lightly shaken to ensure thorough mixing of the well contents, and is read after standing for approximately 50 minutes at room temperature or when the antigen titration is reading 4 HA units. For reading, the plate should be tilted and only those wells in which the RBCs 'stream' at the same time as those from wells with RBCs and diluent only, should be considered to be inhibited. The serum control should show a clear button of RBCs and the other controls should react as expected. The HI titre is the highest serum dilution exhibiting complete inhibition of HA.

Sera giving nonspecific HA must be adsorbed to remove all nonspecific haemagglutinins so that a clear button is obtained in the control well without HA antigen. The adsorption is carried out by incubating 1 ml of the serum dilution with 6–8 drops of packed washed chicken or turkey RBCs. The cells are removed after incubation at 37°C for 10 minutes, and the supernatant is tested for haemagglutinating activity.

c) Enzyme-linked immunosorbent assay

Several commercial MG antibody ELISA kits are marketed. The sensitivity is determined to some extent by the manufacturer's recommendations for the cut-off levels for positive and suspicious reactions. Sensitivity may sometimes be 'damped down', to avoid the well-known cross-reaction between MG and *M. synoviae*. One recently described blocking ELISA uses a monoclonal antibody (MAb) that recognises an epitope on a 56 kDa polypeptide of MG (7). In this system, ELISA plates are coated with whole cell MG antigen and the sera under test are added just as in the conventional indirect ELISA, but the reaction is assessed by the extent of blocking that occurs when the conjugated MAb is added. One advantage is that the system can be used for sera from any avian species without adaptation.

- **Preparation of *Mycoplasma gallisepticum* and *M. synoviae* antigens**

i) *Mycoplasma gallisepticum* antigens

Antigens are usually prepared from the S6 strain (32). Antigens prepared from other strains may also be used when necessary.

MG antigen for the RSA test: The methods of quality control described below apply solely to suspensions of MG stained with a suitable dye and containing preservative and intended for use in the rapid plate agglutination test with serum. Such antigens are available commercially.

On microscopic examination, the antigen should appear as a homogeneous suspension without floccules or precipitates. It must be free from contamination with bacteria and fungi. The pH must be between 6.5 and 7. It must be stored at 5±3°C and be warmed to room temperature before use.

The sensitivity and specificity of the antigen is determined with respect to its reaction with known positive sera of high and low titre and known negative sera. A positive reaction is recognised by the formation of coloured floccules and the clearing of the suspending medium. The criteria described above continue to apply until the expiry date declared by the manufacturer.

MG antigen for the HI test: The test is preferably performed with live, actively growing cultures. The antigen must be free from contamination with bacteria and fungi.

MG antigen for the ELISA: It may be difficult to prepare satisfactory antigen for use in the indirect ELISA without considerable prior experimentation and confirmation of sensitivity and specificity. Use of a reliable commercial kit is probably the best approach for most diagnostic laboratories. Some kits are now USDA-licensed and approved for use in the NPIP in the United States of America.

ii) *Mycoplasma synoviae* antigens

Antigens prepared from the WVU 1853 (23) strain or other suitable strains should be used.

Mycoplasma synoviae antigen for the RSA test: The specifications apply as for MG antigen for the RSA test.

Mycoplasma synoviae antigen for the HI test: The same specifications apply as for MG antigen for the HI test.

iii) Additional comments

Sera giving nonspecific reactions to the RSA test do not usually give a positive reaction in the HI test using live HA antigen. Positive RSA reactions can be confirmed by a HI test with sera taken after the first 2–3 weeks of infection (the time taken for HI antibodies to develop). However, the HI test tends to be strain specific (15) and therefore may lack sensitivity. ELISA may be a useful alternative.

Samples of serum should not be frozen before use in RSA tests. They should be free from haemolysis and contamination to avoid nonspecific reactions. The use of inactivated vaccines for other diseases may result in nonspecific reactions. Samples should be tested as soon as possible (within 72 hours) because mycoplasma antibodies may deteriorate on storage, even at –20°C. Sera may be inactivated at 56°C for 30 minutes.

B. REQUIREMENTS FOR VACCINES AND DIAGNOSTIC BIOLOGICALS

The preferred method of control is to maintain MG-free flocks. Vaccination should be considered only in situations where field exposure is inevitable, such as on multi-age sites. Potential exposure of neighbouring poultry flocks should also be carefully considered.

Two types of vaccines are available for the control of MG. These are mild to avirulent MG strains used as live vaccines, or inactivated oil-emulsion bacterins. The subject of MG vaccination has been reviewed by Whithear (28). Although there is antigenic variability among MG strains, it is thought that vaccination with a single strain is sufficient.

- **Live vaccines: methods of use**

The use of live vaccines is equivalent to 'controlled exposure'. The objective is to infect the flock with a mild, immunogenic MG strain at an age when little or no significant damage occurs. Such exposure results in resistance to challenge later in life, such as on multi-age commercial sites. Vaccinated birds are resistant to respiratory disease, airsacculitis, and egg-production drops caused by MG. Vaccination also results in reduced levels of egg transmission in breeders.

The F strain of MG has been the most commonly used vaccine strain (4). It is a naturally occurring strain of mild to moderate virulence for chickens, but it is virulent for turkeys. It ordinarily spreads slowly from bird to bird. When administered to healthy chickens via the upper respiratory tract, little or no respiratory reaction is observed. However, when administered by aerosol or in the presence of other respiratory disease agents, such as Newcastle disease or infectious bronchitis virus, respiratory signs and airsacculitis may result. Vaccinated chickens are permanent carriers, so a single dose is adequate. Use of F strain vaccine in each replacement flock on a multi-age site will eventually result in displacement of the field strain with the vaccine strain. Strains ts-11 and 6/85 (8, 29) are avirulent and spread to unvaccinated birds does not occur or occurs very poorly when birds are in very close contact (19).

Commercial pullets are usually vaccinated between 12 and 16 weeks of age, but vaccination of younger or older birds is permissible. It is essential that vaccination occurs before the flock is naturally infected. Vaccination in cases of probable early field exposure can be carried out in birds as young as 2–4 weeks of age. For the F strain, intranasal or eyedrop administration is preferred. Administration in the drinking water may result in some birds being missed unless the procedure is carried out properly. Aerosol administration should also be done carefully, so that all birds are exposed. A respiratory reaction should be expected at approximately 5–7 days after vaccination if aerosol administration is used. Vaccinated flocks should be tested with the agglutination test approximately 3–4 weeks post-vaccination to be sure that all birds were properly exposed. It is desirable that birds be vaccinated at an age when there is no reaction to other respiratory vaccines. Strain ts-11 should be administered by eyedrop, and 6/85 is given as a fine spray. Vaccination with ts-11 results in a low but distinctive serological response by RSA, HI and ELISA, but vaccination with 6/85 does not ordinarily result in a serological response. No post-vaccination reaction should be observed with 6/85 or ts-11. Flocks vaccinated with F strain or ts-11 are culture positive for the life of the flock, but 6/85 may be difficult to recover later than 4–6 weeks after vaccination.

Commercial live vaccines should be used within 1–2 hours after reconstitution. Lyophilised vaccine should be stored at 4°C. Some manufacturers supply the vaccine frozen. Such vaccine should be stored in liquid nitrogen, dry ice, or at –70°C or colder. Live MG vaccine is not stable for long periods at ordinary freezer temperatures. Storage for more than a few days at –20°C should be avoided.

Strains 6/85 and ts-11 are inherently safer than F strain, although the level of protection may be somewhat less, and may be useful as the primary vaccine strain on a multi-age site or as a 'second generation vaccine' on sites previously using F strain vaccine. They may also be preferred in situations where inadvertent exposure of neighbouring poultry flocks is of concern. F strain displaces wild-type MG more efficiently than either ts-11 or 6/85, but ts-11 has been used to eradicate F strain MG from a multi-age commercial egg production site (26). Multi-age sites where strain 6/85 is consistently used often test MG-negative, suggesting that it has displaced the wild-type strain.

Although no published information is available, live vaccines have also been used in some countries in broiler breeder pullets. In Australia, ts-11 live vaccine is being extensively used in broiler breeder pullets as well as in commercial layers. F strain vaccine has been used in broiler breeder pullets raised under multi-age conditions in some Latin American countries for several years; more recently there has been limited use of strains ts-11 and 6/85. Anecdotal evidence and personal experience regarding the performance of the breeders and respiratory disease in their broiler progeny, show that such vaccines have been useful and effective when properly applied. There has been limited use of the 6/85 strain as a vaccine for commercial turkeys in the United States of America. However, no good data on its effectiveness or safety are available; generally, vaccination of turkeys with live vaccines is not recommended. Vaccination of broilers with either live or inactivated vaccines has not been successful.

- **Inactivated vaccines: method of use**

MG bacterins are prepared from a concentrated suspension of whole cells that is emulsified into an oil adjuvant. A high antigen content is essential.

Bacterins are ordinarily used in commercial pullets to provide protection against egg-production drops, which occur after MG exposure on multi-age layer sites (11). They may also be used to reduce the level of egg transmission in breeder pullets (30). Use of bacterins in broilers is limited by the fact that birds vaccinated before 1–2 weeks of age are not protected. Although bacterins may provide protection against respiratory signs, airsacculitis, and egg-production losses, vaccinated flocks are readily infected. The duration of immunity is not known, but most flocks are exposed within 1–2 months after vaccination.

Administration is by the intramuscular or subcutaneous route, usually with a dose of 0.5 ml per bird. There is a risk that a persistent reaction at the site of vaccination will require trimming of carcasses of spent fowl vaccinated by the intramuscular route, so subcutaneous administration in the upper dorsal part of the neck is the most commonly used route. Two doses are preferred, but cost and labour considerations may dictate the use of a single dose, usually between 16 and 18 weeks of age for commercial pullets. A multidose syringe may be used.

All equipment should be cleaned and sterilised between flocks, and vaccination crews should exercise proper methods of biosecurity when travelling between flocks. Vaccine should be stored at 2–8°C up to the time of use. It should not be frozen or exposed to strong light.

1. Seed management

a) Characteristics of the seed

- **Live vaccine**

The vaccine strain should be immunogenic, have the ability to readily colonise the upper respiratory tract, and cause minimal damage to the respiratory system. A strong antibody response does not necessarily correlate with immunity.

The seed culture should be free from all extraneous agents. The culture should be cloned to ensure purity. If desired, restriction endonuclease patterns of the mycoplasmal DNA on agarose gels can be run to be sure of the identity and purity of the strain.

The seed culture should be stable with no tendency to revert to virulence. This can be confirmed with ten back passages in susceptible chickens. Contact chickens can be introduced at weekly intervals. If necessary, tracheal swabs can be taken from infected chickens and can then be inserted into the trachea of contact chickens. Transmission of the organism should be proven. The resulting isolate can then be used to challenge susceptible chickens.

- **Killed vaccine**

For killed vaccines the most important characteristics are high yield and good antigenicity. It is assumed, but not proven, that virulent strains are desirable. The seed culture should be free from all extraneous organisms.

b) Method of culture

The seed culture may be propagated in a medium similar to that described above. For live vaccines, the broth culture is lyophilised or frozen at –70°C or colder. For bacterins the culture must be concentrated and resuspended in a small volume of saline or PBS before the emulsion is prepared.

c) Validation as a vaccine

Data on efficacy should be obtained before bulk manufacture of vaccine begins. Chickens should be vaccinated by the same route that will be used in the field. Vaccinated birds should be challenged, and protection should be determined against respiratory signs, nasal discharge, and/or airsacculitis. Ideally, protection against egg-production losses should be evaluated, but such challenge trials are expensive and cumbersome.

Efficacy test: Groups of 20 specific pathogen free (SPF) or at least mycoplasma-free chickens, 2 weeks of age or older, are vaccinated by eyedrop or other route of administration with one field dose of live vaccine, or subcutaneously or intramuscularly with one dose (usually 0.5 ml) of bacterin. A similar group of unvaccinated chickens is maintained separately as controls. All chickens should be challenged with a 24-hour broth culture of a virulent strain of MG, 2–3 weeks post-vaccination. A simple challenge method is inoculation of 0.1 ml of the challenge culture into the posterior thoracic air sac. All birds are necropsied 7–10 days post-challenge, and air-sac lesions are scored. An alternative method is to challenge by inoculating 0.1 ml into the infraorbital sinus and examining the birds for nasal discharge from 7 to 14 days post-challenge.

2. Method of manufacture

The vaccine must be manufactured in suitable clean and secure accommodation, well separated from diagnostic facilities or commercial poultry. Special care must be taken to avoid MG contamination of other products manufactured in the same facility.

Production of vaccine should be on a seed-lot system, using a suitable MG strain of known origin, passage history, and purity. The growth medium is similar to that given above. The serum used in the growth medium should be inactivated at 56°C to prevent contamination with any mycoplasmal organism that may be present, and filter sterilised. A source of SPF serum is desirable.

Broth medium is inoculated, with a rapidly growing inoculum, at a rate of approximately 5% (v/v). Incubation is at 37°C. Production can be in batches using large flasks or in a fermenter. In batch cultures, harvest is approximately 24 hours after inoculation. Live vaccines are preserved by lyophilisation or by freezing at –70°C, in liquid nitrogen, or on dry ice.

For bacterin production, the antigen must be concentrated, usually by centrifugation, ultrafiltration, or other suitable method. Bacterins are made as water-in-oil emulsions, typically 80% mineral oil, 20% aqueous, with suitable emulsifying agents.

3. In-process control

Antigen content: At harvest, the titre should be from 10^8 to 10^9 CFU/ml. The antigen concentration of bacterins is difficult to standardise but may be based on packed cell volume, which is typically 1% (v/v) packed cells in the final product.

Inactivation of killed vaccines: Inactivation is frequently done with either beta-propiolactone or formaldehyde. The inactivating agent and the inactivation procedure must be shown under the conditions of vaccine manufacture to inactivate the vaccine organism and potential contaminants.

Prior to inactivation, care should be taken to ensure a homogeneous suspension free from particles that may not be penetrated by the inactivating agent. A test for inactivation should be carried out by culture in mycoplasma broth on each batch of both the bulk harvest after inactivation and the final product. No evidence of growth of mycoplasma should be observed.

Sterility of killed vaccines: Oil used in the vaccine must be sterilised by heating at 160°C for 1 hour, or by filtration, and the procedure must be shown to be effective. Tests appropriate to oil-emulsion vaccines are carried out on each batch of final vaccine as described, for example, in the British Pharmacopoeia (Veterinary) 1985.

4. Batch control

a) Sterility

Tests for sterility and freedom from contamination of biological materials may be found in Chapter I.4.

b) Safety

- **Live vaccine safety test**

The birds vaccinated in the efficacy test given above can be used to evaluate the safety of the vaccine.

- **Killed vaccine safety test**

Birds vaccinated in the efficacy test described above may be observed for adverse local or systemic effects.

c) Potency

Potency tests for both live and killed vaccine can be conducted by the procedures given above for the efficacy test. The titre of live vaccines should be sufficient to induce infection by the route recommended; 10^5 CFU/dose is sufficient for eyedrop administration of live F strain vaccine. The recommended dose of ts-11 is $\geq 10^{7.7}$ colour changing units (CCU)/dose; with 6/85, a dose of 10^4 organisms/dose was ineffective, but a dose of 10^7 live organisms or 10^8 organisms from a lyophilised preparation provided significant protection (8).

d) Duration of immunity (killed vaccine)

Because flocks are generally exposed within 1–2 months after vaccination, duration of immunity is not a primary consideration. After field challenge, resistance is considered to be permanent.

e) Stability

Evidence should be provided on three batches of vaccine to show that the vaccine passes the batch potency test at 3 months beyond the requested shelf life.

f) Preservatives

A preservative is normally required for vaccine in multidose containers. The concentration of the preservative in the final vaccine and its persistency throughout the shelf life should be checked.

A suitable preservative that has already been established for such purposes should be used. Mycoplasmas are susceptible to many antibacterials except for penicillins; such antibiotics should not be included as preservatives.

g) Precautions (hazards)

Oil-emulsion vaccines cause serious injury to the vaccinator if accidentally injected into the hand or other tissues. In the event of such an accident, the person should go at once to a hospital, taking the vaccine package with him or her. Each vaccine bottle and package should be clearly marked with a warning of the serious consequences of accidental self-injection. Such wounds should be treated by the casualty doctor as a 'grease gun injury'.

5. Tests on the final product

a) Safety

See Section B.4.b.

b) Potency

See Section B.4.c.

REFERENCES

1. ALLAN W.H. & GOUGH R.E. (1974). A standard haemagglutination test for Newcastle Disease. 1. A comparison of macro and micro methods. *Vet. Rec.*, **95**, 120–123.

2. BRADBURY J.M., ALDUL-WAHAB O.M.S., YAVARI C.A., DUPIELLET J.P. & BOVE J.M. (1993). *Mycoplasma imitans* sp. nov. is related to *Mycoplasma gallisepticum* and found in birds. *Int. J. Syst. Bacteriol.*, **43**, 721–728.

3. BROWN M.B., DAVIS J.K. & BRADBURY J.M. (1996). ELISA: in small animal hosts, rodents, birds. *In:* Molecular and Diagnostic Procedures in Mycoplasmology. Volume II, Diagnostic Procedures, Tully J.G. & Razin S., eds. Academic Press, New York, USA and London, UK, 93–104.

4. CARPENTER T.E., MALLINSON E.T., MILLER K.F., GENTRY R.F. & SCHWARTZ L.D. (1981). Vaccination with F-strain *Mycoplasma gallisepticum* to reduce production losses in layer chickens. *Avian Dis.*, **25**, 404–409.

5. CASSELL G.H. & BROWN M.B. (1983). Enzyme-linked immunosorbent assay (ELISA) for detection of antimycoplasmal antibody. *In:* Methods in Mycoplasmology, Vol. 1, Razin S. & Tully J.G., eds. Academic Press, New York, USA and London, UK, 457–469.

6. CLYDE W.A. Jr. (1983). Growth inhibition tests. *In:* Methods in Mycoplasmology, Vol. 1, Razin S. & Tully J.G., eds. Academic Press, New York, USA and London, UK, 405–410.

7. CZIFRA G., SUNDQUIST B., TUBOLY T. & STIPKOVITS L. (1993). Evaluation of a monoclonal blocking enzyme-linked immunosorbent assay for the detection of *Mycoplasma gallisepticum*-specific antibodies. *Avian Dis.*, **37**, 680–688.

8. EVANS R.D. & HAFEZ Y.S. (1992). Evaluation of a *Mycoplasma gallisepticum* strain exhibiting reduced virulence for prevention and control of poultry mycoplasmosis. *Avian Dis.*, **36**, 197–201.

9. FREUNDT E.A. (1983). Culture media for classic mycoplasmas. *In:* The Mycoplasmas, Vol 1, Razin S. & Tully J.G., eds. Academic Press, New York, USA and London, UK, 127–135.

10. GANAPATHY K. & BRADBURY J.M. (1998). Pathogenicity of *Mycoplasma gallisepticum* and *Mycoplasma imitans* in red-legged partridges *(Alectoris rufa)*. *Avian Pathol.*, **27**, 455–463.

11. HILDEBRAND D.C., PAGE D.E. & BERG J.R. (1983). *Mycoplasma gallisepticum* (MG). Laboratory and field studies evaluating the safety and efficacy of an inactivated MG bacterin. *Avian Dis.*, **27**, 792–802.

12. JORDAN F.T.W. (1979). Avian mycoplasmas. *In:* The Mycoplasmas, Vol. II, Tully J.G. & Whitcob R.F., eds. Academic Press, New York, USA, and London, UK, 1–48.

13. JORDAN F.T.W. (1996). Avian mycoplasmosis. *In:* Poultry Diseases, Fourth Edition, Jordan F.T.W. & Pattison M., eds. W.B. Saunders, London, UK, 81–93.

14. KEMPF I. (1998). DNA amplification methods for diagnosis and epidemiological investigations of avian mycoplasmosis. *Avian Pathol.*, **27**, 7–14.

15. KLEVEN S.H., MORROW C.J. & WHITHEAR K.G. (1988). Comparison of *Mycoplasma gallisepticum* strains by hemagglutination-inhibition and restriction endonuclease analysis. *Avian Dis.*, **32**, 731–741.

16. KOTANI H.& MCGARRITY G.J. (1985). Rapid and simple identification of mycoplasmas by immunobinding. *J. Immunol. Methods*, **85**, 225–267.

17. LAUERMAN L.H. (1998). Nucleic Acid Amplification Assays for Diagnosis of Animal Diseases. American Association of Veterinary Laboratory Diagnosticians, 39–66.

18. LEY D.H., BERKHOFF J.E. & MCLAREN J.M. (1996). *Mycoplasma gallisepticum* isolated from house finches *(Carpodacus mexicanus)* with conjunctivitis. *Avian Dis.*, **40**, 480–483.

19. LEY D.H., MCLAREN J.M., MILES A.M., BARNES H.J., HEINS MILLER S. & FRANZ G. (1997). Transmissibility of live *Mycoplasma gallisepticum* vaccine strains ts-11 and 6/85 from vaccinated layer pullets to sentinel poultry. *Avian Dis.*, **41**, 187–194.

20. LEY D.H. & YODER H.W. Jr. (1997). *Mycoplasma gallisepticum* infection. *In:* Diseases of Poultry, Tenth Edition, Calnek B.W., Barnes H.J., Beard C.W., McDougald L.R. & Saif Y.M., eds. Iowa State University Press, USA, 194–207.

21. LUTTRELL M.P., FISCHER J.R., STALLKNECHT D.E. & KLEVEN S.H. (1996). Field investigation of *Mycoplasma gallisepticum* infections in house finches *(Carpodacus mexicanus)* from Maryland and Georgia. *Avian Dis.*, **40**, 335–341.

22. MALLINSON E.T., ECKROADE R.J. & KLEVEN S.H. (1981). *In vivo* bioassay and supplemental serological techniques for the detection of mycoplasma in suspect breeding chickens. *Avian Dis.*, **25**, 1077–1082.

23. OLSON N.O., KERR K.M. & CAMPBELL A. (1964). Control of infectious synovitis. 13. The antigen study of 3 strains. *Avian Dis.*, **8**, 209–215.

24. ROSENDAL S. & BLACK F.T. (1972). Direct and indirect immunofluorescence of unfixed and fixed mycoplasma colonies. *Acta Pathol. Microbiol. Scand. [B]*, **80**, 615–622.

25. TULLY J.G. (1995). Culture medium formulation for primary isolation and maintenance of mollicutes. *In:* Molecular and Diagnostic Procedures in Mycoplasmology. Volume 1, Molecular Characterization, Razin S. & Tully J.G., eds. Academic Press, New York, USA, and London, UK, 29–32.

26. TURNER K.S. & KLEVEN S.H. (1998). Eradication of live F strain *Mycoplasma gallisepticum* vaccine using live ts-11 on a multiage commercial layer farm. *Avian Dis.*, **42**, 404–407.

27. WANG H., FADL A.A. & KHAN M.I. (1997). Multiplex PCR for avian pathogenic mycoplasmas. *Mol. Cell. Probes*, **11**, 211–216.

28. WHITHEAR K.G. (1996). Control of avian mycoplasmoses by vaccination. *Rev. sci. tech. Off. int. Epiz.*, **15**, 1527–1553.

29. WHITHEAR K.G., SOERIPTO, HARRICAN K.E. & GHIOCAS E. (1990). Immunogenicity of a temperature sensitive mutant *Mycoplasma gallisepticum* vaccine. *Aust. Vet. J.*, **67**, 168–174.

30. YODER H.W. Jr. (1979). Serologic response of chickens vaccinated with inactivated preparations of *Mycoplasma gallisepticum*. *Avian Dis.*, **23**, 493–506.

31. ZAIN M.Z. & BRADBURY J.M. (1996). Optimising the conditions for the isolation of *Mycoplasma gallisepticum* collected on applicator swabs. *Vet. Microbiol.*, **49**, 45–57.

32. ZANDER D.V. (1961). Origin of the S6 strain of mycoplasma. *Avian Dis.*, **5**, 154–156.

*

* *

CHAPTER 2.7.4.

AVIAN CHLAMYDIOSIS

SUMMARY

Avian chlamydiosis (AC) is caused by the bacterium Chlamydophila psittaci. *AC occurring in humans and all birds was originally called psittacosis, but later the term ornithosis was introduced to differentiate the disease contracted from or occurring in domestic and wildfowl from the disease contracted from or occurring in psittacine birds. These diseases are similar when contracted by humans. The genus* Chlamydia *was recently divided into two genera,* Chlamydia *and* Chlamydophila. *All known avian strains are now in the species* Chlamydophila psittaci. *Chlamydiosis is still the term used for diseases produced by both genera. The avian strains include at least six serotypes that correlate with the avian species from which they are usually isolated. Chlamydiosis as it occurs naturally in mammalian species and not contracted from avian species, is caused by distinctly different strains of the organism.*

Depending on the chlamydial serovar and the avian host, chlamydiae cause pericarditis, airsacculitis, pneumonia, lateral nasal adenitis, peritonitis, hepatitis, and splenitis. Generalised infections result in fever, anorexia, lethargy, diarrhoea, and occasionally shock and death. Special laboratory handling is recommended because avian chlamydial strains can cause serious illness and possibly death in humans in both laboratory and natural conditions. The disease in ducks and turkeys is of particular concern as transmission to humans is common during handling and slaughter of the birds. Chlamydiosis contracted from these sources can cause severe pneumonia and even death. The diagnosis of AC requires the isolation and identification of the organism, the demonstration of chlamydiae in tissues, or the demonstration of a four-fold increase in specific humoral antibody, as well as typical clinical signs. A tentative diagnosis can be made in a flock that includes birds with clinical signs of AC as well as a high incidence of birds with high antibody levels.

Identification of the agent: *Isolation of chlamydiae requires the inoculation of embryonated eggs, laboratory animals, or cell cultures, and testing for chlamydiae by cytochemical stains or immunohistochemical methods. The isolation of avian chlamydiae has been done by the yolk sac inoculation of 6–7-day-old developing chick embryos; the yolk sac membranes from dead embryos are examined for chlamydiae. This is often done either by using impression smears stained with cytochemical stains, or by repassage in tissue culture and subsequent testing for chlamydial inclusions by immunofluorescence or immunoperoxidase techniques. Samples must be blind passaged three times in eggs before being considered negative.*

The direct inoculation of samples into cell cultures of buffalo green monkey (BGM), African green monkey kidney (Vero), McCoy, or L cells is preferable. Cell cultures are as sensitive for the isolation of most avian strains of chlamydiae as are chicken embryos. To enhance the infectivity of samples, a preferred method is the centrifugation of the inoculum on to monolayers and addition of cell-division inhibitors, such as cycloheximide. The cell cultures are then stained by direct immunofluorescence or by other appropriate stains at appropriate times to demonstrate the presence of inclusions. One or two blind passages are usually done before the sample is considered to be negative.

Enzyme-linked immunosorbent assays (ELISAs) developed for detecting trachomatis antigen in humans have been used for diagnosing chlamydiae in birds. Many of the earlier tests were developed using monoclonal or polyclonal antisera against lipopolysaccharide epitopes, some of which were shared with other Gram-negative bacteria. Their use when screening individual birds is questionable, as their sensitivity and specificity for use with avian samples has not been proven.

Their main value is in confirming chlamydiosis in a bird showing signs of disease. However, these tests have not been approved and licensed for use in testing birds.

Polymerase chain reaction/restriction fragment length polymorphism (PCR-RFLP) and immunohistochemical staining of histological sections are two new techniques showing much promise for the future. Both of these are very rapid, can be readily performed, and do not require the live agent. The current PCR tests for avian strains target the MOMP gene, which allows species differentiation. However, PCR targeting ribosomal RNA genes (16S–23S) may provide a system that will amplify all chlamydial strains and allow identification at the level of the chlamydial species. PCR has the potential to be highly specific and sensitive, and it can be performed on most tissues, including retrospective PCR testing of formalin-fixed sections. There has been an increase in the use of immunohistochemical staining of histological sections because of the recent development and availability of automated staining equipment. It has the advantage that most diagnostic laboratories routinely collect materials for H&E (haematoxylin and eosin)-stained sections, and extra sections can easily be cut at the time or retrospectively be cut for immunohistochemical staining.

***Serological tests:** The standard serological test for chlamydial antibodies is the complement fixation (CF) test. The antigen is a group-reactive lipopolysaccharide antigen present in all strains. The CF test is often used to examine a flock for chlamydial infection. The occurrence of high CF titres in the majority of individuals in a flock with clinical signs is presumptive evidence of active infection. The demonstration of a four-fold increase in titre in an individual bird is considered to be diagnostic of a current infection.*

Other serological tests, such as the ELISA, latex agglutination, elementary body agglutination, micro-immunofluorescence, and the agar gel immunodiffusion tests are available. These tests are of value in specific cases and may replace the CF test; however, comparisons of reliability and reproducibility are not yet available.

***Requirements for vaccines and diagnostic biologicals:** There are no commercial vaccines available for chlamydiosis control in poultry. Antibiotics are the only current means of control.* Chlamydophila psittaci *is susceptible to a number of antibiotics. The drug of choice varies from country to country. Chlortetracyclines and doxycycline are the antibiotics most commonly used in the pet bird industry.*

A. DIAGNOSTIC TECHNIQUES

Avian chlamydiosis (AC) is caused by the bacterium *Chlamydophila psittaci*. The disease in birds was originally called psittacosis, but the term ornithosis was introduced later to differentiate the disease in domestic and wild fowl from the disease in psittacine birds. The two syndromes are currently considered to be the same (5). Their earlier separation was based on the assumption that in humans ornithosis was a milder disease than psittacosis. However, it should be noted that the disease in humans contracted from turkeys and ducks is often as severe as that contracted from psittacine birds.

Chlamydophila psittaci produces a systemic and occasionally fatal disease in birds. The clinical signs vary greatly in severity and depend on the species and age of the bird and the strain of chlamydia. AC can produce lethargy, hyperthermia, abnormal excretions, nasal and eye discharges, and reduced egg production. Mortality rates will vary greatly. In pet birds the most frequent clinical signs are anorexia and weight loss, diarrhoea, yellowish droppings, sinusitis and respiratory distress (25). Many birds, especially older psittacine birds, may show no clinical signs; nevertheless, they may often shed the agent for extended periods. Necropsy of affected birds will often reveal spleen and liver enlargement, fibrinous airsacculitis, pericarditis and peritonitis (5, 38).

The severity of disease in turkeys depends on the chlamydial strain and the presence of other diseases. Serovar D strains are usually the most severe and are particularly hazardous for poultry workers. At the peak of disease in a flock infected with serovar D strains, 50–80% of the birds can show clinical signs and mortality is often 10–30% (5). In broiler turkeys, mortality rates as high as 80% have been reported (39). Strains of other serovars, such as serovars B and E, often have morbidity rates of 5–20% and mortality rates of under 50%.

Clinical signs and necropsy lesions in turkeys vary greatly. Turkeys infected with the highly virulent strains show cachexia, anorexia, and elevated temperatures. The birds will excrete yellow-green gelatinous droppings. In laying hens, egg production will drop rapidly and remain low until recovery is complete. In broiler turkeys, a respiratory syndrome having the characteristics of rhinotracheitis has been reported. Signs included are conjuctivitis, swelling of the infra-orbital sinuses and sneezing. In turkeys infected with strains of low virulence, the disease signs are milder and usually include anorexia and, in some birds, loose green droppings. Characteristic lesions on necropsy of birds infected with the virulent strain include enlarged spleen and liver, and a fibrinous to fibropurulent exudate on respiratory, peritoneal, and pericardial surfaces. The lesions can include sinusitis, tracheitis, airsacculitis, pneumonia, and enteritis. Pneumonia is usually seen only in birds that die of the infection. The lesions in birds infected with the low virulence strains are similar, but not as extensive or severe.

Chlamydiosis in ducks is important both economically and as a public health hazard in a number of parts of the world. The disease is usually severe with morbidity as high as 80% and mortality ranging from 0 to 40% depending on the age of the ducks and the presence of concurrent infections (5). Clinical signs include head tremors, unsteady gait, conjunctivitis, serous to purulent nasal discharge, depression and death. On necropsy, enlarged spleens, focal necrosis of the liver, fibrinous polyserositis, and pneumonia are common. In recent years, a mild form has been recognised in which disease signs are minimal or absent, and death is associated only with stress of handling or with other disease. Human infections have been known to occur following handling or slaughter of both clinically and inapparently infected birds.

The family Chlamydiaceae was recently reclassified into two genera and nine species based on sequence analysis of its 16s and 23s rRNA genes (15). The two new genera, *Chlamydia* and *Chlamydophila*, correlate with the former species *C. trachomatis* and *C. psittaci.* The genus *Chlamydia* includes *C. trachomatis* (human), *C. suis* (swine), and *C. muridarum* (mouse, hamster). The genus *Chlamydophila* includes *C. psittaci* (avian), *C. felis* (cats), *C. abortus* (sheep, goats, cattle), *C. caviae* (guinea pigs), and the former species *C. pecorum* (sheep, cattle) and *C. pneuminiae* (human).

The two genera and nine species have merit both molecularly and for classification of host range and clinical disease. The species show a high degree of correlation with host range, disease syndrome, and virulence, and thus provide an understanding of the epidemiology of the various species and serovars affecting livestock and birds. The terms 'chlamydiosis' and 'chlamydia(e)' are used as generic terms to refer to members of either and both genera. However, the new scientific names are used when referring to a specific chlamydial species.

The avian strains all belong to the species *Chlamydophila psittaci.* This species includes six known avian serovars, and two mammalian serovars, M56 from muskrats and WC from cattle. M56 and WC were each isolated from a single outbreak. The six avian serovars are labelled A through F and each shows host specificity. The hosts that each serovar has been associated with are: A, psittacine birds; B, pigeons; C, ducks and geese; D, turkeys; E, pigeons and ratites; and F is a single isolate from a psittacine bird. What is not known is how many of these birds and mammals are the natural hosts of the serovars.

The strains of avian chlamydiae can infect humans and should be handled carefully under conditions of biocontainment (12). Most infections occur through inhalation of infectious aerosols. Post-mortem examinations of infected birds and handling of cultures should be done in laminar flow hoods or with proper protective equipment. Human infection can result from transient exposures. The incubation period is usually 5–14 days; however, longer incubation periods are known. Human infections vary from inapparent to severe systemic disease with pneumonia and encephalitis. The disease is rarely fatal in properly treated patients; therefore, awareness of the danger and early diagnosis are important. Infected humans typically develop headache, chills, malaise and myalgia, with or without signs of respiratory involvement. Pulmonary involvement is common; auscultatory findings, however, may appear to be normal or to underestimate the extent of involvement. Diagnosis can be difficult and is usually established through testing paired sera for antibodies to chlamydia by the complement fixation (CF) test. In humans tetracycline, doxycycline, or azithromycin are usually the drugs of choice unless contraindicated. The length of treatment will vary with the drug, but should be continued for at least 14 days for tetracycline.

1. Identification of the agent

The preferred method for the identification of AC is the isolation and identification of the organism. Because of the time involved, the need for high quality samples, and the hazard to laboratory personnel, other techniques are often used. These include histochemical staining of smears of exudate and faeces, and impression smears of tissues, immunohistochemical staining of cytological and histological preparations, antigen-capture enzyme-linked immunosorbent assays (ELISA), PCR and PCR-RFLP.

a) Collection and treatment of samples

The samples to be collected will depend on the disease signs in evidence. They must be taken aseptically. Contaminant bacteria may interfere with the isolation of the chlamydiae. Specimens from acute cases should include inflammatory or fibrinous exudate in or around organs that display lesions, ocular and nasal exudates, whole blood and tissue samples from kidney, lung, pericardium, spleen, and liver. In cases with diarrhoea, colon contents or excrement should be cultured. In live birds, the preferred samples are pharyngeal and nasal swabs (2). Intestinal excrement, cloacal swabs, conjunctival scrapings, and peritoneal exudate can also be taken.

Proper handling of clinical samples is necessary to prevent loss of infectivity of chlamydiae during shipping and storage. A special medium consisting of sucrose/phosphate/glutamate (SPG) was developed for rickettsiae and has proven to be satisfactory for transport of chlamydial field samples. The medium as recommended for chlamydiae (34) consists of SPG buffer: sucrose (74.6 g/litre); KH_2PO_4 (0.512 g/litre); K_2HPO_4 (1.237 g/litre); and L-glutamic acid (0.721 g/litre), which can be sterilised by autoclaving or filtering. Added to this are fetal calf serum (10%), vancomycin and streptomycin (200–500 µg/ml), nystatin and gentamicin (50 µg/ml). The addition of antibiotics reduces the effect of contamination, even when samples are shipped at ambient temperatures. This medium can also be used as a laboratory diluent and for freezing of chlamydiae.

Contaminated samples must be pretreated before being used to inoculate animals or cell cultures. There are three basic methods: treatment with antibiotics (7, 8), treatment with antibiotics together with low speed centrifugation (4, 5), and treatment with antibiotics with filtration (4, 7, 8, 11). A number of antibiotics that do not inhibit chlamydia can be used. Samples are homogenised in phosphate buffered saline (PBS), pH 7.2, containing a maximum of the following: streptomycin (1 mg/ml), vancomycin (1 mg/ml), and kanamycin (1 mg/ml). Gentamicin (200 µg/ml) can be used. Amphotericin B (50 µg/ml) can be added to control yeast and fungal growth. Other antibiotic solutions are often used. Penicillin, tetracycline and chloramphenicol should be avoided, as these inhibit the growth of chlamydiae.

When contamination is light, samples should be homogenised in an antibiotic solution prior to inoculation into chicken embryos, guinea-pigs, mice or tissue cultures. Samples are often left to stand in the antibiotic solution for 24 hours at 5°C before inoculation. Heavily contaminated samples, such as faecal samples, should be homogenised in antibiotics and then centrifuged at 500 ***g*** for 20 minutes. The surface layer and the bottom layer are discarded. The supernatant fluid is collected and recentrifuged. The final supernatant fluid is used for inoculation. Samples should be passed through a filter of 450–800 µm average pore size if contamination persists.

b) Isolation in cell culture

Cell cultures are the most convenient method for the isolation of *C. psittaci*. Cell lines are satisfactory, the more common ones being buffalo green monkey (BGM), McCoy, HeLa, African green monkey kidney (Vero), and L cells (37). The cells are grown as monolayers, using standard tissue culture media containing 5–10% fetal calf serum and antibiotics that are not inhibitory to chlamydia (see above).

When selecting cell culture equipment, it is important to remember that:

i) Chlamydiae can be identified by direct immunofluorescence or some other appropriate staining technique;

ii) The inoculum is usually centrifuged on to the monolayer to enhance its infectivity;

iii) The sample may need to be blind passaged at 5–6 days to increase sensitivity of isolation;

iv) The sample will need to be examined from two to three times during any one passage; and

v) Chlamydia can be infectious to humans.

Small flat-bottomed vials, such as 1 dram (3.7 ml, 15 × 45 mm) shell vials or bottles containing cover-slips that are 12 mm in diameter, will meet these requirements (7, 8, 11). A number of vials, often four to six, are inoculated with each sample to permit fixing and staining at various intervals, and to permit repassaging of apparently negative samples 6 days after inoculation. When testing multiple samples, 96-well multiwell dishes can also be used as they have a labour-saving advantage. However, it should be noted that cross-contamination between samples can be a problem.

Chlamydiae can be isolated from cells that are replicating normally, but the use of nonreplicating cells is preferable as these may provide increased nutrients for the growth of chlamydiae. Suppressed cells can also be observed for longer periods. Host cell division can be suppressed either by irradiation or, more commonly, by cytotoxic chemicals. The latter include 5-iodo-2-deoxyuridine, cyto-cholasin B, cycloheximide, and emetine hydrochloride (30). Cycloheximide is the most commonly used and can be added to the medium at the rate of 0.5–2.0 µg/ml at the time of inoculation of the monolayer. Emetine is removed after treatment and replaced by medium (4, 5, 7, 8). The monolayer is first treated for 5 minutes with emetine (0.5 µg/ml), after which the emetine is removed and replaced with culture medium; the monolayer is then ready for use. The growth of most chlamydial strains will be enhanced by the treatment of the monolayer by one of these drugs; the treatment will have no effect on the growth of other strains.

Attachment of chlamydia to cells is increased by centrifuging the inoculum on to the monolayer at 500–1500 *g* for 30–90 minutes at 37°C. The inoculum is removed and replaced with tissue culture medium containing a cell-division inhibitor, and then incubated at 37–39°C. Cultures must be examined for chlamydiae at regular intervals using an appropriate staining method. This is usually done on day 2 or 3, as well as on day 5 or 6. Cultures that appear to be negative at the sixth day are harvested and repassaged. When repassaging chlamydiae, freeze–thawing should not be used to disrupt cells as this may destroy the chlamydiae.

Before staining the cultures, the medium is first removed, the cultures are washed with PBS and fixed with acetone for 2–10 minutes. The fixation time will depend on the tissue culture vessel used. As acetone will soften most plastics, the use of a mixture of 50% acetone and 50% methyl alcohol may be preferable. A number of staining methods can be employed to demonstrate chlamydial inclusions. The preferred method is direct immunofluorescence (4, 7, 26). A chlamydial fluorescein-conjugated antiserum is applied to the infected cells and incubated in a humid chamber for 30 minutes at 37°C. The cover-slips are then washed three times with PBS, air-dried, mounted, and examined. Chlamydial inclusions fluoresce a green colour. Commercial conjugate preparations using MAbs are available and are highly specific. Conjugates may also be prepared from polyclonal sera, but it is important to obtain specific, high-titred antisera. Polyclonal antisera can be prepared in rabbits, guinea-pigs, sheep or goats. Sheep and goats are excellent sources because of the volume and high titres that are readily obtained following infection. Conjugates are then prepared using standard techniques (4, 5, 7).

Chlamydial inclusions can also be demonstrated by indirect fluorescent antibody and immunoperoxidase techniques (4, 6, 26). Direct staining can be done with Gimenez, Giemsa, Ziehl–Neelsen, or Macchiavello's stains. Except for immunofluorescence, all these stains have the advantage that standard light microscopes can be used.

c) Isolation in eggs

Chicken embryos are still used for the primary isolation of chlamydiae. The standard procedure is to inject up to 0.5 ml of inoculum into the yolk sac of a 6–7-day-old embryo (5). The eggs are then incubated in a humid atmosphere at 39°C, rather than at 37°C, as multiplication of chlamydia is greatly increased at the higher temperature. Replication of the organism usually causes the death of the embryo within 3–10 days. If no deaths occur, two additional blind passages are usually made before designating any sample as negative. Chlamydial infections will give rise to a typical vascular congestion of the yolk sac membranes. These are harvested and homogenised as a 20% (w/v) suspension in SPG buffer, and can be frozen to preserve the strain, or inoculated into eggs or on to cell cultures.

The organism can be identified by preparing an antigen from an infected yolk sac and testing it by direct staining of smears using appropriate stains or by using the antigen in a serological test. Cell culture monolayers can be inoculated with the yolk sac suspension and examined by direct immunofluorescence 48–72 hours later for the presence of chlamydial inclusions. Typical inclusions are intracytoplasmic, round, or hat-shaped bodies. With some virulent strains, the inclusions rapidly break up and the chlamydial antigen is dispersed throughout the cytoplasm.

d) Differentiating among species/strains

All avian isolates are in the *Chlamydophila psittaci* group, as discussed earlier (15). The avian strains can be differentiated from other chlamydiae by PCR-RFLP of either the MOMP gene or the 16S–23S rDNA operon. A provisional *C. psittaci* determination can be made using the source of the isolate and serovar-specific MAbs.

The avian strains of *C. psittaci* contain a number of specific serotypes (1, 3, 4). The syndromes caused by the various strains are quite specific; the natural host range of a particular strain may also be fairly specific. There are at least six serotypes that infect birds. These are labelled A through F. The hosts from which they are mainly isolated are: serotype A, psittacine birds; serotype B, pigeons; serotype C, ducks; serotype D, turkeys; serotype E, pigeons and ratites; and one isolate of serotype F from a psittacine bird.

Serovar-specific MAbs to the six serotypes have been developed and are being used by a limited number of laboratories to serotype new isolates (1, 3). PCR-RFLP techniques have been developed that will also differentiate the strains (33, 36). Again the use is mainly experimental with only a limited number of laboratories using either the PCR-RFLP technique or serovar-specific MAbs. Serotyping is relatively easy to perform and laboratories that need it can easily set up the procedures.

e) Histochemical staining

Giemsa, Giminez, Ziehl–Neelsen and Macchiavello's stains are commonly used to detect chlamydiae in smears of liver and spleen. The following modified Giminez technique is used by several laboratories (4).

- **Modified Giminez technique or (Pierce-van der Kamp) stain**
- *Reagents:*

  Solution 1: Distilled H_2O (450.0 ml) and phenol (5.0 ml) added to basic fuchsin (2.5 g) and 95% ethanol (50.0 ml). Incubate at 37°C for 48 hours. Filter and store in the dark at room temperature.

  Solution 2: Na_2HPO_4 (11.65 g); $NaH_2PO_4 \cdot H_2O$ (2.47 g); distilled H_2O, pH 7.5 (to 1.0 litre).

  Solution 3: Solution 1 (20.0 ml); and solution 2 (25.0 ml). Let stand for 10 minutes, filter and use.

  Solution 4: 0.5% citric acid.

  Solution 5: Fast green (0.2 g); distilled H_2O (100.0 ml); and glacial acetic acid (0.2 ml).

  Solution 6: Solution 5 (20.0 ml); and distilled H_2O (50.0 ml).

- *Procedure for smears is as follows:*

i) Fix in methanol for 5 minutes.

ii) Stain in Solution 3 for 10 minutes and rinse in tap water.

iii) Counterstain in Solution 6 for 2 minutes.

iv) Rinse in tap water and air-dry.

- *Procedure for paraffin sections is as follows:*

i) Deparaffinise and hydrate with distilled H_2O.

ii) Stain in Solution 3 for 10 minutes and rinse in tap water.

iii) Dip in Solution 4 until no more red runs out of the section. Rinse in tap water.

iv) Counterstain in Solution 6 for 20 dips.

v) Dip in two changes of 95% alcohol, for five dips each. Dehydrate, clear, and mount.

Chlamydiae will appear red against a green background.

f) Immunohistochemical staining

Immunohistochemical staining can be used to detect chlamydiae in cytological and histological preparations. The technique is more sensitive than histochemical staining, but some experience is necessary as cross-reactions with some bacteria and fungi require that morphology must be considered.

Most widely used immunohistochemical staining procedures can be adapted to give satisfactory results. The selection of the primary antibody is very important. Both polyclonal and monoclonal antibodies have been used. Because formalin does affect chlamydial antigens, it is recommended that polyclonal antibodies be made to purified formalin-inactivated chlamydiae. The chlamydial strain used is not important as the antibodies will be mainly to the group-reactive antigens. MAbs should also be selected for reactions to formalin-fixed chlamydia. A pool of group-reactive MAbs can be used.

g) Enzyme-linked immunosorbent assays

The ELISA is a relatively new technique that has been extensively promoted as kits for use in the diagnosis of human chlamydiosis. These test kits detect the lipopolysaccharide (LPS) antigen (group reactive) and will detect all species of chlamydiae. A number of these kits have been tested for use in detecting chlamydia in birds (40), but none of the kits has been licensed for detection of *C. psittaci*. One problem with some of these tests is that the chlamydial LPS shares some epitopes with other Gram-negative bacteria, and these epitopes can cross-react, resulting in a high number of false-positive results. This problem has been reduced or eliminated in more recently developed kits by careful selection of the MAbs used. These kits, however, still lack sensitivity because a few hundred organisms are still needed to give a positive reaction. Most diagnosticians believe that a diagnosis of AC can be made when a strong positive ELISA reaction is obtained from birds with signs of psittacosis. Because of the number of false-positive results, a positive in an individual bird without signs of disease is not considered to be significant.

h) Polymerase chain reaction

PCR techniques have been reported for the detection of chlamydiae in animals. The technique has promise for a rapid low-cost diagnostic test; however, it is still too early to recommend any specific procedures for general use. The PCR test used to detect *C. trachomatis* in humans is highly specific and sensitive. This test detects a plasmid that is not present in other chlamydiae, and therefore, cannot be used to detect chlamydia in birds. Current tests for species-specific detection of *C. psittaci* are based on target sequences in the MOMP gene region. These tests are very specific, but efficient pre-PCR sample processing may be required to attain high sensitivity. Sensitivity is being increased by targeting a relatively short DNA fragment (21) or by using a nested procedure (24, 35). Other tests are being developed that target the intergenic spacer region between the 16S and 23S rRNA genes. A further problem is the need for developing improved procedures for processing the wide variety of veterinary samples (faecal material, swabs, tissues, etc.).

2. Serological tests

a) Modified direct complement fixation test for *Chlamydia*

The following is a widely used modified direct CF test for the detection of antibody. The reagents are relatively easy to prepare and standardise. There are other CF tests; each has advantages. The modified direct CF test is performed in 96-well round-bottom multiwell dishes. Incubation steps are usually done by floating the plates in a 37°C water bath. The chlamydial antigen can be prepared from either infected yolk sacs or cell culture preparations. The modified direct CF test differs from the direct CF test in that normal, unheated chicken serum from chickens without chlamydial antibody is added to the complement dilution. The normal serum increases the sensitivity of the CF procedure so that it can be used to test sera from avian species whose antibodies do not normally fix guinea-pig complement.

- **Test procedure**

i) *Dilution of sera*

Figure 1 gives a suggested pattern for performing the test in round-bottom, 96-well multiwell dishes. All sera must be heat-inactivated at 60°C for 30 minutes prior to use. The sera are diluted in Veronal (barbiturate) buffer saline (VBS) as shown in Figure 1. The dilutions are made in the multiwell dish by adding 100 µl of VBS to each well of rows A and E, and then adding 25 µl of the undiluted sera, positive serum, or negative serum to each of three wells. This gives a starting dilution of 1/5. Then, 25 µl of VBS is added to each well in row B through to D and row F through to H. Twofold dilutions are made, using a 25 µl micropipette, from row A through to D and row E through to H. Appropriate volumes are discarded from the starting and finishing rows to give 25 µl per well. Diluters are rinsed twice in distilled H_2O and once in VBS between each serum.

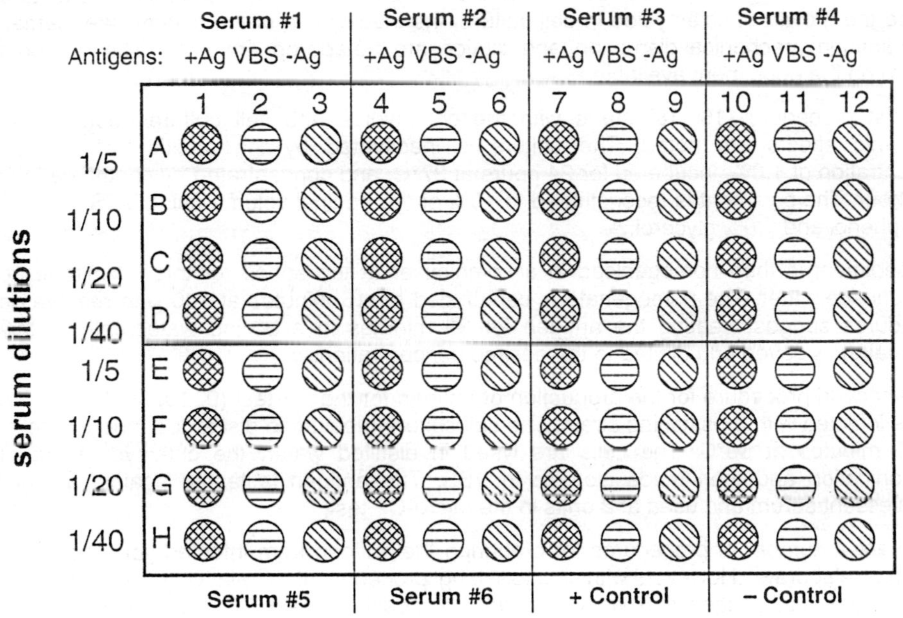

Fig. 1. Suggested test pattern for the modified direct complement fixation test when using 96-well dishes.

ii) *Addition of antigen*

To each well in columns 1, 4, 7, and 10, add 25 µl of positive chlamydial antigen. In columns 2, 5, 8, and 11, add 25 µl of VBS (anticomplementary control wells), and in columns 3, 6, 9, and 12, add 25 µl of negative antigen (normal yolk sac or cell culture prepared the same as the chlamydial antigen). The chlamydial antigens are stored undiluted at 4°C and diluted to proper concentration in VBS prior to use.

iii) *Addition of complement*

Complement (C') is stored at –70°C and should be thawed and diluted in VBS prior to the addition of the antigen. Fresh chicken serum is added before diluting the C' to give a 5% concentration in the complement. Dilutions of C' are made as in previous tests or from titrations. C' should be allowed to stand in an ice bath to stabilise for 15 minutes. The diluted C' should be stored at 4°C following stabilisation and should be used within 2 hours: 50 µl of the C' are added to each well immediately following the addition of the antigens. The plates are incubated uncovered in a 37°C water bath for 2 hours.

iv) *Addition of sheep red blood cells*

Mix 4% standardised sheep red blood cells (SRBCs) with an equal volume of VBS. To this add an equal volume of haemolysin diluted in VBS. The final dilution is incubated in a 37°C water bath for 15 minutes to sensitise the SRBCs. To each well add 50 µl of sensitised SRBCs. The plates are then incubated for 1 hour in a 37°C water bath. The plates can be centrifuged at 400 ***g*** for 5 minutes before reading or they can be refrigerated at 4°C overnight prior to reading.

v) *Interpretation of the results*

The wells are often scored 1+, 2+, 3+, or 4+ corresponding to reduction of haemolysis of 25, 50, 75, or 100%. A positive reaction is 2+ or higher, which is equivalent to 50% or less lysis of the SRBCs. This indicates that the C' was fixed by antibody prior to the addition of the SRBCs. Negative wells are indicated by the complete lysis of the cells: the C' remains unbound and reacts with the SRBCs and the haemolysin to produce lysis of the SRBCs.

Invalid tests occur when the serum is anticomplementary and a positive reaction occurs in the dilution with VBS as the antigen. Nonspecific serum reactions give positive reactions in both the positive and negative wells.

• **Reagents**

i) *Antigen preparation*

The simplest methods start with the growth of chlamydiae in cell culture. The two methods described below produce antigens that can be used in the micro-CF test. The procedures are quite similar: both include the growth of chlamydiae in cell culture, the inactivation of the chlamydiae, partial purification of the antigen, mechanical disruption, and dilution into the appropriate buffer. The method selected will depend on the equipment available.

The first procedure (16, 18) starts with the chlamydiae and cell culture debris harvested when cytopathic effects are noted. The culture is inactivated by the addition of phenol to a final concentration of 1.0%, incubated for 24 hours at 37°C, and concentrated by centrifugation at 10,000 ***g*** for 1 hour. The sediment is reconstituted to 10% of the original volume using VBS, pH 7.2, containing 1.0% phenol and 1.0% glycerol.

The sediment is then homogenised in an omnimixer at top speed for three 1-minute periods while cooled in ice water. The homogenate is centrifuged for 15 minutes at 100 ***g*** to remove debris. Some procedures suggest heating the antigen for 30 minutes in a boiling water bath at this time. The supernatant is saved and diluted to the desired concentration.

In the second procedure for the production of antigen for the CF test (9, 10), antigen is prepared from L cells infected with a psittacine strain. The cell culture medium is discarded, and the cells are heated for 40 minutes at 56°C. The cells are lysed in distilled water, the chlamydiae are disrupted by ultrasonication and then made isotonic in VBS. The antigen is tested against a standard sheep convalescent serum and used at 2 units in the micro-CF test.

There are a number of procedures for preparing the antigen from infected yolk sacs, some of which are quite elaborate. However, with the following procedure it is relatively easy to prepare a crude infected yolk sac antigen that works well in the modified direct CF test. An egg-adapted strain of chlamydia is used to inoculate 6–7-day-old embryonated chicken eggs via the yolk sac. The yolk sacs are harvested from embryos that die between 3 and 7 days post-inoculation. The yolk-sac harvest is diluted 1/3 in PBS, Tris buffer, or cell culture medium, and then autoclaved for 20 minutes. The suspension is cooled and then homogenised thoroughly. The use of a high speed tissue homogeniser for 3–5 minutes is recommended. After homogenisation, phenol is added to make a final concentration of 0.5% phenol (prepare a 5% phenol stock solution and add 1 ml for every 9 ml of antigen). The antigen preparation is prepared, held for 3 days, and then used after centrifugation for 20 minutes at 1000 ***g***. The antigen can be stored for long periods of time at 4°C.

ii) *Preparation of sensitised SRBCs*

Defibrinated SRBCs are preserved by mixing in an equal volume of Alsever's solution. These can be stored at 4°C for up to 4 weeks. Wash 25 ml of the stock SRBCs with 25 ml of VBS. Centrifuge at 400 ***g*** for 10 minutes. Aspirate off the VBS and resuspend in 50 ml of VBS. Repeat the wash a total of three times. Following the final wash, dilute the SRBCs at a ratio of 2.2 ml of packed SRBCs to 98 ml of VBS. The SRBCs can then be standardised by optical density: mix 1 ml of the diluted, washed SRBCs with 14 ml distilled H_2O, determine the absorbance using a spectrophotometer, and standardise to 0.25 at a wave length of 550 mm. The reading obtained can be used in the following formula to determine the dilution needed:

$$\text{Final volume of SRBCs} = \frac{(\text{absorbance reading x current volume})}{0.25 \text{ desired absorbance}}$$

The SRBCs are sensitised by rapidly adding an equal volume of VBS containing the appropriate dilution of haemolysin (dilution determined by titration). Incubate at 37°C for 15 minutes prior to use.

iii) *Veronal buffer saline*

VBS is prepared as a 5 × stock solution and diluted 1/5 with distilled H_2O prior to use. The following formula makes 4 litres. To distilled water add sodium barbital (7.5 g); barbital H_2O (dissolve in boiling H_2O) (11.5 g); $MgSO_4.7H_2O$ (4.056 g); NaCl (170.0 g); and $CaCl_2$ (0.078 g). Add distilled H_2O to make to 4 litres.

iv) *Complement titration*

Complement (C') is unstable and will deteriorate if improperly handled. Normally it should be kept frozen at –70°C in aliquots that are used at one time to eliminate refreezing. To obtain the desired working concentration (2 units per test well) first add 5% normal chicken serum for the modification to enhance sensitivity as described earlier. Then estimate a starting point based on previous lots. A good starting point is a dilution of 1/30 after the chicken serum has been added. Set up a series of tubes with various amounts of complement in VBS. The VBS should contain the antigen to be used in the reaction and take into account any anticomplementary properties of the antigen. A common method is to dilute 0.10 ml C' + 0.90 ml VBS; 0.12 ml complement + 0.88 ml VBS, etc. through 0.25 ml C' + 0.75 ml VBS. Incubate the tubes for 2 hours in a 37°C water bath. Add 0.5 ml of sensitised SRBCs to each tube. Incubate for 1 additional hour in the 37°C water bath. The highest dilution giving complete haemolysis equals 1 unit. Twice that amount equals 2 units. The following formula can be used to obtain 2 units/0.05 ml:

$$x = (di)\,(v)/2dh$$

where:

x = reciprocal of C' dilution desired to yield 2 units C'/well
di = reciprocal of C' initial dilution used in titration (1/30)
v = volume of diluted C' to be added
dh = twice the volume of C' giving complete haemolysis in titration

v) *Titration of haemolysin*

Haemolysin can be obtained from commercial sources. It must be standardised by titration. The following procedure is recommended:

Prepare a 1/100 dilution of the stock haemolysin in VBS. From this, prepare 1/300, 1/400, and 1/500 dilutions in tubes. From each of these dilutions, make 0.5 ml of twofold dilutions in VBS for a block titration.

To determine haemolysin concentration, add the following to 0.5 ml of each dilution: 0.5 ml of C' at 1/30 dilution, 0.5 ml of unsensitised SRBCs at 0.25 optical density, and 1.5 ml of VBS. Incubate for 1 hour at 37°C, and then centrifuge at 400 ***g*** for 5 minutes. One unit of the haemolysin is the dilution that gives complete lysis of the SRBCs. The haemolysin solution is prepared in VBS at the dilution containing 2 units of haemolysin. This is then added to an equal volume of SRBCs at the proper concentration.

vi) *Titration of antigen and positive control serum*

In order to standardise the CF test, it is also necessary to have titres of both the antigen and the positive control serum. If the titre is known for either the positive serum or antigen, the titre of the other component can be determined by performing the CF test using dilutions of the component being titred. If titres of both the positive serum and antigen are unknown, a block titration (chequerboard) can be used to determine the limiting dilutions of both the antigen and the antibody where haemolysis starts. It is very critical to obtain these titres accurately.

For both the antigen and the positive control serum, 4 units are used. A unit is the highest dilution that will give a positive test. That is, if a dilution of 1/160 gives a positive test, then a 1/40 dilution has 4 units and is used for the test.

Complement-fixing antibodies usually appear within 7–10 days of infection. For a positive diagnosis, a four-fold rise in CF antibody titre is required. A presumptive diagnosis by serological tests on a flock can only be made if typical clinical signs are present and a majority of the birds have antibody titres of ≥1/64.

b) Other tests

Other serological tests have been developed, but their specificity has not yet been sufficiently evaluated. The ELISA for group-specific chlamydial antibodies is more rapid and sensitive than the CF test; it can be automated. Evaluations of ELISA for the detection of antibodies to both *C. trachomatis* and *C. psittaci* (14, 22, 31, 32) indicate that it can be substituted for the CF test in most cases. However, it has yet to be tested extensively, standards for its use have not been established, and conjugates are not commercially available for all species of birds.

Other tests include the agar gel immunodiffusion test (27), the latex agglutination (LA) test, the elementary body agglutination (EBA) test (17, 20) and the micro-immunofluorescence test (MIFT). Immunodiffusion is less sensitive than the CF test. The LA test will detect antibodies to *C. psittaci*, and is easy and rapid to perform (19). Latex beads are coated with purified chlamydial antigen, mixed thoroughly with the test serum on a glass plate, and rotated for 2 minutes to enhance agglutination. The test is read against a dark background. Sera giving positive reactions should be retested with uncoated beads to eliminate possible nonspecific agglutination. The LA and direct CF tests correlate in 72.5% of tests with paired sera. The LA test has a sensitivity of 39.1% and a specificity of 98.8% relative to the direct CF test (19). The test detects both IgM and IgG, but it is best at detecting IgM. It has been suggested for use in detecting recent or active infections. The EBA test detects only IgM, and it is indicative of a current infection. The MIFT is rapid and easy to perform; however, fluorescence-conjugated anti-species sera are not always available.

B. REQUIREMENTS FOR VACCINES AND DIAGNOSTIC BIOLOGICALS

There are no commercial vaccines available for chlamydiosis in poultry. Attempts to produce a vaccine have met with limited success, and most have been based on bacterins produced by formalin inactivation of concentrated suspensions of chlamydiae. There is evidence that immunity involves cell-mediated immune responses (28, 29), but vaccine manufacture has not been directed towards reactions of this type.

Antibiotics are the only current means of control. *Chlamydophila psittaci* is susceptible to a number of antibiotics: the drug of choice varies from country to country. Chlortetracycline, doxycycline, and other tetracyclines are the most commonly used. Fluoroquinolone antibiotics have also proven their value (23). Treatment needs to be maintained for extended periods of time. For pet birds, 45 days is often recommended (13, 38).

REFERENCES

1. ANDERSEN A.A. (1991). Serotyping of *Chlamydia psittaci* isolates using serovar-specific monoclonal antibodies with the micro-immunofluorescence test. *J. Clin. Microbiol.*, **29**, 707–711.

2. ANDERSEN A.A. (1996). Comparison of pharyngeal, fecal, and cloacal samples for the isolation of *Chlamydia psittaci* from experimentally infected cockatiels and turkeys. *J. Vet. Diagn. Invest.*, **8**, 448–450.

3. ANDERSEN A.A. (1997). Two new serovars of *Chlamydia psittaci* from North American birds. *J. Vet. Diagn. Invest.*, **9**, 159–164.

4. ANDERSEN A.A. (1998). Chlamydiosis. *In:* A Laboratory Manual for the Isolation and Identification of Avian Pathogens, Fourth Edition. Kendall/Hunt Publishing, Dubuque, Iowa, USA.

5. ANDERSEN A.A., GRIMES J.E. & WYRICK P.B. (1997). Chlamydiosis (Psittacosis, Ornithosis). *In:* Diseases of Poultry, Tenth Edition. Iowa State University Press, Ames, Iowa, USA, 333–349.

6. ANDERSEN A.A. & VAN DUSEN R.A. (1988). Production and partial characterization of monoclonal antibodies to four *Chlamydia psittaci* isolates. *Infect. Immun.*, **56,** 2075–2079.

7. BEVAN B.J. & BRACEWELL C.D. (1986). Chlamydiosis in birds in Great Britain. 2. Isolations of *Chlamydia psittaci* from birds sampled between 1976 and 1984. *J. Hyg. (Camb.),* **96,** 453–458.

8. BEVAN B.J., CULLEN G.A. & READ W.M.F. (1978). Isolation of *Chlamydia psittaci* from avian sources using growth in cell culture. *Avian Pathol.,* **7,** 203–211.

9. BRACEWELL C.D. & BEVAN B.J. (1982). *Chlamydia* infections in ducks: Preliminary communication. *J. R. Soc. Med.,* **75,** 249–252.

10. BRACEWELL C.D. & BEVAN B.J. (1986). Chlamydiosis in birds in Great Britain. 1. Serological reactions to chlamydia in birds sampled between 1974 and 1983. *J. Hyg. (Camb.),* **96,** 447–451.

11. BROWN S. & WHITE J. (1982). Diagnosis of avian psittacosis using cell culture techniques. *Proc. Am. Assoc. Vet. Lab. Diagnosticians,* **25,** 151–158.

12. CENTERS FOR DISEASE CONTROL AND PREVENTION (1997). Compendium of psittacosis (chlamydiosis) control, 1997. *Morb. Mortal. Weekly Rep.*, **46** (Rr-13), 1–13.

13. EIDSON M., STOBIERSKI M.G., SMITH K.A. & WILLIAMS L.P. (1997). Compendium of chlamydiosis (psittacosis) control, 1995. *J. Vet. Med. Assoc.,* **206,** 1874–1879.

14. EVANS R.T., CHALMERS W.S.K., WOOLCOCK P.R., FARMER H. & TAYLOR ROBINSON D. (1983). An enzyme-linked immunosorbent assay (ELISA) for detection of chlamydial antibody in duck sera. *Avian Pathol.,* **12,** 117–124.

15. EVERETT K.D.E., BUSH R.M. & ANDERSEN A.A. (1999). Emended description of the order Chlamydiales, proposal of Parachlamydiaceae fam. nov. and Simkaniaceae fam. nov., each containing one monotypic genus, revised taxonomy of the family Chlamydiaceae, including a new genus and five new species, and standards for the identification of organisms. *Int. J. Syst. Bacteriol.,* **49,** 415–440.

16. GRIMES J.E. (1985). Direct complement fixation and isolation attempts for detecting *Chlamydia psittaci* infection of psittacine birds. *Avian Dis.*, **29,** 837–877

17. GRIMES J.E. & ARIZMENDI F. (1996). Usefulness and limitations of three serologic methods for diagnosing or excluding chlamydiosis in birds. *J. Am. Vet. Med. Assoc.*, **209,** 747–750.

18. GRIMES J.E., GRUMBLES L.C. & MOORE R.W. (1970). Complement fixation and haemagglutination antigens from a chlamydial (ornithosis) agent grown in cell cultures. *Can. J. Comp. Med.,* **34,** 256–260.

19. GRIMES J.E., PHALEN D.N. & ARIZMENDI F. (1993). *Chlamydia* latex agglutination antigen and protocol improvement and psittacine bird anti-chlamydial immunoglobulin reactivity. *Avian Dis.,* **37,** 817–824.

20. GRIMES J.E., TULLY I.N. JR, ARIZMENDI F. & PHALEN D.N. (1994). Elementary body agglutination for rapidly demonstrating chlamydial agglutinins in avian serum with emphasis on testing cockatiels. *Avian Dis.,* **38,** 822–831.

21. HEWINSON R.G., GRIFFITHS P.C., BEVAN B.J., KIRWAN S.E.S., FIELD M.E., WOODWARD M.J. & DAWSON M. (1997). Detection of *Chlamydia psittaci* DNA in avian clinical samples by polymerase chain reaction. *Vet. Microbiol.,* **54,** 155–166.

22. LANG G.H. (1984). La chlamydiose du dindon : Diagnostic serologique par la methode ELISA. *Rec. Med. Vet.,* **160,** 763–771.

23. LINDESTRUTH H. & FROST J.W. (1993). Enrofloxacin (Baytril) – eine Alternative in der Psittakoseprophylaxe und -therapie beim importierten Psittacidien. *Dtsch Tierarztl. Wochenschr.*, **100,** 364–368.

24. MESSMER T.O., SKELTON S.K., MORONEY J.F., DAUGHARTY H. & FIELDS B.S. (1997). Application of a nested, multiplex PCR to psittacosis outbreaks. *J. Clin. Microbiol.*, **35**, 2043–2046.

25. MOHAN R. (1984). Epidemiologic and laboratory observations of *Chlamydia psittaci* infection in pet birds. *J. Am. Vet. Med. Assoc.*, **184**, 1372–1374.

26. MOORE F.M. & PETRAK M.L. (1985). *Chlamydia* immuno reactivity in birds with psittacosis: Localization of chlamydiae by the peroxidase antiperoxidase method. *Avian Dis.*, **29**, 1036–1042.

27. PAGE L.A. (1974). Application of an agar gel precipitin test to the serodiagnosis of avian chlamydiosis. *Proc. Am. Assoc. Vet. Lab. Diagnosticians*, **17**, 51–61.

28. PAGE L.A. (1975). Studies on immunity to chlamydiosis in birds, with particular reference to turkeys. *Am. J. Vet. Res.*, **36**, 597–600.

29. PAGE L.A. (1978). Stimulation of cell-mediated immunity to chlamydiosis in turkeys by inoculation of chlamydial bacterin. *Am. J. Vet. Res.*, **39**, 473–480.

30. PAUL I.D. (1982). The growth of chlamydia in McCoy cells treated with emetine. *Med. Lab. Sci.*, **39**, 15–32.

31. PEPIN M., BAILLY L., SOURIAU A. & RODOLAKIS A. (1985). An enzyme-linked immunosorbent assay (ELISA) for the detection of chlamydial antibodies in caprine sera. *Ann. Rech. Vet.*, **16**, 393–398.

32. RUPPANER R., BEHYMER D.E., DELONG W.J. III, FRANTI C.E. & SCHULTZ T.E. (1984). Enzyme immunoassay of chlamydia in birds. *Avian Dis.*, **28**, 608–615.

33. SAYADA C., ANDERSEN A.A., STOREY C., MILON A., EB F., HASHIMOTO O.N., HIRAI K., ELION J. & DENAMUR E. (1995). Usefulness of *omp1* restriction mapping for avian *Chlamydia psittaci* isolate differentiation. *Res. Microbiol.*, **146**, 155–165.

34. SPENCER W.N. & JOHNSON F.W.A. (1983). Simple transport medium for the isolation of *Chlamydia psittaci* from clinical material. *Vet. Rec.*, **113**, 535–536.

35. TAKASHIMA I., IMAI Y., KARIWA H. & HASHIMOTO N. (1996). Polymerase chain-reaction for the detection of *Chlamydia psittaci* in the feces of budgerigars. *Microbiol. Immunol.*, **40**, 21–26.

36. VANROMPAY D., BUTAYE P., SAYADA C., DUCATELLE R. & HAESEBROUCK F. (1997). Characterization of avian *Chlamydia psittaci* strains using *omp1* restriction mapping and serovar-specific monoclonal antibodies. *Res. Microbiol.*, **148**, 327–333.

37. VANROMPAY D., DUCATELLE R. & HAESEBROUCK F. (1992). Diagnosis of avian chlamydiosis; specificity of the modified Gimenez staining on smears and comparison of the sensitivity of isolation in eggs and three different cell cultures. *J. Vet. Med. [B]*, **39**, 105–112.

38. VANROMPAY D., DUCATELLE R. & HAESEBROUCK F. (1995). *Chlamydia psittaci* infections: a review with emphasis on avian chlamydiosis. *Vet. Microbiol.*, **45**, 93–119.

39. VANROMPAY D., DUCATELLE R., HAESEBROUCK F. & HENDRICKX W. (1993). Primary pathogenicity of an European isolate of *Chlamydia psittaci* from turkey poults. *Vet. Microbiol.*, **38**, 103–113.

40. VANROMPAY D., VAN NEROM A., DUCATELLE R. & HAESEBROUCK F. (1994). Evaluation of five immunoassays for detection of *Chlamydia psittaci* in cloacal and conjunctival specimens from turkeys. *J. Clin. Microbiol.*, **32**, 1470–1474.

*

* *

CHAPTER 2.7.5.

FOWL TYPHOID AND PULLORUM DISEASE

SUMMARY

Pullorum disease of chickens is caused by Salmonella pullorum[1] *and, in its acute form, is almost exclusively a disease of young chickens. However, the organism is also associated with disease in turkey poults. Game birds and 'backyard' poultry flocks may act as reservoirs of infection, and wild birds may act as vectors for the organism and as such are important in the epidemiology of the disease.*

Fowl typhoid in chickens and turkeys is caused by S. gallinarum *and is more often observed in the later growing period and in mature stock. The clinical signs resemble those of septicaemia, with inappetence and, eventually, death. Diagnosis depends on the demonstration of the organism or specific antibodies.*

Samples should not originate from birds or eggs that have recently been treated with antimicrobial drugs. They can be swabs or aseptically collected samples from affected tissues, or intestinal and cloacal contents. Other materials to sample include eggs, eggshell surfaces, embryos, faecal droppings and hatcher debris, especially fluff, dust and broken eggshells. The nature and quantity of the sample will depend on whether it is taken from live poultry or carcasses, and whether lesions or faecal contamination are present.

***Identification of the agent:** Tissue and faeces samples should be inoculated into nonselective and selective enrichment broth and into selective agar medium, such as deoxycholate–citrate agar, brilliant green agar, etc., as soon as possible after collection. In case of delay, samples should be stored at 0–4°C. Typical colonies can be identified by serological and biochemical tests. Molecular tests, including nucleic acid probes and a polymerase chain reaction, are being developed.*

***Serological tests:** These are satisfactory for establishing the presence and estimating the prevalence of infection within a flock. The test used in the field is the rapid whole blood plate agglutination test (WBT). This test is unreliable in turkeys and ducks and many uninfected birds may give positive reactions. In the laboratory a serum agglutination test is used, either as a rapid plate test or as a tube test. These can be applied as macro- or microagglutination tests. Any positive reactors should be confirmed as being infected by culture at post-mortem examination. Enzyme-linked immunosorbent assays are undergoing validation and show promise for the future.*

It is likely that the increasing use of vaccines to control S. enteritidis *infections in chickens may cause problems in the interpretation of serological results.*

***Requirements for vaccines and diagnostic biologicals:** Live and inactivated vaccines are available for fowl typhoid in some countries. The most commonly used vaccine is a live vaccine derived from the stable rough strain of* S. gallinarum *known as '9R'.*

1 Special note on nomenclature of the genus *Salmonella*: See the note on nomenclature in Chapter X.4. Salmonellosis for the principles followed concerning the nomenclature of *Salmonella*.

A. DIAGNOSTIC TECHNIQUES

A distinction is usually made in veterinary literature between infections caused by the two nonmotile host-adapted serovars: *Salmonella pullorum* (pullorum disease)[2], *S. gallinarum* (fowl typhoid) and the remainder of the salmonellae (salmonellosis, paratyphoid). These separations are made because of important differences in epidemiology, host range, virulence and diagnostic and control measures. The two host-adapted serovars, *S. pullorum* and S. *gallinarum,* are highly pathogenic for chickens and turkeys, but have negligible public health significance. Long-standing control programmes have substantially reduced the occurrence of *S. pullorum* in poultry production in many countries. *Salmonella gallinarum* has been eradicated from many western countries but is still a major problem in areas of Central and South America, Africa, and the Middle East.

For the above reason, the two nonmotile salmonellae will be treated as two separate serovars, although the current Kauffman–White scheme refers to them as one serotype, namely *S. gallinarum.*

In its acute form, pullorum disease is almost exclusively a disease of young chickens, and the agent can be recovered from almost all chicken organs, tissues and faeces. In older birds that have become carriers, *S. pullorum* is most commonly recovered from the ova, and only exceptionally from other organs and tissues, including the alimentary tract. In contrast, fowl typhoid is more often observed in the later growing period and in mature stock. However, it may occur in young chickens where it is indistinguishable clinically from pullorum disease. In carrier birds, the organism is found most often in the liver and faeces.

To recover the organisms, the birds should not have been treated with antimicrobial drugs for approximately the previous 2–3 weeks.

Samples may be obtained from live birds, fresh or freshly frozen carcasses, egg materials, fresh faeces, poultry food, or any contaminated materials from housing, hatchers or transport boxes. Swabs may be taken from the cloaca of live birds. Carcasses or conjunctiva can be swabbed or aseptic samples can be taken from the spleen, liver, gall-bladder, kidneys, lungs, heart, ova, testes, alimentary tract or joint lesions. The surface is seared with a hot spatula and a sample is obtained by inserting a sterile cotton swab or wire loop through the heat-sterilised surface. The demonstration of infection in serological reactor birds that are apparently normal may require the culture of large volumes of homogenised tissues with or without direct swabbing. Tissue pools may be made from tissues collected from a number of birds.

When floor litter is sampled, it should be remembered that *S. pullorum and S. gallinarum* are more difficult to isolate from faecal and environmental samples than other salmonellae. Samples should include moist and dry litter and swabs from open drinkers.

If poultry feed is to be examined for salmonellae, representative samples should be taken from the widest practicable distribution within the load. Where possible, this should include the finest particulate material. These samples must be taken aseptically from feed stores or delivery vehicles. Several aliquots should be collected, making a total quantity of 25–100 g.

• Culture media

Both *S. pullorum* and *S. gallinarum* grow well on nonselective media, but selective and enrichment media have been described that contain substances to inhibit the growth of extraneous organisms. The efficiency of recovery of these bacteria varies according to circumstances, and experience in the use of a medium is an important but unquantifiable factor. Some complex media may have an inhibitory effect on these organisms, so that it is advisable to use both nonselective and selective media for isolation. Both solid media and broth can be employed. As the toxic properties of selective media may vary, it is preferable to monitor these by comparing growth of control cultures on both types of medium. The inhibitory media should grow at least 75% of the colonies of the corresponding noninhibitory medium (3, 4, 7, 8).

All the media mentioned below are examples of commonly used media, but there are many others found to be equally satisfactory.

Noninhibitory media include nutrient agar and blood agar, on which colonies are seen to be smooth, translucent, slightly raised, and about 2 mm in diameter. Broths include nutrient and meat infusion broth.

2 Although *S. pullorum* is nonmotile in normal laboratory media, it has been shown that the organism can be induced to produce flagellae and display motility (Holt P.S. & Chaubal L.H. [1997]. Detection of motility and putative synthesis of flagellar proteins in *Salmonella pullorum* cultures. *J. Clin. Micorbiol.,* **35**, 1016–1020.).

- **Selective media include:**

MacConkey agar: inhibitory to nonenteric organisms, differentiates lactose fermenters (pink colonies) from nonlactose fermenters (colourless colonies). NaCl is omitted to limit the spread of *Proteus* colonies. Salmonella colonies are smooth and colourless. *Salmonella pullorum* produces smaller colonies than other salmonellae.

Desoxycholate citrate agar: inhibitory to nonenteric organisms. *Salmonella pullorum* grows sparsely as very small colourless colonies; *S. gallinarum* colonies are 2–3 mm in diameter, dome-shaped, with a central black spot. *Proteus* grow readily, as does *Pseudomonas.*

Brilliant green agar: inhibitory to coliforms and most *Proteus* strains; useful for distinguishing enteric organism colonies. Salmonellae form low, convex, pale red, translucent colonies of 1–3 mm in diameter, similar to *Citrobacter. Proteus* forms pin-point colonies, *Pseudomonas aeruginosa* appears as small red colonies, and lactose fermenters are green. *Salmonella pullorum* produces smaller colonies than other salmonellae.

Brilliant green sulphapyridine agar: inhibitory to coliforms and *Proteus* strains. The sulphapyridine is added to stabilise selectivity in the presence of egg materials. *Salmonella pullorum* produces small colonies.

- **Liquid enrichment and selective media include:**

Selenite F broth: inhibitory to coliforms but not *Proteus,* improved by addition of brilliant green. Loss of activity after 24 hours. Selenite cysteine broth is more stable.

Tetrathionate/brilliant green broth: inhibitory to coliforms and *Proteus*, but may also inhibit *S. pullorum/ gallinarum.*

Rappaport–Vassiliadis Soya Peptone broth: for selective enrichment following pre-enrichment, use 1 part inoculum to 100 parts medium.

- **Recovery of salmonellae**

The methods for recovering *S. pullorum* and *S. gallinarum* vary according to the origin of the samples. Although their isolation from cloacal swabs and faeces may be unrewarding, examination of tissues taken at post-mortem is usually more successful. The methods are as follows:

Cloacal swabs and fresh faeces from live birds: swabs dipped in nutrient broth are suitable, small swabs being used for young chickens. The swabs are streaked on to nonselective and selective media, and placed in enrichment broth. The plates and the broth are incubated at 37°C. At this temperature, some *Proteus* and *Pseudomonas* organisms tend to be inhibited. Higher temperatures may be used with some broths, e.g. 41.5°C for Rappaport–Vassiliadis, but care needs to be exercised because some enrichment media may be too inhibitory. Subcultures are made on to selective media after 24 and 48 hours.

Gall-bladder contents: swabs of gall-bladder contents are streaked on to nonselective and selective agars and placed in inhibitory and noninhibitory broths, followed by incubation at 37°C and subculture on to inhibitory agar after 24 and 48 hours.

Organs and tissues: swabs are taken from individual tissues and lesions and cultured on to nonselective and selective media, and into similar broths. These are incubated at 37°C and subcultured on to selective agar after 24 and 48 hours. Intestinal material in inhibitory broths should be incubated at 40°C; *S. gallinarum* grows well but there may be some inhibition of *S. pullorum* at this temperature.

Carrier birds: here larger amounts of material are required. The ova should be tested for *S. pullorum*, and the liver and gall-bladder should be tested for *S. gallinarum.* Tissues are homogenised in a small volume of broth and directly plated out. Approximately 10 ml is added to 100 ml of enrichment broth (e.g. selenite F broth, brilliant green broth), and incubated at 37°C; this is subcultured on to nonselective and selective agar after 24 hours.

Alimentary canal, including the intestinal contents: after grinding or homogenisation in a small volume of broth, 10 ml of the homogenate is incubated in 100 ml of enrichment broth at 37°C. If Rappaport–Vassiliadis is to be used, the ratio should be 1:100. This is incubated at 40°C and subcultured on to selective agar after 24 and 48 hours.

Eggshell surfaces: the eggs are placed in plastic bags containing 25–50 ml of enrichment broth (e.g. selenite F broth) and their surfaces are massaged through the walls of the bags. The broth is incubated at 37°C and subcultured on to selective agar after 24 and 48 hours.

Egg contents: homogenised contents of fresh eggs are mixed with about 100–200 ml of nutrient broth, incubated at 37°C, and subcultured on to nonselective and selective agar after 24 and 48 hours. Incubated eggs, whether infertile or containing small embryos, can be similarly treated; or 10 ml of homogenised contents can be mixed with 100 ml of enrichment broth, incubated at 37°C, and subcultured on to selective agar after 24 and 48 hours.

Embryos: swabs should be taken from the yolk sacs of well developed embryos and streaked on to nonselective and selective agar, one swab being placed in 10 ml of nonselective and enrichment broth (e.g. selenite F broth, brilliant green broth). Incubation is carried out at 37°C, and subcultures are made on to nonselective and selective agars after 24 and 48 hours.

Hatchery fluff and dust: a few grams are mixed with 50–100 ml of nonselective and enrichment broth (e.g. selenite F broth), incubated at 37°C, and subcultures are made on to nonselective and selective agars after 24 and 48 hours.

Floor and nest litter: 2–3 g are mixed with 50–100 ml of enrichment broth (e.g. selenite F broth, brilliant green broth), incubated at 40°C, and subcultured on to selective agar after 24 and 48 hours.

Poultry feed: 25 g are mixed with 225 ml of buffered peptone water, incubated overnight at 37°C, subcultured in enrichment broth and, after 24 and 48 hours, subcultured on to selective agar. Poultry feed may also be examined by electrical conductance methods.

1. Identification of the agent

Typical salmonella colonies on noninhibitory media are round, glistening, domed, smooth, and 1–2 mm in diameter after 24–48 hours' incubation. On selective media their appearance varies with the medium. Suspect colonies can be investigated serologically and biochemically, and observed for motility.

After incubation for 20–24 hours, the plates with subcultures streaked on to nutrient agar, blood agar or selective agars should be examined carefully for the presence of typical *S. pullorum* and *S. gallinarum* colonies. If growth is slight after 24 hours' incubation, the plates should be reincubated for a further 24 hours and examined again for the presence of typical *S. pullorum* or *S. gallinarum* colonies. For biochemical and serological confirmation from each plate, five typical or suspect colonies should be chosen for further examination. If there are fewer than five typical or suspect colonies, all of them should be taken for further examination. Selected colonies should be streaked on to the surface of nutrient agar, in a manner that allows the growth of separate colonies. For biochemical confirmation, only pure cultures should be used. By means of an inoculating loop the following media should be streaked: triple sugar iron (TSI) agar; lysine iron agar (or L-lysine decarboxylation medium); urea agar according to Christensen; tryptone/tryptophan medium for indole reaction; glucose with an inverted Durham tube for acid and gas production; dulcitol, maltose, ornithine decarboxylation medium and semisolid agar, for motility. The reactions shown in Table 1 occur.

Table 1. Biochemical investigation of Salmonella pullorum *and* S. gallinarum

	Salmonella pullorum	*Salmonella gallinarum*
TSI glucose (acid formation)	+	+
TSI glucose (gas formation)	v	–
TSI lactose	–	–
TSI saccharose	–	–
TSI hydrogen sulphide	v	v
Gas from glucose (medium with Durham tube)	+	–
Urea splitting	–	–
Lysine decarboxylation	+	+
Ornithine decarboxylation	+	–
Maltose fermentation	– or late +	+
Dulcitol	–	+
Motility	–	–

+ = 90% or more positive reaction within 1 or 2 days; – = No reaction (90% or more); v = Variable reactions.

Identification kits are commercially available, for example Analytical Profile Index (API) system for Enterobacteriaceae. However, care must be taken when using API because *S. pullorum* may be misidentified as *Hafnia* spp. Molecular tests using DNA hybridisation techniques and polymerase chain reaction are being developed.

For serological confirmation, colonies from nonselective media (nutrient or blood agar) are used. The first stage is elimination of autoagglutinable strains. For this, material taken from a single colony of pure culture is transferred to a glass slide and mixed with a drop of sterile saline. The slide is rocked gently for 30–60 seconds and observed for agglutination against a dark background, preferably with the aid of a magnifying glass. If the bacteria have clumped into more or less distinctive units, the strain is considered to be autoagglutinable and must not be submitted to the following tests. If the bacterial sample is recognised as nonautoagglutinable, it is tested with a polyvalent 'O' (A–G) antiserum. For this purpose, the material from a single colony is dispersed in the drop of polyvalent 'O' antiserum on the glass slide to obtain a homogenous and turbid suspension. After gently rocking for 30–60 seconds, the reaction is observed against a dark background for agglutination. If the reaction is positive, the single colony is tested further in the same manner using group-specific sera for *S. pullorum* and *S. gallinarum* serotypes (D antiserum). After serogrouping, isolates may be sent to a reference laboratory for serotyping.

2. Serological tests

The tests that are most readily applied include rapid whole blood agglutination, rapid serum agglutination, tube agglutination and micro-agglutination (10).

Both *S. pullorum* and *S. gallinarum* possess 'O' antigens 1, 9 and 12. However, in the case of *S. pullorum*, there is a variation in the ratio of 12_1, 12_2 and 12_3; the standard strain contains more 12_3 than 12_2, while the reverse is true of the variant form. Intermediate forms also exist. (There appears to be no such form variation in the case of *S. gallinarum*.) As this variation occurs, it is necessary to use a polyvalent antigen in the agglutination tests. The same antigen is used to detect both *S. pullorum* and *S. gallinarum*.

a) Rapid whole blood agglutination test

The rapid whole blood agglutination test can be used under field conditions for detecting both *S. pullorum* and *S. gallinarum*, and the reactors can be identified immediately. However, it is not reliable in turkeys. Chickens can be tested at any age, although some authorities specify a minimum age of 4 months (10, 11).

- **Preparation of stained antigen for the rapid whole blood or rapid serum agglutination test**

One standard form strain of *S. pullorum* (antigenic structure 9, 12_1, 12_3) and one variant form (antigenic structure 9, 12_1, 12_2) are grown and harvested separately until final mixing for the complete antigen. All incubations are at 37°C.

Sow strains on to separate agar slopes, incubate at 37°C for 24 hours, emulsify growth with sterile normal saline and spread an inoculum over an agar plate to produce easily selected discrete colonies. For this the plates are incubated for 48 hours, a number of colonies are marked out and each is tested for agglutination on a slide with 1/500 acriflavine in saline. Smooth phase colonies do not produce agglutination. Pick off typical colonies that do not produce any agglutination, seed on to agar slopes, and incubate for 24 hours. Emulsify the growth in saline and evenly distribute 2 ml over the surface of the medium (200 ml) in a Roux or similar flask. Incubate the flasks for 60 hours.

For harvesting the bacterial growth, flood the surface of each flask with enough sterile buffered formol saline, pH 6.5, to give dense cell suspensions (about 10 ml per flask). Add 12–15 sterile glass beads of 3–5 mm diameter and rock the flasks until all the growth is in even suspension; leave in a vertical position for at least 15 minutes. Check the morphology and purity of the suspensions by preparing and examining Gram-stained films. Bulk the suspension from each flask containing the same strains. To each 100 ml of suspension, add 200 ml of absolute alcohol. Shake the mixture and allow to stand for 36 hours or until precipitation is complete. Check the agglutinability of the standard and variant precipitate by first centrifuging a sample to separate the alcohol, which is removed, dilute with normal saline and test with a known positive and negative serum. If satisfactory, remove the clear supernatant alcohol (centrifugation at 2000 ***g*** for 10 minutes may be helpful in precipitation), and add sufficient phosphate buffered saline (PBS) containing 10% (v/v) glycerol to standardise the density to 75 × no. 1 Wellcome opacity tube (or 50 × tube no. 1.0 on the McFarland scale). Add equal volumes of standard and variant strains, and add 1% (v/v) of 3% (w/v) alcoholic crystal violet solution to the final mixture, and allow to stand for 48 hours at room temperature. Store in a tightly closed container at 0–4°C for up to 6 months. To assess safety, a culture test is made on agar for nonviability of the unwashed antigen before standardisation. Each bottle of antigen must be tested after alcoholic precipitation and before standardisation against standard titre antisera for

S. pullorum and *S. gallinarum*, and against a negative serum. If possible, also test with known positive and negative serum and **blood** from positive and negative chickens.

Stained antigen for the whole blood plate agglutination test is available commercially, but there does seem to be some slight differences in their sensitivity (5), although it is unlikely that birds infected with the different variants of *S. pullorum* would be missed.

- **Test procedure**

i) Use a clean white tile marked into squares of about 3 × 3 cm. If a tile with 3 × 4 squares is used, up to 12 blood samples can be tested at the same time.

ii) Place 1 drop (about 0.02 ml) of crystal-violet-stained antigen in the centre of each square.

iii) Obtain a sample of fresh whole blood. This is conveniently done by making a stab of a wing vein, using a needle with a triangular point.

iv) Place an equal size drop of fresh whole blood next to a drop of antigen.

v) Mix the drops of antigen and blood using a fine glass rod, which is wiped clean between samples.

vi) Use a gentle rocking motion to keep the drops agitated for up to 2 minutes. The drops should not be allowed to dry out during this time. In very warm conditions, larger drops may be required to avoid drying out.

vii) A positive reaction is indicated by easily visible clumping of the antigen within 2 minutes.

viii) A negative reaction is indicated by absence of clumping of the antigen within 2 minutes.

ix) Include known positive and negative control sera on each testing occasion, using them in the same way as the blood.

x) On completion of a set of tests, the tile is washed and dried, ready for further use.

In the absence of positive reactions, any doubtful reactions can only be interpreted in the light of the previous salmonella-testing history of the flock. Where there are positive reactors, any doubtful reactor should be regarded as positive. Also, recently infected birds may not show a typical positive reaction until they are retested after 3–4 weeks.

b) Rapid serum agglutination test

The rapid serum agglutination test is performed in the same manner, except that serum is substituted for whole blood.

c) Tube agglutination test

Fresh serum from chickens, turkeys or other birds is used at an initial dilution of 1/25, obtained by mixing 0.04 ml of serum with 1.0 ml of antigen[3]. Positive and negative control sera are included in each test. The antigen is prepared from unstained *S. pullorum* or *S. gallinarum* cultures diluted to a concentration of no. 1 on the McFarland scale (as described above). The mixture is incubated at 50°C for 18–24 hours before reading. A positive reaction consists of a granular white deposit with a clear supernatant fluid; a negative reaction shows uniform turbidity. Samples positive at a dilution of 1/25 are retested at a higher range of dilutions and a titre of 1/50 is usually considered to be positive, although there does seem to be variation in the literature.

d) Micro-agglutination test

This resembles the tube agglutination test, but requires much smaller volumes of reactants. The test is performed in microtest plates. Sera are first diluted by adding 10 µl of serum to 90 µl of normal saline, and then adding 100 µl of previously standardised stained microtest antigen to give a final dilution of 1/20. By titrating the serum in doubling dilutions and adding an equal volume of standardised stained antigen, an end-point (titre) can be obtained. The plates are sealed and incubated at 37°C for 18–24 or 48 hours. A positive reaction consists of a fine diffuse precipitation, whereas a negative reaction shows a button-like precipitate. Titres of 1/40 are usually considered to be positive.

Other serological tests include micro-antiglobulin (Coombs), immunodiffusion, haemagglutination and enzyme-linked immunosorbent assay (ELISA).

3 For preparation of small volumes of somatic antigens see Chapter X.4. Salmonellosis.

It seems probable that once standardisation of the method and the interpretation of results have been agreed, the indirect ELISA using polysaccharide antigen is likely to become the most sensitive and specific serological flock test for *S. gallinarum* and *S. pullorum*. It is relatively easy to perform with serum or yolk, and can be used for quantifying the titre of antibody (1, 2, 11).

B. REQUIREMENTS FOR VACCINES AND DIAGNOSTIC BIOLOGICALS

Although both live and inactivated vaccines have been prepared for use against *S. gallinarum*, the vaccine most widely used is made from the rough 9R strain (6). It has only been employed in chickens. The number of viable organisms per dose is important; these organisms can survive in vaccinated birds for many months and may be transmitted through the egg (and perhaps from bird to bird). Vaccination may reduce flock losses, but will not prevent infection with field strains. In addition, vaccination with 9R may sometimes precipitate high mortality in infected birds (9), and may stimulate the production of transient antibodies. It is usual to vaccinate at 8 weeks and again at 16 weeks of age. Antimicrobials should be avoided before and after vaccination.

Current vaccines, however, have only a minor role to play in the control of fowl typhoid. This can best be achieved by hygiene in management, monitoring and removal of infected stock, and the careful use of antimicrobials.

1. Seed management

a) Characteristics of the seed

Live fowl typhoid vaccine is a suspension of suitably attenuated living organisms of a rough strain of *S. gallinarum*, e.g. 9R. The organisms in the vaccine give the biochemical reactions characteristic of *S. gallinarum*. Colonies of a 24-hour culture prepared from the vaccine on nutrient agar plates are rough when examined by the acriflavine slide test. The culture does not contain the somatic antigens characteristic of the smooth forms of *S. gallinarum*.

b) Method of culture

Salmonella gallinarum is grown on or in a suitable medium, such as nutrient agar or broth, for 24 hours at 37°C.

c) Validation as a vaccine

There is no satisfactory method of assessing the protection afforded by the vaccine in the field. However, experience has shown that the vaccine can provide some benefit in situations where control cannot be achieved by hygiene and management alone.

2. Method of manufacture

The vaccine may be prepared by inoculation of a suitable medium, such as nutrient broth, with a fresh culture of *S. gallinarum* (9R) and incubation at 37°C for 24 hours, with or without aeration. The organisms are harvested by sedimentation or centrifugation.

Alternatively the organisms may be grown on and harvested from a solid medium, such as nutrient agar. In either case, the suspension is diluted in PBS solution, pH 7.0, and may be freeze-dried. The dose used per bird is between 5×10^6 and 5×10^7 organisms.

3. In-process control

The culture used for inoculation of the production cultures and the harvested cells are examined microscopically using Gram staining to check for purity.

4. Batch control

a) Sterility

Tests for sterility and freedom from contamination of biological materials may be found in Chapter I.4.

b) Safety

Six healthy, susceptible (preferably specific pathogen free [SPF]) chickens, 8–16 weeks of age, are each injected subcutaneously with ten doses of vaccine, and are observed for at least 7 days; no local or systemic reaction should develop.

c) **Potency**

First, 15 healthy chickens, 8–16 weeks of age, of the Light Sussex or Rhode Island Red breeds, or crosses of these, and taken from a stock that is free from *S. pullorum* infection, are each injected subcutaneously with a quantity of vaccine corresponding to one field dose, i.e. 5×10^7 viable organisms. After an interval of 21–28 days, the vaccinated chickens and an equal number of similar unvaccinated chickens are deprived of food for approximately 18 hours. The chickens are then challenged by oral administration of 1 ml of a broth suspension containing 5×10^7 organisms of a virulent strain of *S. gallinarum* mixed with 300 mg of a powder consisting of chalk (40%), light kaolin (43%) and magnesium trisilicate (17%). All the chickens are observed for 14–21 days. The vaccine passes the test if at the end of this period the number of surviving vaccinated chickens that show no macroscopic lesions of fowl typhoid at post-mortem exceeds by eight or more the number of similarly defined control chickens.

d) **Duration of immunity**

The vaccine should provide protection throughout the laying period, and this can be measured by potency tests at stages during lay. A booster dose during lay may be required.

e) **Stability**

Shelf life of the vaccine can be measured by conducting potency tests at periods after manufacture. These should be done on at least six samples. Potency should remain satisfactory for at least 1 year.

f) **Preservatives**

No preservatives are used

g) **Precautions (hazards)**

The organism is not known to be pathogenic to humans, and there are no special risks associated with the manufacture of either the vaccine or the antigen. However, the vaccine may establish a persistent infection in carrier birds and can precipitate disease in already infected chickens.

5. Tests on the final product

a) **Safety**

The safety test described in Section B.4.b. should be used on a representative sample from each batch of final product.

b) **Potency**

The potency test described in Section B.4.c. should be used on a representative sample from each batch of final product.

REFERENCES

1. BARROW P.A. (1992). ELISAs and the serological analysis of salmonella in poultry: a review. *Epidemiol. Infect.*, **109**, 361–369.

2. BARROW P.A. (1994). Serological diagnosis of *Salmonella* serotype *enteritidis* infections in poultry by ELISA and other tests. *Int. J. Food Microbiol.*, **21**, 55–68.

3. ELLIS E.M., WILLIAMS J.E., MALLINSON E.T., SNOEYENBOS G.H. & MARTIN W.J. (1976). Culture Methods for the Detection of Animal Salmonellosis and Arizonosis. Iowa State University Press, Ames, Iowa, USA.

4. FRICKER C.R. (1987). The isolation of salmonellas and campylobacters. *J. Appl. Bacteriol.*, **63**, 99–116.

5. GAST R.K. (1997). Detecting infections of chickens with recent *Salmonella pullorum* isolates using standard serological methods. *Poult. Sci.*, **76**, 17–23.

6. HARBOURNE J.F., WILLIAMS B.M., PARKER W.H. & FINCHAM I.H. (1963). The prevention of fowl typhoid in the field using a freeze-dried 9R vaccine. *Vet. Rec.*, **75**, 858–861.

7. HARVEY R.W.S. & PRICE T.H. (1975). Isolation of Salmonellas. Public Health Laboratory Service, London, UK.

8. MALLINSON E.T. & SNOEYENBOS G.H. (1989). Salmonellosis. *In:* Isolation and Identification of Avian Pathogens, Third Edition, Purchase H.G. *et al.*, eds. American Association of Avian Pathologists, Kendall Hunt Publishing, Iowa, USA, 3–11.

9. SILVA E.N., SNOEYENBOS G.H., WEINACK O.M. & SMYSER C.F. (1981). Studies on the use of 9R strain *Salmonella gallinarum* as a vaccine in chickens. *Avian Dis.*, **25**, 38–52.

10. UNITED STATES DEPARTMENT OF AGRICULTURE (1996). Auxiliary Provisions on National Poultry Improvement Plan. Code of Federal Regulations, Title 9, Part 147, 717–727.

11. WRAY C. & WRAY A. (EDS) (2000). Salmonella in Domestic Animals. CAB International, Wallingford, Oxon, UK, 407–427.

*

* *

CHAPTER 2.7.6.

AVIAN INFECTIOUS BRONCHITIS

SUMMARY

Infectious bronchitis (IB) is usually defined as an acute, contagious disease of chickens characterised primarily by respiratory signs. However, infections with the causative virus may also lead to nephritis (acute or chronic) and egg production problems in laying hens. The severity of respiratory infections with IB virus can be greatly enhanced by the presence of other pathogens of the respiratory tract. Clinical signs are indicative, but not diagnostic, of IB, and confirmation requires the isolation or direct demonstration of the presence of IB virus, although serology may also be useful in some circumstances. The widespread use of both live and inactivated vaccines may complicate both virus isolation and serology in the diagnosis of IB. The natural occurrence of antigenic variant strains may overcome any immunity induced by conventional vaccines.

Laboratory diagnosis is made by virus isolation in chicken embryos or in tracheal organ cultures. This can be supplemented by immunofluorescence, electron microscopy, polymerase chain reaction techniques, haemagglutination inhibition tests (HI) or enzyme-linked immunosorbent assays (ELISA).

Identification of the agent: *IB virus may be isolated from tracheal mucosa during the acute phase of the respiratory form of the disease. Faeces or caecal tonsillar tissue are better sources of virus at other times.*

Chicken embryos originating from specific pathogen free flocks or tracheal organ cultures (TOCs) from 20-day-old embryos are used for virus isolation. The inoculation of the allantoic cavity of chicken embryos of 9–11 days' incubation with IB virus results in embryo stunting or death within about three serial passages. TOCs have the advantage that IB virus produces stasis of the tracheal cilia on initial inoculation. The virus can be identified by neutralisation tests using specific antiserum. The antigen may be visualised in infected allantoic cells by immunofluorescence, or by electron microscopy after concentration by ultracentrifugation.

Antigenic typing of IB virus is difficult and controversial. Within the same laboratory, a limited range of strains can be shown to be antigenically related or different by using various serological methods. The use of monoclonal antibodies may prove to be a useful method of distinguishing vaccine strains from field strains, and for defining serotypes.

Serological tests: *Regular monitoring of sera from flocks for IB antibody titres may help to indicate the level of vaccine response. Because many chicken sera, especially from older birds, contain antibodies that are highly cross-reactive against antigenically unrelated strains, sero-diagnosis of suspected disease outbreaks of IB cannot be used with a high degree of confidence. The HI test is rapid, inexpensive, practicable and under some circumstances may allow identification of infection with antigenic variant virus. Commercially produced kits that are very sensitive and suitable for monitoring immune response to vaccine are available for ELISAs. They appear to lack type specificity.*

A positive diagnosis of IB is made by virus isolation together with tests to demonstrate a significant rise in specific antibody. Following preparation of antiserum to a virus isolate, a serological comparison can be made with existing strains to allow antigenic serotype identification.

Requirements for vaccines and diagnostic biologicals: *Both live attenuated and oil emulsion inactivated vaccines are available. Live vaccines have been attenuated by serial passage in chicken embryos and confer a better local immunity of the respiratory tract. The use of some live* *vaccines carries the risk of residual pathogenicity, and this consideration may be avoided by using inactivated vaccines instead.*

Inactivated vaccines have to be given to birds individually, and a single inoculation does not confer protection unless preceded by the administration of a live vaccine. Both types of vaccine are available in combination with Newcastle disease vaccine; in some countries inactivated multivalent vaccines are available that include Newcastle disease, infectious bursal disease, reovirus and egg-drop syndrome 76 antigens.

A. DIAGNOSTIC TECHNIQUES

Avian infectious bronchitis (IB) was first described in the United States of America (USA) in the 1930s as an acute respiratory disease mainly of young chickens. A viral aetiology was established, and the agent was termed avian infectious bronchitis virus. IB virus, a single positive-strand RNA virus, is a member of the genus *Coronavirus*, of the family Coronaviridae.

IB virus affects chickens of all ages, which, apart from pheasants, are the only species reported to be naturally affected. IB occurs world-wide and assumes a variety of clinical forms, the principal one being a classical respiratory syndrome. Infection of the oviduct can lead to permanent damage in young birds lacking maternal antibodies, and, in older birds, can lead to cessation of egg-laying or production of thin-walled and misshapen shells with loss of shell colour. IB can be nephrotropic causing acute nephritis, urolithiasis and mortality (1). After apparent recovery, chronic nephritis can produce sudden death some time later, especially in brown birds. The virus persists in the intestinal tract and is excreted in the faeces for long periods. This occurs with vaccine strains as well as natural field strains (2).

Extensive use is made of live and inactivated vaccines, but this does not completely prevent IB infections. Vaccination may complicate diagnosis by serological methods as vaccinal immunity and field infections cannot always be distinguished. Persistence of live vaccine virus may also confuse attempts at recovering the causative agent.

There have been no reports of human infection with IB virus.

1. Identification of the agent

a) Sampling

Samples taken from birds should relate to the disease under investigation. For acute respiratory disease, swabs made from the trachea, or tracheal and lung tissues from recently killed birds should be kept on ice in transport medium containing penicillin (10,000 international units [IU]/ml) and streptomycin (10 mg/ml). For birds showing nephritis or egg-production problems, samples may also be selected from the kidneys or oviduct, but the highest success rate of virus recovery has been reported from samples of large intestine, particularly the caecal tonsillar tissue, or faeces (2). However, isolates from the intestinal tract may have no relevance to the latest infection or clinical disease, and samples from the respiratory tract must be taken in all investigations.

Suspensions of tissues (20% [w/v]) are prepared in sterile broth with antibiotics for egg inoculation, or in tissue culture medium for tracheal organ culture (TOC) inoculation (17). The suspensions are clarified by low speed centrifugation and filtration through bacteriological filters before inoculation of eggs or TOCs.

b) Culture

Embryonated hens' eggs and TOCs are widely used to titrate the virus or to make primary isolations of virus. Cell cultures are not used for primary isolation as it is usually necessary to adapt IB virus isolates to growth in chicken embryos before cytopathic effects (CPE) of virus infection are seen.

Eggs used in all culture work with IB virus must originate from birds that have been neither infected nor vaccinated. Such eggs should preferably be from specific pathogen free (SPF) hens. Most commonly, 0.1–0.2 ml of sample supernatant is inoculated into the allantoic cavity of 9–11-day-old embryos. Embryos should be examined daily thereafter. Any deaths that occur within 24 hours are assumed to be nonspecific and the eggs are discarded. True effects take up to 1 week to be apparent. The initial inoculum usually has no effect on the embryo unless the strain is already egg adapted. Normally, the allantoic fluids of all eggs are pooled after harvesting 3–7 days after infection; this pool is diluted 1/5 or 1/10 in antibiotic broth and further passaged into another set of eggs. This is repeated as desired. Typically, a field strain will induce teratological changes in the embryo at the second or third passage with some mortality in later passages. Infective allantoic fluids are kept at –60°C or below for long-term storage, or at 4°C after lyophilisation.

TOCs prepared from 20-day-old embryos can be used to isolate IB virus directly from field material (14). An automatic tissue-chopper is desirable for the large-scale production of suitable transverse sections or rings of the trachea for this technique (17). The rings are about 0.5–1.0 mm thick, and are maintained in a medium consisting of Eagle's N-2-hydroxyethylpiperazine N'-2-ethanesulphonic acid (HEPES) in roller drums (15 rev/hour) at 37°C. Infection of tracheal organ cultures usually produces ciliostasis within 24–48 hours.

c) Methods for identification

The virus neutralisation (VN) test in embryonated eggs and the immunodiffusion technique are useful for identification purposes (see below). Fluorescent antibody tests on cells present in the allantoic fluid of infected eggs may also demonstrate the presence of IB virus (9) and direct negative-contrast electron microscopy will reveal particles with typical coronavirus morphology in allantoic fluid or TOC fluid concentrates. The specific presence of IB virus in infective allantoic fluid may be detected by polymerase chain reaction (PCR) amplification and use of a DNA probe in a dot hybridisation assay (23). Direct immunofluorescence staining of infected TOCs for the rapid detection of the presence of IB virus has been described (4).

d) Serotype identification

Antigenic and biological variation among IB virus strains is well reported (13, 18–21), but at present there is no agreed definitive classification system. Nevertheless, antigenic relationships and differences among strains are important, as vaccines based on one particular subtype may show little or no protection against viruses of a different antigenic group. As a result of the regular emergence of antigenic variants, the viruses, and hence the disease situation and vaccines used, may be quite different in different geographical locations. Constant assessment of the viruses present in the field is necessary to produce vaccines that will be efficacious in the face of antigenic variants that may arise. Serotyping of IB virus isolates and strains has been done using VN tests in embryonated eggs (19), TOCs (18) and cell cultures (21). Neutralisation of fluorescent foci has also been applied to strain differentiation (15). The haemagglutination inhibition (HI) test has been employed for serotyping IB virus (6, 26) and has proved useful providing early response sera are used.

Monoclonal antibodies (MAbs), usually employed in enzyme-linked immunosorbent assays (ELISA), have proven useful in grouping and differentiating strains of IB virus (22, 27). The limitations of MAb analysis for IB serotype definition are the lack of availability of MAbs or hybridomas and the need to produce new MAbs with appropriate specificity to keep pace with the ever-growing number of emerging IB-variant serotypes (24).

e) Genotype identification

The molecular basis of antigenic variation has been investigated, usually by nucleotide sequencing of the gene coding for the spike (S) protein or, more specifically, nucleotide sequencing of the gene coding for the S1 subunit of the S protein (7, 29) where most of the epitopes to which neutralising antibodies bind are found (28). An exact correlation with VN results has not been seen, in that while different serotypes generally have large differences (20–50%) in the deduced amino acid sequences of the S1 subunit (29), other viruses that are clearly distinguishable in neutralisation tests show only 2–3% differences in amino acid sequences (7). However, there is in general good agreement between data represented by the S1 sequence and the VN serotype, and it may eventually be possible to select vaccine strains on the basis of sequence data.

Nucleotide sequencing has also produced evidence that recombination between IB virus strains occurs often (8, 38) and this may be a consideration in assessing the validity of using DNA probes (23) or restriction fragment length polymorphism analysis (30) in the differentiation of IB virus serotypes. Using the latter technique, however, clear distinction could be made between antigenic reference strains (30), and this may represent a method for rapid assessment of probable serotype for field isolates. Further advantages include the use of inactivated virus for reverse-transcriptase PCR using primers to identify and amplify the peplomer (S-1) gene of specific serotypes (25).

2. Serological tests

A number of tests have been described. Those considered here include VN (19), agar gel immunodiffusion (AGID) (37), HI (3) and ELISA (31). Each test has advantages and disadvantages in terms of practicality, specificity, sensitivity and cost. In general, for routine serological testing, the VN tests are too expensive and impractical, and AGID tests lack sensitivity. HI test and ELISAs are suitable for routine serology although they differ in their specificity. As ELISAs are available in kit form with detailed instructions for their use, the HI test is described in detail below. Regular monitoring of sera from flocks for IB antibody titres may help to indicate the level of vaccine response. Because many chicken sera, especially from older birds, contain antibodies that are highly cross-reactive against antigenically unrelated strains, serodiagnosis of suspected disease outbreaks of IB cannot be used with a high degree of confidence.

a) Virus neutralisation

In VN tests, all sera should first be heated to 56°C for 30 minutes. Virus is mixed with serum and incubated for 30–60 minutes at room temperature. Chicken embryos are most often employed, but antibodies can be measured using TOC or cell culture systems. Two methods have been used to estimate neutralising antibodies. One employs a constant serum concentration reacted with varying dilutions of virus (the alpha method) and the other employs a constant amount of virus and varying dilutions of serum (the beta method).

In the alpha method, tenfold dilutions of egg-adapted virus are reacted with a fixed dilution (usually 1/5) of antiserum, and the mixtures are inoculated into groups of from five to ten eggs. The virus alone is titrated in parallel. End-points are calculated by the Kärber or the Reed and Muench methods. The results are expressed as a neutralisation index (NI) that represents the $\log_{10}$ difference in the titres of the virus alone and that of the virus/antiserum mixtures. The NI values may reach 4.5–7.0 in the case of homologous virus/serum mixtures; values of <1.5 are not specific, but a heterologous virus will give a value as low as 1.5.

The beta method is the more widely used neutralisation test for antibody assay with chicken embryos. Two- or four-fold dilutions of antiserum are reacted in equal volumes with a dilution of virus, usually fixed at 100 or 200 EID_{50} (50% embryo-infective doses) per 0.05 ml and 0.1 ml of each mixture inoculated into the allantoic cavity of each of from five to ten embryonated eggs. A control titration of the virus is performed simultaneously to confirm that the fixed virus dilution in the virus/serum mixtures was between $10^{1.5}$ and $10^{2.5}$ EID_{50}. End-points of the serum titres are determined by the Kärber or Reed and Muench method as before, but here are expressed as reciprocals of $\log_2$ dilutions. This fixed virus-varying serum method is also employed for neutralisation tests in tracheal organ cultures using five tubes per serum dilution, as is conventional with other viruses (18). The results are calculated according to Reed and Muench, and the virus titres are expressed as median ciliostatic doses per unit volume ($\log_{10}$ CD_{50}). Serum titres are again expressed as $\log_2$ dilution reciprocals. This test is more sensitive than others, but technical logistics hamper its more widespread adoption.

b) Haemagglutination inhibition

A standard protocol for an HI test for IB virus has been described (3), and the test procedure detailed below is based on that standard. Many strains and isolates of IB virus have been shown to agglutinate chicken red blood cells (RBCs) after enzyme treatment. The virus selected to produce antigen may be varied, depending on the requirements of diagnosis.

- **Preparation of antigen**

Infective allantoic fluid is centrifuged at 30,000 ***g*** for 3 hours and the pellet is resuspended at 100-fold concentration in 0.01 M Tris-HCl buffer, pH 6.5. IB virus antigen requires enzyme treatment to acquire haemagglutination (HA) activity. Originally this was shown to be facilitated by commercial phospholipase C type 1 enzyme, and it was recommended that the virus suspension be mixed with an equal volume of this enzyme to a final concentration of 1 unit/ml in the same buffer. However, it was found to be more efficient to use crude filtrate from *Clostridium perfringens* culture, and it seemed most likely that a contaminating enzyme rather than phospholipase was the constituent responsible for the activity. Subsequent work has indicated that this enzyme is most probably neuraminidase (33). The mixture is incubated at 37°C for 2 hours.

For HA and HI tests, procedures are best carried out at 4°C.

- **Haemagglutination test**

i) Dispense 0.025 ml of phosphate buffered isotonic saline (PBS), pH 7.0–7.4, into each well of a plastic microtitre plate (V-bottomed).

ii) Place 0.025 ml of virus antigen in the first well. For accurate determination of the HA content, this should be done from a close range of an initial series of dilutions, i.e. 1/3, 1/4, 1/5, 1/6, etc.

iii) Make twofold dilutions of 0.025 ml volumes of the virus antigen across the plate.

iv) Dispense a further 0.025 ml of PBS into each well.

v) Dispense 0.025 ml of 1% (v/v) chicken RBCs to each well.

vi) Mix by tapping the plate gently and allow the RBCs to settle for about 40 minutes, when control RBCs should be settled to a distinct button.

vii) HA is determined by tilting the plate and observing the presence or absence of tear-shaped streaming of the RBCs. The titration should be read to the highest dilution giving complete HA in which there is no streaming; this is 100% HA and represents 1 HA unit (HAU) and can be calculated accurately from the initial range of dilutions.

- **Haemagglutination inhibition test**

The HI test is widely used in the diagnosis and routine flock monitoring of vaccine responses.

i) Dispense 0.025 ml of PBS into each well of a plastic microtitre plate (V-bottomed).

ii) Place 0.025 ml of serum into the first well of the plate.

iii) Make twofold dilutions of 0.025 ml volumes of the serum across the plate.

iv) Add 4 HAU of virus antigen in 0.025 ml to each well and leave for 30 minutes.

v) Add 0.025 ml of 1% (v/v) chicken RBCs to each well and, after gentle mixing, allow the RBCs to settle for about 40 minutes when control RBCs should be settled to a distinct button.

vi) The HI titre is the highest dilution of serum causing complete inhibition of 4 HAU of antigen. The agglutination is assessed more exactly by tilting the plates. Only those wells in which the RBCs 'stream' at the same rate as the control wells (containing 0.025 ml RBC and 0.05 ml PBS only) should be considered to show inhibition.

vii) The validity of results should be assessed against a negative control serum, which should not give a titre $>2^2$, and a positive control serum, for which the titre should be within one dilution of the known titre.

viii) Sera are usually regarded as positive if they have a titre of 2^4 or more. However, it should be noted that even in SPF flocks, a very small proportion of birds may show a nonspecific titre of 2^4, but usually in birds over 1 year of age.

c) Enzyme-linked immunosorbent assay

The ELISA technique is the most sensitive serological method and gives earlier reactions and higher antibody titres than other tests (31). It lacks type or strain specificity, but is suitable for monitoring vaccination responses under field conditions. Commercial kits for ELISAs are available – these are based on several different strategies for the detection of IB virus antibodies. Usually, such tests have been evaluated and validated by the manufacturer, and it is therefore important that the instructions specified for their use be followed carefully.

d) Agar gel immunodiffusion

Immunodiffusion can be used in diagnosis (36, 37). The antigen is prepared from a homogenate of the chorioallantoic membranes of infected chicken embryos. The Beaudette embryo-lethal strain is often employed to produce antigen. The test lacks sensitivity and is liable to yield inconsistent results as the presence and duration of precipitating antibodies may vary with individual birds.

B. REQUIREMENTS FOR VACCINES AND DIAGNOSTIC BIOLOGICALS

All viruses in live virus vaccines must be attenuated or naturally apathogenic. At present, many countries only permit live vaccines based on the Massachusetts type. A single inoculation of an inactivated IB vaccine is unlikely to confer full protection to the end of lay unless preceded by a primary response, usually to a live vaccine. Inactivated vaccines have to be administered to birds individually, using intramuscular or subcutaneous injection, whereas live vaccines can be given as aerosols or in the drinking water, or by eyedrop. Live vaccines confer a better local immunity on the respiratory tract and may protect against a wider antigenic spectrum of field strains (14, 32).

The more recent oil emulsion inactivated vaccines are now more efficacious, especially when preceded by a live virus vaccine. They also stimulate a more persistent antibody response. There are prospects for genetically engineered vaccines (5), and *in-ovo* vaccination is under development (35).

National and international standards that apply in the country in which IB vaccines are manufactured should be complied with. The licensing authority should provide information and guidance on requirements. These are now often presented in general terms, as applying to all vaccines - avian and mammalian, live and inactivated, or viral and bacterial vaccines. There may also be specific requirements applying to IB vaccines, live and inactivated. As examples, references are given to the European and USA regulations (10–12, 34).

The list of extraneous agents that must be shown to be absent continues to grow. Manufacturers must be familiar with those that currently apply in their country. Recent additions are avian nephritis virus and turkey rhinotracheitis virus.

For IB vaccines, important differences among countries may arise regarding the challenge virus to be used for potency tests, and its validation. Traditionally, a virulent M-41 strain of the Massachusetts type has been used for challenge tests of both live and inactivated vaccines. Although this type is still common, it is often not the only or the dominant type in many countries, and it may be advisable to prepare vaccines from other types. It is logical for challenges to be made by the same type as present in the vaccine. Establishing criteria for validating the challenge virus may be more difficult for non-Massachusetts types, because of their lower virulence in general. Inactivated vaccines are usually expected to protect against drops in egg production. The traditional M-41 challenge, as described in this chapter, should cause a drop of at least 67% in the unvaccinated controls, but when using other types much lower drops may be regarded as satisfactory, depending on published evidence of the effects of these strains in the field. There is also a tendency to relax the criteria for Massachusetts type challenges, and the European Pharmacopoeia now defines a satisfactory drop for Massachusetts types to be at least 35%, and for non-Massachusetts types to be at least 15%, provided that the drop is 'commensurate with the documented evidence' (12).

1. Seed management

a) Characteristics of the seed

The seed-lot system should be employed for whatever type of vaccine is produced, and for challenge strains. Each virus must be designated as to strain and origin and must be free from contamination with other strains of IB virus. Separate storage facilities should be provided between the strains of virus intended for vaccines or for challenge.

For live virus vaccines, many countries permit only strains of the Massachusetts type. Some countries allow other strains, usually on the basis that those strains are already present in their national flocks. The antigenic type incorporated in both live and inactivated vaccines requires justification if there is doubt as to its existence in a country.

b) Method of culture

All seed viruses are grown in the allantoic sac of developing chicken embryos or in suitable cell cultures. The eggs should be from an SPF flock.

c) Validation as a vaccine

- **Purity**

Every seed lot must be free from bacterial, fungal, mycoplasmal and viral contamination.

For the detection of extraneous viruses, the seed is first treated with a high-titred monospecific antiserum prepared against the strain under examination or against one of identical type. This mixture is cultured in a variety of ways, designed to confirm the absence of any viruses considered from past experience to be potential contaminants. The serum must not contain antibodies to adenovirus, avian encephalomyelitis virus, avian rotavirus, chicken anaemia virus, fowl pox virus, infectious laryngotracheitis virus, influenza A virus, Newcastle disease virus, infectious bursal disease virus, leukosis virus, reovirus, Marek's disease virus, turkey herpesvirus, adeno-associated virus, egg-drop syndrome 76 (EDS76) virus, avian nephritis virus, turkey rhinotracheitis virus or reticulo-endotheliosis virus. The inoculum given to each unit of the culture system used should contain a quantity of the neutralised IB virus component under test that had an initial infectivity of at least ten times the minimum field dose. These systems include:

1. SPF chicken embryos, incubated for 9–11 days, inoculated via both allantoic sac and chorioallantoic membrane (two passages);
2. Chicken embryo fibroblast cultures, for leukosis virus subgroups A and B. The COFAL test (test for avian leukosis using complement fixation) or double-antibody sandwich ELISA for group-specific

leukosis antigen is performed on cell extracts harvested at 14 days. An immunofluorescence test for reticulo-endotheliosis virus is done on cover-slip cultures after two passages.

3. SPF chicken kidney cultures that are examined for CPEs, cell inclusions and haemadsorbing agents passaged at intervals of no fewer than 5 days for up to 20 days' total incubation.

4. SPF chickens of minimum vaccination age inoculated intramuscularly with 100 field doses, and on to the conjunctiva with ten field doses; this is repeated 3 weeks later when the chickens are also inoculated both into the foot pad and intranasally with ten field doses. Observations are made for 6 weeks overall, and serum is collected for tests for avian encephalomyelitis, infectious bursal disease, Marek's disease, Newcastle disease and *Salmonella pullorum* infection.

- **Potency**

Vaccines intended to protect against loss of egg production should be tested for duration of antibody response. Mean HI titres should be >6 $\log_2$ up to at least 60 weeks of age. Serological tests should be done at intervals frequent enough to show that titres have not been boosted by extraneous IB virus infection.

Vaccines intended for protection of broiler chickens or rearing chickens against the respiratory form of the disease should be similarly tested for duration of antibody responses; in the case of broilers this would be up to the normal age for slaughtering, and in the case of rearers up to the age when a booster vaccination would be administered (often at 16–18 weeks of age).

- **Safety**

Tests on seed virus should include a test for any potential ability to revert to virulence. Live and inactivated vaccine seed must be tested for safety as in Section B.4.b.

- **Efficacy**

To demonstrate efficacy, a trial vaccine must be made from the master seed and the working seed at five passages from the master seed and subjected to tests that demonstrate their protective effect.

For live vaccines, a minimum of ten SPF chickens aged 3–4 weeks are vaccinated intranasally or by eyedrop with the recommended dose. Ten unvaccinated control birds from the same age and source are retained separately. All birds of both groups are challenge inoculated intranasally or by eyedrop 3–4 weeks later, each with $10^{3.0}$–$10^{3.5}$ EID_{50} of the virulent Massachusetts M-41 strain. A swab of the trachea is taken from each bird 4–7 days after challenge and placed in 3 ml of antibiotic broth. Each fluid is tested for IB virus by the inoculation (0.2 ml) of five embryonated eggs after 9–11 days of incubation. An alternative test to that of taking swabs is to kill birds at 4–6 days after challenge and examine microscopically the tracheal rings for ciliary activity (16). Failure to resist challenge is indicated by an extensive loss of ciliary motility. The live vaccine is suitable for use if at least 80% of the challenge vaccinated birds show no evidence of IB virus in their trachea, while 80% or more of the control birds should have evidence of the presence of the virus.

To assess an inactivated vaccine intended to protect laying birds, 30 or more SPF chickens are vaccinated as recommended at the earliest permitted age. If a primary vaccination with live vaccine is first undertaken, an additional group of birds is given only the primary vaccination. In both cases, these primary vaccinations should be done at no later than 3 weeks of age. A further group of 30 control birds are left unvaccinated. All groups are housed separately until 4 weeks before peak egg production, and then are housed together. Individual egg production is monitored and once it is regular, all birds are challenged, egg production being recorded for a further 4 weeks. The challenge should be sufficient to ensure loss of production during the 3 weeks after challenge. The loss in the control group should be at least 67%; the group that received primary live virus vaccine followed by inactivated vaccine should remain at the previous level, and the group given only a primary vaccination should show an intermediate drop in production. Sera are collected from all birds at vaccination, 4 weeks later, and at challenge; there should be no response in the control birds.

To assess an inactivated vaccine intended to protect birds against respiratory disease, 20 SPF chickens aged 4 weeks are vaccinated as recommended. An additional 20 control birds of the same age and origin are housed with this first group. Antibody responses are determined 4 weeks later; there should be no response in the control birds. All birds are then challenged with 10^3 CID_{50} (50% chick infective dose) of virulent virus, killed 4–7 days later, and tracheal sections are examined for cilial motility. At least 80% of the unvaccinated controls should display complete ciliostasis, whereas the tracheal cilia of a similar percentage of the vaccinated birds should remain unaffected.

Both live and inactivated vaccines are available in combination with Newcastle disease virus; inactivated vaccines containing Newcastle disease, infectious bursal disease, reovirus and EDS76 viruses are also available in some countries. The efficacy of the different components of these vaccines must each be established independently.

2. Method of manufacture

All virus strains destined for live vaccines are cultured in the allantoic sac of SPF chicken embryos or in suitable cell cultures. For inactivated vaccines, hens' eggs from healthy flocks may be used. The pooled fluid is clarified and then titrated for infectivity. For live vaccines this fluid is lyophilised in vials, and for inactivated vaccines it is blended with high-grade mineral oil to form an emulsion to which a preservative is added.

3. In-process control

The required antigen content is based on initial test batches of vaccine of proven efficacy in laboratory and field trials. Infectivity titrations are done in chicken embryos.

Live vaccine should contain not less than $10^{3.5}$ EID_{50} per dose per bird until the expiry date indicated, and not less than $10^{2.5}$ EID_{50} per dose per bird after incubation at 37°C for 7 days at the time of issue. For inactivated vaccine, the inactivating agent and inactivation procedure must be shown under manufacture to be effective on both IB virus and potential contaminants. With the use of beta-propiolactone or formalin, any live leukosis viruses and *Salmonella* species must be eliminated; and with other inactivating agents, the complete range of potential contaminants must be rendered ineffective. Before inactivation procedures, it is important to ensure homogeneity of suspensions, and a test of inactivation should be conducted on each batch of both bulk harvest after inactivation and the final product.

Tests of inactivation should be appropriate to the vaccine concerned and should consist of two passages in cell cultures, embryos or chickens, using inoculations of 0.2 ml and ten replicates per passage.

4. Batch control

a) Sterility

Every batch of live vaccine should be tested for the absence of extraneous agents as for the seed virus.

b) Safety

- **For live vaccines**

Use no fewer than ten chickens from an SPF flock that are of the minimum age stated on the label for vaccination. Administer by eyedrop to each chicken ten doses of the vaccine reconstituted so as to obtain a concentration suitable for the test. Observe the chickens for 21 days. For vaccines intended for chickens that are 2 weeks old or more, use the chickens inoculated in the 'test for extraneous agents using chickens' (see Section B.1.c.4.). If during the period of observation, more than two chickens die from causes not attributable to the vaccine, repeat the test. The vaccine complies with the test if no chicken shows serious clinical signs, in particular respiratory signs, and no chicken dies from causes attributable to the vaccine.

- **For inactivated vaccines**

Inject a double dose of vaccine by the recommended route into each of ten 14–28-day-old chickens from an SPF flock. Observe the chickens for 21 days. Ascertain that no abnormal local or systemic reaction occurs.

c) Potency

The potency test is developed from the results of efficacy tests on the master seed virus. Live vaccines are tested for potency by titration of infectivity, and inactivated vaccines by measuring antibody production. The potency test for a batch of inactivated vaccine consists of vaccinating 20 SPF chickens, 4 weeks of age, and showing that their mean HI titre 4 weeks later is not less than 6 $\log_2$.

d) Duration of immunity

Vaccine must be shown to have the required potency to achieve the claimed duration of immunity at the end of the claimed shelf life.

e) Stability

At least three batches should be tested for stability and must give satisfactory results for 3 months beyond the claimed shelf life.

The stability of a live vaccine must be measured by maintenance of an adequate infectivity titre.

The stability of an inactivated vaccine is measured at intervals by batch potency tests. The concentration of preservative and persistence through the shelf life should be assessed. There should be no physical change in the vaccine and it should regain its former emulsion state after one quick shake.

f) **Preservatives**

There are maximum level requirements for the use of antibiotics, preservatives and residual inactivating agents.

g) **Precautions (hazards)**

IB virus itself is not known to present any danger to staff employed in vaccine manufacture or testing. Extraneous agents may be harmful, however, and the initial stages of handling a new seed virus should be carried out in a safety cabinet. It is a wise precaution with all vaccine production to take steps to minimise exposure of staff to aerosols of foreign proteins. Persons allergic to egg materials must never be employed in this work.

5. Tests on the final product

a) **Safety**

A safety test must be carried out on each batch of final product, as in Section B.4.b.

b) **Potency**

A potency test must be carried out on each batch of final product, as in Section B.4.c., at manufacture and at the end of the stated shelf life.

REFERENCES

1. ALBASSAM M.A., WINTERFIELD R.W. & THACKER H.L. (1986). Comparison of the nephropathogenicity of four strains of infectious bronchitis virus. *Avian Dis.*, **30**, 468–476.

2. ALEXANDER D.J., GOUGH R.E. & PATTISON M. (1978). A long-term study of the pathogenesis of infection of fowls with three strains of avian infectious bronchitis virus. *Res. Vet. Sci.*, **24**, 228–233.

3. ALEXANDER D.J. *et al.* (The Poultry Disease Group) (1983). A standard technique for haemagglutination inhibition tests for antibodies to avian infectious bronchitis virus. *Vet. Rec.*, **113**, 64.

4. BHATTACHARJEE P.S., NAYLOR C.J. & JONES R.C. (1994). A simple method for immunofluorescence staining of tracheal organ cultures for the rapid identification of infectious bronchitis virus. *Avian Pathol.*, **23**, 471–480.

5. BINNS M.M., BOURSNELL M.E.G., TOMLEY F.M., MOCKETT A.P.A., CAVANAGH D. & BROWN T.D.K. (1986). Prospects for a genetically engineered vaccine against infectious bronchitis. *Israel J. Vet. Med.*, **42**, 124–127.

6. BROWN A.J. & BRACEWELL C.D. (1985). Application of the haemagglutination inhibition test to typing of infectious bronchitis virus. *Vet. Rec.*, **116**, 47–48.

7. CAVANAGH D. (1991). Sequencing approach to IBV antigenicity and epizootiology. *In:* Proceedings of the Second International Symposium on Infectious Bronchitis. Rauischholzhausen, Germany, June 1991, 147–160.

8. CAVANAGH D., DAVIS, P.J. & COOK J.K.A. (1992). Infectious bronchitis virus: evidence for recombination within the Massachusetts serotype. *Avian Pathol.*, **21**, 401–408.

9. CLARKE J.K., MCFERRAN J.B. & GAY F.W. (1972). Use of allantoic cells for the detection of avian infectious bronchitis virus. *Arch. Gesamte Virusforsch.*, **36**, 62–70.

10. COMMISSION OF THE EUROPEAN COMMUNITIES (Interim Publication Nov. 1993). The Rules Governing Medicinal Products in the European Community. Volume VII: Guidelines for the Testing of Veterinary Medicinal Products.

11. COUNCIL OF EUROPE (1997). European Pharmacopoeia, Third Edition. Vaccinum bronchitidis infectivae aviariae vivum cryodesiccatum. Editions of the Council of Europe, Strasbourg, France, 1795–1796.

12. COUNCIL OF EUROPE (1997). European Pharmacopoeia, Third Edition. Vaccinum bronchitidis infectivae aviariae inactivatum. Council of Europe, Strasbourg, France, 1745–1746.

13. COOK J.K.A. (1984). The classification of new serotypes of infectious bronchitis virus isolated from poultry flocks in Britain between 1981 and 1983. *Avian Pathol.*, **13**, 733–741.

14. COOK J.K.A., DARBYSHIRE J.H. & PETERS R.W. (1976). The use of chicken tracheal organ cultures for the isolation and assay of avian infectious bronchitis virus. *Arch. Virol.*, **50**, 109–118.

15. CSERMELYI M., THIJSSEN R., ORTHEL F., BURGER A.G., KOUWENHOVEN B. & LUTTICKEN D. (1988). Serological classification of recent infectious bronchitis virus isolates by the neutralisation of immunofluorescent foci. *Avian Pathol.*, **17**, 139–148.

16. DARBYSHIRE J.H. (1985). A clearance test to assess protection in chickens vaccinated against avian infectious bronchitis virus. *Avian Pathol.*, **14**, 497–508.

17. DARBYSHIRE J.H., COOK J.K.A. & PETERS R.W. (1978). Growth comparisons of avian infectious bronchitis virus strains in organ cultures of chicken tissues. *Arch. Virol.*, **56**, 317–325.

18. DARBYSHIRE J.H., ROWELL R.G., COOK J.K.A. & PETERS R.W. (1979). Taxonomic studies on strains of avian infectious bronchitis virus using neutralisation tests in tracheal organ cultures. *Arch. Virol.*, **61**, 227–238.

19. DAWSON P.S. & GOUGH R.E. (1971). Antigenic variation in strains of avian infectious bronchitis virus. *Arch. Gesamte Virusforsch.*, **34**, 32–39.

20. HOFSTAD M.S. (1958). Antigenic differences among isolates of avian infectious bronchitis virus. *Am. J. Vet. Res.*, **19**, 740–743.

21. HOPKINS S.R. (1974). Serological comparisons of strains of infectious bronchitis virus using plaque purified isolates. *Avian Dis.*, **18**, 231–239.

22. IGNJATOVIC J., MCWATERS P. & GALLI L. (1991). Antigenic relationship of Australian infectious bronchitis viruses: analysis using polyclonal and monoclonal antibodies. *In:* Proceedings of the Second International Symposium on Infectious Bronchitis. Rauischholzhausen, Germany, June 1991, 161–167.

23. JACKWOOD M.W., KWON H.M. & HILT D.A. (1992). Infectious bronchitis virus detection in allantoic fluid using the polymerase chain reaction and a DNA probe. *Avian Dis.*, **36**, 403–409.

24. KARACA K., NAGI S.L. & GELF J. JR (1992). Production and characterisation of monoclonal antibodies to three infectious bronchitis virus serotypes. *Avian Dis.*, **36**, 903–995.

25. KEELER C.L. JR, REED K.L., NIX W.A. & GELB J. Jr (1998). Serotype identification of avian infectious bronchitis virus (IBV) by RT-PCR of the peplomer (S-1) gene. *Avian Dis.*, **42**, 275–284.

26. KING D.J. & HOPKINS S.R. (1984). Rapid serotyping of infectious bronchitis virus isolates with the haemagglutination inhibition test. *Avian Dis.*, **28**, 727–733.

27. KOCH G., HARTOG L., KANT A., VAN ROOZELAAR D. & DE BOER G.F. (1986). Antigenic differentiation of avian bronchitis virus variant strains employing monoclonal antibodies. *Israel J. Vet. Med.*, **42**, 80–97.

28. KOCH G., KANT A., COOK J.K.A. & CAVANAGH D. (1992). Location of antigenic sites defined by neutralising monoclonal antibodies on the S1 avian infectious bronchitis virus glycopolypeptide. *J. Gen. Virol.*, **73**, 591–596.

29. KUSTERS J.G., NIESTERS H.G.M., LENSTRA J.A., HORZINEK M.C. & VAN DER ZEIJST B.A.M. (1989). Phylogeny of antigenic variants of avian coronavirus IBV. *Virology*, **169**, 217–221.

30. KWON H.M., JACKWOOD M.W. & GELB J. (1993). Differentiation of infectious bronchitis virus serotypes using polymerase chain reaction and restriction fragment length polymorphism analysis. *Avian Dis.*, **37**, 194–202.

31. MOCKETT A.P.A. & DARBYSHIRE J.H. (1981). Comparative studies with an enzyme-linked immunosorbent assay (ELISA) for antibodies to avian infectious bronchitis virus. *Avian Pathol.*, **10**, 1–10.

32. PICAULT J.P., DROUIN P., GUITTET M., BENNEJEAN G., PROTAIS J., L'HOSPITALIER R., GILLET J.P., LAMANDE J. & LE BACHELIER A. (1986). Isolation, characterisation and preliminary cross-protection studies with a new pathogenic avian infectious bronchitis virus (strain PL-84084). *Avian Pathol.*, **15**, 367–383.

33. SCHULTZE B., CAVANAGH D. & HERRLER G. (1992). Neuraminidase treatment of avian infectious bronchitis coronavirus reveals a haemagglutinating activity that is dependent on sialic acid-containg receptors on erythrocytes. *Virology*, **189**, 792–794.

34. UNITED STATES DEPARTMENT OF AGRICULTURE (USDA), ANIMAL AND PLANT HEALTH INSPECTION SERVICE (APHIS) (1 January, 1994). Code of Federal Regulations. § 113. 327 Bronchitis Vaccine. US Government Printing Office, Washington D.C., USA

35. WAKENELL P. (1991). Vaccination of chicken embryos against infectious bronchitis virus. *In:* Proceedings of the Second International Symposium on Infectious Bronchitis. Rauischholzhausen, Germany, June 1991, 239–240.

36. WITTER R.L. (1962). The diagnosis of infectious bronchitis of chickens by the agar gel precipitin test. *Avian Dis.*, **6**, 478–492.

37. WOERNLE H. (1959). Diagnose der infektiösen Bronchitis der Huöhner mit Hilfe der Prazipitationsreaktion im festen Agarmedium. *Monatsh. Tierheilkunde (Stuttgart)*, **11**, 154–167.

38. ZWAAGSTRA K.A., VAN DER ZEIJST B.A.M. & KUSTERS J.G. (1992). Rapid identification and identification of avian bronchitis virus. *J. Clin. Microbiol.*, **30**, 79–84.

*

* *

CHAPTER 2.7.7.

AVIAN INFECTIOUS LARYNGOTRACHEITIS

SUMMARY

Avian infectious laryngotracheitis (ILT) is a respiratory disease caused by an alphaherpesvirus. It is principally a disease of chickens, although it can also affect pheasants, partridges and peafowl. The clinical signs and pathological reactions may vary from extremely severe, with some birds dying due to asphyxiation, to very mild, indistinguishable from other mild respiratory diseases of chickens. The principal lesion is tracheitis.

Laboratory diagnosis depends on isolation of the virus, demonstration of the presence of the virus or viral antigens, and detection of specific antibodies in the serum. Histopathological examination of the trachea for characteristic intranuclear inclusions may be of value.

***Identification of the agent:** Virus isolation may be done by inoculation of suspected material on to the dropped chorioallantoic membrane of embryonated eggs, or into avian embryonic cell cultures. These methods are time-consuming but sensitive. Rapid methods include direct electron microscopy on tracheal exudate, Immunofluorescence on tracheal exudate or frozen sections, agar gel immunodiffusion (AGID) to detect viral antigens in tracheal samples or infected egg material, and an enzyme-linked immunosorbent assay (ELISA) to demonstrate viral antigen in mucosal scrapings. Molecular techniques using polymerase chain reaction methodology have been reported to be more sensitive than virus isolation for the examination of clinical material and are likely to be used increasingly in future. Virus isolation may be needed if these tests are negative or inconclusive.*

***Serological tests:** Antibodies to ILT virus can be detected by virus neutralisation tests conducted in eggs or in cell cultures, or by AGID reactions, indirect immunofluorescence, or ELISA.*

***Requirements for vaccines and diagnostic biologicals:** Vaccines against ILT are usually prepared from attenuated live virus. Those available at present afford some degree of protection, but are not completely satisfactory.*

A. DIAGNOSTIC TECHNIQUES

Avian infectious laryngotracheitis (ILT) is a respiratory disease of chickens caused by an alphaherpesvirus. It can also affect pheasants, partridges and peafowl. In the acute form, the history, clinical signs and very severe tracheal lesions are highly suggestive, but the mild form may be indistinguishable from other mild respiratory diseases. Laboratory diagnosis depends on the demonstration of the presence of the virus or viral antigens or of specific antibodies in the serum (13).

Clinically, the disease may appear in three forms, namely peracute, subacute, and chronic or mild. In the peracute form, onset of disease is sudden with a rapid spread. The morbidity is high and mortality may exceed 50%. Some birds may die in good body condition before the appearance of signs, which are characteristic and comprise difficulty in breathing with extension of the neck and gasping in an attempt to inhale. There is also gurgling, rattling and coughing when birds try to expel obstructions in the trachea. Clots of blood may be coughed up and can be found on the floor and walls of the house. Post-mortem changes are confined to the upper respiratory tract and are also characteristic, consisting of haemorrhagic tracheitis with blood clots and blood-stained mucus along the length of the trachea.

In the subacute form, the onset of illness is slower and respiratory signs may extend over some days before deaths are seen. The morbidity is high but the mortality is lower than in the peracute form, between 10% and 30%. Post-mortem findings are less severe and consist of mucoid exudate with or without blood in the trachea. Yellow caseous diphtheritic membranes may be found adherent to the larynx and upper tracheal mucosa.

Chronic or mild ILT may be seen among survivors of either of the above forms of the disease, although some outbreaks themselves may be entirely mild. Incidence within a flock may be only 1–2%, but most affected birds will die of suffocation. An outbreak of mild ILT may extend over months with deaths occurring at irregular intervals. Signs include spasms of coughing and gasping with nasal and oral discharge and reduced production. Birds may fail to grow well and vigorously. On post-mortem examination, diphtheritic and caseous necrotic plaques and plugs are found in the trachea, larynx and mouth.

1. Identification of the agent

The virus may be isolated in chicken embryo liver (12), chicken embryo kidney (6) or in chicken kidney (16) cell cultures. Of these, monolayers of chicken embryo liver cells have been found to be the most sensitive (7). The virus can also be grown on the dropped chorioallantoic membrane (CAM) of 10–12-day-old embryonated chicken eggs (8).

The causative herpesvirus may be demonstrated directly in tracheal exudate by electron microscopy (16). Viral antigens may be detected by immunofluorescence (4, 17), agar gel immunodiffusion (AGID) (9), or enzyme-linked immunosorbent assay (ELISA), using tracheal mucosal scrapings (19). Histopathological examination of the trachea for typical herpesvirus intranuclear inclusions may also be helpful (3, 14). Methods of detecting ILT virus using polymerase chain reaction (PCR) have been described and PCR has been reported to be generally more sensitive than virus isolation (2, 10, 11, 18).

a) Virus isolation

When samples are taken from live birds for virus isolation, tracheal swabs are superior to oropharyngeal or conjunctival swabs. These are placed in transport medium containing antibiotics. The whole head and neck from dead birds may be submitted, or only the trachea and larynx after their removal with minimal contamination. Tracheas should be transported in antibiotic broth for virus isolation, but wrapped in moist tissue paper if destined for electron microscopy. Any prolonged storage of infected tissues should be at –70°C or below to minimise loss of virus titre. Repeated freezing and thawing must be avoided as this reduces virus infectivity.

Exudate and epithelial cells are scraped from the tracheas, diluted approximately 1/5 in nutrient broth containing penicillin and streptomycin, and agitated vigorously. The resulting suspension is centrifuged at low speed to remove debris, and 0.1 ml of the supernatant fluid is inoculated on to the dropped CAM of at least three embryonated chicken eggs of 10–12 days' incubation. The eggs are sealed with paraffin wax and incubated at 37°C for up to 7 days. They are candled daily and the CAMs of dead embryos or of those surviving for 7 days are examined for typical pocks. Alternatively, at least two confluent chicken embryo liver or chicken embryo kidney cell monolayers, with their medium removed, are inoculated and allowed to adsorb for 1–2 hours. Cultures are overlaid with fresh medium, incubated for up to 7 days and examined daily under the microscope for evidence of a typical syncytial cell cytopathic effect (CPE).

In each instance, up to three passages of material may be necessary before a specimen is considered to be negative. The identity of a virus isolate needs confirmation as ILT virus by a neutralisation test in eggs or cell culture using hyperimmune antiserum to ILT virus. Alternatively, virus particles may be identified rapidly in cell culture fluid or in pocks on CAMs by electron microscopy, and viral antigens may be detected by immunofluorescence in acetone-fixed ILT-virus-infected cell cultures or in frozen sections of CAM.

b) Electron microscopy

To demonstrate the presence of virus by electron microscopy, tracheal exudate or epithelial scrapings from the trachea are smeared on to a microscope slide and mixed with a few drops of distilled water. One drop of suspension is placed on a carbon and formvar-coated grid and left for 2 minutes, after which excess moisture is removed using filter paper. One drop of 4% phosphotungstic acid, pH 6.4, is added and the excess removed after a further 3 minutes. The grid is allowed to dry thoroughly and examined using the electron microscope at a magnification of ×30–45,000 for typical herpesvirus particles.

c) Immunofluorescence

In immunofluorescence tests for viral antigens, epithelial cell scrapings from the trachea are smeared on to a glass slide. Alternatively, snap-frozen 5 µm thick sections of trachea may be used. The preparations are fixed in acetone at room temperature for 10 minutes. These can be stained directly by applying chicken anti-ILT virus immunoglobulin labelled with fluorescein isothiocyanate (FITC) for 1 hour, followed by rinsing for 15 minutes in a bath of phosphate buffered saline (PBS), pH 7.2, agitated with a magnetic stirrer. Otherwise, they can be stained indirectly by applying an appropriate dilution of chicken anti-ILT serum for 1 hour. The slide is rinsed thoroughly with PBS for 15 minutes as above, and an FITC-labelled anti-chicken immunoglobulin is applied for 30 minutes. After a final rinse, cover-slips are applied over nonfade mountant. The preparations are examined for specific intranuclear fluorescence in the epithelial cells using a microscope with epifluorescent ultraviolet illumination. Suitable controls include the use of known uninfected specimens and, for the indirect method, the application of nonimmune chicken serum. Particular care should be taken in the reading of indirect immunofluorescence preparations, as endogenous chicken IgG in the trachea may cause unwanted attachment of FITC-labelled anti-chicken IgG.

d) Agar gel immunodiffusion

ILT viral antigens may be demonstrated by AGID tests on tracheal exudate, infected CAMs and infected cell culture material using hyperimmune ILT virus antiserum. The gel is made with Noble agar (1.5%) containing sodium chloride (8%) and sodium azide (0.02%) – as preservative – in distilled water. The ingredients are autoclaved at 15 lb/sq. inch (2.4 bar) for 15 minutes; 5 ml of the molten agar is poured into a 5 cm diameter Petri dish. When the agar has set, a pattern of wells is punched in the agar, consisting of a central well and six surrounding wells. The wells are usually 8 mm in diameter and 4 mm apart. The hyperimmune serum is pipetted into the central well, while the surrounding wells are filled with suspect virus samples under test, but with at least one well containing positive viral antigen. Dishes are incubated in a humid atmosphere at room temperature or at 37°C, and examined 24–48 hours later by oblique illumination for lines of precipitation (reactions of identity). Tests should include uninfected material as negative antigen and known negative antiserum as controls. For economy of materials, the test can be done on a microscale – the agar being poured in a thin layer on to a microscope slide and holes punched of 4 mm diameter and 2 mm apart.

e) Enzyme-linked immunosorbent assay

When the monoclonal antibody (MAb) ELISA is used for detecting viral antigens (15), tracheal exudate is mixed with an equal volume of PBS containing 1% (v/v) of a detergent, such as Nonidet P40 (BDH Chemicals, Poole, United Kingdom), then vortexed for 30 seconds and centrifuged at 10 ***g*** for 1 minute. The supernatant fluid is dropped in 50 µl volumes in wells of microtitre plates previously coated with rabbit IgG against ILT virus, diluted 1/200 in 0.05 M carbonate/bicarbonate buffer, pH 9.0, and incubated for 1 hour. Next, 50 µl of MAb against major glycoproteins of ILT virus, diluted 1/50 in PBS, is added to each well, followed by 50 µl of a 1/1000 dilution of affinity-purified goat anti-mouse IgG conjugated to horseradish peroxidase. The substrate, 5-aminosalicylic acid (6.5 mM), is added to the wells in 100 µl volumes. After 30 minutes, the plates are read at 450 nm on a spectrophotometer and the absorbance reading for each well is corrected by subtracting the reading obtained for wells containing diluting buffer instead of tracheal exudate. The positive/negative cut-off point is taken as the mean absorbance value for several negative (i.e. tracheal material without ILT virus) samples plus 3 standard deviations.

f) Histopathology

Tracheas for histopathological examination should be placed in formol saline immediately after removal from the birds and embedded in paraffin wax. Intranuclear inclusions may be seen in the epithelial cells in longitudinal sections after staining by haematoxylin and eosin. They are the classical Cowdry type A inclusions of herpesviruses, but they may be present for only 3–5 days after infection. In severe cases where most infected cells have detached from the tracheal lining, inclusions may be seen in intact cells among the cellular debris in the lumen of the trachea.

g) Molecular methods

Molecular methods for identifying ILT virus DNA in clinical samples have been reported (10, 11, 18). Dot-blot hybridisation assays and cloned virus DNA fragments were shown to be highly sensitive for detecting virus when isolation and ELISA were negative (10, 11).

The PCR has been found to be more sensitive than virus isolation for clinical samples, especially when other contaminant viruses such as adenoviruses are present (18). Alexander & Nagy (2) found that during the middle to the end of the infection phase, PCR and virus isolation were similar in sensitivity, but PCR was superior in the recovery phase.

A problem of detection methods for ILT virus has been that hitherto, they have not been able to differentiate between field strains and vaccine strains. This seems to have been overcome by Chang *et al.* (5), who used PCR in conjunction with restriction fragment length polymorphism. This approach would also seem to offer promise for a better understanding of ILT virus epidemiology and evolution.

2. Serological tests

Antibodies to ILT virus in chicken serum can be detected by virus neutralisation (VN), AGID, indirect immunofluorescence tests and ELISA (1).

a) **Virus neutralisation**

VN tests may be conducted on the dropped CAMs of embryonating chicken eggs that have been incubated for 9–11 days, where antibody specifically neutralises pock formation due to ILT virus. Alternatively, the tests can be performed in cell cultures, where antibody specifically neutralises the ILT virus thus preventing CPE. Doubling dilutions of serum are added to equal volumes of a constant concentration of virus. This concentration may either be 100 median egg infectious doses (EID_{50}) for egg inoculations, or 100 median tissue culture infectious doses ($TCID_{50}$) for the inoculation of cultures. The mixtures are incubated at 37°C for 1 hour to allow any neutralisation to occur.

When the test is performed in eggs, the virus/serum mixtures are inoculated on to the dropped CAMs, using at least five eggs per dilution. Eggs are sealed and incubated at 37°C for 6–7 days. The end-point is recorded as the highest dilution of the serum where no pocks are present on the CAMs. When the tests are done in cell cultures, serum dilutions are prepared in 96-well microculture plates and virus is then added. After the period allowed for neutralisation, freshly prepared chicken embryo liver or kidney cells are added to each well. The plates are incubated at 37°C in an atmosphere of 5% CO_2 and examined daily for CPE; 50% end-points are read after approximately 4 days when the virus control titre indicates that 30–300 $TCID_{50}$ of virus have been used in the test.

b) **Agar gel immunodiffusion**

For AGID tests, antigen is prepared from virus-infected CAMs or infected cell cultures. For the former, at least 10^4 $TCID_{50}$ of ILT virus is inoculated into the allantoic cavity of a batch of 10-day-old embryonating specific pathogen free (SPF) chicken eggs. The CAMs are harvested after 4 days' incubation, and those with large pocks are homogenised and sonicated in a small amount of PBS, pH 7.1. Alternatively, heavily infected monolayers of chicken embryo liver or kidney, or chicken kidney cells are incubated at 37°C until the CPE is maximal. Any remaining attached cells are scraped from the culture vessel into the medium. Total culture harvests may be concentrated up to 100-fold by dialysis against polyethylene glycol (PEG 20,000 or PEG 30,000). For the test, the agar is prepared as described previously for antigen detection, but this time the CAM or cell culture antigen is placed in the central well with test sera in the surrounding wells. Known positive and negative antisera are incorporated in the test, which is read after 24–48 hours' incubation at room temperature or at 37°C. AGID tests are simple, economical to perform, and useful for flock screening, although they are less sensitive than the other methods.

c) **Indirect fluorescent antibody test**

For indirect fluorescent antibody tests, the antigen consists of ILT-virus-infected cell culture monolayers grown on teflon-coated multispot slides. When CPE is beginning to develop, the cultures are fixed in acetone for 10 minutes. Dilutions of test sera prepared in PBS are applied to each spot culture and the slides are incubated at 37°C for 1 hour. The slides are washed in PBS as described previously, drained and treated with an appropriate dilution of a commercial FITC-labelled rabbit anti-chicken IgG. After incubation at 37°C for 1 hour, the slides are rewashed and cover-slips are applied over a nonfade mountant. They are examined by epifluorescence with ultraviolet illumination, and end-point titres are read as the highest serum dilutions giving specific fluorescent staining. This test is more sensitive than AGID, but the interpretation of results may be subjective.

d) **Enzyme-linked immunosorbent assay**

The antigen for ELISA is obtained by sonication of heavily infected cell cultures at the time of maximum CPE, which is then absorbed on to the wells of microtitre plates. A negative antigen is provided by uninfected cell culture material treated in the same way. The test consists essentially of the addition of 0.1 ml of 1/10 dilutions of test sera to duplicate wells coated with positive or negative antigen. After incubation at 37°C for 2 hours, the plates are washed four times and a 1/4000 dilution of a rabbit anti-chicken IgG conjugated with peroxidase is added. After incubation at 37°C for 1 hour, the slides are washed again four times. Finally a substrate consisting of 5-aminosalicylic acid is added to each well followed by hydrogen peroxide to a final concentration of 0.0005%, and the absorbance of the fluid in each well is read at 450 nm on a spectrophotometer. The result for each serum is expressed as the difference between the mean absorbance produced with the positive and negative antigens. The positive/negative cut-off point is taken as the mean absorbance value for numerous negative sera plus 3 standard deviations. The test is very sensitive and possibly the best available for surveillance purposes. A fowl laryngotracheitis antibody ELISA kit is also available commercially.

B. REQUIREMENTS FOR VACCINES AND DIAGNOSTIC BIOLOGICALS

ILT is usually controlled with live vaccines, although inactivated vaccines have also been used for safety reasons. The live virus seed is a suitably attenuated or naturally avirulent strain of ILT virus. Vaccines may be administered by eye-drop, spray or in the drinking water. Young chickens may require vaccinating in endemic areas, but show more severe reactions to the vaccine. Repeated doses may be required to afford good protection. The level of virulence of the vaccine virus is critical. Strains of low virulence may not be effective, and those of higher virulence may cause severe disease. The spray route of administration requires care over droplet size and uniformity of application. It can be more effective with low virulence strains, but may be more dangerous with high virulence strains. At present, the available vaccines attempt to make a compromise between lack of efficacy and poor safety. Because of persistence of virulent vaccine virus on a site, it may be difficult to discontinue vaccination once it has been started. Subclinical mixed infections of vaccine and field virus, in vaccinated birds, can cause severe disease in unvaccinated in-contacts.

1. Seed management

a) Characteristics of the seed

The master seed virus (MSV) is selected and propagated in SPF chicken embryos. Initial tests are performed to demonstrate safety and efficacy. The safety test on the MSV must include tests to show lack of reversion to virulence on serial passage (six passes). Evidence of spread is also required. The MSV is stored in aliquots at –70°C. The MSV should not cause mortality or a severe respiratory reaction in chickens following ocular instillation, although pheasants are more susceptible. Administration by spray is convenient but may cause quite severe respiratory disease in some flocks.

b) Method of culture

In large-scale vaccine production, the virus is propagated in SPF chicken embryos, up to the fourth embryo passage from the MSV.

c) Validation as a vaccine

A test must be carried out to establish the efficacy of the vaccine. A suitable test is as follows:

Ten SPF chickens, 1–4 weeks old, are vaccinated with one dose of vaccine. This is repeated in further batches of chickens for each of the recommended routes of administration. Three weeks later, the birds, together with ten controls of the same age and source, are challenged by intratracheal administration of approximately 10^3 EID_{50} of a strain of ILT virus of known high virulence. To be satisfactory, none of the vaccinated birds should die or show severe signs of ILT. No more than four should show mild signs of ILT. At least eight of the controls should die or show severe signs of ILT.

2. Method of manufacture

The vaccine is made by inoculation of the production seed virus into 11-day-old chicken embryos derived from SPF flocks. Eggs are inoculated through a hole in the shell, on to the dropped CAM. They are sealed and incubated at 37°C for 4–6 days. All eggs are candled before harvest and only those with living embryos are used. To harvest the virus, the eggs are chilled, then cleansed and opened aseptically. The CAMs and fluids are pooled in sterile, cooled containers. The CAMs should show the thick grey plaques typical of ILT virus growth. They are then homogenised in a sterile tissue blender. The resulting homogenate is then pooled and tested.

3. In-process control

The infected tissue homogenate is tested for purity, potency, safety and virus content, mixed with a stabiliser (usually beef peptone and sucrose) and then lyophilised and stored at 4°C.

4. Batch control

a) Sterility

Tests for sterility and freedom from contamination of biological materials may be found in Chapter I.4.

b) Safety

Using the recommended route of administration, each batch of vaccine is tested in ten SPF chickens, or ten birds of other target species, using ten doses per bird. The birds are observed for at least 21 days for adverse effects attributable to the vaccine.

c) **Potency**

Once the *in-vivo* efficacy of the vaccine has been established, the batch potency may be determined by measurement of virus content. Serial dilutions of the vaccine are inoculated on to the dropped CAM of 10-day-old SPF chicken embryos, using at least seven eggs per dilution, in a volume of 100 µl. The eggs are incubated for 5 days and the virus titre is calculated by observing characteristic lesions on the CAMs. The virus content shall be at least 10^3 EID_{50} per field dose, for each bird, until the expiry date shown on the label.

d) **Duration of immunity**

The results of vaccination will depend on many factors, including dose schedule and route of administration. Some degree of protection should be given, over a period of several months.

e) **Stability**

This is tested by taking samples of correctly stored vaccine at intervals and measuring virus content. Tests should be carried out on at least six batches of the vaccine, and be continued for 3 months after the claimed shelf-life.

f) **Preservatives**

These should not be required, but some antibiotics may be added to the tissue harvest during manufacture.

g) **Precautions (hazards)**

Care should be taken over diluting and administering the vaccine, and over the proper disposal of unused vaccine.

5. Tests on the final product

a) **Safety**

Tests of virus content should be carried out. The virus titre shall normally be no higher than one-tenth of the dose at which the vaccine has been shown to be safe.

b) **Potency**

The test of virus content (see above) may also be used as a measure of potency. It must be no lower than the agreed minimum release titre.

REFERENCES

1. ADAIR B.M., TODD D., MCKILLOP E.R. & BURNS K. (1985). Comparison of serological tests for the detection of antibodies to infectious laryngotracheitis virus. *Avian Pathol.*, **14**, 461–469.

2. ALEXANDER H.S. & NAGY E. (1997). Polymerase chain reaction to detect infectious laryngotracheitis virus in conjunctival swabs from experimentally infected chickens. *Avian Dis.*, **41**, 646–653.

3. ARMSTRONG W.H. (1959). A slide smear technique for the diagnosis of laryngotracheitis. *Avian Dis.*, **3**, 80–84.

4. BRAUNE M.O. & GENTRY R.F. (1985). Standardization of the fluorescent antibody technique for the detection of avian respiratory viruses. *Avian Dis.*, **9**, 535–545.

5. CHANG P.C., LEE Y.L., SHIEN J.H. & SHIEH H. K. (1997). Rapid differentiation of vaccine strains and field isolates of infectious laryngotracheitis virus by restriction fragment length polymorphism of PCR products. *J. Virol. Methods*, **66**, 179–186.

6. CHANG P.W., YATES V.J., DARDIRI A.H. & FRY D.E. (1960). Some observations of the propagation of infectious laryngotracheitis virus in tissue culture. *Avian Dis.*, **4**, 484–490.

7. HUGHES C.S. & JONES R.C. (1988). Comparison of methods of isolation of infectious laryngotracheitis from field material. *Avian Pathol.*, **17**, 295–303.

8. JORDAN F.T.W. (1964). Diagnosis of infectious laryngotracheitis by chick embryo inoculation. *J. Comp. Pathol.*, **74**, 119–128.

9. JORDAN F.T.W. & CHUBB R.C. (1962). The agar gel diffusion technique in the diagnosis of infectious laryngotracheitis (ILT) and its differentiation from fowl pox. *Res. Vet. Sci.*, **3**, 245–255.

10. KEAM L., YORK J.J., SHEPPARD M. & FAHEY K.J. (1991). Detection of infectious laryngotracheitis virus in chickens using a non-radioactive DNA probe. *Avian Dis.*, **35**, 257–262.

11. KEY D.W., GOUGH B.C., DERBYSHIRE J.B. & NAGY E. (1994). Development and evaluation of a non-isotypically labeled DNA probe for the diagnosis of infectious laryngotracheitis. *Avian Dis.*, **38**, 467–474.

12. MCNULTY M.S., ALLAN G.M. & MCCRACKEN R.M. (1985). Infectious laryngotracheitis in Ireland. *Irish Vet. J.*, **39**, 124–125.

13. MEULEMANS G. & HALEN P. (1978). A comparision of three methods of diagnosis of infectious laryngotracheitis. *Avian Pathol.*, **7**, 433–436.

14. PIROZOK R.P., HELMBOLDT C.F. & JUNGHERR E.L. (1957). A rapid histological technique for the diagnosis of avian infectious laryngotracheitis. *J. Am. Vet. Med. Assoc.*, **130**, 406–407.

15. SCHOLZ E., PORTER R.E. & GUO P.X. (1994). Differential diagnosis of infectious laryngotracheitis from other avian respiratory diseases by a simplified PCR procedure. *J. Virol. Methods*, **50**, 313–321.

16. VAN KAMMEN A. & SPADBROW P.B. (1976). Rapid diagnosis of some avian virus diseases. *Avian Dis.*, **20**, 748–751.

17. WILKS C.R. & KOGAN V.G. (1979). An immunofluorescence diagnostic test for avian infectious laryngotracheitis. *Aust. Vet. J.*, **55**, 385–388.

18. WILLIAMS R.A., SAVAGE C.E. & JONES R.C. (1994). A comparison of direct electron microscopy, virus isolation and a DNA amplification method for the detection of avian infectious laryngotracheitis virus in field material. *Avian Pathol.*, **23**, 709–720.

19. YORK J.J. & FAHEY K.J. (1988). Diagnosis of infectious laryngotracheitis using a monoclonal antibody ELISA. *Avian Pathol.*, **17**, 173–182.

*

* *

CHAPTER 2.7.8.

AVIAN TUBERCULOSIS

SUMMARY

Avian tuberculosis is a bacterial disease of birds caused by the slow-growing nonphotochromogenic, acid-fast, rod-shaped Mycobacterium avium. *The disease has a world-wide distribution and occurs in many kinds of birds, but all varieties are not equally susceptible. Tuberculous lesions are mostly found in the intestinal tract, liver and spleen. The organism causes tuberculosis in chickens and other fowl and avian species, but can also infect an extensive range of different animal species such as swine, cattle, deer, sheep, goats, horses, cats, dogs, and exotic species (15).*

In humans, M. avium *is capable of inducing a progressive disease that is refractory to treatment. All operations involving the handling of open live cultures of* M. avium, *or of material from infected birds, must be carried out with adequate biohazard containment.*

Diagnosis of tuberculosis in birds depends on the demonstration of M. avium *in the dead bird, or the detection of an immune response, cellular or humoral, in the live bird.*

Identification of the agent: *Where clinical signs of tuberculosis are seen in the flock, or typical lesions of tuberculosis are present in birds at necropsy, the demonstration of acid-fast bacilli in smears or sections made from affected organs is sufficient for a positive diagnosis. If acid-fast bacilli are not found, but typical signs or lesions are present in the birds, culture of the organism must be attempted. This can be done on artificial media. Any acid-fast organism isolated should be identified by biochemical, nucleic acid relatedness, serological or chromatographic (thin-layer chromatography of lipids) criteria. In selected cases (namely if the isolate is not serotype 1, 2, or 3), the virulence of the isolate for the species of bird affected should be demonstrated by inoculation.*

Tuberculin test and serological tests: *These tests are normally used to determine the prevalence of disease in a flock, or to detect infected birds. When used to detect the presence of tuberculosis in a flock, they should be supported by the necropsy of any birds that give positive reactions.*

In domestic fowl, the tuberculin test in the wattle has been the test of choice. This test is less useful in other species of bird. A better test, especially for waterfowl, is the whole blood stained-antigen agglutination test (Rozanska). It is more reliable and has the advantage that it will give a result within a few minutes, while the bird is still being held. The tests are not reliable in cage birds.

Requirements for vaccines and diagnostic biologicals: *No vaccines are available for use in birds. An antigen preparation stained with 1% malachite green is available for the whole blood agglutination test. Avian tuberculin purified protein derivative is the standard preparation for use in the tuberculin test of domestic poultry*

A. DIAGNOSTIC TECHNIQUES

Tuberculosis in birds is caused by *Mycobacterium avium.* It is most prevalent in chickens and in many wild birds raised in captivity. Turkeys are quite susceptible, but duck and geese are comparatively resistant. The practice of allowing poultry to roam at large on the farm and of keeping the breeders for several years is conducive to the spread of tuberculosis among them. In most cases, infected birds show no clinical signs, but they may eventually become lethargic and emaciated. Under intensive husbandry conditions, sudden death may occur, often associated with severe lesions in the liver; such lesions are easily observed at post-mortem examination.

The primary lesions of tuberculosis in birds are nearly always in the intestinal tract. Such lesions take the form of deep ulcers filled with caseous material containing many organisms, and these are discharged into the lumen and appear in the faeces. Before the intestinal tract is opened, the ulcerated areas appear as tumour-like masses attached to the gut wall, but when the intestine is opened, the true nature of the mass becomes evident. Typical caseous lesions are nearly always found in the liver and spleen, and these organs usually are greatly enlarged because of the formation of new tuberculous tissue. The lungs and the other tissues are ordinarily free from lesions even in advanced cases.

It is essential to bear in mind that *M. avium* is capable of giving rise to a progressive disease in humans that is refractory to treatment, especially in immunocompromised individuals. All manipulations involving the handling of open live cultures or of material from infected birds must be performed with adequate biohazard containment.

1. Identification of the agent

If there is a characteristic history of tuberculosis in the flock and typical lesions are found in birds at post-mortem, the detection of acid-fast bacilli in smears or sections from affected organs, stained by the Ziehl–Neelsen method, is normally sufficient to establish the diagnosis. Occasionally a case will occur, presumably as a result of large infecting doses giving rise to acute overwhelming disease, in which affected organs, most obviously the liver, have a 'morocco leather' appearance with fine greyish or yellowish mottling. In such cases acid-fast organisms may not be found, but careful inspection will reveal parallel bundles of brownish refractile bacilli. Prolongation of the hot carbol fuchsin stage of Ziehl–Neelsen staining to 10 minutes will usually reveal that these are indeed acid-fast bacilli, with unusually high resistance to penetration of the stain. Recently, DNA probes and polymerase chain reaction (PCR) techniques have been used to identify the agent. Traditionally, *M. avian* is separated from common nonchromogenic slow-growing organisms by their ability to grow at 42°C and biochemical tests such as the Tween hydrolysis test, pyrazinamidase, growth on thiophen-2-carboxylic acid hydrazide (TCH)-containing media and tellurite reduction.

If there is a characteristic flock history and suggestive lesions are found at necropsy, but no acid-fast bacilli are seen in smears or sections, an attempt must be made to isolate *M. avium* from the necropsy material. Liver or spleen are usually the best organs to use, but if the carcass is decomposed, bone marrow may prove more satisfactory as it could be less contaminated. *Mycobacterium avium* grows best on media such as Lowenstein–Jensen, Herrold's medium, Middlebrook 7H10 and 7H11 or Coletsos, with 1% sodium pyruvate added. It may occasionally be necessary to incorporate mycobactin, as used for the isolation of *M. paratuberculosis*. Growth may be confined to the edge of the water of condensation. Typically *M. avium* produces 'smooth' colonies, but rough variants do occur.

Typing of mycobacteria to the species and subspecies level requires a specialised laboratory. Conventional biochemical tests for species identification are lengthy and fail to distinguish between *M. avium* and *M. intracellulare*. Thus, a miscellaneous group of mycobacteria that includes both species is usually classified under the denomination of *M. avium* complex (MAC). Seroagglutination, which is based on sugar residue specificity of surface gylcopeptidolipids, allows classification of MAC organisms into 28 serovars. More sophisticated typing methods directed at cell-wall-specific targets are currently available, such as enzyme-linked immunosorbent assays with monoclonal antibodies to major serovars, and thin-layer chromatography of lipids. Serovars 1 to 6, 8 to 11 and 21 are currently ascribed to *M. avium*, and serovars 7, 12 to 20 and 25 to *M. intracellulare*. However, no consensus was achieved on other serovars, and some isolates cannot be typed (7). Tuberculosis in birds is usually caused by *M. avium* types 1, 2, or 3. If one of these is found, it may be assumed to be the cause of the disease. If the isolate is not one of these, but is still suspected of being the cause of the disease, pathogenicity tests must be carried out. However, it should be borne in mind that superficial tuberculosis lesions in cage birds, especially psittacines, may be caused by *M. tuberculosis*. Hence, if rough colonies of mycobacteria are isolated from such birds, they should be tested for growth at 42°C. If the isolate will not grow at 42°C, *M. tuberculosis* should be suspected.

Specific and reliable genetic tests for speciation are currently available (12). Commercial nucleic acid hybridisation probes have become a 'gold standard' for distinction between *M. avium* and *M. intracellulare* cultures[1]. A further probe that covers the whole MAC was also developed, as genuine MAC strains have been described that fail to react with specific *M. avium* and *M. intracellular* probes (13). These tests use a chemiluminescent-labelled, single-stranded DNA probe that is complementary to the ribosomal RNA of the target organism. The labelled DNA–RNA hybrids are measured in a luminometer. Various in-house molecular methods have been reported for the identification of mycobacterial cultures, including MAC. The latter include 16S rRNA sequencing (8) to PCR amplification followed by either hybridisation with species-specific probes or restriction enzyme analysis (4, 14). Even though some of these methods would allegedly detect the agent directly in tissue samples, none of them has been validated for this use. Therefore, molecular identification of MAC is currently performed on organisms previously isolated by culture.

---

1 Accuprobe, Gen-Probe, Gen-Probe Inc., San Diego, California, United States of America.

Regarding intraspecies genotyping, pulsed-field gel electrophoresis of large DNA restriction fragments proved to be highly sensitive (9). Also, a number of DNA mobile elements have been identified that may be exploited for this purpose. Insertion sequence IS*1245*, which is virtually *M. avium* specific, was shown to be the most discriminative for the analysis of strain relatedness (2, 5). A standardised method consisting of IS*1245* restriction fragment length polymorphism (RFLP) analysis was recently proposed (16). Bird infection was found to be caused by a particular subset of *M. avium* strains that are characterised by specific, highly conserved RFLP patterns with IS*1245* and IS*901*, in addition to serovars 1, 2 or 3 (10).

If specialised typing facilities are not available, the likelihood that the organism isolated is the cause of the disease may be established by pathogenicity tests. It is preferred that these be carried out on the species of bird being investigated, but failing that, domestic fowl or Japanese quail may be used. Young adult birds are best. An inoculum is prepared by putting a small square of aluminium foil and some glass beads in a screw-capped container, which is then sterilised and weighed. A loopful of culture is then placed on the foil and the whole is reweighed. Finally, sufficient sterile normal saline solution is added to suspend the culture at 0.1 mg/ml. Birds are then inoculated intravenously with 1 ml of the suspension. If the organism is virulent, the bird will die in 5–6 weeks or, by that time, the bird will have extensive lesions filled with acid-fast bacilli.

2. Tuberculin and serological tests

a) Tuberculin test

The most widely used test in domestic fowl, and the only test for which an international standard for the reagent exists, is the tuberculin test. The tuberculin is the standard avian purified protein derivative (PPD). Birds are tested by intradermal inoculation in the wattle with 0.05 ml or 0.1 ml of tuberculin (containing approximately 2000 International Units [IU]), using a very fine needle of approximately 10 mm × 0.5 mm. The test is read after 48 hours and a positive reaction is any swelling at the site, from a small firm nodule approximately 5 mm in diameter to gross oedema extending into the other wattle and down the neck. With practice, even very small wattles on immature birds can be inoculated successfully. However, in immature birds the comb may be used, although results are not so reliable. Tuberculin testing of the wattle in turkeys is much less reliable than in the domestic fowl. Inoculation in the wing web has been recommended as being more efficient, but this is still not as good as for domestic fowl. Other birds may also be tested in the wing web, but results are not generally satisfactory. The bare ornamental skin areas on Muscovy ducks and some species of pheasant can be used, but reliability is doubtful and interpretation difficult. Testing in the foot web of waterfowl has also been described; the test is not very sensitive and is often complicated by infections of the inoculation site.

In pheasants, the tuberculin test can be performed in either of two ways. In the first, 0.05 ml or 0.1 ml of tuberculin is injected into the skin of the lower eyelid. A positive result is indicated by marked swelling at the site of injection after 48 hours. Alternatively, 0.25 ml of tuberculin is injected into the thoracic muscles and the birds are observed for 6–10 hours. Infected birds will show signs of depression and keep aside from the flock, and there may be cases of sudden death. No clinical signs will be provoked in uninfected birds.

b) Stained antigen test

- **Preparation of the antigen**

An antigen stained with 1% malachite green is used for the rapid whole blood plate agglutination test (11). The strain used for preparation of the stained antigen must be smooth and not autoagglutinate in saline suspension. It must conform to the characteristics of the *M. avium* species.

Although at first sight it might appear that it would be best to use a strain of the serotype that is most likely to be encountered (in Europe serotype 2 for domestic fowl, serotype 1 for waterfowl), in practice it is often better to use a strain that will detect infection with any serotype. For special purposes, however, it may be preferable to use a strain that is highly specific for the serotype it detects. The specificity of strains can be determined only by testing them as antigens, although in general a serotype 2 antigen will always detect serotype 3 infection and vice versa. Serotype 1 strains appear to detect more often a wide spectrum of infection, and will often also detect infections with mycobactin-dependent mycobacteria or *M. silvaticum*. There is no reason not to use a culture containing more than one strain of *M. avium*, provided that it shows the desired properties of sensitivity and specificity. Consistency of results between batches will be easier with the use of pure cultures.

The organism should be grown in a suitable liquid medium, such as Middlebrook 7H9 medium; better growth will be obtained if the medium contains 1% sodium pyruvate. Good growth should be obtained in approximately 7 days. The liquid culture is used as seed for bulk antigen preparation.

Antigen for agglutination tests is best grown on solid medium, such as Lowenstein–Jensen or 7H11, in Roux flasks or large bottles; again the incorporation of 1% sodium pyruvate (rather than glycerol in Lowenstein–Jensen medium) is beneficial. The use of solid medium maximises the chance of detecting any contamination, and antigens grown in some liquid media are not agglutinated by specific antibody. Liquid seed culture should be diluted (on the basis of experience) to give discrete colonies on the solid medium. This will usually give the best yield, and again increases the chance of detecting contamination. About 10 ml of inoculum will usually be enough to allow it to wash over the whole surface, and provide sufficient moisture to keep the air in the bottle near 100% humidity.

The bottles are incubated at 37°C, and good growth should be obtained in 14–21 days with most strains. The antigen is harvested by the addition of sterile glass beads and twice the volume of sterile normal saline (containing 0.3% formalin) as was used to inoculate the bottle. The bottle is then shaken gently to wash off all the growth and the washing is collected into a sterile bottle and reincubated at 37°C for 7 days. The killed bacilli are then washed twice in sterile normal saline with 0.2% formalin by centrifugation and resuspension. This sequence is safer than the original method in which the washing was carried out before the incubation that kills the organisms. Finally the organisms are again centrifuged and resuspended in sterile normal saline containing 0.2% formalin and 0.4% sodium citrate, to a concentration of about 10^{10} bacteria per ml. This corresponds to a concentration ten times that which matches tube no. 4 on McFarland's scale.

Cultures for antigen should be inspected for contamination daily for the first 5 days of incubation. The suspension made from the culture washings is also re-examined microscopically (for likely contaminants such as yeasts), and rechecked by culture to ensure that the formalin has killed the mycobacteria.

- **Validation of the antigen**

Cultures should be checked by Gram staining for the presence of organisms other than mycobacteria.

One or more batches for agglutinating antigen must be tested for efficacy in naturally or artificially infected tuberculous birds by comparison with a standard preparation of known potency. The potency relative to that of the standard preparation must not differ significantly from that declared on the label. Each bottle of antigen must be tested with normal chicken serum (to detect autoagglutination) and *M. avium* positive chicken serum of low and high antibody content. This should be done, where possible, alongside a previous batch of stained antigen. Those bottles that give satisfactory agglutination reactions with the antisera can now be pooled and the antigen stained. This is done by the addition of 3 ml of 1% malachite green solution per 100 ml of suspension. If possible, the stained antigen should now be checked using whole blood just as the unstained antigen was tested with serum. The agglutinating antigen should keep for at least 6 months in the refrigerator at 4°C, and much longer if frozen at -20°C or below. If a batch has not been used for a long time it should be rechecked, especially for autoagglutination.

The only safety test needed is the culture test of the unwashed antigen after 7 days of incubation, to ensure that all the bacilli are dead.

- **Test procedure**

The stained-antigen agglutination test has been used with good results, especially in both domestic and ornamental waterfowl. A drop (0.05–0.1 ml) of the antigen is mixed with the same volume of fresh whole blood, obtained by venipuncture, on a white porcelain or enamel tile. The mixture is rocked for 2 minutes and examined for agglutination. The agglutination may be coarse, in which case it is obvious, or quite fine, in which case it may be most clearly seen as an accumulation of the malachite-green-stained antigen around the edge of the drop, leaving the centre a normal blood-red colour. This test is especially useful for screening large flocks for immediate culling, and therefore has advantages over the tuberculin test for the control of the disease, even in domestic fowl. It has also been claimed that in domestic fowl it is more reliable than the tuberculin test.

Note on limitation of use

Neither the tuberculin test with avian tuberculin nor the stained-antigen agglutination test is likely to be of any value in cases of *M. tuberculosis* infection in cage birds.

B. REQUIREMENTS FOR VACCINES AND DIAGNOSTIC BIOLOGICALS

No vaccines are available.

Avian tuberculin is a preparation made from the heat-treated products of growth of *M. avium*. It is used by intradermal injection to reveal delayed hypersensitivity as a means of identifying birds infected with or sensitised to the same species of tubercle bacillus.

1. Seed management

a) Characteristics of the seed

Strains of *M. avium* used to prepare seed cultures should be identified as to species by appropriate tests. They should be shown to be free from contaminating organisms and to be capable of yielding a product of satisfactory quality. The strains recommended by the European Union (EU), for example, are D4ER and TB56. Reference may also be made to the World Health Organization (17).

b) Method of culture

The seed material is kept as a stock of freeze-dried cultures. If the cultures have been grown on solid media, it will be necessary to adapt the organism to grow as a floating culture. This is most easily accomplished by incorporating a piece of potato in the flasks of liquid medium (e.g. Watson Reid's medium). When the culture has been adapted to liquid medium, it can be maintained by passage at 2–4-week intervals (1, 6).

The production culture substrate must be shown to be capable of producing a product that conforms to the standards of the European Pharmacopoeia or other international standards (3). It must be free from ingredients known to cause toxic or allergic reactions.

c) Validation

The strains of *M. avium* used as seed cultures must be shown to be free from contaminating organisms.

Seed lots must be shown to be efficacious in producing tuberculin with sufficient potency. The necessary tests are described in Section B.4. below.

2. Method of manufacture

Avian tuberculin may be made by the following three methods:

a) Old tuberculin

The organism is cultivated in glycerol broth medium, killed by heating in flowing steam, and filtered to remove cells. The filtrate is concentrated by heat and sterilised by filtration.

b) Heat-concentrated synthetic-medium tuberculin

As for old tuberculin but the glycerol broth medium is replaced by a synthetic medium.

c) Purified protein derivative

As for heat-concentrated synthetic-medium (HCSM) tuberculin but, instead of being concentrated by heat, the protein in the filtrate is precipitated chemically (ammonium sulphate or trichloroacetic acid [TCA] are used), washed and resuspended. PPD tuberculin is recommended as it gives fewer false-positive reactions and can be standardised more precisely. An antimicrobial preservative that does not give rise to false-positive reactions, such as phenol (not more than 0.5% [w/v]), may be added. Mercurial derivatives should not be used. Glycerol (not more than 10% [w/v]) or glucose (2.2% [w/v]) may be added as a stabiliser. The product is dispensed aseptically into sterile neutral glass containers, which are then sealed to prevent contamination. The product may be freeze-dried.

3. In-process control

The production flasks, inoculated from suitable seed cultures, are incubated for the appropriate time period. Any flasks showing contamination or grossly abnormal growth should be discarded after autoclaving. As incubation proceeds, the surface growth of many cultures becomes moist and may sink into the medium or to the bottom of the flask. In PPD tuberculins, the pH of the dissolved precipitate (the so-called concentrated tuberculin) should be pH 6.6–6.7. The protein level of the PPD concentrate is determined by the Kjeldahl method. Total nitrogen and trichloroacetic acid precipitable nitrogen are usually compared.

4. Batch control

a) Sterility

Sterility testing is generally performed according to the European Pharmacopoeia or other guidelines (see also Chapter I.4.).

b) Safety

Two guinea-pigs, each weighing not less than 250 g and that have not been treated previously with any material that will interfere with the test, are injected subcutaneously with 0.5 ml of the tuberculin under test. No abnormal effects should occur within 7 days.

Tests on tuberculin for living mycobacteria may be performed either on the tuberculin immediately before it is dispensed into final containers or on samples taken from the final containers themselves. A sample of at least 10 ml must be taken and this must be injected intraperitoneally or subcutaneously into at least two guinea-pigs, dividing the volume to be tested equally between the guinea-pigs. It is desirable to take a larger sample, 50 ml, and to concentrate any residual mycobacteria by centrifugation or membrane filtration. The guinea-pigs are observed for at least 42 days, and are examined macroscopically at post-mortem. Any lesions found are examined microscopically and by culture.

Each filled container must be inspected before it is labelled, and any showing abnormalities must be discarded.

c) Sensitising effect

To test the sensitising effect, three guinea-pigs that have not previously been treated with any material that could interfere with the test are each injected intradermally on each of three occasions with the equivalent of 500 IU of the preparation under test in a 0.1 ml volume. Each guinea-pig, together with each of three control guinea-pigs that have not been injected previously, is injected intradermally 15–21 days after the third injection with the same dose of the same tuberculin. The reactions of the two groups of guinea-pigs should not be significantly different when measured 24–28 hours later.

d) Potency

The potency of avian tuberculin is determined in guinea-pigs sensitised with *M. avium*, by comparison with a standard preparation calibrated in IU.

Use no fewer than nine albino guinea-pigs, each weighing 400–600 g. Sensitise the guinea-pigs by administering to each, by deep intramuscular injection, a suitable dose of inactivated or live *M. avium*. The test is performed between 4 and 6 weeks later as follows: Shave the guinea-pigs' flanks so as to provide space for three-to-four injections on each side. Prepare at least three dilutions of the tuberculin under test and at least three dilutions of the standard preparation in isotonic buffer solution containing 0.0005% (w/v) polysorbate 80 (Tween 80). Choose the dilutions so that the reactions produced have diameters of not less than 8 mm and not more than 25 mm. Allocate the dilutions to the injection sites randomly according to a Latin square design. The dilutions are injected intradermally in volumes of 0.1 or 0.2 ml.

After 24–28 hours, the diameters of the reactions are measured and the results are calculated using standard statistical methods, taking the diameters to be directly proportional to the logarithms of the concentrations of the tuberculins. The estimated potency must be not less than 75% and not more than 133% of the potency stated on the label. The test is not valid unless the fiducial limits of error ($p = 0.95$) are not less than 50% and not more than 200% of the estimated potency. If the batch fails a potency test, the test may be repeated one or more times provided that the final estimate of potency and of fiducial limits is based on the combined results of all the tests.

It is recommended that avian tuberculin should contain the equivalent of at least 20,000 IU/ml, giving a dose for practical use of 2000 IU/0.1 ml.

e) **Specificity**

One or more batches of tuberculin may be tested for specificity along with a standard preparation of bovine tuberculin by comparing the reactions produced in guinea-pigs sensitised with *M. bovis* using a procedure similar to that described in Section B.4.d. In guinea-pigs sensitised with *M. bovis,* the potency of the preparation of avian tuberculin must be shown to be not more than 10% of the potency of the standard preparation of bovine tuberculin used in the potency test.

f) **Stability**

During storage, liquid avian tuberculin should be protected from the light and held at a temperature of 5°C (±3°C). Freeze-dried preparations may be stored at higher temperatures (but not exceeding 25°C) protected from the light. During use, periods of exposure to higher temperatures or to direct sunlight should be kept at a minimum.

Provided the tuberculins are stored at a temperature between 2°C and 8°C and protected from light, they may be used up to the end of the following periods subsequent to the last satisfactory potency test: Liquid PPD tuberculins: 2 years; lyophilised PPD tuberculins: 8 years; HCSM tuberculins diluted: 2 years.

g) **Preservatives**

Antimicrobial preservatives or other substances that may be added to a tuberculin, must have been shown not to impair the safety and effectiveness of the product. The maximum permitted concentrations for phenol is 0.5% (w/v) and for glycerol it is 10% (v/v). The pH should be between 6.5 and 7.5.

h) **Precautions (hazards)**

Experience both in humans and animals led to the observation that appropriately diluted tuberculin injected intradermally results in a localised reaction at the injection site without generalised manifestations. Even in very sensitive persons, severe, generalised reactions are extremely rare and limited.

5. Tests on the final product

a) **Safety**

A test for the absence of toxic or irritant properties must be carried out according to the specifications of the European Pharmacopoeia (see also Section B.4.b.).

b) **Potency**

The potency of tuberculins must be estimated by biological methods. These methods must be used for HCSM and PPD tuberculins; they are based on the comparison with standard tuberculins of the tuberculins to be tested (see also Section B.4.d.).

REFERENCES

1. ANGUS R.D. (1978). Production of Reference PPD tuberculins for Veterinary use in the United States. *J. Biol. Stand.*, **6**, 221.

2. BONO M., JEMMI T., BERNASCONI C., BURKI D., TELENTI A. & BODMER T. (1995). Genotypic characterisation of *Mycobacterium avium* strains recovered from animals and their comparison to human strains. *Appl. Environ. Microbiol.*, **61**, 371–373.

3. COUNCIL OF EUROPE (1997). Purified protein derivative (avian). *In:* European Pharmacopoeia, Third Edition. Editions of the Council of Europe, Strasbourg, France, 1694.

4. DEVALLOIS A., PICARDEAU M., GOH K.K., SOLA C., VINCENT V. & RASTOGI N. (1996). Comparative evaluation of PCR and commercial DNA probes for detection and identification to species level on *Mycobacterium avium* and *Mycobacterium intracellulare. J. Clin. Microbiol.*, **34**, 2756–2759.

5. GUERRERO C., BERNASCONI C., BURKI D., BODMER T. & TELENTI A. (1995). A novel insertion element from *Mycobacterium avium*, IS*1245*, is a specific target for analysis of strain relatedness. *J. Clin. Microbiol.*, **33**, 304–307.

6. HAAGSMA J. & ANGUS R.D. (1995). Tuberculin production. *In: Mycobacterium bovis* Infections in Humans and Animals, Steele J.H. & Thoen C.O., eds. Iowa State University Press, Ames, USA, 73–84.

7. INDERLIED C.B., KEMPER C.A. & BERMUDEZ L.E.M. (1993). The *Mycobacterium avium* complex. *Clin. Microbiol. Rev.*, **6**, 266–310.

8. KIRSCHNER P., MEIER P.A. & BOTTGER E.C. (1993). Genotypic identification and detection of mycobacteria. *In:* Diagnostic Molecular Microbiology, Persing D.H., Smith T.F., Tenover F.C. & White T.C., eds. American Society for Microbiology, Washington DC, USA, 173–190.

9. MAZUREK G.H., HARTMAN S., ZHANG Y., BROWN B.A., HECTOR J.S.R., MURPHY D. & WALLACE R.J. (1993). Large DNA restriction fragment polymorphism in the *Mycobacterium avium, M. intracellulare* complex: a potential epidemiological tool. *J. Clin. Microbiol.*, **31**, 390–394.

10. RITACCO V., KREMER K., VAN DER LAAN T., PIJNENBURG J.E.M., DE HAAS P.E.W. & VAN SOOLINGEN D. (1997). Use of IS*901* and IS*1245* in RFLP typing of *Mycobacterium avium* complex: relatedness among serovar reference strains, human and animal isolates. *Int. J. Tuberculosis Lung Dis.*, **2**, 242–251.

11. ROZANSKA M. (1965). Preparation of antigen for whole blood rapid agglutination test and its specificity for diagnosis of avian tuberculosis. *Bull. Vet. Inst. Pulawy*, 9 (1), 20–25.

12. SAITO H., TOMIOKA H., SATO K., TASAKA H. & DAWSON D.J. (1990). Identification of various serovar strains of *Mycobacterium avium* complex by using DNA probes specific for *Mycobacterium avium* and *Mycobacterium intracellulare. J. Clin. Microbiol.*, **28**, 1694–1697.

13. SOINI H., EEROLA E. & VILJANEN M.K. (1996). Genetic diversity among *Mycobacterium avium* complex Accu-Probe-positive isolates. *J. Clin. Microbiol.*, **34**, 55–57.

14. TELENTI A., MARCHESI F., BALZ M., BALLY F., BOTTGER E.C. & BODMER T. (1993). Rapid identification of mycobacteria to the species level by polymerase chain reaction and restriction enzyme analysis. *J. Clin. Microbiol.*, **31**, 175–178.

15. THOREL M.F., HUCHZERMEYER H., WEISS R. & FONTAINE J.J. (1997). *Mycobacterium avium* infections in animals. Literature review. *Vet. Res.*, **28**, 439–447.

16. VAN SOOLINGEN D., BAUER J., RITACCO V., CARDOSO LEAO S., PAVLI I., VINCENT V., RASTOGI N., GORI A., BODMER T., GARZELLI C. & GARCIA M.J. (1998). IS*1245* restriction fragment length polymorphism typing of *Mycobacterium avium* isolates: proposal for standardization. *J. Clin. Microbiol.*, **36**, 3051–3054.

17. WORLD HEALTH ORGANIZATION (WHO) (1987). Requirements for Biological Substances No. 16, Annex 1: Requirement for Tuberculins. Technical Report Series No. 745, WHO, Geneva, Switzerland, 31–59.

*

* *

CHAPTER 2.7.9.

DUCK VIRUS HEPATITIS

SUMMARY

Hepatitis in ducks can be caused by at least three different viruses. The more common and internationally widespread is duck hepatitis virus (DHV) type I, an enterovirus, which causes a highly lethal, acute, contagious infection in ducklings under 6 weeks of age and, frequently, under 3 weeks of age. It does not occur in older birds. This infection is often referred to simply as duck virus hepatitis (DVH).

DHV type II has been reported in the United Kingdom only. It occurred in ducklings from 10 days to 6 weeks of age, and caused pathological changes similar to those of DHV type I. From electron microscopy studies it is considered to be an astrovirus.

DHV type III has been reported only in the United States of America. It causes similar liver lesions in young ducklings, but is less virulent than DHV type I. It is believed to be a picornavirus, serologically unrelated to type I virus.

Diagnosis of hepatitis in ducklings is based on the characteristic disease pattern in the flock, gross pathological changes, the recovery of virus from dead ducklings, and the reproduction of the disease in susceptible ducklings.

***Identification of the agent:** It is not possible to distinguish among DHV types I, II and III on the basis of clinical findings and pathology, but distinctions can be made from the responses of ducklings, embryonated eggs and cell cultures to the isolated viruses.*

***Serological tests:** Serological tests have little value in the diagnosis of the acute infections caused by DHV types I, II and III.*

Serum neutralisation tests in ovo *have been used with all three viruses and in-vitro tests have been developed for DHV type 1. These tests have been used for virus identification, assay of immune responses to vaccination and epidemiological surveys.*

***Requirements for vaccines and diagnostic biologicals:** DHV type I infections can be controlled by the use of live attenuated virus vaccines and an inactivated virus vaccine. They are administered to breeder ducks to confer passive immunity to ducklings. Live attenuated virus vaccines may also actively immunise DHV type-I-susceptible day-old ducklings.*

Ducklings susceptible to DHV type I may also be passively protected with a chicken egg yolk antibody preparation.

DHV type III infections can be controlled by the use of a live attenuated virus vaccine given to breeder ducks to confer passive immunity to ducklings.

A. DIAGNOSTIC TECHNIQUES

Duck hepatitis is caused by at least three different viruses, namely duck hepatitis virus (DHV) types I, II and III. The most common is DHV type I, which is an enterovirus. DHV type II is an astrovirus, and DHV type III is considered to be a picornavirus.

These viruses, which cause acute infections, should not be confused with duck hepatitis B virus, a hepadnavirus classified in the same group as mammalian hepatitis B virus. The significance of this infection for the duck is not fully understood.

1. Identification of the agent

a) DHV type I

DHV type I causes a highly contagious infection of ducks. It is of no known public health significance. The disease is an acute, rapidly spreading, often fatal virus infection of young ducklings. It usually affects ducklings under 6 weeks of age and often much younger. The clinical disease is characterised by lethargy and ataxia. Ducklings lose their balance, fall on their sides and kick spasmodically prior to death. At death the head is usually drawn back in the opisthotonos position. The whole disease sequence is rapid and can take as little as 1–2 hours. Practically all mortality in a flock will occur within 3–4 days, with most deaths on the second day. Gross pathological changes appear chiefly in the liver, which is enlarged and displays distinct punctate and ecchymotic haemorrhages. Spleen enlargement and swelling of the kidneys with some congestion of renal blood vessels may also be apparent. Microscopic changes in the liver are characterised by extensive hepatocyte necrosis and bile duct hyperplasia, together with varying degrees of inflammatory cell response and haemorrhage.

The clinical and pathological observations are highly indicative of DHV type I infection. The virus can readily be recovered from liver tissue by homogenisation as a 20% (w/v) suspension in buffered saline. The suspension is clarified, and can then be treated further (if desired) with 5% chloroform (v/v) for 10–15 minutes at ambient temperature. DHV type I is resistant to this treatment.

The presence of DHV type I is usually confirmed by one or more of the following procedures:

i) By subcutaneous or intramuscular inoculation of the isolate into ducklings between 1 and 7 days of age that are susceptible to DHV type I. The characteristic clinical disease should follow, with deaths occurring within 18–48 hours of inoculation, often in under 24 hours. The ducklings should show the gross pathology attributable to DHV type I. Virus should be re-isolated from the livers.

ii) By inoculation of serial dilutions of the liver homogenate into the allantoic sac of embryonated duck eggs (10–14 days) or chicken eggs (8–10 days). Duck embryos die between 24 and 72 hours later, whereas chicken embryos are more variable and erratic in their response and usually take 5–8 days to die. Gross pathological changes in the embryos include stunting and subcutaneous haemorrhages over the whole body, with oedema particularly of the abdominal and hind limb regions. The embryo livers may be red and yellowish, swollen and may show some necrotic foci. In embryos that take longer to die, the greenish colour of the allantois is more pronounced, and both the liver lesions and stunting become more evident.

iii) By inoculation of primary cultures of duck embryo liver (DEL) cells, which are particularly sensitive (10). Dilutions of the liver homogenate containing DHV type I cause a cytopathic effect (CPE), which is characterised by a cell rounding and necrosis. When overlaid with a maintenance medium containing 1% agarose (w/v), the CPE gives rise to plaques approximately 1 mm in diameter.

- **Immunological tests**

Such tests have not been used extensively for the routine identification of DHV type I infection. Various virus neutralisation (VN) assays have been described, which may assume greater significance if DHV types II and III infections become more widespread. The tests that have been described (2, 10–12) include:

i) Passive subcutaneous immunisation of 1–7-day-old ducklings susceptible to DHV type I with 1–2 ml specific hyperimmune serum or specific egg yolk antibody. These ducklings are then challenged intramuscularly or subcutaneously, 24 hours later with at least $10^{3.0}$ LD_{50} (50% lethal dose) of the virus isolate. A control group of uninoculated ducklings is similarly challenged. Identification of infection is based on 80–100% survival in the passively immune ducklings and 80–100% mortality in the controls.

ii) 1-7-day old DVH type-I-susceptible and DVH type I maternally immune ducklings are challenged intramuscularly or subcutaneously with at least $10^{3.0}$ LD_{50} of the virus isolate. Identification is based on 80–100% losses in the susceptible ducklings and 80–100% survival in the maternally immune ducklings.

iii) Serial tenfold dilutions of the virus isolate are mixed with equal volumes of DHV type-I-specific hyperimmune serum diluted between 1/5 and 1/10. The mixtures are allowed to react at room temperature for 1 hour and are then inoculated (0.2 ml) subcutaneously into susceptible ducklings, via the allantoic cavity (0.2 ml) of embryonated duck eggs, and on to primary DEL cell monolayer cultures. Controls in each case consist of the virus isolate mixed with control serum.

There is little evidence for antigenic variation among DHV type I isolates. However, a variant, DHV type Ia, isolated in the United States of America (USA) only partially reacts with the classical type I virus in cross-SN (serum neutralisation) tests (7, 13). Other variants have been reported from India and Egypt, but nothing further is known about them.

b) **DHV type II**

DHV type II infection of ducks has only been reported from the United Kingdom (1, 4). It is an acute, fatal infection of ducklings producing clinical and pathological signs similar to DHV type I. Affected birds may show signs of polydypsia and usually die within 1–2 hours of appearing sick.

Gross pathological changes include multiple haemorrhages, both punctate and confluent bands in the liver, swollen pale kidneys with congested blood vessels, and enlarged spleens. The alimentary tract is often empty although the small intestine may contain mucus and haemorrhagic areas are occasionally seen. Petechial haemorrhages are also occasionally seen on the heart. Histologically, changes in the liver are similar to DHV I, the extent of bile duct hyperplasia may be greater than with DHV I, but this is relative. Electron microscopy of liver and faecal preparations have revealed viral particles 28–30 nm in diameter with a morphology resembling that of astroviruses (4).

The virus may be recovered in 20% (w/v) homogenised liver suspensions in buffered saline. This can be used to inoculate:

i) Susceptible ducklings, in which the response can be variable. A mortality rate of up to 20% may occur within a period of 2–4 days. The gross pathology is similar to that observed in field cases (4). This is in contrast to the findings with DHV type I infection, which is more virulent and rapid in its effect.

ii) Embryonated chicken or duck eggs, either via the amniotic cavity or yolk sac. These may respond, erratically, after four passages, but no deaths may be seen during earlier passages. Embryos take 6–10 days to show evidence of infection; when this occurs there is stunting with green necrotic livers.

- **Immunological tests**

Immunological tests have not been employed routinely as the serological response to infection of both ducklings and duck embryos is poor. However, a neutralisation assay has been applied (4) for virus identification by inoculating chicken embryos via the amniotic cavity with constant serum/varying virus mixtures.

Cross protection tests have been performed in 2–4-day old ducklings (4); these are inoculated with antisera to types I or II, then challenged 3 days later with the virus isolate. This technique could distinguish DHV type II from types I and III.

c) **DHV type III**

This has been reported in the USA only. Losses of up to 20% occur in ducklings immune to DHV type I (5, 8). DHV type III causes an acute infection of young ducklings with clinical signs similar to those seen in type I infections.

The gross pathology is also similar to type I infection. The liver surface is pale and mottled with many red bands and some petechial haemorrhages. The spleen is paler, but not noticeably enlarged, and the kidneys may show patchy congestion.

The virus can be recovered from homogenised liver suspensions and is resistant to treatment with 5% chloroform. The virus can be isolated by:

i) Inoculating the isolate intramuscularly into susceptible ducklings. The mortality rate may reach 20% with 60% morbidity. No deaths occur in the first 24 hours and all losses ensue between day 2 and day 4 after inoculation. Intravenous inoculation is more effective; type III infection is less virulent than type I.

ii) Inoculating the isolate on to the chorioallantoic membrane (CAM) of 10-day-old embryonated duck eggs. The response is erratic, but some embryo mortality always occurs within 7–10 days. The membranes assume a dry crusty appearance, beneath which they are oedematous. The embryos may be stunted and oedematous with skin haemorrhages. The liver, kidneys and spleen are enlarged.

Attempts to cultivate the virus in hens' eggs have not been successful.

Attempts to induce a CPE with the virus in tissue cultures have not been successful, but the virus has been detected by direct immunofluorescence in experimentally infected DEL and duck embryo kidney (DEK) cell monolayer cultures (5).

2. Serological tests

These do not apply to diagnosis as the clinical disease is too acute.

All three DHV types have been used in virus neutralisation tests *in ovo*, but their success depends on the expression of the virus in the assay system used; with type II and III viruses this can be a problem. *In-vitro* tests have been developed for DHV type I; these include a plaque reduction assay and a microtitre assay (10, 11). The plaque reduction assay may be performed using either primary DEK or DEL cells. Primary cell culture monolayers are prepared in Eagle's Minimal Essential Medium (MEM) containing 5–10% fetal calf serum (FCS), 2 mM glutamine, 0.17% sodium bicarbonate and gentamicin. Trypsinised cells are seeded into 5 cm diameter Petri dishes, then incubated at 37°C in a 5% CO_2 atmosphere. Monolayers should be nearly confluent at 24–48 hours post-seeding. The monolayers are washed twice with serum-free MEM or Hank's Balanced Salt Solution to remove all traces of FCS before infecting with DHV type I. Equal volumes of DHV type I suspended in serum-free MEM, adjusted to 200 plaque-forming units (PFU)/0.1 ml, are mixed with equal volumes of serially diluted duck sera (twofold dilutions in MEM). The serum samples should be heat inactivated at 56°C for 30 minutes before testing. The virus/serum mixtures are incubated at 37°C for 1 hour, then 0.1 ml aliquots are added to the confluent cell monolayers, three dishes per dilution. The plates are left for 30 minutes at room temperature (20–22°C), then overlaid with agarose maintenance medium (MEM containing 2% chicken serum and 0.1–0.2% FCS to which agarose had been added to a final concentration of 1% [w/w]). The plates are then placed at 37°C in a 5% CO_2 atmosphere. The number of plaques produced is recorded after 48 hours' incubation. Plaques may be observed using an oblique light source, or alternatively monolayers may be fixed with 10% formol-buffered saline and stained with 1% crystal violet. Serum antibody titres are expressed as the reciprocal of the highest serum dilution that reduces the plaque count by 50%.

A microtitre neutralisation assay may be performed using primary DEK cells. Serial twofold dilutions of each serum sample (heat-inactivated) are prepared in 50 µl of serum-free Eagle's Basal Medium (BME) in microtitre plates. Approximately $10^{2.0}$ $TCID_{50}$ (50% tissue culture infective dose) of DHV type I in 50 µl of BME is added to each well and the mixtures are allowed to react at 37°C for 1 hour. Primary DEK cells are suspended in BME supplemented with 10% tryptose phosphate broth, 2 mM L-glutamine, 0.17% sodium bicarbonate and 2–4% chicken serum, and are adjusted to contain 3×10^5 cells/ml. Cells are next added to the plates at 100 µl per well and the plates are then incubated for up to 96 hours at 37°C in a humidified 5% CO_2 atmosphere. Following incubation, cells are fixed with 10% formol-buffered saline and stained with 1% crystal violet. The plates are read macroscopically. The titre for virus neutralising activity is expressed as the reciprocal of the highest dilution of serum at which a monolayer grew, i.e., there is no evidence of CPE and therefore complete virus neutralisation has occurred. A titre of less than 4 log_2 is considered to be negative.

These neutralisation tests have been used to assay humoral immune responses to vaccination and for epidemiological surveys, as well as for virus identification.

B. REQUIREMENTS FOR VACCINES AND DIAGNOSTIC BIOLOGICALS

DHV type I can be controlled by the use of a live attenuated virus vaccine. This is given to breeder ducks so that immunity is transferred via the yolk to newly hatched birds. Live vaccine virus can also be used to actively immunise newly hatched DHV type-I-susceptible ducklings (3). An inactivated DHV type I vaccine is also effective when administered to breeder ducks, that have been primed with live vaccine or previously field exposed to live DHV type I; progeny from these breeders have maternal immunity (11). Ducks may also be passively protected by inoculation of antibodies in chicken egg yolk.

An attenuated live virus DHV type II vaccine has been used to protect ducklings only under experimental conditions (4).

DHV type III infections have been controlled by the use of attenuated live virus vaccines given to breeder ducks, so that the immunity is transferred via the yolk sac to the hatching ducklings.

1. Seed management

a) Characteristics of the seed

The type I virus vaccine seed used most commonly in Europe is derived from an isolate passaged in embryonated chicken eggs 53–55 times, that in the USA for live and inactivated vaccines has been passaged 84–89 times.

The type II virus vaccine seed originated from an isolate attenuated by 25 serial passages in embryonated chicken eggs (1), and has been employed only experimentally under field conditions (R.E. Gough, personal communication).

The type III vaccine seed has been attenuated by 30 serial passages in embryonated duck eggs inoculated via the CAM.

b) Method of culture

The seed viruses of types I and II are handled similarly. They should be prepared in 8–10-day-old specific pathogen free (SPF) embryonated chicken eggs inoculated via the allantoic route and incubated at 37°C. They can be stored as embryo homogenates in buffered saline at –70°C or below for several years.

The type III seed virus is prepared in 10-day-old SPF duck embryos, inoculated on to the CAM, and incubated for 6–10 days at 37°C. It may be stored as a homogenate of CAM and embryos at –70°C or below.

c) Validation as a vaccine

All seed viruses should be shown to be free from extraneous viruses that are pathogenic for ducks, chickens or turkeys. The seeds should be free from all microbiological and fungal contamination.

In the case of newly hatched ducklings, attenuated live DHV type I replicates rapidly and results in an immunity within 48–72 hours of vaccination. This immunity persists throughout the susceptible period of life (3). However in ducklings protected by vaccination of their parents, the level of maternally derived immunity decreases over the first 2 weeks of life, but such ducklings can be actively re-immunised with attenuated virus given subcutaneously or orally at about 7–10 days of age (6, 9). Alternatively, the immunity can be enhanced by the administration of specific hyperimmune serum or of egg yolk antibody prepared from eggs laid by chickens actively hyperimmunised against DHV type I.

Breeder ducks primed with live DHV type I and then given, intramuscularly, a single dose of inactivated type I vaccine produced maternally immune progeny through a complete laying cycle (11).

2. Method of manufacture

DHV types I and II viruses are treated similarly. The vaccine is produced in 8–10-day-old SPF embryonated chicken eggs inoculated via the allantoic route, and incubated at 37°C. Most embryo deaths occur within 2–3 days in the case of DHV type I, but with type II, the deaths do not occur until 6–10 days after inoculation, although they are harvested at 3–5 days for maximum virus yield. The embryo harvests are homogenised in buffered saline and clarified by low speed centrifugation. The preparation is diluted as appropriate and dispensed into vials, which are preferably frozen rapidly at –70°C or below. Subsequently, they may be stored satisfactorily between –20°C and –40°C. DHV type I attenuated vaccine is also available as a lyophilised preparation that may be stored at 2–8°C. The reconstituted vaccine may be used with or without the incorporation of aluminium hydroxide in the diluent.

In the case of inactivated DHV type I vaccine, the embryo harvests are homogenised and clarified by low speed centrifugation and then further purified by treatment with chloroform (final concentration 10% [v/v]). This preparation is then inactivated with freshly prepared binary ethylenimine (BEI). The inactivated virus is then blended with an adjuvant such as LES-STM[1]; 0.2 % (v/v) formalin is added as a preservative (11).

The type III vaccine is prepared in 10-day-old SPF duck eggs inoculated via the CAM with attenuated DHV type III and incubated at 37°C. Most embryo deaths occur between 6 and 10 days. Eggs containing dying embryos,

1 A preparation of *Salmonella typhimurium* (STM), a B cell mitogen, in a lipid emulsion system (LES). Available from Ribi Immunochem Research, Hamilton, Montana 59840, USA.

together with their CAMs, are harvested and homogenised in buffered saline and clarified by low speed centrifugation. The preparation is diluted as appropriate and dispensed into vials, which are preferably frozen rapidly at –70°C or below.

- **Egg yolk antibody**

  Virulent DHV type I prepared from duckling livers or attenuated virus may be used to hyperimmunise SPF chickens for egg-yolk antibody production. Eggs are collected from the hyperimmunised birds and stored at 4°C until time of production. The yolks are separated, pooled and blended with an antifoaming agent. The mixture is diluted with buffered saline containing no more than 0.2% (v/v) formalin as a preservative. The dispensed product is stored at 4°C and has a shelf life of 1 year. Tests are carried out for sterility in the usual way for the absence of contaminants.

3. In-process control

Any embryo deaths within the first 24 hours of inoculation should be discarded as nonspecific deaths.

The identity of the virus type should be confirmed by a VN test conducted with specific antiserum by a constant serum/varying virus method. In the case of types I and II viruses, the tests are performed in embryonated chicken eggs; with type III virus the tests are done in embryonated duck eggs. The antiserum should reduce the titre of the respective virus by at least $10^{2.0}$ ELD_{50} (50% embryo lethal dose).

4. Batch control

a) Sterility

Tests for sterility and freedom from contamination of biological materials may be found in the Chapter I.4.

b) Safety

A group of 1–3-day-old ducklings susceptible to the type of virus concerned, should be inoculated subcutaneously or intramuscularly (in the case of types I and II), or subcutaneously (in the case of type III), with the attenuated vaccine at ten times the recommended dose, and kept under observation for between 10 and 21 days for any adverse reactions. Attenuated live vaccines should be stable and not revert to virulence on back passages in susceptible ducklings.

A safety test on the inactivated DHV type I vaccine is performed by inoculating the recommended dose (0.5 ml) intramuscularly into a group of day-old ducklings; no adverse effects should be observed during the period of testing.

Safety tests on yolk antibody are done by inoculating 1 ml subcutaneously into each of a group of ducklings, which are then kept under observation for 3 days for signs of adverse effects.

c) Potency

For DHV types I and II viruses, the virus titre of the vaccine should be determined in 8–10-day-old embryonated chicken eggs inoculated into the allantoic cavity and incubated at 37°C. The immunogenicity, of the vaccine for ducklings susceptible to type I or II virus can be assessed by inoculating subcutaneously a minimum of $10^{3.3}$ ELD_{50} per duckling of the vaccine virus and challenging subcutaneously with $10^{3.0}$ LD_{50} per duckling of virulent DHV virus type I or II 72 hours later (3). At least 80% of the vaccinated birds should survive and, in the case of type I, at least 80% of the controls should die; in the case of type II, a 20% mortality in the controls is more realistic.

The immunogenicity of the inactivated vaccine is considered to be satisfactory if a four-fold or greater increase in neutralising antibody titre can be demonstrated following administration to ducklings that have been previously primed with live attenuated DHV type I.

For type III virus, the titre of the vaccine should be determined in 10-day-old embryonated duck eggs inoculated on to the CAM. Immunogenicity tests in ducklings have proved difficult because of the variable pathogenicity of the challenge virus for ducklings.

Potency tests on yolk antibody are done by determining the neutralising index (NI) for the product in embryonated hens' eggs using the constant yolk/varying virus method. A minimum NI of $10^{3.0}$ is considered to be satisfactory. The efficacy of the product is determined by inoculating a group of susceptible ducklings with the recommended dose of egg yolk antibody. A second group is left untreated. After 24 hours each group is challenged with virulent DHV type I virus. The product is adjudged efficacious if at least 80% of the treated ducklings survive and at least 80% of the controls die.

d) **Duration of immunity**

Breeder ducks given live attenuated DHV type I vaccine two or three times at 12, 8 and 4 weeks before coming in to lay, and breeder ducks given live attenuated DHV type III vaccine twice at 12 and 4 weeks before coming in to lay should produce passively immune progeny throughout a breeding season. However, it is usually recommended to revaccinate every 3 months with DHV type I vaccine and every 6 months with DHV type III vaccine after the onset of lay. DVH type I attenuated vaccine can also be supplied as a lyophilised preparation that is blended with a diluent containing aluminium hydroxide, just before administration. This is given at 7 weeks of age with a second dose 2 weeks before onset of lay. This should provide maternally immune progeny throughout a complete laying cycle. No information on the use of DHV type II vaccine in breeder ducks is available.

Live attenuated DHV type I or type II vaccine given subcutaneously or intramuscularly to 1-day-old ducklings protects against the disease for the duration of their susceptibility. No information is available on the use of DHV type III vaccine to actively immunise 1-day-old ducklings.

Breeder ducks primed with live DHV type I and then given a single dose of inactivated DHV type I vaccine intramuscularly, should produce maternally immune progeny through a complete laying cycle (11).

Egg-yolk antibody offers passive immunisation in the face of an outbreak. The duration of its efficacy is short-lived.

e) **Stability**

Aqueous preparation of live attenuated DHV type I, II and III vaccines when stored frozen at –70°C or lower should remain stable for at least 1 year. Once thawed these vaccines should be held at 4°C and used within 1 week. Live lyophilised vaccines may be stored at 2–8°C and should retain their potency for at least 1 year.

The inactivated DHV type I vaccine is blended with adjuvant and can be stored at 4°C for at least 20 months without loss of immunogenicity.

Egg-yolk antibody can be stored for up to 1 year at 4°C.

f) **Preservatives**

No preservatives are added to the live attenuated DHV type I, II and III vaccines.

Formalin (up to 0.2% [v/v]) is added to the DHV type I inactivated vaccine, and to the egg-yolk antibody preparation.

g) **Precautions (hazards)**

The inactivated DHV type I vaccine should be shaken well to ensure that it is completely blended before use.

5. Tests on the final product

The live attenuated DHV type I and III vaccines are issued as vials of lyophilised or frozen concentrated vaccine virus together with bottles of sterile diluent, on which standard sterility checks have been made (see Section B.4.a.). The DHV type II live attenuated vaccine has only been made experimentally.

a) **Safety**

No additional testing is performed after the batch testing on any of the products.

b) **Potency**

No additional testing is performed after the batch testing on any of the products.

REFERENCES

1. ASPLIN F.D. (1965). Duck hepatitis. Vaccination against two serological types. *Vet. Rec.*, **77**, 1529–1530.

2. CHALMERS W.S.K. & WOOLCOCK P.R. (1984). The effect of animal sera on duck hepatitis virus. *Avian Pathol.*, **13**, 727–732.

3. CRIGHTON G.W. & WOOLCOCK P.R. (1978). Active immunisation of ducklings against duck virus hepatitis. *Vet. Rec.*, **102**, 358–361.

4. GOUGH R.E., BORLAND E.D., KEYMER I.F. & STUART J.C. (1985). An outbreak of duck hepatitis type II in commercial ducks. *Avian Pathol.*, **14**, 227–236.

5. HAIDER S.A. & CALNEK B.W. (1979). *In-vitro* isolation, propagation and characterisation of duck hepatitis virus type III. *Avian Dis.*, **23**, 715–729.

6. HANSON L.E. & TRIPATHY D.N. (1976). Oral immunisation of ducklings with an attenuated hepatitis virus. *Dev. Biol. Stand.*, **33**, 357–363.

7. SANDHU T.S., CALLNEK B.W. & ZEMAN L. (1992). Pathologic and serologic characterisation of a variant of duck hepatitis type I virus. *Avian Dis.*, **36**, 932–936.

8. TOTH T.E. (1969). Studies of an agent causing mortality among ducklings immune to duck virus hepatitis. *Avian Dis.*, **13**, 834–846.

9. TRIPATHY D.N. & HANSON L.E. (1986). Impact of oral immunisation against duck viral hepatitis in passively immune ducklings. *Prev. Vet. Med.*, **4**, 355–360.

10. WOOLCOCK P.R. (1986). An assay for duck hepatitis virus type I in duck embryo liver cells and a comparison with other assays. *Avian Pathol.*, **15**, 75–82.

11. WOOLCOCK P.R. (1991). Duck hepatitis virus type I: Studies with inactivated vaccines in breeder ducks. *Avian Pathol.*, **20**, 509–522.

12. WOOLCOCK P.R. (1998). Duck virus hepatitis. *In:* A Laboratory Manual for the Isolation and Identification of Avian Pathogens, Fourth Edition, Swayne D.E., Glisson J.R., Jackwood M.W., Pearson J.E. & Reed W.M., eds. American Association of Avian Pathologists, Kennett Square, Pennsylvania, USA, 200–204.

13. WOOLCOCK P.R. & FABRICANT J. (1997). Duck hepatitis. *In:* Diseases of Poultry, Tenth Edition, Calnek B.W., Barnes H.J., Beard C.W., McDougald L.R. & Saif Y.M., eds. Iowa State University Press, Ames, Iowa, USA, 661–673.

*

* *

CHAPTER 2.7.10.

DUCK VIRUS ENTERITIS

SUMMARY

Duck virus enteritis (DVE) or duck plague is an acute contagious infection of ducks, geese and swans (order Anseriformes) caused by a herpesvirus. Diagnosis is based on a combination of assessing the clinical signs, gross pathology and histopathology supported by the isolation and identification of the virus.

Identification of the agent: *The virus may be isolated from the liver, spleen and kidneys of birds dying from this infection. Virus may be recovered by infecting susceptible ducklings, in which the disease can be reproduced; by inoculating embryonated Muscovy duck eggs on the chorioallantoic membrane; or by inoculating cell cultures of duck embryo or Muscovy duck embryo origin. The identity of the virus can be confirmed by neutralisation tests using specific antiserum to inhibit pathological changes in the duck embryos or the cytopathological effects in the cell cultures, or by direct or indirect immunofluorescence tests on infected cell cultures. Alternatively the DVE DNA may be detected by the polymerase chain reaction from at least the liver and spleen of DVE-infected birds as well as from the Muscovy duck embryos or cells used for virus isolation.*

Serological tests: *Immunological tests have little value in the diagnosis of acute DVE infection. Serum neutralisation tests* in ovo *and* in vitro *have been used to monitor exposure to DVE in wildfowl.*

Requirements for vaccines and diagnostic biologicals: *A live attenuated virus vaccine is available to control DVE in birds over 2 weeks of age. Ducks are vaccinated subcutaneously or intramuscularly for active immunity. Vaccine virus is not thought to spread from vaccinated to unvaccinated stock. An inactivated vaccine has been reported to be efficacious in laboratory tests, but has not been developed or licensed for large-scale use.*

A. DIAGNOSTIC TECHNIQUES

Duck virus enteritis (DVE) is an acute, sometimes chronic, contagious virus infection that occurs naturally only in ducks, geese and swans, all members of the family Anatidae of the order Anseriformes. The aetiological agent, a herpesvirus, is a member of the Alphaherpesvirinae subfamily of the Herpesviridae. DVE may also be referred to as duck plague, anatid herpes, eendenpest, entenpest and peste du canard. The infection has not been reported in other avian species, mammals or humans.

In domestic ducks and ducklings, DVE has been reported in birds ranging from 7 days of age to mature breeders. In susceptible flocks the first signs are often sudden, high and persistent mortality with a significant drop in egg production. In chronically infected partially immune flocks, only occasional deaths occur. Recovered birds may be carriers and may shed the virus in faeces or on the surface of eggs over a period of years.

Clinical signs and gross pathology associated with a DVE outbreak vary with the species, age and sex of the affected birds, and the virulence of the virus. In breeder ducks the range of signs include eye watering and pasted eye-lids associated with photophobia, polydypsia, loss of appetite, ataxia, watery diarrhoea and nasal discharge. Birds often have ruffled feathers and soiled vents. Sick birds may maintain an upright stance by using their wings for support, but their overall appearance is one of weakness and depression. In ducklings 2–7 weeks of age, losses may be lower than in older birds and the signs associated with DVE infection include dehydration, loss of weight, a blue coloration of the beaks and bloodstained vents.

At necropsy, there is little evidence of emaciation in adult ducks that have died. In mature males, prolapse of the penis may occur. In mature females, haemorrhages may be observed in ovarian follicles. The gross lesions are characterised by vascular damage, with tissue haemorrhages and free blood in the body cavities, eruptions, or annular haemorrhages and diphtheroid lesions of the mucosal surfaces of the digestive tract, lesions of the lymphoid organs and retrograde changes of the parenchymatous organs. Collectively, these lesions are pathognomonic for DVE. The pathology and histopathology of DVE in White Pekin ducks has been reviewed (15). Microscopic lesions are characterised by vascular damage and its consequences in visceral organs. Eosinophilic intranuclear inclusions and cytoplasmic inclusions in epithelial cells of the digestive tract are typically present.

1. Identification of the agent

Primary isolation of the virus is best achieved from samples of liver, spleen or kidney tissue, which have been homogenised in buffered saline containing antibiotics and clarified by low speed centrifugation (1800 ***g***). Isolation may be attempted by inoculating such homogenates into cell cultures, ducklings or duck embryos.

a) Cell cultures

Cell culture is reported as the method of choice for isolation of DVE virus, but may not always be successful. Isolations may be made in primary duck embryo fibroblasts (DEF) (18) or, preferably, primary Muscovy duck embryo fibroblasts (MDEF) (7, 11). Muscovy duck embryo liver (MDEL) cells are thought to be even more sensitive, (R.E. Gough, pers. comm.). Cell monolayers grown in medium consisting of Eagle's Minimal Essential Medium (MEM), containing 10% fetal calf serum (FCS), 2 mM glutamine and 0.17% sodium bicarbonate and gentamicin, are washed with serum-free MEM and then inoculated with the clarified sample homogenate suspected to contain DVE virus. After 1 hour at 37°C to allow for virus adsorption, the cultures are maintained on MEM containing 2% FCS, 2 mM glutamine and 0.17% sodium bicarbonate and gentamicin, and incubated in an atmosphere containing 5% CO_2. The cytopathic effect is characterised by the appearance of rounded clumped cells, which enlarge and become necrotic 2–4 days later. Cultures should be stained with a fluorescent antibody conjugate using a direct or indirect method to identify the virus. Cells can also be fixed and then stained with haematoxylin and eosin to show syncytial formation, intranuclear inclusions and marked cytoplasmic granulation. It has been reported (1) that the isolation of DVE in MDEF cells is favoured by incubation at temperatures between 39.5°C and 41.5°C. However, an elevated temperature does not appear to be essential for isolation, which is often carried out at 37°C. More than one passage in cell culture may be necessary to isolate the virus. This virus isolation method in cell cultures may be modified to a plaque assay by overlaying the cell monolayer with maintenance medium containing 1% agarose. As the virus can be cell associated, sequential passaging should be carried out by trypsinising potentially infected cells and replanting them, as well as inoculating fresh cells with infected culture supernatant from the previous passage.

b) Ducklings

When inoculated intramuscularly, 1-day-old susceptible ducklings die within 3–12 days. Muscovy ducklings *(Cairina moschata)* are more susceptible than White Pekin ducklings. Both macroscopical and microscopical lesions typical of DVE should be seen at post-mortem examination. At the same time uninoculated ducklings, housed separately, should be maintained as controls. The diagnosis may be confirmed either by vaccinating ducklings against DVE and challenging them subsequently with the virus isolate or by immunofluorescence. However, virulent strains of the virus exist, against which the vaccine may be ineffective (10). In the author's recent experience of natural infections occurring in Muscovy ducks, this method of virus isolation has proved more sensitive than cell culture methods.

c) Duck embryos

Primary virus isolations can be made by inoculating on to the chorioallantoic membrane (CAM) of 9–14-day-old embryonated Muscovy duck eggs. The embryos may die, showing characteristic extensive haemorrhages 4–10 days after inoculation. Two to four serial blind passages of the homogenised CAMs may be necessary before an isolation can be effected. This method is not as sensitive as that using susceptible day old ducklings.

Embryonated chicken eggs are not very susceptible to infection with field strains of DVE. The virus can nevertheless be adapted to chicken embryos by serial passages. Pekin duck embryos vary in their susceptibility to strains of DVE virus.

d) Immunological methods

Serological tests used to confirm the identity of newly isolated virus include neutralisation assays performed in either embryonated eggs or cell cultures. A plaque assay for DVE in duck embryo cell cultures has been described (3). In the author's laboratory a microtitre assay using primary MDEF or MDEL cells is used. Provided a hyperimmune antiserum of sufficiently high titre is used, a fluorescent antibody test (direct or indirect) for DVE in DEF, MDEF or MDEL cells is the next most sensitive assay after isolation in 1–9-day-old ducklings (6). A reverse passive haemagglutination test for DVE has been described (4), but it is reported to be less sensitive than immunofluorescence and plaque assays. An avidin–biotin–peroxidase method of immunoperoxidase staining to detect DVE antigen in formalin-fixed, paraffin-embedded sections of liver and spleen from experimentally infected birds has been described (9); this method could have diagnostic potential. The identity of the virus may also be confirmed by negative-stain electron microscopy, but this alone is not positive confirmation that the herpesvirus observed is DVE virus. Immunoelectron microscopy has been developed recently using DVE hyperimmune serum (12).

e) Nucleic acid recognition methods

Recently detection of DVE virus by polymerase chain reaction has been reported (8, 13). Primers have been identified that are able to amplify DNA from DVE virus present in tissues from an original outbreak and after passage through Muscovy duck embryos.

f) Strain variation

Although strains of DVE differ considerably in virulence, there is little reported evidence of serological variation.

2. Serological tests

Serological tests have little value in the diagnosis of acute DVE infections, but assays based on serum neutralisation in embryonated eggs and cell cultures have been used to monitor antibodies following exposure to DVE in wildfowl. The humoral response to natural infection with DVE virus is often low and antibodies may be short-lived (5); it is assumed that cell-mediated immunity also plays a role in the infection (14). However, detection of neutralising antibodies to DVE virus in serum is possible. Virus neutralisation (VN) assays using a constant serum/varying virus method may be performed in chicken or duck embryos by using embryo-adapted virus, or in cell cultures. Neutralisation indices (NI) (17) between 0 and 1.5 were detected in domestic and wild waterfowl that had not been exposed to DVE; an NI of 1.75 or greater was considered to be evidence of prior exposure to DVE virus (2). Alternatively, sera may be screened using a constant virus/varying serum method. In the author's laboratory a microtitre neutralisation assay using primary MDEF of DEF is used. Serial twofold dilutions of each serum sample (heat-inactivated at 56°C) are prepared in 50 µl of serum-free MEM in microtitre plates. Approximately $10^{2.0}$ $TCID_{50}$ (50% tissue culture infective dose) of DVE virus in 50 µl of MEM is added to each well and the mixtures are allowed to react at 37°C for 1 hour. A suspension of primary MDEF or DEF in MEM supplemented with 2 mM L-glutamine, 0.17% sodium bicarbonate and 10% FCS, is adjusted to contain 3×10^5 cells per ml. Cells are added to the plates at 100 µl per well and the plates are then incubated for up to 96 hours at 37°C in a humidified 5% CO_2 atmosphere. Following incubation, cells are observed daily by light microscopy and finally fixed with 10% formol-buffered saline and stained with 1% crystal violet. The plates are read macroscopically. The titre for virus neutralising activity is expressed as the reciprocal of the highest dilution of serum at which a monolayer grew, i.e. there is no evidence of cytopathic effect and therefore complete virus neutralisation has occurred. A titre of less than 3 log_2 is usually considered to be negative. A VN titre of 8 or greater is considered to be significant and is evidence of exposure to DVE virus (5). VN antibody may also be detected using cell cultures by mixing sera at a single dilution, e.g. 1/10, with 100–200 $TCID_{50}$ virus and then testing inoculated cell cultures for non-neutralised virus by immunofluorescence. Although this method is not quantitative, it can be useful for screening large numbers of sera. These latter methods, using constant virus/varying serum, are much more economical on sera than the NI methods.

B. REQUIREMENTS FOR VACCINES AND DIAGNOSTIC BIOLOGICALS

A live attenuated virus vaccine can be used to control DVE in birds over 2 weeks of age. Fattening or breeding ducks may be vaccinated subcutaneously or intramuscularly to produce an active immunity. The vaccine virus is thought not to spread by contact from vaccinated to unvaccinated ducks, as the unvaccinated birds remain susceptible to infection.

An inactivated vaccine has been reported to be as efficacious as modified live vaccine (16). This vaccine has been tested only under laboratory conditions; it has not been tested on a large scale and is not licensed.

1. Seed management

a) Characteristics of the seed

DVE vaccine can be prepared from a strain of the virus that has been attenuated by serial passage in embryonated chicken eggs. In the USA the vaccine strain seed was originally imported from Holland and has been serially passaged 41–46 times.

b) Method of culture

The seed virus should be prepared in 8–11-day-old specific pathogen free (SPF) embryonated chicken eggs by inoculating on to the CAM followed by incubation at 37°C. The seed may be stored at –70°C or lower in the form of a homogenate of the embryo-CAM in buffered saline.

c) Validation as a vaccine

The seed virus should be shown to be free from extraneous viruses pathogenic to ducks, chickens and turkeys. It should also be free from bacterial, fungal and mycoplasmal contaminants:

The identity of the virus should be confirmed by a virus neutralisation test conducted with specific antiserum using the constant serum/varying virus method. This test should be performed in embryonated chicken eggs. The antiserum should reduce the virus titre by at least $10^{1.75}$ ELD_{50} (50% embryo lethal dose).

The immunogenicity of the vaccine can be assessed in DVE-susceptible ducks or ducklings by inoculating the recommended vaccine dose intramuscularly and challenging intramuscularly 21 days later with virulent DVE virus. The vaccinated birds should survive challenge while unvaccinated control birds should die. This test should be carried out on the master seed, but need not be done routinely on each vaccine batch produced. For release of subsequent batches, the titre of the virus should be a sufficient indication of vaccine potency.

2. Method of manufacture

The vaccine is produced in 8–11-day-old SPF embryonated chicken eggs inoculated on to the CAM and incubated at 37°C. Most embryo deaths occur between 48 and 96 hours after inoculation. The embryos, their CAMs and chorioallantoic fluids are harvested, pooled and homogenised in buffered saline and clarified by low-speed centrifugation (1800 *g*). The preparation is diluted as appropriate, and a stabiliser is incorporated. It is then dispensed into vials and preferably frozen rapidly to –70°C or lower.

3. In-process control

Eggs that have been inoculated should be candled 24 hours later to identify any embryos that have died from nonspecific causes.

4. Batch control

a) Sterility

Tests for sterility and freedom from contamination of biological materials may be found in chapter I.4.

b) Safety

A group of 1-day-old ducklings susceptible to DVE should be inoculated subcutaneously or intramuscularly with the vaccine at 10 times the recommended dose, and observed for 7–14 days for any signs of adverse reactions.

The final product should be free from contamination by bacteria, fungi, and mycoplasma as well as extraneous viruses potentially pathogenic to poultry.

c) Potency

The virus titre of the vaccine should be determined in 9–11-day-old embryonated chicken eggs inoculated on to the CAM and incubated at 37°C. The vaccine should contain a minimum of $10^{3.0}$ ELD_{50} per dose at time of use.

d) Duration of immunity

Immunity in vaccinated ducks should last throughout a breeding season. Annual revaccination is recommended (15).

e) Stability

When stored at –70°C or lower the vaccine is stable for at least 1 year. Potency testing should be repeated after this time on an aliquot of vaccine to determine whether the virus titre has been maintained. Once thawed the vaccine should not be refrozen, it should be maintained at 4°C in a refrigerator, but for no longer than 1 week. Lyophilised vaccine should be stored at 4–8°C and used before the stated expiry date.

f) Preservatives

No preservatives are added to the vaccine.

g) Precautions (hazards)

None.

5. Tests on the final product

The vaccine is issued as a vial of frozen or lyophilised concentrated vaccine virus together with a bottle of sterile diluent (phosphate buffered saline), on which standard sterility checks have been made (see Section B.4.a.).

a) Safety

No additional testing is performed after the batch testing.

b) Potency

No additional testing is performed after the batch testing.

REFERENCES

1. BURGESS E.C. & YUILL T.M. (1981). Increased cell culture incubation temperatures for duck plague virus isolation. *Avian Dis.*, **25**, 222–224.

2. DARDIRI A.H. & HESS W.R. (1967). The incidence of neutralizing antibodies to duck plague virus in serums from domestic ducks and wild waterfowl in the United States of America. Proceedings of the 71st Annual Meeting of the United States Livestock Sanitary Association, USLSA, Phoenix, Arizona, USA, 225–237.

3. DARDIRI A.H. & HESS W.R. (1968). A plaque assay for duck plague virus. *Can. J. Comp. Med.*, **32**, 505–510.

4. DENG M.Y., BURGESS E.C. & YUILL T.M. (1984). Detection of duck plague virus by reverse passive haemagglutination test. *Avian Dis.*, **28**, 616–628.

5. DOCHERTY D.E. & FRANSON C.J. (1992). Duck Virus Enteritis. *In:* Veterinary Diagnostic Virology, Castro A.E. & Heuschele W.P., eds. Mosby Year Book, St Louis, Missouri, USA, 25–28.

6. ERICKSON G.A., PROCTOR S.J., PEARSON J.E. & GUSTAFSON G.A. (1975). Diagnosis of duck virus enteritis (duck plague). 17th Annual Proceedings of American Association of Veterinary Laboratory Diagnosticians. Roanoake, Virginia, USA. AAVLD, Madison, Wisconsin, USA, 85–89.

7. GOUGH R.E. & ALEXANDER D.J. (1990). Duck virus enteritis in Great Britain, 1980 to 1989. *Vet. Rec.*, **126**, 595–597.

8. HANSEN W.R., BROWN S.E., NASHOLD S.W. & KNUDSON D.L. (1999). Identification of duck plague virus by polymerase chain reaction. *Avian Dis.,* **43**, 106–115.

9. ISLAM M.R., NESSA J. & HALDER K.M. (1993). Detection of duck plague virus antigen in tissues by immunoperoxidase staining. *Avian Pathol.,* **22**, 389–393.

10. KISARY S. & ZSAK L. (1983). Comparative studies on duck viral enteritis (DVE) virus strains in geese. *Avian Pathol.,* **12**, 395–408.

11. KOCAN R.M. (1976). Duck plague virus replication in Muscovy duck fibroblasts. *Avian Dis.,* **20**, 574–580.

12. PEARSON G.L. & CASSIDY D.R. (1997). Perspectives on the diagnosis, epizootiology and control of the 1973 duck plague epizootic in wild waterfowl at Lake Andes, South Dakota. *J. Wildl. Dis.,* **33**, 681–705.

13. PLUMMER P.J., ALEFANTIS T., KAPLAN S., O'CONNELL P., SHAWKY S. & SCHAT K.A. (1998). Detection of duck enteritis virus by polymerase reaction. *Avian Dis.,* **40**, 554–564.

14. RICHTER J.H.M. & HORZINEK M.C. (1993). Duck Plague. *In:* Virus Infections of Birds, McFerran J.B. & McNulty M.S., eds. Elsevier Science Publishers B.V., Amsterdam, the Netherlands, 77–90.

15. SANDHU T.S. & LEIBOVITZ L. (1997). Duck plague (duck virus enteritis). *In:* Diseases of Poultry, Tenth Edition, Calnek B.W., Barnes H.J., Beard C.W., McDougald, L.R. & Saif Y.M., eds. Iowa State University Press, Ames, Iowa, USA, 675–683.

16. SHAWKY S.A. & SANDHU T.S. (1997). Inactivated vaccine for protection against duck virus enteritis. *Avian Dis.,* **41**, 461–468.

17. THAYER G.S. & BEARD C.W. (1998). Serological procedures. *In:* A Laboratory Manual for the Isolation and Identification of Avian Pathogens, Fourth Edition, Swayne D.E., Glisson J.R., Jackwood M.W., Pearson J.E. & Reed W.M., eds. American Association of Avian Pathologists, Kennett Square, Pennsylvania, USA, 255–266.

18. WOLF K., BURKE C.N. & QUIMBY M.C. (1976). Duck viral enteritis: a comparison of replications by CCL-141 and primary cultures of duck embryo fibroblasts. *Avian Dis.,* **20**, 447–454.

*

* *

CHAPTER 2.7.11.

FOWL CHOLERA (avian pasteurellosis)

SUMMARY

Fowl cholera (avian pasteurellosis) is a commonly occurring avian disease that can affect all types of birds and is distributed world-wide. It usually occurs as an acute septicaemia and is often fatal. Diagnosis depends on identification of the causative bacterium, Pasteurella multocida, *following isolation from birds with signs and lesions consistent with this disease. Presumptive diagnosis may be based on the occurrence of typical signs and lesions and/or on the microscopic demonstration of bacteria with typical morphology and staining in tissue smears, such as blood, liver, or spleen. Mild forms of the disease may occur.*

Identification of the agent: Pasteurella multocida *is a facultative anaerobic bacterium that grows best at 35–37°C. Primary isolation is usually accomplished using media such as dextrose starch agar, blood agar, and trypticase soy agar. Isolation may be improved by the addition of 5% heat-inactivated serum. Colonies range from 1 to 3 mm in diameter after 18–24 hours' incubation. They are usually discrete, circular, convex, and butyraceous. The cells are coccobacillary or short rod-shaped, usually 0.2–0.4 × 0.6–2.5 µm in size, stain Gram negative, and generally occur singly or in pairs. Recent isolates show bipolar staining.*

Isolation of the organism from visceral organs, such as liver, bone marrow, spleen or heart blood of birds that succumb to the acute form of the disease, and from exudative lesions of birds with the chronic form of the disease, is generally easily accomplished.

Identification of P. multocida *is based on the results of biochemical tests, which include carbohydrate fermentation, enzyme production, and selected metabolite production.*

Serological characterisation of strains of P. multocida *includes capsular serogrouping and somatic serotyping. DNA fingerprinting can differentiate among* P. multocida *having the same capsular serogroup and somatic serotype. These characterisations require a specialised laboratory with appropriate diagnostic reagents.*

Serological tests: *Serological tests are rarely used for diagnosis of fowl cholera. The ease of obtaining a definitive diagnosis through isolation and identification of the causative organism generally precludes the need for serodiagnosis.*

Requirements for vaccines and diagnostic biologicals: *Vaccination plays a significant role in the control of this disease. The* P. multodica *vaccines in general use are bacterins, containing aluminium hydroxide or oil as adjuvant, prepared from serotypes selected on the basis of epidemiological information. At least two doses of the killed vaccine are required. Live vaccines are seldom used, except in North America.*

A. DIAGNOSTIC TECHNIQUES

Fowl cholera (avian pasteurellosis) is a commonly occurring avian disease that can affect all types of birds and is often fatal (3, 6). In the peracute form, fowl cholera is one of the most virulent and infectious diseases of poultry. Diagnosis depends on identification of the causative bacterium, *Pasteurella multocida*, following isolation from birds with signs and lesions consistent with this disease. Presumptive diagnosis may be based on the occurrence of typical signs and lesions and/or on the microscopic demonstration of bacteria showing bipolar staining in smears of tissues, such as blood, liver, or spleen. Mild forms of the disease may occur.

All avian species are susceptible to *P. multocida*, although turkeys may be particularly severely affected. Often the first sign of disease is dead birds. Other signs include: fever, anorexia, depression, mucous discharge from the mouth, diarrhoea, ruffled feathers, increased respiratory rate, and cyanosis at the time of death. Lesions that are often observed include: passive hyperaemia, haemorrhages, enlarged liver and spleen, focal necrotic areas in the liver and/or spleen, pneumonia, and slightly increased amounts of peritoneal and pericardial fluids. Birds that survive the acute septicaemic stage or those infected with organisms of low virulence may develop chronic fowl cholera, characterised by localised infections. These infections often involve joints, foot pads, tendon sheaths, sternal bursa, conjunctivae, wattles, pharynx, lungs, air sacs, middle ears, bone marrow, and meninges. Lesions resulting from these infections are usually characterised by fibrino-suppurative exudate, necrosis, and varying degrees of fibroplasia.

Other bacterial diseases, including salmonellosis, colibacillosis and listeriosis in chickens, and pseudo-tuberculosis, erysipelas and chlamydiosis in turkeys, often have signs and lesions similar to those of fowl cholera. Differential diagnosis depends on isolation and identification of the causative organisms.

1. Identification of the agent

Pasteurella multocida is a facultative anaerobic bacterium that grows best at 35–37°C. Primary isolation is usually accomplished using media such as blood agar, trypticase soy agar or dextrose starch agar, and isolation may be improved by supplementing these media with 5% heat-inactivated serum. Maintenance media usually do not require supplemental serum. Colonies range from 1 to 3 mm in diameter after 18–24 hours' incubation. They usually are discrete, circular, convex, and butyraceous. Capsulated organisms usually produce larger colonies than those of noncapsulated organisms. The watery mucoid colonies, often observed with mammalian respiratory tract isolates, are very rare with avian isolates. The cells are coccobacillary or short rod-shaped, usually 0.2–0.4 × 0.6–2.5 µm in size, stain Gram negative, and generally occur singly or in pairs. Recently isolated organisms or those found in tissue smears show bipolar staining with Wright's or Giemsa stains or methylene blue, and are usually encapsulated.

Isolation of the organism from visceral organs, such as liver, bone marrow, spleen, or heart blood of birds that succumb to the acute form of the disease, and from exudative lesions of birds with the chronic form of the disease, is generally easily accomplished. Isolation from those chronically affected birds that have no evidence of disease other than emaciation and lethargy is often difficult. In this condition or when host decomposition has occurred, bone marrow is the tissue of choice for isolation attempts. The surface of the tissue to be cultured is seared with a hot spatula and a specimen is obtained by inserting a sterile cotton swab or wire loop through the heat-sterilised surface. The specimen is then inoculated into tryptose or another broth medium, incubated for a few hours, transferred to agar medium, and incubated again

Identification is based primarily on the results of biochemical tests. Carbohydrate fermentation reactions are essential. Those carbohydrates that are fermented include: glucose, mannose, galactose, fructose, and sucrose. Those not fermented include: rhamnose, cellobiose, raffinose, inulin, erythritol, adonitol, m-inositol, and salicin. Mannitol is usually fermented. Arabinose, maltose, lactose, and dextrin are usually not fermented. Variable reactions occur with xylose, trehalose, glycerol, and sorbitol. *Pasteurella multocida* does not cause haemolysis, is not motile, and does not grow on MacConkey's agar. It produces catalase, oxidase, and ornithine decarboxylase, but does not produce urease, lysine decarboxylase, beta-galactosidase, or arginine dihydrolase. Phosphatase production is variable. Nitrate is reduced; indole and hydrogen sulphide are produced, and methyl red and Voges-Proskauer tests are negative. Commercial biochemical test kits are available.

Differentiation of *P. multocida* from other avian *Pasteurella* and *Riemerella anatipestifer* can usually be accomplished using the tests and results indicated in Table 1. (*Pasteurella anatipestifer* has recently been reclassified as *Riemerella anatipestifer.*) Laboratory experience has shown that *P. multocida* is most easily identified by its colony morphology and appearance in Gram stains. Positive reactions to indole and ornithine decarboxylase are the most useful biochemical indications.

Antigenic characterisation of *P. multocida* is accomplished by capsular serogrouping and somatic serotyping. Capsular serogroups are determined by a passive haemagglutination test (1, 2). Serogroups A, B, D, E, and F have been reported; all but serogroup E have been isolated from avian hosts. A nonserological disk diffusion test that uses specific mucopolysaccharidases to differentiate serogroups A, D, and F has been developed (7).

Somatic serotypes are usually determined by an agar gel immunodiffusion (AGID) test (4, 5). Serotypes 1–16 have been reported; all but serotypes 8 and 13 have been isolated from avian hosts. The most effective characterisation involves determination of both serogroup and serotype. These determinations require a specialised laboratory with appropriate diagnostic reagents.

a) Agar gel immunodiffusion test procedure

i) Heavily seed *P. multocida* on a dextrose starch agar plate and incubate for 18–24 hours.

ii) Scrape the growth from the agar surface and resuspend in 1.0 ml of phosphate buffered saline (PBS) that contains 0.3% formalin.

iii) Heat the bacterial cell suspension in a boiling water bath for 1 hour.

iv) Remove the cells by centrifugation and use the supernatant fluid as test antigen.

v) Suspend Noble agar to a 0.9% concentration in 8.5% sodium chloride solution, heat to dissolve, and cast gels on to standard microscope slides using 4 ml per slide.

vi) Cut opposing 3 mm diameter immunodiffusion wells 3 mm apart into the Noble agar gel slide.

vii) Fill wells with test antigen and fill opposing wells with serotype-specific chicken antiserum. Incubate gel slides at 37°C for 24 hours.

viii) A somatic serotype is determined by a precipitin line that occurs between a test antigen well and opposing well of any of 16 serotype-specific antisera.

DNA fingerprinting of *P. multocida* by restriction endonuclease analysis (REA) has proved valuable in determining the epidemiology of fowl cholera in poultry flocks. Isolates of *P. multocida* having both capsular serogroup and somatic sertoype in common are capable of being distinguished by REA. The method is accomplished by analysis of ethidium-bromide-stained fingerprint profiles in agarose gels following electrophoresis of DNA digested with either *Hha*I or *Hpa*II endonuclease (8).

Table 1. *Tests used to differentiate* Pasteurella multocida *from other avian* Pasteurella *species and* Riemerella anatipestifer

Test*	*Pasteurella*			
	multocida	***haemolytica***	***gallinarum***	***R. anatipestifer***
Haemolysis on blood agar	–	+	–	V
Growth on MacConkey's agar	–	+u	–	–
Indole production	+	–	–	–
Gelatin liquefaction	–	–	–	+u
Catalase production	+	+u	+	+
Urease production	–	–	–	V
Glucose fermentation	+	+	+	–
Lactose fermentation	–u	+u	–	–
Sucrose fermentation	+	+	+	–
Maltose fermentation	–u	–	+	–
Ornithine decarboxylase	+	–	–	–

* Test reaction results: – = no reaction; + = reaction; V = variable reactions; –u = usually no reaction; +u usually a reaction.

2. Serological tests

Serological tests for the presence of specific antibodies are not used for diagnosis of fowl cholera. The ease of obtaining a definitive diagnosis through isolation and identification of the causative organism precludes the need for serodiagnosis. Serological tests, such as agglutination, AGID, and passive haemagglutination, have been used experimentally to demonstrate antibody against *P. multocida* in serum from avian hosts; none were highly sensitive. Determinations of antibody titres using enzyme-linked immunosorbent assays have been used with varying degrees of success in attempts to predict immunity in vaccinated poultry, but not for diagnosis

B. REQUIREMENTS FOR VACCINES AND DIAGNOSTIC BIOLOGICALS

Fowl cholera or avian pasteurellosis may be caused by any 1 of 16 Heddleston serotypes of *P. multocida*, although certain serotypes appear to be more often associated with disease. The *P. multocida* vaccines in general use are bacterins, containing aluminium hydroxide or oil as adjuvant, prepared from inactivated cells of serotypes selected on the basis of epidemiological information. Vaccination plays a significant role in the control of this disease. Live vaccines containing modified *P. multocida* are not generally used except in North America. This chapter is concerned only with killed vaccines. Vaccine is normally administered by intramuscular injection in the leg or breast muscles, or subcutaneously at the back of the neck. Two doses are required with an interval of 2–4 weeks. As with most killed vaccines, full immunity cannot be expected until approximately 2 weeks after the second dose of a primary vaccination course. Vaccination of birds in the presence of disease or poor nutritional status should be avoided as a satisfactory immune response would not be expected in such circumstances.

1. Seed management

a) Characteristics of the seed

The strains of *P. multocida* to be incorporated in a vaccine should be pure, of known serotype, virulent, of avian origin and of proven antigenicity.

b) Method of culture

Each strain is cultivated separately in a suitable liquid medium, then lyophilised. Ampoules are preferably kept at –70°C for long-term storage. Seed cultures are normally produced in a seed-lot system. One ampoule of the stock culture is used to produce a number of secondary ampoules (e.g. 100) and each one of these is in turn used to produce a number of working ampoules. One working ampoule is used to produce the seed culture for each batch of *P. multocida* vaccine.

Subcultures are made in a suitable liquid medium (e.g. brain–heart infusion broth), which is checked for purity before inoculation of a larger volume of medium, for the final seed. Seed cultures are checked microscopically before use and by cultural techniques for retrospective confirmation of purity.

c) Validation as a vaccine

i) Efficacy

Candidate vaccine strains should be shown to be effective as monovalent vaccines against homologous challenge infection in a suitable animal model. Final vaccines may be tested according to the methods outlined under potency testing.

ii) Safety

Safety must be tested in the target species, which may include turkeys, ducks, chickens or others. For example, ten healthy turkey poults aged 1–2 weeks are injected intramuscularly with twice the recommended dose and observed for at least 15 days. The birds should show no systemic reaction and only a slight local reaction.

In addition, safety may be tested by injecting ten healthy mice, each weighing 18–20 g, subcutaneously with 0.5 ml of the vaccine under test. The mice should show no significant local or systemic reactions during the subsequent 10-day observation period.

2. Method of manufacture

For each strain to be included in a vaccine, the contents of a freeze-dried ampoule from the working (daughter) stock are reconstituted in a small volume of seed medium. The seed medium should be the same as that used in the main batch and would typically be a rich nutrient broth that gives good cell yields. The reconstituted cultures are used to inoculate several flasks containing approximately 100 ml of medium, which are incubated at 37°C overnight. These cultures are then used to inoculate 5–20-litre volumes of medium, which may be in seed fermenter vessels or glass bottles, followed by incubation at 37°C until satisfactory growth is achieved. The number required will depend on the volume of the main batch, for which an inoculum size of 2–5% should be used, e.g. a 2000-litre batch would be inoculated with 40–100 litres of an actively growing culture. The main culture is grown at 37°C until the stationary phase of growth is reached, which can be monitored by following culture absorbance. At this stage, the culture is inactivated by the addition of formalin to the vessel. The contents are mixed thoroughly, transferred to a fresh sterile vessel, and maintained at 37°C for a further period of time that has been demonstrated to inactivate the strain, plus at least a further 33% to establish a margin of safety. The inactivated cells are harvested by centrifugation and resuspended in formol saline typically to a volume of one-tenth of the culture volume. The cells are stored in sterile containers at 2–8°C until required for vaccine blending. A total cell count is done on the cell harvest either by microscopic assessment or by turbidometric measurements where these have been correlated with cell numbers.

Vaccine blending is achieved by sterilisation of vaccine base (e.g. aluminium hydroxide gel) in a suitable vessel followed by the aseptic addition of appropriate volumes of each strain to give the final required cell concentration. Sterile buffer is used to make up the final vaccine volume as necessary. Bulk vaccine is agitated to ensure homogeneity of the product. The vaccine is filled into suitable containers, normally collapsible plastic packs or glass bottles with rubber septae, under sterile conditions. This would normally be achieved using an automatic filling line that accurately dispenses the required volume into each container.

3. In-process control

The purity of the cultures is determined at each stage from the opening of the ampoule until immediately prior to inactivation of the main batch. This is achieved by microscopic examination (e.g. phase-contrast microscopy, Gram strain) and by culture on sheep blood agar. Seed cultures and the main batch culture are checked for identity to confirm that the strain being grown is the correct serotype. A test for complete inactivation is performed following incubation with formalin. This test should involve the neutralisation of residual formalin with sodium metabisulphite and the inoculation of a medium that is most likely to support the growth of any remaining viable cells. This would normally be the same medium as that used for production. Analytical assays to determine the levels of aluminium, formaldehyde, pH, and preservatives are done on bulk vaccine and should be within specified limits.

4. Batch control

a) Sterility

Sterility tests are done on the cell harvests, vaccine base, bulk vaccine and filled vaccine. For further information see Chapter I.4.

b) Safety

Safety testing of the final vaccine may be done according to the method outlined in Section B.1c.ii.

c) Potency

Potency testing of avian *P. multocida* vaccines is not described in either the British or European Veterinary Pharmacopoeia. A suitable potency test would be to infect vaccinated and unvaccinated turkeys, ducks or chickens with one or more of the serotypes of *P. multocida* most commonly associated with the disease. The vaccination schedule would preferably, but not necessarily, be that recommended for the vaccine in the field, and the challenge infection may be achieved by any suitable means, e.g. intramuscular injection, subcutaneous injection, swabbing of nasal cleft. Challenge infection should be done no fewer than 2 weeks after the second vaccination. A satisfactory vaccine is one that protects a specified number or more of turkeys against fatal infection. For the test to be valid, a minimum number of nonvaccinates must die following infection. In the United States of America's Code of Federal Regulations, the specifications are that at least 14/20 vaccinates should survive and at least 16/20 nonvaccinates must die.

It may be acceptable to perform potency tests in other small animal models based on vaccination and challenge infection. Mice may be used in passive protection tests, but tests involving vaccination of mice should be given careful consideration as the immune response to certain *Pasteurella* antigens may be poor.

d) Duration of immunity

Duration of immunity is demonstrated by the vaccination of birds according to the recommended schedule followed by challenge infection with a representative virulent strain of *P. multocida*. The timing of the challenge infection should reflect the period of susceptibility to natural infection. For example, where birds are typically slaughtered at 24 weeks of age, the vaccination schedule should be demonstrated to afford protection through to this age. It would not be appropriate to test each vaccine batch in this way as the potency test is used to show batch-to-batch consistency in terms of efficacy. The first vaccination may be at 1 week of age (3).

e) **Stability**

Vaccine stability is demonstrated by repeating the tests on sterility, safety, potency, and preservatives after blending of the vaccine. Three batches of vaccine should pass the requirements of these tests 3 months beyond the proposed shelf life. This would not be an appropriate test to apply to each vaccine batch. Vaccines are stored at 2–8°C and protected from freezing. Partly used packs should be discarded at the end of a day's operations.

f) **Preservatives**

Any preservatives added should be analysed and levels shown to fall within specified limits. Preservatives are generally added to vaccines to limit the growth of any contaminants introduced during the course of a day's operations when the rubber cap is pierced with a needle. Ideally, multidose vaccination equipment should be used whereby the vaccine pack is entered only once with a sterile needle. This may preclude the need for preservatives to be added and manufacturers ought to consider whether preservatives are really necessary, as mercuric and phenolic compounds are generally used and are hazardous to people handling raw materials.

g) **Precautions (hazards)**

Vaccines based on aluminium hydroxide gel will cause temporary nodules at the site of injection. Operator self-injection poses no immediate problems, but medical advice should be sought as there is a risk of infection via a contaminated needle.

Vaccines that are oil based will cause more severe reactions at the site of injection, which may be manifested as large nodules. Care should be taken to administer these vaccines correctly. Operator self-injection requires immediate medical attention, involving prompt incision and irrigation of the site.

5. Tests on the final product

a) **Safety**

Safety testing is performed on the bulk vaccine and on the final filled product according to the method outlined in Section B.1.c. The final filled vaccine is also tested for safety or, perhaps more correctly, freedom from abnormal toxicity: five mice are each injected with 0.5 ml and two guinea-pigs with 2 ml, and monitored for 7 days for abnormal local or systemic reactions. If two turkeys poults given twice the recommended dose are used in the test, then it is not necessary to perform the test in mice and guinea-pigs.

b) **Potency**

The final filled vaccine is not usually tested for potency as this would have already been demonstrated on the bulk vaccine according to Section B.4.c.

REFERENCES

1. Canter G.R. (1972). Improved hemagglutination test for identifying type A strains of *Pasteurella multocida*. *Appl. Microbiol.*, **24**, 162–163.

2. Canter G.R. (1995). Studies on *Pasteurella multocida*. 1. A hemagglutination test for the identification of serological types. *Am. J. Vet. Res.*, **16**, 481–484.

3. Derieux W.T. (1978). Response of young chickens and turkeys to virulent and avirulent *Pasteurella multocida* administered by various route. *Avian Dis.*, **22**, 131–139.

4. Heddleston K.L. (1962). Studies on pasteurellosis. V. Two immunogenic types of *Pasteurella multocida* associated with fowl cholera. *Avian Dis.*, **6**, 315–321.

5. Heddleston K.L., Gallagher J.E. & Rebers P.A. (1972). Fowl cholera: Gel diffusion precipitin test for serotyping *Pasteurella multocida* from avian species. *Avian Dis.*, **16**, 925–936.

6. RHOADES K.R. & RIMLER R.B. (1991). Fowl cholera. *In:* Diseases of Poultry, Ninth Edition, Calnek B.W., Barnes H.J., Beard C.W., Reid W.M. & Yoder Jr H.W., eds. Iowa State University Press, Ames, Iowa, USA, 145–162.

7. RIMLER R.B. (1994). Presumptive identification of *Pasteurella multocida* serogroups A, D, and F by capsule depolymerisation with mucopolysaccharidases. *Vet. Rec.*, **134**, 191–192.

8. WILSON M.A., RIMLER R.B. & HOFFMAN L.J. (1992). Comparison of DNA fingerprints and somatic serotypes of serogroups B and E *Pasteurella multocida* isolates. *J. Clin. Microbiol.*, **30**, 1518–1524.

*

* *

SECTION 2.8.

LAGOMORPH DISEASES IN LIST B

CHAPTER 2.8.1.

MYXOMATOSIS

SUMMARY

Myxomatosis is a disease of the European rabbit caused by the myxoma virus, a member of the Poxviridae. The diagnosis of myxomatosis, regardless of its clinical form, depends on the isolation and identification of the virus or the demonstration of its antigens. The presence of a humoral immune response facilitates a retrospective diagnosis of a mild form of the disease, and can provide an indication of the prevalence of infection in a rabbit population. The disease is characterised by gross myxomatous skin lesions.

Identification of the agent: *When skin lesions are present on a dead rabbit, the viral antigen may be demonstrated by immunodiffusion tests on lesion fragments. Monolayer cell cultures of rabbit kidney inoculated with lesion material will show the characteristic cytopathic effects of poxviruses. The presence of virus can be confirmed by immunofluorescence and negative-staining electron microscopy.*

The inoculation of rabbits with suspect material takes longer to identify infection, but this will serve to confirm the presence of infective virus and indicate its pathogenicity.

Serological tests: *Identification and titration of specific antibodies arising from natural infection or from immunisation are done by traditional complement fixation or by a recently developed and more sensitive enzyme-linked immunosorbent assay (ELISA), which is not affected by pro- or anti-complementary factors. The difficulty in obtaining blood samples from representative members of a population can be obviated by collecting blood dried on filter paper; this can later be extracted and examined by the indirect fluorescent antibody test or ELISA.*

Qualitative agar gel immunodiffusion tests have the advantage of detecting antigen and humoral antibodies simultaneously.

Requirements for vaccines and diagnostic biologicals: *Modified live virus vaccines prepared from fibroma virus or modified myxoma virus strains are available for immunisation of rabbits. There are no standard requirements for diagnostic biologicals.*

A. DIAGNOSTIC TECHNIQUES

Myxomatosis is a virus disease of the European rabbit *(Oryctolagus cuniculus)* caused by the myxoma virus, a member of the Poxviridae. The virus has a characteristic tropism for skin, causing a nodular skin form, or has an oculo-respiratory tract tropism, the nonmyxomatous form. It affects rabbits of all ages, and strains, which vary in virulence, give rise to inflammatory skin lesions, generalisation and, possibly, eventual death of the animal by secondary bacterial infections or through inanition. The virus is transmitted to susceptible rabbits by biting insects, such as fleas, mosquitoes, etc. Limited transmission from rabbit to rabbit is possible if they are closely confined.

A primary myxoma lesion arises at the site of infection after 2–5 days, followed by conjunctivitis as a sign of systemic infection, infection of the anogenital region, and the formation of secondary skin lesions at various other sites. In the oculo-respiratory form, the primary lesion is usually an inflammatory pink macule followed by oculonasal catarrh. Virulent strains can kill a rabbit within 10–15 days. There is no health risk to humans working with the myxoma virus.

As the signs of the disease become less distinct with the attenuation of virus strains, the submission of samples for laboratory diagnosis becomes more important. The different techniques available vary in their ability to detect myxoma virus in typical myxomatous lesions, oedema of the eyelids or genital oedema. With atypical lesions, these techniques distinguish myxoma virus infection from that with Shope's fibroma virus.

1. Identification of the agent

A portion of lesion is excised with scissors and separated from the epidermis and superficial dermis. This is washed with phosphate buffered saline (PBS) with antibiotics as defined below and homogenised with ground glass at a dilution rate of 1 g tissue/4.5–9.0 ml of PBS. Cells are disrupted by two freeze–thaw cycles, or by ultrasonication to liberate virions and viral antigens. This suspension is centrifuged for 5–10 minutes at 1500 ***g***. The supernatant fluid is used for the tests.

a) Culture

Isolation of the virus in cell culture is accomplished using primary cultures of rabbit kidney (RK) cells, or with established cell lines, such as RK-13, in minimal essential medium (MEM) containing 5% calf serum, 100 international units (IU)/ml penicillin; 100 µg/ml streptomycin; 100 µg/ml gentamycin; 50 IU/ml nystatin (mycostatin); and 5 µg/ml amphotericin (fungizone). The inoculum consists of the supernatant fluid from a homogenised lesion or oculo-respiratory discharge in Opti-MEM with 2% calf serum and antibiotics. This is removed from the cell layer after 2 hours. The cell layer is washed in a small volume of medium and then replenished with maintenance medium (Opti-MEM).

A cytopathic effect (CPE) typical of poxviruses (10) develops after 24–48 hours (37°C and 5% CO_2). Groups of cells with a confluent cytoplasm form syncytia that vary in size from 2 to 50 or even 100 nuclei together, according to the strain of virus. The nuclei of some cells change, the chromatin forming basophilic aggregations that vary in size and number and give the culture a leopard-skin appearance. Eosinophilic intracytoplasmic inclusions remain discrete, if present at all. Affected cells round up, contract and become pyknotic. They then lyse and become detached from the glass or plastic support. Later, all cells are affected and the cell monolayer detaches completely.

Shope's fibroma virus at first produces well-defined voluminous masses of rounded cells, which proliferate and pile up (10). At the edge, cells just becoming infected show discrete nuclear changes and acidophilic cytoplasmic inclusions that are numerous at an early stage. The cell layer is destroyed after several days.

b) Immunological methods

Agar gel immunodiffusion (AGID) tests are simple and rapid to perform – results can be obtained within 24 hours. Agar plates are prepared with Noble agar (0.6 g), ethylene diamine tetra-acetic acid (EDTA) (2.5 g), sodium chloride (4.5 g), and distilled water (500 ml) containing thiomersal (merthiolate) at 1/100,000 dilution. Standard antiserum (see below), and the test sample are placed in opposing wells that are 6 mm in diameter and 5 mm apart. Another technique is to deposit a small portion of the lesion directly into the agar, 5 mm away from a filter paper disk impregnated with the antiserum. A number of lines of precipitation, usually up to three, appear within 48 hours, indicating the presence of myxoma viral antigens. Only one line forms in the presence of heterologous reactions with Shope's fibroma virus.

Indirect fluorescent antibody (IFA) tests can be applied to cultures from 24 hours onwards. IFA tests reveal intracytoplasmic multiplication of virus, without being able to distinguish myxoma virus from fibroma virus. The inoculation of chicken embryo cells (trypsinised at day 11 of egg incubation) does not result in CPE, but it is useful for detecting the viral antigens by IFA tests.

c) Electron microscopy

Negative-staining electron microscopy (EM) can be applied to a portion of skin lesion. The technique is simple and rapid to perform, giving results in 1 hour. About 1 mm^3 of the tissue is laid in a watch glass and 3 drops of distilled water are added. After 1–2 minutes at room temperature an EM grid coated with formvar and carbon is laid over the liquid. After 1 minute any excess liquid is removed with filter paper and immediately a 2% aqueous solution of ammonium molybdate, pH 7.0, is dropped on to the grid. After 10 seconds the excess liquid is removed with filter paper and the grid is prepared for the electron microscope. In a positive case, typical poxvirus particles can be seen. Myxoma virus cannot be distinguished from fibroma virus using this method.

d) Inoculation tests

Rabbit intradermal inoculation also offers a means of identifying the virus through its special characteristics and pathogenicity, namely cutaneous tropism (nodular form) and oculo-respiratory tropism (nonmyxomatous form). It has the advantage of being a gauge of virulence, from the type of inflammation in lesions (local or systemic infection) to the extent of lesions and survival time, and can distinguish fibroma virus (with its simple fibromatous local lesion) from myxoma virus (capable of causing generalised infection in adults). Rabbits should be of a domestic breed, weighing approximately 2 kg, unvaccinated and previously tested for the absence of antibodies (10).

The inoculum may be the supernatant fluid from a homogenised lesion (with antibiotics) or the product of a cell culture. Between 0.1 and 0.2 ml is administered intradermally behind the ear or into the dorso-lumbar region, which has previously been depilated. The inoculum may be assayed by injecting serial dilutions in saline buffer at one site for each dilution. A primary lesion will appear at the sites within 2-5 days, followed by conjunctivitis. Using five sites for each dilution allows a 50% infective dose (ID_{50}) to be obtained. If the animal survives, the disease can be confirmed serologically after 15 days.

2. Serological tests

Antibodies develop within 8–13 days. In the nonlethal forms and in vaccinated rabbits, the titre, which is an indicator of virulence, is highest after 20–60 days; it declines thereafter, disappearing after 6–8 months in the absence of reinfection (11).

Various serological tests may be used, but complement fixation (CF), IFA and enzyme-linked immunosorbent assay (ELISA) (in order of increasing sensitivity) are the most appropriate tests for international trade and other applications. These tests require standard antigens and antisera. The antigen can be prepared from the Lausanne strain, or some antigenically related strain, propagated in rabbits or cell cultures.

- **Preparation of standard reagents**

Myxomatous lesions are removed from rabbits at 6–7 days after inoculation and homogenised in veronal buffer to a dilution of 1/5. The antigen is the supernatant fluid that is obtained following centrifugation. Any anticomplementary activity is abolished by adding 0.6% chloroform. The antigen fluid can be frozen at –30°C or –70°C for stock purposes or used directly in CF tests after titration against a standard antiserum.

Antigen is made from cell cultures using the RK-13 lines. The virus is harvested as a suspension of cells 48 hours after infection, and is centrifuged. The supernatant fluid is retained. The cell deposit is homogenised (gently) or ultrasonicated (for 3 minutes continuously or for 5 minutes, 50% pulse 100 watts) resuspended and recentrifuged, and the supernatant is added to the former fluid. The final supernatant fluid is the antigen, and is stored at –20°C or –70°C (for longer conservation). It is titrated in cell cultures before use in virus neutralisation (VN) tests.

For the standard antiserum, an adult serologically negative rabbit is vaccinated with an attenuated strain of myxoma virus, or with the Shope's fibroma virus. After 3–4 weeks, the rabbit is inoculated with myxoma lesion material derived from the Lausanne strain of virus. Serum is obtained 3 weeks later and titrated by the CF test. If the titre is 1/640 or more, the animal is bled out and the serum is stored at –20°C.

- **Titration of standard reagents**

i) Inactivate standard antiserum for 30 minutes in a water bath at 56°C. No international standard serum for myxomatosis is available, but internal positive standards should be prepared and titrated in the appropriate range, using the CF test. After this, the following procedure is used to standardise batches of antigen.

ii) Make doubling dilutions of standard serum in calcium/magnesium/veronal buffer (CMV), pH 7.2, from 1/2 to 1/4096, using a 96-well round-bottomed microtitre plate, one well per dilution and 25 µl volume in each line.

iii) Using tubes, make doubling dilutions of antigen in CMV, from 1/10 to 1/1280.

iv) Add 25 µl per well of the same dilution of antigen, (transferred from the tubes) to each dilution on one line of the plate, from 1/10 to 1/1280, vertically.

v) Add 25 µl (6 H_{50} units [50% haemolysis]) per well of complement.

vi) Incubate the plate, covered with a plastic film, for 1 hour at 37°C or 14 hours at 4°C.

vii) Add 50 µl per well of the haemolytic system (2.5% sheep red blood cells [RBCs] and an equal volume of anti-sheep RBC serum 1/2000, both in CMV).

viii) Cover the plate again and incubate for 30 minutes at 37°C.

ix) Read the highest dilution of antigen giving complete haemolysis (H_{100}) with the highest dilution of standard serum. There is 1 antigenic unit (AgU) in 25 µl of antigen of this dilution.

VN tests (11) can be carried out in flat-bottomed cell-culture grade microtitre plates using the constant virus/varying serum method with 100 $TCID_{50}$ (50% tissue culture infective dose) of virus.

CF tests (11) are done in tubes or in microtitre plates (4) by conventional methods, recording 100% or 50% haemolysis. This is the standard method at the present time.

a) Complement fixation test

i) Titrate the complement in haemolysis tubes, in the presence of 1 AgU, in order to determine the H_{50} unit.

ii) Inactivate the positive and negative control sera in a water bath for 30 minutes at 56°C.

iii) Make doubling dilutions of test and control sera in CMV, from 1/4 to 1/1024, using a 96-well round-bottomed microtitre plate and 25 µl per well. Use the first well for the initial 1/4 dilution and the second as a serum control (anticomplementary control at 1/4 dilution). Prepare antigen, complement, and RBC control wells (two wells of each).

iv) Add 1 AgU in 25 µl per well (except to serum, complement and RBC control wells), then add 6 H_{50} of complement in 25 µl per well (except to RBC control wells).

v) Incubate the plates, covered with plastic film, for 14 hours (overnight) at 4°C.

vi) Add 50 µl haemolytic antiserum per well.

vii) Cover the plates again and incubate for 30 minutes at 37°C.

viii) Prepare H_{100}, H_{75}, H_{50}, H_{25} haemolysis controls using complement controls (H_{100}) and CMV.

ix) Read after centrifugation or passive sedimentation at 4°C. The test sera results are determined as the highest dilution of serum that gives at least 50% haemolysis inhibition.

x) A negative serum should give haemolysis inhibition <50% at 1/4 dilution.

b) Indirect fluorescent antibody test

IFA test (7) is carried out using chicken embryo cell cultures in flat-bottomed wells of microtitre plates: 200 µl of a cell suspension, diluted 1/1000 in medium, is distributed into all wells and a confluent cell sheet is formed within 24 hours. The medium is discarded and 100 µl of viral suspension containing 10^4 $TCID_{50}$ is added to each well. After 2 hours, 100 µl of MEM containing 2% calf serum is added. After 48 hours of incubation, the plates are washed with PBS and fixed with acetone containing 15% water for 30 minutes at –20°C. The plates are then dried at 37°C for 15 minutes. The plates can be stored at –30°C or –70°C for 3 months. Sera are tested by IFA using anti-rabbit IgG conjugated to fluorescein isothiocyanate. The test results may be qualitative with sera diluted 1/10 or 1/20, or quantitative with serial dilutions of serum.

c) Enzyme-linked immunosorbent assay

A recently developed ELISA (6) uses a semi-purified myxomatosis virus (French hypervirulent T1 strain antigenically related to Lausanne strain) produced in RK-13. The virus is harvested as a suspension of cells 48 hours after infection, and is centrifuged. The cell deposit is homogenised in TL20 (20 mM Tris, pH 8.6, 150 mM NaCl, and 1 mM EDTA), disrupted in ground glass and centrifuged at 1200 ***g*** at 4°C for 10 minutes.

The supernatant fluid is laid down on an equal volume of a 36% sucrose cushion in TL20 and centrifuged at 200,000 ***g*** for 2 hours in an SW 41 rotor at 4°C. The deposit is homogenised in 4–12 ml TL20 and again laid down on a 36% sucrose cushion.

The new deposit is homogenised in 1 ml TL20 and run into a linear 30–65% saccharose gradient by centrifugation at 200,000 ***g*** for 3 hours. The viral disc is harvested and diluted in 10 ml TL20 and then centrifuged at 130,000 ***g*** for 1 hour to concentrate the virus.

The deposit is homogenised in 0.2 ml TL20 and quantified by the Bradford method (colorimetric reaction with Coomassie brilliant blue) (3) or spectrophotometry (viral proteins account for around three-fifths of total protein). It can be stored at –30°C before use.

i) Coat probind assay plates for 16 hours (overnight at 37°C) with 1 µg per well viral proteins in 100 µl PBS, pH 7.6, leaving one column blank (i.e. coat with PBS only). Note that different batches of antigen vary in activity, and should be titrated against known standards to select antigen with high optical densities (OD).

ii) After three washes in PBS, block free binding sites by incubation in 25 mg/ml gelatin in PBS for 1 hour at 37°C.

iii) Wash the plate three times in PBS–0.01% Tween 20, and add 100 µl serial twofold dilutions of serum in PBS–Tween. Include positive and negative serum standards in each plate.

iv) After 60 minutes' incubation at 37°C and three washes in PBS–Tween, add 100 µl of a dilution in PBS–Tween of goat anit-rabbit IgG serum (typically 1/3000) conjugated to alkaline phosphatase for 1 hour at 37°C.

v) After four washes in PBS–Tween add, as substrate, 100 µl of disodium *p*-nitrophenyl phosphate at a concentration of 1 mg/ml in 10% diethanolamine.

vi) After 12 minutes in the dark at room temperature, the enzymatic reaction is stopped by the addition of 50 µl of 2 N NaOH.

vii) Read OD in a spectrophotometer at a wavelength of 405 nm.

viii) Express the serum sample titre as the inverse of the highest dilution for which the OD is greater than three times the OD of the negative serum standard.

The detection of specific myxoma virus antibodies by ELISA has been shown to be a highly sensitive and specific method for kinetic studies in experimental infection (2). Evaluation of the test has shown its great value for diagnostic application in wild rabbit populations (6).

For epidemiological surveys, the IFA test and the indirect ELISA can also be carried out using blood dried on blotting or filter paper: discs are cut (paper punch size) and two discs are placed in each well, to which is added 100 µl PBS to extract the serum. The dilution is about 1/30 and this can be used in another well for testing (7).

d) Agar gel immunodiffusion test

Agar gel immunodiffusion (AGID) (14) is qualitative and can detect antigen or antibody. Agar is prepared as described previously (Section A.1.) using 6 ml per 10 cm Petri dish. Strips of filter paper containing the standard antigen and antiserum, and discs containing test sera are arranged on the surface of the agar (discs between the strips). The plates are incubated in a humid atmosphere at 37°C and read after 24–48 hours. Three precipitation lines should appear. If the test sera contain antibody, at least one of the three lines is bent towards the antigen band; otherwise it remains straight. If sera contain antigen, at least one of the lines is bent towards the standard serum strip. The test can also be carried out in a more conventional manner using liquid reagents in wells cut in the agar..

B. REQUIREMENTS FOR VACCINES AND DIAGNOSTIC BIOLOGICALS

A master seed virus (MSV) must be established and used according to a seed-lot system. A record must be kept of its origin, passage history and characteristics.

Two types of live vaccine are used for vaccination against myxomatosis: a heterologous vaccine prepared from Shope's fibroma virus (5, 9, 13), and a homologous vaccine prepared from an attenuated strain of myxoma virus (1, 8, 12, 15–17). They are administered subcutaneously or intradermally.

Recently a new recombinant myxoma virus expressing rabbit haemorrhagic disease virus (RHDV) capsid protein and conferring double protection against myxomatosis and RHDV (2) has been developed, but is not yet available commercially.

1. Seed management

a) Characteristics of the seed

The viruses employed are fibroma virus or myxoma virus. The strains of *fibroma virus* are usually the original Shope's OA strain (1932), Boerlage's strain or various closely related strains. The strains of *myxoma virus* are modified by passaging in embryonated chicken eggs, rabbit kidney cells at decreasing temperatures, or chicken embryo cells. The strains usually result from several clonings.

b) Method of culture

Fibroma strains are maintained by passage in specific pathogen free (SPF) rabbits or in unvaccinated rabbits from a stock known to be free from myxomatosis. Skin on the backs of healthy adult rabbits is shaved, and multiple sites are inoculated with a 1% suspension of virulent material. Fibromas are fully developed within 8–10 days, at which time the rabbits are killed and the tumours are removed aseptically and homogenised with distilled water. The suspension is stored at –30°C or –70°C in 50% buffered glycerol, or as a 5% dilution in a protein solution. The production of the fibroma virus is also possible in rabbit dermal cell line.

Myxoma virus is grown on chicken embryo cell culture obtained from flocks free from specified pathogens, or on suitable cell lines (rabbit dermal cell line).

c) Validation as a vaccine

i) *Identity*

Specific antigenic characteristics of the *fibroma virus* strains are verified by AGID using sera against fibroma and myxomatosis.

The identity of *myxoma virus* is confirmed by neutralisation tests in RK-13 cells, or in a suitable cell line using a monospecific antiserum.

ii) *Purity*

The Master seed must be free from bacterial, fungal, mycoplasmal and viral contamination.

iii) *Safety*

Samples for safety testing are taken from a batch produced according to the manufacturing process. The dose to be used shall contain the maximum titre or potency established by the manufacturer (release titre).

Several tests are performed, at the Master Seed level, to demonstrate different aspects of safety. The safety of 10 times the normal dose must be demonstrated. Also, it is necessary to examine the dissemination of vaccine virus within the vaccinated animal, the ability of vaccine virus to spread from the vaccinated animal to in-contact animals and to test whether there is reversion-to-virulence of the vaccine virus, following serial passage in rabbits.

The pathogenicity of the *fibroma virus* strains is tested by inoculating rabbits with serial dilutions of supernatant fluids obtained by centrifugation of tumour preparations. Macroscopic and histopathological features and the course of development of fibromas are tested in SPF rabbits periodically. (Numerous serial passages in rabbits may induce mutation to the inflammatory IA strain, which produces severe lesions that are more inflammatory than neoplastic.)

The residual pathogenicity of the *myxoma virus* strains is tested by intradermal inoculation into SPF rabbits or unvaccinated rabbits free from myxomatosis. These rabbits should not develop more than a local reaction with perhaps small secondary lesions on the head that disappear within a few days.

For both strains, the rectal temperature and the body weight should be recorded as additional parameters.

iv) *Efficacy*

Different trials must be undertaken from representative batches of final product containing the minimum titre or potency. The proctective effect is demonstrated as follows:

A minimum of ten adult rabbits are inoculated with a dose of *fibroma vaccine,* and three rabbits serve as unvaccinated controls. After 14 days, all rabbits are inoculated, intradermally into the eyelids, with a pathogenic strain of myxoma virus (example: 0.1 ml inoculum containing 10^3 ID_{50} [median infectious dose]). During the following 21 days, the controls will die from myxomatosis, and at least seven of the ten vaccinated rabbits must present no signs of generalised infection.

Similarly, *myxoma vaccine* is tested in ten rabbits with three controls. After 14 days, all the rabbits are challenged with a sufficient quantity of virulent strain (example: 0.1 ml of the Lausanne virus strain containing 10^3 ID_{50}). After 21 days, seven of ten rabbits must have survived, while controls must have died from myxomatosis.

The manufacturer shall have established a minimum titre or potency taking into account loss in potency during the shelf life.

2. Method of manufacture

Fibroma virus is produced by multiple intradermal inoculations of seed virus into the skin on the back of a number of rabbits. Production is also possible in rabbit dermal cell line. Only the second (and perhaps the third) passage can be used if modification of the virus is to be avoided. The product of fibroma homogenate can be stored by freezing or used immediately. After clarification by centrifugation, the supernatant fluid is mixed with a stabiliser containing antibiotics and is distributed into ampoules or bottles for lyophilisation. Kaolin may be added as an adjuvant (40 mg/ml), in which case the vaccine is administered subcutaneously.

Myxoma virus is produced in chicken embryo cells (derived from SPF eggs) or a suitable cell line, limiting the passage number to a maximum of five. Virus is harvested after 2–6 days. The viral suspension may be stored at –70°C. The vaccine is prepared by diluting in specified proportions the viral preparation with a stabiliser for lyophilisation. After homogenisation, the product is distributed into bottles for lyophilisation, the bottles being sealed under vacuum or in sterile nitrogen.

Each virus can also be produced in RK-13 cells.

3. In-process control

The *fibroma virus* titre is measured by calculating the ID_{50} after intradermal inoculation of serial dilutions of the clarified supernatant fluid into several sites (e.g. five) on up to six rabbits. A dilution of a standard preparation of fibroma virus is also inoculated into each rabbit to confirm the animal's correct response to inoculation. The titration can also be performed in a rabbit cell line. In each case the titre should correlate with the required potency as defined by the test for efficacy, see Section B.1.c.

The identity of *myxoma virus is* checked in RK cells. Titration of each virus can also be done in RK-13 cells ($TCID_{50}$).

Testing for contaminating viruses is done by inoculating a confluent cell sheet of Vero cells. Vaccine, adjusted to the equivalent of 20 doses/ml, is neutralised with an equal volume of monospecific hyperimmune serum for 30 minutes at 37°C. The mixture is filtered through a 0.22 µm membrane filter, and 1 ml volumes are inoculated into five 25 ml bottles of cell cultures. These are kept under observation for 7 days. After harvesting, the cells are suspended in medium and subjected to several freeze–thaw cycles, followed by centrifugation and filtration, and the material is inoculated into fresh cultures and observed for 7 days. There should be no evidence of CPE or haemadsorption to chicken RBCs.

4. Batch control

a) Sterility

Tests for sterility and freedom from contamination of biological materials may be found in Chapter I.4.

b) Safety

After rehydration, ten doses of the lyophilised *fibroma vaccine* are injected subcutaneously into each of three susceptible rabbits, which are then observed for 21 days. Local reactions should be slight, with no generalisation and no effect on general health.

Myxoma vaccine is tested using ten doses injected intradermally into the ears of three susceptible rabbits, which are then observed for 21 days. The primary myxoma lesion should remain mild.

c) Potency

The batch potency is determined by measurement of virus content. Serial dilutions of the vaccine are inoculated into suitable cell cultures. One dose of vaccine shall contain not less than the minimum titre established in Section B.1.c.

If the vaccine strain is not adapted to cultures, an efficacy test in rabbits shall be carried out (see Section B.1.c.).

d) Duration of immunity

Several batches of ten susceptible rabbits are vaccinated. One batch is tested by challenge infection (as in the batch potency test), at 1, 2, 3, etc., months post-vaccination for *fibroma virus,* and at 1, 3, 6, and 9 months for *myxoma virus.* The duration of immunity is deduced from the time during which at least seven of the ten rabbits prove to be resistant to infection.

e) Stability

Titrations of vaccine virus are carried out at intervals until 3 months beyond the requested shelf life on at least three batches of vaccine.

5. Tests on the final product

a) Safety

See Section B.4.b.

b) Potency

See Section B.4.c.

REFERENCES

1. ARGUELLO VILLARES J.L. (1986). Contribución a la profilaxis de la mixomatosis del conejo mediante el uso de una ceba homologa. *Medicina Veterinaria*, **3**, 91–103.

2. BERTAGNOLI S., GELFI J., LEGALL G., BOILLETOT E., VAUTHEROT J.F., RASSCHAERT D., LAURENT S., PETIT F., BOUCRAUT-BARALON C. & MILON A. (1996). Protection against myxomatosis and rabbit viral hemorrhagic disease with recombinant myxoma virus expressing rabbit hemorrhagic disease virus capsid protein. *J. Virol.*, **70**, 5061–5066.

3. BRADFORD M. (1976). A rapid and sensitive method for quantification of microgram quantities of protein utilizing the principle of protein-dye binding. *Anal. Biochem.*, **72**, 248–254.

4. CHANTAL J., BOUCRAUT-BARALON C., GANIERE J.P., PETIT F., PY R. & PICAVET D.P. (1993). Réaction de fixation du complément en plaques de microtitration: application à la sérologie de la myxomatose. Etude comparative des résultats avec la réaction d'immunofluorescence indirecte. *Rev. sci. tech. Off. int. Epiz.*, **12**, 895–907.

5. FENNER F. & WOODROOFE G.M. (1954). Protection of laboratory rabbits against myxomatosis by vaccination with fibroma virus. *Aust. J. Exp. Biol.*, **32**, 653–668.

6. GELFI J., CHANTAL J., PHONG T.T., PY R. & BOUCRAUT-BARALON C. (1999). Development of an ELISA for detection of myxoma virus-specific rabbit antibodies; test evaluation for diagnostic applications on vaccinated and wild rabbit sera. *J. Vet. Diagn. Invest.*, **11**, 240–245.

7. GILBERT Y., PICAVET D.P. & CHANTAL J. (1989). Diagnostic de la myxomatose: mise au point d'une technique d'immunofluorescence indirecte. Utilisation de prélèvements sanguins sur papier buvard pour la recherche d'anticorps. *Rev. sci. tech. Off. int. Epiz.* **8**, 209–220.

8. GORSKI J. & MIZAK B. (1985). Polish vaccine against myxomatosis in rabbits. *Med. Weter.*, **41**, 113–116.

9. JOBERT R. (1983). Contribution à l'étude de la vaccination contre la myxomatose, vaccination à l'aide du virus fibromateux. Thèse Doctorat Vétérinaire Toulouse n° 82.

10. JOUBERT L. (1973). La Myxomatose T.II. Série : Les Maladies Animales à Virus. L'Expansion éditeur, Paris, France.

11. SAURAT P., CHANTAL J., GANIERE J.P., GILBERT Y., PICAVET D.P & LEFORT C. (1980). La réponse immunitaire dans la myxomatose. Etude de la réponse humorale. *Bull. Mens. Off. Nation. Chasse*, **12**, 297–309.

12. SAURAT P., GILBERT Y. & GANIERE J.P. (1978). Etude d'une souche de virus myxomateux modifié. *Rev. Med. Vet.*, **129**, 415–451.

13. SHOPE R.E. (1932). A filtrable virus causing a tumor like condition in rabbits and its relationship to virus myxomatosis. *J. Exp. Med.*, **56**, 803.

14. SOBEY W.R., CONOLLY D. & ADAMS K.M. (1966). Myxomatosis: a simple method of sampling blood and testing for circulating soluble antigens or antibodies to them. *Aust. J. Sci.*, **28**, No. 9, 354.

15. TOZZINI F. & MANI P. (1975). Studio su alcune carratteristiche di crescita del virus della mixomatosi ceppo Pisa 73. *Arch. Vet. Ital.*, **26**, 19–26.

16. TOZZINI F. & POLI A. (1980). Biological characteristics of myxomatosis virus strain P73, after 51 serial passages on RK13 cells. *Arch. Vet. Ital.*, **31**, 48–51.

17. VON DER AHE C., DEDEK J. & LOEPELMANN H. (1981). Ergebnisse und Erfahrungen in der DDR bei der staatlichen Prüfung und Praxiserpropung der aus der CSSR emportierten Myxomatose-Vakzine. *Monatshe. Veterinarmed.*, **36**, 492–495.

*

* *

CHAPTER 2.8.2.

TULAREMIA

SUMMARY

Tularemia is a zoonosis caused by Francisella tularensis. *It occurs naturally in lagomorphs (rabbits and hares), and in rodents, especially microtine rodents (such as voles, vole rats and muskrats), and beavers. A wide variety of other mammals, and several species of birds, have also been reported to be infected.*

Two types of F. tularensis *are recognised on the basis of cultural characteristics, epidemiology, and virulence in some hosts.* Francisella tularensis tularensis *(Type A) is associated with lagomorphs in North America. It is transmitted primarily by ticks and biting flies, is highly virulent for humans and domestic rabbits, and ferments glycerol.* Francisella tularensis palaearctica *(Type B) occurs mainly in aquatic rodents (beavers, muskrats) in northern North America, and in hares and small rodents in northern Eurasia. It may be water- or arthropod-borne, is less virulent for humans and rabbits, and does not ferment glycerol. In addition to vector transmission, tularemia may be spread by direct contact with contaminated animals or material, by inhalation, or by ingestion of the poorly cooked flesh of infected animals or contaminated water.*

The disease is characterised by fever, apathy and septicaemia. In humans, there may be ulcers or abscesses at the site of inoculation (this is rarely seen in animals), and swelling of the regional lymph nodes. On post-mortem examination, lesions may include caseous necrosis of lymph nodes and multiple greyish-white foci of necrosis in the spleen, liver, bone marrow and lungs. The spleen is usually hypertrophied.

It is important to understand that there is a high risk of direct infection of humans by simple contact with this organism. Special precautions, including the wearing of gloves, masks and eyeshields, are therefore recommended when handling infective materials.

Identification of the agent: *The bacteria can be demonstrated in impression smears or in fixed specimens of organs, such as liver, spleen, bone marrow, kidney and lung, as well as in blood smears. Immunological methods, such as the fluorescent antibody test (FAT), are the most reliable way to identify the bacteria. With Gram staining, the bacteria appear as very small punctiform Gram-negative rods, often difficult to distinguish as bacteria. They can also be stained with May–Grunwald–Giemsa or phenol thionin.*

The organism is highly fastidious. For growth it is necessary to use either Francis medium, McCoy and Chapin medium, or glucose cysteine agar supplemented with blood. The colonies are small, round and transparent, and do not appear before 48 hours' incubation at 37°C. On Francis medium, the colonies may be confluent and have a milky appearance. If transportation is necessary, samples should be inoculated into sterile nutrient broth and stored at 4–10°C for a few hours, or at –70°C if transit is likely to be prolonged.

Mice or guinea-pigs can be experimentally inoculated with infected tissue material or with cultures to aid in the diagnosis of tularemia. Infection is fatal within 2–10 days. FAT and capillary tube precipitation tests also demonstrate F. tularensis *in pathological specimens.*

Serological tests: *Serological tests are useful diagnostic aids in human infection, but are of limited value in sensitive animal species as these species usually die before developing antibodies. Epidemiological surveys can be conducted in domestic animals in relatively resistant species, such as sheep, cattle, pigs, dogs and wild ungulates, as these species develop antibodies. Relatively resistant species of rodents and lagomorphs can also be used in epidemiological surveys.*

***Requirements for vaccines and diagnostic biologicals:** A live attenuated vaccine strain is available for vaccination of humans at high risk of exposure to virulent* F. tularensis. *However, the vaccine is only available for restricted use. The outcome of vaccination can be estimated by demonstration of specific antibodies and the ability of lymphocytes to proliferate in the presence of* F. tularensis *antigen.*

A. DIAGNOSTIC TECHNIQUES

Tularemia is a zoonosis caused by *Francisella tularensis.* It occurs naturally in lagomorphs (rabbits and hares) and rodents, especially microtine rodents such as voles, vole rats and muskrats, as well as in beavers. In addition, a wide variety of other mammals, birds, amphibians and invertebrates have been reported to be infected (12). Tularemia occurs endemically in the Northern Hemisphere. The disease can occur as epizootic outbreaks in many countries (in North America, Europe, Russia, Japan), while it occurs only as sporadic cases in some other countries (in Europe and Asia). Some epizootic outbreaks occur as a result of importation of subclinically infected lagomorphs.

Two types of *Francisella tularensis* are recognised on the basis of culture characteristics, epidemiology, and virulence. *Francisella tularensis tularensis* (Type A) is mainly associated with lagomorphs in North America. It is primarily transmitted by ticks or biting flies, or by direct contact with infected lagomorphs. It is highly virulent for humans and domestic rabbits, and ferments glycerol. *Francisella tularensis palaearctica* (Type B) occurs mainly in aquatic rodents (beavers, muskrats) and voles in northern North America, and in lagomorphs (hares) and rodents in northern Eurasia. It is primarily transmitted by direct contact or by mosquitoes, but may be transmitted through inhalation or through infected water or food. It is less virulent for humans and domestic rabbits, and does not ferment glycerol (1, 2, 8, 9).

In sensitive animals, clinical signs of intense apathy are accompanied later by a fatal septicaemia. The course of the disease is approximately 2–10 days in susceptible species, and animals are usually dead when presented for diagnosis. Most domestic species do not usually manifest signs of tularemia infection, but they do develop specific antibodies to the organism following infection. Outbreaks with high mortality caused by the Type A organism have occurred in sheep (1, 2).

At necropsy, animals that have died from acute tularemia are usually in good body condition. There are signs of septicaemia characterised by whitish foci of necrosis randomly distributed in the liver, bone marrow and spleen. In addition, the spleen is usually hypertrophic. Necrotic foci vary in size, and in some cases may be barely visible to the naked eye. The lungs are usually congested and oedematous, and there may be areas of consolidation and fibrinous pneumonia or pleuritis. Fibrin may be present in the abdominal cavity. Foci of caseous necrosis are often present in one or more lymph node(s). The lymph nodes that are most often affected are those in the abdominal and pleural cavities and lymph nodes draining the extremities. In less sensitive species, the histological picture can resemble that of tuberculosis with chronic granulomas in liver, spleen, lungs and kidneys.

There is a high risk of human infection from *F. tularensis.* Infection can occur by simple contact. Suitable precautions, such as the wearing of gloves, masks and eyeshields during any manipulation of pathological specimens or cultures, must be taken in order to avoid human infection. Experimentally inoculated animals and their excreta are especially hazardous to humans.

1. Identification of the agent

Francisella tularensis can be demonstrated in smear preparations or in histological sections. It can also be identified by culture or animal inoculation. However, *F. tularensis* may be difficult to isolate from dead animals and carcasses due to overgrowth of other bacteria. As the post-mortem picture is also not constant, diagnosis is sometimes difficult and immunological or immunohistochemical methods are preferable, although reagents may be difficult to obtain. It can sometimes be recommended, therefore, that fixed specimens be analysed at laboratories equipped with proper reagents or methods.

a) Smear preparations

Smear preparations are made on microscope slides as impression smears of organs such as the liver, spleen, bone marrow, kidney, lung or blood. The bacteria are abundant in such smears, but may be overlooked because of their very small size (0.2–0.7 µm). The bacteria can be demonstrated by direct or indirect fluorescent antibody staining. This is a safe, rapid and specific diagnostic tool (7, 11).

Gram staining of smears reveals a scattering of small, punctiform Gram-negative bacteria near the limit of visibility. The bacteria may be difficult to distinguish from precipitates of stain.

b) **Histological sections**

Bacteria can be demonstrated in sections using immunohistochemical methods such as the fluorescent antibody test (FAT) (10). The test is normally performed on specimens from liver, spleen or bone marrow, fixed in neutral buffered formalin and paraffin embedded. Slides are treated with rabbit anti-tularemia serum, washed and thereafter treated with sheep fluorescein-isothiocyanate-conjugated anti-rabbit serum. The samples are examined under a fluorescence microscope. Large numbers of bacteria can be seen in necrotic lesions and in the blood.

c) **Culture**

Francisella tularensis will not grow on ordinary media, although an occasional strain can sometimes, on initial isolation, grow on blood agar. Incubation is at 37°C. Heart blood, liver, spleen and bone marrow from moribund animals should be used for culture. It is necessary to use special culture media, such as:

i) *Francis medium:* Peptone agar containing 0.1% cystine (or cysteine) and 1% glucose, to which is added, before solidification, 8–10% defribrinated rabbit, horse or human blood.

ii) *McCoy and Chapin medium:* This consists of 60 g egg yolk and 40 ml normal saline solution, carefully mixed and coagulated by heating to 75°C.

iii) *Modified Thayer–Martin agar:* Glucose cysteine agar (GCA)-medium base supplemented with haemoglobin and Iso VitaleX.

Media can be stored for up to 8–10 days at 4°C. Colonies that form on McCoy medium are small, prominent, round and transparent. A more abundant growth is obtained on Francis medium and modified Thayer–Martin agar, with confluent colonies that have a milky appearance and a mucoid consistency. On either medium, colonies do not appear until after 48 hours' incubation at 37°C.

iv) *GCA agar with thiamine (BBL):* When used with added blood, the medium is commonly referred to as GBCA and can be substituted for the original, noncommercial medium described by Down *et al.* (4). Suspend 58 g of the dry material in 1 litre of distilled or demineralised water, and mix thoroughly. Heat with frequent agitation and boil for 1 minute. Dispense into tubes and sterilise by autoclaving at 118–121°C for 15 minutes.

For litre quantities, autoclave at the same temperatures for 30 minutes. Cool to 45–48°C. Aseptically add 25 ml of packed human blood cells or 50 ml of defibrinated rabbit or sheep blood. Mix thoroughly and pour into plates. Incubate at 37°C for 24 hours before use to decrease surface moisture and to test for sterility (4).

Differential criteria for the identification of *F. tularensis* include absence of growth on ordinary media, distinctive cellular morphology, and specific fluorescent antibody and slide agglutination reactions. The bacteria are nonmotile, nonsporulating, bipolar staining, and of uniform appearance in 24-hour cultures, but pleomorphic in older cultures.

Francisella tularensis can be identified in stained smears, by agglutination with tularemia hyperimmune antiserum, or by animal inoculation. In areas of North America where both types of *F. tularensis* may occur, Type A may be distinguished from Type B by the fact that Type A ferments glycerol.

The bacteria can also be identified by hybridisation with probes specific to the 16S rRNA of *F. tularensis*, *F. tularensis* Type A, and *F. tularensis* Type B (5), or by polymerase chain reaction (PCR) with primers targeting specific regions of the 16 rDNA molecules. The PCR will allow identification at the genus, species and subspecies level (6).

d) **Capillary tube precipitation test on pathological samples**

Tissues, such as spleen, liver or bone marrow, are ground with sterile sand in three-to-five times their volume of normal saline. The suspension is transferred to a tube and two volumes of ethyl ether are added. After shaking, the mixture is allowed to stand for 4–5 hours at room temperature. It is again shaken and then allowed to stand overnight.

The aqueous phase is drawn off and centrifuged at 2000 ***g*** for 30 minutes. The supernatant fluid, containing the antigen, is drawn off and distributed into capillary tubes to which tularemia antiserum is added.

The tubes are incubated at 37°C for 3 hours, then kept at 4°C overnight. A positive result is the formation of a ring of precipitate.

e) Animal inoculation

Animal inoculation is extremely hazardous and is not recommended for routine identification. It should only be undertaken where proper biosafety facilities and cages are available. The use of animals for diagnostic purposes must be carefully considered.

Laboratory animals are inoculated with culture material to confirm the nature of an isolate. Pathological specimens may be inoculated for the direct detection of *F. tularensis*. Mice are more sensitive than guinea-pigs, although the latter may be preferred for diagnostic purposes as the lesions are more definitive than in mice. Furthermore, mice usually die before lesions can form.

In infected animals, the only evidence at the onset of infection is a slight anaemia with a lymphocytosis and monocytosis.

Intraperitoneal injection is sufficient for passage of pure cultures. All routes of administration in mice, such as subcutaneous, percutaneous, or intravenous, will lead to an infection that is invariably fatal within 2–10 days.

Inoculation in guinea-pigs may be made into a foot-pad, provoking a lymphadenitis that is detectable after 3–4 days. If this reaction is pronounced, the animal may be killed at 5–6 days. Use of the percutaneous route, by smearing a shaved area of skin with the material, allows the selective isolation of *F. tularensis* from material that contains a mixture of organisms.

Post-mortem examination reveals hypertrophy and periadenitis of regional lymph nodes, and oedema at the inoculation site, which is sometimes haemorrhagic. The spleen contains a scattering of minute nodules and is hypertrophied. The liver is also hypertrophied, but foci of necrosis may not be evident. Smears of blood, spleen and liver may be extremely rich in the bacterium.

The regional lymph nodes show a lymphadenitis, oedema that distends the node capsule, a lymphocytic infiltration and peripheral micro-abscessation. Blood vessels are congested and thrombotic. Later, areas of necrosis become confluent to form multiple abscesses. If the animal survives long enough, these may become surrounded by an epithelioid reaction with giant cells, plasma cells and macrophages.

2. Serological tests

Serology is currently carried out for diagnosis of tularemia in humans, but is of limited value in sensitive animal species, which usually die before specific antibodies can develop. Serology may be employed, either on sera or on lung extracts (11), in epidemiological surveys on animals that are constitutionally more resistant to infection, such as sheep, cattle, pigs, moose, dogs or birds (10, 12).

a) Tube agglutination

The most commonly used serological test is the tube agglutination test. The antigen is a culture of *F. tularensis* on Francis medium. The culture is harvested after 5–6 days. Younger cultures yield a poorer antigen. The colonies are suspended in 96% alcohol, giving a thick suspension that can be stored for 1–7 days at room temperature. The sediment is washed with normal saline and resuspended in an equal volume of normal saline. Crystal violet powder is added to a final concentration of 0.25%. The bacteria are stained by incubation at 37°C for at least 24 hours and at most 7 days.

After the supernatant fluid has been discarded, the deposit is suspended in normal saline with or without thiomersal (merthiolate) at a final concentration of 1/10,000, or formaldehyde at a final concentration of 0.5%. The suspension is calibrated with positive and negative sera, and adjusted by adding normal saline to provide an antigen that when tested on a slide gives readily visible stained agglutination reactions against a clear fluid background.

The test is performed in tubes containing a fixed amount of antigen (0.9 ml) and different dilutions of serum commencing with 1/10, 1/20, 1/40, etc. The results are read after 20 minutes of shaking, or after 1 hour in a water bath at 37°C followed by overnight storage at room temperature. The agglutinated sediment is visible to the naked eye or, preferably, by using a hand lens. The positive tubes are those that have a clear supernatant fluid. Possible cross-reactions with *Brucella abortus* and *B. melitensis* have to be taken into consideration.

b) Enzyme-linked immunosorbent assay

Another serological test, the enzyme-linked immunosorbent assay (ELISA), also allows an early diagnosis of tularemia (3). Following the first report of ELISA for early diagnosis, this method is widely used for clinical purposes. Different antigens, whole bacteria as well as subcellular components, have been used as recall antigens against immunoglobulines IgA, IgM and IgG; 2 weeks after the onset of tularemia, specific antibodies can be detected in the serum. For routine diagnosis, whole heat-killed (65°C for 30 minutes) bacteria can be used as antigen. Bacteria can be coated to plastic plates, using the usual procedures, followed by serial dilutions of serum to be tested. Positive reactions can be visualised by anti-antibodies labelled with enzyme. The test should also be read in a photometer with negative sera as control. The FAT has also been developed for infected tissue samples and to confirm the identity of an isolate in culture (10), but this test is no longer in use.

B. REQUIREMENTS FOR VACCINES AND DIAGNOSTIC BIOLOGICALS

Vaccines have been produce with the aim of protecting humans, but as all vaccine development involves testing in animals, it is clear that some of the vaccines could be used to protect animals.

Before 1940, attempts to vaccinate against tularemia were performed by use of whole killed bacteria or bacterial extracts. None of these vaccines induced protection against highly virulent strains of *F. tularensis.* Instead, viable attenuated vaccines were developed. Attenuation was performed by repeated culture of bacteria on various media with or without antiserum. Such live attenuated vaccines have been used in mass vaccinations of people in the former Soviet Union since 1946, either as monocultures or as a mixture of strains.

An attenuated live vaccine strain of *F. tularensis* biovar palaearctica is available and can be used for restricted vaccination of individuals at high risk (13).

REFERENCES

1. BELL J.F. (1980). Tularaemia. *In:* CRC Handbook Series in Zoonoses. Section A: Bacterial, Rickettsial, and Mycotic Diseases. Vol. 2, Steel J.H., ed. CRS Press, Boca Raton, Florida, USA, 161–193.

2. BELL J.F. & REILLY J.R. (1981). Tularemia. *In:* Infectious Diseases of Wild Mammals, Second Edition, Davies J.W., Karstad L.H. & Trainer D.W., eds. Iowa State Press, Ames, Iowa, USA, 213–231.

3. CARLSSON H.E., LINDBERG A., LINDBERG G., HEDERSTEDT B., KARLSSON K. & AGELL B.O. (1979). Enzyme-linked immunosorbent assay for immunological diagnosis of human tulreamia. *J. Clin. Microbiol.,* **10**, 615–621.

4. DOWN C.M., CORIELL L.L., CHAPMAN S.S. & KLAUBER A. (1947). The cultivation of *Bacterium tularense* in embryonated eggs. *J. Bacteriol.,* **53**, 89–100.

5. FORSMAN M., SANDSTROM G. & JAURIN B. (1990). Identification of *Francisella* species and discrimination of Type A and Type B strains of *F. tularensis* by 16S rRNA Analysis. *Appl. Environ. Microbiol.,* **56**, 949–955.

6. FORSMAN M., SANDSTROM G & SJOSTEDT A. (1995). Analysis of 16S ribosomal DNA sequences of *Francisella* strains and utilization for determination of the phylogeny of the genus and for identification of strains by PCR. *Int. J. Syst. Bacteriol.,* **44**, 38–46.

7. KARLSSON K.A., DAHLSTRAND S., HANKO E. & SODERLIND O. (1970). Demonstration of *Francisella tularensis* in sylvan animals with the aid of fluourescent antibodies. *Acta Pathol. Microbiol. Immunol. Scand. (B),* **78**, 647–651.

8. MARKOWITZ L.E., HYNES N.A., DE LA CRUZ P., CAMPOS E., BARBAREE J.M., PLIKAYTIS B., MOOSIER D. & KAUFMAN A.F. (1985). Tick-borne tularemia. *JAMA,* **254**, 2922–2925.

9. MOLLARET H.H. & BOURDIN M. (1972). Le diagnostique biologique de la tularémie humaine. *Med. Mal. Infect.,* **2**, 419–422.

10. MORNER T. (1981). The use of FA technique of detecting *Francisella tularensis* in formalin fixed material. *Acta Vet. Scand.,* **22**, 296–306.

11. MORNER T., SANDSTROM G. & MATTSON R. (1988). Comparison of sera and lung extracts for surveys of wild animals for antibodies against *Francisella tularensis* biovar *palaearctica. J. Wildl. Dis.,* **24**, 10–14.

12. PHAHLER-JUNG K. (1989). Die globale verbreitungen der tularämie. Diss. Justus. Liebig-Univertsität, Giessen, Germany, 1989.

13. SANDSTROM G. (1994). The tularemia vaccine. *J. Chem. Tech. Biotechn.,* **59**, 315–20.

*

* *

CHAPTER 2.8.3.

RABBIT HAEMORRHAGIC DISEASE

SUMMARY

Rabbit haemorrhagic disease (RHD) is a highly contagious and acute fatal disease of the European rabbit (Oryctolagus cuniculus), *caused by a calicivirus. A similar disease, termed European brown hare syndrome (EBHS), has been described in the hare* (Lepus europaeus); *the aetiological agent is a different calicivirus, antigenically related to the RHD virus (RHVD). RHD is characterised by high morbidity and high mortality (40–90%), and spreads very rapidly by direct and indirect transmission. Infection can occur by nasal, conjunctival or oral routes. Transmission of RHD is facilitated by the high stability of the virus in the environment. The incubation period varies from 1 to 3 days, and death usually occurs 12–36 hours after the onset of fever. The clinical manifestations have been described mainly in the acute infection (nervous and respiratory signs, apathy and anorexia). Clear and specific pathological lesions, both gross and microscopic, are present. There is primary liver necrosis and a massive disseminated intravascular coagulopathy in all organs and tissues. The most severe lesions are in the liver, trachea and lungs. Petechial haemorrhages are evident in almost all organs and are accompanied by poor blood coagulation.*

Identification of the agent: *The liver contains the highest viral titre and is the most suitable organ for viral identification. As no satisfactory growth conditions or sensitive cell substrates have been established,* in-vitro *isolation cannot be employed. The haemagglutination test using human Group O red blood cells was the first test applied for routine laboratory diagnosis of RHD. However, other tests (negative-staining immunoelectron microscopy, sandwich enzyme-linked immunosorbent assay [ELISA], immunohistological staining, polymerase chain reaction and Western blot) have shown a higher level of specificity and sensitivity.*

Serological tests: *Characterisation and titration of specific antibodies arising from natural infection or from immunisation are performed using the haemagglutination inhibition test or the ELISA, either as an indirect or competitive reaction. The following reagents are prepared: antigen from infected rabbit liver, anti-RHDV serum from convalescent or hyperimmunised rabbits, and negative serum from rabbits fully sensitive to RHDV infection. Monoclonal antibodies have been produced in several laboratories. Some laboratories have produced a recombinant antigen, VP60 structural protein expressed in baculovirus, which can also be used as a diagnostic reagent.*

Requirements for vaccines and diagnostic biologicals: *Indirect control of the disease is achieved by vaccination using a killed vaccine prepared from clarified liver suspensions of experimentally infected rabbits and subsequently inactivated and adjuvanted. Experimental data indicate that protection lasts for a long period (over 1 year). Moreover, vaccinated animals quickly produce solid immunity against RHDV infection; vaccination is therefore considered to be effective in protecting nonexposed rabbits and its primary use is in rabbitries after an outbreak of the disease has been diagnosed.*

A. DIAGNOSTIC TECHNIQUES

Rabbit haemorrhagic disease (RHD) is a highly contagious and acute fatal disease of wild and domestic European rabbits *(Oryctolagus cuniculus).*

RHD was first reported in 1984 in the People's Republic of China (31); currently it is endemic in East Asia and Europe. Outbreaks have also been recorded in Cuba, Mexico, Reunion Island, and parts of North Africa. The disease was introduced into Australia in 1995 as a national programme to control rabbits, and has become endemic there. In 1997, it was introduced into New Zealand.

The causative agent of RHD presents features of a calicivirus, including its size (32–35 nm in diameter), morphology as seen by electron microscopy (EM), the presence of a single major capsid polypeptide (60 kDa), a positively stranded RNA genome of 7.437 kb and a subgenomic RNA of 2.2 kb detected in infected tissue and in purified virions (16, 34, 35, 39, 40). In addition, cryo-EM studies showed that RHD virus (RHDV) capsid protein (VP60), similarly to that of Norwalk virus (42), folds in two distinct domains held together by a hinge region (50). The N-terminal 200–250 residues constitute the inner domain and the C-terminal residues beyond 200–250 constitute the protruding domain. In the overall picture of the capsid, these domains make the inner shell and the outer shell, respectively, which is characterised by arch-like structures. This structure also correlates with the antigenic characteristics of RHDV, in fact the main antigenic determinants are located on the C-terminal end of the VP60 (11, 12, 45, 52).

Since 1991, a second type of virus particle was identified as the main component in approximately 5% of the RHDV-positive specimens (15). The characteristics of this particle are: i) a smooth surface and a diameter lower than RHDV; ii) its protein is of 28–30 kDa; iii) it is reactive with the RHDV convalescent rabbit sera and with those anti-RHDV monoclonal antibodies (MAbs) reactive against the N-terminal end of the RHDV VP60; and iv) it is haemaglutination (HA) negative. Such characterisation was then confirmed when this viral particle was purified from the liver of an experimentally infected rabbit showing a protracted course of the disease, and analysed using either specific MAbs as well as hyperimmune antisera (21). Indeed, the smaller viral particle only corresponds to the inner shell of RHDV, but its origin is not fully understood and two hypotheses have been proposed. Granzow *et al.* (21) assumed that the smaller particle, named core-like particles (CLPs), arises from a truncated RHDV genome or defective expression. Differently, Barbieri *et al.* (5) observed the following: i) a strict correlation between the higher prevalence of smooth RHDV (s-RHDV) particles in the organs together with its sharp increase, and the appearance of specific anti-RHDV IgM at 3–4 days post-infection; ii) the presence of large amounts of s-RHDV only in the liver and spleen and not in the bloodstream, as occurs during the viraemic phase of acute RHD; iii) the finding of fragments of the VP60 having different molecular weight (41–30 kDa) during transition from RHDV to s-RHDV. Therefore they concluded that the genesis of the particle, named s-RHDV, is due to a degradative process that is probably the consequence of the physiological clearance of the RHDV-IgM immuno-complex formed in large amounts at the beginning of the humoral response.

Apart from its origin, the identification of this second particle (s-RHDV/CLPs) in the liver of a rabbit can be considered to be a marker of the subacute/chronic form of RHD that usually evolves between 4 and 8 days post-infection and is followed either by the death of the rabbit or, more often, in its recovery (5, 32).

All known isolates appear to belong to one serotype (6). The complete sequence of geographically different RHD isolates has been reported. Their comparison reveals close overall homology in terms of genome sequence with few or no consequent predicted changes in amino acid composition. Viruses from all those countries where RHD has been diagnosed differ by between 2% and 5% (9, 23, 36, 38, 43). Nevertheless, isolates that exhibit temperature-dependant differences in haemoagglutinating characteristics (10, 18) have been described, and very recently a consistent genetic and antigenic RHDV variant has been identified at the same time in Italy (11) and Germany (45). This RHDV variant, named RHDVa, presents amino acid changes in the surface-exposed E region (aa 344–434) that contains the main antigenic epitopes of calicivirus, three times higher than in all previously sequenced RHDV isolates. A group of related MAbs, able to protect rabbits from infection by RHDV, was found to be totally negative by enzyme-linked immunosorbent assay (ELISA) with RHDVa. Rabbits experimentally vaccinated with the presently available RHDV vaccine were still protected by the challenge with RHDVa, even if with a lower efficiency (11, 45).

RHD is characterised by high morbidity and a mortality rate between 40% and 90% (1). Infection occurs in rabbits of all ages, but clinical disease is observed only in adults and young animals older than 40–50 days. The pathogenic mechanism of resistance in young animals is still unclear (15).

The European rabbit *(Oryctolagus cuniculus)* is the only species known to be affected by RHD. No other lagomorphs, such as the Volcano rabbit *(Romerolagus diazzi)* of Mexico, the black-tail jackrabbit *(Lepus californicus)* and the cottontail *(Sylvilagus floridanus)* of North America, have been shown to be susceptible (22). A similar disease, termed European brown hare syndrome (EBHS), has been described in the hare *(Lepus europaeus)*, but its aetiological agent, which is also a calicivirus, is different from RHDV, although it is related antigenically. Alignment of the RNA sequences of the EBHS virus (EBHSV) and RHDV genomes shows 71% nucleotide identity, and amino acid alignment shows 78% identity and 87% similarity (29, 52).

Recently a new rabbit calicivirus related to the RHDV was identified in healthy rabbits (13, 14). This virus, provisionally named rabbit calicivirus (RCV), is significantly different from the previously characterised RHDV isolates in terms of pathogenicity, viral titre, tissue tropism, and primary sequence of the structural protein. It is avirulent, replicates in the intestine at a low titre and presents a genomic identity with RHDV of around 92%. Cross-protection experiments, which indicate that the new virus does not infect hares, as well as antigenic data and sequence comparisons demonstrate that it is more closely related to RHDV than to the EBHSV.

RHD spreads very rapidly, and infection can occur by nasal, conjunctival or oral routes. The disease can be transmitted directly from infected animals to healthy ones, indirectly by contact with a carcass, or by the contamination of foodstuffs, water or bedding materials by the excretions and secretions of infected animals (53). The possibility of indirect transmission over short distances or to new areas by passive vectors, such as haematophagous insects (biting flies, fleas and mosquitoes), birds (particularly rabbit predators such as gulls), rodents and wild animals or contaminated utensils and vehicles, should be considered (1, 53). There is evidence that foxes can seroconvert to RHD after ingestion of the virus (30) and, although there is probably no replication within these animals, foxes and dogs may bring the infection to previously unexposed wild rabbits (47). Humans seem to play an important role as a passive vector of the virus by transmitting the disease from one rabbitry to another (54). Dissemination by airborne particles over large distances as a result of meteorological conditions is also not excluded (17). The hair from diseased rabbits has been shown to carry the virus (19).

RHDV is very stable and resistant in the environment; the viral infectivity is not reduced by treatment with ether or chloroform and trypsin, by exposure to pH 3.0, or by heating at 50°C for 1 hour. The virus survives at least 225 days in an organ suspension kept at 4°C, at least 105 days in the dried state on cloth at room temperature, and at least 2 days at 60°C, both in organ suspension and in the dried state (48). It also retains its infectivity at low temperatures, and remains quite stable during freezing and thawing. For this reason, frozen rabbit meat should be considered to be a potential source of infectivity. RHDV is inactivated by 10% sodium hydroxide and by 1.0–1.4% formaldehyde. Even 0.2–0.5% beta-propiolactone at 4°C produces the same effect. Such treatments do not alter the immunogenicity of the virus.

The clinical evolution of the disease can be peracute, acute, subacute or chronic (32). Peracute RHD usually affects highly susceptible rabbits at first introduction of the disease into a disease-free area. The acute form is prevalent in epidemic areas, whereas the subacute form usually occurs in a few animals in the later stages of an epidemic.

The clinical manifestations have been described mainly in the acute infection, as there are usually no clinical signs in the peracute form and the subacute form is characterised by similar but milder signs. The incubation period varies between 1 and 3 days; death may occur 12–36 hours after the onset of fever (>40°C). During this phase, several signs can be observed, although they are not all present in all cases. In particular, rabbits may have elevated temperature (≥41°C) and show anorexia, apathy, dullness, prostration, and congestion of the palpebral conjunctiva. Nervous signs (convulsions ataxia, paralysis, opisthotonos, paddling, groans and cries) are rarely seen, but respiratory signs (dyspnoea, frothy and bloody nasal discharge), and cyanosis of mucous membranes may be seen in the late stages of the disease (32). During an outbreak, a limited number of rabbits (5–10%) may show a chronic or subclinical evolution of the disease, which is characterised by severe and generalised jaundice, weight loss and lethargy. These animals often die 1 or 2 weeks later, probably due to a liver dysfunction. However, in meat animals, the hepatic lesions (degeneration and necrosis) in subclinical and chronic cases may be evident only during meat inspection at slaughter.

The gross pathological lesions are variable and may be subtle. Liver necrosis and splenomegaly are the primary lesions. However, a massive coagulopathy is usually the cause of sudden death and hemorrhages in a variety of organs (22). The liver has a yellowish-brown reticular pattern of peripheral lobular necrosis. Acute congestion in the lungs is the result of venous thrombosis and gives rise to acute oedema and a frothy serous or blood-tinged transudate that fills the trachea with foam and may exude from the nostrils terminally. Infarcts may occur in any organ, and the kidneys are sometimes completely infarcted and very dark brown. Petechial hemorrhages may be seen on the viscera or serosal membranes. A catarrhal enteritis of the small intestine is common but mild (22) and may be more prominent in the chronic disease. Blood may not coagulate due to the coagulopathy. In subacute and chronic disease, an icteric discoloration on the ears, conjuctiva and subcutis is clearly evident.

The microscopic hepatic lesions are quite distinctive. There is diffuse acute peripheral lobular hepatic necrosis (2). Necrosis sometimes involves nearly entire lobules. There are all stages of hepatocyte degeneration, including nuclear pyknosis and karyorrhexis. A few heterophils may be present in areas of acute necrosis. In subacute cases, a mild periportal lymphocytic infiltrate may be present. Chronic cases may also have bile or iron pigment accumulation. In acute cases, there may be microthrombi and infarction in any organ. Major venous thrombosis, rarely seen in other diseases, may be seen in the lungs and kidneys with massive congestion and oedema or, in the case of the kidney, complete infarction (22). More commonly there are microthrombi in many lung alveoli and renal glomeruli (2). Lymphoid necrosis may be seen in the spleen or lymph nodes and is associated with lymphopenia (32).

The clinical signs and the gross and microscopic lesions observed in hares affected by EBHS are very similar to those described in RHD in rabbits. The behaviour of affected hares during the disease has been observed in animals in captivity because wild hares are most often found dead due to the rapid course of the infection. Sick animals show abnormal behaviour or true neurological signs, such as loss of balance and coordination, paralysis and dullness. At necropsy, oedema and congestion of tracheal mucosa with foamy haemorrhagic contents, liver degeneration, enlargement of the spleen and generalised jaundice are the principal findings (15).

The disease in hares lasts slightly longer and causes a lower mortality rate (around 50%) than RHD in rabbits; the peak of mortality in experimentally infected hares is commonly observed between 60 and 90 hours post-infection.

1. Identification of the agent

The liver contains the highest viral titre (from 10^3 LD_{50} [50% lethal dose] to $10^{6.5}$ LD_{50}) and is the organ of choice to submit for viral identification both for RHDV and EBHSV. The amount of virus present in other parts of the body is directly proportional to vascularisation; thus spleen and serum are quite rich in virus and can serve as alternative diagnostic materials. In particular, higher levels of subviral particles could be detected in the spleen than in the liver of those animals that died from a subacute/chronic form of the disease (5). The initial treatment of the diagnostic samples is almost identical irrespective of the diagnostic method to be applied, with the exception of immunostaining techniques. An organ fragment is mechanically homogenised in 5–20% (w/v) phosphate buffered saline solution (PBS), pH 7.2, filtered through cheesecloth and clarified by centrifugation at 5000 ***g*** for 15 minutes. At this stage, the supernatant can be directly examined by HA test or ELISA. If the sample is to be observed by EM, it is advisable to perform a second centrifugation at 12,000 ***g*** for 15 minutes, before the final ultracentrifugation.

As no satisfactory growth conditions and sensitive cell substrates have been established, *in-vitro* isolation of RHDV or EBHSV cannot be included among the virological methods. Rabbit inoculation therefore remains the only way of isolating, propagating and titrating the infectivity of the virus.

Large quantities of viral antigen are prepared for diagnostic reagents and to produce inactivated tissue-derived vaccines. Experimental infection is not practical as a routine diagnostic method, although it is useful in the case of samples that give equivocal test results (e.g. HA negative/ELISA positive) or for the initial diagnosis of the disease in countries where RHD is not known to exist.

Natural hosts are the only species in which the two diseases can be reproduced. Inoculations of tissue suspensions from infected rabbits failed to produce disease in guinea-pigs, hamsters, rats, mice, chicken embryos, chinchillas, or piglets (48, 53). To perform successful experimental trials, the animals involved must be fully susceptible to the virus. Susceptibility depends on both the age of animals (which should be over 40–50 days), and the absence of specific antibodies, even at low titres. RHD can be reproduced by using filtered and antibiotic-treated liver suspension, inoculated either by the intramuscular, intravenous or oro-nasal route. When the disease is clinically evident, the signs and post-mortem lesions are similar to those described after natural infection. A rise in body temperature is registered between 18 and 24 hours post-infection, followed, in around 70–90% of cases, by death between 24 and 72 hours post-infection. A few individuals may survive until 6 days after infection. Animals that overcome the disease show only a transient hyperthermia, depression and anorexia, but present a striking seroconversion, that can be easily detected 4–6 days post-infection.

a) Haemagglutination test

HA was the first test to be used for routine laboratory diagnosis of RHD (31). It should be performed with human Group O red blood cells (RBCs), freshly collected, stored overnight in Alsever's solution, and washed in 0.85% PBS at pH 6.5 (range 6–7.2). HA is less evident or nonexistent when RBCs of other species are used. Washed RBCs are suspended at 0.75% in PBS. A twofold dilution of the clarified supernatant of a 10% tissue homogenate of liver or spleen is incubated with an equal volume of washed RBCs in a sealed round-bottom microtitre plate at, preferably, 4°C. After 1 hour (range from 20 minutes to 2 hours) of incubation, agglutination at an end-point dilution of >1/160 is considered to be positive. Lower titres should be regarded as suspicious, and should be checked using other methods. Around 10% of samples found to be positive by ELISA or EM give negative results in HA (HA false-negative). Some RHD isolates may exhibit temperature-dependant differences in haemoagglutinating characteristics (10, 18) and could show HA activity only when the test is performed at 4°C. Nevertheless, the HA false negativity is mainly detected in organs of rabbits showing a subacute/chronic form of the disease and it depends on the characteristics of the s-RHDV/CLPs particles.

Hare organs rarely give a significant titre when the same HA protocol employed for RHDV is applied. To show the presence of HA activity in EBHSV-positive organs, a modified procedure should be adopted: all steps are carried out at 4°C, the organ suspension is treated with an equal volume of chloroform, and RBCs are used at a pH not higher than 6.5 (15). Even using this method, only 50% of the samples usually give positive results. This is because the disease of hares more frequently shows a subacute/chronic character and therefore the examined virus, similarly to RHDV, has the antigenic and structural characteristics typical of the s-RHDV/CLPs particles (15).

Because of the practical difficulty of obtaining and keeping human Group O blood cells, and because of the difficulty in obtaining consistent results, this test is being superseded by the virus-detection ELISA.

b) Electron microscopy

Negative-staining EM can be performed using the so-called 'drop method'. A formvar/carbon-coated grid is placed on a drop of organ suspension (prepared as described in Section A.1.a.), and left for 5 minutes. After removing excess fluid with the edge of a torn piece of filter paper, the grid is put to float on a drop of 2% sodium phosphotungstate (NaPT), pH 6.8, for 1.5 minutes. Excess stain is removed and the grid is finally observed at ×25,000.

Due to the lower sensitivity of the drop method, it is advisable to ultracentrifuge the sample in order to concentrate the viral particles. The pellet obtained after ultracentrifugation (at least 100,000 ***g*** for 30 minutes or, alternatively, using Beckman Airfuge at 21 psi for 15 minutes) is resuspended in PBS or distilled water, put on to a grid for a few minutes, and then stained as described. RHD virions are visible as uncoated particles, 32–35 nm in diameter, presenting an inner shell (25–27 nm in diameter), delineated by a rim from which radiate ten short regularly distributed peripheral projections. s-RHDV/CLPs particles are identified by the complete loss of external portions, becoming perfectly hexagonal and smaller, with only the capsid rim visible (5, 15, 21).

For diagnostic purposes and especially when other methods give doubtful results, the best EM method is an immuno-EM technique (IEM). This method uses either a hyperimmune anti-RHDV serum, obtained from rabbit or other species, or specific MAbs, which are incubated with an equal volume of the sample for 1 hour at 37°C before ultracentrifugation. The immunological reaction induces the clumping of the viral particles into aggregates that are quickly and easily identified by EM. Immunogold methods can also be applied to better identify virions and viral proteins (28).

EM examination allows the identification of EBHSV in diagnostic samples. Valid results can be obtained when performing the IEM method using convalescent anti-EBHSV serum or specific anti-EBHS MAbs. By using heterologous antisera, it is possible to differentiate between EBHSV and RHDV.

c) Enzyme-linked immunosorbent assay

Virus detection by ELISA relies on a 'sandwich' technique and several variations of this have been described. One procedure uses the reagents, solutions, times and temperature that are used in the competitive ELISA for serology (see Section A.2.b.), except that the Tween 20 concentration is twofold (0.1% [v/v]). The microplate used should be of high adsorption capability (e.g. Nunc Maxisorp immunoplate). The liver homogenate is a 10% (w/v) solution in standard PBS; 50 µl/well is the standard volume to use in each step. The ELISA buffer used for all steps is PBS with 1% yeast extract (or bovine serum albumin [BSA]), and 0.1% Tween 20, pH 7.4. All incubation steps are for 50–60 minutes at 37°C with gentle agitation. After all steps three washes of 3–5 minutes must be performed using PBS with 0.05% Tween 20. A positive and negative RHD rabbit liver homogenate must be used as controls. The horseradish peroxidase (HRP) conjugate could be purified IgG from a specific polyclonal serum or MAbs (see Section A.2.b.).

- **Test procedure (example)**

For steps that are not specifically indicated see the procedure of the competitive ELISA for serology (Section A.2.b.)

i) Adsorb the plate with anti-RHDV hyperimmune serum and the negative RHDV serum. The latter serves as control for nonspecific reactions (false-positive samples). For each sample, 4 wells must be sensitised with the positive serum and 4 wells with the negative one.

ii) Dilute the liver extract to 1/5 and 1/30 (two replicates for each dilution) in ELISA buffer (see above), directly in the wells of the plate (e.g. add 45 µl of the buffer into all the wells of the plate, add 10 µl of the sample to the first two wells and then, after rocking, transfer 9 µl to the second wells). Treat the controls, both positive and negative, in the same way as the samples.

iii) After incubation and washing (see above), incubate with the HRP conjugate.

iv) After a last series of washing, add the chromogenic substrate. Orthophenylene-diamine (OPD) must be used as peroxidase substrate for the final development of the reaction. Use 0.15 M citrate phosphate buffer, pH 5.0, with 0.5 mg/ml OPD and 0.02% H_2O_2. The reaction is stopped after 5 minutes by addition of 50 µl of 1 M H_2SO_4.

v) Absorbance is read at 492 nm. Positive samples are those showing a difference in absorbance >0.3, between the wells coated with RHDV-positive serum and wells coated with the negative serum. Usually, at the dilution 1/30, positive samples taken from rabbits showing the classical acute form of RHD give an absorbance value >0.8, while the absorbance value of the negative sample, at the dilution 1/5, ranges from 0.1 to 0.25.

For diagnosis of EBHSV, it is possible to use this RHDV-specific sandwich ELISA, but, due to the high antigenic difference existing between the two viruses, there is a risk of obtaining false-negative results. Therefore, the adoption of an EBHSV-specific sandwich ELISA technique using either a high-titre positive anti-EBHSV hare serum, or cross-reacting RHDV MAbs (12, 15), or specific EBHSV MAbs, instead of rabbit serum, is highly recommended (15).

d) Immunostaining

Tissue fixed in 10% buffered formalin and embedded in paraffin can be immunostained using an avidin-biotin complex (ABC) peroxidase method. The sections are first deparaffinised in xylene and alcohol, counter-stained with haematoxylin for 1 minute and rinsed in tap water. They are then put in a methanol bath containing 3% H_2O_2 and washed in PBS three times for 5 minutes. To limit background interference due to nonspecific antibody binding, the samples are incubated with normal rabbit serum for 1 hour at room temperature prior to the addition of biotin. The slides are incubated overnight in a humid chamber at room temperature with biotinylated rabbit anti-RHDV serum or MAbs, washed as before and incubated again for 30 minutes at 37°C with an ABC peroxidase. The slides are washed three times. Amino-ethyl-carbazole is used as substrate. Finally, the slides are rinsed in tap water and mounted (49).

Intense nuclear staining and diffuse cytoplasmic staining of necrotic cells in the liver, mainly in the periportal areas, are characteristic and specific. Positive staining of macrophages and Kupffer's cells is also observed, as well as hepatocellular reactions. Positive reactions can also be detected in the macrophages of the lungs, spleen and lymph nodes, and in renal mesangial cells (2, 49).

Tissue cryosections fixed in methanol can be directly immunostained by incubation for 1 hour with fluorescein-conjugated rabbit anti-RHDV serum or MAbs. Specific fluorescence can be detected in the liver, spleen, and renal glomeruli.

e) Western blotting

When other tests such as HA or ELISA give doubtful results (low positivity) or the samples are suspected of containing s-RHDV/CLPs particles, western blotting analysis is useful for determining the final diagnosis.

The samples are prepared as described above (see Section A.1.), and are further treated in order to concentrate viral particles (tenfold) by ultracentrifugation (100,000 ***g*** for 90 minutes) through a 20% (w/w) sucrose cushion.

Both the supernatant and the pellet can be examined to detect, respectively, the RHDV 6S subunits (12) and the denatured VP60 structural protein of RHDV or its proteolytic fragments, which can range in size from 50 to 28 kDa. A positive and negative control sample should be used on each occasion.

Proteins could be detected with polyclonal or MAbs. If MAbs are used, they should recognise continuous epitopes. RHDV-specific MAbs recognising internal or buried epitopes could be used also to detect EBHSV. Rabbit anti-RHDV hyperimmune sera are less efficient than MAbs at recognising the same band patterns (13).

The proteins are denatured for 2 minutes at 100°C in the presence of 60 mM Tris, pH 6.8, 2% sodium dodecyl sulphate (SDS), 2% beta-mercaptoethanol, and 5% glycerol, separated on 10% SDS/PAGE (polyacrylamide gel electrophoresis), and then transferred by electroblotting to nitrocellulose filters, at 0.3 Å for 60 minutes in 25 mM Tris, pH 8.3, 192 mM glycine, and 20% (v/v) methanol. After transfer the filters are saturated overnight at 4°C with 2% bovine serum albumin (BSA), dissolved in phosphate buffer, pH 7.4, and incubated for 2 hours at room temperature with the appropriate serum diluted in phosphate buffer, pH 7.4, and 1% BSA. The filters are washed thoroughly with PBS and incubated for 1.5 hours at room temperature with anti-species alkaline phosphatase-labelled immunoglobulins at a dilution predetermined by titration. Finally, the filters are again washed and the chromogenic substrate – 5-bromo 4 chloro-3-indolylphosphate nitro blue tetrazolium – is added (25).

Positive test samples and the positive control will produce a pattern consistent with reaction to proteins of molecular weights, respectively, 60 kDa (the single structural protein of RHDV) or 41–28 kDa (the fragments of the VP60 associated with the transition from RHDV to s-RHDV/CLPs), when examining the pellet, and 60 kDa (the subunits) when examining the supernatant.

Western blot analysis can also be used to identify EBHSV. The test procedure is identical. The pattern of protein bands, detected using either an anti-EBHSV polyclonal serum or cross-reacting anti-RHDV MAbs, is similar. However, the percentage of samples showing viral degradation is higher and therefore several fragments of lower molecular weight, originating from the VP60 structural protein, are often observed.

f) Nucleic acid recognition methods

The application of the reverse-transcription polymerase chain reaction (RT-PCR) to the detection of RHDV-specific nucleic acid has recently been described (23). This method is carried out on liver specimens by using two different oligonucleotide primers, derived from the capsid region of the RHDV genome (N-terminal portion). cDNA obtained from the RT reaction is amplified as described by Baginski *et al.* (4). To reveal the PCR product, the amplified DNA reaction mixture is subjected to electrophoresis on agarose gel. If needed, specificity of the PCR product can be determined by sequencing or by transfer of the agarose gel on to a nylon filter that can be finally hybridised with a labelled internal probe, and examined by autoradiography.

A similar RT-PCR method has been used to identify the nonpathogenic RCV (11). Several primers, specific for the RHDV RNA polymerase gene and complementary to the VP60 and ORF2 genes, are used and the amplified fragments are subjected to Southern blot analysis.

RT-PCR appears to be an extremely sensitive method for the detection of RHDV, and is 10^4-fold more sensitive than ELISA (23). It is not always necessary for routine diagnosis, but is more appropriate for studies on molecular epidemiology (29, 38) and to study the early stages of RHDV infection (24).

An *in situ* hybridisation technique using either sense or antisense DNA probes has been developed for investigating the presence of RHDV in tissue samples (20). This method is highly sensitive and can be used for early diagnosis of RHD as it gives positive results as soon as 6–8 hours post-infection. However, it is expensive and difficult to carry out, and thus it is mainly indicated for research studies.

2. Serological tests

Infection by RHDV can be diagnosed through detection of a specific antibody response. As the humoral response has great importance in protecting animals from RHD, determination of the specific antibody titre after vaccination or in convalescent animals is predictive of the ability of rabbits to resist RHDV infection. It should be noted that some epidemiological data suggest the existence of an 'apathogenic' viral strain antigenically related to RHDV. In fact, the presence of so called 'naturally acquired' antibodies that confer full protection against virulent RHDV infection was shown in colonies where no previous outbreak had been reported or vaccination performed (48). The existence of the nonpathogenic RCV (13, 14) provides an explanation for the early discrepancies found in the course of serological surveys of the rabbit populations in European countries.

Three basic techniques are applied for the serological diagnosis of RHDV: haemagglutination inhibition (HI) (31), indirect ELISA and competitive ELISA (15).

Each of these methods has advantages and disadvantages. With respect to the availability of reagents and the technical complexity of carrying out the test, HI is the most convenient method, followed by the indirect ELISA and competitive ELISA, respectively. On the other hand, both ELISAs are more easily and quickly performed, particularly when a large number of samples are tested. The sensitivity and specificity of the competitive ELISA are markedly higher than those achieved with the other two methods (15).

a) Haemagglutination inhibition

Antigen: The antigen is prepared using infected rabbit liver collected freshly at death. The liver is homogenised in 10% (w/v) PBS, pH 6.4, and clarified by two consecutive low speed centrifugations (500 *g* for 20 minutes and 6000 *g* for 30 minutes). The supernatant, drawn from the tube so as to avoid the superficial lipid layer, is filtered through a 0.22 µm pore size mesh, titrated by HA, and divided into aliquots, which are stored at –70°C.

Serum samples: Before testing, sera are inactivated by incubation at 56°C for 30 minutes. The sera are then treated with 25% kaolin (serum final dilution: 1/10) at 25°C for 20 minutes and centrifuged. This is followed by another treatment, also at 25°C for 20 minutes, this time with 1/10 volume of approximately 50% packed human Group O RBCs. These are freshly collected, stored overnight in Alsever's solution and washed in 0.85% PBS, pH 6.5. The sera are clarified by centrifugation.

- **Test procedure**

i) Dispense 0.05 ml of serum into the first well of a round-bottom microtitre plate and make double dilutions into wells 2–8 using PBS with 0.05% BSA.

ii) Add 0.025 ml of RHDV antigen containing 8 HA units to each well and incubate the plate at 25°C for 30–60 minutes.

iii) Add 0.025 ml of human Group O RBCs at 2–3% concentration to each well and allow to settle at 25°C for 30–60 minutes.

iv) Titrate the antigen with each test to ensure that 8 HA/0.025 ml were used, and include positive and negative serum controls.

The serum titre is the end-point dilution showing inhibition of HA. The positive threshold of serum titres is correlated to the titre of the negative control sera; it usually is in the range 1/20–1/80.

Because of the practical difficulty of obtaining and keeping human Group O blood cells, and because of the difficulty in obtaining consistent results, this test is being superseded by the serological or antibody-detection ELISA.

b) **Competitive enzyme-linked immunosorbent assay**

Antigen: An international standard strain is not yet available; however, as only one serotype has been identified world-wide so far (indicative of the high antigenic stability of virulent RHDV), reliable results can be obtained by different laboratories each using its own standard virus. Preliminary results indicate that even the antibodies induced by the recently identified RHDV variants are recognised by the standard method described here. In addition, the test can also easily detect antibodies originating from infection of rabbits with the nonpathogenic RCV; this is because of its high genetic correlation with RHDV (13, 14).

The antigen can be prepared as described above for HI (Section A.2.a.), taking care to store it at –20°C in the presence of glycerol at 50% (v/v) to prevent freezing. If necessary, the virus can be inactivated before the addition of glycerol, using 0.1% formaldehyde at 4°C for 24 hours. Antigen must be pretitrated in ELISA and then used as the limiting reagent: i.e. the dilution that corresponds to 60–70% of the plateau height (absorbance value at 492 nm in the range 1.1–1.3).

Anti-RHDV serum: specific polyclonal sera with high anti RHDV titre can be obtained in different ways. Two possible and currently used methods are as follows:

i) Rabbits are infected with a RHDV-positive 10% liver extract diluted 1/100 in PBS to obtain convalescent sera (21–25 days) containing a high level of anti-RHDV IgG. Due to the high mortality rate associated with RHDV, it is necessary to infect at least 10–15 seronegative rabbits or to infect rabbits that are only partially protected (e.g. 4–8 rabbits infected from 3 to 7 days post-vaccination). Rabbits that survive the infection must be bled 21–25 days post-infection to obtain the convalescent sera. Alternatively, convalescent rabbits can be re-infected 3–4 months post-infection and bled 10–15 days later to obtain RHDV hyperimmune sera.

ii) RHDV is purified from the livers of experimentally infected rabbits that died from an acute form of the disease (between 28 and 40 hours post-infection), using one of the methods that has been published (12, 15, 16, 34, 39, 40). The purified RHDV can then be used to immunise sheep or goats according to classical protocols using oil adjuvants. The same procedure can also be used to inoculate rabbits, but, of course, the purified virus must be inactivated before the inoculation.

Anti-RHDV MAbs have been produced in several laboratories (12, 15, 44) and can be used instead of rabbit polyclonal sera. Purification of rabbit IgG and conjugation to HRP can be done following the standard protocol (51). The conjugated antibody is titred in a sandwich ELISA in the presence and absence of RHDV antigen (negative rabbit liver). It is then used at the highest dilution showing maximum (plateau high) absorbance (if the serum had a good anti-RHDV titre, the value of the HRP-conjugate should range from 1/1000 to 1/3000).

Control sera: Negative serum is taken from rabbits fully susceptible to RHDV infection. Positive serum is either a convalescent serum diluted 1/100 in a negative serum or a serum taken from a vaccinated animal.

- **Test procedure (example)**

i) The rabbit anti-RHDV serum diluted to a predetermined titre, e.g. 1/5000 in 0.1 M carbonate/bicarbonate buffer, pH 9.6, should be adsorbed to an ELISA microplate of high adsorption capability (e.g. Nunc Maxisorb Immunoplate) at 4°C overnight.

ii) Wash the plate three times for 3–5 minutes each time, in PBS, pH 7.4, with 0.05% Tween 80 (PBST). When the plates are not immediately used, they can be stored, closed in a plastic bag, for at least 3 months at –20°C.

iii) Distribute 0.025 ml/well PBST with 1% yeast extract (PBSTY) or 1% BSA (PBST-BSA) to all the wells needed on the plate (see below). Add 0.007 ml of the first serum sample to the first two wells (A1 and B1), 0.007 ml of the second serum to the second two wells (C1 and D1), and continue with the third

(E1 and F1) and the fourth (G1 and H1) sera, thus completing the first column. If qualitative data (positive/negative) are needed, repeat the operation in the second column with sera samples from 5 to 8, and in the third column with sera samples from 9 to 12, and so on. If the titre of the serum needs to be determined, the serum must be diluted further. Agitate the plate and then use an eight-channel micropipette to transfer 0.007 ml from the wells in column 1 to the wells in column 2. This corresponds to a four-fold dilution of the sera. This last operation can be repeated once (titre 1/160), twice (titre 1/640), or four times (titre 1/10,240). Complete each plate leaving 12 wells free for the control sera. Add 0.007 ml of positive sera to wells G6 and H6, and 0.007 ml of negative sera to wells G9 and H9, then dilute them twice (1/160).

iv) Add 0.025 ml/well antigen suspended in PBSTY to all the wells on the plate, at a dilution that is double the decided dilution, as described above in the antigen section (see the first part of this ELISA method description).

v) Incubate the plate at 37°C on a rocking platform for 50 minutes.

vi) Wash the plate as described in step ii.

vii) Add 0.05 ml/well rabbit IgG anti-RHDV conjugated with HRP at the decided dilution, as described above in the 'anti-RHDV serum' section (see the first part of this ELISA test description).

viii) Incubate the plate at 37°C on a rocking platform for 50 minutes, and wash as described in step ii, adding a fourth wash of 3 minutes duration.

ix) Use 0.05 ml/well OPD as hydrogen donor under the following conditions: 0.5 mg/ml OPD in 0.1 M phosphate/citrate buffer, pH 5, and 0.02% H_20_2. Stop the reaction after 5 minutes by addition of 0.05 ml/well 1 M H_2SO_4.

x) Read the plate on a spectrophotometer using a 492 nm filter.

The serum titre corresponds to the dilution giving an absorbance value equal to 50% (±10) of the value of the negative serum at dilution 1/160 (reference value).

The serum is considered to be negative when the absorbance value of the first dilution (1/10) decreases by less than 20% of the reference value, while it is positive when the absorbance value decreases by 30% or more. When the absorbance value of the 1/10 dilution decreases by between 20% and 30% of the reference value, the sera is considered to be doubtful. A wide range of titres will be found, depending on the origin of the sample. Positive sera range from 1/640 to 1/10,240 in convalescent rabbits, from 1/80 to 1/640 in vaccinated rabbits and from 1/10 to 1/160 in 'nonpathogenic' infection. Knowing the origin of the sample allows a choice to be made between testing one or more dilutions. Testing only the first dilution gives a positive or negative result. Testing all dilutions, up to the sixth one, will indicate the titre.

Due to the significant antigenic differences existing between RHDV and EBHSV (15, 52), the serological techniques described above, which use RHDV as antigen, are not recommended for the serological diagnosis of EBHS. However, a direct ELISA method could be employed for the detection of positive and negative EBHSV hare sera; in fact, the adsorption of RHDV on to the solid phase of an ELISA microplate exposes cross-reactive antigenic determinants. Alternatively, a specific competitive ELISA for EBHSV can be arranged in a similar way, using specific reagent (antigen and antisera) prepared as described above for RHDV.

B. REQUIREMENTS FOR VACCINES AND DIAGNOSTIC BIOLOGICALS

In all the countries where RHD is endemic, indirect control of the disease is achieved by vaccination using the same type of vaccine, prepared from clarified liver suspension of experimentally infected rabbits, and subsequently inactivated and adjuvanted. The methods of inactivation (formaldehyde, beta-propiolactone or other substances) and the adjuvants used (incomplete mineral oil or aluminium hydroxide), can vary according to the protocol used by the different manufacturers.

Several studies have been carried out recently on the expression of RHDV capsid protein in *Escherichia coli* (9), in vaccinia virus (8) and in attenuated myxoma virus (7). Moreover, it has been shown that a recombinant capsid protein VP60 expressed in the baculovirus/Sf9 cell expression system, self assembled into virus-like particles (VLPs), structurally and antigenically identical to RHD virions (27, 33, 37, 41, 46). While the fusion protein expressed in *E. coli* is highly insoluble and of low immunogenicity, active immunisation can be achieved with VLPs obtained in the baculovirus system or using recombinant vaccinia and myxoma virus, administered either intramuscularly or orally (8, 41): vaccinated rabbits have been found to be totally protected after virus challenge. Indeed, the immunogenicity of VLPs administered by the oral route as an alternative to parenteral immunisation offers an economical and practical way to administer a vaccine for mass immunisation of wild animals. However, at the present time, recombinant vaccines are not yet registered and commercially available.

The usual programme is to administer the inactivated vaccine twice with an interval of at least 2 weeks. Normally, a 1 ml dose is inoculated subcutaneously in the neck region. In those units with no history of disease, where the anamnesis for RHD is negative, it is advisable to vaccinate only the breeding stock; the first injection should be done at 2–3 months of age. Annual revaccination is strongly recommended to ensure a good level of protection, although experimental data indicate that protection usually lasts for a long time (over 1 year) (3). The vaccination of meat animals is not necessary if disease has not occurred on the farm. Following an outbreak of RHD, even if strict hygiene and sanitary measures are adopted, including cleaning and disinfection, safe disposal of carcasses and an interval before repopulation, it is strongly recommended to vaccinate meat animals at the age of 40 days, because the incidence of re-infection is very high. Only after several production cycles is it advisable to stop vaccination of meat animals. In order to verify the persistence of infective RHD inside the unit, a variable number of rabbits, starting with a small sentinel group, should not be vaccinated.

Vaccinated animals quickly produce strong immunity against RHDV infection, therefore vaccination is considered to be effective in protecting nonexposed rabbits and its primary use is in rabbitries after an outbreak of the disease has been diagnosed; once RHD has been confirmed in some sick or dead rabbits, the remaining healthy animals are immediately vaccinated.

The administration of immune serum is also effective in producing a rapid, but short-lived, protection against RHDV infection (26).

Vaccine should be stored at 2–8°C and it should not be frozen, or exposed to bright light or high temperatures.

1. Seed management

a) Characteristics of the seed

The source of seed virus for the production of inactivated tissue vaccines is infected liver homogenates obtained by serial passages in rabbits that have been inoculated with a partially purified RHD viral suspension. The latter is obtained by centrifuging the 1/5 liver suspension (w/v) in PBS at 10,000 ***g*** for 20 minutes at 4°C. The resulting supernatant is treated with 8% (v/v) polyethylene glycol – PEG 6000 – overnight at 4°C. The pellet is resuspended at a dilution of 1/10 in PBS, and subsequently centrifuged at 10,000 ***g*** for 10 minutes at 4°C. The supernatant is ultracentrifuged at 80,000 ***g*** for 2 hours at 4°C through a 20% cushion of sucrose. The pellet is resuspended in PBS (1/100 of the starting volume). This viral suspension is then characterised by negative-stain EM examination, determination of reactivity in ELISA, and capability of HA at room temperature with slow elution (HA titre against RBCs of human Group O higher than 1/1280).

Seed virus is titrated before use and should contain at least 10^5 LD_{50}. It should be stored frozen (–70°C) or freeze-dried.

b) Method of culture

At present, RHDV replication can be obtained exclusively in susceptible animals (3). The rabbits used for inoculation are selected from colonies shown to be susceptible to the disease by periodic serological testing. The animals (at least 4 months old) must be kept in strict quarantine on arrival, in a separate area and reared under satisfactory health conditions (see 'Laboratory animal facilities' in Chapter I.5). Seed virus propagation and production of vaccine batches relies on the same protocol of experimental infection, involving intramuscular injection of a dose of at least 100 LD_{50}.

c) Validation as a vaccine

The seed virus used for vaccine production must be shown to be free from other viruses, bacteria, mycoplasma and fungi. Seed virus is controlled by direct inoculation into susceptible rabbits followed by evaluation of the clinical signs in the course of the experimental infection. Suitable seed virus should cause the death of 70–80% of the rabbits within 24–72 hours post-inoculation, with the internal organ lesions characteristic of RHD. To validate the test, gross and histopathological examination of all rabbits should be performed to exclude intercurrent diseases.

2. Method of manufacture

Following inoculation of susceptible rabbits, the liver, spleen and sometimes kidney of those rabbits that die between 24 and 72 hours post-inoculation are collected. The organs are minced in 1/10 (w/v) sterile PBS, pH 7.2–7.4, and the mixture is homogenised for 10 minutes in a blender in a refrigerated environment. The mixture is then treated with 2% chloroform (18 hours at 4°C), followed by centrifugation at 6000 ***g*** for 1 hour at

4°C. The supernatant is collected by high pressure continuous pumping and is subsequently inactivated. The viral suspension is assayed by HA test and ELISA (see Section B.3.) and, once the number of HA units from the initial titration is known, more sterile PBS is added in sufficient volume to provide, after inactivation and adsorption on adjuvant, a concentration of 640–1280 HA units/dose in the commercial product (3). Various agents have proved effective at abolishing viral infectivity. The most frequently used are formaldehyde and beta-propiolactone, which can be used at different concentrations and temperatures, for variable periods of time and also in combination (3, 26). During inactivation, it is advisable to continuously agitate the fluid. Aluminium hydroxide, Freund's incomplete adjuvant or another oil emulsion is then incorporated into the vaccine as adjuvant. A preservative, thiomersal (merthiolate), is finally added at a dilution of 1/10,000 (v/v) before distribution into bottles.

3. In-process control

Antigen content: The RHD titre is determined before inactivation by calculating the HA titre, which should be higher than 1/1280, and the ELISA reactivity. Both values are again determined after inactivation and adsorption on adjuvant. Negative-staining EM confirms the identity of RHD.

Sterility: The organs are tested for the presence of viable bacteria, viruses, fungi or mycoplasma according to the protocol used for testing master seed virus. PBS solution and aluminium hydroxide gel are sterilised by autoclaving; oil emulsion is sterilised by heating at 160°C for 1 hour.

Inactivation: Before incorporation of the adjuvant, the inactivating agent and the inactivation process must be shown to inactivate the vaccine virus under the conditions of manufacture. Thus, a test is carried out on each batch of the bulk harvest as well as on the final product. Five rabbits are inoculated with a 2 ml dose of the suspension and five unvaccinated rabbits are kept as controls. After 10 days, adequate inactivation and absence of undesirable side-effects are demonstrated by the absence of clinical signs and by similar weight increments in the two groups. At the end of the trials, the animals are slaughtered and liver extracts are tested by HA, ELISA and EM.

4. Batch control

Sterility, safety and potency tests should be carried out on each batch of final vaccine; tests for duration of immunity should be carried out once using a typical batch of vaccine, and stability tests should be carried out on three batches.

a) Sterility

Each batch of vaccine must be tested for the presence of viable bacteria, viruses, fungi or mycoplasma according to the same protocol recommended for testing master seed virus.

b) Safety

Ten rabbits should be inoculated by the recommended routes with three times the vaccinal dose. The rabbits are observed for 3 weeks. No abnormal local or systemic reaction should develop.

c) Potency

Ten seronegative adult rabbits that are at least 4 months old are vaccinated with one full dose of vaccine given by the recommended route. Two other groups of five animals each are vaccinated with 1/4 and 1/16 of the full dose, respectively. A fourth group of ten unvaccinated rabbits is maintained as controls. All animals are challenged at 4 weeks post-vaccination by intramuscular inoculation of a dose of RHDV containing at least 100 LD_{50} or presenting a HA titre higher than 1/2560. No vaccinated rabbits should show signs of infection, while the mortality rate among control animals should be higher than 70%. The antibody response of each vaccinated animal is then determined with reference to titrated standard antisera; the mean antibody level should not be significantly less than the level recorded in the protection test performed using as vaccine the inactivated seed virus.

d) Duration of immunity

The data reported in the literature (3) indicate a long-term duration of immunity induced by a single vaccination (up to 15 months). However, it is advisable to carry out the following test: 20 rabbits vaccinated once are divided into four groups and are serologically tested at monthly intervals over a period of 1 year. Each group is inoculated with virulent RHDV at either 3, 6, 9 months or 1 year post-vaccination (see Section B.4.c.). Challenge infection should produce increasing seroconversion, which is directly related to the time that has elapsed since vaccination. The absence of clinical signs and of mortality proves that the RHDV has not multiplied.

e) **Stability**

Evidence should be provided to show that the vaccine passes the batch potency test at 3 months beyond the suggested shelf life.

f) **Preservatives**

A suitable preservative is normally required for vaccine in multidose containers (see Section B.2.). Its persistence throughout shelf life should be checked.

g) **Precautions (hazards)**

When oil-emulsion vaccines are prepared, vaccinators should be warned against the risk and consequences of accidental self-injection, which must be treated urgently as a 'grease-gun' injury.

5. Tests on the final product

The tests for safety, potency and sterility of the final product must be performed after bottling and packaging. Thus, it is important that these two last manufacturing steps be performed following standardised good manufacturing procedures. The tests are conducted by removing samples from a statistically determined number of randomly taken multidose containers (20 or 100 doses) of vaccine.

a) **Safety**

See Section B.4.b.

b) **Potency**

See Section B.4.c.

c) **Sterility**

See Section B.4.a.

REFERENCES

1. ALLEGRANZA G., VANZETTI T., LAVAZZA A., CAPUCCI L. & SCICLUNA M.T. (1990). Malattia emorragica virale del coniglio: indagine epidemiologica nel Canton Ticino, Svizzera. *Sel. Vet.*, **31**, 847–858.

2. ALONSO C., OVIEDO J.M., MARTIN-ALONSO J.M., DIAZ E., BOGA J.A. & PARRA F. (1998). Programmed cell death in the pathogenesis of rabbit haemorrhagic disease. *Arch. Virol.*, **143**, 321–332

3. ARGUELLO VILLARES J.L. (1991). Viral haemorrhagic disease of rabbits: vaccination and immune response. *Rev. sci. tech. Off. int. Epiz.*, **10**, 471–480.

4. BACINSKI I., CHEMIN I., BOUFFARD P., HANTZ O. & TREPO C. (1991). Detection of polyadenilated RNA in hepatitis B virus infected peripheral blood mononuclear cells by polymerase chain reaction. *J. Infect. Dis.*, **161**, 996–1000.

5. BARBIERI I., LAVAZZA A., BROCCHI E., KONIG M. & CAPUCCI L. (1997). Morphological, structural and antigenic modifications of rabbit haemorrhagic disease virus in the course of the disease. Proceedings of the 1st Symposium on Calicivirus of the European Society of Veterinary Virology (ESVV), Reading, UK, 15–17 September 1996, 182–193.

6. BERNINGER M.L. & HOUSE C. (1995). Serologic comparison of four isolates of rabbit hemorrhagic disease virus. *Vet. Microbiol.*, **47**, 157–165.

7. BERTAGNOLI S., GELFI J., LE GALL G., BOILLETOT E., VATHEROT J.F., RASSCHAERT D, LAURENT S., PETIT F., BOUCRAT-BARALON C. & MILON A. (1996). Protection against myxomatosis and rabbit viral haemorrhagic

disease with recombinant myxoma viruses expressing rabbit hemorrhagic disease virus capsid protein. *J. Virol.*, **70**, 5061–5066.

8. BERTAGNOLI S., GELFI J., PETIT F., VATHEROT J.F., RASSCHAERT D., LAURENT S., LE GALL G., BOILLETOT E., CHANTAL J. & BOUCRAT-BARALON C. (1996). Protection of rabbits against rabbit viral haemorrhagic disease with a vaccinia-RHDV recombinant virus. *Vaccine*, **14**, 506–510.

9. BOGA J.A., CASAIS R., MARIN M.S., MARTIN-ALONSO J.M., CARMENES R.S., PRIETO M. & PARRA F. (1994). Molecular cloning, sequencing and expression in *Escherichia coli* of the capsid protein gene from rabbit haemorrhagic disease virus (Spanish isolate AST/89). *J. Gen. Virol.*, **75**, 2409–2413.

10. CAPUCCI L., CHASEY D., LAVAZZA A. & WESTCOTT D. (1996). Preliminary characterisation of a non-haemagglutinating strain of rabbit haemorrhagic disease virus from the United Kingdom. *J. Vet. Med. [B]*, **43**, 245–250.

11. CAPUCCI L., FALLACARA F., GRAZIOLI S., LAVAZZA A., PACCIARINI M.L., BROCCHI E. (1998). A further step in the evolution of rabbit hemorrhagic disease virus: the appearance of the first consistent antigenic variant. *Virus Res.*, **58**, 115–126.

12. CAPUCCI L., FRIGOLI G., RONSHOLT L., LAVAZZA A., BROCCHI E. & ROSSI C. (1995). Antigenicity of the rabbit hemorrhagic disease virus studied by its reactivity with monoclonal antibodies. *Virus Res.*, **37**, 221–238.

13. CAPUCCI L., FUSI P., LAVAZZA A., PACCIARINI M.L. & ROSSI C. (1996). Detection and preliminary characterization of a new rabbit calicivirus related to rabbit hemorrhagic disease virus but nonpathogenic. *J. Virol.*, **70**, 8614–8623.

14. CAPUCCI L., NARDIN A. & LAVAZZA A. (1997). Seroconversion in an industrial unit of rabbits infected with a non-pathogenic rabbit haemorrhagic disease-like virus. *Vet. Rec.*, **140**, 647–650.

15. CAPUCCI L., SCICLUNA M.T. & LAVAZZA A. (1991). Diagnosis of viral haemorrhagic disease of rabbits and European brown hare syndrome. *Rev. sci. tech. Off. int. Epiz.*, **10**, 347–370.

16. CAPUCCI L., SCICLUNA M.T., LAVAZZA A. & BROCCHI E. (1990). Purificazione e caratterizzazione dell'agente eziologico della malattia emorragica virale del coniglio. *Sel. Vet.*, **31**, 301–312.

17. CHASEY D. (1994). Possible origin of rabbit haemorrhagic disease in the United Kingdom. *Vet. Rec.*, **15**, 496–499.

18. CHASEY D., LUCAS M.H., WESTCOTT D.C., SHARP G., KITCHING A. & HUGHES S.K. (1995). Development of a diagnostic approach to the identification of rabbit haemorrhagic disease. *Vet. Rec.*, **137**, 158–160.

19. CHEN K.Y. (1986). Rabbit Plague. *Infect. Dis. Dom. Anim.*, **3**, 53–55.

20. GELMETTI D., GRIECO V., ROSSI C., CAPUCCI L. & LAVAZZA A. (1998). Detection of rabbit haemorrhagic disease virus (RHDV) by in situ hybridization with a digoxigenin labelled RNA-probe. *J. Virol. Methods*, **72**, 219–226.

21. GRANZOW H., WEILAND F., STREBELOW H.-G., LIU C.M. & SCHIRRMEIER H. (1996). Rabbit hemorrhagic disease virus (RHDV): ultrastructure and biochemical studies of typical and core-like particles present in liver homogenates. *Virus Res.*, **41**, 163–172.

22. GREGG D.A., HOUSE C., MEYER R. & BERNINGER M. (1991). Viral haemorrhagic disease of rabbits in Mexico: epidemiology and viral characterization. *Rev. sci. tech. Off. int. Epiz.*, **10**, 435–451.

23. GUITTRE C., BAGINSKI I., LE GALL G., PRAVE M., TREPO C. & COVA L. (1995). Detection of rabbit haemorrhagic disease virus isolates and sequence comparison of the N-terminus of the capsid protein gene by the polymerase chain reaction. *Res. Vet. Sci.*, **58**, 128–132.

24. GUITTRE C. RUVOUEN-CLOUET N., BARRAUD L., CHEREL Y., BAGINSKI I., PRAVE M., GANIERE J.P., TREPO C. & COVA L. (1995). Early stages of rabbit haemorrhagic disease virus infection monitored by the polymerase chain reaction. *J. Vet. Med. [B]*, **43**, 109–118.

25. HARLOW E. & LANE D. (1988). Antibodies: a Laboratory Manual. Cold Spring Harbor Laboratory Press. Cold Spring Harbor. New York, USA

26. HUANG H. (1991). Vaccination against and immune response to viral haemorrhagic disease of rabbits: a review of research in the People's Republic of China. *Rev. sci. tech. Off. int. Epiz.*, **10**, 481–498.

27. LAURENT S., VAUTHEROT J.F., MADELAINE M.F., LE GALL G. & RASSCHAERT D. (1994). Recombinant rabbit haemorrhagic disease virus capsid protein expressed in baculovirus self-assembles into virus like particles and induces protection. *J. Virol.*, **68**, 6794–6798.

28. LAVAZZA A. & CAPUCCI L. (1993). Detection of haemorrhagic disease virus by using an immuunogold-labelling electron microscopy method. Proceedings of a Multinational Congress on Electron Microscopy, Parma, Italy, 455–456.

29. LE GALL G., HUGUET S., VENDE P., VAUTHEROT J. & RASSCHAERT D. (1996). European brown hare syndrome virus: molecular cloning and sequencing of the genome. *J. Gen. Virol.*, **77**, 1693–1697.

30. LEIGHTON F.A., ARTOIS M, CAPUCCI L., GAVIER-WIDEN D. & MORISSE J.P. (1995). Antibody response to rabbit viral haemorrhagic disease virus in red foxes *(Vulpes vulpes)* consuming livers of infected rabbits *(Oryctolagus cuniculus)*. *J. Wildl. Dis.*, **31**, 541–544.

31. LIU S.J., XUE H.P., PU B.Q. & QUIAN N.H. (1984). A new viral disease in rabbits. *Anim. Hus. Vet. Med.*, **16**, 253–255.

32. MARCATO P.S., BENAZZI C., VECCHI G., GALEOTTI M., DELLA SALDA L., SARLI G. & LUCIDI P. (1991). Clinical and pathological features of viral haemorrhagic disease of rabbits and the European brown hare syndrome. *Rev. sci. tech. Off. int. Epiz.*, **10**, 371–392.

33. MARIN M.S., ALONSO J.M.M., GARCIA L.I.P.O., BOGA J.A., ARGUELLO-VILLARES J.L., CASAIS R., VENUGOPAL K., JIANG W., GOULD E.A. & PARRA F. (1995). Immunogenic properties of rabbit haemorrhagic disease virus structural protein VP60 expressed by a recombinant baculovirus: an efficient vaccine. *Virus Res.*, **39**, 119–128.

34. MEYERS G., WIRBLICH C. & THIEL H.J. (1991). Rabbit haemorrhagic disease virus – molecular cloning and nucleotide sequencing of a calicivirus genome. *Virology*, **184**, 664–676.

35. MEYERS G., WIRBLICH C. & THIEL H.J. (1991). Genomic and subgenomic RNAs of rabbit haemorrhagic disease virus are both protein-linked and packaged into particles. *Virology*, **184**, 677–686.

36. MILTON I.D., VLASAK R., NOWOTNY N., RODAK L. & CARTER M.J. (1992). Genomic 3' terminal sequence comparison of three isolates of rabbit haemorrhagic disease virus. *FEMS Microbiol. Lett.*, **93**, 37–42.

37. NAGESHA H.S., WANG L.F., HYATT A.D., MORRISSY C.I., LENGHAUS C. & WESTBURY H.A. (1995). Self-assembly, antigenicity, and immunogenicity of the rabbit haemorrhagic disease virus (Czechoslovakian strain V-351) capsid protein expressed in baculovirus. *Arch. Virol.*, **140**, 1095–1108.

38. NOWOTNY N., ROS BASCUNANA C., BALLAGI-PORDANY A., GAVIER-WIDEN D., UHLEN M. & BELAK S. (1997). Phylogenetic analysis of rabbit haemorrhagic disease and European brown hare syndrome viruses by comparison of sequences from the capsid protein gene. *Arch. Virol.*, **142**, 657–673.

39. OHLINGER R.F., HAAS B., MEYERS G., WEILAND F. & THIEL H.J (1990). Identification and characterization of the virus causing rabbit haemorrhagic disease. *J. Virol.*, **64**, 3331–3336.

40. PARRA F. & PRIETO M. (1990). Purification and characterization of a calicivirus as the causative agent of lethal hemorrhagic disease in rabbits. *J. Virol.*, **64**, 4013–4015.

41. PLANA DURAN J., BASTONS M., RODRIGUEZ M.J., CLIMENT I., CORTES E., VELA C. & CASAL I. (1996). Oral immunization of rabbits with VP60 particles confers protection against rabbit hemorrhagic disease. *Arch. Virol.*, **141**, 1423–1436.

42. PRASAD B.V.V., ROTHNAGEL R., JIANG X. & ESTES M.K. (1994). Three-dimesional structure of baculovirus-expressed Norwalk virus capsids. *J. Virol.*, **68**, 5117–5125.

43. RASSCHAERT D., HUGUET S., MADELAINE M.F. & VAUTHEROT I.F. (1994). Sequence and genomic organization of a rabbit hemorrhagic disease virus isolated from a wild rabbit. *Virus Genes*, **9**, 121–132.

44. RODAK L., GRANATOVA M., VALICEK L., SMID B., VESELY T. & NEVORANKOVA Z. (1990). Monoclonal antibodies to rabbit haemorrhagic disease virus and their use in the diagnosis of infection. *J. Gen. Virol.*, **71**, 2593–2598.

45. SCHIRRMAIER H., REIMANN I., KOLLNER B. & GRANZOW H. (1999). Pathogenic, antigenic and molecular properties of rabbit haemorrhagic disease virus (RHDV) isolated from vaccinated rabbits: detection and characterization of antigenic variants. *Arch. Virol.*, **144**, 719–735.

46. SIBILIA M., BONIOTTI M.B., ANGOSCINI P., CAPUCCI L. & ROSSI C. (1995). Two independent pathways of expression lead to self-assembly of the rabbit hemorrhagic disease virus capsid protein. *J. Virol.*, **69**, 5812–5815.

47. SIMON M.C., MUGURUZA R., ALONSO I.L., MUZQUIZ I.L., GIRONES O. & HAFFAR A. (1994). Recherche du virus de la maladie hémorragique virale du lapin (RHD) chez le renard et role des canides domestiques dans la transmission de la maladie. *Rec. Med. Vet.*, **170**, 841–845.

48. SMID B., VALICEK L., RODAK L., STEPANEK J. & JURAK E. (1991). Rabbit haemorrhagic disease: an investigation of some properties of the virus and evaluation of an inactivated vaccine. *Vet. Microbiol.*, **26**, 77–85.

49. STOERCKLE-BERGER N., KELLER-BERGER B., ACKERMANN M. & EHRENSPERGER F. (1992). Immunohistological diagnosis of rabbit haemorrhagic disease (RHD). *J. Vet. Med. [B]*, **39**, 237–245.

50. THOUVENIN E., LAURENT S., MADELAINE M.F., RASSCHAERT D., VAUTHEROT J.F. & HEWAT E.A. (1997) Bivalent binding of a neutralising antibody to a calicivirus involves the tortional flexibility of the antibody hinge. *J. Mol. Biol.*, **270**, 238–246.

51. TIJSSEN P. (1985). Practice and Theory of Enzyme Immunoassays. *In:* Laboratory Techniques and Molecular Biology, Vol. 15. Elsevier, Amsterdam, The Netherlands.

52. WIRBLICH C., MEYERS G., OHLINGER V.F., CAPUCCI L., ESKENS U., HAAS B. & H.-J. THIEL (1994). European Brown Hare Syndrome virus: relationship to Rabbit Hemorrhagic Disease virus and other caliciviruses. *J. Virol.*, **68**, 5164–5173.

53. XU Z.J. & CHEN W.X. (1989). Viral haemorrhagic disease in rabbits: a review. *Vet. Res. Commun.*, **13**, 205–212.

54. XU Z.J., CHEN W.X., CHEN J.X. & YU J.Y. (1985). Studies on control and prevention of a new rabbit disease. *Zhejiang J. Anim. Husb. Vet. Med.*, **10**, 12–13.

*

* *

SECTION 2.9.

BEE DISEASES IN LIST B

INTRODUCTORY NOTE ON BEE DISEASES

Bees are insects that are closely related to ants and wasps. There are many thousands of species of bee, most of which are not social insects, living solitary lives. The honey bee, Apis *species, lives as a colony, which is a family of social insects. There are many species, subspecies, races and subraces of honey bees that are adapted to their environment.*

Two species are important for bee keeping – the western honey bee Apis mellifera, *and the eastern honey bee* A. cerana. *The Africanised bee, which is found in South and Central America and some states of the United States of America, is a cross between two subspecies of the western honey bee, the European bees and the Central African bee.* Apis cerana *is important in South and South-East Asia. The colonies are small and docile, but the honey yields are low. In a suitable climate, the western honey bee,* A. mellifera, *is sometimes preferred for its greater honey production.*

It is thought that all bees are susceptible to the known diseases of bees, but different races may have varying susceptibility. For example, A. cerana *is less susceptible to varroosis. When sampling a colony of bees for diagnosis of diseases, live bees must first be killed with diethyl ether or in a deep freezer (–20°C) overnight. Larval and pupal smears must be made when testing for brood diseases or a piece of comb containing brood showing visible signs of disease may be sent to the laboratory.*

*

* *

CHAPTER 2.9.1.

ACARIOSIS OF BEES

SUMMARY

Acariosis or acarine disease is a disease of the adult honey bee Apis mellifera *L. and other* Apis *species. It is caused by the Tarsonemid mite, known as the tracheal mite,* Acarapis woodi *(Rennie). The mite is approximately 150 µm in size, and is an internal parasite of the respiratory system, living and reproducing mainly in the large prothoracic trachea of the bee. Sometimes they are also found in the head, thoracic and abdominal air sacs. The mites feed on the haemolymph of their host.*

The pathogenic effects found in infected bees depend on the number of parasites within the trachea and are attributable both to mechanical injuries and to physiological disorders consequent to the obstruction of the air ducts, lesions in the tracheal walls, and the depletion of haemolymph. As the parasite population increases, the tracheal walls, normally white and translucent, become opaque and discoloured with blotchy black areas, probably due to melanin crusts.

The mortality rate may range from moderate to high. Early manifestations of infection normally go unnoticed, and only when infection is heavy does it become apparent. This is generally in the early spring. The infection spreads by direct contact. Generally, only newly hatched bees under 10 days old are susceptible. Reproduction occurs within the tracheae of adult bees, where female mites may lay 8–20 eggs, with 2–4 times as many females as males. Development takes 11–12 days for males and 14–15 days for females.

Identification of the agent: *The parasites are demonstrated only by laboratory methods and under the microscope. The mites need to be observed inside the tracheae or removed from them to be observed microscopically. Several techniques are available for demonstrating the mites, such as dissection, grinding and staining.*

The thoraces of suspect bees are dissected to expose the trachea. Each trachea is examined under a dissecting microscope (×18–20), where the mites will be seen through the transparent wall as small oval bodies.

Alternatively, larger samples of suspect bees can be ground or homogenised in water, followed by coarse filtration of the suspension, and centrifugation. The deposit is treated with undiluted lactic acid for 10 minutes. This is then mounted for microscopic examination.

The parasites may be stained by histological techniques so that they can be observed within the bee trachea. The tracheae are separated out, cleared with 8% potassium hydroxide, and stained with 1% methylene blue. This is the best method for large numbers of samples.

Serological tests: *Serological tests are not available.*

Requirements for vaccines and diagnostic biologicals: *There are no biological products available. Menthol crystals or oil patties made with vegetable oil (not animal fat) and white granulated sugar will keep mite levels under control.*

A. DIAGNOSTIC TECHNIQUES

Acariosis is a disease of the adult honey bee *Apis mellifera* L. and other *Apis* species, caused by the microscopic Tarsonemid mite *Acarapis woodi* (Rennie). The mite is approximately 150 µm in size, and it is an internal parasite of the respiratory system (Figure 1). These tracheal mites enter, live, and reproduce mainly in the large prothoracic tracheae of all bees, feeding on the haemolymph of their host. Sometimes they are also found in the head, thoracic and abdominal air sacs (5).

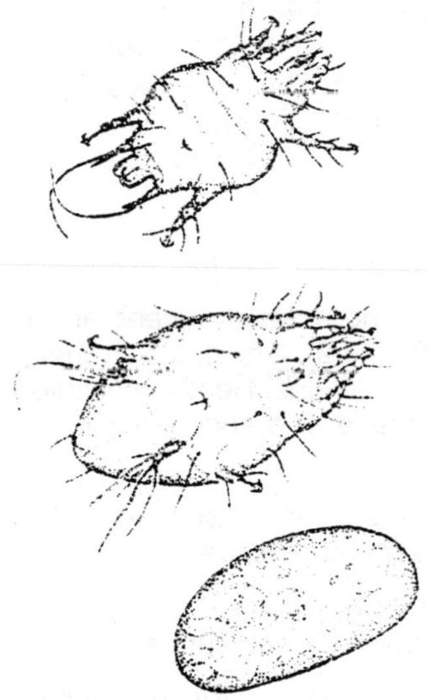

Fig. 1. Acarapis woodi *Rennie. Top: Adult male, Centre: Adult Female, Bottom: Egg.*

The pathogenic effects on individual bees depend on the numbers of parasites within the tracheae, and are attributable both to mechanical injuries and to physiological disorders consequent to the obstruction of the air ducts, lesions in the tracheal walls, and to the depletion of haemolymph. As the parasite population increases, the tracheal walls, which are normally whitish and translucent, become opaque and discoloured with blotchy black areas, probably due to melanin crusts (4).

The mortality rate may range from moderate to high. Early signs of infection normally go unnoticed, except for a slow dwindling in the colony size. Only when infection is heavy does it become apparent. This is generally in the early spring after the winter clustering period when the mites have bred and multiplied undisturbed into the longer-living winter bees.

Infection spreads from one bee to another by direct contact. Generally, only newly hatched bees under 10 days old, are susceptible. Attempts to rear *A. woodi* on artificial and synthetic diets have been unsuccessful, while culturing them on immature stages of the honey bee itself has been only partially successful (6). The life span of the mites in dead bees is approximately 1 week. Reproduction occurs within the tracheae of adult bees, where female mites may lay 8–20 eggs. There are 2–4 times as many females as males; development takes 11–12 days for males and 14–15 days for females.

There are no reliable clinical signs for the diagnosis of acariosis as the signs of infection are not specific and the bees behave in much the same way as do bees affected by other diseases or disorders. They crawl around in the front of the hive and climb blades of grass, unable to fly. Dysentery may be present.

1. Identification of the agent

Acariosis can be detected only in the laboratory using microscopic examination or an enzyme-linked immunosorbent assay (ELISA). There is no reliable method for detection of very low levels of infection. The number of bees sampled determines the detection threshold of the method. It has been shown that a 2% rate of infection can be detected by sampling 50 bees, while a 1% rate of infection is detected using 100 bees (confidence limit is 80% for a colony of average size in spring). Because of the high level of manual work involved, it is suitable to examine 50 bees. Sequential sampling data are given in ref. 15. The best time to take bee samples is in the early spring or late autumn (Northern hemisphere), when *Acarapis* populations are high. Visualisation of mites is easier in older bees that have more mites. Samples of queens, drones or workers can be used, but *Acarapis* prefer drones.

a) **Dissection (7)**

A sample of 50 bees is collected at random from the suspected colony. These are mainly bees crawling and unable to fly, found within about 3 metres of the front of the hive. This is preferable to random collection from within the colony. The bees may be living, dying, or dead. Live bees must first be killed with ethyl alcohol or in a deep freezer (–20°C); bees must not have been dead for over 2–3 days unless kept at 4°C for up to 4 weeks or –20°C for up to 2 months. They may be preserved indefinitely in a preservative such as Oudemann solution: glacial acetic acid (80 ml); glycerol (50 ml); 70% ethanol (870 ml).

- **Test procedure**

i) Lay and secure bees on their backs or hold with thumb and first finger..

ii) Remove the heads and forelegs using a small forceps and remove the collar surrounding the neck opening to expose the tracheae (Figure 2). Check the tracheae nearest to the spiracle (as mites enter through the spiracle) to see light infestations. Heavy infestations are easily visible as shadows or dark objects in clear to dark brown tracheae. Old and heavy infestations will make the tracheae brown to black.

iii) Cut through the thorax in front of the middle pair of legs and the base of the forewings. These thin disks can be further treated to clear muscle tissue.

iv) Macerate either by gentle heating in an 8% solution of potassium hydroxide for approximately 20 minutes or by leaving to stand overnight without heating.

v) Examine the first pair of tracheae – which are covered by muscle tissue – under a dissecting microscope at a magnification of ×18–20, or transfer the tracheae to another slide, add glycerin or water and observe at higher magnification.

vi) Mites are easily seen through the transparent wall as small, oval bodies.

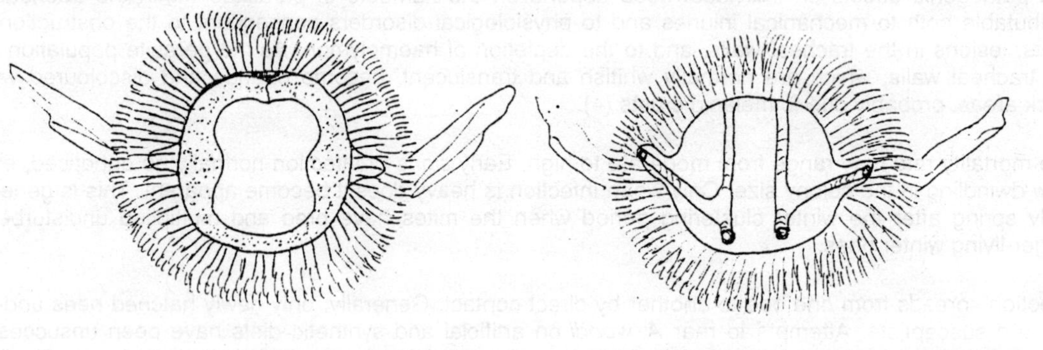

Fig. 2. Left: front view of bee thorax with head removed and collar intact.
Right: Collar removed and tracheae exposed to spiracle openings.

This is the simplest and most reliable technique for the laboratory diagnosis of acariosis, allowing the detection of early infections and enabling the infection rate to be established. Even light infections can be detected by the use of a dissecting microscope with this technique. Only in very exceptional instances will it be necessary to employ higher magnifications in order to make a diagnosis. However, this is a demanding technique, especially when a large number of acariosis diagnoses have to be made. If it is necessary only to distinguish between heavily infected and lightly or non-infected colonies, dissection can be stopped at step ii and the colour of the tracheae observed.

b) **Grinding (3)**

A sample of about 200 bees is collected at random from the suspect colony. The wings and legs of each bee are removed from the thorax, and the bodies are pooled in a 100 ml container that has been one-quarter filled with water. This suspension is homogenised three times, each time for several seconds, in a homogeniser at 10,000 rpm with the addition of more water. The resulting suspension is strained through a sieve (mesh 0.8 mm) and rinsed with water to a final volume of approximately 50 ml. The filtrate is centrifuged at 1500 ***g*** for 5 minutes and the supernatant fluid is discarded. A few drops of undiluted lactic acid solution are added to the debris of the deposit, which will contain the mites. This is left for 10 minutes to allow the muscle fibres to dissolve, and is then mounted under a cover-slip for microscopic examination. This technique is quicker than dissection, but may be less accurate. External mites *A. externus, A. vagans* and *A. dorsalis,* all of which are morphologically similar to *A. woodi,* are often found on the thorax of healthy bees and can very easily be mistaken for *A. woodi* (Table 1). It seems, however, that they do not cause any serious threat to bees or beekeeping. This method should therefore only be chosen if all that is required is a rough estimation of the degree of infection in a region. It is not suitable for determining a first outbreak.

Table 1. *Differential diagnosis of* Acarapis *species (13)*

Character	*A. dorsalis*	*A. externus*	*A. woodi*
Notch of the coxal plate	Deep	Short	Flat
Space between stigmata	16.7 µm	16.8 µm	13.9 µm
Length of tarsal limb (IV leg pair)	7.6 µm	11.4 µm	7.5 µm

c) **Staining (9)**

Both pathogen and trachea can be stained specifically, rendering them easily visible by microscopy.

- **Test procedure**

i) Make a transverse cut through the membranous areas behind the forelegs.

ii) Remove the head and forelegs.

iii) Make a second transverse cut in front of the middle pair of legs at the base of the forewings.

iv) To clear the sections (1–1.5 mm thick), place them in an 8% solution of potassium hydroxide.

v) Stir gently and heat near to boiling point for approximately 10 minutes until the soft internal tissues are dissolved and cleared, leaving the chitinous tissues intact.

vi) Retrieve sections by filtration and wash with tap water.

vii) Stain and mount the sections.

viii) Examine for mites by low-power microscopy.

Permanent mounts are prepared by the usual histological techniques.

Cationic stains are the most suitable and specific as they stain the mites intensely but the tracheae only weakly. A solution of 1% aqueous methylene blue is the most suitable, prepared by dissolving the methylene blue first and then adding sodium chloride to make a 0.85% NaCl solution.

- **Test procedure**

i) Stain in 1% aqueous methylene blue.

ii) Differentiate sections in distilled water for 2–5 minutes.

iii) Rinse the sections in 70% alcohol.

When kept in 95% ethanol, the mites will retain the stain for 6 hours (1). It is essential with this technique to macerate the tissues effectively in the potassium hydroxide solution. Using this method, it is possible to process a large number of samples rapidly and conveniently.

d) **Enzyme-linked immunosorbent assay**

An ELISA for trachea mites has been developed (8, 11, 12). This test may produce false-positive results, and is therefore only recommended for survey examinations. Another method is the visualisation of guanine, a nitrogenous waste product of mites (10).

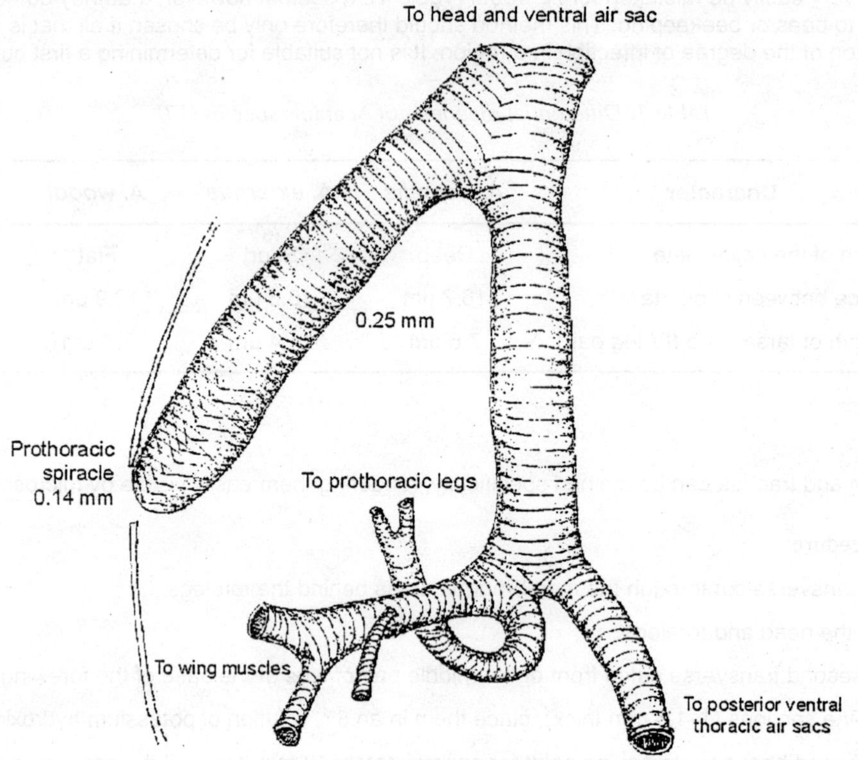

Fig. 3. *Main thoracic tracheae of honey bee where* Acarapis *is commonly found; light infestations are near the spiracle opening.*

B. REQUIREMENTS FOR VACCINES AND DIAGNOSTIC BIOLOGICALS

There are no biological products available. Menthol crystals (50 g for a two story colony) control mites if left in the colony for 28 days, providing the ambient temperature is at least 18°C. The optimum temperature range for the vapours to work is 27–29°C. Small cakes made with vegetable shortening (e.g. margarine, not animal fat) and white granulated sugar will keep mite levels to 10%. The cake (about 100 g in weight) should be placed on the top bars of the frames in the broodnest (14).

Some races of bees, such as Buckfast bees (2) and some hygienic strains, are less susceptible to attack by *Acarapsis.*

- **Acknowledgements**

Illustrations by Diana Sammataro and are reproduced with her permission.

Parts of this chapter were taken from or based on the chapter on acariosis of bees in previous editions of the *Manual.*

REFERENCES

1. BANCROFT J.D. & STEVENS A. (1982). Theory and Practice of Histological Techniques. Churchill Livingstone, Edinburgh, UK.

2. BROTHER A. (1968). 'Isle of Wight' or acarine disease: its historical and practical aspects. *Bee World*, **49**, 6–18.

3. COLIN M.A., FAUCON J.P., GIANFERT A. & SARRAZIN C. (1979). A new technique for the diagnosis of Acarine infestation in honey bees. *J. Apic. Res.*, **18**, 222–224.

4. GIORDANI G. (1964). Recherches au laboratoire sur *Acarapis woodi* (Rennie), agent de l'acariose des abeilles (*Apis mellifera* L.). Note 3. *Bull. Apic.*, **7**, 43–60.

5. GIORDANI G. (1965). Recherches au laboratoire sur *Acarapis woodi* (Rennie), agent de l'acariose des abeilles (*Apis mellifera* L.). Note 4. *Bull. Apic.*, **8**, 159–176.

6. GIORDANI G. (1970). Ricerche di laboratorio su *Acarapis woodi* (Rennie), agente dell'acarosi delle api mellifiche (*Apis mellifera* L.) Nota 6. *Ann. Acc. Naz. Agric.*, **90**, 69–76.

7. GIORDANI G. (1974). Méthodes de diagnostic des maladies des abeilles adultes. Diagnostic de l'acariose. *Bull. Apic.*, **17**.

8. GRANT G., NELSON D., OLSEN P. & RICE W.A. (1993). The ELISA detection of tracheal mites in whole honey bee samples. *Am. Bee J.*, **133**, 652–655.

9. PENG Y. & NASR M.E. (1985). Detection of honey bee tracheal mites *(Acarapis woodi)* by simple staining techniques. *J. Invertebr. Pathol.*, **46**, 325–331.

10. MOZES-KOCH R. & GERSON U. (1997). Guanine visualization, a new method for diagnosing tracheal mite infestation of honey bees. *Apidologie*, **28**, 3–9.

11. RAGSDALE D. & FURGALA B. (1987). A serological approach to the detection of *Acarapis woodi* parasitism in honey bees using an enzyme-linked immunosorbent assay. *Apidologie*, **18**, 1–10.

12. RAGSDALE D. & KJER K.M. (1989). Diagnosis of tracheal mite *(Acarapis woodi* Rennie*)* parasitism of honey bees using a monoclonal based enzyme-linked immunosorbent assay. *Am. Bee J.*, **129**, 550–553.

13. RITTER W. (1996). Diagnostik und Bekämpfung der Bienenkrankheiten (Diagnosis and control of bee diseases). Gustav Fischer Verlag, Jena, Stuttgart, Germany.

14. SAMMATARO D. & NEEDHAM G.R. (1996). Host-seeking behaviour of tracheal mites (Acari: Tarsonemidae) on honey bees (Hymenoptera: Apidae). *Exp. Appl. Acarol.*, **20**, 121–136.

15. TOMASKO M., FINLEY J., HARKNESS W. & RAJOTTE E. (1993). A sequential sampling scheme for detecting the presence of tracheal mite *(Acarapis woodi)* infestations in honey bee *(Apis mellifera* L.*)* colonies. *Penn. State Agric. Exp. Stn Bull.*, 871.

*

* *

CHAPTER 2.9.2.

AMERICAN FOULBROOD

SUMMARY

American foulbrood affects the larval stage of the honey bee Apis mellifera *and other* Apis *spp., and occurs throughout the world.* Paenibacillus larvae[1] *(White), the causative organism, is a bacterium that can produce over one billion spores in each infected larva. The spores are extremely resistant to heat and chemical agents, and only the spores are capable of inducing the disease.*

Identification of the agent: *Combs of infected colonies have a mottled appearance due to a mixture of healthy capped brood, uncapped cells containing the remains of diseased larvae, and empty cells. This is not characteristic only of American foulbrood. Cell cappings of a diseased larva appear moist and darkened, becoming concave and possibly punctured as infection progresses. The larval or pupal colour changes to creamy brown and then to a dark brown with a ropy appearance when drawn out. A very unpleasant odour develops in the advanced stage. The diseased brood eventually dries out to form characteristic brittle scales that adhere tightly to the lower sides of the cell. The formation of a pupal tongue is one of the most characteristic signs of the disease and precedes the formation of the scales.*

American foulbrood can usually be diagnosed in the field, but laboratory tests are available for its confirmation. Most cases are diagnosed by light microscopy. A simple stain, such as Gram, is used for diagnosis. This differentiates the bacteria by their morphology. The modified hanging drop technique will differentiate American foulbrood from other brood diseases; this technique and the characteristic morphology of the spores permit almost immediate diagnosis.

Immunofluorescence may be used, but it should be noted that cross-reactions with Bacillus alvei *can occur.* Paenibacillus larvae *can be distinguished biochemically from other spore-forming bacilli because it reduces nitrate to nitrite and is negative for catalase production; these characteristics and the bacterium's growth requirements will give a positive identification.*

Paenibacillus larvae *spores can be recovered from honey by centrifugation or by dialysis. Spores similar to those of* P. larvae *have also been recovered from contaminated beeswax.*

Serological tests: *There are no serological tests available.*

Requirements for vaccines and diagnostic biologicals: *There are no biological products available.*

A. DIAGNOSTIC TECHNIQUES

American foulbrood is a disease of the larval stage of the honey bee *Apis mellifera* and other *Apis* spp., and occurs throughout the world where such bees are kept. *Paenibacillus larvae*[1] (White), the causative organism, is a bacterium that can produce over one billion spores in each infected larva. The bacterium is a slender rod with slightly rounded ends and a tendency to grow in chains. It varies greatly in size from 2.5 to 5.0 µm long and 0.5 µm wide (Figure 1). The spores are oval, approximately twice as long as they are wide, and about 0.6 × 1.3 µm. They are extremely heat stable and resistant to chemical agents. Only spores are capable of inducing the disease.

1 *Paenibacillus larvae* is now known as *Paenibacillus larvae* subsp. *larvae*, as distinct from *P. larvae* subsp. *pulvifaciens*. Heyndrickx M. *et al.* (1996). *Int. J. Syst. Bacteriol.*, **46**, 270–279.

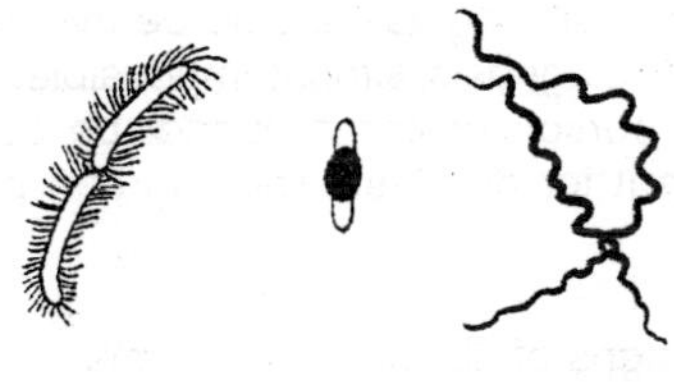

Fig. 1. Diagram of Paenibacillus larvae *subsp.* larvae: *(a) Vegetative cells (2.5–5 × 0.7–0.8 µm) with flagella specially stained. (b) Sporulating* P. larvae *subsp.* larvae. *(c) Flagella bundles also called giant whips, sometimes used for diagnosis. (These features require a microscope with oil immersion objectives to be seen. All drawings are approximately proportional.)*

The infection can be transmitted to a larva from nurse bees or by spores remaining at the base of a brood cell. Although the larval stages of worker bees, drones and queen are susceptible to infection, under natural conditions infected queen and drone larvae are rarely seen. The susceptibility of larvae to American foulbrood disease decreases with increasing age (13); larvae cannot be infected later than 53 hours after the egg has hatched. The mean infective dose (ID_{50}) needed to initiate infection is about 35 spores in 1-day-old bee larvae, though very variable (2). Exchanging combs containing the remains of diseased larvae is the most common means of spreading the disease from colony to colony. In addition, feeding or robbing of spore-laden honey, artificial swarms and the introduction of queens from infected colonies can also spread the disease. The early detection of American foulbrood helps to prevent further spread.

1. Identification of the agent

A healthy larva has a glistening, pearly white appearance. It first develops at the base of the cell in the shape of the letter 'C' and subsequently grows upright to fill the cell. Infected larvae die in this erect position.

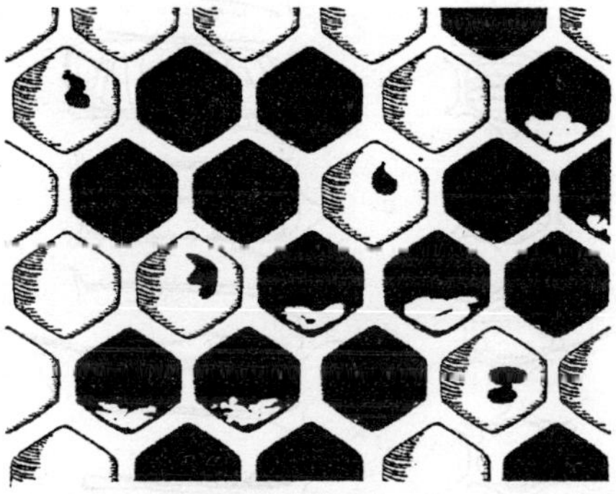

Fig. 2. External appearance of affected comb: cappings with moist and sunken appearance, some punctured with larval remains.

In severely infected colonies, the combs appear to be mottled due to a pattern of healthy capped brood, uncapped cells containing the remains of diseased larvae, and empty cells. The capping of a cell that contains a diseased larva appears moist and darkened and becomes concave and punctured as the infection progresses (Figure 2). Also, the larva or pupa changes colour, first to a creamy and eventually to a dark brown. The larvae become glutinous in consistency and can be drawn out as threads when a probe is inserted into the larval remains and removed from the cell. A very unpleasant foul odour develops at this stage, resembling that of animal glue. Finally, after 1 month or more, the remains of the diseased brood dry out to form typical hard, dark scales that are brittle and adhere strongly to the lower sides of the cell (Figure 3). If death occurs in the pupal stage, the formation of the pupal tongue, a protrusion from the pupal head that traverses the top of the brood cell, is one of the most characteristic signs of the disease. The tongue may persist also on the dried scale.

In most cases, American foulbrood can be diagnosed in the field by visual inspection. When diagnosis requires confirmation, several laboratory tests are available.

a) Sample preparation

The correct diagnosis of any bee disease depends on the sample submitted. The sample of comb should be about 9 cm^2 and contain as much of the dead or discoloured brood as possible. Little or no honey should be present in the sample. The sample can be loosely wrapped in paper, and wrappings such as plastic bags, aluminium foil, waxed paper, tin or glass should be avoided as these materials allow samples to become mouldy, making an accurate diagnosis almost impossible. The sample can be dispatched in a heavy cardboard or wooden box. If a portion of comb cannot be sent, the probe used to examine cell contents may have enough material on it for any test. This too can be wrapped in paper and sent to the laboratory in a paper envelope.

The sample is then checked for typical signs of disease. Sometimes, the larval remains are difficult to locate because of the condition of the comb. Scale material can be conveniently located by using ultra-violet or near ultra-violet light. Exposure between 3100 and 4000 Å will cause any scale material to fluoresce. Some discretion must be used when using this technique as both honey and pollen will also fluoresce.

b) Microscopy

In most cases, American foulbrood disease can be diagnosed by observing *P. larvae* by light microscopy. The modified hanging drop technique (9) can be used to differentiate between American foulbrood and other brood diseases. Suspect material is mixed with water, and a drop of this suspension is placed on a cover-slip, dried and fixed by heat, and stained with carbol fuchsin or a suitable spore stain for 30 seconds. Any excess stain is washed off with water. While the preparation is still wet, the cover-slip is inverted on to a slide on which there is a very thin layer of immersion oil. Excess water will emerge. The slide is gently blotted dry and examined by high-power microscopy. By examining fields where pockets of water have formed in the oil, the spores of *P. larvae* will be seen exhibiting Brownian movement. This is a valuable diagnostic technique as the spores formed by other members of the genus *Paenibacillus* associated with known bee diseases remain fixed. This, taken together with the characteristic morphology of the spores, permits a diagnosis. If the infection is under 10 days old, long vegetative forms of the bacterium are present and some newly formed spores may be seen (9).

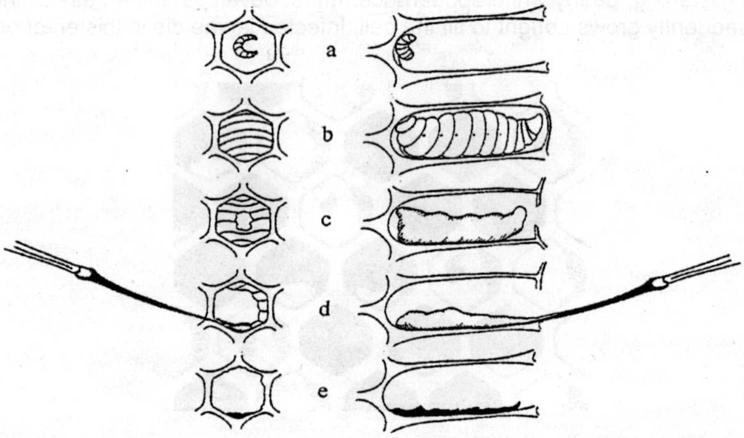

Fig. 3. Progression of the disease: (a) Point of infection. (b) Larval development to the prepupal stage. (c) Cell contents reduce and capping is drawn inwards or is punctured. (d) Cell contents become glutinous. (e) Residual scale tightly adherent to bottom of cell.

In some laboratories, a simple stain, such as Gram, is used for diagnosis. This relies solely on differentiating the bacterium by its morphology. A further refinement is the fluorescent antibody technique.

c) Fluorescent antibody technique

This technique is preferable and requires the preparation of specific antibodies labelled with a fluorescent dye. Rabbits are injected with pure cultures of *P. larvae* and the antiserum is conjugated with a fluorochrome dye. The resulting fluorescent antibody is reacted with a bacterial smear on a slide. Any excess antiserum is washed off and the smear is examined by fluorescence microscopy. *Paenibacillus larvae* stains specifically as brightly fluorescing bacteria on a dark background (10, 12, 14), but cross-reactions with *P. alvei* can occur.

d) The Holst milk test

The Holst Milk test (5) uses the fact that a high level of proteolytic enzymes is produced by sporulating *P. larvae*. The test is performed by suspending a suspect scale, or a smear of a diseased larva, in a tube containing 1–4 ml of 1% powdered skim milk in water. The tube is then incubated at 37°C. If *P. larvae* is present, the suspension will clear in 10–20 minutes.

e) Culture techniques

Absolute identification and further biochemical tests require that *P. larvae* be grown in the laboratory. The bacterium requires complex media for growth, such as Difco brain–heart infusion (BHI) medium that has been fortified with thiamin hydrochloride (0.2 mg/litre). Other media used contain yeast extract, soluble starch, glucose and potassium phosphate buffer, pH 6.6 (1), and yet another medium uses sheep blood agar (6). The medium can be liquid, semisolidified by the addition of 0.3% agar, or solidified with 2% agar.

To culture *P. larvae*, spore suspensions are prepared by mixing diseased material in 9 ml of sterile water in test tubes. The suspension is heated at 80°C for 10 minutes to kill nonsporulating bacteria. A sterile cotton swab is used to transfer a portion of the suspension on to the surface of Petri dishes containing solid BHI agar, which are then incubated for 2–3 days at 35–37°C. Individual colonies are small and opaque. If the inoculum contains large numbers of spores, a solid layer of growth will cover the plate. Difficulties can occur when the spore suspensions contain other spore-forming bacteria, which may completely overgrow the culture.

f) Nitrate reduction

Paenibacillus larvae almost invariably reduces nitrate to nitrite (8). It can be grown on a medium such as BHI containing potassium nitrate (1–2 mg/litre of medium). When growth has occurred, the addition of a drop of sulphanilic acid-alpha-naphthyl reagent produces a red colour if any nitrate has been reduced to nitrite. This test should be used for confirmation and should not be employed alone.

g) Catalase

A drop of 3% hydrogen peroxide is placed on an actively growing culture on solid medium. Most aerobic bacteria break down the peroxide to water and oxygen, producing a bubbly foam, but *P. larvae* is almost always negative for this reaction (4).

h) Detection of spores in honey

Occasionally, it may be necessary to examine honey for the presence of *P. larvae*. The classical method (Sturtevant, 1932) is to dilute the honey with water and centrifuge at high speed to deposit the spores. The following method has been developed to detect *P. larvae* spores in honey (11). Samples of honey to be examined for spores are heated to 45°C and shaken to distribute any spores that may be present. Honey (25 ml) from each sample is diluted with 25 ml of water to permit easier handling. The diluted honey is transferred into 44 mm width dialysis tubing that has been tied at one end. The open end is tied after filling. The tubes are submerged in running water for 18 hours or in a water bath with 3–4 water changes over the same time period. After dialysis, the contents are centrifuged at 2000 ***g*** for 15 minutes. The supernatant liquid is discarded and the deposit is resuspended in 9 ml of water. The suspension is heated at 80°C for 10 minutes to kill nonspore-forming bacteria and plated on to BHI as previously described.

Another method is direct streaking of diluted honey on to an agar plate. One part of honey is diluted with two parts of buffer and then centrifuged. The sediment is dissolved in 0.5 ml of water, heat shocked at 80°C for 15 minutes and streaked on a sheep blood agar plate supplemented with 3 µg/ml nalidixic acid to inhibit the growth of *P. alvei* (6).

Spores similar to *P. larvae* have also been recovered from contaminated beeswax by chloroform extraction (7) and from pollen by filtration of a suspension through filter paper (3).

2. Serological tests

No serological tests are available.

B. REQUIREMENTS FOR VACCINES AND DIAGNOSTIC BIOLOGICALS

No vaccines or diagnostic biological products are available.

• **Acknowledgement**

Illustrations by Karl Weiss, extracted from Bienen-Pathologie, 1984. Reproduced with the kind permission of the author and Ehrenwirth-Verlag, Munich (Germany).

REFERENCES

1. BAILEY L. & LEE D.C. (1962). *Bacillus larvae:* Its cultivation *in vitro* and its growth *in vivo. J. Gen. Microbiol.*, **29**, 711-717.

2. BUCHER G.E. (1958). General summary and review of utilisation of disease to control insects. *Proceedings of the Tenth International Congress of Entomology*, **4**, 695–701.

3. GOCHNAUER T.A. & CORNER J. (1987). Detection and identification of *Bacillus larvae* in a commercial pollen sample. *J. Apic. Res.*, 13, 264–267.

4. HAYNES W.C. (1972). The catalase test. An aid in the identification of *Bacillus larvae. Am. Bee J.*, **112**, 130–131.

5. HOLST E.C. (1946). A single field test for American foulbrood. *Am. Bee J.*, **86**, 14–34.

6. HORNITZKY M.A.Z. (1993). Honey bee diseases. *In:* Australian Standard Diagnostic Techniques for Animal Diseases. Commonwealth Scientific and Industrial Research Organization (CSIRO) Information Services, Victoria, Australia, 3–7 (pages in each chapter numbered individually).

7. KOSTECKI R. (1969). Studies on improvement of control of American foulbrood of the honey bee (in Polish). *Pszczelnicze Zeszyty Naulcowe*, **13**, 97-135.

8. LOCHHEAD A.G. (1937). The nitrate reduction test and its significance in the detection of *Bacillus larvae. Can. J. Res.*, **C15**, 79–86.

9. MICHAEL A.S. (1957). Droplet method for observation of living unstained bacteria. *J. Bacteriol.*, **74**, 831-832.

10. OTTE E. (1973). A contribution of the laboratory diagnosis of American foulbrood of the honey bee with a particular reference to the immunofluorescence method. *Apidologie*, **4**, 331–339.

11. SHIMANUKI H. & KNOX D.A. (1988). Improved method for the detection of *Bacillus larvae* spores in honey. *Am. Bee J.*, **128**, 353–354.

12. TOSHKOV A., VALARIANOV T. & TOMOV A. (1970). The immunofluorescence method and the quick and specific diagnosis of American foulbrood of beebrood (in German). *Bull. Apic.*, **13**, 13–18.

13. WOODROW A.W. (1941). Susceptibility of honey bee larvae to American foulbrood. Gl. *Bee Cult.*, **69**, 148–151.

14. ZHAVNENKO V.M. (1971). Indirect method of immunofluorescence in the diagnosis of foulbrood (American and European) (in Russian). *Veterinariia*, **8**, 109–111.

*
* *

CHAPTER 2.9.3.

EUROPEAN FOULBROOD

SUMMARY

The causal organism of European foulbrood of honey bees is the bacterium Melissococcus pluton. *The identification of its presence by the observation of signs of disease in the field is unreliable. The most usual and obvious sign is the death of larvae shortly before they are due to be sealed in their cells, but this may be for reasons other than European foulbrood. Most infected colonies display few visible signs, which themselves often quickly abate spontaneously before the end of each active season. Infection remains enzootic within individual colonies because of mechanical contamination of the honeycombs by the durable organism. Recurrences of disease can therefore be expected in subsequent years.*

Identification of the agent: *Examination, by high-power microscopy, of suitable preparations of larval remains for the presence of numerous lanceolate cocci is adequate for most practical purposes, especially when it is done by experienced individuals.*

The only certain means of making a diagnosis is by isolating and identifying the causative organism. This can be differentiated quite readily from all other bacteria associated with bees by its fastidious cultural requirements.

The isolated bacterium can be identified and differentiated by means of simple tube agglutination tests.

Serological tests: *No tests for detecting antibodies in bees are available.*

Requirements for vaccines and diagnostic biologicals: *There are no biological products available.*

A. DIAGNOSTIC TECHNIQUES

Bee larvae usually die of European foulbrood 1–2 days before being sealed in their cells, or sometimes shortly afterwards, and always before transformation to pupae. The disease is caused by *Melissococcus pluton* and occurs mostly during the period when colonies are growing quickly. Most sick larvae become displaced from their coiled position in the bottom of their cells before they die. Many are quickly detected and removed by nurse bees, leaving empty cells scattered randomly among the remaining brood.

Infected larvae that escape detection by adult bees and then die, first become flaccid and turn a light yellow colour that becomes increasingly brown, and at the same time they dissolve into a semiliquid mass. They then become dry and form a dark brown scale that can easily be removed from the cells. Severely affected brood may have a very stale or sour odour, sometimes acidic, like vinegar, but often there is no smell.

Signs of disease usually disappear spontaneously from infected colonies before the end of the active season, but are likely to return in subsequent years (3, 8).

1. Identification of the agent

a) Microscopy

Freshly dead larvae are best for diagnosis. Before any decomposition occurs, diseased larvae can be smeared on a microscope slide or pulled apart by pinching the cuticle about the centre of the body with two pairs of forceps, which are then pulled apart. The mid-gut contents are left exposed on the slide, still within the gelatinous, transparent peritrophic membrane. This is partially or almost completely filled with bacteria, which are easily seen as opaque chalk-white clumps. The contents of the mid-guts of healthy larvae, which are less easily dissected, have a golden-brown colour. Apparently healthy larvae may contain a mixture of bacteria and pollen. The mid-guts of healthy larvae that contain much light-coloured pollen may resemble those that are filled with bacteria.

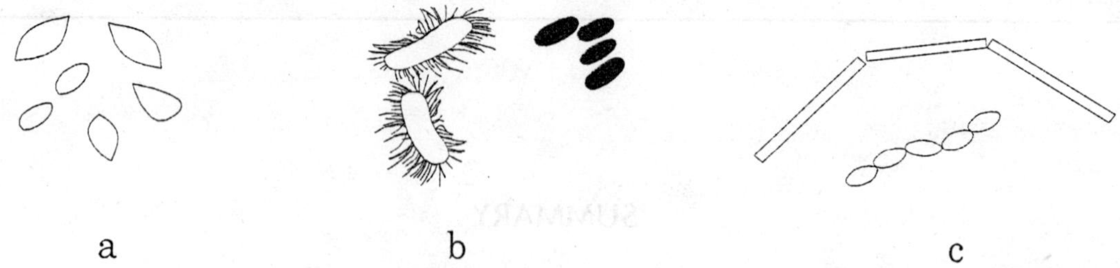

Fig. 1. Bacteria associated with European foulbrood.
(a) Melissococcus pluton*: The cause of European foulbrood. Occurs singly, in longitudinal chains or in clusters. Morphologically resembles* Enterococcus faecalis*, a common secondary invader.*
(b) Paenibacillus alvei*: Vegetative rods 2.0–7.0 × 0.8–1.2 µm with flagella; sporulating with spores lying adjacently. Both rods and spores are larger than those of* Paenibacillus larvae *(see American foulbrood).*
(c) Bacterium eurydice*: Slender, square-ended rods* in vivo *but can form chains of cocci* in vitro *in certain media.*

For a bacteriological investigation, a loopful of a dilute aqueous suspension of the mid-gut contents is transferred to a clean microscope slide and mixed with a loopful of 5% aqueous nigrosin. This is spread over one or two square centimetres, dried gently over a flame, and examined directly by high-power microscopy. The presence of numerous lanceolate cocci, about 0.5 × 1.0 µm in size, occurring either singly or in clusters, and arranged end to end in pairs or short chains, is almost certainly diagnostic of European foulbrood. Some very slender square-ended rod-like bacteria are also usually present (Figure 1). The cocci are Gram positive and the rods are Gram negative. Similar preparations made from aqueous suspensions of whole dead or decomposing larvae are likely to present a confusing array of bacteria in which *M. pluton* will be difficult to distinguish.

b) Culture methods

Melissococcus pluton (type strain NCDO 2443) is the most abundant bacterium during the early stages of an infection (4, 5). *Melissococcus pluton* can be cultivated on a medium (expressed in g/litre or ml/litre) comprising: yeast extract or certain peptones, 10 (4); cysteine or cystine, 0.2–2.0; glucose or fructose, 10; soluble starch, 10; 1 M KH_2PO_4, 100 at pH 6.6; and agar, 2. The medium is preferably autoclaved in 100 ml lots in screw-capped bottles at 116°C for 20 minutes and poured into Petri plates immediately before use. These plates are streaked with dilute aqueous suspensions of diseased larvae, or ideally, of diseased larval mid-guts. The latter can be prepared beforehand by allowing them to dry on a slide, which may then be kept, for years if necessary, at 4°C or –20°C.

This treatment also eliminates most secondary organisms after a few weeks without affecting the viability of *M. pluton*. This organism is isolated most efficiently by inoculating decimal dilutions of the aqueous suspension into agar that has been maintained molten at 45°C and which is then poured into plates. The plates must be incubated anaerobically, such as in McIntosh and Fildes jars in an atmosphere of approximately 5–10% carbon dioxide (CO_2) at 35°C. Small white opaque colonies of *M. pluton* usually appear within 4 days. This bacterium is somewhat pleomorphic *in vitro*, often appearing in rod-like forms. The final pH of the medium may reach 5.5. Decreasingly fastidious strains become selected *in vitro*. Simplified or modified forms of the medium then support multiplication, especially of a serologically distinct *M. pluton* group from Brazil (1) that will multiply on chemically defined media (2). CO_2 remains essential. Inoculated slopes should be sealed when bacterial growth is apparent and may then be kept at 4°C for up to 6 months. Alternatively, the cultures can be suspended in a medium of 10% sucrose, 5% yeast extract and 0.1 M KH_2PO_4, pH 6.6, and then lyophilised.

A number of other bacteria are often associated with and may be confused with *M. pluton*. *Bacterium eurydice* inhabits the alimentary tract of adult bees and occurs commonly in the gut of healthy larvae in small numbers. It is more numerous in larvae infected with *M. pluton*. The incidence of *B. eurydice* in healthy bees is very low in winter and early spring, but it increases in summer. It forms thin square-ended rods, which can grow either singly or in chains. When grown in certain media, it sometimes resembles streptococci and has been confused with *M. pluton*. However, its cultural characteristics closely resemble those of *Corynebacterium pyogenes* (7), and it multiplies poorly in the form of thin rods, under the conditions necessary for the cultivation of *M. pluton*.

Enterococcus (= Streptococcus) faecalis closely resembles *M. pluton* morphologically and has often been confused with it, although they are both culturally and serologically distinct. Unlike *M. pluton,* it does not remain viable for long when dried, or persist as mechanical contamination within bee colonies. It is probably brought into the hive by foraging adult bees, and is responsible for the sour smell sometimes encountered with European foulbrood.

Enterococcus faecalis grows well *in vitro* under the conditions suitable for *M. pluton,* but it may be readily differentiated by its ability to grow aerobically. It forms small transparent colonies within 24 hours and is a facultative anaerobe. It multiplies on a variety of the more common media with or without carbohydrates or CO_2. The final pH in the presence of glucose is 4.0. *Enterococcus faecalis* rarely exceeds the number of *M. pluton* in bee larvae, and can usually be diluted out. When it is not diluted out it produces sufficient acid to prevent the *in-vitro* multiplication of *M. pluton.*

Enterococcus faecalis does not multiply in bee larvae in the absence of *M. pluton,* so its presence in large numbers can be taken as presumptive evidence of European foulbrood.

Paenibacillus (= Bacillus) alvei is generally more common than *E. faecalis* in bee colonies affected with European foulbrood, but it is not invariably associated with the disease and so cannot act as a reliable indicator of it. In bee colonies, it multiplies only in the decomposing remains of larvae, and then its spores often predominate over all other bacteria, even to their apparent exclusion. *Paenibacillus alvei* forms very resistant spores and becomes well established in bee colonies with enzootic European foulbrood. It causes a characteristic stale odour. *Paenibacillus alvei* multiplies poorly under the conditions necessary for the *in-vitro* growth of *M. pluton.* It produces a spreading growth of transparent colonies, some of which are motile and move in arcs over the surface of the agar. Cultures have the characteristic stale odour that is associated with European foulbrood when the bacillus is present. Spores are formed rapidly.

c) Tube agglutination test

For the identification of *M. pluton*, antisera can be prepared in rabbits against washed cultures of *M. pluton* either by intravenous injections (6) or by a single intramuscular injection of 1 ml of antigen suspension mixed with an equal volume of Freund's incomplete adjuvant.

Assays are made by agglutination tests in tubes containing suspensions of bacteria equivalent to 0.25 mg dry weight/ml. End-points are noted after tubes have been incubated for 4 hours at 37°C.

2. Serological tests

No tests for detecting antibodies in bees are available.

B. REQUIREMENTS FOR VACCINES AND DIAGNOSTIC BIOLOGICALS

There are no biological products available.

• Acknowledgment

Illustrations by Karl Weiss, extracted from Bienen-Pathologie, 1984. Reproduced with the kind permission of the author and Ehrenwirth-Verlag, Munich (Germany).

REFERENCES

1. ALLEN M.F. & BALL B.V. (1993). The cultural characteristics and serological relationships of isolates of *Melissococcus pluton. J. Apic. Res.*, **32**, 80–88.

2. BAILEY L. (1984). A strain of *Melissococcus pluton* cultivable on chemically defined media. *FEMS Microbiol. Lett.*, **25**, 139–141.

3. BAILEY L. & BALL B.V. (1991). Honey Bee Pathology. Academic Press, London, UK, and New York, USA.

4. BAILEY L. & COLLINS M.D. (1982). Taxonomic studies on *Streptococcus pluton. J. Appl. Bacteriol.*, **53**, 209–213.

5. Bailey L. & Collins M.D. (1982). Reclassification of *Streptococcus pluton* (White) in a new genus *Melissococcus*, as *Melissococcus pluton* nom. rev.; Comb. nov. *J. Appl. Bacteriol.*, **53**, 215–217.

6. Bailey L. & Gibbs A.J. (1962). Cultural characters of *Streptococcus pluton* and its differentiation from associated enterococci. *J. Gen. Microbiol.*, **28**, 385–391.

7. Jones D. (1975). A numerical taxonomic study of Coryneform and related bacteria. *J. Gen. Microbiol.*, **87**, 52–96.

8. Ministry of Agriculture, Fisheries and Food (MAFF). (1996). Foul Brood Disease of Honey Bees: Recognition and Control. P.B. 3053, HMSO London, UK.

*

* *

CHAPTER 2.9.4.

NOSEMOSIS OF BEES

SUMMARY

The microsporidium Nosema apis *(Zander) is a parasite of the honey bee that invades the epithelial cells of the ventriculus. Infections are acquired by the uptake of spores during feeding or grooming. The disease occurs throughout the world and testing of bees can help in preventing the spread of infection to unaffected bee colonies.*

The parasite invades the posterior region of the ventriculus, giving rise to large numbers of spores within a short period of time. The parasite is ubiquitous and occurs in greatest numbers in the spring when there is an increase in the brood. Spores can persist for up to 2 years in faecal droppings and up to 1 year in honey and in bee carcasses. They are inactivated by acetic acid or by heating to 60°C for 15 minutes.

***Identification of the agent:** In the acute form, brown faecal marks are seen on the comb, with sick or dead bees in the vicinity of the hive. During winter, there may be an increase in the mortality rate. In milder cases, there may be no special signs, only poor colonies with large quantities of brood and few adult bees. In affected bees, the ventriculus, which is normally brown, is white and very fragile. Microscopic examinations of homogenates of the abdominal contents of affected bees will reveal the oval spores of* Nosema, *which are approximately 5–7 × 3–4 µm with a dark edge. Their internal contents cannot be distinguished. Staining is usually not necessary.*

The appearance of Nosema *spores can be confused with yeast cells, fungal spores, fat and calciferous bodies or cysts of* Malpighamoeba mellificae. *The latter are similar in size to* Nosema *spores, being 6–7 µm in diameter, but are completely spherical instead of oval.*

Positive identifications can be made only by observation of typical spores in the ventriculus or faeces. Very mild infections may not be demonstrable. The extent of infection is determined by counting the spores on a microscope grid and calculating the average number of spores per area.

***Serological tests:** There are no applicable serological tests.*

***Requirements for vaccines and diagnostic biologicals:** There are no biological products available.*

A. DIAGNOSTIC TECHNIQUES

The microsporidium *Nosema apis* (Zander) is a protozoan parasite exclusive to the epithelial cells of the ventriculus of adult bees. Infection occurs by the ingestion of the spores in the feed or after the grooming of the body hairs of the bee (2, 4, 6).

The polar tube of the spore is everted and penetrates the peritrophal membrane of the intestine, particularly in the posterior region of the ventriculus. The sporoplasm passes down the tube and enters the cytoplasm of the epithelial cells, where it reproduces. Autoinfections can occur at the same time as new infections. After a short interval, spores develop in large quantities. Infected bees are unable to fly and have been shown to be infected with up to 500 million spores.

The parasite is ubiquitous and multiplies at a specific rate throughout the year, with maximum numbers occurring during spring, coinciding with the increase in the brood (6, 8). In winter, spores are rarely to be found, or are only found in heavily infected bees. The development stages necessary for hibernation are difficult to find microscopically because of their very small size.

Any inherent natural defence by a bee colony against a heavy infection with the parasite depends on the colony size as well as on the prevailing weather conditions during the early part of the autumn of the previous year (7). If these conditions are unfavourable, the overall life expectancy of the colony is reduced. This may lead to the premature death of bees during winter or early spring. In a typical case of a colony being depleted because of a *Nosema* infection, the queen can be observed surrounded by a few bees, confusedly attending to brood that is already sealed.

The spores have a variable viability. In faecal droppings, spores may persist for up to 2 years, and in honey or in the carcasses of dead bees, they may be viable for 1 year. Mostly, the comb is infected. Spores may be killed by heating to a temperature of at least 60°C for 15 minutes. Fumes from a solution of at least 60% acetic acid will inactivate any spores within a few hours, depending on the concentration; higher concentrations are even more effective and will kill spores within a few minutes. Such procedures come under the jurisdiction of national control authorities with protocols that vary from country to country. Disinfection can be carried out, for example, by putting acetic acid solution into bowls or on to sponges that can soak up the liquid. Following disinfection after an outbreak, all combs should be well ventilated for at least 14 days prior to use.

1. Identification of the agent

In acute forms of infection, especially in early spring, brown faecal marks will be noted on the comb (1). At the entrance of the hive, both sick and dead bees will be seen, and during winter there will be an increased mortality rate in the colony. In milder infections, there may be no special signs except for colonies of weak appearance with large numbers of brood, but only a few adult bees.

To diagnose a *Nosema* infection, the posterior pair of abdominal segments are removed with a forceps to reveal the ventriculus, complete with the malpighian tubules, the small intestine and rectum. The ventriculus is normally brown but, following a *Nosema* infection, becomes white and very fragile. However, this appearance is given by other causes of intestinal disturbance, for example, feeding on indigestible food stores, such as syrup containing actively growing yeast. For a reliable diagnosis, a number of bees in a sample should be examined.

a) Microscopy

It is necessary to attempt to distinguish between a *Nosema* infection and that of *Malpighamoeba mellificae* (5). There is quite often an indication of dysentery in a *Nosema* infection. In an *M. mellificae* infection, there may be a diarrhoea, often of a sulphur-yellow colour and with a distinct odour. Characteristics of *Amoeba* cysts are described later. Secondary mixed infections may occur (6). A simple, nonquantitative method for detecting *Nosema* infection is as follows: A sample of about 20 dead bees is collected from a suspect colony. The abdomens are separated and ground up in 2–3 ml of water. Three drops of the suspension are placed on a slide under a cover-slip and examined microscopically at ×400 magnification. This is a slight simplification of Cantwell's original method (3). The spores are about 5–7 µm long and 3–4 µm wide. They are completely oval with a dark edge. Their contents, consisting of nucleus, sporoplasm and polar tube, cannot be seen. Dyes are usually not necessary.

Nosema spores must be differentiated from yeast cells, fungal spores, fat and calciferous bodies, and from *M. mellificae* cysts, which are spherical and approximately 6–7 µm in diameter.

In order to obtain accurate, reliable and meaningful quantification of levels of *Nosema* infections in honey bees, a standardised procedure must be used. A suitable protocol is as follows:

A sample of older worker honey bees is taken, from which the abdomens of ten individuals are macerated in 5 ml of water using a mortar and pestle. When tissue pieces have become quite fine, the suspension is filtered through two layers of muslin (thin loosely woven cotton fabric) in a funnel leading to a graduated centrifuge tube. A second 5 ml of water is used to rinse the pestle, swirl around the inside of the mortar and pour through the subsample in the funnel. Water levels are equalised in the tubes and the suspensions are centrifuged for six minutes at 800 *g*. The supernatants are decanted and the tubes are refilled to the 10 ml level. Using disposable pipettes and a rubber bulb, the pellets are resuspended by repeated uptake and forcible ejection through the pipette tips. When the solution appears to be homogenous, a sample is taken to fill the calibrated volume under the cover-slip of a haemocytometer (blood cell counting chamber). After a few minutes the spores will have settled to the bottom of the chamber. *Nosema* spores appear transparent but with a very distinct dark edge and are 5–7 µm long and 3–4 µm wide. They are best seen using a magnification of ×400. The number of spores in each square is counted. Where a spore lies over the edge of a square, count only those spores that straddle the left and upper edges of the square, not the right and bottom edges. One *Nosema* spore, observed in the area that covers the entire etched grid (4000 small squares), is equal to an average of 4 million spores per bee. If no spores are seen, the result should be designated 'not detected', but that does not mean that the bees are not infected. Regulatory agencies will decide on the level of infection useful for their purposes.

A laboratory method for the simultaneous detection of *Nosema* spores and *M. mellificae* cysts consists of the individual examination of the colonies using 30–60 bees per colony. A suspension of the abdomens of dead bees is prepared by grinding with 5–10 ml water; the volume of water depending on the number and condition of the bees. The suspension must be filtered to remove debris that would interfere with the examination, first through a 100 µm and then a 40 µm filter. Parts of the malpighian tubules pass through the 100 µm filter, but are collected on the 40 µm filter. They are placed on a slide or bacterial counting chamber and examined at ×400 magnification. Only a few tubules are filled with cysts after an *M. mellificae* infection. The normal structure of malpighian tubules is not visible in this case. Only cysts inside the malpighian tubules can be taken as a positive result, because *M. mellificae* cysts are often confused with fungal spores and yeast cells.

b) Culture

There are no cultural methods for growing these organisms.

2. Serological tests

There are no serological tests available.

B. REQUIREMENTS FOR VACCINES AND DIAGNOSTIC BIOLOGICALS

No biological products are available.

• Acknowledgement

The authors would like to thank Dr F. Gnädinger for his valuable advice.

REFERENCES

1. BAILEY L. (1967). *Nosema apis* and dysentery of the honey bee. *J. Apic. Res.*, **6**, 121–125.

2. BULLA (1977). *In:* Comparative Pathobiology. Vol. 1: Biology of *Microsporidia* (1976); Vol. 2: Systematics of the *Microsporidia*, Lee A. & Cheng T.C., eds. Plenum Press, New York, USA, and London, UK.

3. CANTWELL G.E. (1970). Standard methods for counting nosema spores. *Am. Bee J.*, **110**, 222–223.

4. FRIES I. (1988). Contribution to the study of *Nosema* disease (*Nosema apis* Z.) in honey bee (*Apis mellifera* L.) colonies. Rapport 166, Sveriges Landbruksuniversitet, Institutionen för husdjurens utfodring och värd, Uppsala, Sweden.

5. MINISTRY OF AGRICULTURE, FISHERIES AND FOOD (1984). *Nosema* and *Amoeba*. Advisory Leaflet 473, HMSO, UK.

6. MORGENTHALER D. (1939). Die ansteckende Frühjahrsschwindsucht (*Nosema-Amoeben*-Infection) der Bienen. Erweiterter Sonderdruck aus der Scheizerischen Bienenzeitung Heft 2, 3 und 4.

7. STECHE W. (1985). Revision of ZANDER & BÖTTCHER. Nosematose. *In:* Krankheiten der Biene, Handbuch der Bienenkunde.

8. WEISER J. (1961). Die Mikrosporidien als Parasiten der Insekten. Verlag Paul Pavey, Hamburg and Berlin, Germany.

*
* *

CHAPTER 2.9.5.

VARROOSIS

SUMMARY

The mite Varroa destructor *(formerly* Varroa jacobsoni*) is a parasite of adult bees and their brood. It penetrates the intersegmental skin between the abdominal sclera of adult bees to ingest haemolymph. It can sometimes be found between the head, thorax and abdomen. The number of parasites steadily increases with increasing brood activity and the growth of the bee population, especially late in the season when clinical signs of infestation can first be recognised. The life span of the mite depends on temperature and humidity but, in practice, it can be said to last from some days to a few months.*

Identification of the agent: *The clinical signs of varroosis can only be recognised at a late stage of infestation, so that diagnosis entails the examination of the hive debris. The debris produced during the summer is especially useful for diagnosis. The earliest and most precise diagnosis can be made only after the application of a medication that forces the mites to drop off the bees or kills them directly. Larger amounts of debris can be examined using a flotation procedure. Bees are washed in petroleum spirit, alcohol or detergent solution. However, this method is less accurate due to the unequal distribution of mites and the usually small sample sizes.*

Serological tests: *No serological tests are applicable.*

Requirements for vaccines and diagnostic biologicals: *No biological products are available.*

A. DIAGNOSTIC TECHNIQUES

The mite *Varroa destructor* (formerly *Varroa jacobsoni*) (Oudemans) is a parasite of adult bees and their brood (Figure 1), and is responsible for the condition of varroosis or varroatosis. The mite inserts itself between the abdominal sclera in adult bees (8) where it penetrates the intersegmental membranes in order to ingest haemolymph. Sometimes it can also be found between the head and thorax. For reproduction, the mite enters the cells with the bee brood shortly before the cells are sealed. They prefer drone brood to worker brood. After the brood cell is sealed, the mite lays up to seven eggs in intervals of about 1–2 days. These hatch into nymphs, but only two to three reach the adult stage.

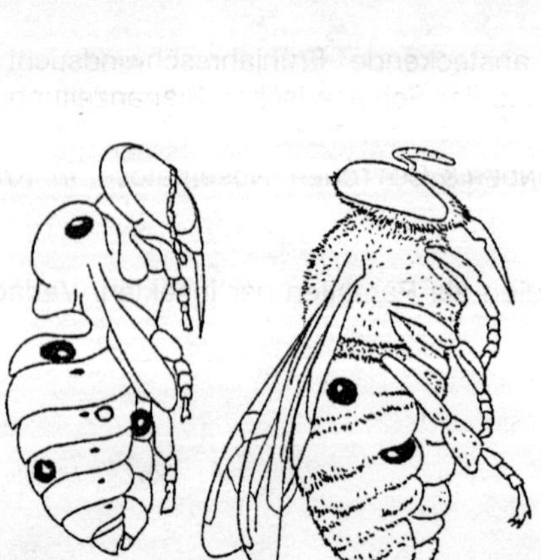

Fig. 1. Varroa *on pupa and adult bee. Left: pupa with four* Varroa *female mites. Right: worker bee with two female mites.*

The number of mites usually increases slowly at the beginning of the season. Clinical signs may be seen at any time during the active season, although usually maximum numbers are reached late in the season (Figure 2), when the first clinical signs of infestation can be recognised. The course of this parasitism is usually lethal, except in tropical Latin America (4, 10). The life span of mites on larval or adult bees depends on temperature and humidity. Under practical conditions, the life span may vary from some days to a few months.

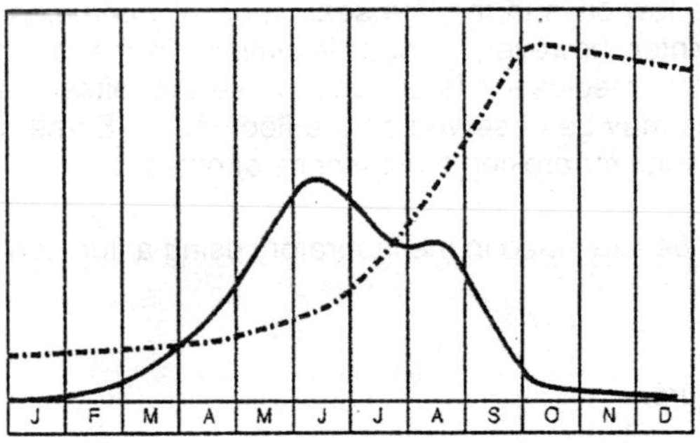

Fig. 2. Graph of populations of bees and mites over 1 year in a temperate Northern Hemisphere climate: brood numbers (solid line); mite numbers (broken line).

In heavily infested bee colonies, clinical signs of varroosis can often first be seen in the latter part of the season when the brood is reduced (10). Heavy infestations are usually reached 3–4 years after the primary invasion, but can occur within weeks if infested by bees from nearby colonies that are collapsing.

Essentially, the brood is damaged by the parasitic mites. Bees and their offspring that have been infected during the brood phase by only one parasitic mite show various ill effects, such as a shortened life span, changes in behaviour and an increased disease susceptibility (6). The parasitism is critical if more than one mite penetrates the brood cell for reproduction. Only in the lethal stage immediately before the collapse of the colonies do clinical signs, such as shrunken wings and shortened abdomen, appear (Figure 3). This is due to an increased susceptibility to deformed wing and acute paralysis virus, as well as to the infection of wounds and loss of haemolymph (1, 2). If the brood dies shortly before or after sealing, clinical signs of European foulbrood appear without the presence of the specific agent *Melissococcus pluton*. If the brood survives, the emerging bees show various behavioural changes and their life span is considerably shortened (5, 9).

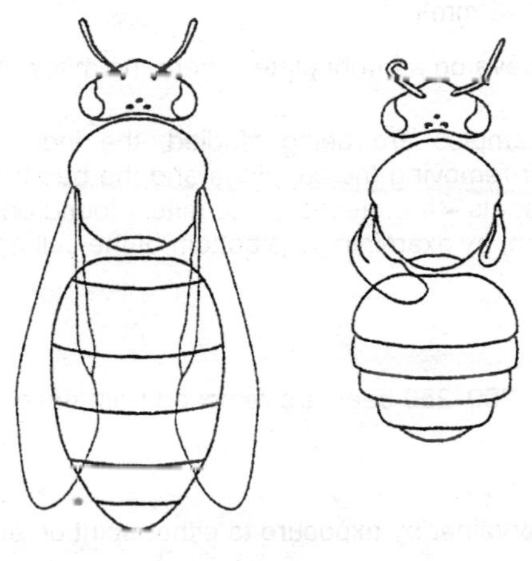

Fig. 3. Effect of Varroa *on bee morphology. Left: normal bee appearance. Right: bee heavily attacked by mites. This newly emerged bee has a deformed wing and reduced abdominal volume.*

1. Identification of the agent

The female mite is a dark reddish/brown colour and has a flat, oval-shaped body approximately 1.1 mm × 1.5 mm. It is the only common parasite of honey bees that can be seen with the naked eye (11).

a) Debris examination

An easy method of diagnosis of varroosis is by the examination of the debris generated by bees themselves. An insert covered with a screen mesh is placed on the floor of the hive. Unless this insert is covered with such a gauze, or smeared with grease, the bees will dispose of the mites outside the hive.

The debris produced within a few days in the late season usually contains little other than visible mites (7, 9). The debris collected in winter, however, must be examined in the laboratory. An insert is placed in the hive as before, but an effective medication is used to cause the mites to fall off the bees, so that after a given time, a number of mites may be observed on the floor insert. Some countries demand the diagnostic application of certain medications for proving the absence of mites.

Large amounts of debris can be examined in the laboratory using a flotation procedure (3).

- **Test procedure**

i) Dry the debris for 24 hours.

ii) Flood the debris with industrial alcohol.

iii) Stir continuously for around 1 minute or, if debris contains wax or propolis particles, stir for 10–20 minutes.

iv) Identify and observe the mites that float to the surface.

b) Brood examination

For the second method, drone brood is examined, if available, otherwise worker brood is examined.

When a large number of samples are examined, a rough determination of the degree of infection can be obtained.

- **Test procedure**

i) Remove the cappings of the brood cells with a knife.

ii) Wash the brood cells directly into a sieve system with warm water from a hand-held shower.

iii) Collect the mites in the lower fine sieve (mesh width 1 mm) while the brood is gathered in the upper coarse sieve (mesh width 2–3 mm).

iv) Place the contents of the sieve on a bright plate, where the mites can be easily identified and counted.

When a smaller number of samples are being studied, the individual cells are examined using an appropriate source of light. After removing the cappings and the bee brood, infected cells can be identified by the presence of small white spots – the faeces of the mite – found on the cell wall. The mites themselves should be sought for confirmation, by examining the bottom of the cell and the bee brood for attached mites.

c) Bee examination

In a third method, approximately 200–250 bees are removed from unsealed brood combs.

- **Test procedure**

i) Kill the bees in a special container by exposure to either spirit or alcohol.

ii) Stir the container for 10 minutes.

iii) Separate the bees from the mites by means of a sieve with a mesh size of approximately 2–3 mm.

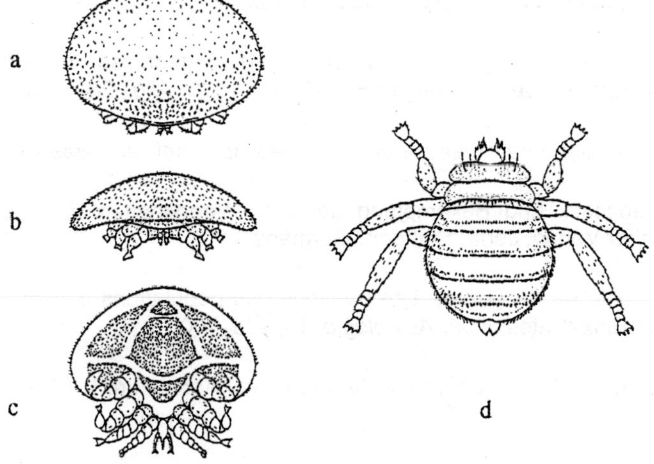

Fig. 4. Diagram of Varroa destructor (formerly *Varroa jacobsoni*) *Oudemans (female).*
a) Dorsal aspect
b) Anterior aspect — *Note the flat shell-like back and four pairs of legs.*
c) Ventral aspect
*d) The bee louse (*Braula coeca*, female). Note the lack of shell-like back and only three pairs of legs.*

Under some circumstances, the *Varroa* mite may be confused with the bee louse, *Braula coeca* (Figure 4). The latter is round, not oval, and being an insect, has only three pairs of legs. A number of different species of mite may be associated with *Varroa* mites on bees, but these are easily distinguished. In addition, other parasitic mites, such as those of the *Tropilaelaps* spp., are known to cause similar damage to bee colonies as the *Varroa* mites.

2. Serological tests

No serological tests are available for diagnosis.

B. REQUIREMENTS FOR VACCINES AND DIAGNOSTIC BIOLOGICALS

There are no biological products available.

• Acknowledgement

Illustrations by Karl Weiss, extracted from Bienen-Pathologie, 1984. Reproduced with the kind permission of the author and Ehrenwirth-Verlag, Munich (Germany).

REFERENCES

1. BAILEY L. (1981). Honey Bee Pathology. Academic Press, London, UK.

2. BALL B.V. (1985). Acute paralysis virus isolated from honey bee colonies infested with *Varroa jacobsoni*. *J. Apic. Res.*, **24**, 115–119.

3. BREM S. (1980). Laboruntersuchungen von Wintergemull. *In:* Diagnose und Therapie der Varroatose. Apimondia Publishing House, Bucharest, Romania, 116–117.

4. DE JONG D. (1997). Varroa and other parasites of brood. *In:* Pests, Predators and Diseases of Honey Bees, Third Edition, Morse R.A., ed. A. I. Root, Medina, Ohio, USA, 231–279.

5. DE JONG D. & DE JONG P.H. (1983). Longevity of Africanized honey bees *(Hymenoptera Apidae)* infested by *Varroa jacobsoni* (Parasitiformes Varroidae). *J. Econ. Entomol.*, **76**, 766–768.

6. DE JONG P.H. & GONCALVES L.S. (1982). Weight loss and other damage to developing worker honey bees from infestation with *Varroa jacobsoni*. *J. Apic. Res.*, **21**, 165–167.

7. LIEBIG G., SCHLIPF U., FREIMUT W. & LUDWIG W. (1984). Ergebnisse der Untersuchungen über die Befallsentwicklung der Varroamilben in Stuttgart Hohenheim 1983. *Allg. Dtsch Imkerztg.*, **6**, 185–190.

8. RITTER W. (1980). Varroatosis: A new disease of honey bee *Apis mellifera*. *Bee World*, **6**, 141–153.

9. RITTER W. (1996). Diagnostik und Bekämpfung der Bienenkrankheiten (Diagnosis and control of bee diseases). Gustav Fischer Verlag, Jena, Stuttgart, Germany.

10. RITTER W., LECLERQ E. & KOCH W. (1984). Observations des populations d'abeilles et de *Varroa* dans les colonies à différents niveaux d'infestation. *Apidologie*, **14**, 389–400.

11. SHIMANUKI H. & KNOX D.A. (1991). United States Department of Agriculture (USDA) Handbook No. 690. 53p.

*

* *

PART 3

OTHER DISEASES OF IMPORTANCE IN INTERNATIONAL TRADE

SECTION X

DISEASES NOT COVERED IN THE *CODE*

CHAPTER X.1.

LEISHMANIOSIS

SUMMARY

Leishmaniosis is not a single entity but comprises a variety of syndromes due primarily to at least 16 species and subspecies of Leishmania. *Dogs are commonly affected by* L. infantum *and* L. chagasi, *but infections with* L. tropica, L. major *and* L. braziliensis braziliensis *have been reported. In humans, the clinical spectrum ranges from asymptomatic infections to those with high mortality, with three distinct forms being classically described: visceral (VL), cutaneous (CL) and mucocutaneous (MCL). The vectors of these diseases are phlebotomine sandflies belonging to the genera* Phlebotomus *and* Lutzomyia.

Identification of the agent: *When clinical signs and characteristic lesions are present in affected humans and animals, the demonstration of the parasites in stained smears of splenic, bone marrow and lymph node aspirates, and of skin scrapings, gives a positive diagnosis. If the infection is low grade, detection of parasites is possible only by attempting* in-vitro *or* in-vivo *isolation. As there are very few morphological differences among various species, any isolated* Leishmania *organism must be identified by biochemical and/or immunological methods. Several centres throughout the world are presently using isoenzyme, DNA and antigen characterisation to identify the agent.*

Serological tests: *Serology is the preferred method for diagnosis of VL and canine leishmaniosis, even during the early stages of the disease. In subclinical forms, seropositive cases are confirmed by parasitic diagnosis. Serology is of less value for CL and MCL. Of the several techniques available, the indirect fluorescent antibody test and the enzyme-linked immunosorbent assay are the most suitable. Serodiagnostic antigens need to be prepared in the laboratory, though some commercial products are now under evaluation.*

Delayed hypersensitivity test: *The leishmanin skin test is useful for determining the distribution of human infections, distinguishing immune from nonimmune cases. The test is positive in CL, MCL and cured VL, but negative in active VL.*

Requirements for vaccines and diagnostic biologicals: *There is no effective vaccine available at present for use in humans and dogs. Leishmanin, no longer available commercially, needs to be standardised.*

A. DIAGNOSTIC TECHNIQUES

Leishmaniosis is caused by the vector-borne protozoan parasite, *Leishmania*. Various forms of clinical manifestations of human leishmaniosis have been described (30) and divided into three entities: visceral leishmaniosis (VL, kala azar), cutaneous leishmaniosis (CL, oriental sore, uta, pian bois, chiclero's ulcer) and mucocutaneous leishmaniosis (MCL, espundia). In the New World[1], leishmanioses are caused by *L. braziliensis* complex (MCL and CL), *L. mexicana* complex (CL), *L. peruviana* (CL) and *L. chagasi* (VL); in the Old World,

1 In this chapter, the term 'New World' refers to the Americas, and the term 'Old World' refers to Europe, Africa and Asia.

leishmanioses are caused by *L. donovani* (VL), *L. infantum* (VL and CL), *L. tropica* (CL), *L. major* (CL) and *L. aethiopica* (CL). The diseases are mainly zoonoses with a few exceptions. Canine leishmaniosis (CanL) is a chronic viscero-cutaneous disease caused by *L. infantum* and *L. chagasi*, of which the dog acts as the source reservoir. In some instances, parasites belonging to *L. braziliensis* complex, *L. major* and *L. tropica* have been isolated from this host (21). The vectors of leishmanioses are phlebotomine sandflies belonging to the genera *Lutzomyia* (New World) and *Phlebotomus* (Old World).

1. Identification of the agent

Clinical examination of suspected cases, parasitological diagnosis and immunodiagnosis are the routine methods available for the diagnosis of leishmaniosis. However, the demonstration of the parasite is the only way to confirm the disease conclusively (19). In VL, isolation and identification of the parasite from biopsies (bone marrow, spleen aspirate) coupled with immunodiagnostic tests are recommended. Parasitological diagnosis is necessary for confirmation of CL (through lesion scraping or needle aspiration from the edge of the lesions) as neither clinical examination nor serology are adequate. Smears of biopsy material are stained with Giemsa stain and examined microscopically at ×600–1000 magnification. Material should also be cultured in appropriate media at 22–26°C.

Morphological characteristics of amastigotes (in humans and mammalian hosts) and promastigotes (in invertebrate hosts and in cultures) are the following:

- Amastigote: small intracellular rounded or oval body, 1.5–3 × 2.5–6.5 µm in size, found in the cytoplasm of the macrophages. There is no free flagellum. The organism has a relatively large nucleus and a kinetoplast consisting of a rod-like body and a dot-like basal body;

- Promastigote: elongated extracellular organism, body size 15–20 × 1.5–3.5 µm with a single flagellum 15–28 µm long, arising close to the kinetoplast at the anterior. The nucleus is situated centrally.

The choice of the isolation and culture methods will depend on the immediate circumstances and on the technical capability and experience of the laboratory staff (27). *In-vitro* isolation offers certain advantages over the *in-vivo* methods: cultures become positive more rapidly – 5–30 days compared with months for lesions to appear on an animal – and the materials are less expensive. However, for *in-vitro* isolation, the techniques used should be carried out in strict sterile conditions; hence, it is not always feasible in the field. Unfortunately, there is still no 'universal' culture medium in which all the different leishmanias will grow easily, and it is almost impossible to predict which medium will be best suited to the growth of a particular isolate of *Leishmania*. Individual laboratories have to find the most suitable medium among biphasic blood agar media and tissue culture media supplemented with fetal calf serum (6). When attempting primary isolation of unknown organisms, a blood agar-based medium should be used – preferably NNN medium (Novy, McNeil and Nicolle), otherwise brain–heart infusion (BHI) agar medium or EMTM (Evan's modified Tobie's medium) should be used. For bulk cultivation of established isolates, suitable media are reported below in Section A.1.a. (see ref. 6 for media composition). The organisms from patients with VL and MCL can be very difficult to cultivate. Sometimes, even when the initial isolation is successful, the parasites may die when subcultured. This seems especially common when the initial isolation has been into a rich medium. Often this can be overcome if subcultures are made into less nutritionally rich media, such as NNN, or one of the semisolid media such as 'sloppy Evans' or semisolid Locke blood agar.

Hamster *(Mesocricetus auratus)* is the most commonly used animal for *in-vivo* isolation (21). Tissue suspensions or aspirates are inoculated intradermally into the nose and/or feet in the case of detection of dermotropic parasites. When the material is suspected to be infected with parasites causing VL, the inoculation should preferably be made by the intraperitoneal route. The resulting infection becomes apparent, weeks or months later, by the development of a nodule or ulcer at the site of inoculation, and in case of viscerotropic parasites, the infection becomes apparent, some months later, by massive infection of internal organs. The examination of Giemsa-stained smears of hamster tissue suspension/aspirate will show amastigotes. BALB/c mice are commonly used for the diagnosis of *L. major.*

Several techniques are now being used in many centres to identify the different *Leishmania* species, subspecies or strains.

a) Isoenzyme characterisation is the most commonly used method (1, 11, 21, 27). This technique requires a large number of parasites (5×10^9–1×10^{10}). The principles of enzyme electrophoresis are as follows: soluble enzymes are extracted from the organisms grown in media for bulk cultivation (BHI medium, MEM/FCS/EBLB [minimal essential medium/fetal calf serum/Evans' blood lysate broth] medium, Schneider's *Drosophila* medium). A small amount of the extract is then placed in an inert supporting substance, the matrix, containing a buffer at a fixed pH. The matrix is usually starch gel, but it could equally well be absorbent cellulose acetate, acrylamide or agarose. The pH of the buffer in the matrix is usually chosen so that the isoenzymes are negatively charged. A direct current is passed through the matrix carried by the ions in the buffer. When electrophoresis is completed, most proteins will have moved in the matrix towards the anode, depending on the amount of negative charge. If stained at this stage with a general protein stain, many bands will be seen. However, the high substrate and cofactor specificity of enzymes make it possible to stain only these proteins. Hence, the electrophoretic mobility of one particular enzyme can be compared among several organisms. The stained matrix with its collection of stained isoenzyme bands is known as a zymogram. Normally one or more extracts from reference organisms, in which the enzyme banding patterns are well documented, are included in the gel to aid the interpretation of results. Most enzymes used for characterisation purposes are stained by methods incorporating a dehydrogenase reaction. At least 12 enzymes should be examined.

b) The monoclonal antibody (MAb) technique is applied to the analysis and classification of both New and Old World *Leishmania* species and subspecies (11, 21, 25). For the production of the antibodies, BALB/c mice are immunised with membrane preparations from either promastigotes or amastigotes. Antibody-secreting hybridoma cultures are then selected and cloned by limiting dilutions. Specificity to *Leishmania* strains is assessed through immunofluorescence or immunoradiometric assays. This analysis seems to be quantitative rather than qualitative, as the amount of the same surface antigen may vary among *Leishmania* species.

c) Kinetoplast DNA restriction endonuclease analysis is based on the analysis, through gel electrophoresis, of fragments generated by endonucleases on the abundant mitochondrial DNA, which constitutes the kinetoplast (8, 11, 13, 21, 25). The electrophoretic pattern obtained, known as a restriction 'fingerprint', is a biochemical marker at the organelle genotype level that allows the identification and classification of *Leishmania* strains into schizodemes – populations having similar kinetoplast DNA sequences. This technique also requires a large number of parasites (1×10^{10}).

d) DNA hybridisation probes are a promising tool the principle of which is to allow labelled, single-stranded nuclear or kinetoplast DNA sequences from well characterised standard strains to find and hybridise with homologous DNA sequences from or within unknown *Leishmania* isolates (11, 26). Only complementary DNA sequences will form double-stranded DNA, which can be detected by autoradiography if the probe is radiolabelled, or by immunoenzymatic reaction. These techniques are sensitive enough to identify 10^2–10^3 organisms spotted on to nylon filters. Much fewer parasites (<10) are required for identification through the *in situ* hybridisation technique.

e) Polymerase chain reaction (PCR)-based methods are now available for diagnosis and/or identification of *Leishmania* from human and canine samples. Essentially, techniques developed either to detect organisms from fresh or frozen biopsies, or to identify established isolates of *Leishmania* include: (a) digestion of material with proteinase K and DNA extraction; (b) standard PCR amplification using oligonucleotide sequences selected from the small-subunit rRNA gene as primers (17), kinetoplast DNA minicircles (14) or other highly repetitive genomic DNA sequence (20); (c) analysis of amplification products by 1–2% agarose gel. In human VL, PCR has a sensitivity comparable with that of culture-based methods, but gives results much faster. In American CL and MCL, PCR appears to be consistently more sensitive than any previously recommended method of diagnosis (4).

2. Serological tests

Several serological tests are now used for detecting anti-leishmanial antibodies (2, 10, 11, 22). Sensitivity values reported below for each test, however, apply only to individuals who are not immunocompromised. A high percentage of patients with VL co-infected with human immunodeficiency virus (HIV) have recently been reported to be seronegative for anti-leishmanial antibodies (7).

a) Indirect fluorescent antibody test

The indirect fluorescent antibody (IFA) test is widely used because it is easy to perform. The test is genus-specific, although significant cross-reactions have been reported in individuals infected with *Trypansoma cruzi*. The IFA test is a more sensitive (96%) and specific (98%) test than the enzyme-linked immunosorbent assay (ELISA) for the detection of VL. Although amastigotes from frozen sections or smears of infected organs can be used as antigen, cultured promastigotes represent the commonest antigen source.

- **Antigen preparation**

i) Harvest 3–4 ml of the liquid phase of a 3-day-old culture medium showing flourishing promastigote growth (see Section A.1. for culture media).

ii) Wash the organisms three times with phosphate buffered saline (PBS), pH 7.2–7.4, by centrifugation at 350 *g* for 15 minutes at room temperature.

iii) Resuspend the final cell pellet in PBS and adjust the promastigote concentration to approximately 4 × 10^6/ml with the aid of a haemocytometer.

iv) Distribute 30 µl of the promastigote suspension on to each circle of a multispot slide and allow to dry at room temperature.

v) Fix the promastigotes in cold acetone for 10 minutes, then put the slides into a plastic box and keep in a deep freezer (–35°C) for no longer than 2–3 months.

- **Test procedure**

i) Wash the frozen antigen-coated slides in PBS and allow to dry at room temperature.

ii) Inactivate the sera for 30 minutes in a water bath at 56°C.

iii) Make doubling dilutions of test sera from 1/80 to 1/10,240 for human VL, and from 1/40 to 1/5120 for CanL. Positive and negative control sera, at dilutions of 1/80 and 1/160 for human VL, and of 1/40 and 1/80 for CanL, are also included in the test. No standard sera are available, but internal standards should be prepared and titrated.

iv) Distribute 30 µl of diluted serum samples on to each slide circle and incubate for 30 minutes at 37°C.

v) Remove the serum samples by vigorous washing in PBS, followed by immersion of the slides in PBS for 10 minutes. Allow the slides to dry.

vi) Distribute 30 µl of diluted fluorescein isothiocyanate (FITC)-conjugated anti-immunoglobulin on to each slide circle and incubate for 30 minutes at 37°C. FITC-conjugated anti-human and anti-dog immunoglobulins are commercially available. Follow the instructions for the appropriate dilution.

vii) Repeat step v and mount with a cover-slip in a few drops of PBS/glycerol (50% [v/v] of each).

viii) Read the slides under a fluorescent microscope. The highest dilution showing fluorescent promastigotes is taken to be the antibody titre. In human VL, the threshold titre usually ranges from 1/80 to 1/60, in CanL it ranges from 1/40 to 1/60. As IFA test performance may vary in different laboratories, it is better for each laboratory to define its own threshold titre using defined positive and negative reference sera.

b) Enzyme-linked immunosorbent assay

The ELISA can be carried out on serum or on a measured volume of blood. The blood is collected by needle-prick on to suitable absorbent paper strips and allowed to dry. The sample is eluted and tested at a single dilution previously determined to give an acceptable sensitivity and specificity. This test can be used for seroepidemiological surveys under field conditions.

In the classical method, the antigen is prepared as follows: promastigotes harvested from cultures are washed four times with PBS, pH 7.2, at 4000 *g* for 15 minutes. The packed promastigotes are resuspended in twice their volume of distilled water, and then sonicated at medium amplitude in an ice bath. The suspension is left at 4°C overnight to allow the proteins to come into solution. After a final centrifugation at 4000 *g* for 10 minutes to eliminate the cellular debris, the overlay, representing the concentrated soluble antigen, is dispensed into vials and stored at –20°C until required. For use in the test, it is reconstituted with PBS to the predetermined optimal protein concentration (around 20 µg/ml) as measured by Lowry's method. The ELISA is useful for the diagnosis of Old and New World leishmanioses. There is little or no cross-reaction with other diseases and, according to the *Leishmania* strain used, sensitivity can range from 86% to 99%.

A recent version of the ELISA, which is called the Falcon assay screening test and enzyme-linked immunosorbent assay (FAST-ELISA) and uses antigen-coated beads, is considered to be a sensitive, specific and field-adaptable test for canine visceral leishmaniosis with comparable sensitivity and specificity to the IFA test and ELISA. Whole blood or plasma can be evaluated quickly without the use of a microscope or spectrophotometer (2).

A detergent-soluble promastigote antigen has been used in ELISA instead of the crude lysate, for the diagnosis of canine leishmaniosis. The detergent was Triton X-100 and the proteic extract was protected with protease inhibitors. Using this method, ELISA sensitivity increased to 99.5%, while its specificity was comparable with that of the IFA test (97%) (15).

The ELISA methods described above are all based on crude antigenic preparations. More recently, a recombinant antigen from a cloned protein of *L. chagasi*, called rK39, has been reported to be highly reactive to sera from human and canine visceral leishmaniosis cases when run in an ELISA format. Using 25–50 ng of the antigen, 99% specificity and sensitivity was consistently found for immunocompetent human patients with clinical VL and for dogs with parasitologically proven disease. In HIV-positive patients, K39-ELISA showed higher sensitivity (82%) than the IFA test (54%) (3, 12). The K39 antigen, which shows remarkable stability and reproducibility, is now produced commercially.

c) **Direct agglutination test**

This test has been introduced for the diagnosis of VL and CanL, but needs further evaluation and standardisation. The antigen consists of promastigotes harvested from cultures, washed in PBS, pH 7.2, treated with 0.4% trypsin (for 45 minutes at 37°C and then washed again), and stained with 0.02% Coomassie brilliant blue. Two-fold serial dilutions of serum in PBS are made in V-bottomed microtitre-plate wells; 50 µl of antigen preparation is added to each well, and the plate is then carefully shaken by hand and left for 18 hours at room temperature. The test is read visually against a white background. Positive reactions are indicated by a clear sharp-edged blue spot.

A modified direct agglutination test for detection of specific anti-leishmanial antibodies in canine reservoir hosts is considered to be highly suitable for wide-scale epidemiological and ecological field work and diagnosis of canine leishmaniosis, having 100% sensitivity and 98.9% specificity (9, 10). The reliability of the test was improved by treating the test sera with 0.2 M 2-mercaptoethanol and incubating them at 37°C.

d) **Counter immunoelectrophoresis (CIEP)**

The general principle of this test is that the movement of most of the protein molecules is towards the anode, except for gamma-globulins, which move towards the cathode. This property is used in the counter immunoelectrophoresis (CIEP) test. The antibody moves towards the cathode under electroendosmotic flow and negatively charged antigen moves towards the anode and precipitates on contact with antiserum. The procedure is as follows: 3–5 ml of agarose are poured on to slides, and wells are punched when the agarose has set. Serum is placed in the anodal well and leishmanial antigen, prepared as for ELISA, in the cathodal well. The slide is placed in an electrophoresis tank filled with barbitone buffer, pH 8.2, and connected to the buffer chambers with filter-paper strips. A current of approximately 8 mAmp (milli-Ampere) is applied and after 2–3 hours the slide is examined for precipitation lines. The CIEP test is a reliable diagnostic test and in CanL has given better results than ELISA.

3. Delayed hypersensitivity test

Delayed hypersensitivity is an important feature of all forms of human leishmaniosis and can be measured by the leishmanin test, also known as the Montenegro reaction (16). Leishmanin is a killed suspension of whole (0.5–1 × 10^7/ml) or disrupted (250 µg protein/ml) promastigotes in pyrogen-free saline containing phenol. The dose is 0.1 ml given intradermally in the forearm. Promastigotes of any species of *Leishmania* are suitable as antigen, as are other kinetoplastid parasites. A delayed reaction develops and is read at 48–72 hours. The reaction is an indurated nodule with some surrounding erythema, and can be measured and graded according to the 'ballpoint pen' method. By applying moderate pressure, a line is slowly drawn with a ballpoint pen from a point approximately 1–2 cm from the margin of the skin reaction towards its centre. When resistance to further movement is first felt, indicating the margin of the reaction, the pen is lifted from the skin. By repeating the procedure on the opposite side of the skin reaction, this technique gives a visual record of the margins of the induration, the diameter of which can then be accurately determined by measuring the distance between the opposing lines.

The false-positive reaction rate in otherwise healthy people is approximately 1%, but this can be higher in areas where there is a background of leishmaniosis, as many of the healthy population may show quite high rates of leishmanin sensitivity. There is complete cross-reactivity among all strains of *Leishmania,* although heterologous antigens often give smaller reactions, but this may be caused by difficulty in standardisation. No cross-reactions occur with Chagas' disease, but some cross-reactions are found with cases of glandular tuberculosis and lepromatous leprosy. The leishmanin skin test has no value for the diagnosis of CanL. It is used in the clinical diagnosis of CL and MCL. In VL it will only measure past infections because during active disease, a complete anergy is found. Leishmanins are no longer available commercially and need to be standardised.

B. REQUIREMENTS FOR VACCINES AND DIAGNOSTIC BIOLOGICALS

1. Vaccine

There is no effective vaccine available for prophylactic immunisation against leishmaniosis. Until now, the only dependable vaccination against *Leishmania* has been limited to the protection of individuals from both *L. tropica* and *L. major* by prior syringe-induced infection with *L. major* organisms. The promastigotes are injected into the arm or other parts of the body. The living promastigotes used must either be freshly extracted from cultures or may be preserved in liquid nitrogen. The infection is allowed to run a natural course and after recovery, the individual is firmly immune to subsequent infection with both leishmaniae. This type of immunisation has been practised on a limited scale in hyperendemic areas of CL (caused by *L. major*) in Israel, Iran and the former Union of Soviet Socialist Republics (23). The immunising preparations consist of living, virulent and infective promastigotes. However, a killed *L. major* vaccine plus bacille Calmette-Guérin (BCG) against zoonotic cutaneous leishmaniosis has recently undergone a randomised, double-blind controlled trial in Iran (24).

Leishmania major causes cross-protection against *L. tropica*, but the reverse is not true. However, this species cannot be considered to be totally safe and may convert the immunised host into a reservoir that will be a potential source of infection as long as the lesion remains unhealed. Therefore, this type of immunisation should be used only for those moving into high-risk areas. Moreover, it is not beneficial in highly endemic areas as individuals contract infection long before this type of preparation confers protection. It takes approximately 3 months before immunity is acquired. Standardisation and quality control of such vaccines, presently not available, are urgently needed. At present, a number of promising anti-leishmanial vaccines are under development (33). First generation vaccines consist of killed *Leishmania* organisms mixed with a low concentration of BCG as adjuvant. Different preparations using either whole (autoclaved) or ultrasonic-disrupted promastigotes are currently undergoing phase I–II and phase III trials for immunisation against CL *Leishmania* agents in humans and against VL in humans and in dogs (5, 18). Therapeutic candidate subunit vaccines, consisting of several cloned antigens, one of which is a powerful adjuvant, have recently been used to treat drug-resistant mucosal *L. braziliensis* in humans in Brazil (24).

Second generation vaccines, which are currently at the predevelopment stage, consist of genetically reconstructed *Leishmania* parasites incapable of producing disease, recombinant molecules or their corresponding DNAs, or recombinant organisms carrying leishmanial genes and expressing parasite antigens.

2. Immunodiagnostic antigens

Neither the leishmanin used for skin tests nor the antigens employed in serodiagnosis in leishmaniosis are internationally standardised. The leishmanin test is group-specific, not species-specific, and the leishmanin prepared from one clinical type of leishmaniosis will cause the development of delayed hypersensitivity to the same or other clinical types. Similarly, serological cross-reactions are common among leishmanial species.

a) Leishmanin

The leishmanin test is described in Section A.3. Sterility, safety and potency tests are required for leishmanin preparations.

b) Antigens for serological tests

Antigens for the IFA tests and ELISAs are now produced commercially, but they are still under evaluation. The main reason for unsatisfactory results is the poor stability of leishmanial antigens. They can be obtained in the laboratory by growing a *Leishmania* strain in a suitable culture medium. For the IFA and direct agglutination tests, crude particulate antigens, i.e. intact promastigotes, are required, whereas for ELISAs and the CIEP test a soluble form of the antigen is needed.

3. Seed management

a) Characteristics of the seed

Strains of *Leishmania* species used to prepare biological products should be identified at species and subspecies level by appropriate identification tests given in Section A.1. Once the organisms have been isolated and established in the laboratory, they must be assigned an International Code (21, 27, 30). This code should consist of four elements separated by oblique strokes: (a) the type of host from which the strain was isolated (M for Mammalia and I for Insecta followed by three letters indicating the generic name of the host); (b) the country where isolation was made, indicated by a two-letter code; (c) the year of isolation indicated by the last two digits, and (d) the original laboratory code given to the isolate (for example, MHOM/IN/80/DD8). The parasites must be free from contaminating organisms and should be capable of yielding a product that conforms to the norms. Standard strains are available on request from the World Health Organization (WHO) Collaborating Centres in London, Montpellier and Jerusalem. A list of Identification Centres has been published by WHO (32).

b) Method of culture

The strain of the parasite used for preparing leishmanin should be capable of producing a product that conforms to national/international norms. It should be free from ingredients causing toxic or allergic reactions. There is no single specific antigen standardised for use in serodiagnostic tests, but when these antigens are prepared in the laboratory, they must be standardised for their sensitivity depending on the requirement. For the preparation of leishmanin as well as serodiagnostic antigens, the organisms should be grown in a suitable culture medium (such as those recommended in Section A.1. for *Leishmania* isolation and bulk cultivation). Normally, good growth of parasites is obtained 7 days after inoculation, and care must be taken that leishmanial stocks are not lost by overgrowth of the flagellates, which may occur after approximately 10 days.

c) Cryopreservation

Promastigote cultures and tissue infected with amastigotes may easily be conserved in the living state at low temperatures. Both forms can be cryopreserved for years at low temperatures in mechanical freezers (–70°C), in solid carbon dioxide containers (–76°C), or in liquid nitrogen containers (–196°C) (27). A sterile cryoprotectant is required – glycerol, to give a final concentration of 7.5–10%, or dimethyl sulphoxide (DMSO), to a final concentration of 5–7.5%. The cryoprotected samples are transferred to the sterile containers in which they are to be frozen. These may be 2 ml plastic freezing tubes with airtight screw caps, hard glass, heat-sealed ampoules, or glass/plastic capillaries. A slow cooling rate (approximately 1°C/minute) is essential for the cryopreservation of *Leishmania*. This can be obtained by cooling samples to 4°C and keeping them at this temperature for a minimum of 1 hour; they are then transferred to a -20°C freezer and left for 24 hours, then removed to a –70°C freezer for at least 24 hours. They can be permanently stored at this temperature, or else transferred into liquid nitrogen or solid carbon dioxide. If possible, a programmable freezing unit should be used. When the cryopreserved material is required, the sample is taken out and thawed rapidly in a water bath at 37°C.

d) Validation

Cultures for leishmanin or serodiagnostic antigens should be checked for sterility before use. Leishmanin is stored at 4°C and serodiagnostic antigens at –20°C or –70°C until required. The latter should be reconstituted with PBS, pH 7.2, before use. Viable *Leishmania* cultures can be kept at –70°C for 3–4 years or at –196°C indefinitely. Because of nonavailability of suitable vaccine, it has not been possible to validate the currently developed immunising agents. Live or attenuated promastigotes of *L. major* used in some areas are far from being satisfactory. Leishmanin should be tested for allergenicity in guinea-pigs before use. Serodiagnostic antigens should be tested for their efficacy and sensitivity by proper standardisation for a particular test. If a batch of antigen has not been used for a long time, it should be rechecked before being used in the test.

4. Method of manufacture

As the immunodiagnostic antigens are either not available commercially or, if so, are still under evaluation, they need to be prepared in the laboratory. Workers in the laboratory can be at risk of laboratory acquired infection, especially by injection. Appropriate biosafety precautions are therefore essential to minimise the risks.

a) Leishmanin

Leishmania species are grown, preferably in blood-free liquid media such as Schneider's *Drosophila* medium and RPMI (Rosewell Park Memorial Institute) medium, in order to avoid blood–antigen contamination. The promastigotes are harvested during the log phase, washed four times in pyrogen-free saline at 1000 *g* for 15 minutes, and resuspended in pyrogen-free saline containing 0.5% phenol (w/v) to obtain a final concentration of 0.5–1 × 10^7/ml. Leishmanin can also be made with disrupted promastigotes obtained as above and sonicated. The filtrate is adjusted to a final protein concentration of 250 µg/ml with pyrogen-free saline containing Tween 80 (0.0005% [v/v]) and phenol (0.28% [w/v]).

b) Antigens for serological tests

Methods of antigen preparation for various tests are given in Section A.2.

5. In-process control

One or more batches of leishmanin should be tested in guinea-pigs by allergic test. Sensitivity and specificity of the leishmanin should preferably be determined by performing the test in appropriate animal models (different inbred mice according to the *Leishmania* species), or in patients who have recovered from leishmanial infections, and in an unexposed control population.

6. Batch control

The WHO has suggested guidelines for the production of leishmanin (29, 31). It is recommended that the source material be controlled by using isoenzyme analysis to type the *Leishmania* strains used in preparing leishmanin.

a) Sterility

Each filling lot should be tested for bacterial and mycotic sterility according to WHO (28). Absence of live leishmaniae is checked by inoculating one sample of each lot in an appropriate blood-agar medium, which is then incubated at 23°C for at least 15 days. One sample is injected intradermally (for dermotropic leishmaniae) or intraperitoneally (for viscerotropic leishmaniae) in mice or hamsters. These animals are observed during a period of 30–90 days.

b) Safety

Samples from each filling lot should be tested for abnormal toxicity by appropriate tests in guinea-pigs and mice. For each lot, five mice weighing 17–22 g and two guinea-pigs weighing 250–350 g are injected subcutaneously and intraperitoneally with one human dose of the product. The animals are then observed for at least 7 days for death or signs of disease.

c) Potency

The leishmanin is tested on animal models (according to the *Leishmania* species involved) that have been previously infected by the same strain used for leishmanin production. Lots of at least five infected animals and control animals are injected intradermally into one of the posterior footpads with 50 µl of leishmanin. After 2–3 days, all the infected animals should show a significant enlargement of the footpad compared with control animals.

An international standard preparation has yet to be established. The Leishmaniosis Section of WHO's Tropical Disease Research Programme is funding programmes aimed at reaching a satisfactory standardisation of leishmanin production.

7. Tests on the final product

a) Safety

See Section B.6.b.

b) Potency

See Section B.6.c.

REFERENCES

1. ANDREWS R.H., HANDMAN E., ADAMS M., BEVERSTOCK P.R. & MITCHELL G.F. (1988). Genetic characterization of *Leishmania* isolates at 37 enzyme loci. *Int. J. Parasitol.*, **18**, 445–452.

2. ASHFORD D.A., BADARO R., EULALIO C., FREIRE M., MIRANDA C., ZALIS M.G. & DAVID J.R. (1993). Studies on the control of visceral leishmaniasis: validation of the Falcon assay screening test-enzyme linked immunosorbent assay (FAST-ELISA) for field diagnosis of canine visceral leishmaniasis. *Am. J. Trop. Med. Hyg.*, **48**, 1–8.

3. BADARO R., BENSON D., EULALIO M.C., FREIRE M., CUNHA S., NETTO E.M., PEDRAL-SAMPAIO D., MADUREIRA C., BURNS J.M., HOUGHTON R.L., DAVID J.R. & REED S.G. (1996). rK39: a cloned antigen of *Leishmania chagasi* that predicts active visceral leishmaniasis. *J. Infect. Dis.*, **173**, 758–761.

4. DE BRUJIN M.H.L., LABRADA L.A., SMYTH A.J., SANTRIC C. & BARKER D.C. (1993). A comparative study of diagnosis by the polymerase chain reaction and by current clinical methods using biopsies from Colombian patients with suspected leishmaniasis. *Trop. Med. Parasitol.*, **44**, 201–207.

5. DUBE A., SHARMA P., SRIVASTAVA J.K., MISRA A., NAIK S. & KATIYAR J.C. (1998). Vaccination of langur monkeys *(Presbytis entellus)* against *Leishmania donovani* with autoclaved *L. major* plus BCG. *Parasitology*, **116**, 21–221.

6. EVANS D.A. (1987). Leishmania. *In: In-Vitro* Methods for Parasite Cultivation, Taylor A.E. & Baker J.R., eds. Academic Press, London, UK, 52–75.

7. GRADONI L., SCALONE A. & GRAMICCIA M. (1993). HIV-*Leishmania* co-infections in Italy: serological data as an indication of the sequence of acquisition of the two infections. *Trans. R. Soc. Trop. Med. Hyg.*, **87**, 94–96.

8. GRAMICCIA M., SMITH D.F., ANGELICI M.C., READY P.D. & GRADONI L. (1992). A kinetoplast probe diagnostic for *Leishmanis infantum. Parasitology*, **107**, 509–517.

9. HARITH A.E., KOLK A.H.J., LEEUWENBURGH J., MUIGAI R., HUIGEN E., JELSMA T. & KAGER P.A. (1988). Improvement of a direct agglutination test for field studies of visceral leishmaniasis. *J. Clin. Microbiol.*, **26**, 1321–1325.

10. HARITH A.E., SLAPPENDEL R.J., REITER I., VAN KNAPEN F., KORTE P.D., HUIGEN E. & KOLK A.H.J. (1989). Application of a direct agglutination test for detection of specific anti-*Leshmania* antibodies in the canine reservoir. *J. Clin. Microbiol.*, **27**, 2252–2257.

11. HART D.T. (1989). Leishmaniosis. The Current Status and New Strategies for Control. NATO ASI Series. Ser. A: Life Sciences, Vol. 163. Plenum Press, New York, USA, 1041 pp.

12. HOUGHTON R.L., PETRESCU M., BENSON D.R., SKEIKY Y.A.W., SCALONE A., BADARO R., REED S.G. & GRADONI L. (1998). A cloned antigen (recombinant K39) of *Leishmania chagasi* diagnostic for visceral leishmaniasis in human immunodeficiency virus type 1 patients and a prognostic indicator for monitoring patients undergoing drug therapy. *J. Infect. Dis.*, **177**, 1339–1344.

13. KREIER J.P. & BAKER J.R. (1987). Parasitic Protozoa. Allen & Unwin, Boston, USA, 49–59.

14. MAARTEN H.L., DE BRUJIN M.H.L. & BARKER D.C. (1992). Diagnosis of New World leishmaniasis: specific detection of species of the *Leishmania braziliensis* complex by amplification of kinetoplast DNA. *Acta Trop.*, **52**, 45–58.

15. MANCIANTI F., FALCONE M.L., GIANNELLI C. & POLI A. (1995). Comparison between and enzyme-linked immunosorbent assay using a detergent-soluble *Leishmania infantum* antigen and indirect immunofluorescence for the diagnosis of canine leishmaniosis. *Vet. Parasitol.*, **59**, 13–21.

16. MANSON-BAHR P.C. (1987). Diagnosis. *In:* The Leishmaniases in Biology and Medicine. Vol. II. Clinical Aspects and Control, Peters W. & Killick-Kendrick R., eds. Academic Press, London, UK, 703–729.

17. MATHIS A & DEPLAZES P. (1995). PCR and *in vitro* cultivation for detection of *Leishmania* spp. in diagnostic samples from humans and dogs. *J. Clin. Microbiol.*, **33**, 1145–1149.

18. MAYRINK W., GENARO O., FRANCA SILVA J.C., DA COSTA R.T., TAFURI W.L., PEIXOTO TOLEDO V.P.C., DA SILVA A.R., BARBOSA REIS A., WILLIAMS P. & DA COSTA C.A. (1996). Phase I and II open clinical trials of a vaccine against *Leishmania chagasi* infections in dogs. *Mem. Inst. Oswaldo Cruz*, **91**, 695–697.

19. MOLYNEUX D.H. & ASHFORD R.W. (1983). The Biology of *Trypanosoma* and *Leishmania*. Parasites of Man and Domestic Animals, Taylor & Francis, London, UK, 185–250.

20. PIARROUX R., AZAIEZ R., LOSSI A.M., REYNIER P., MUSCATELLI F., GAMBARELLI F., FONTES M., DUMON H. & QUILICI M. (1993). Isolation and characterization of a repetitive DNA sequence for *Leishmania infantum*: development of a visceral leishmaniosis polymerase chain reaction. *Am. J. Trop. Med. Hyg.*, **49**, 364–369.

21. RIOUX J.A. (1986). Leishmania. Taxonomie – Phylogenèse. IMEEE, Montpellier, France, 537 pp.

22. SEHGAL S., MITTAL V. & BHATIA R. (1987). Manual on Laboratory Techniques in Leishmaniosis. National Institute of Communicable Diseases, Delhi, India.

23. SHUIKINA E.E., SERGIEV V.P., TRIERS I.I., SHCHERBAKOV V.A. & DIVEEV S.KH. (1968). Experience of antileishmaniasis vaccination with cultures of *Leishmania tropica major* grown in various types of media. *Med. Parazitol. (Mosk.)*, **37**, 648–651 (in Russian).

24. TDR NEWS (1999). UNDP/World Bank/WHO Special Programme for Research and Training in Tropical Diseases. No. 58, p. 4 and 12.

25. UNITED NATIONS DEVELOPMENT PROGRAMME/WORLD BANK/WORLD HEALTH ORGANIZATION (1984). Genes and Antigens of Parasites. A Laboratory Manual, Morel C.M., ed. Fundaao Oswaldo Cruz, Rio de Janeiro, Brazil, 93–135.

26. UNITED NATIONS DEVELOPMENT PROGRAMME/WORLD BANK/WORLD HEALTH ORGANIZATION (1985). Characterization of *Leishmania* spp. by DNA Hybridization Probes. A Laboratory Manual, D.C. Barker, ed. WHO, Geneva, Switzerland, 1–57.

27. UNITED NATIONS DEVELOPMENT PROGRAMME/WORLD BANK/WORLD HEALTH ORGANIZATION (1989). Handbook on Isolation, Characterization and Cryopreservation of *Leishmania*, Evans D., ed. WHO, Geneva, Switzerland, 1–45, pp.

28. WORLD HEALTH ORGANIZATION (WHO) (1972). General Requirements for Sterility of Biological Substances. Technical Report Series 530. WHO, Geneva, Switzerland.

29. WORLD HEALTH ORGANIZATION (WHO) (1982). Report of the Fourth Meeting of the Scientific Working Group on Immunology of Leishmaniases. TDR/LEISH SWG(4)/82.3.

30. WORLD HEALTH ORGANIZATION (WHO) (1984). The Leishmaniases. Technical Report Series 701. WHO, Geneva, Switzerland, 1–140.

31. WORLD HEALTH ORGANIZATION (WHO) (1985). Proposed Requirements for Tuberculins. WHO/BS/85.1463 Rev. 1.

32. WORLD HEALTH ORGANIZATION (WHO) (1988). Guidelines for Leishmaniosis Control at Regional and Subregional Levels. PDP. WHO/LEISH/88.25.

33. WORLD HEALTH ORGANIZATION (WHO) (1997). 13th Programme Report, Special Programme for Research and Training in Tropical Disease, WHO, Geneva, Switzerland.

*

* *

CHAPTER X.2.

MALIGNANT CATARRHAL FEVER

SUMMARY

Malignant catarrhal fever (MCF) is an acute, generalised and usually fatal disease affecting many species of Artiodactyla. The disease has been most often described as affecting species of the subfamily Bovinae and family Cervidae, but is also recognised in domestic pigs as well as giraffe and species of antelope belonging to the subfamily Tragelaphinae. MCF is defined by the recognition of characteristic lymphoid cell accumulations in nonlymphoid organs, vasculitis and T-lymphocyte hyperplasia in lymphoid organs, and can be caused by either of two gammaherpesviruses. The alcelaphine herpesvirus-1 (AlHV-1), the natural host of which – the wildebeest – is infected inapparently, causes the disease in cattle in regions of Africa and in a variety of ruminant species in zoological collections world-wide. Ovine herpesvirus-2 (OvHV-2), which is prevalent in all varieties of domestic sheep as a subclinical infection, is the cause of MCF in most regions of the world. This form of the disease was formerly referred to as sheep-associated MCF. In both forms of the disease, animals with clinical disease are not a source of infection as virus is only excreted by the natural hosts – wildebeest and sheep, respectively.

MCF usually appears sporadically and affects few animals, though both viruses can give rise to epizootics. There is a marked gradation in susceptibility to the OvHV-2 form of MCF ranging from the relatively resistant Bos taurus *and* B. indicus, *through water buffalo and many species of deer, to the extremely susceptible Pere David's deer and Bali cattle. The disease may present a wide spectrum of clinical manifestations ranging from the acute form, when minimal changes are observed prior to death, to the more florid cases characterised by high fever, bilateral corneal opacity, profuse catarrhal discharges from the eye and nares, necrosis of the muzzle and erosion of the buccal epithelium. Infectivity from animals with the AlHV-1 form of MCF can be recovered only by employing techniques that retain the viability of host cells, while OvHV-2 has never been recovered from affected animals. Diagnosis is normally achieved by observing the characteristic histopathological changes, though detection of viral DNA in either form of the disease has become the preferred method.*

Identification of the agent: *AlHV-1 may be recovered from clinically affected animals using peripheral blood leukocytes or cell suspensions prepared from lymph nodes and spleen, but cell viability must be preserved during processing, as infectivity cannot be recovered from dead cells. Virus can also be recovered from wildebeest, either from peripheral blood leukocytes or from cell suspensions of other organs. Most monolayer cultures of ruminant origin are probably susceptible and develop cytopathic effect (CPE), although bovine thyroid cell cultures have been used extensively for recovery of virus. Primary isolates typically produce multinucleated CPE in which viral antigen can be identified by immunofluorescence or immunocytochemistry using suitable antisera or monoclonal antibodies. The OvHV-2 agent has never been identified formally, although lymphoblastoid cell lines propagated from affected animals contain OvHV-2-specific DNA.*

Viral DNA has been detected in clinical material from MCF caused by both AlHV-1 and OvHV-2 using the polymerase chain reaction, and this is becoming the method of choice for diagnosing the OvHV-2 form of the disease.

Serological tests: *Infected wildebeest, the natural host, consistently develop antibody to AlHV-1, which can be detected in a variety of assays including virus neutralisation, immunoblotting, enzyme-linked immunosorbent assay, immunofluorescence, and immunocytochemistry. However, the antibody response of clinically affected animals is limited, with no neutralising antibody developing, so that detection relies on the use of immunofluorescence or immunoblotting. Antibody to OvHV-2 has only been detected by using AlHV-1 as the source of antigen. Domestic sheep* *consistently have antibody that can be detected by immunofluorescence or immunoblotting. While antibody often can be detected in cattle with MCF by immunofluorescence, in more acutely affected animals, such as deer, antibody is not always present.*

Requirements for vaccines and diagnostic biologicals: *No vaccine has been developed and there has been no attempt to standardise diagnostic reagents.*

A. DIAGNOSTIC TECHNIQUES

Malignant catarrhal fever (MCF) is a generally fatal disease of cattle and many other species of Artiodactyla, which occurs following infection with either alcelaphine herpesvirus-1 (AIHV-1) or ovine herpesvirus-2 (OvHV-2). Wildebeest (*Connochaetes* spp. of the subfamily Alcelaphinae), the natural hosts of AIHV-1, experience no clinical disease following infection. Likewise, infection of domestic sheep, the natural host of OvHV-2, has not been associated with any clinical reaction. Disease caused by AIHV-1 is restricted to those areas of Africa where wildebeest are present and to zoological collections elsewhere, and formerly has been referred to as wildebeest-derived MCF. The OvHV-2 form of the disease occurs world-wide wherever sheep husbandry is practised and has been described as sheep-associated (SA) MCF. Both forms of the disease may present a wide spectrum of clinical entities, though the characteristic histopathological changes are very similar in all cases.

• Clinical and pathological changes

The clinical signs of MCF are highly variable and range from peracute to chronic with, in general, the most obvious manifestations developing in the more protracted cases. In the peracute form, either no clinical signs are detected, or depression followed by diarrhoea and dysentery may develop for 12–24 hours prior to death. In general, the onset of signs is associated with the development of a fever, increased serous lachrymation and nasal exudate, which progresses to profuse mucopurulent discharges. Animals may be inappetent and milk yields may drop. Characteristically, progressive bilateral corneal opacity develops, starting at the periphery. In some cases skin lesions appear (characterised by ulceration and exudation), which may form hardened scabs associated with necrosis of the epidermis, and are often restricted to the perineum, udder and teats. Salivation associated with hyperaemia may be an early sign, progressing to erosions of the tongue, hard palate, gums and, characteristically, the tips of the buccal papillae. Superficial lymph nodes may be enlarged and limb joints may be swollen.

Nervous signs such as hyperaesthesia, incoordination, nystagmus and head pressing may be present in the absence of other clinical signs or as part of a broader more characteristic syndrome.

There is a wide spectrum of susceptibility to OvHV-2-induced disease, ranging from *Bos taurus* and *B. indicus* which are relatively resistant, through most species of deer and water buffalo *(Bubalus bubalis)*, which are much more susceptible, to the extremely susceptible Bali cattle *(Bos javanicus)* and Pere David's deer *(Elaphurus davidianus)*. The more resistant species tend to experience a more protracted infection and florid lesions, while in the more susceptible species the disease course tends to be shorter and the clinical signs less dramatic.

Reports from several countries, and in particular from Norway, that the disease affects domestic pigs have recently been confirmed (8). Signs are very similar to those seen in acutely affected cattle.

A mild form of the disease described in 1930 was regarded with some scepticism because the disease could be confirmed only by histological changes observed post-mortem. However, recent investigations using molecular and serological methods would appear to confirm that a few infected animals may recover following mild or even quite severe clinical reactions (9).

• Pathology

Gross pathological changes reflect the severity of clinical signs, but are generally widespread and may involve most organ systems. Erosions and haemorrhages may be present throughout the gastrointestinal tract, and in the more acute cases can be associated with haemorrhagic intestinal contents. In general, lymph nodes are enlarged, although the extent of lymph node involvement varies within an animal. Lymph nodes can often be firm and white when cross-sectioned, while others, in particular submandibular and retropharyngeal, may be haemorrhagic and even necrotic. Catarrhal accumulations, erosions and the formation of a diphtheritic membrane are often observed in the respiratory tract.

Within the urinary tract characteristic echymotic haemorrhages of the epithelial lining of the bladder are often present, while the renal cortex may be affected with multiple raised white foci, each 1–5 mm in diameter and sometimes surrounded by a thin zone of haemorrhage.

Histological changes have been the basis for confirming cases of MCF and are characterised by epithelial degeneration, vasculitis, hyperplasia and necrosis of lymphoid organs, and widespread interstitial accumulations of lymphoid cells in nonlymphoid organs. Epithelial lesions may be present at all epithelial surfaces and are characterised by erosion and ulceration, frequently with subepithelial and intraepithelial lymphoid cell infiltration, which may be associated with vasculitis and haemorrhages.

Vasculitis is generally present and may be pronounced in the brain, affecting veins, arteries, arterioles and venules. It is characterised by lymphoid cell infiltration of the tunica adventitia and media, often associated with fibrinoid degeneration. In the lumen there may be 'pavementing' by lymphoid cells, and in severe cases, endothelial damage and subendothelial accumulations by lymphoid cells can sometimes lead to occlusion.

Lymph-node hyperplasia is characterised by an expansion of lymphoblastoid cells in the paracortex, while degenerative lesions are generally associated with the follicles. Oedema with lymphoid inflammation often affects the perinodal tissue.

The interstitial accumulation of lymphoid cells in nonlymphoid organs, in particular the renal cortex and periportal areas of the liver, is typical, and in the case of the kidney may be very extensive. In the brain there may be a nonsuppurative meningoencephalitis with lymphocytic perivascular cuffing and a marked increase in the cellularity of the cerebrospinal fluid.

The macroscopic lesions observed in the cornea are reflected histologically by lymphoid cell infiltration originating in the limbus and progressing centrally, with oedema and erosion developing in the more advanced cases. Vasculitis, hypopyon and iridocyclitis also may be present.

The pathological features of MCF caused by either agent are essentially similar. However, apart from histological examination, the methods available for diagnosing AIHV-1- and OvHV-2-induced disease are very different and are thus considered separately.

A1. Alcelaphine herpesvirus-1

This form of the disease occurs in the cattle-raising regions of eastern Africa where pastoralists use areas grazed by wildebeest, and in southern Africa in areas where wildebeest and cattle are grazed together. The disease, however, can also affect a variety of other ruminant species in zoological collections world-wide and so, apart from antelope of the subfamilies Alcelaphinae and Hippotraginae, it is advisable to regard all ruminants as susceptible. Most laboratory-based tests have relied on one attenuated isolate – WC11 – that has been subjected to many laboratory passages as a source of viral antigen and DNA (11). The recent publication of the full nucleotide sequence of the virulent low passage virus – C500 – will form the basis of further studies of this virus (4).

1. Identification of the agent

- **Clinically affected animals**

a) Isolation

The striking feature of AIHV-1-induced MCF is the lack of detectable viral antigen or herpesvirus-specific cytology within lesions. Confirmation of infection thus relies on virus recovery. Generally, infectivity is strictly cell associated and thus isolation can be achieved only from cell suspensions either of peripheral blood leukocytes, lymph nodes or other affected tissues. Cell suspensions are prepared in tissue culture fluid, approximately 5×10^6 cells/ml, and inoculated into preformed cell monolayer cultures. Bovine thyroid cells have been used extensively, but most primary and low passage cell monolayer cultures of ruminant origin will probably provide a suitable cell substrate for isolating the virus. Following 36–48 hours' incubation, culture medium should be changed and monolayers should be examined microscopically (×40) for evidence of cytopathic effects (CPE). These appear characteristically as multinucleate foci within the monolayers, which then progressively retract forming dense bodies with cytoplasmic processes that may detach. This is followed by regrowth of normal monolayers. A CPE may take up to 21 days to become visible and is seldom present before day 7. Infectivity at this stage tends to be largely cell associated and thus any further passage or storage must employ methods that ensure that cell viability is retained. Specificity of the isolate should be determined using specific antisera or monoclonal antibodies (MAbs) in fluorescence or immunocytochemical tests.

b) Viral DNA

Characteristically, very little viral DNA can be detected within affected tissues, hence it is necessary to amplify the viral genome either by conventional culture or the polymerase chain reaction (PCR).

A restriction map of the standard laboratory strain (WC11) using the restriction enzymes *Hin*dIII, *Eco*RI, *Bam*HI and *Sma*I has been published and most of the genome has been cloned (2). Such clones can be used to identify and characterise other bovid gammaherpesvirus isolates. Sequence data on the WC11 isolate of AIHV-1 have been generated and primers suitable for use in the PCR have been identified (6). None, however, has been established as appropriate for use as diagnostic aids. In addition, the complete genome of the virulent C500 isolate has been published (4).

- **Natural hosts**

It is almost certain that all free-living wildebeest are infected by 6 months of age, virus having been spread as an intense epizootic during the perinatal period. The species *Connochaetes taurinus taurinus*, *C.t. albojubatus* and *C. gnu* are all assumed to be infected with the same virus. Infection also appears to persist in most groups of wildebeest held in zoological collections. However, it is possible that infection may be absent in animals that have been isolated during calf-hood or that live in small groups. Natural infection has been successfully demonstrated by *in-situ* hybridisation on lung sections from blue wildebeest calves in South Africa (10).

Virus isolation will seldom be contemplated. Following infection there is a brief period when virus is excreted in a cell-free form and can be isolated from nasal swabs. Virus can also be isolated from blood leukocytes at this time, but in older animals this is less likely to be successful unless the animal is immunosuppressed either through stress or pharmacological intervention. In addition, virus may be isolated by establishing cultures of tissues from apparently normal animals, and this has been achieved in monolayer cultures of both kidney and thyroid cells from adult animals.

Other large antelope of the subfamilies Alcelaphinae and Hippotraginae are also infected with antigenically closely related gammaherpesviruses, but there is no evidence that they can spread to other species and cause MCF.

2. Serological tests

- **Clinically affected animals**

The antibody response of clinically affected animals is limited, with no neutralising antibody developing. Antibody in clinical cases can be demonstrated consistently by immunofluorescence or the immunoperoxidase test (IPT) employing WC11-infected cell cultures as substrate. Although other methods of antibody detection have been described, none has proved to be satisfactory.

- **Natural hosts**

Antibody appears to develop consistently in wildebeest following infection and can be identified by neutralisation assays using the cell-free isolate WC11, or by immunofluorescence, again using the WC11 isolate and anti-bovine IgG, which has been shown to react with wildebeest IgG.

There has been no attempt so far to standardise the indirect fluorescent antibody (IFA) test and IPT, but the two methods below are given as examples.

a) Indirect fluorescent antibody test

The IFA is less specific than virus neutralisation (VN); it can be used to demonstrate several varieties of 'early' and 'late' antigens in AIHV-1-infected cell monolayers. Antibodies reacting in IFA or IPT develop in cattle and experimentally infected rabbits during the incubation period, and later in the clinical course of the disease though cross-reactions with some other bovine herpesviruses, as well as OvHV-2, reduces the differential diagnostic value. Detection of such cross-reacting antibodies can sometimes be useful in supporting a diagnosis of SA-MCF.

- **Preparation of fixed slides**

Inoculate nearly or newly confluent cell cultures (see Section A1.2.c.) with AIHV-1 (strain WC11). Uninoculated control cultures should be processed in parallel. At about 4 days – when the first signs of CPE are expected to appear but before overt CPE is visible – treat the cultures as follows: discard the medium, remove the cells with trypsin–versene solution, spin down cells at approximate 800 ***g*** for 5 minutes, discard the supernatant fluid, and resuspend the cells in 10 ml of phosphate buffered saline (PBS) for each 800 ml plastic bottle of cell culture.

Make test spots of the cell suspension on two wells of a polytetrafluoroethylene-coated multiwell slide; air-dry and fix in acetone. Stain the spots with positive standard serum and conjugated anti-IgG to the appropriate species. Examine the incidence of positive and negative cells under a UV microscope. Adjust the cell suspension by adding noninfected cells and/or PBS to give a suitable concentration that will form a single layer of cells when spotted on to the slide, with clearly defined positive cells among a background of negative cells.

Spot the adjusted positive cell suspension and the control negative suspensions on to multiwell slides in the desired pattern, and air-dry. Fix in acetone for 10 minutes. Rinse, dry and store over silica gel in a sealed container at –70°C.

An alternative procedure, which is easier to evaluate, is to prepare monolayers of infected and noninfected cells in Leighton tubes or chamber slides. The cell monolayers are infected with from 150 to 200 $TCID_{50}$ (50% tissue culture infective dose) of virus that has been diluted in cell culture medium. The infected and noninfected slides are fixed in acetone and stored, as above, at –70°C.

- **Test procedure**

i) Rehydrate the slides for 5 minutes with PBS, rinse in distilled water and air-dry.

ii) Dilute sera 1/20 in PBS. Samples that give high background staining may be retested at higher dilutions. Apply diluted fluids to one MCF virus-positive cell spot and one negative control spot for each sample. Include positive and negative serum controls. Ideally, the test should be validated by titrating the control positive to determine its end-point.

iii) Incubate at 37°C for 30 minutes in a humid chamber.

iv) Drain the fluids from the spots. Wash the slides in two changes of PBS, for 5 minutes each.

v) Wash in PBS for 1 hour with stirring, and then air-dry the slides.

vi) Apply rabbit anti-bovine IgG fluorescein isothiocyanate (FITC) conjugate at a predetermined working dilution.

vii) Incubate at 37°C for 20 minutes, drain the slides, and wash twice in PBS for 10 minutes each.

viii) Counterstain in Evans blue $1/10^4$ for 30 seconds, and wash with PBS for 2 minutes. Dip in distilled water, dry and mount in PBS/glycerol (50/50).

ix) Examine by fluorescence microscopy for specific binding of antibody to the infected cells.

h) Immunoperoxidase test

A 1/800 dilution of bovine turbinate (BT) cell-cultured AlHV-1 is made in a freshly trypsinised suspension of BT cells and seeded into Leighton tubes containing glass cover-slips, 1.6 ml per tube, or four-chambered slides, 1.0 ml per chamber.

Observe the cell cultures at 4–6 days for CPE and fix the cultures with acetone when signs of CPE begin. Remove the plastic chambers, but not the gaskets, from the slide chambers before fixation, and use acetone (e.g. UltimAR) that will not degrade the gasket. Store the fixed cells at –70°C.

- **Test procedure**

i) Prepare IPT diluent (21.0 g NaCl and 0.5 ml Tween 20 added to 1 litre of 0.01 M PBS, pH 7.2) and washing fluid (0.5 ml Tween 20 added to 1 litre of 0.01 M PBS, pH 7.2).

ii) Dilute the serum to be tested 1/20 in IPT diluent and overlay 150–200 µl on to a fixed virus-infected cover-slip or slide chamber.

iii) Incubate the cover-slip in a humid chamber at 37°C for 30 minutes.

iv) Dip the cover-slip three times in washing fluid.

v) Overlay 150–200 µl of diluted (1/5000 in IPT diluent) peroxidase-labelled anti-bovine IgG on to the cover-slip or slide chamber.

vi) Incubate the cover-slip or slide chamber in a humid chamber at 37°C for 30 minutes.

vii) Dip the cover-slip three times in washing fluid.

viii) Dilute the AEC substrate (3-amino-9-ethylcarbazole) in distilled water (5 ml of distilled water, 2 drops buffer, 2 drops hydrogen peroxide, and 3 drops AEC) and apply to the cover-slip or slide chamber.

ix) Incubate in a humid chamber at 37°C for 8–10 minutes.

x) Dip the cover-slip in distilled water, air-dry, and mount on a glass slide. Slide chambers are read dry.

xi) The slide is read on a light microscope. The presence of a reddish-brown colour in the nuclei of the infected cells indicates a positive reaction.

c) Virus neutralisation

Tests have been developed for detecting antibodies to AIHV-1 in both naturally infected reservoir and indicator hosts. The first of these is a VN test using cell-free virus of the WC11 strain, and another uses a hartebeest isolate (AHV-2). The test is laborious, but can be performed in microtitre plates using low passage cells or cell lines. The main applications have been in studying the range and extent of natural infection in wildlife, captive species in zoos and, to a lesser extent, sheep populations. It has also been useful in attempts to develop vaccines, all of which have had very limited success. High-titre VN antibodies can be induced, but these are evidently not protective.

AIHV-1 stock (strain WC11) is grown in primary or secondary cell cultures of bovine kidney, bovine thyroid, low passage bovine testis, or other permissive cell type, and stored in aliquots at –70°C. The stock is titrated to determine the dilution that will give 100 $TCID_{50}$ in 25 µl under the conditions of the test.

- **Test procedure**

i) Inactivate the sera for 30 minutes in a water bath at 56°C.

ii) Make doubling dilutions of test sera in cell culture medium from 1/2 to 1/16 using a 96-well flat-bottomed cell-culture grade microtitre plate, four wells per dilution and 25 µl volumes per well. Positive and negative control sera are also included in the test. No standard sera are available, but internal positive standards should be prepared and titrated in an appropriate range.

iii) Add 25 µl per well of WC11 virus stock at a dilution in culture medium calculated to provide 100 $TCID_{50}$ per well.

iv) Incubate for 1 hour at 37°C. The residual virus stock is also incubated.

v) Back titrate the residual virus in four tenfold dilution steps, using 25 µl per well and at least four wells per dilution.

vi) Add 50 µl per well of bovine kidney cell suspension at 3×10^5 cells/ml.

vii) Incubate the plates in a humidified CO_2 atmosphere at 37°C for 7–10 days.

viii) Read the plates microscopically for CPE. Validate the test by checking the back titration of virus (which should give a value of 100 $TCID_{50}$ with a permissible range 30–300) and the control sera. The standard positive serum should give a titre within 0.3 $\log_{10}$ units of its predetermined mean.

ix) The test serum results are determined by the Spearman–Kärber method as the dilution of serum that neutralised the virus in 50% of the wells.

x) A negative serum should give no neutralisation at the lowest dilution tested (1/2 equivalent to a dilution of 1/4 at the neutralisation stage).

A2. Ovine herpesvirus-2

This form of the disease occurs world-wide in cattle and other species, normally appearing sporadically and affecting only one or a few animals. However, on occasion, incidents occur in which several animals become affected, and this appears to be associated with certain sheep flocks that may continue to transmit disease for a number of years. The disease can also spread more readily to red deer *(Cervus elaphus)* and other deer species, water buffalo *(Bubalus bubalis)* and even more readily to Pere David's deer *(Elaphurus davidianus)* and Bali cattle *(Bos javanicus)*. OvHV-2 is also responsible for causing MCF in zoological collections, where disease has been reported in a variety of species including giraffe. Disease in pigs has been reported from several countries, but is most frequently recognised in Norway where incidents involving several animals regularly occur.

Diagnosis based on clinical signs and gross pathological examination cannot be relied on as these can be extremely variable. Histological examination of a variety of tissues including, by preference, kidney, liver, urinary bladder, buccal epithelium, cornea/conjunctiva and brain, has been the only method of reaching a more certain diagnosis. However, detection of antibody to the virus and/or viral DNA can now also be attempted and is rapidly becoming the method of choice.

It must be emphasised that the viral cause of SA-MCF has not been isolated and evidence for OvHV-2 relies on: (a) the presence of antibody in sera of all domestic sheep that cross-reacts with AIHV-1 antigens in the IFA test and immunoblots (5), but not in neutralisation assays; (b) the development of antibody that cross-reacts with AIHV-1 in the IFA test in a proportion of cattle with SA-MCF and in all experimentally infected hamsters: (c) the detection and cloning of DNA from lymphoblastoid cell lines derived from natural cases of SA-MCF that cross-hybridises with, but is distinct from, AIHV-1 DNA.

1. Identification of the agent

• Clinically affected animals

Attempts to recover the disease-causing virus from clinical cases have failed consistently. There are, however, several reports of the recovery of different viral agents from clinical cases, none of which has established any causal relationship; their isolation is certainly fortuitous or due to laboratory contamination. However, lymphoblastoid cell lines have been generated from affected cattle and deer, some of which transmit disease following inoculation into experimental animals (12). Such cell lines contain viral sequences that hybridise with clones of AlHV-1 DNA (3). Several viral fragments have been cloned from a genomic library of one such line and have been the subject of further characterisation. A subclone that did not hybridise with AlHV-1 was chosen for sequencing and found to code for a protein very similar to the tegument protein of Epstein–Barr virus. Primers were identified within this sequence that were suitable for use in the PCR, and a sensitive protocol was designed in which a fragment of 422 base pairs (bp) is amplified initially, followed by amplification of a truncated internal fragment of 238 bp. It has been proven that this test is able to detect as few as 35 viral genome equivalents and that no product is amplified from AlHV-1 or other bovid herpesviruses (1). This PCR is thus both highly specific and sensitive for OvHV-2 and has been employed world-wide in studies of the disease in clinically affected animals and the natural host. It is emerging as a robust test that can be employed to detect viral DNA in peripheral blood leukocytes of clinically affected animals as well as fresh tissues and paraffin-embedded samples collected at post-mortem. The use of magnetic particles to purify DNA prior to amplification has been reported to be an additional improvement to the test, but is yet to be evaluated.

• Polymerase chain reaction

Amplification reactions are performed in 50 µl volumes containing 2 µg test DNA in 10 mM Tris HCl, pH 8.3, 50 mM KCl, 2 mM $MgCl_2$, 0.01% (v/v) gelatine, 10% (v/v) dimethyl sulphide, 200 µm dATP, dCTP, dGTP and dTTP (Pharmacia), 1 µM of each primer and 2 units Taq DNA-polymerase overlaid with 50 µl mineral oil (Sigma) to prevent evaporation.

The programme consists of a precycle at 99°C for 3 minutes, after which dNTP and enzyme mix are added. This is followed by 25 cycles of 94°C for 20 seconds, 60°C for 30 seconds and 72°C for 30 seconds. A 2 µl aliquot of the primary amplification product, specified by the primer pair 556/755, is transferred directly to a new reaction mixture and amplified using the primer pairs 556/555 under identical conditions for a further 25 cycles with a final extension at 72°C for 5 minutes.

Final amplification products (10 µl) are analysed directly by 1.8% agarose gel electrophoresis and ethidium bromide fluorescence. With each batch of test samples a known positive control and distilled water are also amplified and analysed.

• Natural hosts

The domestic sheep is the natural host of OvHV-2 and all animals tested have been shown to be seropositive for AlHV-1. Furthermore, it would appear that some lambs become infected *in utero*, rendering it very difficult to identify uninfected animals. Neonatal lambs are often the source of infection, though sheep of all ages can transmit disease. Virus has never been recovered from sheep, but the PCR developed for detecting OvHV-2 DNA in clinical cases of MCF has also been employed to detect virus in the peripheral blood leukocytes of normal adult sheep and in nasal secretions and the oropharynx of lambs during the first months of life. Thus it would appear that, as with AlHV-1 infection in wildebeest, sheep become infected with OvHV-2 at a young age and thereafter remain latently infected for life.

Factors that predispose to virus shedding and transmission to MCF-susceptible hosts remain speculative.

In addition to domestic sheep, domestic goats and other members of the subfamily Caprinae have antibody that reacts with AlHV-1 in a similar pattern to sheep serum. This implies that these species are infected with viruses similar to OvHV-2, and some goats have been found to be positive to an OvHV-2 PCR, though their potential role in causing MCF is not known.

2. Serological tests

Antibody to OvHV-2 has only been detected by using AlHV-1 as the source of antigen. Antibody to AlHV-1 can be detected in 70–80% of affected cattle by IFA or IPT procedures, but generally is not present in affected deer or animals that develop acute or peracute disease. Antibody is detected by IFA using tissue culture cells infected with AlHV-1. Cell monolayers grown on cover-slips exhibiting 10–50% CPE are harvested, washed, fixed in acetone and used in the assay. Cover-slips are mounted with DPX, the side containing the cells facing uppermost, on microscope slides and treated with 10% normal horse serum before progressing with a conventional IFA test. The IPT procedure can be carried out as for AlHV-1. The only virus of cattle that has been reported to cross-react with AIHV-1 is bovine herpesvirus-4 (BHV-4). Thus the negative control for this test should be similarly infected monolayers of BHV-4. Sera are only considered to be positive when foci show characteristic intranuclear distribution of antigen with little or no cytoplasmic staining being detected in the AIHV-1-infected cells and no reaction in the BHV-4-infected cells. Sera that react to antigens of both viruses are considered to be inconclusive. A competitive inhibition enzyme-linked immunosorbent assay (CI-ELISA) has been developed for detecting antibody to OvHV-2 (7) using an MAb (15-A) raised against the so-called Minnesota isolate of virus, which is indistinguishable from AIHV-1. The test has been employed to detect antibody in serum of wild and domestic ruminants in North America and appears to have some merit. However, there was poor correlation between the development of antibody detected in serum of lambs and the acquisition of infection with OvHV-2 as indicated by the presence of viral DNA detected by PCR, and only a proportion of sheep were found to be positive. This is in marked contrast to other studies employing IFA, which indicate that most if not all domestic sheep are serologically positive. In a study on the reaction of sheep serum to the structural proteins of AIHV-1 in immunoblots, the reactivity of different sera varied strikingly, indicating that individual sheep responded differently with regard to antibody recognition of cross-reacting epitopes of AIHV-1. Thus it is likely that some of the negative results obtained by CI-ELISA are due to the extreme epitope specificity of such an MAb-based test that fails to detect antibody in a proportion of sera. Results from such a test should therefore be interpreted with caution.

A3. Control

Control at present relies on segregating natural hosts from susceptible species, the extent to which this is enforced depending on the species involved. With AIHV-1, it would appear that MCF-affected animals never or rarely transmit infection, hence it is only the natural hosts that can act as a source of infection. Wildebeest would appear to be relatively efficient transmitters of infection to most other categories of ruminant, and hence their segregation in mixed collections is important. Likewise, pastoralists must ensure that cattle are entirely segregated from the vicinity of wildebeest and pastures recently grazed by them, particularly around the time of wildebeest calving.

With OvHV-2, the requirement to segregate sheep depends on the susceptibility of the species involved. Thus with Pere David's deer and Bali cattle, strict separation and avoidance of contact through fomites must be ensured. Equally, with farmed deer every reasonable effort must be taken to segregate the management of sheep and deer, although fallow deer *(Dama dama)* appear to be more resistant to MCF. Cattle only rarely develop SA-MCF, and thus are generally managed with sheep without taking precautions to guard against disease transmission. However, if multiple cases do occur, it is essential to segregate the sheep flock as far as possible from cattle. As such flocks may continue to be sources of infection for some years, disposal of these flocks for slaughter should be considered.

The possibility that very long incubation periods may occur, up to 9 months, further necessitates a guarded prognosis when advising on the control of such outbreaks.

B. REQUIREMENTS FOR VACCINES AND DIAGNOSTIC BIOLOGICALS

No successful vaccination regimen has been identified. However, most investigations have employed isolates of AIHV-1 that are adapted to tissue culture and that are generally avirulent. Recent studies of the molecular changes in the virus have shown that in the course of adaptation to *in-vitro* culture, a specific deletion occurs in the viral DNA that appears to be consistent among different isolates during the process of attenuation. Thus, it is proposed that this deleted segment codes for a virulence factor(s). The omission of this product from previously tested vaccines may have contributed to the poor success with these experiments. A sequence homologous to this deletion is also present in OvHV-2, suggesting that it is conserved and thus provides further weight to the hypothesis that it may have an important role in the pathobiology of MCF (4).

Future vaccine strategies should therefore consider incorporating these viral components that may protect against both forms of MCF.

REFERENCES

1. BAXTER S.I.F., POW I., BRIDGEN A. & REID H.W. (1993). PCR detection of the sheep-associated agent of malignant catarrhal fever. *Arch. Virol.*, **132**, 145–159.

2. BRIDGEN A. (1991). The derivation of a restriction endonuclease map for Alcelaphine herpesvirus-1 DNA. *Arch. Virol.*, **117**, 183–192.

3. BRIDGEN A. & REID H.W. (1991). Derivation of a DNA clone corresponding to the viral agent of sheep-associated malignant catarrhal fever. *Res. Vet. Sci.*, **50**, 38–44.

4. ENSSER A., PFLANZ R. & FLECKSTEIN B. (1997). Primary structure of the alcelaphine herpes virus 1 genome. *J. Virol.*, **71**, (9) 6517–6525.

5. HERRING A.J., REID H.W., INGLIS N. & POW I. (1989). Immunoblotting analysis of the reaction of wildebeest, sheep and cattle sera with the structural antigens of Alcelaphine herpesvirus-1 (malignant catarrhal fever virus). *Vet. Microbiol.*, **19**, 205–215.

6. HSU D., SHIH L.N., CASTRO A.E .& ZEE Y.C. (1990). A diagnostic method to detect Alcelaphine herpesvirus-1 of malignant catarrhal fever using the polymerase chain reaction. *Arch. Virol.*, **114**, 259–263.

7. LI H., SHEN D.T., KNOWLES D.P., GORHAM J. & CRAWFORD T. (1994). Competitive inhibition enzyme-linked immunosorbent assay for antibody in sheep and other ruminants to a conserved epitope of malignant catarrhal fever virus. *Clin. Microbiol.*, **32**, 1674–1679.

8. LOKEN T., ALEKSANDERSEN M., REID H. & POW I. (1998). Malignant catarrhal fever caused by ovine herpesvirus-2 in pigs in Norway. *Vet. Rec.*, **143**, 464–467.

9. MICHEL A.L. & ASPELING I.A. (1994). Evidence of persistent malignant catarrhal fever infection in a cow, obtained by nucleic acid hybridisation. *J. S. Afr. Vet. Assoc.*, **65**, 26–27.

10. MICHEL A.L., VAN DER LUGT J.J., BENGIS R.G. & DE VOS V. (1997). Detection of AHV-1 DNA in lung sections from blue wildebeest *(Connochaetes taurinus)* calves by *in situ* hybridisation. *Ondesterpoort J. Vet. Res.*, **64**, 169–172.

11. PLOWRIGHT W., FERRIS R.D. & SCOTT G.R. (1960). Blue wildebeest and the aetiological agent of bovine catarrhal fever. *Nature*, **188**, 1167–1169.

12. REID H.W., BUXTON D., POW I. & FINLAYSON J. (1989). Isolation and characterisation of lymphoblastoid cells from cattle and deer affected with 'sheep-associated' malignant catarrhal fever. *Res. Vet. Sci.*, **47**, 90–96.

*

* *

CHAPTER X.3.

Q FEVER

SUMMARY

Q fever is a zoonosis that occurs in most countries. Humans acquire infection from animal reservoirs, especially from ruminants. Q fever is a contagious disease, which is due to the proliferation in the body of a rickettsia, Coxiella burnetii, *a small bacterium measuring 0.3–1.5 µm × 0.25 µm. It can be stained by Stamp's or Giemsa or Gimenez methods, and it occurs in two forms: the pathogenic phase I, recovered from animals or humans, and the less pathogenic phase II, obtained by repeated passages in eggs or in cell cultures. As an obligate intracellular bacterium,* C. burnetii *can be grown only in embryonated eggs or cell cultures, or if unavoidable in inoculated laboratory animals.*

In humans, Q fever occurs in either an acute form (pneumonia, hepatitis, influenza-like symptoms, headache) or a severe chronic form (endocarditis) following an early infection, which may have passed unnoticed. The first form resolves quite quickly after appropriate antibiotic therapy, but the chronic form requires prolonged antibiotic therapy (for 2 years or more), coupled with constant serological monitoring. In some countries, a vaccine is available for laboratory and abattoir workers.

In animals, cattle develop a subacute form with abortion, retained placentitis, endometritis, infertility and low birth weight. In small ruminants, Q fever is often associated with an acute form inducing outbreaks of abortions followed by recovery without complications. Recurrences over many successive years are quite common. Domestic animals, such as cats, rabbits, etc., can present the same type of disease, and should be regarded as sources of infection for humans.

Laboratory personnel handling C. burnetii *must remember that this microorganism is extremely hazardous, and isolation of* C. burnetii *must be done only in biosafety level 3 laboratories.*

Identification of the agent: *For laboratory diagnosis, samples can be taken from the placenta, vaginal discharges, stomach contents of the aborted fetuses and, when necessary, from milk and colostrum (although* C. burnetii *is irregularly present in these fluids).*

The bacteria can be visualised by microscopy with an oil-immersion objective lens applied to placental smears stained with 2% basic fuchsin and counterstained with methylene blue, where it appears as a red-stained body (Stamp's staining). This finding, coupled with serological tests and clinical findings, is sufficient to establish a diagnosis at the flock or herd level. Coxiella burnetii *can be isolated by inoculation of specimens into conventional cell cultures or into embryonated chicken yolk sacs or laboratory animals. Inoculation of laboratory animals (guinea-pig, mouse, hamster) is helpful in cases requiring isolation from tissues contaminated with various bacteria or in order to obtain phase I* Coxiella *antigens from phase II cells. Demonstration of the agent by the polymerase chain reaction can be done in suitably equipped laboratories.*

Serological tests: *A number of tests can be used, particularly the indirect immunofluorescence test, the enzyme-linked immunosorbent assay, and the complement fixation test.*

Requirements for vaccines and diagnostic biologicals: *Vaccines against Q fever are inactivated vaccines prepared from infected yolk sacs following the inoculation of embryonated hens' eggs. The vaccine may be in the form of an aqueous suspension of rickettsias, and may contain an adjuvant (aluminium hydroxide or a mineral oil emulsion). Annual revaccination is recommended. The vaccine can be combined with other antigens, particularly with chlamydial antigen, to provide a polyvalent vaccine for use in sheep, goats and cattle.*

Localised adverse reactions may occur, particularly in heavily infected herds of cattle. Verification of the vaccine efficacy is done by testing for complement-fixing antibody in vaccinated rabbits. The presence of complement-fixing antibody in vaccinated ruminants is erratic. Vaccines causing milder reactions can be prepared, but they are expensive.

A. DIAGNOSTIC TECHNIQUES

Q fever is an infectious disease that occurs in most countries. The aetiological agent, *Coxiella burnetii,* has been classified in the Rickettsiaceae family; however, recent phylogenetic investigations, based mainly on 16s rRNA sequence analysis, have shown that the *Coxiella* genus belongs to the gamma subdivision of Proteobacteria with the genera *Legionella, Francisella* and *Rickettsiella* as its closest relatives. The other rickettsiae have been placed in the alpha 1 subdivision of Proteobacteria (23) Unlike other rickettsias, *C. burnetii* produces a small, dense, highly resistant spore-like form, whose stability in the environment is important for transmission (9, 12). Q fever is a zoonosis, and in humans the infection has two forms: acute and chronic. The acute form is manifested by pneumonia, prolonged fever, granulomatous hepatitis and, rarely, meningoencephalitis. The main clinical manifestation of chronic Q fever is endocarditis. The epidemiology of Q fever suggests that the disease can be transmitted through contact with infected animals, blood transfusions, inhalation of infectious aerosol, the digestive tract, skin trauma, and sexual contact, and, rarely, by vertical transmission (7, 12). In cows, ewes and goats, Q fever can induce abortion and reproductive disorders (4). Domestic animals, such as cats, rabbits, etc., can present the same type of disease, and should be regarded as sources of infection for humans (14).

Serological evidence of the disease has been obtained in most countries. The presence of serological reactions in a given species and a given country does not necessarily correlate with expression of the clinical disease. Moreover, the isolation of *C. burnetii* does not automatically mean that there is a clinical manifestation of the disease. In sheep flocks or cattle herds in which abortion may or may not have occurred, the rickettsia can be recovered (though rarely) from the placenta after a normal parturition. It may be present exceptionally and in small numbers in milk from infected animals (5). Ticks might be involved in transmitting the disease, but it is more likely to be transmitted by the respiratory route, by inhaling dust contaminated with the Q fever agent, derived from the large numbers present in the placenta of animals that have aborted.

It is important to remember that *C. burnetii* is extremely hazardous to humans, and laboratory infections are common. Appropriate precautions must be taken when the microorganism is handled and isolation of *C. burnetii* must be done only in biosafety level 3 laboratories.

1. Identification of the agent

Samples should be collected from the fetus, placenta and vaginal discharges soon after abortion. Milk or colostrum samples can also be taken. *Coxiella burnetii* can be demonstrated in various ways, depending on the type of sample and the purpose of diagnosis (7, 18).

Smears are prepared on microscope slides of placental tissue from a case of abortion suspected of being caused by a rickettsial infection. These are stained by a rapid method (Stamp) using 2% basic fuchsin solution, followed by rapid decoloration with 0.5% acetic acid solution, and counterstaining with 1% methylene blue or malachite green solution. The smears are examined microscopically (×500). A very large number of thin, pink-stained bacillary bodies will be seen against a blue or green background. These may sometimes be difficult to detect because of their small size (0.3–1.5 µm long × 0.25 µm wide), which is compensated for by their large numbers; the organisms can often be visualised as inclusions within the host cells where they appear as red masses against the blue or green background. Microscopically, *C. burnetii* can be confused with *Chlamydia psittaci* or *Brucella* spp. However, by the same staining procedure, *Chlamydia* have sharper outlines, are round, small and may resemble globules. *Brucella* are larger (0.6–1.5 µm long × 0.5–0.7 µm wide), more clearly defined and stained more intensely. Diagnosis made on the basis of microscopy, coupled with positive serological results, is usually adequate for routine purposes. In cases where biological staining is inconclusive, indirect immunofluorescence may be employed as a confirmatory test. Human positive control serum or positive guinea-pig serum is used to detect the *Coxiella* organisms on acetone-fixed placental smears. An anti-species (human or guinea-pig) anti-IgG fluorescein isothiocyanate is then used to visualise the organisms. Control positive slides of *C. burnetii, Chlamydia psittaci* and *Brucella* should be available for comparison.

For specific laboratory investigations, it may be necessary to isolate the agent. Where microscopic examination has revealed large numbers of *C. burnetii* combined with a low contamination rate with other bacteria, direct isolation by inoculation of embryonated chicken eggs is possible. For this a portion of placenta is homogenised in phosphate buffered saline (PBS) containing antibiotics (streptomycin and penicillin). After low speed centrifugation, dilutions of the supernatant fluid are inoculated into 5-day-old embryonated chicken eggs via the yolk sac. Any embryos that die during the first 5 days after inoculation are discarded. The yolk sacs are harvested after 10–15 days of incubation. Stained smears of the yolk sac wall are examined to ensure the absence of bacterial contamination and to determine the presence of *C. burnetii*. Further passages may be required to obtain an isolate in pure culture.

In the case of a more heavily contaminated sample, such as a placenta, or where there is only a small number of *C. burnetii* in a body fluid, such as in milk, the inoculation of laboratory animals may be necessary. Mice and guinea-pigs are the most appropriate laboratory animals for this purpose. Guinea-pigs should be used in preference as they are approximately tenfold more susceptible than mice. Following intraperitoneal inoculation, body temperature and antibody status are monitored. If pyrexia develops, the animal is killed and the spleen is removed for recovery of the agent by inoculation into embryonated chicken eggs. This method should always be performed in conjunction with serological tests on other guinea-pigs that have been inoculated with the same samples. These sera are collected 21 days after inoculation. Any positive results will confirm a diagnosis of *C. burnetii* infection.

In human medicine, the recent development of a cell microculture system from a commercially available method for virus culture, the 'shell vial cell culture[1]', has improved the method for isolating intracellular bacteria, such as *C. burnetii*. The shell vial cell culture system is described in ref. 7. Samples are inoculated into human embryonic lung fibroblasts grown on a 1 cm^2 cover-slip within a shell vial. A 1-hour centrifugation step enhances the attachment and penetration of bacteria into the cells. After an incubation period of 6 days, detection of *C. burnetii* within the cells is achieved by microscopic examination after staining, and the identification can be performed by a direct immunofluorescence assay with polyclonal or monoclonal anti-*C.-burnetii* antibodies conjugated to fluorescein isothiocyanate (7). This method of detection could be adapted in veterinary medicine for numerous cases. A detailed description of isolation of *C. burnetii* in cell culture is given in refs 7 and 15.

Detection of *C. burnetii* in samples can be achieved by other methods, such as immunodetection in tissues (capture enzyme-linked immunosorbent assay [ELISA], immunohistology), or DNA amplification. Immunohistology, using immunoperoxidase staining, may be used with paraffin-embedded tissues to reveal the presence of *C. burnetii* in tissues such as cardiac valve (17). Polymerase chain reaction (PCR) has been used successfully to detect *C. burnetii* DNA in cell cultures and clinical samples, and has proven to be more sensitive than standard culture techniques. This technique can be performed by suitably equipped laboratories using primers derived from the *htpAB*-associated repetitive element or from an intervening sequence of the 23S rRNA gene (8, 22).

2. Serological tests

Various techniques can be employed, but the three most often used are: indirect immunofluorescence (IFA) test, the ELISA and the complement fixation (CF) test. A few older serological tests are no longer used in routine diagnosis: the microagglutination technique, the capillary agglutination test and the allergic test.

a) Indirect immunofluorescence test

In human medicine, the immunofluorescence assay adapted as a microimmunofluorescence technique is the reference method for the serodiagnosis of Q fever (7). In order to exclude nonspecific fluorescence, it is preferable to use a highly purified antigen. Some commercial CF test antigens are suitable, but antigens prepared for the diagnosis of human Q fever are preferred. These can be adapted by replacing the human conjugate by a fluorescent conjugate adapted to the animal species. Both phase I and phase II *C. burnetii* antigens are used; phase II antigen is obtained by growing *C. burnetii* in cell culture, while phase I antigen is obtained from spleens of infected mice. The two forms of the infection, acute and chronic, have different serological profiles: during acute Q fever, IgG antibodies are elevated only against phase II whereas during chronic Q fever, high levels of IgG antibodies to both phases I and II of the bacteria are observed (15).

Twofold dilutions of the serum under test are placed on immunofluorescence slides with wells previously coated with the antigen. If specific antibodies are present, they are fixed by the antigen on the slide. The complex is then detected by examination with a fluorescence microscope following the addition of the fluorescent conjugate recognising the species immunoglobulins.

- **Materials and reagents**

Microscope equipped for fluorescence, humidified incubator, washing basin, and slides to support the antigen are necessary. The latter may be purchased from a supplier or prepared in the laboratory (12 wells each of 7 mm diameter per slide, coated with antigen and stored at 4°C or –20°C).

Concentrated fluorescent conjugate, to be diluted when required with PBS + 0.1 p1000 Evans blue at the dilution recommended by the manufacturer.

1 Sterilin, Bibby Sterilin Ltd, Stone, Staffordshire ST15 O5A, United Kingdom.

PBS, buffered glycerine, Evans blue dye 1% solution.

- **Test procedure**

i) Inactivate the sera under test for 30 minutes at 56°C, then dilute from 1/20 to 1/2560.

ii) Allow the previously antigen-coated slides to warm to room temperature. Do not touch the wells.

iii) Add 30 µl of each serum dilution to the wells. Add negative and positive control sera. To one well, add 30 µl of PBS to serve as antigen control.

iv) Incubate in a humid chamber for 30 minutes at 37°C. Wash the slide twice with PBS for 10 minutes each. Rinse with distilled water and air dry.

v) Add to the wells, including the controls, 30 µl of the conjugate, freshly diluted in PBS + Evans blue. Incubate in a humid chamber for 30 minutes at 37°C. Rinse with distilled water and air-dry. Add a few drops of buffered glycerine and cover with a cover-slip. Examine under a fluorescence microscope at magnification ×40 or more.

- **Interpretation of the results**

A positive reaction will consist of small brilliant points against a dark background. In a negative reaction, small brilliant points will not be present.

Verify that the conjugate by itself and the negative control serum give a negative result. Nonspecific fluorescence usually takes the form of spots of irregular shape.

The reaction is considered to be positive if there is obvious immunofluorescence at 1/20 or 1/40. Values of 1/160–1/320 or above may occur during acute infection or following *C. burnetii* abortion. In human medicine, this method is used to determine antibodies to phases I and II in the IgG, IgM, and IgA fractions allowing acute and chronic Q fever to be differentiated.

b) Enzyme-linked immunosorbent assay

This is the most sensitive technique. It is easy to perform in laboratories that have the necessary equipment (particularly a spectrophotometer) and reagents. The ELISA is beginning to replace the IFA and CF tests as the test of choice. It requires a relatively pure antigen. Antigens prepared for the CF test may be used for coating the plates. Ready-to-use kits are commercially available. Both anti-phase I and II antibodies are detected by ELISA (2, 6, 7, 21).

Wells of the microplate are coated with inactivated antigen. Diluted serum samples are added to the wells and react to antigens bound to the solid support. Unbound material is removed by washing after a suitable incubation period. Conjugate (horesradish-peroxidase-labelled anti-ruminant Ig) reacts with specific antibodies bound to the antigen. Unreacted conjugate is removed by washing after a suitable incubation period. Enzyme substrate is added. The rate of conversion of substrate is proportional to the amount of bound antibodies. The reaction is terminated after a suitable time and the amount of colour development is measured spectrophotometrically.

- **Materials and reagents**

Microtitre plates with 96 flat-bottomed wells, freshly coated or previously coated with Q fever antigen; photometer; microplate reader (spectrophotometer; 405 and/or 490 nm filters); 37°C humidified incubator; 8- and 12-channel pipettes with disposable plastic tips; microplate shaker (optional).

Positive and negative control sera; conjugate (ruminant anti-immunoglobulin labelled with peroxidase); tenfold concentration of diluent (PBS–Tween); distilled water; substrate or chromogen (OPD [orthophenylene diamine], ABTS [2,2'-Azino-bis-(3-ethylbenzothiazoline-6-sulphonic acid)] for peroxidase); hydrogen peroxide.

- **Test procedure**

i) Prepare the required volume of diluent by adding nine volumes of distilled water to one volume of concentrated diluent. Reconstitute freeze-dried components, if required, while equilibrating other reagents.

ii) Allow the microplates and the chromogen solution to equilibrate to room temperature.

iii) Dilute the serum samples, including control sera, to the appropriated dilution (usually 1/100) and distribute 0.1 ml per well in duplicate.

iv) Cover the plate with a lid and incubate at room temperature for 30–90 minutes. Shake out the contents and wash three times in washing solution at room temperature.

v) Add the appropriate dilution of freshly prepared conjugate to the wells (0.1 ml per well).

vi) Cover each plate and incubate as in step iv. Wash again three times.

vii) Add 0.1 ml of freshly prepared chromogen substrate solution to each well (for example: OPD [0.1 mg/ml] in 0.1 M acetic acid, 0.2 M Na_2HPO_4, pH 4.8, and 30% H_2O_2 solution [0.2 µl/ml]; or 0.25 mM ABTS in citrate phosphate buffer, pH 5.0, and 30% H_2O_2 solution [0.1 µl/ml]).

viii) Shake the plate; after incubation, stop the reaction by adding stopping solution to each well, e.g. 0.05 ml 3 M sulphuric acid for peroxidase or 10% sodium dodecyl sulphate (SDS) for ABTS.

ix) Read the absorbance of each well with the microplate reader at 405 nm (ABTS) or 490 nm (OPD). The absorbance values will be used to calculate the results.

- **Interpretation of the results**

For commercial kits, interpretations and values are provided with the kit.

For example: calculate the mean absorbance (Ab) of the sample serum and of the positive (Ab_{pos}) and negative (Ab_{neg}) control sera, and for each serum, calculate the percentage:

$$\frac{Ab - Ab_{neg}}{Ab_{pos} - Ab_{neg}} \times 100$$

Interpret the results as follows:

Ab <30%	negative serum
Ab 30–40%	doubtful serum
Ab >40%	positive serum

c) Complement fixation test (18)

This is a cold fixation micromethod of the type developed by Kolmer, and is performed using 96-well U-bottomed microtitre plates. The test detects serum antibodies (e.g. of vaccinated rabbits or for diagnosis of abortion in epidemiological surveys). The CF test is very specific but less sensitive than the ELISA or indirect immunofluorescence test; it still gives excellent results for routine diagnosis at the flock level for abortive diseases (18, 19). This method detects both anti-phase I and II antibodies. Seroconversion is detected later by the CF test than by the immunofluorescence test or ELISA. The CF test is still largely used by many laboratories in many countries.

The reaction is done in two stages. Antigen and complement-fixing antibody are first mixed, and sheep erythrocytes, sensitised by the anti-sheep erythrocyte serum, are added. Fixation of the complement by the antigen/antibody complex during the first step does not permit lysis of erythrocytes; in contrast, if there are no complement-fixing antibodies, the complement induces the lysis of the sensitised erythrocytes. Then the haemolysis rate is inversely proportional to the level of specific antibodies present in the sample serum.

- **Reagents**

Veronal/calcium/magnesium buffer (VB), pH 7.2.

The haemolytic system: a mixture of equal parts of a 2% suspension of sheep erythrocytes in VB; and haemolytic serum diluted to a specified titre in VB.

Complement: commercial freeze-dried preparation or fresh guinea-pig serum.

Antigen: use commercial antigens at the titre recommended by the manufacturer if the antigen titration is performed with this method. Results may vary from one antigen to another, and antigens prepared from various strains (ovine, bovine, human) or from indigenous strains should be preferred.

Positive and negative control sera.

- **Pretitrations**

i) Dilute the sheep erythrocytes to a final concentration of 2% in VB.

ii) Titrate the haemolytic serum on a microplate: 25 µl of complement at a known haemolytic concentration (e.g. 1/30); 25 µl of increasing dilutions of haemolytic serum + 2% sheep erythrocytes.

Include controls without complement. Incubate for 30 minutes at 37°C. Establish the dilution equivalent to 2 haemolytic units.

iii) Dilute the antigen as recommended by the manufacturer. The antigen may also be titrated: make increasing dilutions of antigen (25 µl; horizontally) and a positive serum of known titre (25 µl, vertically). Add 25 µl of the suspension of sensitised erythrocytes and incubate for 30 minutes at 37°C. The antigen titre is the highest dilution producing a positive reaction with the highest serum dilution. Verify the absence of anticomplementary activity of the antigen at different dilutions.

iv) Titrate the complement on a microplate: serially dilute the complement or guinea-pig serum in VB, for example from 1/15 to 1/200. To each well containing 25 µl of this dilution, add 25 µl of antigen and 25 µl of the haemolytic system. Incubate for 30 minutes at 37°C and establish the dilution equivalent to 2 haemolytic units of complement.

- **Test procedure**

i) Make twofold dilutions of decomplemented sample sera from 1/10 to 1/320 in six wells and in four additional wells at dilutions from 1/10 to 1/80 to detect anticomplementary activity (25 µl per well).

ii) Add 25 µl of diluted antigen or 25 µl of VB to control serum wells.

iii) Add 25 µl diluted complement to all wells. Cover the plate with plastic adhesive film and incubate for 18 hours at 4°C.

iv) Remove the plates from the refrigerator, allow them to reach room temperature, and add 25 µl of freshly prepared haemolytic system. Incubate at 37°C for 30 minutes. Centrifuge the plates at 500 ***g*** for 5 minutes at 4°C. Examine the controls and read the results.

- **Interpretation of the results**

Titres between 1/10 and 1/40 can be considered to be a latent infection. Titres of 1/80 or above in one or more sera from a group of from five to ten animals signify active infection. As Q fever is a zoonosis, an appropriate intervention is desirable when several titres reach 1/40.

B. REQUIREMENTS FOR VACCINES AND DIAGNOSTIC BIOLOGICALS

Inactivated vaccines against Q fever are prepared from strains of *C. burnetii* that have been cultured in the yolk sacs of embryonated chicken eggs, preferably from specific pathogen free (SPF) hens (phase II vaccines). Vaccines are presented as an aqueous suspension or an adjuvant preparation. Vaccine emulsified with mineral oil (oil/water emulsion) are the most active. Vaccine strains must be analysed and selected carefully because recent studies of molecular epidemiology have demonstrated an antigenic variation among *C. burnetii* strains independent of phase variation. However, recent phylogenetic analysis indicates that *C. burnetii* is a highly homogeneous species and does not support the existence of previously defined subgroups of strains based either on genotypic heterogeneity or on susceptibility (13, 16).

The ideal situation is to prepare national vaccines from local strains. Serological surveys have shown that ovine and caprine sera react best with the Henzerling strain (ATCC VR 145), while bovine sera react best with the Nine Mile strain (ATCC VR 146). If no local strain is available, a vaccine prepared from these two strains is recommended.

In general, the clinical efficacy of vaccination has been recognised, but it is less effective in preventing excretion of the organism in milk (5). Vaccination failure has been observed among sheep and goats. In an infected environment, annual revaccination is recommended. A phase I vaccine has been developed for human use, with good results (11).

The preparation of a *C. burnetii* vaccine must be reserved for trained staff only working in adequate conditions of protection (at a minimum in a level 3 biosecurity laboratory).

1. Seed management

a) Characteristics of the seed

The standard strain used for vaccine production is often the Nine Mile strain (ATCC VR 146). It is a phase II bovine strain of lower virulence for laboratory personnel than the more recently isolated phase I strains. For vaccination of small ruminants, local or ovine strains are indicated.

b) Method of culture

Culture of *C. burnetii* in SPF embryonated eggs converts it to phase II. On the other hand, passage in animals can restore any loss of virulence and maintain it in phase I. Seed stocks of *C. burnetii* are either freeze-dried or placed in ampoules for storage at –80°C or in liquid nitrogen.

c) Validation as a vaccine

The vaccine is injected subcutaneously behind the shoulder in sheep or goats, and into the neck of cattle. Vaccination reduces but does not suppress excretion of *C. burnetii* after parturition (1, 3, 20). In infected herds of cattle, vaccination reduces considerably the number of cases of endometritis, infertility and weak calves (10).

2. Method of manufacture

SPF eggs must be used for vaccine production. At 5–6 days of incubation, the microorganism is inoculated into the yolk sac of the embryonated eggs, which are harvested after death of the embryo at 12–15 days. Infected yolk sacs have a characteristic straw-yellow colour. Uninfected yolk sacs are orange in colour and have a viscous consistency. Any embryos that die between 5 and 10 days of incubation are discarded.

The virulent strain used for egg inoculation is a 1/100 homogenate of yolk sac in PBS containing penicillin (500 International Units/ml) and streptomycin (0.5 mg/ml). The yolk sacs are pooled and homogenised with three parts PBS.

The suspension is inactivated with 1.6% formaldehyde for 24 hours at 37°C. It is stored at 4°C until tests for safety, inactivation and sterility have been completed. The lipid supernatant fluid is discarded. The suspension is then centrifuged at moderate speed (~500 *g*) for 30 minutes. After removal of the supernatant fluid, more PBS is added and centrifugation is repeated. The final suspension is diluted with PBS to provide 20 vaccine doses per egg, or 20 ml per egg in the case of an oil emulsion vaccine used in a dose of 2 ml. Thiomersal is added as an antibacterial preservative at a final dilution of 1/10,000.

Q fever vaccine may be used by itself or in combination with other antigens, for example *Chlamydia* vaccine, to give a combination suitable for preventing outbreaks of abortion and reproductive disorders in cows, ewes and goats.

Q fever vaccine may be prepared as an oil emulsion containing one volume of inactivated *C. burnetii* suspension and one volume of oil phase (e.g. Montanide 80® or Marcol 82® and a water-dispersible emulsifier). It may also be prepared in aluminium hydroxide adjuvant.

3. In-process control

The abundance of *C. burnetii* and the absence of bacterial contaminants in homogenate of yolk sacs suspended in PBS is verified by microscopic examination of a smear on a microscope slide, stained by Stamp's method.

4. Batch control

a) Sterility and confirmation of identity

Tests for sterility and freedom from contamination of biological materials may be found in Chapter I.4.

Observation by microscopy with an oil-immersion lens of numerous thin and short bacilli, of homogeneous appearance, in a slide smear stained by Stamp's method is sufficient to confirm that the suspension does contain rickettsias of the species *C. burnetii*.

b) Safety

The inactivated yolk sac homogenate is inoculated into the yolk sac of batches of ten embryonated eggs at 5 days of incubation. The eggs must remain alive, and are opened after a week of incubation. The yolk sacs must not have the appearance or colour of eggs infected with *C. burnetii*. A second subculture is carried out, and there must be no abnormalities when the eggs are opened. In addition, a double dose of the final vaccine is inoculated into two animals of the target species.

c) Potency

It is difficult to titrate homogenised yolk sac suspension by egg inoculation because embryonic mortality is not related directly to the degree of dilution. However, titration is made easier by using SPF eggs. Simple microscopic observation provides an approximate indication of the strength of a suspension.

Tests on the target species are generally ruled out because of the difficulties of the test and the potential risk to personnel. Testing of the serological response of the target animal to vaccination is also ruled out because the appearance of complement-fixing antibody is irregular in ruminants.

The activity of the vaccine can be confirmed in laboratory animals by the kinetics and titre of complement-fixing antibodies. Rabbits give a good response to vaccination. Blood samples are taken from five or ten rabbits before and 3 weeks after vaccination with 2 ml of vaccine. There should be an increase in the titre of complement-fixing antibodies to approximately 1/20–1/80.

d) Duration of immunity

The vaccination protocol usually consists of one subcutaneous injection in a nonpregnant animal, preferably 15 days before insemination or mating. In a heavily infected environment, a second inoculation may be given a month later.

e) Stability

Fluid inactivated vaccine, ready for immediate use, maintains its antigenicity and can be stored for 2 years at 2–6°C.

f) Preservatives

Formaldehyde-inactivated vaccine contains thiomersal at a final concentration of 1/10,000.

g) Precautions (hazards)

Sterile equipment is essential for vaccinal injections. Vaccine is inoculated subcutaneously in order to avoid severe local reactions. Such reactions, occasionally seen in cattle, are due to the oil adjuvant, to an existing infection that has sensitised the herd, or to faulty purification of the rickettsial suspension.

The best results are obtained by primary vaccination of uninfected heifers.

Vaccines causing a reduced reaction can be prepared after purification with chloroform/methanol. However, they may be less antigenic and are more expensive.

5. Tests on the final product

a) Safety

Sterility is tested on a sample of bottles from each batch. As the safety of the stock vaccine has been tested already, it does not need to be repeated.

b) Potency

As potency in rabbits is verified for the stock vaccine, it does not have to be repeated for each production batch.

REFERENCES

1. BEHYMER D.E., BIBERSTEIN E.L., RIEMANN H.P., FRANTI C.E., SAWYER M., RUPANNER R. & CRENSHAW G.L. (1976). Q fever *(Coxiella burnetii)* investigations in dairy cattle: challenge of immunity after vaccination. *Am. J. Vet. Res.*, **37**, 631–634.

2. BEHYMER D., RUPPANER R., BROOKS D. & WILLIAMS J. (1985). Enzyme immunoassay for surveillance of Q fever. *Am. J. Vet. Res.*, **46**, 2413–2417.

3. BROOKS D.L., ERMEL R.W., FRANTI C.E., RUPANNER R., BEHYMER D.E., WILLIAMS J.C. & STEPHENSON J.C. (1986). Q fever vaccination of sheep: challenge of immunity in ewes. *Am. J. Vet. Res.*, **47**, 1235–1238.

4. CHARTIER C., BEZIAUD E., BUZONI-GATEL D., BOUT D., CALAMEL M., RUSSO P., PEPIN M., MALLEREAU M.P., LENFANT D. & DUFOUR P. (1997). Enquête séro-épidémiologique sur les avortements infectieux des caprins en région Poitou-Charentes. *Rev. Med. Vet.*, **148**, 489–496.

5. DURAND M.P. & DURAND J.L. (1993). La fièvre Q. Epidémiologie et prophylaxie humaine et animale. *Bull. Soc. Vet. Prat. de France*, **77**, 269–297.

6. FIELD P.R., HUNT J.G. & MURPHY A.M. (1983). Detection and persistence of specific IgM antibody to *Coxiella burnetii* by enzyme linked immunosorbent assay: a comparison with immunofluorescence and complement fixation tests. *J. Infect. Dis.*, **148**, 477–187.

7. FOURNIER P.E., MARRIE T.J. & RAOULT D. (1998). Diagnosis of Q fever. J. *Clin. Microbiol.*, **36**, 1823–1834.

8. IBRAHIM A., NORLANDER L. MACELLARO A. & SJOSTEDT A. (1997). Specific detection of *Coxiella burnetii* through partial amplification of 23S rDNA. *Eur. J. Epidemiol.*, **13**, 329–334.

9. LA SCOLA B. & RAOULT D. (1997). Laboratory diagnosis of rickettsioses: current approaches to diagnosis of old and new rickettsial diseases. *J. Clin. Microbiol.*, **35**, 2715–2727.

10. LUOTO L., WINN J. & HUEBNER R. (1952). Q fever studies in southern California: vaccination of dairy cattle against Q fever. *Am. J. Hyg.*, **55**, 190–202.

11. MARMION B.P., ORMSBEE R.A. & KYRKOV N.V. (1990). Vaccine prophylaxis of abattoir associated Q fever. Eight years experience in Australian abattoirs. *Epidemiol. Infect.*, **104**, 275–287.

12. MARRIE T.J. (1990). Q fever – a review. *Can. Vet. J.*, **31**, 555–563.

13. MASUZAWA T. SAWAKI K., NAGAOKA H., AKIYAMA M., HIRAI K. & YANAGIHARA Y. (1997). Identification of rickettsiae isolated in Japan as *Coxiella burnetii* by 16S rRNA sequencing. *Int. J. Syst. Bacteriol.*, **47**, 883–884.

14. MATTHEWMAN L., KELLY P., HAYTER D., DOWNIE S., WRAY K., BRYSON N., RYCROFT A. & RAOULT D. (1997). Exposure of cats in southern Africa to *Coxiella burnetii*, the agent of Q fever. *Eur. J. Epidemiol.*, **13**, 477–480.

15. MAURIN M. & RAOULT D. (1999). Q fever. *Clin. Microbiol. Rev.*, **12**, 518–553.

16. MOLLET C., DRANCOURT M. & RAOULT D. (1998). Determination of *Coxiella burnetii rpoB* sequence and its use for phylogenetic analysis. *Gene*, **207**, 97–103.

17. RAOULT D., LAURENT J.C. & MULTILLOD M. (1994). Monoclonal antibodies to *Coxiella burnetii* for antigenic detection in cell cultures and in paraffin embedded tissues. *Am. J. Clin. Pathol.*, **101**, 318–320.

18. RUSSO P. (1997). Infection à *Coxiella burnetii* ou Fièvre Q. *In:* Manuel pratique de diagnostic de laboratoire des avortements infectieux des petits ruminants, Rodolakis A. & Nettleton P., eds. L'Espace Vétérinaire, Casablanca, Morocco, 79–88.

19. SANCHIS R., RUSSO P., CALAMEL M. & PEPIN M. (1997). Diagnostic différentiel des avortements infectieux des petits ruminants. *In:* Manuel pratique de diagnostic de laboratoire des avortements infectieux des petits ruminants, Rodolakis A. & Nettleton P., eds. L'Espace Vétérinaire, Casablanca, Morocco, 25–34.

20. SCHMEER N., MULLER P., LANGEL J., KRAUSS H., FROST S. & WIEDA J. (1987). Q fever vaccines for animals. *Zentralbl. Bakteriol. Mikrobiol. Hyg. A.*, **267**, 79–88.

21. SOLIMAN A.N., BOTROS B.A. & WATTS D.M. (1992). Evaluation of a competitive immunoassay for detection of *Coxiella burnetii* antibody in animal sera. *J. Clin. Microbiol.*, **30**, 1595–1597.

22. STEIN A. & RAOULD D. (1992). Detection of *Coxiella burnetii* by DNA amplification using polymerase chain reaction. *J. Clin. Microbiol.*, **30**, 2462–2466.

23. WEISBURG W.G., DOBSON M.E., SAMUEL J.E., DASCH G.A., MALLAVIA L.P., BACA O., MANDELCO L., SECHREST J.E., WEISS E. & WOESE C.R. (1989). Phylogenetic diversity of the Rickettsiae. *J. Bacteriol.*, **171**, 4202–4206.

*

* *

CHAPTER X.4.

SALMONELLOSIS

SUMMARY

Salmonellosis is an infectious disease of humans and animals caused by organisms of the two species of salmonella (Salmonella enterica *and* S. bongori). *Although primarily intestinal bacteria, salmonellae are widespread in the environment and commonly found in farm effluents, human sewage and in any material subject to faecal contamination. Salmonellosis has been recognised in all countries, but appears to be most prevalent in areas of intensive animal husbandry, especially of poultry or pigs and dairy cattle reared in confinement.*

The disease can affect all species of domestic animals; young animals and pregnant and lactating animals are the most susceptible. Enteric disease is the commonest clinical manifestation, but a wide range of clinical signs, which include acute septicaemia, abortion, arthritis and respiratory disease, may be seen. Many animals, however, may also be infected but show no clinical illness. Such animals may be important in relation to the spread of infection between flocks and herds and as causes of human food poisoning.

Identification of the agent: *Diagnosis is based on the isolation of the organism either from tissues collected aseptically at necropsy or from faeces, rectal swabs or environmental samples. When infection of the reproductive organs or conceptus occurs, it is necessary to culture fetal stomach contents, placenta and vaginal swabs and, in the case of poultry, egg contents.*

Salmonellae may be isolated by a variety of techniques, which may include pre-enrichment to resuscitate sublethally damaged salmonellae, enrichment media that contain inhibitory substances to suppress non-salmonella organisms, and selective plating agars to differentiate salmonellae from other enterobacteria.

Various biochemical and serological tests can be applied to the pure culture to provide a definitive confirmation of an isolated strain. Salmonellae possess antigens designated somatic (O), flagellar (H) and virulent (Vi), which may be identified by specific typing sera, and the serovar may be determined by reference to the antigenic formulae in the Kauffman–White scheme. Many laboratories may need to send isolates to a reference laboratory to confirm the full serological identity.

Serological tests: *These are preferably conducted on a representative sample of the population and may be of limited value except in endemic situations. In poultry, the whole blood test is used for rapid diagnosis of* S. pullorum/gallinarum *on the farm. In the laboratory, the tube agglutination test is the method of choice for export and diagnostic purposes for samples from all species of farm animals. Enzyme-linked immunosorbent assays are available for some serovars and may be used for serological diagnosis and surveillance.*

Requirements for vaccines and diagnostic biologicals: *Many inactivated vaccines are used against salmonellosis and some live vaccines are available commercially. While inactivated vaccines have been used successfully in a number of circumstances, the efficacy of some may be low, and therefore oil or alhydrogel adjuvants have been used. Field efficacy data are often lacking, although laboratory testing may provide a useful indication. Innocuity tests are performed in laboratory animals and, in the case of inactivated vaccines, sterility tests using bacteriological enrichment media are carried out. Further reassurances, such as environmental impact and stability, are necessary for vaccines produced using genetic manipulation.*

SPECIAL NOTE ON THE NOMENCLATURE OF THE GENUS *SALMONELLA*

The classification of salmonellae has been controversial for many years. According to the latest nomenclature, which reflects recent advances in salmonella taxonomy[1], the genus *Salmonella* consists of only two species: *S. enterica* and *S. bongori* (9, 13). *Salmonella enterica* is divided into six subspecies, which are distinguishable by certain biochemical characteristics and some of which correspond to the previous subgenera. These subspecies are:

- Subspecies I = subspecies *enterica*
- Subspecies II = subspecies *salamae*
- Subspecies IIIa = subspecies *arizonae*
- Subspecies IIIb = subspecies *diarizonae*
- Subspecies IV = subspecies *houtenae*
- Subspecies VI = subspecies *indica*

For the serovars of *S. bongori*, the symbol V was retained to avoid confusion with the serovar name of *S. enterica* subsp. *enterica*. Strains of salmonella are classified into serovars on the basis of extensive diversity of lipopolysaccharide (LPS) (O) antigens and flagellar protein (H) antigens in accordance with the Kauffmann–White scheme; currently 2463 serovars are recognised (13, 14). This number is constantly being increased. The most common serovars that cause infections in humans and food animals belong to subspecies I. The serovars of the other subspecies are common in poikilothermic (cold blooded) animals and in the environment, although some serovars of *S. arizonae* are associated with disease in poultry and sheep.

In this chapter, the previous conventions are followed, using the older terminology; i.e. *S. typhimurium* rather than the more complete nomenclature *S. enterica,* subsp. *enterica* serovar Typhimurium.

A. DIAGNOSTIC TECHNIQUES

Salmonellosis is an infectious disease of humans and animals caused by organisms of the two species of salmonella *(Salmonella enterica* and *S. bongori).* Although primarily intestinal bacteria, salmonellae are widespread in the environment and commonly found in farm effluents, human sewage and in any material subject to faecal contamination. Salmonellosis has been recognised in all countries, but appears to be most prevalent in areas of intensive animal husbandry, especially of poultry or pigs.

The disease can affect all species of domestic animals; young animals and pregnant animals are the most susceptible. Enteric disease is the commonest clinical manifestation, but a wide range of clinical signs, which include acute septicaemia, abortion, arthritic and respiratory disease, may be seen. Many animals, however, may also be infected but show no clinical illness. Such animals may be important in relation to the spread of infection between flocks and herds and as causes of human food poisoning.

The course of infection, the clinical signs, the post-mortem findings and epidemiological patterns vary according to the serovar and the animal species involved. Some serovars only affect certain hosts, e.g. *S. choleraesuis* in pigs, although most serovars may cause disease in a wide range of animal species (15). Many serovars (including some that are host adapted) have been shown to cause human food poisoning, and animal attendants, veterinarians and abattoir workers may be infected directly during the course of their work, as may laboratory personnel.

The most common clinical manifestation is enteritis, although septicaemia, genital infection with abortion, and arthritis often occur. The signs and lesions are not pathognomonic and in many cases, especially in poultry and pigs, salmonella infections may be inapparent (15).

Disease is usually referred to as salmonellosis, although the term paratyphoid may be used, e.g. swine paratyphoid. In poultry, pullorum disease or bacillary white diarrhoea and fowl typhoid are often used to describe infections caused by *S. pullorum* and *S. gallinarum,* respectively (15).

---

1 *Note on nomenclature :*
New terminology for *Salmonella* serovars has been proposed by Popoff M.Y. & LeMinor L. (1997). Antigenic Formulas of the *Salmonella* Serovars. World Health Organization Collaborating Centre for Reference and Research on *Salmonella*. Pasteur Institute, Paris, France. This states 'Names are retained only for subspecies *enterica* serovars. These names must no longer be italicised. The first letter is a capital letter. In clinical practice the subspecies name does not need to be indicated as only serovars of subspecies *enterica* bear a name, e.g. Typhimurium, London or Montevideo are serovars of subspecies enterica. The name *Salmonella* Typhimurium may be used for routine practice'. As this proposal has not yet achieved universal agreement, the old *Salmonella* nomenclature has been retained in this chapter.

For detailed epidemiological investigations, strain identification is necessary and such investigations have traditionally relied on biochemical and serological methods, phage typing of some serovars, and occasionally antibiograms. Genotypic analysis of the organism by plasmid profiles and chromosomal DNA has been used to good effect in recent years. Plasmid profile analyses supply a quick and relatively easy method to fingerprint strains, and have been used in both human and veterinary medicine to study the spread of salmonella. Not all strains of salmonella harbour several plasmids, and alternative genetic techniques have been used to genotype plasmid-free strains (16). Genotyping is a rapidly expanding field and many new methods have been developed in recent years. It should be remembered that a single method may not work for all isolates and it may be necessary to evaluate a number of different techniques to find a method or combination of methods that are satisfactory and capable of differentiating isolates of a particular serovar or phage type.

The isolation and subsequent identification of salmonellae depend not only on the quality of the sample but also on the culture medium and growth characteristics of the serovar, particularly those adapted to a host species. A comprehensive review of *Salmonella* infection in domestic animal has recently been published (20).

National schemes have been implemented in some countries to control salmonella infections in animals in order to protect the consumer. In the European Union, the Zoonoses Directive 92/117/EEC requires the monitoring of breeding flocks of more than 250 birds and hatcheries for *S. enteritidis* and *S. typhimurium* (4). Culture of chicken delivery-box liners and dead or culled chickens is carried out on the day of arrival. At 4 weeks of age and 2 weeks prior to laying, pooled faeces of up to 60 samples, depending on the flock size, are cultured. Subsequently, adults are sampled every 2 weeks. At the hatchery, the meconium and dead-in-shells are cultured every 2 weeks. There is also the possibility that serological monitoring will be permitted if the serological tests can offer guarantees equivalent to the system of inspection at the hatchery.

1. Identification of the agent

The frequency of sampling and the type of samples obtained will depend largely on the clinical findings, laboratory facilities, epidemiological data and the objectives.

Individual samples for bacteriological tests are collected as aseptically as possible and before any antibiotic treatment has commenced. Samples are collected preferably during the acute phase of the disease or as soon as possible after death. In the case of intensively housed poultry flocks, environmental samples, such as litter or swabs from internal surfaces, may be the most cost-effective way to identify infected flocks. Precautions should be taken to avoid cross-contamination of samples during transit and at the laboratory. Packages should be kept cool and accompanied by adequate information. For smaller animal species, it may be preferable to submit a representative number of sick or recently dead animals to the laboratory, if that is possible (19).

Particular attention should be given to the isolation of salmonellae from animals with subclinical infection, as these only excrete bacteria intermittently and in low numbers. An increased sample size, increased number of samples representing more individuals combined with pooling of samples and repeat sampling can provide an increased diagnostic sensitivity. In such situations bacteriological methods should be used to identify infected flocks or herds rather than to identify infected individual animals.

• Isolation media for salmonellae (3, 6, 8, 11, 19)

a) Pre-enrichment media

The number of salmonellae in faeces from asymptomatic animals, environmental samples, animal feed and food is usually low, and it is necessary to use pre-enrichment media, such as buffered peptone water, to assist isolation. This may allow the small numbers of salmonellae, which may otherwise be killed by the toxic effect of enrichment media, to multiply, or it may help to resuscitate salmonellae that have been sublethally damaged, e.g. by freezing, heating or desiccation.

b) Enrichment media

These are liquid or semisolid agar media that contain additives that selectively permit salmonellae to grow while inhibiting the growth of other bacteria. Some, however, are also toxic to certain serovars of salmonella, e.g. selenite is toxic to *S. choleraesuis*, and brilliant green is toxic to *S. dublin*. Elevated temperatures have also been used to increase the selectivity of enrichment medium, and a temperature of 43°C is used in many laboratories, although this may be inhibitory with some media, e.g. tetrathionate and Rappaport–Vassiliadis at 43°C inhibit *S. dublin*. Selective motility enrichment may also be used to increase the sensitivity of salmonella isolation, and passage of a mixed growth of salmonellae and other organisms through 0.1–0.15% nutrient agar increases the proportion of salmonellae to other bacteria. Semisolid enrichment media, e.g. Rappaport–Vassiliadis, may provide greater sensitivity. The formulation of the medium, temperature and duration of incubation, and the volume of the samples used to inoculate the medium, may all serve to improve the isolation rate, and these variables should always be taken into account. Examples of selective enrichment medium are sodium tetrathionate, as in Muller–Kauffman broth, selenite F, brilliant green and Rappaport–Vassiliadis broths, or semisolid Rappaport's medium.

c) **Selective plating media**

These are solid, selective agars that permit differential growth to varying degrees. They inhibit growth of other bacteria and give information on some of the principal differential biochemical characteristics – usually non-lactose fermentation and hydrogen sulphide (H_2S) production. The results are read after 24 and 48 hours of culture at 37°C. Salmonellae form characteristic colonies on such media that are usually distinguishable from the colonies of other bacteria on the plate, with the possible exceptions of *Proteus, Pseudomonas* and *Citrobacter.* Lactose-fermenting salmonellae may occasionally be isolated and H_2S production may be variable. *Salmonella abortusovis* is a slow-growing serovar and it is usual to incubate plates for up to 72 hours and to use the nonselective blood agar. Examples of selective media are brilliant green agar, deoxycholate–citrate agar, Rambach agar, and bismuth sulphite agar, although many more will be found in the literature and media catalogues.

• Identification of suspect colonies

Suspect colonies are subcultured on to selective and nonselective agars to ensure that possible contaminants, such as *Proteus* spp., are absent. If there is an abundant pure growth, suspect colonies may be tested by slide agglutination with polyvalent salmonella-typing sera (10, 13). In some cases, the suspect colony may not agglutinate and it is necessary to use biochemical tests to confirm the identity. These tests can be performed with peptone water sugars or commercial systems, such as the Analytical Profile Index (API) system, or composite media, such as triple sugar iron agar, can be used to screen organisms (5).

The determination of the O factor(s) and the H antigen(s), and in special circumstances the Vi antigen, are performed by direct slide agglutination using specific antisera. In the case of biphasic organisms, it is necessary to determine both phases by phase inversion by passage through semisolid agar containing antiserum to the known phase. Screening is facilitated by the availability of antisera directed against several factors, which can be pursued further by the use of monovalent typing sera. While most laboratories can identify the more common serotypes, it is necessary to use the facilities of a reference laboratory to confirm the identity of an isolate and possibly to obtain information on the phage type, if there is a scheme available, and genetic profile.

Additional biochemical tests may be necessary to identify some serotype variants, e.g. maltose and dulcitol, can be used to differentiate *S. pullorum* from *S. gallinarum*. Isolates should also be tested for their sensitivity to a range of antimicrobial agents.

2. Serological tests

• Serological identification of infected animals, flocks and herds

A number of serological tests have been developed for the diagnosis of salmonella infections in animals. In poultry, the whole blood test, which uses a stained antigen, and the serum agglutination test (SAT) have been used successfully for over 50 years for the identification of flocks infected with *S. pullorum/gallinarum.* Because *S. enteritidis* possesses the same group D somatic antigen as *S. pullorum/gallinarum*, the whole blood test and related tests can be used for the diagnosis of infection. In recent years, other tests, such as the enzyme-linked immunosorbent assay (ELISA) (1, 17) have been developed for the diagnosis of *S. enteritidis* infections in poultry and for other serovars in farm animals. The ELISA has been used effectively to identify serologically *S. dublin* carrier cattle. The mix-ELISA (for serum or meat-juice ELISA) is used in Denmark to detect salmonella infections in pigs (12).

Some ELISAs are now in routine use and a number are available commercially. The purpose of this section is to consider the serological tests that have been fully evaluated and are in routine use for the diagnosis of salmonellosis in animals. Other tests that are still in the development stage will therefore not be considered.

• Factors affecting serological diagnosis

1. Serological methods should be used to identify infected flocks/herds rather than to identify infected individual animals.

2. It is well recognised that some animals with a positive serological response may no longer be infected with salmonella organisms. Likewise, animals that are actively excreting salmonellae may be serologically negative. Similar considerations may also apply to bacteriological culture methods, and negative faecal

culture results may not necessarily indicate that an animal is not infected. However, neither of these situations should be considered to be a major problem. Animals that are serologically positive may have ceased to excrete salmonellae although circulating immunoglobulin concentrations may remain high. Other animals on the farm may still be infected. Serologically negative animals may result from a recent infection causing excretion before immunoglobulin production is maximal, or infection with less invasive serotypes. Animals that have been infected recently would, in all probability, eventually be detected serologically by an appropriate monitoring programme throughout the life of the flock/herd.

3. Newborn animals are immunologically immature and do not respond serologically to the somatic, LPS antigen until 2–3 weeks of age. They do, however, produce a serological response to the flagellar protein antigens. Cattle may be unresponsive until about 10–12 weeks of age.

   Chickens may also acquire salmonella antibodies passively from their parents via the yolk sac; this may indicate an infected parent flock. Mammals can acquire maternally derived antibodies via the colostrum.

4. Following salmonella infections, immunoglobulin concentrations remain elevated for 2–3 months. An IgM response indicates recent infection.

5. Immunisation has been used for many years to control salmonella infections in farm animals, and if diagnostic serology is to be used, it is necessary to differentiate the vaccine response from that of actual infection.

6. The effect of antibiotic therapy on the serological response remains unclear. Some workers found reduced titres following therapy whereas others found no effect. Serology, however, may be more useful diagnostic technique for salmonellosis than culture if antimicrobial therapy has been used.

7. More than 2400 different salmonella serovars exist. Depending on the antigen and test used, serological cross-reactions between different serovars may occur, e.g. *S. typhimurium* and *S. enteritidis.*

8. In poultry, egg yolk may be tested for immunoglobulins to salmonella and eggs may provide a method to screen flocks. In cattle, milk may be tested for salmonella antibodies to screen dairy herds.

9. The use of filter-paper discs for serum collection obviates the necessity to separate serum. The discs also provide long-term storage and reduce transport costs to the laboratory.

a) The whole blood test

The whole blood test provides a rapid test for fowl typhoid and pullorum disease that can be used on the farm. The sensitivity of the whole blood test is low and in inexperienced hands false-positive and false-negative results may be recorded.

For a detailed description of the whole blood test, see Chapter 2.7.5. Fowl typhoid and Pullorum disease.

b) Rapid slide agglutination test

Serum (0.02 ml) is mixed with polyvalent crystal-violet-stained antigen (0.02 ml). The tile is rocked gently for 2 minutes, after which the test is read. The test components are stored at 4°C and must have reached room temperature before being used.

Test sera should be free from contamination and haemolysis. It may be helpful to centrifuge serum samples that have been stored for any period.

Due to transient, nonspecific reactions, positive/suspicious sera should be retested after heat-inactivation at 56°C for 30 minutes.

c) Serum agglutination test

The SAT is relatively insensitive, and many older animals have low levels of agglutinins in their sera caused by enterobacteria other than salmonella. Single samples are of little value; paired samples are needed as the minimal requirement. The test is relatively cheap; the antigens can be readily prepared and expensive equipment is not necessary. The SAT can be adapted to the microtitre format and can be readily used to determine somatic and flagellar titres. It is advisable to have standard sera for quality control of SAT antigen preparation(s).

- **Preparation of somatic antigen**

i) Plate out the salmonella culture from the appropriate stock culture on to a blood agar base (BAB) plate, or other suitable medium, for single colony growth. Incubate overnight at 37°C (±2°C).

ii) Select a smooth colony and carry out a slide agglutination test to ensure that the required somatic antigen is present.

iii) Using a sterile loop, inoculate a nutrient agar slope in a universal container from the selected colony.

iv) Incubate the culture for 8–12 hours at 37°C (±2°C).

v) Using a Pasteur pipette, wash off the culture, preferably inside a safety cabinet, with approximately 2 ml of absolute alcohol, and transfer into a sterile universal container.

vi) Leave the antigen for 4–6 hours at room temperature to enable the alcohol to kill the bacteria and detach flagellae.

vii) Spin the universal container in a bench-top centrifuge for 5 minutes at 1000 ***g***. Pour off the liquid and add enough phenol saline to make the antigen up to an opacity equivalent to Brown's tube no. 2 (approximately 10^8 colony-forming units/ml) or other appropriate standard.

viii) Carry out standard titration with known serum to ensure that the antigen is positive for the required factor.

ix) Store in a refrigerator at 4°C until required.

- **Preparation of flagellar antigens**

i) Plate out the appropriate salmonella stock culture on to a BAB plate, or other appropriate medium. Incubate overnight at 37°C (±2°C).

ii) Passage in semisolid agar (about 0.3%) in a Craigie's tube, or other suitable container, to induce optimum expression of the appropriate flagellar antigen. If the serovar is biphasic, H antiserum corresponding to the phase to be suppressed is added to the agar.

iii) Use slide agglutination to check that the salmonella is in the required phase. If this is correct, inoculate a loop of culture into 20 ml of nutrient broth. Incubate for 12–18 hours at 37°C (±2°C) for optimum growth. (If the phase is incorrect, repassage through semisolid agar.)

iv) Pipette 250 µl of 40% formaldehyde into the antigen suspension (use gloves and preferably work in a safety cabinet), and leave overnight.

v) Test the antigen by SAT using the appropriate typing serum.

- **Test procedure**

i) It is easiest to screen the sera at a dilution of 1/20; 0.25 ml of antigen is added to 0.25 ml of serum prediluted to 1/10 in normal saline.

ii) The tests are incubated in a water bath at 50°C, for 24 hours in the case of somatic antigens and for 4 hours for the flagellar antigens.

iii) Sera that give a positive reaction are then diluted from 1/20 to 1/320 and retested with the appropriate antigen.

d) Enzyme-linked immunosorbent assays for *Salmonella enteritidis*

Two main basic systems are available for detection of IgG (IgY) specific for *S. enteritidis:* the indirect ELISA (1) and the competitive 'sandwich type' ELISA (17).

The indirect ELISA involves the use of a detecting antigen coated on to the wells of a microtitre plate. After the application of a blocking reagent to reduce nonspecific binding, test samples are applied to the wells. Specifically bound antibody in the sample is detected by an antibody/enzyme conjugate. A variety of antigens, including LPS, flagella, SEF14 fimbriae, outer membrane proteins and cruder antigen preparations have been used.

The competitive sandwich ELISA employs a specific reagent – a monoclonal antibody (MAb) – for coating antigen to wells. This is then followed by a pure or crude antigen preparation. Test samples are applied followed by conjugated MAb, which will not bind to the antigen if the sample contained specific antibodies. The assay time can be shortened by adding both test sample and conjugate together. MAbs have been prepared for LPS, flagella and SEF14 for *S. enteritidis.*

There are advantages and disadvantages to both systems. The indirect assay is simpler and reagents are available for all salmonella serotypes of chickens, turkeys, ducks and mammalian hosts. The competitive ELISA can be applied to all animal species and in general shows higher specificity. However, reagents are not available commercially for all serotypes. There are also some affinity problems and it may be less sensitive than the indirect assays. In the field, both systems have produced false-positive reactions.

Both types of assay may be used with serum, yolk or reconstituted dried blood eluted from filter paper discs, which may be treated with some antibacterial agents without loss of antibody titre. A mix-ELISA (or meat-juice ELISA, is used in Denmark to detect salmonella infections in pigs (12). This ELISA contains the O antigens 1, 4, 5, 6, 7 and 12, which enables it to detect serologically 95% of the salmonella serogroups found in Danish pigs. Serum is used to screen breeding and multiplying herds, whereas for pigs in the abattoir, the assay is performed on the juice that is liberated when a frozen 10 g muscle sample is thawed.

With some ELISAs a differentiation can be made between infections produced by salmonella serotypes from different serogroups. Some cross-reaction occurs between groups B and D that, ideally, should be reduced. The optimal method for choosing a 'cut-off' absorbance value, above which sera are designated as having come from an *S.-enteritidis*-infected flock, without producing an unacceptable level of false-positive tests, has not yet been decided on and agreed internationally.

ELISAs are readily adapted to automation and hence to large-scale testing programmes. A major problem is that expensive equipment is necessary and many of the reagents are also expensive.

An example of an ELISA is the one developed at the OIE Reference Laboratory at VLA Weybridge (see Table given in Part 4 of this *Manual*). The requirements are given below.

- **Equipment**

Falcon microtest III PVC plates; appropriate pipettes and measuring cylinders; ultrawash microtest plate washer; ELISA plate reader; test filter of 405–410 nm and reference filter of 630 nm.

- **Antigen**

i) Phenol-extracted *S. enteritidis* LPS is available commercially (Sigma Cat. No. L6011). This is reconstituted in 1 ml deionised water and stored at –20°C in 100 µl aliquots in phosphate buffered saline (PBS), pH 7.2, at a concentration of 2.5 mg/ml. For use, the antigen should be thawed in coating buffer at the appropriate concentration.

ii) The LPS antigen can also be prepared by the technique of Westphal & Luderitz (18) and standardised as to its carbohydrate concentration by the method of Gerhardt (7), and adjusted to 1000 µg/ml.

- **Serum and conjugate diluent**

Add bovine serum albumin (BSA) (2 g) and Tween 20 (0.05 ml) to PBS (100 ml). (Alternatively, powdered milk [1 g] can replace the BSA.) Store at 4°C and make fresh solutions every week.

Coating buffer: add sodium carbonate (1.59 g) and sodium bicarbonate (2.93 g) to deionised water (1 litre) and adjust to pH 9.6. (Alternatively, dissolve one tablet of 0.05 M Sigma carbonate–bicarbonate buffer [Cat. No. C-3041] in deionised water [100 ml].) Store at 4°C and renew every 2 weeks.

Substrate buffer: make a 10% (v/v) solution of diethanolamine in deionised water. The diethanolamine should be prewarmed to 37°C before dispensing, and the pH of the solution should be adjusted to pH 9.8 with 1 M hydrochloric acid. Store at 4°C and renew every 2 weeks.

Enzyme conjugate: goat anti-chicken immunoglobulin conjugated to alkaline phosphatase (e.g. ICN Immunobiologicals, alternative supply Sigma: A9171) or other species anti-chicken globulin. Store at 4°C diluted in diluent at the appropriate concentration and renew every week.

Enzyme substrate: dissolve one tablet of *p*-nitrophenyl phosphate disodium (5 mg) in substrate buffer (5 ml) no earlier than 30 minutes before dispensing, and store in the dark.

- **Standards**

i) Positive control antiserum prepared by intramuscular inoculation of four 1-week-old specific pathogen free (SPF) chickens with an inoculum containing 10^6 *S. enteritidis*. The serum is subsequently obtained 3–4 weeks later when antibody titres are maximal.

ii) Negative control serum A from four 1-week-old SPF birds.

iii) Negative control serum B from 58 1-week-old breeders known to be free from salmonella infections. Pool the sera and store in 100 µl volumes at –20°C.

B. REQUIREMENTS FOR VACCINES AND DIAGNOSTIC BIOLOGICALS

Many inactivated vaccines are used against salmonellosis caused by different serovars in different animal species, including *S. enteritidis* and *S. typhimurium* vaccine for use in poultry. Inactivation is usually achieved by either heating or the use of formalin. Live vaccines have also been used in a number of countries; these include the semi-rough strains, such as 9R for fowl typhoid and HWS51 for *S. dublin* infections. Other methods of attenuation include auxotrophic mutants, which are used to prevent salmonella infections in farm animals in Germany. Mutant vaccines attenuated rationally by molecular biological techniques are now becoming available for evaluation in poultry and other species; these include aroA mutants and strains with mutations in the genes encoding adenylate cyclase (cya) and the cyclic adenosine monophosphate receptor protein (crp) (2), which is now available in the United States of America.

1. Seed management

a) Characteristics of the seed

For killed or living vaccines, the bacterial strain (or each bacterial strain) should be identified by historical records and characterised by stable phenotypic and/or genetic markers. Living vaccinal strains should be marked by stable characters allowing distinction from wild strains. Markers and attenuation of virulence should be stable, and preferably obtained by two independent mutations.

b) Method of culture

The seed culture is propagated and maintained using suitable media, of which many have been described (in textbooks) for growth of salmonella. The media used must not contain serum or animal tissues. Culture may be on solid medium, in Roux flasks, or in liquid medium, in which case large-scale fermentation equipment may be used.

c) Validation as a vaccine

i) *Purity*

The vaccine strain must be checked as follows:

- Staining of a smear of bacterial suspension on a glass slide using Gram stain.
- Homogeneity of culture on nonselective media.
- Metabolic requirements as indicated by biochemical tests.
- Detection of markers and phage type.
- Agglutination with specific antiserum.

ii) *Safety*

The LD_{50} (50% lethal dose) or ID_{50} (50% infectious dose) may be determined in mice. Ten times the field dose of live vaccine or twice the dose for killed vaccines must be given to the target species at the recommended age and by the recommended route. The animals are observed for absence of adverse reactions. Stability and nonreversion to virulence after serial passages in susceptible species should be shown for live vaccines. It is also necessary to consider repeat vaccination.

iii) *Efficacy*

Laboratory experiments and field trials should be used to show that the vaccine is effective. The laboratory experiments consist of vaccination-challenge tests in the target species at the recommended dose and age. The efficacy data can also be used as the basis for a batch potency test. Field trials are more difficult to undertake with respect to testing efficacy, and many problems are encountered in their implementation.

iv) *Environmental aspects*

Live vaccine strains should be tested for their ability to persist in the environment and infect nontarget species that are likely to be exposed.

2. Method of manufacture

Vaccine must be made in suitable clean rooms to which only approved personnel have access. Care must be taken to avoid cross-contamination between infected and uninfected areas and contamination from operators and/or the environment. Operators must not be ill. Personnel must be provided with protective clothing in production areas and in animal rooms.

Seed-lot cultures are prepared from the primary seed-lot, and the number of passages is dependent on the validation of the process. The vaccine may be prepared by inoculation of a suitable medium, such as nutrient broth, with a fresh culture and incubation at 37°C for 24 hours, with or without aeration. The organisms are harvested by sedimentation or centrifugation. Alternatively, the organisms may be grown on and harvested from a solid medium, such as nutrient agar. In the case of live vaccines, the suspension is diluted in PBS, pH 7.0, and may be freeze-dried.

The time of inactivation of dead vaccines should be at least 33% more than that taken to reduce the viable number to an undetectable level. The inactivation process must be applied to the whole volume of the vaccine cell harvest.

Preservatives, excipient for lyophilisation, stabiliser for multidose containers or other substances added to or combined with a vaccinal preparation must have no deleterious effect on the immunising potency of the product.

3. In-process control

The following points require attention:

- Visual control of the suspension, homogeneity by Gram stain, culture on nonselective medium.
- Slide agglutination with specific antisera.
- Titration of bacteria by turbidimetry and/or plate count.
- Test of effective inactivation (dead vaccine) by plating on nonselective medium or use of a medium that gives optimum chance of recovery e.g. production medium with neutralisation of the inactivating compound.
- Titration of viable bacteria (living vaccine) before and after lyophilisation.

4. Batch control

a) Sterility

Tests for sterility and freedom from contamination of biological materials may be found in Chapter I.4.

b) Safety

A laboratory test in mice that has previously shown a correlation with safety in the target species may be used to determine the LD_{50} and/or ID_{50}. Each batch should be tested in the target species at the recommended age and route, using at least twice the field dose for killed vaccines and ten times the dose for live vaccines.

c) Potency

Potency is tested using vaccination-challenge assay in mice and/or other species, including (if practicable) the target species and immunological response in target species.

d) Duration of immunity

It has not been possible to find any data on the duration of immunity. Consultation among colleagues suggests that killed vaccines will provide protection for 6 months, while live vaccines elicit stronger immunity, which may persist for 1 year or more. It should be remembered, however, that a strong challenge may overwhelm vaccinal immunity.

e) Stability

Information is lacking on the stability of killed vaccines. Stability is affected by storage conditions and by the presence of contaminating microorganisms growing in the product. The stability is assessed by potency tests repeated at appropriate time intervals. The stability of live vaccines can be assessed by performing counts of the number of viable organisms repeated at appropriate time intervals.

f) Preservatives

Thiomersal is probably the most widely used preservative.

g) Precautions

Killed vaccines may cause abortion in pregnant animals because of their LPS content, and likewise live vaccines should not be used parenterally in pregnant animals. It is useful to include endotoxin assay so that the levels can be compared with those shown to be safe in the double dose tests. Vaccines may also cause swelling at the site of injection.

5. Tests on the final product

a) Safety

Killed vaccines are assessed in a double-dose test, and live vaccines are assessed in a test using ten times the dose, in the target species.

b) Potency

If possible, the potency test should relate to the efficacy of the vaccine in the target species, and suitable criteria should be applied for passing batches. It may be possible to assess killed vaccines by the O-H antibody response produced, although it should be remembered that serum antibodies are only part of the host's protective mechanism against salmonella. Alternatively, the potency of the vaccine may be assessed by its effect on the LD_{50} in mice.

• Acknowledgement

Parts of this chapter were taken from or based on the chapter on salmonellosis in previous editions of the *Manual*.

REFERENCES

1. BARROW P.A. (1994). Serological diagnosis of *Salmonella* serotype Enteritidis infections in poultry by ELISA and other tests. *Int. J. Food Microbiol.*, **21**, 55–68.

2. COOPER G.L. (1994). Salmonellosis – infections in man and the chicken: pathogenesis and the development of live vaccines – a review. *Vet. Bull.*, **64**, 123–143.

3. ELLIS E.M., WILLIAMS J.E., MALLINSON E.T., SNOEYENBOS G.H. & MARTIN W.J. (1976). Culture Methods for the Detection of Animal Salmonellosis and Arizonosis. Iowa State University Press, Ames, USA.

4. EUROPEAN UNION (1992). Council Directive 92/117/EEC of 17 December 1992 concerning measures for protection against specified zoonoses and specified zoonotic agents in animals and products of animal origin in order to prevent outbreaks of food-borne infections and intoxications.

5. EWING W.H. (1986). Edwards and Ewing's Identification of Enterobacteriaceae, Fourth Edition. Elsevier, New York, USA, London, UK, and Amsterdam, The Netherlands.

6. FRICKER C.R. (1987). The isolation of salmonellas and campylobacters. *J. Appl. Bacteriol.*, **63**, 99–116.

7. GERHARDT P. (1981). Manual of Methods for General Microbiology. American Society for Microbiology, Washington DC, USA, 332–334.

8. HARVEY R.W.S. & PRICE T.H. (1974). Isolation of Salmonellas. Public Health Laboratory Service. Monograph Series 8. Her Majesty's Stationery Office, London, UK.

9. LE MINOR L. & POPOFF M.Y. (1987). Request for an opinion. Designation of *Salmonella enterica* sp. *nov. nom. rev*, as the type and only species of the genus *Salmonella*. *Int. J. Syst. Bacteriol.*, **37**, 465–468.

10. LINDBERG A.A. & LE MINOR L. (1984). Serology of Salmonella. *In:* Methods in Microbiology, Vol. 15, Bergman T.E., ed. Academic Press London, UK, 1–14.

11. MALLINSON E.T. & SNOEYENBOS G.H. (1989). Salmonellosis. *In:* Isolation and Identification of Avian Pathogens, Third Edition, Purchase H.G. *et al.*, eds. American Association of Avian Pathologists. Kendall Hunt Publishing, Iowa, USA, 3–11.

12. NIELSEN B., BAGGESEN D.L., LIND P., FELD N. & WINGSTRAND A. (1996). Serological surveillance of *Salmonella* infections in swine herds by use of an indirect LPS ELISA. Proceedings of the 14th International Pig Veterinary Society Congress, Bologna, Italy, 7–10 July 1996, p.169.

13. POPOFF M.Y., BOCKEMUHL J. & MCWHORTER-MURLIN A. (1994). Supplement 1993 (No. 37) to antigenic formulas of the salmonella serovars. World Health Organization Collaborating Centre for Reference and Research on Salmonella. Institute Pasteur, Paris. Kauffmann–White scheme. *Res. Microbiol.*, **145**, 711–716.

14. POPOFF M.Y. & LE MINOR L. (1997). Antigenic Formulas of the *Salmonella* Serovars. World Health Organization Collaborating Centre for Reference and Research on Salmonella. Pasteur Institute, Paris, France.

15. SNOEYENBOS G.H. (1994). Avian salmonellosis. *In:* Handbook of Zoonoses, Second Edition, Beran G.W., ed. CRC Press, Boca Raton, Florida, USA.

16. THRELLFALL E.J. & FROST J.A. (1990). The identification, typing and fingerprinting of salmonellae: laboratory aspects and epidemiological applications. *J. Appl. Bacteriol.*, **68**, 5–16.

17. VAN ZIJDERVELD F.G., VAN ZIJDERVELD-VAN BEMMEL A.M. & ANAKOTTA J. (1992). Comparison of four different enzyme-linked immunosorbent assays for serological diagnosis of *Salmonella enteritidis* infections in experimentally infected chickens. *J. Clin. Microbiol.*, **30**, 2560–2566.

18. WESTPHAL O. & LUDERITZ O. (1954). Chemische Erforschung von Lipopolysacchariden gramnegativer Bakterien. *Angew. Chem.*, **66**, 407–417.

19. WORLD HEALTH ORGANIZATION (WHO) (1994). Guidelines on Detection and Monitoring of Salmonella Infected Poultry Flocks with Particular Reference to *Salmonella enteritidis*, Wray C. & Davies R.H., eds. WHO, Geneva, Switzerland.

20. WRAY C. & WRAY A., EDS (2000). *Salmonella* in Domestic Animals. CABI, Wallingford, Oxon, UK.

*
* *

CHAPTER X.5.

BOVINE VIRAL DIARRHOEA[1]

SUMMARY

Cattle of all ages are susceptible to infection with bovine viral diarrhoea virus (BVDV). Distribution of the virus is world-wide. The clinical signs range from subclinical to the fulminating fatal condition called mucosal disease. Acute infections may result in transient diarrhoea or pneumonia, usually in the form of group outbreaks. Acute forms of the disease associated with high mortality have also been described often, but not always, associated with a haemorrhagic syndrome. However, most infections in the young calf are mild and go unrecognised clinically. The virus spreads mainly by contact between cattle. Vertical transmission plays an important role in its epidemiology and pathogenesis.

Infections of the bovine fetus may result in abortions, stillbirths, teratogenic effects or persistent infection in the neonatal calf. Persistently viraemic animals may be born as weak, unthrifty calves or may appear as normal healthy calves and be unrecognised clinically. Some of these animals may later develop mucosal disease with anorexia, gastrointestinal erosions, and profuse diarrhoea, leading invariably to death. Mucosal disease can arise only in persistently infected animals.

It is important to avoid the trade of viraemic animals. It is generally considered that serologically positive, nonviraemic cattle are 'safe', providing that they are not pregnant. Antibody-positive pregnant cattle carrying persistently infected fetuses are important transmitters of the virus between herds. About 15% of persistently viraemic animals have antibody to the NS/2 protein and a lower percentage to the E2 glycoprotein. Therefore, seropositivity cannot be equated with 'safety'. Latent infections are not known to occur in recovered animals.

***Identification of the agent:** BVDV is a pestivirus in the Flaviviridae and is closely related to classical swine fever and ovine border disease viruses. BVDV occurs in two forms, noncytopathogenic and cytopathogenic. There are two antigonically distinct genotypes (types 1 and 2), and virus isolates within these groups exhibit considerable biological and antigenic diversity.*

Persistently viraemic healthy animals resulting from congenital infection can be readily identified by isolation of noncytopathogenic virus in cell cultures from blood or serum. It is necessary to use an immune-labelling method to detect the growth of virus in the cultures. Alternative methods based on direct detection of viral antigen or viral RNA in leukocytes are also available. Persistence of virus should be confirmed by resampling after an interval of at least 3 weeks. These animals will usually have no or low levels of antibodies to BVDV.

Viraemia in acute cases is transient and can be difficult to detect. In fatal cases of haemorrhagic disease, virus can be isolated from tissues post mortem. Confirmation of mucosal disease can be made by isolation of the cytopathogenic biotype of BVDV, particularly from intestinal tissues. Noncytopathogenic virus should also be detected, especially in blood.

***Serological tests:** Acute infection with BVDV is best confirmed by demonstrating seroconversion using sequential paired samples from several animals in the group. The testing of paired (acute and convalescent) samples should be done a minimum of 14 days apart and samples should be tested side by side. The enzyme-linked immunosorbent assay for antibody and the virus neutralisation test are the most widely used.*

***Requirements for vaccines and diagnostic biologicals:** There is no standard vaccine for BVD, but a number of commercial preparations are available. Modified live virus vaccine should not be administered to pregnant cattle (or to their sucking calves) due to the risk of transplacental*

1 See also Append x 3.2.1. in the *Code*.

infection. There is also a risk of inducing mucosal disease in persistently infected animals. Killed virus vaccines generally require booster vaccinations. An ideal vaccine should be able to prevent transplacental infection in pregnant cows.

BVDV is a particularly important hazard to the manufacture of biological products for other diseases due to the high frequency of contamination of batches of fetal calf serum used as a culture medium supplement.

A. DIAGNOSTIC TECHNIQUES

Bovine viral diarrhoea virus (BVDV) is a pestivirus in the Flaviviridae and is closely related to classical swine fever and ovine border disease viruses (18). Two antigenically distinct genotypes of BVDV exist, types 1 and 2. They may be differentiated from each other, and from other pestiviruses, by monoclonal antibodies (MAbs) directed against the E2 major glycoprotein, or by genetic analysis (46, 49). A multiplex polymerase chain reaction (PCR) has been described that enables virus typing direct from blood samples (26). Type 1 virus is generally more common although the prevalence of type 2 is reported to be almost as high as type 1 in North America. BVDV of both genotypes may occur in noncytopathogenic and cytopathogenic forms (biotypes), classified according to whether or not it produces visible change in cell cultures. Usually, it is the noncytopathogenic biotype that circulates in the environment. Each biotype has a specific role in a variety of clinical syndromes – acute, congenital and chronic infections (4, 10). Type 2 viruses are usually noncytopathogenic and have been associated with outbreaks of severe acute infection (15). Clinically inapparent infections are common with both genotypes.

a) Acute infections

Acute infections of cattle occur particularly in young animals, and may be clinically inapparent or associated with diarrhoea (1). Affected animals may be predisposed to concurrent infections, for example respiratory disease, perhaps due to an immunosuppressive effect of the virus. Bulls may suffer a temporary depression of fertility and can show transient shedding of virus in the semen (43). During acute infections, a brief viraemia may be detectable and nasal shedding of virus may occur. There may also be a transient leukopenia or temperature response, but these can vary greatly among animals. A serological response is the most certain means of diagnosing a previous infection. Outbreaks of a severe form of acute disease with haemorrhagic lesions, thrombocytopenia and high mortality have been reported sporadically from some countries (1, 5). Other acute outbreaks may show fever, pneumonia, diarrhoea and sudden death in any age group, with haemorrhagic signs (15).

b) Congenital infection

If noncytopathogenic virus infects the bovine fetus, this may result in abortion, stillbirth, teratogenic effects or a congenital infection that persists in the neonatal calf (1, 10, 20, 39). Confirmation that an abortion is caused by BVDV is often difficult to establish (50), but virus may be isolated from fetal tissue in some cases. An attempt should be made to detect specific antibody in samples of fetal fluids or serum, or in the supernatant fluid from a tissue suspension. Stillbirths or teratogenic effects may be associated with an active fetal immune response to the virus during mid-to-late gestation.

Although congenital infection with BVDV often leads to abortion, it is not always recognised in the field. Infection during the first third of the gestation period can result in the abortion of a conceptus that is small and goes unnoticed by the farmer. The cow would return to service and the failure to maintain pregnancy would be classified as an example of early embryonic death. Another possible outcome of infection is the death and subsequent resorption of fluids from the fetus that results in mummification. It is frequently observed that aborted fetuses have subcutaneous oedema and copious pleural and peritoneal effusions. There may also be congenital abnormalities that result in growth retardation and in selective central nervous system (CNS) defects, such as cerebellar hypoplasia and dysmyelination (51), and eye defects, such as cataracts. Sometimes there are skeletal defects, the most advanced of which is arthrogryposis.

Stillborn calves are a common sequel to congenital infection. The calves usually appear to be fully developed at parturition, but fail to survive. After day 150 of pregnancy, the immune system of the fetus will be developed and infection of the fetus will usually result in an antibody response and the birth of a normal calf.

c) Persistent viraemia

When infections of the fetus occur before approximately 110 days of gestation and before immunocompetence, the calf may be born with a persistent viraemia. Identification of these animals is readily made by detection of noncytopathogenic BVDV in blood. Furthermore, animals with a persistent viraemia will also lack specific antibody, but diagnosis in the young calf, up to approximately 3 months of age, may be confused by the presence of maternal antibody to BVDV. Maternal antibody may also interfere with virus isolation. In older animals with persistent viraemia, low levels of antibody may be present due to their ability to seroconvert to strains of BVDV (including vaccines) 'heterologous' (antigenically different) from the persisting virus (11). To confirm a diagnosis of persistent viraemia, animals should be retested after an interval of at least 3 weeks.

There are no pathognomonic lesions in the viraemic calf. The clinical signs vary from the apparently normal healthy animal to the weak, unthrifty calf that has difficulty in standing and sucking. These latter calves can show CNS defects, such as muscular tremors, incoordination and blindness. They often die within days of birth, thus contributing to the 'weak calf syndrome'.

Some viraemic animals survive to sexual maturity and are retained for breeding. Calves born to these infected dams are always persistently viraemic, and are often weak at birth and fail to thrive. Persistently viraemic animals are a continual source of infective virus to other cattle, and thus their rapid identification and removal from the herd are required. Animals being traded should first be screened for the absence of persistent BVD viraemia.

Bulls that are persistently infected usually have poor quality, highly infective semen and, as a result, reduced fertility (34, 48). All bulls used for natural or artificial insemination should be screened for persistent BVD infection.

Female cattle used as embryo recipients should always test negative for BVD viraemia before first use. Donor cows that are persistently infected with BVDV also represent a potential source of infection, as oocysts without an intact zona pellucida are shown to be susceptible to infection *in vitro* (54). However, a limited study of two persistently infected animals revealed that the majority of oocysts were BVDV-negative (52). Embryos may also become contaminated following acute infection of the donor (2). Biological materials used for *in-vitro* fertilisation techniques (bovine serum, bovine cell cultures) have a high risk of contamination and should be screened for BVDV (8).

d) Mucosal disease

It is well established that persistently viraemic animals may later succumb to mucosal disease (10). This syndrome has been shown to be associated with the presence of the cytopathogenic biotype, which can arise either through superinfection (4, 13), recombination between noncytopathogenic biotypes, or mutation of the persistent biotype (36). Consequently, confirmatory diagnosis of mucosal disease should include the isolation of cytopathogenic virus from affected cattle. This biotype may sometimes be isolated from blood, but it can be recovered more consistently from a variety of other tissues, in particular intestinal and Peyer's patch tissue (16). Virus isolation is also readily accomplished from spleen. This is easy to collect and is seldom toxic for cell culture after preparation for viral isolation. Isolation from gut samples may be difficult if autolysis has occurred; in this case suspensions from lymph nodes or tonsil should then be tested. Noncytopathogenic virus can also be detected, particularly from blood or blood-associated organs. Cryostat tissue sections from mucosal disease cases can be stained for viral antigen by immunofluorescence or immunoperoxidase labelling.

Mucosal disease is invariably fatal. Its onset may be so rapid that the first signs seen are dead or moribund animals. However, it is more common for animals to become anorexic over a period of several days, to be disinclined to move and to show signs of abdominal pain. They can develop a profuse diarrhoea and rapidly lose bodily condition. Erosions can often be seen in the mouth, particularly along the gingival margin. Lacrimation and excessive salivation occur.

Post-mortem examination reveals erosions in the mucosa at various sites along the gastrointestinal tract. The most noticeable are those overlying the lymphoid Peyer's patches in the small intestine and in the colonic tonsils. On histological examination, there is a clear demonstration of destruction of the lymphoid tissue within the gut-associated lymphoid tissue. Most of the Peyer's patch lymphoid cells have been lysed and replaced by inflammatory cells, debris and cells from the overlying collapsed epithelium.

1. Identification of the agent (the prescribed test for international trade)

All test methods must be validated by testing on known noninfected and infected populations of cattle, including animals with low- and high-titre viraemias. Methods based on MAb-binding assays or on nucleic acid recognition must be shown to detect the full range of antigenic and genetic diversity found among BVD viruses. There are two designated OIE Reference Laboratories for BVD (see Table given in Part 4 of this *Manual*); the reference laboratories for classical swine fever could also be approached to offer advice.

a) Virus isolation

The virus may be isolated in a number of bovine monolayer cell cultures (e.g. kidney, lung, testis or turbinate). Growth of both biotypes is usually satisfactory. Noncytopathogenic BVDV is a common contaminant of fresh bovine tissue, and cell cultures must be checked for freedom from adventitious virus by regular testing (7, 22). Primary or secondary cultures can be frozen as cell suspensions in liquid nitrogen. These can then be tested over a series of passages, or seeded to other susceptible cells and checked before routine use. Such problems may be overcome by the use of continuous cell lines, which can be obtained BVD-free (7). The fetal bovine serum that is selected for use in cell culture must also be free not only from virus, but also and of equal importance, from BVDV neutralising antibody (22). Heat treatment (56°C for 30–45 minutes) is inadequate for the destruction of BVDV in contaminated serum; irradiation at 25 kilograys (2.5 Mrad) is more certain. Commercial batches of fetal bovine serum mostly test positive by PCR even after irradiation. Where appropriate, horse serum can be substituted for bovine fetal serum, although it is often found to have poorer cell-growth-promoting characteristics.

Buffy coat cells, whole blood or serum are suitable for isolation of the virus from live animals. Maternal antibody may interfere with isolation from serum in young calves. Tissue suspensions from post-mortem cases should be prepared by standard methods. Semen can also be examined, but a blood sample from the donor bull is preferable if it can be obtained. Raw semen is cytotoxic and must be diluted in culture medium. Extended semen can usually be inoculated directly on to cell monolayers, but may occasionally cause cytotoxicity. For these reasons, it is important to monitor the health of the cells by microscopic examination at intervals during the incubation.

There are many variations of procedure in use for virus isolation. All should be optimised to give maximum sensitivity of detection of a standard virus preparation. This may include one or more *in-vitro* passage(s). Conventional methods for virus isolation are used, with the addition of a final immune-labelling step (fluorescence or enzymatic) to detect growth of noncytopathogenic virus. Thus tube cultures should include flying cover-slips, while plate cultures can be fixed and labelled directly in the plate. Examples are given below.

- **Microplate immunoperoxidase method for mass screening for virus detection in serum samples (38)**

i) 10 µl of the serum sample is placed into each of four wells of a 96-well tissue-culture grade microplate. This is repeated for each sample. Known positive and negative controls are included.

ii) 100 µl of a cell suspension of 150,000 cells/ml in medium without fetal calf serum (FCS) is added to all wells. *NB:* the sample itself acts as the cell-growth supplement. If testing samples other than serum, use medium with 10% FCS.

iii) The plate is incubated at 37°C for 4 days, either in a 5% CO_2 atmosphere or with the plate sealed.

iv) Each well is examined microscopically for evidence of cytopathic effect (CPE), or signs of cytotoxicity.

v) The plate is emptied by gentle inversion and rinsed in phosphate buffered saline (PBS).

vi) The plate is fixed as follows: the plate is dipped into a bath of 20% acetone in PBS, emptied immediately, and then transferred to a fresh bath of 20% acetone in PBS for 10 minutes. The plate is drained thoroughly and as much fluid as possible is removed by tapping and blotting. The plate is dried thoroughly for at least 3 hours at a temperature of 25–30°C (e.g. using radiant heat from a bench lamp). *NB:* the drying is part of the fixation process.

Alternative fixation methods include paraformaldehyde or heat (see Chapter 2.1.13. Classical swine fever, Section A.2.b.viii).

vii) The fixed cells are rinsed by adding PBS to all wells.

viii) The wells are drained and the BVD antibody (50 µl) is added to all wells at a predetermined dilution in PBS containing 1% Tween 80 (PBST) and 5% horse serum. (Horse serum may be added to reduce nonspecific staining.) The plate is incubated at 37°C for 15 minutes.

ix) The plate is emptied and washed three times in PBST.

x) The plate is then drained and appropriate antispecies serum conjugated to peroxidase is added at a predetermined dilution (50 µl per well) for 15 minutes at 37°C.

xi) The plate is emptied and washed three times in PBST.

xii) The plate is rinsed in distilled water. All fluid is tapped out from the plate.

xiii) Freshly prepared hydrogen peroxide substrate with a suitable chromogen, e.g. 3-amino-9-ethyl carbazole (AEC) is added. The stock solution is: AEC (0.1 g) dissolved in dimethyl formamide (15 ml). For use, the stock (0.3 ml) is added to 0.05 M acetate buffer (5 ml), pH 5.0, and then 30% H_2O_2 (5 µl) is added.

xiv) The plate is examined microscopically. Virus-positive cells show red-brown cytoplasmic staining.

- **Tube method for tissue or buffy coat suspensions, or semen samples**

  NB: this method can also be conveniently adapted to 24-well plastic dishes.

i) Tissue samples are ground up and a 10% suspension in culture medium is made. This is then centrifuged to remove the debris. Raw semen is diluted 1/10 in culture medium.

ii) Test tube cultures (with cover-slips) with newly confluent or subconfluent monolayers of susceptible bovine cells are inoculated with 0.1 ml of the sample. The culture is left to adsorb for 1 hour at 37°C.

iii) The culture is washed with 1 ml of medium; this is then discarded and 1 ml of culture maintenance medium is added.

iv) The culture is incubated for 4–5 days at 37°C, and examined microscopically for evidence of CPE or signs of cytotoxicity.

v) Culture may then either be frozen and thawed for passage to fresh cultures, or the cover-slip may be removed, fixed in acetone and stained with direct immunofluorescent conjugate to BVDV. In this case, examine under a fluorescent microscope for diffuse, cytoplasmic fluorescence characteristic of pestiviruses.

   Alternatively, cultures may be freeze–thaw harvested and passaged on to microtitre plates for culture and immunoperoxidase staining (see section on microplate immunoperoxidase method for mass screening of serum samples above).

b) Enzyme-linked immunosorbent assay for antigen detection

Several methods for the enzyme-linked immunosorbent assay (ELISA) for antigen detection have been published (e.g. ref. 23) and a number of commercial kits are available. Most are based on the sandwich ELISA principle, with a capture antibody bound to the solid phase, and a detector antibody conjugated to a signal system, such as peroxidase. Both monoclonal- and polyclonal-based systems are described. The test is suitable for detection of persistently infected animals, and usually measures BVD antigen in lysates of peripheral blood leukocytes. The best of the methods gives a sensitivity equivalent to virus isolation, and may be preferred in those rare cases where persistent viraemia is combined with seropositivity. The antigen ELISA appears to be less useful for virus detection in acute BVD infections.

c) Immunohistochemistry

Enzyme-labelled methods are useful to detect BVDV antigen in tissue sections (55), particularly where suitable MAbs are available. It is important that the reagents and procedures used be fully validated, and that nonspecific reactivity be eliminated. For persistently infected cattle almost any tissue can be used, but particularly good success has been found with lymph nodes, thyroid gland, skin, brain, abomasum and placenta.

d) Nucleic acid detection

The reverse transcription-polymerase chain reaction (RT-PCR) method can be adapted to the detection of BVD viral RNA for diagnostic purposes (9, 27). This may have a special value where low-level virus contamination is suspected, for example in screening batches of FCS, or biological products such as vaccines (28). Caution is needed in the interpretation of results, as the detection of viral RNA does not imply *per se* that infective virus is present. Testing for virus after inoculation of cell cultures using PCR should be avoided as it may give positive results if commercial bovine fetal serum has been used in the growth medium. Primers should be selected in conserved regions of the genome, such as the 5'-noncoding region, or the NS3 (p80) gene. The usual precautions should be taken to avoid DNA contamination in the test system, and rigorous controls must be mounted (see Chapter I.7. Biotechnology in the diagnosis of infectious diseases and vaccine development). A multiplex PCR can be used to amplify and type virus from cell culture, or direct from blood samples, by producing different sized PCR products (26).

The RT-PCR technique is also sensitive enough to enable the detection of persistently infected lactating cows in a herd of up to 100 animals or more, by testing the somatic cells within bulk milk (19, 47). A positive result indicates that at least one such animal is present in the milking herd. Follow-up virus isolation or antigen detection tests are required to identify the individual(s).

Viral nucleic acid in tissues can be detected by *in situ* hybridisation with enzyme-linked riboprobes (17). This is a sensitive technique that can be applied to formalin-fixed paraffin-embedded tissue, thereby allowing a retrospective analysis.

2. Serological tests

Antibody to BVDV can be detected in cattle sera by a standard virus neutralisation (VN) test or by ELISA, using one of several published methods (21, 30, 33, 44). Control positive and negative standard sera must be included in every test. These should give results within predetermined limits for the test to be considered valid. ELISA for antibody in bulk milk samples can give a useful indication of the BVD status of a herd (41). A high ELISA value of 1.0 or more absorbance units indicates a high probability of the herd having been exposed to BVDV in the recent past, most likely through one or more persistently viraemic animals being present. In contrast, a very low or negative value (≤0.2) indicates that it is unlikely that persistently viraemic animals are present. Further categorisation has been suggested for intermediate values, but this is dependent on the husbandry system in use. Determination of the antibody status of a small number of young stock (9–18 months) has also been suggested as an indicator of recent exposure to BVDV (29). Rapid 'spot tests' can be used for initial screening as part of BVD control and eradication schemes (35).

a) Virus neutralisation test

Because it makes the test easier to read, most laboratories use highly cytopathogenic laboratory-adapted strains of BVDV for VN tests, although immune-labelling techniques are now available that allow simple detection of the growth or neutralisation of noncytopathogenic strains where this is considered desirable. No single strain is likely to be ideal for all circumstances, but in practice one should be selected that detects the highest proportion of serological reactions in the local cattle population. Two widely used cytopathogenic strains are 'Oregon C24V' and 'NADL'. Low levels of antibody to BVD type 2 virus may not be detectable by a neutralisation test that uses type 1 strain of the virus, and vice versa (25).

An outline protocol for a microtitre VN test is given below (21):

i) The test sera are heat-inactivated for 30 minutes at 56°C.

ii) From a starting dilution of 1/5, serial twofold dilutions of the test sera are made in a cell-culture grade flat-bottomed 96-well microtitre plate, using cell culture medium as diluent. For each sample, two or four wells are used at each dilution depending on the degree of precision required. Control positive and negative sera should also be tested.

iii) An equal volume (e.g. 50 µl) of a stock of cytopathogenic strain of BVDV containing 100 $TCID_{50}$ (50% tissue culture infective dose) is added to each well. A back titration of virus stock is also done in some spare wells to check the potency of the virus (acceptance limits 30–300 $TCID_{50}$).

iv) The plate is incubated for 1 hour at 37°C.

v) A flask of suitable cells (e.g. bovine turbinate, bovine testis) is trypsinised and the cell concentration is adjusted to 3×10^5/ml. 50 µl of the cell suspension is added to each well of the microtitre plate.

vi) The plate is incubated at 37°C for 4 days, either in a 5% CO_2 atmosphere or with the plate sealed.

vii) The wells are examined microscopically for CPE. The VN titre for each serum is the dilution at which the virus is neutralised in 50% of the wells. This can be calculated by the Spearman–Kärber method. A seronegative animal will show no neutralisation at the lowest dilution (1/5, equivalent to a final dilution of 1/10).

b) Enzyme-linked immunosorbent assay

Both indirect and blocking types of test can be used (30, 33, 44). A number of commercial kits are available. The chief difficulty in setting up the test lies in the preparation of a viral antigen of sufficient potency. The virus must be grown under optimal culture conditions using a highly permissive cell type. Any serum used in the medium must not inhibit growth of BVDV. The optimal time for harvest should be determined experimentally for the individual culture system. The virus can be concentrated and purified by density gradient centrifugation. Alternatively, a potent antigen can be prepared by treatment of infected cell cultures with detergents, such as Nonidet P40, Mega 10, Triton X-100 or 1-octyl-beta-D-glucopyranoside (OGP). Some workers have used fixed, infected whole cells as antigen. In future, increasing use may be made of artificial antigens manufactured by expressing specific viral genes in bacterial or eukaryotic systems (53). Such systems should be validated by testing sera specific to a wide range of different virus strains. In the future, this technology should enable the production of serological tests complementary to subunit or marker vaccines, thus enabling differentiation between vaccinated and naturally infected cattle.

An example outline protocol for an indirect ELISA is given below (21).

i) Roller cultures of secondary calf testis cells with a high multiplicity of infection (about one), are inoculated with BVDV strain Oregon C24V, overlaid with serum-free medium and incubated for 24 hours at 37°C.

ii) The cells are scraped off and pelleted. The supernatant medium is discarded. The pellet is treated with two volumes of 2% OGP in PBS for 15 minutes at 4°C, and centrifuged to remove the cell debris. The supernatant antigen is stored in small aliquots at –70°C, or freeze-dried. Noninfected cells are processed in parallel to make a control antigen.

iii) The antigen is diluted to a predetermined dilution in 0.05 M bicarbonate buffer, pH 9.6. Alternate rows of an ELISA-grade microtitre plate are coated with virus and control antigens overnight at 4°C. The plates are then washed in PBS with 0.05% Tween 20 (PBST) before use in the test.

iv) Test sera are diluted 1/50 in serum diluent (0.5 M NaCl; 0.01 M phosphate buffer; 0.05% Tween 20; 0.001 M ethylene diamine tetra-acetic acid; 1% polyvinyl pyrrolidone, pH 7.2) and added to virus- and control-coated wells for 1 hour at 37°C. The plates are then washed five times in PBST.

v) Rabbit anti-bovine IgG peroxidase conjugate is added at a predetermined dilution (in serum diluent) for 1 hour at 37°C, then the plates are again washed five times in PBST.

vi) A suitable enzyme substrate is added, such as hydrogen peroxide/tetramethyl benzidine. After colour development, the reaction is stopped with sulphuric acid and the absorbance is read on an ELISA plate reader. The value obtained with control antigen is subtracted from the test reaction to give a net absorbance value for each serum.

vii) It is recommended to convert net absorbance values to sample:positive ratio (or percentage positivity) by dividing net absorbance by the net absorbance on that test of a standard positive serum that has a net absorbance of about 1.0. This normalisation procedure leads to more consistent and reproducible results.

B. REQUIREMENTS FOR VACCINES AND DIAGNOSTIC BIOLOGICALS

Infection via the oropharynx and respiratory tract is probably the most important route of transmission of BVDV on farms. Protection against spread in this way would have a beneficial effect on controlling disease due to the virus, particularly in the young animal. The formulation of a vaccine that will provide protection to the fetus is also required in order to prevent the wide range of syndromes that result from *in utero* infection (12).

A standard vaccine for protection against infection has not yet been developed, but a number of commercial preparations are available in, for example, Europe and North America. Traditionally, BVD vaccines have been based on a cytopathogenic strain of the virus and fall into two classes: modified live virus or inactivated vaccines.

Although live virus vaccines are available in some countries, they should be used under careful veterinary control because a cytopathogenic strain may precipitate mucosal disease by superinfection of persistently viraemic animals, while in pregnant cattle, a noncytopathogenic component of the vaccine may cross the placenta and infect the fetus as described in Section A.b. Live virus vaccine may also be immunosuppressive and precipitate other infections. On the other hand, modified live virus vaccines may only require a single dose. Properly constituted vaccines containing killed virus are safe to use but, to obtain satisfactory levels of immunity, they usually require booster vaccinations, which may be inconvenient. A combined vaccination protocol using inactivated followed by live vaccine may reduce the risk of adverse reaction to the live strain (24).

Experimental inactivated vaccines based on baculovirus-expressed BVD viral glycoprotein E2 have been described. They offer a future prospect of 'marker vaccines' when used in connection with a complementary serological test (14).

BVDV is particularly important as a hazard in the manufacture of biological products for other diseases because of the high frequency of contamination of batches of FCS used as a culture medium supplement (28).

1. Seed management

a) Characteristics of the seed

An ideal vaccine should contain a strain (or strains) of virus that has been shown to give protection against the wide diversity of antigenicity that has been demonstrated by BVDV. A good appreciation of the antigenic characteristics of individual strains can be obtained by screening with panels of MAbs (45). Genetic sequencing can also contribute to virus characterisation (49).

Isolates of cytopathogenic virus are often mixed with the noncytopathogenic biotype. The separation and purification of the two biotypes from an initial mixed culture depends on either three cycles of a limiting dilution technique for the noncytopathogenic virus, or three cycles of plaque selection for the cytopathogenic virus. Purity of the cytopathogenic virus should be confirmed by at least one additional passage at limiting dilution. When isolates have been cloned, their identity should be confirmed by direct or indirect staining with specific antibody linked to fluorescein or enzyme.

b) **Method of culture**

Both biotypes will grow in a variety of cell cultures of bovine origin. Standard procedures may be used, with the expectation for harvesting noncytopathogenic virus on days 5–7 and cytopathogenic virus on days 2–4. The details for optimal yield depend on several factors, including the cell culture and isolate used and the initial seeding rate of virus (32).

c) **Validation as a vaccine**

All vaccines should pass standard tests for safety and efficacy. It is crucial to ensure that the cell cultures and fetal bovine serum included in culture medium be free from adventitious BVDV and antibody (described in Section A), and other microorganisms. Live vaccines must either be demonstrated to be safe in pregnant cattle (i.e. no transmission to the fetus), or should be licensed with a warning not to use them in pregnant animals. Live vaccines containing cytopathogenic strains should have an appropriate warning of the risk of inducing mucosal disease in persistently infected cattle.

Efficacy tests of BVD vaccines in nonpregnant cattle are limited by the difficulty of establishing a satisfactory challenge model. Tests should include as a minimum the demonstration of seroconversion following vaccination, a reduction in virus shedding after challenge in vaccinated cattle, and a diminution in measurable clinical parameters, such as rectal temperature response and leukopenia (3, 12, 32). Vaccines intended for use in adult breeding cattle should be evaluated for their efficiency in reducing transplacental transmission, ideally achieving complete prevention. In this case, a suitable challenge system can be established by intranasal inoculation of noncytopathogenic virus into pregnant cows at under 90 days gestation (12). Usually this system will reliably produce persistently viraemic offspring in nonimmune cows.

2. Method of manufacture

There is no standard method for the manufacture of a BVD vaccine, but conventional laboratory techniques with stationary, rolled or suspension (micro-carriers) cell cultures may be used. Inactivated vaccines can be prepared by conventional methods, such as binary ethylenimine or beta-propiolactone inactivation (32, 42). A variety of adjuvants may be used (32, 40).

3. In-process control

Cultures should be inspected regularly to ensure that they are free from contamination, and to monitor the health of the cells and the development or absence of CPE, as appropriate.

4. Batch control

a) **Sterility**

Tests for sterility and freedom from contamination of biological materials may be found in Chapter I.4.

b) **Safety**

It is essential that all the infectivity be removed during preparation of an inactivated vaccine, and samples should be subjected to several passages in cell culture to ensure the absence of live BVDV. It may also be necessary to ensure the absence of various proscribed agents (prior to inactivation) before use of the vaccine is permitted.

c) **Potency**

Ideally, the potency of the vaccine should be determined by inoculation into seronegative and virus negative calves, followed by monitoring of the antibody response; however, this is prohibitively expensive for batch control. Antigen content can be assayed by ELISA and adjusted as required to a standard level for the particular vaccine (3, 37). Standardised assay protocols applicable to all vaccines do not exist. Live vaccine batches may be assayed by infectivity titration.

d) Duration of immunity

There are few published data on the duration of antibody following vaccination with a commercial product. Protocols for their use usually recommend a primary course of two inoculations and boosters at yearly intervals. Only limited data are available on the antibody levels that correlate with protection against respiratory infections (6, 31) or *in utero* infection (12).

e) Stability

There are no accepted guidelines for the stability of BVD vaccines, but it can be assumed that attenuated virus vaccine (freeze-dried) should remain potent for at least 1 year if kept at 4°C. Inactivated virus vaccine could have a longer shelf life at 4°C. Lower temperatures could prolong shelf life for either type, but adjuvants in killed vaccine may preclude this.

f) Precautions

BVDV is not considered to be a human health hazard. Standard good microbiological practice should be adequate for handling the virus in the laboratory.

5. Tests on the final product

a) Safety tests

The safety of the final product formulation of both live and inactivated vaccines should be assessed in susceptible calves for any local reactions following administration, and in pregnant cattle for their effects on the unborn calf. Tests for individual batches are described in Section B.4.b.

b) Potency tests for antigenicity

BVD vaccines must be demonstrated to produce adequate immune responses, as outlined in Section B.4.c. above, when used in their final formulation according to the manufacturer's published instructions. *In-vitro* assays (Section B.4.c.) may be used to monitor individual batches.

REFERENCES

1. BAKER J.C. (1995). The clinical manifestations of bovine viral diarrhea infection. *Vet. Clin. North. Am.*, **11**, 425–445.

2. BIELANSKI A., SAPP T. & LUTZE WALLACE C. (1998). Association of bovine embryos produced by *in vitro* fertilization with a noncytopathic strain of bovine viral diarrhea virus type II. *Theriogenol.*, **49**, 1231–1238.

3. BOLIN S.R. (1993). Immunogens of bovine viral diarrhea virus. *Vet. Microbiol.*, **37**, 263–271.

4. BOLIN S.R. (1995). The pathogenesis of mucosal disease. *Vet. Clin. North. Am.*, 11, 489–500.

5. BOLIN S.R. & RIDPATH J.F. (1992). Differences in virulence between two noncytopathic bovine viral diarrhea viruses in calves. *Am. J. Vet. Res.*, **53**, 2157–2163.

6. BOLIN S.R. & RIDPATH J.F. (1995). Assessment of protection from systemic infection or disease afforded by low to intermediate titers of passively acquired neutralizing antibody against bovine viral diarrhea virus in calves. *Am. J. Vet. Res.*, **56**, 755–759.

7 BOLIN S.R., RIDPATH J.F., BLACK J., MACY M. & ROBLIN R. (1994). Survey of cell lines in the American Type Culture Collection for bovine viral diarrhea virus. *J. Virol. Methods*, **48**, 211–221.

8. BOOTH P.J., STEVENS D.A., COLLINS M.E. & BROWNLIE J. (1995). Detection of bovine viral diarrhoea virus antigen and RNA in oviduct and granulosa cells of persistently infected cattle. *J. Reprod. Fertil.*, **105**, 17–24.

9. BROCK K.V. (1995). Diagnosis of bovine viral diarrhea virus infections. *Vet. Clin. North. Am.*, **11**, 549–561.

10. BROWNLIE J. (1985). Clinical aspects of the bovine virus diarrhoea/mucosal disease complex in cattle. *In Practice*, **7**, 195–202.

11. BROWNLIE J. (1990). The pathogenesis of bovine virus diarrhoea virus infections. *Rev. sci. tech. Off. int. Epiz.*, **9**, 43–59.

12. BROWNLIE J., CLARKE M.C., HOOPER L.B. & BELL G.D. (1995). Protection of the bovine fetus from bovine viral diarrhoea virus by means of a new inactivated vaccine. *Vet. Rec.*, **137**, 58–62.

13. BROWNLIE J., CLARKE M.C. & HOWARD C.J. (1984). Experimental production of fatal mucosal disease in cattle. *Vet. Rec.*, **114**, 535–536.

14. BRUSCHKE C.M., VAN OIRSCHOT J.M. & VAN RIJN P.A. (1999). An experimental multivalent bovine virus diarrhea virus E2 subunit vaccine and two experimental conventionally inactivated vaccines induce partial fetal protection in sheep. *Vaccine*, **17**, 1983–1991.

15. CARMAN S., VAN DREUMEL T., RIDPATH J., HAZLETT M., ALVES D., DUBOVI E., TREMBLAY R., BOLIN S., GODKIN A. & ANDERSON N. (1998). Severe acute bovine viral diarrhea in Ontario, 1993–1995. *J. Vet. Diagn. Invest.*, **10**, 27–35.

16. CLARKE M.C., BROWNLIE J. & HOWARD C.J. (1987). Isolation of cytopathic and non-cytopathic bovine viral diarrhoea virus from tissues of infected animals. *In:* Pestivirus Infections of Ruminants, Harkness J.W., ed. Commission of the European Communities, Brussels, Belgium, EUR10238, 3–12.

17. DESPORT M., COLLINS M.E. & BROWNLIE J. (1994). Detection of bovine virus diarrhoea virus RNA by *in situ* hybridisation with digoxigenin-labelled riboprobes. *Intervirology*, **37**, 269–276.

18. DONIS R.O. (1995). Molecular biology of bovine viral diarrhea virus and its interactions with the host. *Vet. Clin. North. Am.*, **11**, 393–423.

19. DREW T.W., YAPP F. & PATON D.J. (1999). The detection of bovine viral diarrhoea virus in bulk milk samples by the use of a single-tube RT-PCR. *Vet. Microbiol.*, **64**, 145–154.

20. DUFFELL S.J. & HARKNESS J.W. (1985). Bovine virus diarrhoea-mucosal disease infection in cattle. *Vet. Rec.*, **117**, 240–245.

21. EDWARDS S. (1990). The diagnosis of bovine virus diarrhoea-mucosal disease in cattle. *Rev. sci. tech. Off. int. Epiz.*, **9**, 115–130.

22. EDWARDS S. (1993). Bovine viral diarrhea virus. *In:* Cell & Tissue Culture: Laboratory Procedures, Doyle A., Griffiths J.B. & Newell D.G., eds. John Wiley & Sons, Chichester, UK. Module 7B:5, 1–8.

23. ENTRICAN G., DAND A. & NETTLETON P.F. (1995). A double monoclonal antibody ELISA for detecting pestivirus antigen in the blood of viraemic cattle and sheep. *Vet. Microbiol.*, **43**, 65–74.

24. FREY H.R. & EICKEN K. (1995). Untersuchungen über die Wirksamkeit einer inaktivierten BVD-Vakzine sur Erhöhung der Sicherheit einer BVD-Lebendvakzine. *Tierarztl. Umsch.*, **50**, 86– 93.

25. FULTON R.W., SALIKI J.T., BURGE L.J., DOFFAY J.M., BOLIN S.R., MAES R.K., BAKER J.C. & FREY M.L. (1997). Neutralizing antibodies to type-1 and type-2 bovine viral diarrhea viruses – detection by inhibition of viral cytopathology and infectivity by immunoperoxidase assay. *Clin. Diagn. Lab. Immunol.*, **4**, 380–383.

26. GILBERT S.A., BURTON K.M., PRINS S.E. & DEREGT D. (1999). Typing of bovine viral diarrhea viruses directly from blood of persistently infected cattle by multiplex PCR. *J. Clin. Microbiol.*, **37**, 2020–2023.

27. HAMEL A.L., WASYLYSHEN M.D. & NAYAR G.P.S. (1995). Rapid detection of bovine viral diarrhea virus by using RNA extracted directly from assorted specimens and a one-tube reverse transcription PCR assay. *J. Clin. Microbiol.*, **33**, 287–291.

28. HARASAWA R. (1995). Adventitious pestivirus RNA in live virus vaccines against bovine and swine diseases. *Vaccine,* **13,** 100–103.

29. HOUE H., BAKER J.C., MAES R.K., RUEGG P.L. & LLOYD J.W. (1995). Application of antibody titers against bovine viral diarrhea virus (BVDV) as a measure to detect herds with cattle persistently infected with BVDV. *J. Vet. Diagn. Invest.,* **7**, 327–332.

30. HOWARD C.J., CLARKE M.C. & BROWNLIE J. (1985). An enzyme-linked immunosorbent assay (ELISA) for the detection of antibodies to bovine viral diarrhoea virus (BVDV) in cattle sera. *Vet. Microbiol.,* **10**, 359–369.

31. HOWARD C.J., CLARKE M.C. & BROWNLIE J. (1989). Protection against respiratory infection with bovine virus diarrhoea virus by passively acquired antibody. *Vet. Microbiol.,* **19,** 195–203.

32. HOWARD C.J., CLARKE M.C., SOPP P. & BROWNLIE J. (1994). Systemic vaccination with inactivated bovine virus diarrhoea virus protects against respiratory challenge. *Vet. Microbiol.,* **42**, 171–179.

33. KATZ J.B. & HANSON S.K. (1987). Competitive and blocking enzyme-linked immunoassay for detection of fetal bovine serum antibodies to bovine viral diarrhea virus. *J. Virol. Methods,* **15**, 167–175.

34. KIRKLAND P.D., MACKINTOSH S.G. & MOYLE A. (1994). The outcome of widespread use of semen from a bull persistently infected with pestivirus. *Vet. Rec.,* **135**, 527–529.

35. LINDBERG A.L.E. & ALENIUS S. (1999). Principles for eradication of bovine viral diarrhoea virus (BVDV) infections in cattle populations. *Vet. Microbiol.,* **64**, 197–222.

36. LOEHR B.I., FREY H.R., MOENNIG V. & GREISER WILKE I. (1998). Experimental induction of mucosal disease: consequences of superinfection of persistently infected cattle with different strains of cytopathogenic bovine viral diarrhea virus. *Arch. Virol.,* **143**, 667–679.

37. LUDEMANN L.R. & KATZ J.B. (1994). Enzyme-linked immunosorbent assay assessment of bovine viral diarrhea virus antigen in inactivated vaccines using polyclonal or monoclonal antibodies. *Biologicals,* **22**, 21–27.

38. MEYLING A. (1984). Detection of BVD virus in viremic cattle by an indirect immunoperoxidase technique. *In:* Recent Advances in Virus Diagnosis, McNulty M.S. & McFerran J.B., eds. Martinus Nijhoff, Boston, The Hague, Dordrecht, Lancaster, 37–46.

39. MOENNIG V. & LIESS B. (1995). Pathogenesis of intrauterine infections with bovine viral diarrhea virus. *Vet. Clin. North. Am.,* **11**, 477–487.

40. NEATON H.J. (1986). Which BVD vaccine should I use? *Vet. Med.,* **81**, 876–881.

41. NISKANEN R. (1993). Relationship between the levels of antibodies to bovine viral diarrhoea virus in bulk tank milk and the prevalence of cows exposed to the virus. *Vet. Rec.,* **133**, 341–344.

42. PARK B.K. & BOLIN S.R. (1987). Molecular changes of bovine viral diarrhea virus polypeptides treated with binary ethylenimine, beta-propiolactone and formalin. *Res. Rep. Rural Dev. Admin. (L&V) Korea,* **29**, 99–103.

43. PATON D.J., GOODEY R., BROCKMAN S. & WOOD L. (1989). Evaluation of the quality and virological status of semen from bulls acutely infected with BVDV. *Vet. Rec.,* **124**, 63–64.

44. PATON D.J., IBATA G., EDWARDS S. & WENSVOORT G. (1991). An ELISA detecting antibody to conserved Pestivirus epitopes. *J. Virol. Methods,* **31**, 315–324.

45. PATON D.J., SANDS J.J. LOWINGS J.P., SMITH J.E., IBATA G., EDWARDS S. (1995). A proposed division of the pestivirus genus using monoclonal antibodies, supported by cross-neutralisation assays and genetic sequencing. *Vet. Res.,* **26**, 92–109.

46. PELLERIN C., VANDENHURK J., LECOMTE J. & TIJSSEN P. (1994). Identification of a new group of bovine viral diarrhea virus strains associated with severe outbreaks and high mortalities. *Virology,* **203**, 260–268.

47. RADWAN G.S., BROCK K.V., HOGAN J.S. & SMITH K.L. (1995). Development of a PCR amplification assay as a screening test using bulk milk samples for identifying dairy herds infected with bovine viral diarrhea virus. *Vet. Microbiol.*, **44**, 77–91.

48. REVELL S.G., CHASEY D., DREW T.W. & EDWARDS S. (1988). Some observations on the semen of bulls persistently infected with bovine virus diarrhoea virus. *Vet. Rec.*, **123**, 122–125.

49. RIDPATH J.F. BOLIN S.R. & DUBOVI E.J. (1994). Segregation of bovine viral diarrhea virus into genotypes. *Virology*, **205**, 66–74.

50. RUTH G.R. (1987). Bovine viral diarrhea: a difficult infection to diagnose. *Vet. Med.*, **81**, 870–874.

51. TRAUTWEIN G., HEWICKER M., LIESS B., ORBAN S. & GRUNERT E. (1986). Studies on transplacental transmissibility of a bovine virus diarrhoea (BVD) vaccine virus in cattle. III. Occurrence of central nervous system malformations in calves born from vaccinated cows. *J. Vet. Med.*, **B33**, 260–268.

52. TSUBOI T. & IMADA T. (1998). Detection of BVDV in bovine embryos derived from persistently infected heifers by PCR. *Vet. Rec.*, **142**, 114–115.

53. VANDERHEIJDEN N., DEMOERLOOZE L., VANDENBERGH D., CHAPPUIS G., RENARD A. & LECOMTE C. (1993). Expression of the bovine viral diarrhoea virus osloss-p80 protein: its use as ELISA antigen for cattle serum antibody detection. *J. Gen. Virol.*, **74**, 1427–1431.

54. VANROOSE G., NAUWYNCK H., VAN SOOM A., VANOPDENBOSCH E. & DE KRUIF A. (1998). Replication of cytopathic and noncytopathic bovine viral diarrhea virus in zona-free and zona-intact *in vitro*-produced bovine embryos and the effect on embryo quality. *Biol. Reprod.*, **58**, 857–866.

55. WILHELMSEN C.L., BOLIN S.R., RIDPATH J.F., CHEVILLE F.N. & KLUGE J.P. (1991). Lesions and localization of viral antigen in tissues of cattle with experimentally induced or naturally acquired mucosal disease, or with naturally acquired chronic bovine viral diarrhea. *Am. J. Vet. Res.*, **52**, 269–275.

*

* *

CHAPTER X.6.

TRYPANOSOMOSIS (tsetse-transmitted)

SUMMARY

Tsetse-transmitted trypanosomosis[1] *is a disease complex caused by several species of protozoan parasites of the genus* Trypanosoma, *transmitted cyclically by the genus* Glossina *(tsetse flies). The disease can affect various species of mammals but, from an economic point of view, tsetse-transmitted trypanosomosis, is particularly important in cattle. It is mainly caused by* Trypanosoma congolense, T. vivax *and, to a lesser extent,* T. brucei brucei.

Identification of the agent: *Several parasite detection techniques can be used, including the microscopic examination of the wet and stained thick or thin blood films. Diagnostic sensitivity is increased significantly by concentrating the parasites prior to examination in combination with a phase-contrast or dark-ground microscope. The parasite concentration techniques have the added advantage that the packed cell volume, and hence the level of anaemia, can be determined at the individual animal and/or herd level. A highly sensitive test, used on a more experimental basis, is the polymerase chain reaction.*

Serological tests: *Two trypanosomal antibody detection tests, the indirect fluorescent antibody test and the antibody-detection enzyme-linked immunosorbent assay (ELISA), are routinely used for the detection of antibodies in cattle. They have high sensitivity and specificity but can only be used for the presumptive diagnosis of trypanosomosis. The antibody-detection ELISA, in particular, lends itself to automation and a high degree of standardisation.*

Requirements for vaccines in diagnostic biologicals: *No biological products are in use at the present time.*

A. DIAGNOSTIC TECHNIQUES

Tsetse-transmitted trypanosomosis[1] is a disease complex caused by several species of protozoan parasites of the genus *Trypanosoma*, transmitted cyclically by the genus *Glossina* (tsetse flies). Tsetse infest 10 million square kilometres and affect 37 mostly African countries. The disease infects various species of mammals but, from an economic point of view, tsetse-transmitted trypanosomosis is particularly important in cattle (in southern Africa referred to as nagana or tsetse-fly disease). It is mainly caused by *Trypanosoma congolense, T. vivax* and, to a lesser extent, *T. brucei brucei. Trypanosoma uniforme, T. simiae* and *T. suis* are other, less common tsetse-transmitted species. *Trypanosoma vivax* is also transmitted mechanically by biting flies, as exemplified by its presence in South and Central America. Tsetse-transmitted trypanosomosis also affects humans, causing sleeping sickness, through infection with either *T. brucei gambiense* or *T. brucei rhodesiense.*

Clinical signs of tsetse-transmitted trypanosomosis may include intermittent fever, oedema, and emaciation. Anaemia usually develops in affected animals and this is followed by loss of body condition, reduced productivity and often mortality. Post-mortem signs may include emaciation, enlarged lymph nodes, enlarged liver, excessive fluid in the body cavities, and petechial haemorrhages. Neither clinical nor post-mortem signs of tsetse-transmitted trypanosomosis are pathognomonic. Therefore, diagnosis must rely on direct techniques that confirm the presence of trypanosomes either by microscopic visualisation or by indirect serological techniques.

1 *Note on nomenclature of parasitic diseases:*
The World Association for Advances in Veterinary Parasitology has recommended a 'Standardised Nomenclature of Animal Parasitic Diseases' (Kassai T., Cordero del Campillo M., Euzeby J., Gaafar S., Hiepe Th. & Himonas C.A. [1988]. Vet. Parasitol., ***29,*** *299–326). In principle, the disease name is constructed by adding the suffix '-osis' to the stem of the name of the parasite taxon. This terminology has been followed in this* Manual, *and 'trypanosomosis' therefore replaces tho old term of 'trypanosomiasis'.*

A variety of diagnostic tests are available (19) and researchers are still trying to improve existing tests and to develop new ones. Current diagnostic tests vary in their sensitivity and specificity, the ease with which they can be applied and their cost (16). The choice of a particular test will be guided by economic principles and the availability of expertise, but especially by the diagnostic requirement. For example, different degrees of sensitivity and specificity are applicable to individual animals compared with herds. Similarly, the diagnostic test(s) to establish the parasitological prevalence of trypanosomosis are different from those required to establish the presence or absence of the disease in an area. Reliable diagnosis may be achieved by combining appropriate diagnostic tests. Reliable interpretation of results from diagnostic tests will depend, to a large extent, on proper sample selection/collection, the sample size, and the way the diagnostic tests are conducted.

1. Identification of the agent

Parasite detection techniques are highly specific, but their sensitivity is relatively low (i.e. the proportion of false-negative results recorded is high). Sensitivity is especially low when results are considered at the individual animal level rather than the herd level. Due to this low sensitivity, the apparent parasitological prevalence of trypanosomosis is generally lower than the true parasitological prevalence. The low diagnostic sensitivity also makes it difficult to detect trypanosomosis when present at low parasitological prevalence and it is impossible to establish the absence of the disease with a high degree of confidence. Moreover, in areas where trypanocidal drugs are used extensively, parasites may not be detected.

Several parasite detection techniques are available, each with varying sensitivity. The choice will depend on the laboratory facilities available and the aim of the diagnosis.

• Direct examination techniques

The simplest techniques are examination of wet, thick or thin films of fresh blood, usually obtained from the ear vein, jugular vein or the tail.

a) Wet blood films

These are made by placing a drop of blood (about 2 µl) on a clean microscope slide and covering with a cover-slip (22 × 22 mm). The blood is examined microscopically using a ×40 objective lens with reduced condenser aperture or by phase-contrast. Approximately 50–100 fields are examined. Trypanosomes can be recognised by their movement among the red blood cells (RBCs).

The method is simple, inexpensive and gives immediate results. Depending on the trypanosome size and movements a presumptive diagnosis can be made of the trypanosome species. Final confirmation of the species is made by the examination of the stained preparation.

The diagnostic sensitivity of the method is generally low but depends on the examiner's experience and the level of parasitaemia. Sensitivity can be improved significantly by lysing the RBCs before examination using a haemolytic agent such as sodium dodecyl sulfate (SDS) (15).

b) Thick blood films

These are made by placing a drop of blood (5–10 µl) on a clean microscope slide and spreading it over an area of approximately 2 cm in diameter, using the corner of another slide. The thickness of the resultant film should be such that, when dry, the figures on a wristwatch dial can just be read through it. The film is dried thoroughly by rapidly waving in the air and, without fixation, is dehaemoglobinised by immersion in distilled water for a few seconds and dried before staining. A dry smear should be kept dry and protected from dust, heat, flies and other insects. It is stained for 30 minutes with 4% diluted Giemsa stain in phosphate buffered water, pH 7.2. Staining time and stain dilution may vary with stain and individual technique. Therefore, it is important to start with the manufacturer's directions and to vary staining time and stain concentration to obtain the optimal result. The stained smear is then washed with buffered water and examined with a ×50 or ×100 oil-immersion objective lens.

The method is simple and relatively inexpensive, but results are delayed because of the staining process. Trypanosomes are easily recognised by their general morphology, but may be damaged during the staining process. This may make it difficult to identify the species.

c) Thin blood smear films

Thin blood smears are made by placing a small drop of blood (about 5 µl), for example from a microhaematocrit capillary tube, on a clean microscope slide approximately 20 mm from one end (allowing for space to apply the thick smear) and spreading with the edge of another slide. This slide is placed at an angle of approximately 30° to the first slide and drawn back to make contact with the blood droplet. The blood is allowed to run along the edge of the spreader, which is then pushed to the other end of the slide in a fairly rapid but smooth motion. If the correct amount of blood is used, the slide should be covered with a film of blood with no surplus before the end of the slide is reached. Ideally, thin films should be prepared so that the RBCs are fairly close to each other but not overlapping. The slide is dried quickly by waving in the air and protected from dust, flies and other insects. The slide is fixed for 3 minutes in methanol, and stained as for thick blood smears. After staining, the slide is washed gently under tap water and allowed to dry. A variation of this method is to fix in methanol for 2 minutes, apply May–Grünwald stain for 2 minutes, then add an equal volume of buffered water, pH 7.2, leave for a further 8 minutes and drain off. Approximately 50–100 fields of the stained thin smear are examined, with a ×50 or ×100 oil-immersion objective lens, before the specimen is considered to be negative. Even after a trypanosome has been detected, approximately 20 extra fields are investigated to determine if more than one species is present.

The technique described above can also be used for biopsy samples of lymph obtained from punctured lymph nodes.

Usually, both a thin and thick smear is made from the same sample. Thick smears contain more blood than thin smears and, hence, have a higher diagnostic sensitivity. Thin smears on the other hand allow *Trypanosoma* species identification. Trypanosome species can be identified by the following morphological characteristics:

Trypanosoma vivax: 20–27 µm long, undulating membrane is not obvious, free flagellum present at the anterior end, posterior end rounded, kinetoplast large and terminal.

Trypanosoma brucei is a polymorphic trypanosome species. Two distinctly different forms can be distinguished, i.e. a long slender form and a short stumpy form. Often, intermediate forms, possessing characteristics of both the slender and stumpy forms, are observed. The cytoplasm often contains basophilic granules in stained specimens.

Trypanosoma brucei (long slender form): 17–30 µm long and about 2.8 µm wide, undulating membrane is conspicuous, free flagellum present at the anterior end, posterior end pointed, kinetoplast small and subterminal.

Trypanosoma brucei (short stumpy form): 17–22 µm long and about 3.5 µm wide, undulating membrane is conspicuous, free flagellum absent, posterior end pointed, kinetoplast small and subterminal.

Trypanosoma congolense: 8–25 µm (small species), undulating membrane not obvious, free flagellum absent, posterior end rounded, kinetoplast is medium sized and terminal, often laterally positioned. Although *T. congolense* is considered to be monomorphus, a degree of morphological variation is sometimes observed.

Trypanosoma theileri: 60–70 µm (large species), undulating membrane is conspicuous, long free flagellum present, posterior end pointed, kinetoplast is large and positioned near the nucleus. *Trypanosoma theileri* is normally nonpathogenic, but its presence can confuse the parasitological diagnosis.

- **Parasite concentration techniques**

The probability of detecting trypanosomes in a sample from an infected animal depends largely on the amount of blood examined and the level of parasitaemia. The amount of blood examined with direct examination techniques is low and parasites are often very scanty in the blood of an infected animal. Both of these factors contribute to the low sensitivity of direct examination techniques. Sensitivity can be improved by increasing the volume of blood to be examined and by concentrating the trypanosomes.

a) Microhaematocrit centrifugation technique (Woo method)

The microhaematocrit centrifugation technique, or the Woo method (24), is widely used for the diagnosis of animal trypanosomosis. It is based on the separation of the different components of the blood sample depending on their specific gravity. The method is as follows:

i) Fresh, usually ear vein blood (about 70 µl) is collected into heparinised capillary tubes (75 × 1.5 mm).

ii) One end of the capillary tube is sealed with cristaseal or by heating, ensuring that the column of blood is not charred by the flame.

iii) The sealed capillary tubes are placed in a microhaematocrit centrifuge with the sealed ends pointing towards the outside. To ensure good balance, the tubes are loaded symmetrically.

iv) The rotary cover is screwed on and the centrifuge lid is closed.

v) The capillary tubes are centrifuged at 9000 *g* for 5 minutes.

vi) A tube carrier is made from a slide on which two pieces of glass 25 × 10 × 1.2 mm have been fixed, 1.5 mm apart, to form a groove.

vii) The tube is placed in the groove, a cover-slip is placed on top and the interface is flooded with water.

viii) The plasma/white blood cell interface (buffy coat) is examined by slowly rotating the tube. Trypanosome movement can first be detected using the ×10 objective lens with reduced condenser aperture; the trypanosomes can be seen more clearly using the ×40 objective lens preferably with a long working distance to allow adequate depth of focus through the capillary tube.

The microhaematocrit centrifugation technique is more sensitive than the direct examination techniques (8). Identification of trypanosome species is difficult. As the specific gravity of *T. congolense* is similar to that of RBCs, parasites are often found below the buffy coat in the RBC layer. To improve the separation of RBCs and parasites, and increase the sensitivity for *T. congolense*, the specific gravity of RBCs can be increased by the addition of glycerol (21).

A modification of the Woo method is the quantitative buffy coat method (QBC) (1). The method has been used for the diagnosis of *T. b. gambiense* infections. The method is probably too expensive for the routine large-scale use in animal trypanosomosis surveys.

b) Dark-ground/phase-contrast buffy coat technique

The buffy coat technique or Murray method (13) represents an improved technique for the detection of trypanosomes and is widely used. It is carried out following steps i to v above, after which the capillary tube is cut, with a diamond tipped pencil, 1 mm below the buffy coat, to include the top layer of RBCs. The buffy coat and the uppermost layer RBCs are extruded on to a clean microscope slide and covered with a cover-slip (22 × 22 mm). Approximately 200 fields of the preparation are examined for the presence of motile trypanosomes with a dark-ground or a phase-contrast microscope with a ×40 objective lens. Trypanosome species can be identified by reference to the following criteria:

Trypanosoma vivax: Large, extremely active, traverses the whole field very quickly, pausing occasionally.

Trypanosoma brucei: Various sizes, rapid movement in confined areas.

Trypanosoma congolense: Small, sluggish, adheres to RBCs by anterior end.

Trypanosoma theileri: More than twice the size of pathogenic trypanosomes, tends to rotate

As with the microhaematocrit centrifugation technique, the buffy coat technique is more sensitive than direct examination techniques. The sensitivity of the buffy coat method can be improved by using the buffy coat double centrifugation technique (8). A total amount of 1500–2000 µl of blood is centrifuged, after which the buffy coat is aspired into a microhaematocrit capillary tube and centrifuged again. The buffy coat is examined. Compared with the microhaematocrit centrifugation technique, the buffy coat technique has the added advantage that preparations can be fixed and stained for more accurate identification of species and for retention as a permanent record.

Both the microhaematocrit centrifugation and buffy coat techniques give direct results and can be used for screening large numbers of animals. They require specialised equipment and an electricity supply making the test more expensive compared with the examination of the wet blood film. However, this is compensated for by increased sensitivity. Both parasite concentration techniques rely on the detection of motile, live, trypanosomes. As trypanosomes are heat-sensitive, samples collected in capillary tubes should be kept cool and the microhaematocrit centrifuge should not be allowed to overheat.

The microhaematocrit centrifugation and buffy coat techniques are particularly useful in that the packed cell volume (PCV) can be assessed at the same time. To determine the packed cell volume after centrifugation, the microhaematocrit capillary tube (containing ear vein or jugular vein blood) is placed in a haematocrit reader. The length of the packed RBC column is expressed as a percentage of the total volume of blood. Measuring the PCV is useful for determining the degree of anaemia. Anaemia can be caused by factors other than tsetse-transmitted trypanosomosis. It remains, however, one of the most important indicators of trypanosomosis in cattle. As trypanosomosis is a herd problem, the PCV-profile of a herd is influenced by the number of trypanosome-infected animals and can be used to indicate differences in disease challenge.

c) **Anion exchange**

The miniature anion-exchange chromatography technique (m-AECT) is widely used for the diagnosis of human sleeping sickness caused by *T. b. gambiense* (10). Blood is passed through a diethyl amino-ethyl (DEAE)-cellulose column equilibrated with a phosphate buffered saline (PBS) solution of an ionic strength suited to the blood of the animal species under examination. As the RBCs are more negatively charged than the trypanosomes, they are held in the column and the trypanosomes pass through with the eluate, which is collected, centrifuged to concentrate the trypanosomes and examined under the microscope.

Large volumes of blood can be examined from each animal and, therefore, the method has high sensitivity. However, the technique is cumbersome and is not suitable for the examination of a large number of animals.

d) ***In-vitro* cultivation**

A procedure for the *in-vitro* cultivation of *T. brucei* has been described, but success has been irregular over many years. Moreover, the method needs sophisticated equipment, produces results after a considerable delay and is certainly not suitable for large-scale use. A recently described kit (KIVI) for *in-vitro* isolation of trypanosomes has proven to be promising in isolating and amplifying *T. b. gambiense* in humans, domestic and game animals (20). The test's value in isolating *T. congolense* and *T. vivax* is still unknown. As it is based on the cultivation of procyclic forms of trypanosomes, species differentiation is not possible (7).

• Animal inoculation

The subinoculation of blood into rodents, usually mice or rats, is particularly useful in revealing subpatent infections. The laboratory animals are injected intraperitoneally with 0.2–5 ml (depending on the size of the rodent) of freshly collected blood. They are bled three times a week for at least 2 months. Collected blood is examined using the wet film method.

Animal inoculation is more sensitive than direct examination of the wet blood film. Nevertheless, the method is not practical; it is expensive and diagnosis is not immediate. The method is highly sensitive in detecting *T. brucei* infections. However, some *T. congolense* strains are not easily transmitted and *T. vivax* rarely infects laboratory rodents.

• Tests to detect trypanosomal antigen

An antigen-detection enzyme-linked immunosorbent assay (antigen ELISA) for trypanosomosis has been described (14). Field evaluations of the test have given inconsistent results. Therefore, additional work is needed to discover and overcome the cause of those inconsistencies before the test can be used in the routine diagnosis of trypanosomosis.

• DNA amplification tests

A polymerase chain reaction (PCR) method has been developed as a tool for the diagnosis of infections with African trypanosomes in humans and animals, as well as tsetse flies. Specific repetitive nuclear DNA sequences can be amplified for *T. vivax* and each of the five *T. congolense* subgroups (2, 12). A common primer set is available for detection of the three *T. brucei* subspecies. The primer sets available for different trypanosome species, subspecies and subgroups are referred to as follows: *brucei* subspecies: TBR1 and TBR2 congolense (Savannah subgroup); TCN1 and TCN2 congolense (Forest subgroup); TCF1 and TCF2 congolense (Kenya Coast subgroup); TCK1 and TCK2 *vivax*: TVW1 and TVW2.

Standard PCR amplifications are carried out in a reaction mixture containing Tris-HCl, $MgCl_2$, KCl, each of the four deoxyribonucleotide triphosphates, primers, DNA template and Taq DNA polymerase. Samples are incubated during several cycles at varying temperatures. The PCR products are electrophoresed through agarose. Gels are stained with ethidium bromide.

The procedure is extremely sensitive, but false-positive results may occur as a result of contamination of samples with other DNA. The test requires specialised equipment and highly trained personnel, so it is not suitable for use in many laboratories. False-negative results may occur when the specificity of the primers is too high so that not all types of a particular trypanosome species are recognised. Sample collection has been simplified by adapting the test using blood spotted on to filter paper (5). A large number of samples can be processed at one time, making it potentially suitable for large-scale surveys. However, at the moment, the cost of PCR analyses are prohibitive for the routine use of the test.

2. Serological tests

Several antibody detection techniques have been developed to detect trypanosomal antibodies for the diagnosis of animal trypanosomosis, with variable sensitivity and specificity. The methods of choice are the indirect fluorescent antibody test (IFAT) (6) and the trypanosomal antibody-detection ELISA (4, 9). The development and testing of specific recombinant antigens could, in the near future, allow the detection of species-specific antibodies.

a) Indirect fluorescent antibody test

The original method for this test (23) has been replaced by a new technique for the preparation of trypanosomal antigens (6), which involves fixation of live trypanosomes using a mixture of 80% cold acetone and 0.25% formalin in normal saline (18, 22).

- **Test procedure**

i) Prepare thin smears from heavily parasitaemic blood or from a trypanosome suspension. Air-dry and fix in acetone for 5 minutes.

ii) Mark circles of 5 mm diameter on glass slides using nail varnish.

iii) Using a pipette, place a test serum, diluted 1/40, in each circle, ensuring that the area in each circle is completely covered.

iv) Incubate the antigen/test serum preparation at 37°C for 30 minutes in a humid chamber.

v) Wash the preparation three times in PBS for 5 minutes each time at 4°C, with gentle agitation. Air-dry the slides.

vi) Apply conjugate: rabbit or goat anti-bovine IgG (for tests on bovine sera) conjugated to fluorescein isothiocyanate.

vii) Incubate and wash as above. Rinse in distilled water. Air-dry the slides.

viii) Mount the slides in PBS or buffered glycerol and examine for fluorescence.

b) Antibody-detection enzyme-linked immunosorbent assay

The original antibody ELISA (9) has recently been further developed for use in large-scale surveys of bovine trypanosomosis (4).

- **Test procedure**

Minor modifications are made to the original procedure (9)

i) Dilute antigen in 50 mM carbonate–bicarbonate buffer, pH 9.6, and coat microtitre plates overnight at 4°C.

ii) Wash microtitre plates four times in 2 mM PBS, pH 7.4, containing 0.05% Tween 20.

iii) Dilute sera at 1/400 in PBS, 10 mM, pH 7.4, containing 0.04% Tween 20. Punch 6 mm disks from dried bloodspots on filter paper and elute in 2.0 ml PBS for 2.5 or 5 hours at room temperature or overnight at 4°C.

iv) Incubate diluted sera or bloodspots with anti-bovine IgG peroxidase conjugate in microtitre plate wells at 37°C with orbital shaking for 45 and 30 minutes, respectively.

v) Wash microtitre plates five times in 2 mM PBS, pH 7.4, containing 0.05% Tween 20.

vi) Incubate for 10 minutes in tetramethylbenzidine at 37°C with orbital shaking followed by an H_2SO_4 quench.

vii) Read absorbance at 450 nm.

The standard antigen for trypanosomosis antibody tests is derived from bloodstream-form trypanosomes. Antigens are prepared as a soluble fraction of trypanosomes purified by DEAE anion-exchange chromatography of parasites from whole blood of infected rats, with lysis using seven freeze–thaw cycles and centrifugation at 10,000 ***g*** for 30 minutes. Antigens obtained from *in-vitro* propagated procyclic trypanosome forms can also be used (3). Both the IFAT and antibody-detection ELISA have been adapted for the analysis of blood samples collected on filter paper. Blood contained in one heparinised microhaematocrit centrifuge capillary tube is extruded on to a filter paper (Whatman® No. 4). Samples are air-dried out of direct sunlight and placed in a plastic bag with self-indicating silica gel desiccant. The bag is sealed and should be kept as cool as possible until specimens are refrigerated or frozen.

Each ELISA-microplate is run with strong positive, weak positive and negative reference sera, which are required to comply with pre-set values for quality assurance. The absorbance of each ELISA-sample tested is expressed as a percentage (percentage positivity, PP) of the strong positive reference standard (25). Results are, therefore, quantifiable. The cut-off value is determined using known positive and negative field samples.

Both antibody-detection tests have high sensitivity and specificity. Their species specificity is generally low. They detect immune responses to current and past infections and can, therefore, only provide a presumptive diagnosis of active infection.

Immunodiagnosis needs expensive, sophisticated equipment and expertise, which is not always available. It has to be performed in specialised laboratories and there is a substantial delay between the actual sampling and the availability of the results. Nevertheless, the antibody ELISA lends itself to a high degree of automation and standardisation. Sample collection and storage is made easy through the use of filter papers. All of these factors make the antibody ELISA a very useful test for large-scale surveys to determine the distribution of tsetse-transmitted trypanosomosis.

c) Card agglutination test

This test was originally developed for the diagnosis of human sleeping sickness *(T. b. gambiense)* (11) and has been further adapted for the detection of antibodies against *T. evansi* (17).

B. REQUIREMENTS FOR VACCINES AND DIAGNOSTIC BIOLOGICALS

No biological products are in use at the present time.

REFERENCES

1. BAILEY J.W. & SMITH D.H. (1992). The use of the acridine orange QBC technique in the diagnosis of African trypanosomiasis. *Trans. R. Soc. Trop. Med. Hyg.*, **86**, 630.

2. DESQUESNES M. (1997). Evaluation of a simple PCR technique for the diagnosis of *Trypanosoma vivax* infection in the serum of cattle in comparison to parasitological techniques and antigen-enzyme-linked-immunosorbent assay. *Acta Trop.*, **65**, 139–148.

3. GREINER M., KUMAR S. & KYESWA C. (1997). Evaluation and comparison of antibody ELISAs for serodiagnosis of bovine trypanosomosis. *Vet Parasitol.*, **73**, 197–205.

4. HOPKINS J.S., CHITAMBO H., MACHILA N., LUCKINS A.G., RAE P.F., VAN DEN BOSSCHE P. & EISLER M.C. (1998). Adaptation and validation of the antibody trapping ELISA using dried blood spots on filter paper, for epidemiological surveys of tsetse transmitted trypanosomosis in cattle. *Prev. Vet. Med.*, **37**, 91–99.

5. KATAKURA K., LUBINGA C., CHITAMBO H. & TRADA Y. (1997). Detection of *Trypanosoma congolense* and *T. brucei* subspecies in cattle in Zambia by polymerase chain reaction from blood collected on a filter paper. *Parasitol. Res.*, **83**, 241–245.

6. KATENDE J.M., MUSOKE A.J., NANTULYA V.M. & GODDEERIS B.M. (1987). A new method for fixation and preservation of trypanosomal antigens for use in the indirect immunofluorescence antibody test for diagnosis of bovine trypanosomiasis. *Trop. Med. Parasitol.*, **38**, 41–44.

7. KOMOIN-OKA C., TRUC P., BENGALY Z., FORMENTY P., DUVALLET G., LAUGINIE F., RAATH J.P., N'DEPO A.E. & LEFORBAN Y. (1994). Etude de la prévalence des infections à trypanosomes chez différent espèces d'animaux sauvages du parc national de la Comoé en Côte d'Ivoire : résultats préliminaires sur la comparison de trois méthodes de diagnostic. *Rev. Elev. Med. Vet. Pays Trop.*, **47**, 189–194.

8. KRATZER R.D. & ONDIEK F.O. (1989). The buffy coat double centrifugation technique, an improved method for the diagnosis of African trypanosomiasis. Nairobi:OAU/IBAR (Organization of African Unity/Interafrican Bureau for Animal Resources). International Scientific Committee for Trypanomonosis Research and Control (ISCTRC), Mombassa, Kenya, April 1989.

9. LUCKINS A.G. (1977). Detection of antibodies in trypansome infected cattle by means of a microplate enzyme–linked immunosorbent assay. *Trop. Anim. Health Prod.*, **9**, 53–62.

10. LUMSDEN W.H.R., KIMBER C.D., EVANS D.A. & DOIG S.J. (1979). *Trypanosoma brucei*: miniature anion-exchange centrifugation technique for detection of low parasitaemias: adaptation for field use. *Trans. R. Soc. Trop. Med. Hyg.*, **73**, 312–317.

11. MAGNUS E., VERVOORT T. & VAN MEIRVENNE N. (1978). A card agglutination test with stained trypanosomes (CATT) for serological diagnosis of *T. b. gambiense* trypanosomiasis. *Ann. Soc. Belg. Med. Trop.*, **58**, 169–176.

12. MOSER D.R., COOK G.A., OCHS D.E., BAILEY C.P., MCKANE M.R. & DONELSON J.E. (1989). Detection of *Trypanosoma congolense* and *Trypanosoma brucei* subspecies by DNA amplification using the polymerase chain reaction. *Parasitology*, **99**, 57–66.

13. MURRAY M., MURRAY P.K. & MCINTYRE W.I.M. (1977). An improved parasitological technique for the diagnosis of African trypanosomiasis. *Trans. R. Soc. Trop. Med. Hyg.*, **71**, 325–326.

14. NANTULYA M.V. & LINDQUIST K.J. (1989). Antigen-detection enzyme immunoassays for the diagnosis of *Trypanosoma vivax, T. congolense* and *T. brucei* infections in cattle. *Trop. Med. Parasitol.*, **40**, 267–272.

15. NDAO M., PANDEY V.S., ZINSSTAG J., PFISTER K. & VAN MEIRVENNE N. (1995). Evaluation of sodium dodecyl sulfate (SDS) as a haemolytic agent for the detection of microfilaria and trypanosomes in the blood of cattle. *Ann. Soc. Belg. Med. Trop.*, **75**, 145–148.

16. PARIS J., MURRAY M. & MCODIMBA F. (1982). A comparative evaluation of the parasitological techniques currently available for the diagnosis of African trypanosomiasis in cattle. *Acta Trop.*, **39**, 307–316.

17. PATHAK K.M.L., SINGH Y., VAN MEIRVENNE N. & KAPOOR M. (1997). Evaluation of various diagnostic techniques for *Trypanosoma evansi* infections in naturally infected camels. *Vet. Parasitol.*, **69**, 49–54.

18. PLATT K.B. & ADAMS L.G. (1976). Evaluation of the indirect fluorescent antibody test for detecting *Trypanosoma vivax* in South American cattle. *Res. Vet. Sci.*, **21**, 53–58.

19. TOURE S.M. (1976). Diagnostic des trypanosomiases animales. *Rev. Elev. Med. Vet. Pays Trop.*, **30**, 1–10.

20. TRUC P., AERTS D., MCNAMARA J.J., CLAES Y., ALLINGHAM R., LE RAY D. & GODFREY D.G. (1992). Direct isolation *in vitro* of *Trypanosoma brucei* from man and other animals, and its potential value for the diagnosis of Gambian trypanosomiasis. *Trans. R. Soc. Trop. Med. Hyg.*, **86**, 627–629.

21. WALKER P.J. (1972). Capillary concentration technique applicable to infections of *Trypanosoma congolense* in cattle. *Trans. R. Soc. Trop. Med. Hyg.*, **66**, 348.

22. WELLS E.A., RAMIREZ L.E. & BETANCOURT A. (1982). *Trypanosoma vivax* in Columbia: interpretation of field results. *Trop. Anim. Health Prod.*, **14** 141–150.

23. WILSON A.J. (1969). Value of the indirect fluorescent antibody test as a serological aid to diagnosis of *Glossina*-transmitted bovine trypanosomiasis. *Trop. Anim. Health Prod.*, **1**, 89–95.

24. WOO P.T.K. (1970). The haematocrit centrifuge technique for the diagnosis of African trypanosomiasis. *Acta Trop.*, **27**, 384–386.

25. WRIGHT P.F., NILSSON E., VAN ROOIJ E.M.A., LELENTA M. & JEGGO M.H. (1993). Standardisation and validation of enzyme-linked immunosorbent assay techniques for the detection of antibody in infectious disease diagnosis. *Rev. sci. tech. Off. int. Epiz.*, **12**, 435–450.

*

* *

CHAPTER X.7.

OVINE PULMONARY ADENOMATOSIS

SUMMARY

Ovine pulmonary adenomatosis (OPA), also known as jaagsiekte and sheep pulmonary adenomatosis (SPA), is a contagious tumour of sheep and, exceptionally, of goats. It is a progressive respiratory disease, principally affecting adult animals. The disease occurs in many regions of the world. Two viruses, a herpesvirus and a retrovirus, have been associated with the disease, but only the latter has an aetiological role. The retrovirus of SPA is distinct from the nononcogenic ovine lentivirus, but related to type B and D retroviruses.

Regular inspections and prompt removal of suspected cases may help to limit the spread of infection within affected flocks.

***Identification of the agent:** The retrovirus of OPA cannot yet be propagated* in vitro, *therefore routine diagnostic methods, such as virus isolation, are not available for diagnosis. Diagnosis relies, at present, on clinical history and examination, as well as on the findings at necropsy and by histopathology.*

***Serological tests:** Antibodies to the retrovirus have not been detected in infected sheep and, therefore, serological tests are not available for diagnosis.*

***Requirements for vaccines and diagnostic biologicals:** There are no biological products available.*

A. DIAGNOSTIC TECHNIQUES

Ovine pulmonary adenomatosis (OPA), sometimes called sheep pulmonary adenomatosis (SPA), is also known as jaagsiekte (Afrikaans = driving sickness) and ovine pulmonary carcinoma (OPC), is a contagious lung tumour of sheep and, to a lesser extent, of goats. It is the most common pulmonary tumour of sheep and occurs in many countries of the world. It is absent from Australia and New Zealand and has been eradicated from Iceland.

A number of different viruses have been linked aetiologically to OPA, including a herpesvirus and lentiviruses that have been propagated from tumour tissue. However, the former does not have an aetiological role in OPA and the latter exhibit characteristics of nononcogenic lentiviruses. It was generally accepted, but not formally proven, that OPA is caused by a retrovirus that cannot yet be cultured *in vitro*. The term jaagsiekte sheep retrovirus (JSRV) is used in referring to this virus.

At present, diagnosis of OPA relies on clinical and pathological investigations. In flocks in which the disease is suspected, its presence must be confirmed at least once by histopathological examination of affected lung tissue. For such an examination, it is imperative to take specimens from several affected sites and, if possible, from more than one animal. This is because secondary bacterial pneumonia, which might be the immediate cause of death, often masks the lesions (both macroscopic and microscopic) of the primary disease. There is no vaccine against the disease. In the absence of specific serological tests, which can be used for the diagnosis of OPA in live animals, disease control relies on regular flock inspections and prompt culling of suspected cases and, in the case of ewes, their offspring. This may reduce the prevalence of the disease but it will not eradicate it from an infected flock. Embryo transfer may be useful to obtain animals free from OPA based on clinical and pathological evidence (12).

1. Identification of the agent

- **Herpesvirus**

The association between a herpesvirus and the OPA tumour tissue from which it is isolated probably stems from reactivation of a latent infection coupled with replication of the virus in the numerous alveolar macrophages that characterise cases of OPA. To date, ovine herpesviruses have been isolated only from OPA tumour tissues, and all isolates are antigenically distinct from other members of the Herpesviridae, including herpesviruses of bovine origin, and are designated ovine herpesvirus 1 (OHV-1). A second herpesvirus, provisionally designated ovine herpesvirus 2 (OHV-2), is implicated in the sheep-associated form of malignant catarrhal fever, which occurs in many regions of the world.

Experimental infection of young lambs with OHV-1 results in a subclinical interstitial pneumonia, the pulmonary histiocyte being the main, and perhaps exclusive, site of virus replication (17). These findings imply that the respiratory tract is a predilection site for the virus and account for the readiness with which it can be isolated from cases of OPA. On serological evidence, infection of sheep with OHV-1 is widespread, even in countries where OPA does not occur, which implies that any relationship between the herpesvirus and OPA is coincidental and not causal (18). OHV-2 has not been isolated from sheep, but, by polymerase chain reaction (PCR) amplification of virus-specific DNA, its presence in tissues and peripheral blood leukocytes of normal lambs and adult sheep has been demonstrated. There is no evidence for its association with OPA.

- **Retroviruses**

Association of retroviruses with OPA has been recognised for several years. Ovine lentiviruses have been isolated on a number of occasions, but these viruses have no aetiological role in OPA (13, 14). On the other hand, cumulative morphological, biochemical, immunological and genomic characterisation of JSRV shows that this virus is related to types B and D retroviruses (5, 6, 22, 26) and is associated exclusively with OPA (10).

OPA can be transmitted only with material that contains JSRV, such as tumour homogenates and, more significantly, concentrated cell-free lung fluid from natural cases of OPA. The infectious fraction of the fluid contains JSRV virions and reverse transcription (RT) activity. Following the experimental inoculation of adult sheep, clinical disease develops only after several months or years. Similar inoculation of newborn lambs results in a reduced incubation period of 3–6 weeks, and many of the transformed epithelial cells contain intracytoplasmic retrovirus particles (21, 25). Furthermore, some cell cultures prepared from the tumours occurring in young lambs can support virus replication for a short period (7, 23). Following intratracheal inoculation of concentrated supernatant fluids of such cultures into three lambs within 24 hours of birth, clear histological evidence of OPA was detected in one lamb 6 months later (19).

The inability to culture JSRV, and the lack of antibodies to the virus in affected sheep, have impeded the confirmation of this virus as the aetiological agent and, therefore, development of diagnostic tests. However, alternative approaches using molecular biological techniques are promising. A key advance has been the cloning and sequencing of the 7.5 kb JSRV genome following purification of virions from lung washes of naturally affected sheep (26). JSRV resembles types B and D retroviruses both in its genetic organisation and in its structural proteins. Although cloned JSRV genes, used as hybridisation probes, have revealed a range of homologous endogenous sequences in the genome of both healthy and OPA-affected sheep (1, 5, 26), JSRV is clearly exogenous and associated exclusively with OPA (9). JSRV is detected constantly in the lung fluid, tumour and lymphoid tissues of sheep affected by OPA or unaffected in-contact flockmates, and never in sheep from unaffected flocks with no history of the tumour. Although these findings cannot confirm that JSRV is the aetiological agent, they do demonstrate unequivocally that it must play a major role, even if only as a helper virus. What contribution, if any, the endogenous viral sequences make to the aetiology of OPA remains unclear, but their expression in the fetus may, by induction of tolerance, account for the apparent lack of immune response of mature animals to exogenous JSRV.

Recently, a full-length proviral clone of JSRV has been obtained from OPA tumour DNA. JSRV virus particles, prepared from this clone by transient transfection of a cell line, were used for intratracheal inoculation of neonatal lambs. OPA tumour was induced in two of four lambs, thus demonstrating that JSRV is the causal agent of OPA (11).

Sequencing of JSRV and endogenous sequences in the sheep genome have led to the development of PCRs that specifically detect JSRV (1, 9). Using this sensitive procedure, JSRV has been detected in peripheral blood mononuclear cells of unaffected in-contact sheep from flocks with OPA, as well as experimentally infected lambs. This finding holds promise that it may be possible to develop a molecular test for identifying infected animals during the preclinical stages, thus offering a new way to diagnose OPA.

- **Clinical signs**

As OPA has a long incubation period, clinical disease is encountered most commonly in sheep over 2 years of age, with a peak occurrence at the age of 3–4 years. In exceptional cases, the disease occurs in animals as young as 2–3 months of age. The cardinal signs are those of a progressive respiratory embarrassment, particularly after exercise; the severity of the signs reflects the extent of tumour development in the lungs. Accumulation of fluid within the respiratory tract is a prominent feature of OPA, giving rise to moist râles that are readily detected by auscultation. Raising the hindquarters and lowering the head of affected sheep may cause frothy mucoid fluid to run from the nostrils. Coughing and inappetance are not common but, once clinical signs are evident, weight loss is progressive and the disease is terminal within weeks or months. Death is often precipitated by a superimposed bacterial pneumonia, particularly that due to *Mannheimia haemolytica*. In clinically affected animals, a peripheral lymphopaenia characterised by a reduction in CD4+ T lymphocytes and a corresponding neutrophilia may assist clinical diagnosis, but the changes are not pathognomonic (15).

In some countries, another form of OPA (atypical OPA) occurs, which generally presents as an incidental finding at necropsy or the abattoir (3).

- **Necropsy**

OPA lesions are in most cases confined to the lungs, although intra- and extrathoracic metastases to lymph nodes and other tissues can occur. In typical cases, affected lungs are considerably enlarged and heavier than normal due to extensive nodular and coalescing firm grey lesions affecting much of the pulmonary tissue. Usually lesions are present in both lungs, although the extent on either side does vary. Tumours are solid, grey or light purple with a shiny translucent sheen and often separated from the adjacent normal lung by a narrow emphysematous zone. The presence of frothy white fluid in the respiratory passages is a prominent feature and is obvious even in lesions as small as a few millimetres. In advanced cases, this fluid flows out of the trachea when it is cut or pendant.

Pleurisy may be evident over the surface of the tumour and in some cases abscesses are present in the adenomatous tissue.

In atypical OPA, tumours comprise solitary or aggregated hard white nodules that have a dry cut surface and show clear demarcation from surrounding tissues. The presence of excess fluid is not a prominent feature.

Adult sheep that on post-mortem examination appear to have died from acute pasteurellosis should have their lungs examined carefully as lesions of OPA may be masked by coexisting bronchopneumonia, verminous pneumonia, chronic progressive pneumonia (maedi) or combinations of these. Samples should be taken at necropsy for PCR for retrovirus genome examination. Storage of these samples at –80°C is recommended, prior to RNA extraction and testing.

- **Histopathology**

Histologically, the lesions are characterised by proliferation of mainly type II pneumocytes, a secretory epithelial cell in the pulmonary alveoli. Nonciliated (Clara) and epithelial cells of the terminal bronchioli may be involved. The cuboidal or columnar tumour cells replace the normal thin alveolar cells and sometimes form papilliform growths that project into the alveoli. Intrabronchiolar proliferation may be present. In advanced cases, extensive fibrosis may develop and, occasionally, nodules of loose connective tissue in a mucopolysaccharide substance may be present.

A prominent feature is the accumulation of large numbers of alveolar macrophages in the alveoli adjacent to the neoplastic lesions.

Where maedi is concurrent, perivascular, peribronchiolar and interstitial lymphoid infilrates may be prominent.

The histological appearance of atypical OPA is essentially the same as classical OPA, but with an exaggerated inflammatory response (mostly lymphocytes and plasma cells) and fibrosis (3).

For more detailed accounts of the clinical, post-mortem and histopathological aspects of OPA, the reader is referred elsewhere (16, 20, 24).

There appears to be a synergistic interaction between OPA and maedi. Lateral transmission of maedi-visna virus appears to be enhanced in sheep affected by OPA (2, 4).

2. Serological tests

At present, there are no laboratory tests to support a clinical diagnosis of OPA in the live animal. JSRV has been associated exclusively with both typical and atypical forms of OPA, but antibodies to this virus have not been detected in the sera of affected sheep, even with highly sensitive assays such as immunoblotting (8).

B. REQUIREMENTS FOR VACCINES AND DIAGNOSTIC BIOLOGICALS

There are no vaccines available at the present time.

REFERENCES

1. Bai J., Zhu R.-Y., Stedman K., Cousens C., Carlson J.O., Sharp J.M. & DeMartini J.C. (1996). Unique long terminal repeat U3 sequences distinguish exogenous jaagsiekte sheep retroviruses associated with ovine pulmonary carcinoma from endogenous loci in the sheep genome. *J. Virol.*, **70**, 3159–3168.

2. Dawson M., Venables C. & Jenkins C.E. (1985). Experimental infection of a natural case of sheep pulmonary adenomatosis with maedi-visna virus. *Vet. Rec.* **116**, 588–589.

3. De Las Heras M., Calafat J.J., Jaime J.M., Garcia De Jalon J.A., Ferrer L.M., Garcia Goti M. & Minguijon E. (1992). Sheep pulmonary adenomatosis (jaagsiekte) in slaughtered sheep: variation in pathological characteristics. *Medicina Veterinaria*, 9 (Suppl.), 52–53.

4. Gonzalez L., Juste R.A., Cuervo L.A., Idigoras I. & Saez De Ocariz C. (1993). Pathological and epidemiological aspects of the coexistence of maedi-visna and sheep pulmonary adenomatosis. *Res. Vet. Sci.*, **54**, 140–146.

5. Hecht S.J., Carlson J.O. & De Martini J.C. (1994). Analysis of a type D retroviral capsid gene expressed in ovine pulmonary carcinoma and present in both affected and unaffected sheep genomes. *Virology*, **202**, 480–484.

6. Herring A.J., Sharp J.M., Scott F.M.M. & Angus K.W. (1983). Further evidence for a retrovirus as the aetiological agent of sheep pulmonary adenomatosis (jaagsiekte). *Vet. Microbiol.*, **8**, 237–249.

7. Jassim F.A. (1988). Identification and Characterisation of Transformed Cells in Jaagsiekte, a Contagious Lung Tumour of Sheep. PhD thesis. University of Edinburgh, UK.

8. Ortin A., Minguijon E., Dewar P., Garcia M., Ferrer L.M., Palmarini M., Gonzalez L., Sharp J.M. & De Las Heras M. (1997). Lack of a specific immune response against a recombinant capsid protein of Jaagsiekte sheep retrovirus in sheep and goats naturally affected by enzootic nasal tumour or sheep pulmonary adenomatosis. *Vet. Immunol. Immunopathol.*, **61**, 229–237

9. Palmarini M., Cousens C., Dalziel R.G., Bai J., Stedman K, DeMartini J.C. & Sharp J.M. (1996). The exogenous form of Jaagsiekte retrovirus (JSRV) is specifically associated with a contagious lung cancer of sheep. *J. Virol.*, **70**,1618–1623.

10. Palmarini M., Fan H. & Sharp J.M. (1997). Sheep Pulmonary Adenomatosis: a unique model of a retrovirus-associated cancer. *Trends Microbiol.*, **5**, 478–483

11. Palmarini M., Sharp J.M., De Las Heras M. & Fan H. (1999). Jaagsiekte sheep retrovirus is necessary and sufficient to induce a contagious lung cancer in sheep. *J. Virol.*, **73**, 6964–6972.

12. Parker B.N.J., Wrathall A.E., Saunders R.W., Dawson M., Done S.H., Francis P.G., Dexter I. & Bradley R. (1998). Prevention of transmission of sheep pulmonary adenomatosis by embryo transfer. *Vet. Rec.*, **142**, 687–689.

13. Perk K., De Villiers E.M., Dawson M., Herring H.J., Sharp J.M. & De Martini J.C. (1985). Comparison by Western blotting of the retroviruses associated with sheep adenomatosis (jaagsiekte). *In:* Slow Virus Diseases in Sheep, Goats and Cattle, Sharp J.M. & Hoff-Jorgensen R., eds. CEC Report EUR 8076 EN, Luxembourg, 349–351.

14. QUERAT G., BARBAN V., SAUZE N., VIGNE R., PAYNE A.L., YORK D.F., DE VILLIERS E.M. & VERWOERD D.W. (1987). Characteristics of a novel lentivirus derived from South African sheep with pulmonary adenomatosis (jaagsiekte). *Virology*, **158**, 158–167.

15. ROSADIO R. & SHARP J.M. (1992). Leucocyte frequency alterations in sheep with naturally and experimentally infected lung cancer. *Medicina Veterinaria*, **9** (Suppl.), 49–51.

16. ROSADIO R.H., SHARP J.M., LAIRMORE M.D., DAHLBERG J.E. & DE MARTINI J.C. (1988). Lesions and retroviruses associated with naturally occurring ovine pulmonary carcinoma (sheep pulmonary adenomatosis). *Vet. Pathol.*, **25**, 58–66.

17. SCOTT F.M.M., SHARP J.M., ANGUS K.W. & GRAY E.W. (1984). Infection of specific pathogen-free lambs with a herpesvirus isolated from pulmonary adenomatosis. *Arch. Virol.*, **80**, 147–162.

18. SHARP J.M. (1987). Sheep pulmonary adenomatosis: a contagious tumour and its cause. *Cancer Surv.*, **6**, 73–82.

19. SHARP J.M. & ANGUS K.W. (1990). Sheep pulmonary adenomatosis: studies on its aetiology. *In:* Maedi-Visna and Related Diseases. Developments in Veterinary Virology, Petursson G. & Hoff-Jorgensen R., eds. Martinus Nijhoff, The Hague, The Netherlands, 157–175.

20. SHARP J.M. & ANGUS K.W. (1990). Sheep pulmonary adenomatosis: clinical, pathological and epidemiological aspects. *In:* Maedi-Visna and Related Diseases. Developments in Veterinary Virology, Petursson G. & Hoff-Jorgensen R., eds. Martinus Nijhoff, The Hague, The Netherlands, 177–185.

21. SHARP J.M., ANGUS K.W., GRAY E.W. & SCOTT F.M.M. (1983). Rapid transmission of sheep pulmonary adenomatosis (jaagsiekte) in young lambs. *Arch. Virol.*, **78**, 89–95.

22. SHARP J.M. & HERRING A.J. (1983). Sheep pulmonary adenomatosis: demonstration of a protein which cross reacts with the major core proteins of Mason–Pfizer monkey virus and mouse mammary tumour virus. *J. Gen. Virol.*, **64**, 2323–2327.

23. SHARP J.M., HERRING A.J., ANGUS K.W., SCOTT F.M.M. & JASSIM F.A. (1985). Isolation and *in vitro* propagation of a retrovirus from sheep pulmonary adenomatosis. *In:* Slow Virus Diseases in Sheep, Goats and Cattle, Sharp J.M. & Hoff-Jorgensen R., eds. CEC Report EUR 8076 EN, Luxembourg, 345–348.

24. VERWOERD D.W., TUSTIN R.C. & PAYNE A. (1985). Jaagsiekte: An infectious pulmonary adenomatosis of sheep. *In*: Comparative Pathobiology of Viral Diseases, Vol. II, Olsen R.G., Krakowa S. & Blakeslee J.R., eds. CRC Press, Florida, USA, 53–75.

25. VERWOERD D.W., WILLIAMSON A. & DE VILLIERS E.M. (1980). Aetiology of jaagsiekte: transmission by means of cellular fractions and evidence for the involvement of a retrovirus. *Onderstepoort J. Vet. Res.*, **47**, 275–280.

26. YORK D.F., VIGNE R., VERWOERD D.W. & QUERAT G. (1992). Nucleotide sequence of the jaagsiekte retrovirus, an exogenous and endogenous type D and B retrovirus of sheep and goats. *J. Virol.*, **66**, 4930–4939.

*
* *

CHAPTER X.8.

NAIROBI SHEEP DISEASE

SUMMARY

Nairobi sheep disease (NSD) is caused by a Nairovirus *of the family Bunyaviridae; it is a tick-transmitted disease that is not contagious. It should be suspected when a mortality rate, which may range between 40% and 90%, occurs in a sheep or goat population, especially when this follows movement from free areas into enzootic areas. The disease is characterised by pyrexia (41.5°C), collapse, and diarrhoea. Abortion is also a feature. Animals that die in the early stages of the disease show congestion of most organs and tissues, with enlarged and oedematous lymph nodes; the spleen may also be enlarged. There are likely to be petechial and ecchymotic haemorrhages throughout the carcase on the serous surfaces of organs and especially the lymph nodes. Later in the course of disease, inflammation of the gastrointestinal tract may become evident. Infestation with ticks, notably* Rhipicephalus appendiculatus, *substantiates any suspicion as to the agent involved. There is a low total white cell count in the early febrile stages. Ganjam virus in India is believed to be a strain of NSD and causes a similar syndrome. NSD is an apparently rare zoonotic agent in the field, causing a mild influenza-like disease in humans, but at least seven laboratory aerosol infections by Ganjam virus have been recorded.*

Identification of the agent: *Plasma from febrile animals, mesenteric lymph nodes or spleen are best for virus isolation. Laboratory-reared sheep, 2–4-day-old unweaned mice inoculated intracerebrally, or cell cultures may be used for primary isolation. Sheep are the most sensitive animals for this, whereas a baby hamster kidney cell line and lamb or hamster kidney cell cultures are the most sensitive cells. Subinoculation of plasma from an experimentally infected sheep into cell cultures or mice is also recommended.*

Identification of the virus may be made by direct immunofluorescence of inoculated tissue cultures or of mouse brain smears. The agar gel immunodiffusion test can also be used to demonstrate the presence of NSD antigen in tissues. Infected tissue cultures or mouse brain suspensions may be used as sources of complement-fixing or enzyme-linked immunosorbent assay (ELISA) antigens.

Serological tests: *The most suitable test is the indirect fluorescent antibody test. Complement fixation and indirect haemagglutination tests have also been used to confirm NSD outbreaks in the field. Virus neutralisation tests give equivocal results, a feature that also occurs with other members of the* Nairovirus *group. ELISAs are now being evaluated for NSD. Infected spleen may be used as a source of antigen in immunodiffusion tests.*

Requirements for vaccines and diagnostic biologicals: *An experimental attenuated live virus vaccine has been investigated, and a killed tissue culture vaccine has been shown to be immunogenic.*

A. DIAGNOSTIC TECHNIQUES

Nairobi sheep disease (NSD) is a disease of sheep and goats caused by a *Nairovirus* of the family Bunyaviridae (1). It is characterised by a mortality rate, which may range between 40% and 90%, and should always be suspected when animals have recently been moved from an area free from the disease into one where it is endemic. The clinical signs are similar in both sheep and goats, although there are differences in susceptibility among the various breeds and strains in their response to infection with NSD virus, some being more susceptible than others. The incubation period for the disease varies from 2 to 5 days, when a temperature reaction of 41–42°C develops. There is hyperventilation accompanied by severe depression, anorexia and a disinclination to move. Animals stand with lowered head, and show a conjunctivitis and sero-sanguineous nasal discharge. Some of the superficial lymph nodes, such as the prescapular and/or precrural, become palpable. Diarrhoea usually develops within 36–56 hours of the onset of the febrile reaction. This is at first profuse, watery and foetid, later haemorrhagic and mucoid, and accompanied by colicky pains and tenesmus. Abortion is a common sequel to the infection. Examination of the predilection sites for the attachment of ticks such as the ears, head and body, is likely to reveal the presence of the Ixodid tick *Rhipicephalus appendiculatus.*

Deaths can occur in peracute cases within 12 hours of the onset of the fever and at any time during the febrile reaction, while the animal is acutely ill. Further deaths then follow the fall in temperature for a further 3–7 days, associated with the severe diarrhoea and dehydration.

The gross pathology of NSD can be misleading, for most deaths are likely to occur during the period of viraemia, when the only signs are likely to be lymphadenitis with petechial and ecchymotic haemorrhages on the serous surfaces of the alimentary tract, spleen, heart and other organs. None of these signs allows a specific diagnosis of NSD to be made or even suspected, for they are shared with many other febrile diseases of sheep in NSD-endemic areas. Later in the course of the disease, a haemorrhagic gastroenteritis becomes more obvious, with haemorrhages on the mucosa of the abomasum, especially along the folds, in the region of the ileo-caecal valve, and most commonly in the colon and rectum. Zebra striping of the latter is often seen. The gall bladder is usually enlarged and haemorrhagic. Inflammatory lesions with haemorrhage may be seen in the female genital tract, if there has been abortion. However, in many animals dying from NSD, there may be none of these gastroenteric lesions, and a tentative diagnosis based on post mortem signs can rarely be made. Common histopathological lesions are myocardial degeneration, nephritis and necrosis of the gall bladder.

The post-mortem signs in the early stages are the nonspecific changes associated with death at the viraemic stage of NSD, with congestion and petechial and ecchymotic haemorrhages on serous surfaces, on lymph nodes, the spleen and other organs such as the kidney, lungs and liver. Later, signs of haemorrhagic gastroenteritis become apparent, with ulceration of the abomasum, duodenum, caecum and colon. The virus is principally transmitted by the tick *Rhipicephalus appendiculatus*, and any infestation with such parasites should arouse suspicion of the presence of the disease. NSD virus may also be transmitted by other species of the genus *Rhipicephalus* and by the bont tick *Ambylomma variegatum.*

NSD is an apparently rare zoonotic agent in the field, causing mild influenza-like disease in humans.

1. Identification of the agent

NSD virus may be isolated from material collected from field cases by the use of laboratory animals or cell cultures (5). Safety precautions against aerosol infections should be taken when working with this agent. Uncoagulated blood, mesenteric lymph nodes and spleen tissue submitted on ice are the optimal samples to be collected from febrile or dead animals, respectively. The plasma can be used directly as inoculum, and the lymph nodes or spleen should be homogenised to make an approximate 10% (w/v) suspension in a transport medium. This medium can be Hanks' medium with 0.5% lactalbumin hydrolysate or 0.75% bovine serum albumin, and containing penicillin (500 International Units/ml), streptomycin sulphate (500 µg/ml), and mycostatin (50 units/ml) or fungizone (2.5 µg/ml).

A recommended initial procedure is to inoculate an NSD-susceptible sheep held in isolation with 1–2 ml of the tissue suspensions, or of the plasma. Any pyrexia and clinical disease that develops permits a tentative diagnosis of NSD and, at the same time, furnishes excellent samples for virus isolation. This is especially valuable where the original field samples have been transported in hot climates where some loss of virus has inevitably occurred. Sheep are at least 100 times more sensitive than mice to NSD virus infection.

Infant mice, 2–4 days old, can be inoculated intracerebrally with 0.01 ml of a 1/10 dilution of plasma or of the tissue suspension. Two litters, each of 8–10 suckling mice, should be used for each sample and one blind passage is made routinely. The mice become debilitated and die within 5–9 days post-inoculation. Their brains should be harvested aseptically, pooled and diluted 1/100 for passage into further mice.

Cell cultures may be used in conjunction with mouse inoculation for the primary isolation of NSD virus, as they have shown levels of sensitivity similar to that of the intracerebral inoculation of unweaned mice. The baby hamster kidney (BHK)-21-C13 cell line is especially valuable, and primary and secondary lamb or hamster kidney cells have also been used. Most strains of NSD virus produce a cytopathic effect (CPE) on first passage in BHK cells; others produce a more obvious CPE only after subinoculation. The appearance of a CPE is not such a regular finding with lamb testis and kidney cells, although it is usually seen on the second passage in lamb kidney cells. Tube cultures should be used both with and without flying cover-slips, or if plastic bottles are used for isolation, microwell slide cultures should also be prepared. Approximately 0.2 ml should be inoculated and a period of 1–2 hours allowed for adsorption. The CPE becomes evident in roller cultures as foci of granular rounded cells after 24–48 hours in BHK cells, and in a further 24–48 hours in other cell types. The CPE is not specific for NSD virus, which is identified in cover-slip cultures by immunofluorescence or by staining with haematoxylin and eosin. The latter method reveals pleomorphic eosinophilic intracytoplasmic inclusions peculiarly of a spindle form; other inclusions are bipolar, or surround the nucleus.

The virus can be specifically identified by immunofluorescence staining, which may be positive as early as 24–48 hours after inoculation, when no CPE has yet become evident. Conjugates for direct immunofluorescence may be prepared from hyperimmune mouse ascitic fluids, and from immune rabbit or sheep antisera by standard methods. Some cross-fluorescence may occur with other *Nairoviruses* at low dilutions of the conjugate, but these viruses are not normally associated with disease in sheep or goats.

The agar gel immunodiffusion test can be a valuable primary diagnostic tool for the detection of NSD antigen in tissues. The test can be carried out in laboratories without tissue culture facilities and at field investigation laboratories. The spleen and mesenteric lymph nodes are the tissues of choice to be used in the test. Aliquots of 0.5–1 g should be homogenised with sterile sand in a pestle or a homogeniser to give 10–20% suspensions in phosphate buffered saline (PBS) or saline. The suspension should be centrifuged for 10–15 minutes at approximately 1000 ***g*** and the supernatant fluid used in the test. This test can also be used for the identification of NSD virus antigen in mouse brain harvested from experimentally infected mice (see above). Rabbit hyperimmune serum against NSD can be prepared by repeated inoculations of NSD infected mouse brain. A mouse brain suspension at 2–5 % w/v is prepared as above and centrifuged at 3–5000 ***g*** for 15 minutes. Aliquots are then mixed with an equal volume of Freund's complete adjuvant. Various inoculation regimes may be used but 1 ml volumes may be given subcutaneously and/or intramuscularly at 7-day intervals for 3–5 weeks, or at multiple inoculation sites in 0.1 ml volumes for a similar period. Serum should be collected 5–7 days after the last injection and stored in aliquots at –20°C.

Difco Noble or other suitable agar may be used in the test, using 0.85% sodium chloride at pH 7.2. Slides are prepared to give an agar layer approximately 2 mm in depth. Six wells should be placed hexagonally around a central well. The hyperimmune rabbit serum is placed in the central well and positive control antigen in wells 1 and 4. The tissue under test is placed in wells 2 and 5. Negative control tissue is placed in wells 3 and 6. Wells containing test tissue that give a precipitin line of continuity with the line formed between the positive antigen and the hyperimmune serum are considered to be positive.

The mouse brain suspensions or infective tissue culture fluids can be used as antigens for complement fixation (CF) tests for virus identification. Both have proved satisfactory after partial purification with fluorocarbon; the mouse brain can also be used in the form of a suspension in a borate buffer solution.

An enzyme-linked immunosorbent assay (ELISA) antigen for virus identification purposes can be prepared from an infected tissue culture in a bottle. The cells are removed using a pipette fitted with a rubber bulb when approximately 20% of the monolayer is showing CPEs. They are sedimented and washed three times in borate saline buffer, pH 9. The cells are then lysed and solubilised with SDS (sodium dodecyl sulphate) and 1% Triton X100, diluted approximately 1/5 in borate saline buffer and sonicated to provide an antigen for the ELISA. A control negative antigen is prepared in the same manner from uninfected cells. These are adsorbed directly on to ELISA plates and the test is carried out with NSD immune and normal serum with both antigens.

2. Serological tests

Immunodiffusion, CF, indirect fluorescent antibody tests, haemagglutination and ELISA have all been used with NSD virus. Results of virus neutralisation tests are unreliable, as are those of the same tests on other members of the *Nairovirus* genus.

a) Indirect fluorescent antibody test

This is the most suitable test for use with members of the *Nairovirus* group. There are some cross-reactions, particularly with Dugbe virus and also with other members of the group, such as Congo–Crimean haemorrhagic fever virus (2). The NSD antibody titres by this method range from 1/640 to 1/10,240, and such titres are not obtained with immune sera to other members of the group (3).

The method has been used in epidemiological studies and to study the response to experimental vaccines. There do not appear to be any serological differences among the 40–50 isolates that have been examined. An I-34 strain[1] was the virus usually used to prepare antigen, and this has been adapted to grow in BHK-21-C13 cells, after a series of passages.

The virus antigen in the cell substrate of choice may be grown in loose cover-slips, multiwell slides, Teflon-coated slides or microtitre plates for the test. A method using Teflon-coated slides is described.

- **Preparation of antigen slides**

i) Wash and sterilise Teflon-coated slides. This is done briefly with a hot detergent that is used for tissue culture glassware in the laboratory, then three rinses in tap water for 30 minutes, each followed by similar rinses in distilled/deionised water. Slides are then placed in 70% alcohol for 10 minutes, removed with a sterile forceps and wrapped in greaseproof paper. They will then be found to be sterile, but further sterilisation in a microwave for two cycles of 5 minutes each is recommended.

ii) Place these slides in sterile dishes using a sterile forceps; a square polystyrene type is better than the round variety.

iii) Mix a suspension of BHK cells containing approximately 25,000 cells/ml in BHK growth medium (usually Eagles for BHK cells), and add 1000 $TCID_{50}$ (50% tissue culture infective dose) of NSD I-34 strain per ml. Mix by pipetting. Prepare some uninfected negative control slides.

iv) Add the infected cells in 50 µl volumes (for the 12-well size) or as appropriate to the size of the Teflon wells. Replace the cover on the dishes and put into a humidified CO_2 incubator or anaerobic container.

v) Leave overnight for the monolayer to form. Then remove the plates from the incubator to a laminar flow cabinet, and flood with maintenance medium using a pipette to cover the slides to a depth of 2–3 mm. Return to the incubator.

vi) Harvest the antigen slides just as foci of the CPE become detectable. This will be in 36–56 hours (more accurate determination of the optimal harvesting time may be made by fixing and staining one slide after 24, 36 and 48 hours).

vii) The slides are washed three times in PBS and dried. They are then fixed with dry heat (minimum 80°C) or with ice-cold acetone for 10 minutes. The slides are wrapped and may be stored at 4°C for 2–3 months, or at –20°C for 1–2 years. Slides stored at –20°C must be brought to 4°C overnight before use.

Similar procedures may be followed to prepare antigen on flying cover-slips or multiwell culture slides. When using Nunc tissue culture multiwell plates, however, fixation should be with 75% acetone.

- **Test procedure**

i) The slides are hydrated by adding a drop of PBS to the wells with a Pasteur pipette. Slides are numbered according to the number of sera to be tested. Control positive and negative sera with infected and uninfected cell cultures are included in the series.

ii) Discard the PBS and add the serum dilutions 1/80–1/2560 in a predetermined manner to wells one to six. It is preferable to duplicate each dilution on the same side.

iii) The slides are placed in dishes and held at 37°C in a humid incubator, for 40 minutes.

iv) Wash the slides in racks in three changes of PBS, 5 minutes per wash.

v) Add the fluorescein-conjugated anti-species conjugate (usually anti-sheep or anti-goat) at a predetermined working dilution; one drop can be added to each well with a Pasteur or other pipette.

vi) Incubate as before for 30 minutes.

vii) Wash three times in PBS and dry the slides.

viii) Examine the slides by fluorescent microscopy. NSD virus antigen is found in the cell cytoplasm, and foci of bundles of fluorescing BHK cells will be seen. The antigen is seen mainly in fine fluorescent particles, but larger irregularly shaped antigen clumps occur, often surrounding the nucleus, or in spindle-like masses filling the cytoplasm to the pole of the cells. These particles will not be seen with negative sera or in the uninoculated control culture.

ix) Sera that show this fluorescence at dilutions of 1/640 or 1/1280 are indicative of recent infection with NSD (3).

b) Other tests

CF tests are complicated by the marked anticomplementary activity of many sheep sera.

Immunodiffusion tests have been used successfully with crude antigens prepared from infected sheep tissue, tissue culture fluids or mouse brain material. Hyperimmune sera can be prepared in sheep, mice or rabbits for use in the test, using infected spleen taken from sheep dying from NSD as the source of antigen

1 The I-34 strain was a virulent NSD isolate made in Kenya that was used extensively as a reference strain at the Kabete Laboratory – Kenya Agriculture Research Institute, P.O. Box 58137, Kabete, Nairobi, Kenya.

for immunisation. Control negative test systems should be established using uninfected positive and negative sheep spleens (or other antigen sources), with known NSD-negative sera. Such reagents can be prepared at any laboratory and do not require the support of a virological laboratory. This test is useful although relatively insensitive.

Monoclonal antibodies to the antigens of NSD virus strain I-34 have been developed and are being evaluated for their application as diagnostic reagents.

B. REQUIREMENTS FOR VACCINES AND DIAGNOSTIC BIOLOGICALS

Epidemiological investigations have shown that in a state of enzootic stability, no problems are encountered with NSD. The disease arises from animal movements from free areas into endemic areas and can be avoided when such areas have been defined. Ecological changes that permit spread of the vector tick will result in extensions of these areas.

Experimental vaccines have been prepared for such situations. One vaccine has consisted of virus attenuated by 35 passages in adult mice, but such vaccines can produce severe reactions in some breeds of sheep, and are not considered to be safe for general use. A similar vaccine was developed in Entebbe by further mouse brain passages, but this has not been further developed for use in the field in Uganda or elsewhere.

A tissue-culture-adapted strain of NSD virus has been grown to high titre in rolled culture. When precipitated with methanol, inactivated, and administered with an adjuvant, this was found to give good protection following two inoculations given at an interval of 14 days. Neither of these vaccines are routinely produced, for there has been little demand for their use from the field (4, 6).

REFERENCES

1. DAVIES F.G. (1988). Nairobi sheep disease. *In:* The Ecology of Arboviruses, Vol. 3, Monath T.P., ed. CRC Press, Boca Raton, Florida, USA, 191–203.

2. DAVIES F.G., CASALS J., JESSETT D.M. & OCHIENG P. (1978). The serological relationships of Nairobi sheep disease virus. *J. Comp. Pathol.*, **88**, 519–523.

3. DAVIES F.G., JESSETT D.M. & OTIENO S. (1976). The antibody response of sheep following infection with Nairobi sheep disease virus. *J. Comp. Pathol.*, **86**, 497–502.

4. DAVIES F.G., MUNGAI J. & SHAW T. (1974). A Nairobi sheep disease vaccine. *Vet. Rec.*, **94**, 128.

5. DAVIES F.G., MUNGAI J. & TAYLOR M. (1977). The laboratory diagnosis of Nairobi sheep disease. *Trop. Anim. Health Prod.*, **9**, 75–80.

6. DAVIES F.G., OTIENO S. & JESSETT D.M. (1977). The antibody response in sheep vaccinated with experimental Nairobi sheep disease vaccines. *Trop. Anim. Health Prod.*, **9**, 181–183.

*

* *

CHAPTER X.9.

SCRAPIE

SUMMARY

Scrapie is a naturally occurring infectious neurodegenerative disease of sheep and goats characterised by vacuolar or spongy changes in the central nervous system (CNS). It has been recognised for over two and a half centuries. It is caused by a transmissible agent (the prion), the biochemical nature of which remains unclear.

The disease is endemic in many parts of the world although Australia and New Zealand have maintained freedom from scrapie. The infection in sheep may be passed from ewe to lamb in the period from parturition to weaning and also, possibly, prenatally. Infection can also pass to unrelated sheep or goats, especially when parturition occurs in confined areas. Fetal membranes are thought to be a source of infection. The incubation time between primary infection and clinical disease is nearly always longer than 1 year and may sometimes exceed the commercial life span of the sheep. The majority of cases occur in sheep between 2 and 5 years of age. Clinical disease only develops if the infection enters the CNS.

Scrapie infection can be most easily recognised if it leads to neurological disease. The disease is recognised by the clinical signs, which start insidiously with behavioural abnormalities. These may initially go unrecognised, but usually progress to more obvious neurological signs, including pruritus and incoordination. Loss of bodily condition is also common. The clinical disorder is variable in duration and in the range of signs presented, but it is inevitably fatal.

***Identification of the agent:** No practical definitive diagnostic test for scrapie infection is available. Clinical diagnosis is supported by the histopathological diagnosis of spongiform encephalopathy. This is characterised by bilateral and usually symmetrical neuronal vacuolation and spongiform change of grey matter in the brain stem. The nature of the agent causing scrapie and similar transmissible spongiform encephalopathies (TSEs) is unclear, but during the development of the disease an abnormal form of a host membrane glycoprotein, called prion protein or PrP, accumulates in certain tissues, notably lymphoreticular organs and the CNS. This abnormal isoform (PrP^{Sc}) is a component, perhaps the sole molecule, of the causative agent. Its detection in extracts or tissue sections of diseased brains is therefore a disease-specific diagnostic criterion. PrP^{Sc} can be detected in unfixed brain material by detergent extraction, electrophoresis and immunoblotting, or immunohistochemically in histological brain sections prepared routinely. A morphologically distinctive form of PrP^{Sc} can be visualised in the electron microscope from detergent extracts of unfixed brain tissue, as scrapie-associated fibrils. Detection of the accumulation of the abnormal protein in lymphoreticular tissues during the incubation period of scrapie offers a means of preclinical diagnosis of scrapie infection by proxy and may be particularly useful for surveillance purposes when performed on biopsied tissue.*

Scrapie can be transmitted to laboratory rodents by injecting them with infected tissue, but the variable efficiency of primary isolations coupled with incubation times of 1–2 years preclude this as a practical diagnostic procedure.

***Serological tests:** Scrapie infection is not known to elicit any specific immune response and there is no basis for establishing a diagnosis by detecting specific antibodies.*

***Genetic tests:** Several polymorphisms have been identified within the protein-coding region of the sheep PrP gene. Epidemiological studies have established an association between the occurrence of scrapie and specific polymorphisms in several breeds of sheep. PrP genotyping has the potential to be a valuable tool in the control of clinical scrapie.*

Requirements for vaccines and diagnostic biologicals: *There are no biological products available.*

A. DIAGNOSTIC TECHNIQUES

Scrapie is a naturally occurring progressive, fatal, infectious neurodegenerative disease of sheep and goats. It is characterised by vacuolar or spongy changes in the central nervous system (CNS). In countries of Western Europe, it has been known to occur in sheep for at least the past two and a half centuries. It is therefore, in retrospect, the first transmissible spongiform encephalopathy (TSE) or prion disease of mammals to be recognised.

Scrapie remains endemic in many European countries and has also been reported in several countries throughout most other continents. However, Australia and New Zealand have maintained freedom from the disease through rigorous preventative policies. Because of the absence of procedures for surveillance for scrapie in many countries, their scrapie status is unknown. Within the European Union scrapie has been a notifiable disease since January 1993.

Scrapie, like other TSEs is believed to be caused by a transmissible agent (the prion), the precise biochemical nature of which remains unclear. Reviews of this well known yet enigmatic disease provide details of its clinical signs, epidemiology, pathogenesis, pathology, diagnosis and control (4, 10, 18, 22, 36, 47).

Most cases of clinical scrapie occur in sheep 2–5 years of age (18). Rarely, cases present in sheep under 1 year of age. In some instances the commercial lifespan of the sheep may be too short to allow the clinical disease to develop. Animals incubating the disease and even such animals that never develop clinical signs may still be a source of infection to others. Most breeds are affected, although in some there is a clear genetic basis for resistance or low prevalence of clinical disease (see below). Scrapie has also been described in the moufflon *(Ovis musimon)* a primitive type of sheep (50). The infection in domestic sheep may be passed from ewe to lamb in the period from parturition to weaning and also, possibly, prenatally. Infection can also pass to unrelated sheep or goats, especially when parturition occurs in confined areas. Fetal membranes are thought to be a source of infection. Flock recording indicates that in sheep the disease tends to be linked with certain family lines, but to what extent this represents genetic susceptibility or maternal transmission, or is the influence of both, is uncertain. The clinical disease only develops if the infection enters the CNS.

The clinical signs (4, 11, 21, 30, 31) usually start insidiously, often with behavioural changes that are evident only from repeated inspections. While a flock is being driven, an affected sheep may lead or trail the rest of the flock, it may show abnormal reactions to the sheep dog, appearing, momentarily confused or anxious and may disengage from the flock. Sheep may have a staring gaze. These subtle presenting features progress to a more definite neurological illness frequently characterised by signs of pruritus and an ataxia or incoordination of gait. Either the pruritus or the ataxia usually emerges to dominate the clinical course (49).

Pruritus is seen principally as compulsive rubbing or scraping against fixed objects, nibbling at the skin and scratching with a hind foot. This results in extensive loss of wool, particularly over the lateral thorax, flanks and hindquarters. The persistence of pruritus often causes excoriations with the development of localised self-inflicted skin lesions. These may occur in areas of wool loss and on the poll, face, ears and limbs. A characteristic 'nibbling reflex' can often be elicited by palpation of the lumbar region, and may also be evoked by the sheep's own scraping movements.

Ataxia or incoordination of gait is first apparent as an awkwardness of turning, with difficulty in positioning the hind limbs, swaying of the hindquarters and a high stepping or trotting gait of the forelimbs. Stumbling and falling occur, but the sheep is generally able to quickly regain a standing posture. These signs progress to weakness and recumbency.

Other neurological signs may include teeth grinding (bruxism), an abnormally low carriage of the head and ears, a fine tremor, seizures, and blindness. There may also be apparent hyperaesthesia to sound, movement, or touch. Polydipsia and polyuria may be evident. In most cases, there is also a loss of bodily condition, but significant weight loss may be apparent only in the late clinical stages. This preterminal decline may, it is considered, be associated with the observation of diminished rumination time in sheep with scrapie (2).

The variety of names that have been used among different languages to describe scrapie, for example, la tremblante (trembling), or traberkrankheit (trotting disease), reflect the diversity of the presenting and predominant clinical signs in different sheep populations. Progress of the clinical disease is very variable, lasting for a week or up to several months, with an inevitably fatal outcome. There is also variation in the clinical signs among individual animals and in different breeds of sheep. These variations may be due to the influence of host genotype and strain of agent; variables that in rodent models of scrapie are well known to determine the phenotype of disease observed. Environmental factors may also have an influence on the disease course. The clinical diagnosis of individual cases of scrapie can therefore be difficult. Subtle clinical signs may go unrecognised, and sometimes, irrespective of the degree of supervision of flocks, sheep that are found dead without premonitory signs can be shown to be affected following histopathological examination (7).

The clinical signs may, especially in the early phase of the disease, resemble those of some other conditions of adult sheep. These include: ectoparasitism, pseudorabies (Aujeszky's disease), rabies, encephalic listeriosis, ovine progressive pneumonia (maedi-visna), pregnancy toxaemia (ketosis), hypomagnesaemia and chemical and plant intoxications (10).

1. Identification of the agent

The aetiological agent of scrapie is as yet incompletely characterised. It is known to be a transmissible agent, but the molecular identity remains uncertain. A modified form (PrP^{Sc}) of a host-coded, highly conserved, membrane glycoprotein (PrP^{c}), of unknown function, is the only macromolecular constituent of the infectious agent identified. The protein only or 'prion' hypothesis proposes that the causative agent is composed entirely or principally of the disease-specific isoform of PrP (prion protein) and that the altered form is capable of inducing conversion of the normal form. Other theories as to the nature of the agent suggest that a small portion of nucleic acid is associated with the prion protein, or that the prion protein is merely a by-product of infection caused by another agent.

Transmission from infected tissues, usually to laboratory rodents by injection, is the only available means of detection of infectivity and requires incubation periods of 1–2 years. Although mice have proved the most useful species for this purpose, attempts to transmit natural scrapie to mice are not always successful. It is seldom practical to use the criterion of transmissibility for diagnosis. There is therefore no practical definitive diagnostic test available based on isolation or detection of the agent by culture, nor are there immunological or nucleic acid recognition methods. Subject to proof of the prion hypothesis, demonstration of the pathological form of PrP would constitute identification of the agent.

The known existence of natural scrapie in domestic sheep for the past two and a half centuries and the failure of many investigations to show any epidemiological link between scrapie and the human spongiform encephalopathies, provides a strong indication of low risk to those working with the agent (5). More specifically, Creutzfeldt-Jakob disease has been found to occur at no greater frequency in those with occupations providing closest contact with the agent than in other population groups. However, the extreme chemical and physical resistance of the scrapie agent and the fact that it is experimentally transmissible by injection to a wide spectrum of mammalian species, suggest the prudence of preventing human exposure. Because of the link recently established between bovine spongiform encephalopathy (BSE) and a new variant form of the human TSE, Creutzfeldt-Jakob disease (vCJD), BSE and related agents are now categorised, with respect to biohazard, with the human TSEs (1). Although scrapie is excluded from this categorisation, adoption of containment measures similar to those used for the other TSEs is recommended when dealing with tissues from natural cases of scrapie. This is particularly relevant in those countries that have experienced cases of BSE in their endemic cattle population, as sheep may have been exposed to the same contaminated feedstuffs considered to be the source of infection in cattle, and experimental BSE in sheep is, as yet, clinically and pathologically indistinguishable from scrapie. Those working directly with infected tissues should therefore wear appropriate protective clothing and observe standard decontamination procedures for the spongiform encephalopathy agents (1, 39, 44).

In the absence of *in-vitro* methods for isolation of the causative agent, the diagnosis of scrapie must remain reliant on the demonstration of pathological changes. Historically the only such method was demonstration of the histopathological changes in the CNS. While clinically suspect cases of scrapie should, where suitable samples are available, continue to be investigated initially by histopathological examination, diagnostic criteria should also now include the demonstration of accumulation of the abnormal isoform of PrP. This latter approach not only offers a capability for confirming a clinical diagnosis post-mortem by demonstration of PrP accumulation in the CNS, but can also provide the basis of an ante-mortem diagnosis in the preclinical phase of disease, by detection of abnormal PrP in lymphoid tissues. These include those of the tonsil, regional lymph nodes and nictitating membrane, obtainable by biopsy (29, 37, 38). However, the practicality of collection of such tissue must be considered.

There are no specific gross pathological changes seen in scrapie. The histological lesions are confined to the CNS and most reports of the changes have described those occurring in the brain (13, 47, 51). The lesions are neurodegenerative, with no specific inflammatory changes and no primary degenerative changes of white matter. The most striking change is a vacuolation of neurons. Neuronal perikarya are distended by characteristic single or multiple vacuoles. Vacuolation in neuronal processes produces the distinctive appearance of spongiform change in the neuropil of grey matter. Vacuolar changes are accompanied by variable and usually less conspicuous microscopic features, which include other forms of neuronal degeneration, notably the occurrence of 'dark', shrunken neurons. There may also be neuronal loss, gliosis (particularly an astrocytic reaction), and amyloidosis. Typically, the lesions have a bilaterally symmetrical distribution. There is considerable variation in the distribution pattern of vacuolation and other changes, but lesions are usually most apparent in the brain stem. Nevertheless, there are reports of lesions extending rostrally to involve, in some cases, the cerebral cortex (51).

Although it is principally the vacuolar changes on which the laboratory diagnosis has been based, several factors may contribute to difficulties in making the histopathological diagnosis. Vacuolation of neuronal perikarya of the type seen in scrapie is not pathognomonic because it is present occasionally in the brains of apparently healthy sheep, but in such instances the number of vacuoles is typically very small compared with the numbers usually present in cases of clinical scrapie (13, 52). Furthermore, none of the individual pathological features of scrapie can be considered to be strictly specific, but in combination and with abundant vacuolar changes they are undoubtedly pathognomonic. There is also variation in the prominence of each of the individual pathological features among cases of scrapie, and the severity of the clinical signs is not necessarily reflected in the intensity of the pathology. Incidents of scrapie are recorded in which neuronal vacuolation is virtually undetectable by light microscopy (11, 13). Therefore, a clinical diagnosis of suspected scrapie cannot be refuted by a failure to find significant vacuolar changes in the brain. The absence of lesions is clearly not evidence of the absence of scrapie infection, as this can exist in the absence of either clinical signs or pathological changes. For this reason, immunohistochemistry on tissue sections and/or immunoblotting methods on fresh tissues to demonstrate accumulation of PrP^{Sc} should be carried out in parallel with routine histology in suspected cases.

Despite these reservations, the histological examination of sections of medulla oblongata may be sufficient to confirm a diagnosis in most cases of clinically suspect scrapie (21, 25). While this has been used successfully for routine diagnosis, equivocal findings in the medulla would require examination of additional sections of the brain stem. Where regulatory certification or monitoring for freedom from disease is required, the parties involved must be in agreement on the degree of test sensitivity and specificity required. The absence of lesions can be established with greatest confidence by examining representative areas of the whole brain.

The histological examination of the brain, remains an important method of post-mortem confirmation of clinically suspect scrapie, but methods for the demonstration of accumulation of PrP^{Sc} can now provide independent evidence for the diagnosis (10, 39). PrP^{Sc} can be detected after partial purification from detergent-treated extracts of unfixed, affected brain. The modified protein is demonstrated by electrophoresis and immunoblotting (12, 41). The accumulation of PrP^{Sc} in scrapie-affected brain is also demonstrated immunohistochemically and can be carried out on routinely formalin-fixed material, by the application of a variety of epitope demasking techniques and the use of appropriate antibodies to PrP (17, 26, 27, 46). PrP detection by immunohistochemistry has also been demonstrated in lymphoid tissue (45) and is considered to have potential for the preclinical ante-mortem diagnosis of scrapie in sheep using tonsillar (38) or nictitating membrane (29) lymphoid tissue biopsies. Applications of PrP detection to the preclinical diagnosis of scrapie are promising but preliminary, and require considerable improvements to the knowledge of variability of pathogenesis of the disease before their sensitivity relative to incubation period can be assessed. A morphological form of the pathological PrP can also be demonstrated in unfixed brain extracts in the form of scrapie-associated fibrils (SAF) visualised by negative-stain electron microscopy (14, 40, 41). The latter may be particularly useful when available brain tissue is unsuitable for histological examination due to post-mortem changes (42). The immunoblotting method can also be applied to autolysed material (33). Both immunoblotting and SAF examination can also be applied in circumstances when, at post-mortem, sometimes in error, CNS material intended for fixation and histological examination has been frozen. With modification the method for SAF detection may also be applied successfully to formalin-fixed tissue (6). Caution should be exerted over the use of SAF alone; it should only be used in conjunction with at least one other confirmatory method – either histopathology or immunochemical detection of PrP^{Sc}.

Detection of PrP^{Sc} in spleen and lymph nodes by immunoblotting has also been used in the diagnosis of scrapie at post-mortem (20, 28, 32), but it is not practical under most circumstances to obtain such tissues surgically to effect an ante-mortem diagnosis. The detection of PrP^{Sc} by immunoblotting in placenta (correlating with the presence of infectivity in the tissue) from scrapie-affected sheep, may offer a noninvasive means of ante-mortem diagnosis and disease surveillance in flocks (34).

Methods for the routine laboratory diagnosis of scrapie (39) are summarised and revised as follows. Sheep in which clinical disease is suspected should be killed by intravenous injection of barbiturate, and the brain and a portion of cervical spinal cord should be removed, by standard necropsy procedures, as soon after death as possible. Methods of subdividing the brain and cord tissue for application of PrP detection requiring fresh tissue and for histological techniques are dependent on the optimum sensitivities of each of the tests for different brain areas and the compromise that precisely the same area cannot be used for both techniques. The following protocol is suggested but may be subject to modification to satisfy the particular portfolio of tests applied.

For the detection of PrP (or SAF), fresh tissue samples are taken and stored frozen prior to extraction. Samples should include approximately 3 g of cervical spinal cord and/or medulla, caudal to the obex. Additional samples are advocated to minimise false-negative diagnoses by this method. These can be taken from the cerebellum and cerebral cortex (40, 42, 43). If it is considered necessary to take additional samples also from brain stem areas, it must be accepted that this will be more likely to compromise the histopathological examination. When immunohistochemical examination for PrP is to be employed, it is advisable to select the blocks to be used from the fresh brain and to process these after primary fixation for only 3–5 days. The single medulla block at the obex may well be sufficient for this purpose and indeed, as indicated above, for the morphological diagnosis.

The remaining brain tissue is fixed in 10% formol saline for approximately 1 week and then cut transversely as required to obtain blocks for histological processing to paraffin wax. The initial sampling may be confined to a single block of the medulla (see Chapter 2.3.13. Bovine spongiform encephalopathy, Figure 1) or extended to additional areas of the brain stem and, as necessary, to representative blocks of all major brain regions. Sections, cut at 5 µm thickness, are stained with haematoxylin and eosin and examined for the morphological changes outlined above. A histopathological diagnosis of scrapie is confirmed on the presence of characteristic vacuolar changes in grey matter, which has a bilateral and usually symmetrical distribution. Where such lesions are mild in severity and considered equivocal, it is essential to employ at least one additional (immunohistochemical or immunoblotting) method to confirm the diagnosis. Similarly, if for speed of obtaining a differential diagnosis by histopathological examination, tissues have been fixed for less than 1 week, PrP^{Sc} detection should also be used to resolve possible uninterpretable observations. A diagnosis based on PrP^{Sc} detection by western blotting requires that a wide region of immunostained bands corresponding to proteins of molecular mass 27–30 kDa be present in the proteinase-K-treated scrapie sample lanes only and that control sample lanes provide appropriate results (41). Confirmation by SAF requires the identification of the characteristic fibrils on a systematic search of the specimen grid in the electron microscope (14, 40). Confirmation of scrapie from immunohistochemical preparations must depend not only on the presence of immunologically specific PrP staining, but also on the recognition of morphologically disease-specific patterns of staining.

A wide range of antisera and monoclonal antibodies for PrP detection by immunochemical methods are now in use but not all of them react satisfactorily with ovine PrP. Some (MAb 6H4 and F89/160.1.5) are commercially available. Improved availability and characterisation of antisera, and the further standardisation and validation of the methodologies are required. Positive and negative controls are essential. However, the inclusion of both immunoblotting and immunohistochemical approaches in the tests applied for routine scrapie diagnosis by many laboratories will enable the relative performance of each to be further assessed. Failure to observe characteristic histological changes or to detect PrP/SAF does not provide evidence of the absence of the disease, but agreement between the results of multiple diagnostic approaches provides the best assurance of accuracy. Clearly, in surveillance situations where monitoring is for the purpose of obtaining evidence of freedom from scrapie in small ruminant species, it is necessary to apply multiple diagnostic criteria and to use at least two laboratory methods on CNS tissue (histopathological and immunohistochemical, or immunoblotting) to maintain a high degree of confidence in negative results.

Prospects for more sensitive and specific diagnostic tests for scrapie and other TSEs are mainly directed at present on the development of new approaches to the detection of PrP^{Sc} (35).

2. Serological tests

A serological immune response to the scrapie agent has not been detected.

3. Genetic tests

Common polymorphisms have been identified within the protein-coding region of the sheep *PrP* gene at codons 136 – alanine/valine, 154 – arginine/histidine, and 171 – arginine/glutamine (15, 16, 24). The incidence of scrapie in various breeds of sheep has been associated with some of these polymorphisms (15, 19, 23). The codon 171 polymorphisms are of particular significance in determining overall risk (3, 8, 48). *PrP* genotyping can therefore be used as an aid to the control of scrapie: breeding stock, particularly rams, of appropriate *PrP* genotype can be selected to produce progeny with reduced risk of developing disease (9). Such genotyping services are available on a commercial basis in North America and in several countries in Europe. The test is performed using DNA extracted from white blood cells obtained from ethylene diamine tetra-acetic acid treated blood samples.

B. REQUIREMENTS FOR VACCINES AND DIAGNOSTIC BIOLOGICALS

There are no biological products available.

REFERENCES

1. ADVISORY COMMITTEE ON DANGEROUS PATHOGENS (1998). Transmissible Spongiform Encephalopathy Agents: Safe Working and the Prevention of Infection. Spongiform Encephalopathy Advisory Committee. HMSO Publication Centre, P.O. Box 276, London SW8 DT, UK.

2. AUSTIN A.R, HAWKINS S.A.C., KELAY N.S. & SIMMONS M.M. (1994). New observations on the clinical signs of BSE and scrapie. A Consultation on BSE with the Scientific Veterinary Committee of the Commission of the European Communities held in Brussels, 14–15 September 1993. Bradley R. & Marchant B., eds. Document VI/4131/94-EN. European Commission Agriculture, Brussels, Belgium, 277–287.

3. BELT P.B.G.M., SCHREUDER B.E.C., MUILEMAN I.H., BOSSERS A. & SMITS M.A. (1995). PrP genotype and modulation of disease onset in natural scrapie. *In:* Prion Diseases: Epidemiology, Biochemistry and Molecular Biology. International Symposium, Göttingen, Germany, October 1995, 58 (abstract).

4. BRADLEY R. (1997). Animal prion diseases. *In:* Prion Diseases, Collinge J. & Palmer M.S., eds. Oxford University Press, Oxford, UK, 89–129.

5. BROWN P. (1992). Infectious cerebral amyloidosis: clinical spectrum, risks and remedies. *In:* Transmissible Spongiform Encephalopathies – Impact on Animal and Human Health, Brown F., ed. Basel, Karger, *Dev. Biol. Stand.*, **80**, 91–101.

6. CHAPLIN M.J., ALDRICH A.D. & STACK M.J. (1998) Scrapie associated fibril detection from formaldehyde fixed brain tissue in natural cases of ovine scrapie. *Res. Vet. Sci.* **64**, 41–44.

7. CLARK A.M., DAWSON M. & SCOTT A.C. (1994). Scrapie associated fibrils in found dead sheep. *Vet. Rec.* **134**, 650–651.

8. CLOUSCARD C., BEAUDRY P., ELSEN J.M., MILAN D., DUSSAUCY M., BOUNNEAU C., SCHELCHER F., CHATELAIN J., LAUNAY J.-M. & LAPLANCHE J.M. (1995). Different allelic effects of the codons 136 and 171 of the prion protein gene in sheep with natural scrapie. *J. Gen. Virol.*, **76**, 2097–2101.

9. DAWSON M., HOINVILLE L.J., HOSIE B.D. & HUNTER N. (1998). Guidance on the use of PrP genotyping as an aid to the control of clinical scrapie. *Vet. Rec.* **142**, 623–625.

10. DETWILER L.A. (1992). Scrapie. *Rev. sci. tech. Off. int. Epiz.*, **11**, 491–537.

11. DICKINSON A.G. (1976). Scrapie in sheep and goats. *In:* Slow Virus Diseases of Animals and Man, Kimberlin R.H., ed. North-Holland, Amsterdam, The Netherlands, 209–241.

12. FARQUHAR C.F., SOMERVILLE R.A. & RITCHIE L.A. (1989). Post mortem immunodiagnosis of scrapie and bovine spongiform encephalopathy. *J. Virol. Methods,* **24**, 215–222.

13. FRASER H. (1976). The pathology of natural and experimental scrapie. *In:* Slow Virus Diseases of Animals and Man, Kimberlin R.H., ed. North-Holland, Amsterdam, The Netherlands, 267–305.

14. GIBSON P.H., SOMERVILLE R.A., FRASER H., FOSTER J.D. & KIMBERLIN R.H. (1987). Scrapie associated fibrils in the diagnosis of scrapie in sheep. *Vet. Rec.*, **120**, 125–127.

15. GOLDMANN W., HUNTER N., BENSON G., FOSTER J.D. & HOPE J. (1991). Different scrapie-associated fibril proteins are encoded by lines of sheep selected for different alleles of the *Sip* gene. *J. Gen. Virol.*, **72**, 2411–2417.

16. GOLDMANN W., HUNTER N., FOSTER J.D., SALBAUM J.M., BEYREUTHER K. & HOPE J. (1990). Two alleles of a neural protein gene linked to scrapie in sheep. *Proc. Natl Acad. Sci. USA*, **87**, 2476–2480.

17. HARITANI M., SPENCER Y.I. & WELLS G.A.H. (1994). Hydrated autoclave pretreatment enhancement of prion protein immunoreactivity in formalin-fixed bovine spongiform encephalopathy-affected brain. *Acta Neuropath. (Berlin),* **87**, 86–90.

18. HOINVILLE L.J. (1996). A review of the epidemiology of scrapie in sheep. *Rev. sci. tech. Off. int. Epiz.,* **15** (3), 827–852.

19. HUNTER N., GOLDMANN W., SMITH G. & HOPE J. (1994). The association of a codon 136 PrP gene variant with the occurrence of natural scrapie. *Arch. Virol.*, **137**, 171–177.

20. IKEGAMI Y., ITO, M., ISOMURA H., MOMOTANI E., SASAKI K., MURAMATSU Y., ISHIGURO N. & SHINAGAWA M. (1991). Pre-clinical and clinical diagnosis of scrapie by detection of PrP protein in tissues of sheep. *Vet. Rec.* **128**, 271–275.

21. KIMBERLIN R.H. (1981). Scrapie. *Br. Vet. J.*, **137**, 105–112.

22. KIMBERLIN R.H. (1991) Chapter 29: Scrapie. *In:* Diseases of Sheep, Second Edition, Martin W.B. & Aitken I.D., eds. Blackwell Scientific Publications, Oxford, UK & Boston, USA, 163–169.

23. LAPLANCHE J.L., CHATELAIN J., BEAUDRY P., DUSSAUCY M., BOUNNEAU C. & LAUNAY J.-M. (1993). French autochthonous scrapied sheep without the 136Val PrP polyporhpism. *Mammalian Genome*, **4**, 463–464.

24. LAPLANCHE J.L., CHATELAIN J., WESTAWAY D., THOMAS S., DUSSAUCY M., BRUGERE-PICOUX J. & LAUNAY J.-M. (1993). PrP polymorphisms associated with natural scrapie discovered by denaturing gradient gel electrophoresis. *Genomics*, **15**, 30–37.

25. MCDANIEL H.A. & MOREHOUSE L.G. (1964). The diagnosis of scrapie. *In:* Proceedings of the 67th Annual Meeting of the United States Livestock Sanitary Association, 15–18 October 1963, Albuquerque, New Mexico, USA, 550–564.

26. MILLER J.M., JENNY A.L., TAYLOR W.D., MARSH R.F., RUBENSTEIN R. & RACE R.E. (1993). Immunohistochemical detection of prion protein in sheep with scrapie. *J. Vet. Diagn. Invest.*, **5**, 309–316.

27. MILLER J.M., JENNY A.L., TAYLOR W.D., RACE R.E., ERNST D.R., KATZ J.B. & RUBENSTEIN R. (1994). Detection of prion protein in formalin-fixed brain by hydrated autoclaving immunohistochemistry for the diagnosis of scrapie in sheep. *J. Vet. Diagn. Invest.*, **6**, 366–368.

28. MOHRI S., FARQUHAR C.F., SOMERVILLE R.A., JEFFREY M., FOSTER J. & HOPE J. (1992). Immunodetection of a disease specific PrP fraction in scrapie-affected sheep and BSE-affected cattle. *Vet. Rec.*, **131**, 537–539.

29. O'ROURKE K.I., BASZLER T.V., PARISH S.M. & KNOWLES D.P. (1998). Preclinical detection of PrP^{Sc} in nictitating membrane lymphoid tissue of sheep. *Vet. Rec.*, **142**, 489–491.

30. PALMER A.C. (1976). Scrapie. *In:* Introduction to Animal Neurology, Second Edition, Palmer A.C., ed. Blackwell Scientific Publications, Oxford, UK, 177–178.

31. PARRY H.D. & OPPENHEIMER D.R., eds. (1983). Scrapie Disease in Sheep. Historical, Clinical, Epidemiological, Pathological and Practical Aspects of the Natural Disease, Oppenheimer D.R., ed. Academic Press, London, UK, 192 pp.

32. RACE R.E., ERNST D., JENNY A.L., TAYLOR W., SUTTON D. & CAUGHY, B. (1992). Diagnostic implications of detection of proteinase K-resistant in spleen, lymph nodes and brain of sheep. *Am. J. Vet. Res.*, **53**, 883–889.

33. RACE R.E., ERNST D. & SUTTON D. (1994). Severe autloysis does not prevent scrapie diagnosis in sheep. *J. Vet. Diagn. Invest.*, **6**, 486–489.

34. RACE R., JENNY A. & SUTTON D. (1998). Scrapie infectivity and proteinase K-resistant prion protein in sheep placenta, brain, spleen, and lymph node: Implications for transmission and ante-mortem diagnosis. *J. Infect. Dis.*, **178**, 949–953.

35. SCHMERR M.J., JENNY A. & CUTLIP R.C. (1997). Use of capillary sodium dodecyl sulfate gel electrophoresis to detect the prion protein extracted from scrapie-infected sheep. *J. Chromatogr.* [B], **697**, 223–229.

36. SCHREUDER B.E.C. (1994). Animal Spongiform Encephalopathies: an update. Part 1. Scrapie and lesser known animal spongiform encephalopathies. *Vet. Q.*, **16**, 174–181.

37. SCHREDUER B.E.C., VAN KEULEN L.J.M., VROMANS M.E.W., LANGEVELD J.P.M. & SMITHS M.A. (1996). Preclinical test for prion diseases. *Nature*, **381**, 563.

38. SCHREDUER B.E.C., VAN KEULEN L.J.M., VROMANS M.E.W., LANGEVELD J.P.M. & SMITH M.A. (1998). Tonsillar biopsy and PrP^{Sc} detection in the preclinical diagnosis of scrapie. *Vet. Rec.*, **142**, 564–568.

39. SCIENTIFIC VETERINARY COMMITTEE (1994). Protocols for the Laboratory Diagnosis and Confirmation of Bovine Spongiform Encephalopathy and Scrapie. A report from the Scientific Veterinary Committee, September 1994. European Commission, Directorate General for Agriculture, Unit for Veterinary Legislation and Zootechnics, Brussels, Belgium.

40. SCOTT A.C., DONE S.H., VENABLES C. & DAWSON M. (1987). Detection of scrapie-associated fibrils as an aid to the diagnosis of natural sheep scrapie. *Vet. Rec.*, **120**, 280–281.

41. STACK M.J., KEYES P. & SCOTT A.C. (1996). The diagnosis of bovine spongiform encephalopathy and scrapie by the detection of fibrils and the abnormal protein isoform. *In:* Methods in Molecular Medicine: Prion Diseases, Baker H. & Ridley R.M., eds. Humana Press, Totowa, New Jersey, USA, 85–103.

42. STACK M.J., SCOTT A.C., DONE S.H. & DAWSON M. (1991). Natural scrapie: detection of fibrils in extracts from

43. STACK M.J., SCOTT A.C., DONE S.H. & DAWSON M. (1993). Scrapie associated fibril detection on decomposed and fixed ovine brain material. *Res. Vet. Sci.*, **55**, 173–178.

44 TAYLOR D.M. (1993). Inactivation of SE agents. *In:* Spongiform Encephalopathies. British Medical Bulletin, Vol. 49, Allen I.V., ed. Churchill Livingstone, Edinburgh, UK, 810–821.

45. VAN KEULEN L.J.M., SCHREUDER B.E.C., MELOEN R.H., MOOIJ-HARKES G. VROMANS M.E.W. & LANGEVELD J.P.M. (1996). Immunohistochemical detection of prion protein in lymphoid tissues of sheep with natural scrapie. *J. Clin. Microbiol.*, **34**, 1228–1231.

46. VAN KEULEN L.J.M., SCHREUDER B.E.C., MELOEN R.H., POELEN-VAN DEN BERG M., MOOIJ-HARKES G., VROMANS M.E.W. & LANGEVELD J.P.M. (1995). Immunohistochemical detection and localisation of prion protein in brain tissue of sheep with natural scrapie. *Vet. Pathol.*, **32**, 299–308.

47. WELLS G.A.H. & MCGILL I.S. (1992). Recently described scrapie-like encephalopathies of animals: case definitions. *Res. Vet. Sci.*, **53**, 1–10.

48. WESTAWAY D., ZULIANI V., MIRENDA COOPER C., DA COSTA M., NEUMAN S., JENNY A.L., DETWILER L. & PRUSINER S. (1994). Homozygosity for prion protein alleles encoding glutamine-171 renders sheep susceptible to natural scrapie. *Genes Dev.*, **8**, 959–969.

49. WILESMITH J.W. & WELLS G.A.H. (1991). Bovine spongiform encephalopathy. *Curr. Top. Microbiol. Immunol.*, **172**, 21–38.

50. WOOD J.L.N., LUND L.J. & DONE S.H. (1992). The natural occurrence of scrapie in moufflon. *Vet. Rec.* **130**, 25–27.

51. WOOD J.L.N., MCGILL I.S., DONE S.H. & BRADLEY R. (1997). Neuropathology of scrapie: a study of the distribution patterns of brain lesions in 222 cases of natural scrapie in sheep, 1982–1991. *Vet. Rec.* **140**, 167–174.

52. ZLOTNIK I. & RENNIE J.C. (1958). A comparative study of the incidence of vacuolated neurones in the medulla from apparently healthy sheep of various breeds. *J. Comp. Pathol.*, **68**, 411–415.

*

* *

CHAPTER X.10.

BORDER DISEASE[1]

SUMMARY

Border disease (BD) is a viral disease of sheep first reported in 1959 from the border region of England and Wales. Distribution of the virus is world-wide. Prevalence rates vary in sheep from 5% to 50% between countries and from region to region within countries. Clinical signs include barren ewes, abortions, stillbirths and the birth of small weak lambs. Affected lambs can show tremor, abnormal body conformation and hairy fleeces (so-called 'hairy-shaker' or 'fuzzy' lambs). Vertical transmission plays an important role in the epidemiology of the disease. Infection of fetuses can result in the birth of persistently infected (PI) lambs. These PI lambs are viraemic, antibody negative and constantly excrete virus. The virus spreads from sheep to sheep, with PI animals being the most potent source of infection. Sheep may also be infected following close contact with cattle excreting the closely related bovine viral diarrhoea virus (BVDV).

It is important to identify the viraemic PI animals so that they will not be used for breeding or trading purposes. Serological testing is insufficient. It is generally considered that serologically positive, nonviraemic sheep are 'safe', as latent infections are not known to occur in recovered animals.

***Identification of the agent:** BD virus (BDV) is a pestivirus in the family Flaviviridae and is closely related to classical swine fever virus and BVDV. Nearly all isolates of BDV are noncytopathogenic in cell culture. There are no defined serotypes but virus isolates exhibit considerable antigenic diversity and three distinct antigenic groups have been identified.*

Apparently healthy PI sheep resulting from congenital infection can be identified by isolation of noncytopathogenic virus from blood or serum in laboratory cell cultures. Isolation of virus is unreliable in lambs younger than 2 months of age that have received colostral antibody. The isolation of virus from tissues of aborted or stillborn lambs is difficult, but tissues from PI sheep contain easily detectable levels of virus. To detect the growth of virus in cell cultures, it is essential to use an immunohistochemical-labelling method. Alternative methods based on direct detection of viral antigen or viral RNA in leukocytes are also available. Acute infection is usually subclinical and viraemia is transient and difficult to detect.

***Serological tests:** Acute infection with BDV is best confirmed by demonstrating seroconversion using paired or sequential samples from several animals in the group. The enzyme-linked immunosorbent assay and virus neutralisation are the most commonly used antibody detection methods.*

***Requirements for vaccines and diagnostic biologicals:** There is no standard vaccine for BDV, but a commercial killed whole-virus vaccine has been produced. Ideally, such a vaccine should be suitable for administration to females before breeding for prevention of transplacental infection. The use of BVDV vaccines has been advocated, but the antigenic diversity of BD viruses must be considered.*

BD viruses have contaminated several modified live veterinary vaccines produced in sheep cells or containing sheep serum. This potential hazard should be recognised by manufacturers of biological products.

1 See also Appendix 3.2.2. in the *Code*.

A. DIAGNOSTIC TECHNIQUES

Border disease virus (BDV) is a pestivirus of the family Flaviviridae and is closely related to classical swine fever virus (CSFV) and bovine viral diarrhoea virus (BVDV) (16). There are four principal genotypes of pestiviruses: – CSFV, BVDV types 1 and 2 and BDV. While CSF viruses are predominantly restricted to pigs, examples of the other three genotypes have all been recovered from sheep with the majority of isolates being BD viruses (21). Nearly all isolates of BDV are noncytopathogenic, although occasional cytopathic viruses have been isolated (18). BDV spreads naturally among sheep by the oro-nasal route and by vertical transmission. It is principally a cause of congenital disease in sheep and goats, but can also cause acute and persistent infections. Sheep can become infected from cattle (5). Pigs may also be infected and antibodies to BDV in pigs may interfere with tests for diagnosis of CSF. This chapter describes BDV infection in sheep.

a) Acute infections

Healthy newborn and adult sheep exposed to BDV experience only mild or inapparent disease. Slight fever and a mild leukopenia are associated with a short-lived viraemia detectable between days 4 and 11 post-infection, after which virus neutralising antibody appears in the serum.

Acute infections are best diagnosed serologically using paired sera from a representative number of sheep. Occasional BDV isolates have been shown to produce high fever, profound and prolonged leukopenia, anorexia, conjunctivitis, nasal discharge, dyspnoea and diarrhoea, and 50% mortality in young lambs. One such isolate was recovered from a severe epidemic of BD among dairy sheep in 1984 (6). A second such isolate was a BDV contaminant of a live CSFV vaccine (22).

b) Fetal infection

The main clinical signs of BD are seen following the infection of pregnant ewes. While the initial maternal infection is subclinical or mild, the consequences for the fetus are serious. Fetal death may occur at any stage of pregnancy, but is more common in fetuses infected early in gestation. Small dead fetuses may be resorbed or their abortion pass unnoticed as the ewes continue to feed well and show no sign of discomfort. As lambing time approaches, the abortion of larger fetuses, stillbirths and the premature births of small, weak lambs will be seen. Confirmation that an abortion or stillbirth is due to BDV is often difficult to establish, but virus may be isolated from fetal tissues in some cases. In aborted fetuses, it is also possible to detect virus by immunohistochemistry of brain tissue. Samples of fetal fluids or serum should be tested for BDV antibody.

During lambing, an excessive number of barren ewes will become apparent, but it is the diseased live lambs that present the main clinical features characteristic of BD. The clinical signs exhibited by BD lambs are very variable and depend on the breed of sheep, the virulence of the virus and the time at which infection was introduced into the flock. Affected lambs are usually small and weak, many being unable to stand. Nervous signs and fleece changes are often apparent. The nervous signs of BD are its most characteristic feature. The tremor can vary from violent rhythmic contractions of the muscles of the hind legs and back, to barely detectable fine trembling of the head, ears, and tail. Fleece abnormalities are most obvious in smooth-coated breeds, which develop hairy fleeces, especially on the neck and back. Abnormal brown or black pigmentation of the fleece may also be seen in BD-affected lambs. Blood samples to be tested for the presence of BDV and/or antibody should be collected into anticoagulant from suspect lambs before they have received colostrum. Once lambs have ingested colostrum, it is difficult to detect virus until they are 2 months old and maternal antibody levels have waned.

With careful nursing a proportion of BD lambs can be reared, although deaths may occur at any age. The nervous signs gradually decline and can have disappeared by 3–6 months of age. Weakness, and swaying of the hind-quarters, together with fine trembling of the head, may reappear at times of stress. Affected lambs often grow slowly and under normal field conditions many will die before or around weaning time. In cases where losses at lambing time have been low and no lambs with obvious signs of BD have been born, this can be the first presenting sign of disease.

Some fetal infections occurring around mid-gestation can result in lambs with severe nervous signs, locomotor disturbances and abnormal skeletons. Such lambs have lesions of cerebellar hypoplasia and dysplasia, hydranencephaly and porencephaly resulting from necrotising inflammation. The severe destructive lesions appear to be immune mediated, and lambs with such lesions frequently have high concentrations of serum antibody to BDV. Most lambs infected in late gestation are normal and healthy and are born free from virus but with BDV antibody. Some such lambs can be weak and may die in early life (1).

c) Persistent viraemia

When fetuses survive an infection that occurs before the onset of immune competence, they are born with a persistent viraemia. The ovine fetus can first respond to an antigenic stimulus between approximately

60 and 85 days of its 150-day gestation period. In fetuses infected before the onset of immune competence, viral replication is uncontrolled and 50% fetal death is common. In lambs surviving infection in early gestation, virus is widespread in all organs. Such lambs appear to be tolerant to the virus and have a persistent infection, usually for life. A precolostral blood sample will be virus positive and antibody negative. Typically, there is no inflammatory reaction and the most characteristic pathological changes are in the central nervous system (CNS) and skin. Throughout the CNS, there is a deficiency of myelin, and this causes the nervous signs. In the skin, primary wool follicles increase in size and the number of secondary wool follicles decreases, causing the hairy or coarse fleece.

Persistently viraemic sheep can be diagnosed by virus isolation/detection in a blood sample. Viraemia is readily detectable at any time except within the first 2 months of life, when virus is masked by colostral antibody, and in animals older than 4 years, some of which develop low levels of anti-BDV antibody (11). Although virus detection in blood during an acute infection is difficult, persistent viraemia should be confirmed by retesting animals after an interval of at least 3 weeks.

Some viraemic sheep survive to sexual maturity and are used for breeding. Lambs born to these infected dams are always persistently viraemic. Persistently viraemic sheep are a continual source of infectious virus to other animals and their identification is a major factor in any control programme. Sheep being traded should be screened for the absence of BDV viraemia.

Usually persistently infected (PI) rams have poor quality, highly infective semen and reduced fertility. All rams used for breeding should be screened for persistent BDV infection on a blood sample. Semen samples can also be screened for virus, but they are much less satisfactory than blood due to their toxicity for cell cultures.

d) Late-onset disease in persistently viraemic sheep

Some PI sheep housed apart from other animals spontaneously develop intractable scour, wasting, excessive ocular and nasal discharges, sometimes with respiratory distress. At necropsy such sheep have gross thickening of the distal ileum, caecum and colon resulting from focal hyperplastic enteropathy. Cytopathic BDV can be recovered from the gut of these lambs. With no obvious outside source of cytopathic virus it is most likely that such virus originates from the lamb's own virus pool. Other PI sheep in the group do not develop the disease. This syndrome, which has also been recognised in occasional field outbreaks of BD, has several similarities with bovine mucosal disease (11).

1. Identification of the agent (the prescribed test for international trade)

There is no designated OIE reference laboratory for BDV, but the reference laboratories for BVDV or CSFV will be able to provide advice (see Table given in Part 4 of this *Manual*). The most sensitive proven method for identifying BDV remains virus isolation. Direct immunofluorescence or immunoperoxidase labelling, antigen enzyme-linked immunosorbent assay (ELISA) and reverse-transcription polymerase chain reaction (RT-PCR) methods are also used.

a) Virus isolation

It is essential that laboratories undertaking virus isolation have a guaranteed supply of pestivirus-free susceptible cells and fetal bovine serum (FBS), or equivalent, that contains no anti-pestivirus activity and no contaminating virus. The virus can be isolated in a number of primary or secondary ovine cell cultures (e.g. kidney, testes, lung). Ovine cell lines for BDV growth are rare. Semicontinuous cell lines derived from fetal lamb muscle (FLM) or sheep choroid plexus can be useful, but different lines vary considerably in their susceptibility to the virus. Ovine cells have been used successfully for the isolation and growth of BD viruses and BVDV types 1 and 2 from sheep. In regions where sheep may become infected with BVD viruses from cattle, a virus isolation system using both ovine and bovine cells could be optimal. Several bovine cell cultures may be suggested, including testicular, embryonic tracheal or turbinate cells, or a susceptible continuous kidney cell line. However, bovine cells are insensitive for the primary isolation and growth of some BD viruses, so reliance on bovine cells alone is inadvisable.

From live animals, serum can be tested for the presence of infectious virus, but the most sensitive way to confirm pestivirus viraemia is to wash leukocytes repeatedly (at least three times) in culture medium before co-cultivating them with susceptible cells for 7 days. Cells are frozen and thawed once and an aliquot passaged on to further susceptible cells grown on cover-slips. The cells are stained, 3 days later, for the presence of pestivirus using an immunofluorescence or immunoperoxidase test.

Tissues should be collected from dead animals in virus transport medium (10% [w/v]). In the laboratory, the tissues are ground up, centrifuged to remove debris, and the supernatant passed through 0.45 µm filters. Spleen, thyroid, thymus, kidney, brain, lymph nodes and gut lesions are the best organs for virus isolation.

Semen can be examined for the presence of BDV, but raw semen is strongly cytotoxic and must be diluted, usually at least 1/10 in culture medium. As the major threat of BDV-infected semen is from PI rams, blood is a more reliable clinical sample than semen for identifying such animals.

There are many variations in virus isolation procedures. All should be optimised for maximum sensitivity using a standard reference virus preparation and, whenever possible, recent BDV field isolates. A practical tube isolation procedure is outlined below:

i) Test tube cultures with subconfluent or newly confluent monolayers of susceptible ovine cells are washed at least twice with Hanks balanced salt solution to remove growth medium before being inoculated with 0.2 ml of sample and adsorbed for 2 hours at 37°C.

ii) Cultures are washed with 2 ml medium. This is discarded and 1 ml of culture maintenance medium is added.

iii) Cultures are incubated for 5–7 days at 37°C. They are examined microscopically on a daily basis and evidence of cytopathic effect (CPE) is recorded.

iv) The tubes are frozen at –70°C, and then thawed, as before, for passage to fresh tube cultures containing cells growing on cover-slips.

v) Cover-slips are removed 3–4 days later, fixed in cold acetone for 15 minutes and stained using an indirect or direct immunofluorescence method. Essential controls must include known negative cells and cells growing standard cytopathic and noncytopathic BDV strains.

vi) The cover-slips are examined under a UV microscope for the diffuse cytoplasmic fluorescence that is characteristic of pestiviruses.

Alternatively, frozen and thawed cultures can be added to cells growing on chamber slides and stained by direct immunofluorescence test as above. Immunoperoxidase staining can also be used on cover-slips or chamber slides as well as microtitre plates (see method under virus neutralisation [VN] test below). Frozen and thawed cultures can also be tested in an antigen detection ELISA system.

b) Enzyme-linked immunosorbent assay for antigen detection

The first ELISA for pestivirus antigen detection was described for detecting viraemic sheep. This has now been modified into a double monoclonal antibody (MAb) capture ELISA for use in sheep and cattle. Two capture MAbs are bound to wells in microtitre plates, and two other MAbs, conjugated to peroxidase, serve as detector MAbs (8). The test is most commonly employed to identify PI viraemic sheep using washed, detergent-lysed blood leukocytes. The sensitivity is close to that of virus isolation and it is a practical method for screening high numbers of blood samples. As with virus isolation, high levels of colostral antibody can mask persistent viraemia. The ELISA is more effective than virus isolation in the presence of antibody, but may give false-negative results in viraemic lambs younger than 2 months old. The ELISA is usually not sensitive enough to detect acute BDV infections on blood samples. As well as for testing leukocytes, the antigen ELISA can also be used on tissue suspensions, especially spleen, from suspected PI sheep and, as an alternative to immunofluorescence and immunoperoxidase methods, on cell cultures.

Several pestivirus ELISA methods have been published and a number of commercial kits are now available for detecting BVDV in cattle. While one of these is suitable for use in sheep, further evaluation of other kits may be required.

c) Nucleic acid recognition methods

The complete genomic sequences of two BD viruses have been determined and compared with those of other pestiviruses (3, 14). Phylogenetic analysis shows BD viruses to be more closely related to CSFV than to BVDV (2, 17, 21). Primers for RT-PCR are commonly selected from the conserved 5'- noncoding region (15, 20). While RT-PCR has not yet been evaluated for diagnostic purposes in sheep, it is likely to be of future value. The detection of viral RNA in fetal tissues may yet be an important application, as other methods are insensitive. The exquisite sensitivity of RT-PCR makes it a valuable tool for detecting low level virus contamination, such as in cell culture constituents or vaccines and when BDV-specific antibodies are present. The precautions to be taken with RT-PCR have been covered in Chapter I.7.

2. Serological tests

Antibody to BDV is usually detected in sheep sera using VN or an ELISA. The less sensitive agar gel immunodiffusion (AGID) test may also be used. Control positive and negative reference sera must be included in every test. These should give results within predetermined limits for the test to be considered valid. Single sera can be tested to determine the prevalence of BDV in a flock, region or country. For diagnosis, however, acute and convalescent sera are the best samples for confirming acute BDV infection. Repeat sera from one animal should always be tested alongside each other on the same plate.

a) Virus neutralisation test

A standard cytopathic strain of BDV[2] can be used for the VN test with semicontinuous cells such as FLM. An outline protocol is given below:

i) Test and control sera are heat-inactivated for 30 minutes at 56°C.

ii) From a starting serum dilution of 1/4, serial twofold dilutions of the test sera are made in cell culture growth media in a cell-culture grade flat-bottomed 96 well microtitre plate. For each sample, two or four wells are used at each dilution depending on the accuracy required. The range of dilution can also vary. It is common to screen sera initially at a dilution of 1/4 and titrate out positive sera. To screen sera a minimum of four wells is required. The standard working volume is 25 µl: 25 µl of the diluted serum is added to each well; 25 µl of media is added to each of the lower two control wells; and 25 µl of media containing 100 $TCID_{50}$ (50% tissue culture infective dose) of virus is added to each of the two upper test wells. Control positive and negative sera and a virus titration are included in every test.

iii) Plates are sealed with nontoxic plate sealers or lids, and incubated at 37°C for 1 hour.

iv) 100 µl of a cell suspension with a count of 2×10^5 cells/ml is added to every well. The FBS or equivalent serum used for cell growth must be free from antibody to BDV.

v) The plate is sealed or incubated in a humid chamber in 5% CO_2 for 4 days at 37°C.

vi) The wells are examined microscopically for CPE. In the control wells of the test sera, CPE will be due to toxicity. Further dilution of toxic sera can be attempted, but it may not be possible to obtain reliable results with occasional sera. The VN titre for each serum is the dilution at which the virus is neutralised in 50% of the wells. This can be calculated by the Spearman–Kärber method. A seronegative animal will show no neutralisation at the lowest dilution (i.e. 1/4).

The choice of test virus is difficult due to antigenic diversity among pestiviruses (7, 10, 12). Standard strains of cytopathic BVD viruses and bovine cells can be used. Oregon C24V results correlate better with Moredun BDV than results with the NADL strain. No single strain is ideal. A local strain that gives the highest antibody titre with a range of positive sheep sera should be used. The VN test can also be used with noncytopathic viruses when the following immunoperoxidase staining system is used after step v above:

i) The culture medium is removed and the cells are washed gently with warm phosphate buffered saline (PBS), air-dried and cooled to 4°C.

ii) The cells are fixed by quickly adding to all wells 95% acetone (in water) previously cooled to –20°C. The plates are held at –20°C for 30 minutes and should not be stacked or allowed to warm as etching of the plastic may occur.

iii) The acetone is removed and the plates are dried quickly in a cool environment.

iv) 50 µl of BDV antiserum is added to all wells at a predetermined dilution in PBS with 1% Tween 80 (PBST). Plates are incubated at 37°C for 30 minutes in a humid atmosphere.

v) The plates are emptied and washed three times with PBST.

vi) The wells are drained and an appropriate anti-species serum conjugated to peroxidase at a predetermined dilution is added, and the plates are left for 30 minutes at 37°C in a humid atmosphere.

vii) The plates are emptied and washed three times with PBST.

viii) The plates are drained well and 50 µl of activated substrate e.g. 3-amino-9-ethyl carbazole (AEC) is added. AEC stock solution is: AEC (0.1 g) dissolved in dimethyl formamide (15 ml). For use, add stock (0.3 ml) to membrane-filtered 0.05 M acetate buffer, pH 5.0, (4.7 ml), and then add 30% H_2O_2 (5 µl). NB: This solution is toxic and should be handled with adequate precautions.

ix) The plates are incubated at room temperature and known virus-positive control wells are monitored for development of specific red-brown cytoplasmic staining. When staining is complete, the substrate is removed carefully and the wells are washed thoroughly with tap water. Leaving the tap water in the wells, the plates are examined microscopically for virus-containing wells.

2 For example, Moredun available from Moredun Scientific Limited, Pentlands Science Park, Bush Loan, Penicuik, Edinburgh EH26 0PZ, United Kingdom.

x) The VN titre is calculated as above using the Spearman–Kärber method.

xi) Alternatively, the test can be performed using direct fluorescein isothiocyanate conjugate staining.

Occasionally there may be a need to determine whether antibody in a flock is against a virus belonging to a particular pestivirus serogroup. A differential VN test can be used in which sera are titrated out against representative viruses from each of the four pestivirus groups, i.e. BDV, BVDV types 1 and 2, and CSFV. Maximum titre will identify the infecting serotype and the spectrum of cross-reactivity with the other serotypes will also be revealed.

b) Enzyme-linked immunosorbent assay

An MAb-capture ELISA for measuring BDV antibodies has been described. Two pan pestivirus MAbs that detect different epitopes on the immunodominant nonstructural protein NS 2/3 are used to capture detergent-lysed cell-culture grown antigen. The results correlate qualitatively with the VN test (9).

Antigen is prepared as follows: Use eight 225 cm^2 flasks of newly confluent FLM cells; four flasks will be controls and four will be infected. Wash the flasks and infect four with a 0.01–0.1 m.o.i. (multiplicity of infection) of Moredun cytopathic BDV. Adsorb the virus for 2 hours at 37°C. Add maintenance media containing 2% FBS (free from BDV antibody), and incubate cultures for 4–5 days until CPE is obvious. Pool four control flask supernatants and separately pool four infected flask supernatants. Centrifuge at 3000 ***g*** for 15 minutes to pellet cells. Discard the supernatants. Retain the cell pellets. Wash the flasks with 50 ml of PBS and repeat the centrifugation step as above. Pool all the control cell pellets in 8 ml PBS containing 1% nonidet P40 and return 2 ml to each control flask to lyse the remaining attached cells. Repeat for infected cells. Keep the flasks at 4°C for at least 2 hours agitating the small volume of fluid on the cells vigorously every 30 minutes to ensure total cell detachment. Centrifuge the control and infected antigen at 12,000 ***g*** for 5 minutes to remove the cell debris. Supernatant antigens are stored at –70°C in small aliquots.

- **Test procedure**

i) The two MAbs are diluted to a predetermined dilution (commonly 1/4000) in 0.05 M bicarbonate buffer, pH 9.6. All wells of a suitable ELISA-grade microtitre plate (e.g. Nunc maxisorb, Greiner 129b) are coated overnight at 4°C.

ii) After washing three times in PBST, a blocking solution of PBST containing 10% horse serum (PBSTH) is added to all wells, which are incubated at 37°C for 1 hour.

iii) The antigen is diluted to a predetermined dilution in PBSTH and alternate rows of wells are coated with virus and control antigens for 1 hour at 37°C. The plates are then washed three times in PBST before addition of test sera.

iv) Test sera are diluted 1/50 in PBSTH and added to duplicate virus and duplicate control wells for 1 hour at 37°C. The plates are then washed three times in PBST.

v) Anti-ovine IgG peroxidase conjugate is diluted to a predetermined dilution in PBSTH and added to all wells for 1 hour at 37°C. The plates are washed three times in PBST.

vi) A suitable activated enzyme substrate, such as ortho-phenylene diamine (OPD) or tetramethyl blue (TMB), is added noting the manufacturer's toxicity warning. After colour development, the reaction is stopped with sulphuric acid and the absorbance read on an ELISA plate reader. The mean value of the two control wells is subtracted from the mean value of the two virus wells to give the corrected absorbance for each serum. Results are expressed as corrected absorbance with reference to the corrected absorbance of known positive and negative sera. Alternatively, ELISA titres can be extrapolated from a standard curve of a dilution series of a known positive reference serum.

c) Agar gel immunodiffusion test

The AGID test was first used to demonstrate an immunological relationship between BD, BVD and CSF viruses.

The Oregon C24V strains of BVDV grown on calf testis cells has been used to detect antibody in sheep. Suitable antigen can be prepared using medium harvested from cells showing early CPE. Concentration of the medium approximately 100-fold by dialysis against polyethylene glycol (PEG) is required. Alternatively, PEG 6000 can be added to sonicated virus–cell suspensions at the rate of 8% (w/v). After constant stirring overnight at 4°C, the precipitate is removed by centrifugation at 1800 ***g*** for 1 hour. The supernatant is decanted thoroughly and the precipitate resuspended to 1% of the original virus–cell culture volume in distilled water. The resuspended precipitate is centrifuged at 286,000 ***g*** for 2 hours and the supernatant withdrawn for use as antigen. The precipitate is discarded.

Standard conditions are used for the AGID test with appropriate strong and weak positive, and negative control sera.

B. REQUIREMENTS FOR VACCINES AND DIAGNOSTIC BIOLOGICALS

To be useful, a BDV vaccine should be effective when administered to female sheep before breeding to prevent transplacental infection. Experimental and commercial inactivated whole virus BDV vaccines have been produced in Europe (4, 19).

Pestivirus contaminants of modified live virus vaccines have been found to be a cause of serious disease following their use in pigs, cattle, sheep and goats. Contaminated vaccines have included those used for the control of Aujesky's disease, CSF, rotavirus, coronavirus, rinderpest, sheep pox and contagious pustular dermatitis. The insidious ability of pestiviruses to cross the placenta, and thus establish PI animals, gives them the potential to contaminate vaccines through cells, serum used as medium supplement, or seed stock virus. As nearly all isolates of pestiviruses are noncytopathic, they will remain undetected unless specific tests are carried out.

1. Seed management

a) Characteristics of the seed

An ideal vaccine should contain a strain or strains of virus that gives protection against all sheep pestiviruses. The most recent evidence is that three antigenically distinguishable groups of BD viruses infect sheep. One group is represented by the Moredun reference strain of BDV; the second group contains viruses similar to the majority of cattle BVDV strains (BVDV type 1); the third group contains the less common BVDV (type 2) strains (23). Further cross-protection studies are required to determine the significance of these findings. Nevertheless, it would appear that any BDV vaccine should contain at least a representative of the BDV and BVDV (type 1) groups. Characterisation of the biologically cloned vaccine viruses should include typing with MAbs and genotyping (13).

b) Culture

A variety of ruminant cell cultures can be used. Optimal yields depend on the cell type and isolate used. A commercial BDV vaccine containing two strains of virus is prepared on ovine cell lines (4). Cells must be produced according to a seed-lot system from a master cell seed (MCS) that has been shown to be free from all contaminating microorganisms. Vaccine should only be produced in cells fewer than 20 passages from the MCS. Control cells from every passage should be checked for pestivirus contamination.

c) Validation as a vaccine

All vaccines should pass standard tests for safety and efficacy. Safety testing of inactivated BDV vaccines should include monitoring of all vaccine components for contaminating pestiviruses.

Efficacy tests of BDV vaccines should demonstrate their ability to prevent transplacental spread of virus. Effective challenge of vaccinated pregnant ewes at 50–60 days gestation has been achieved by intranasal installation of virus or by mixing with PI sheep (4).

2. Method of manufacture

Inactivated vaccines have been prepared using conventional laboratory techniques with stationary or rolled cell cultures. Inactivants have included formalin and beta-propriolactone. Adjuvants have included aluminium hydroxide and oil (4, 19).

3. In-process control

Cultures should be inspected daily to ensure they are free from gross bacterial contamination, and that any CPE observed is appropriate to the cytopathic virus being grown. No CPE should be observed in cultures being used to grow noncytopathic strains of virus.

4. Batch control

a) Sterility

Tests for sterility and freedom from contamination of biological materials may be found in Chapter I.4.

b) Safety

Samples from inactivated vaccines should be tested rigorously for viable virus. Samples of the product should be passaged several times in sensitive cell cultures to ensure absence of live BDV. This *in-vitro* monitoring can be augmented by injecting two BDV-seronegative sheep with 20 doses of unformulated antigen, as part of a standard safety test. Presence of live virus will result in the development of a more convincing serological response than will occur with inactivated virus alone. The sheep sera can also be examined for antibody to other prescribed agents.

c) Potency

Vaccine potency is also best tested in seronegative sheep in which the development and level of antibody is measured. An indirect measure of potency is given by the level of virus infectivity prior to inactivation. The antigen content following inactivation can be assayed by MAb-capture ELISA and related to the results of established *in-vivo* potency results. As recommended for potency testing of BVDV vaccine in cattle, it should be demonstrated that the vaccine can prevent transplancental transmission of BDV in pregnant sheep.

d) Duration of immunity

No information is available on duration of immunity following vaccination. Inactivated vaccines are unlikely to provide sustained levels of immunity, and it is likely that after an initial course of two or three injections, annual booster doses may be required. Insufficient information is available to determine any correlation between vaccinal antibody titres in the dam and fetal protection.

e) Stability

There is little information on the stability of BDV vaccines. Inactivated vaccines could be expected to have at least a 1-year shelf life when protected from light and stored at 4°C.

f) Preservatives

Preservatives may be added to multidose vaccine containers subject to the approval of the Control Authority.

g) Precautions (hazards)

BDV is not considered to be a hazard to human health. Standard good microbiological practice should be used when handling the virus.

5. Tests on the final product

a) Safety

In-vitro test only.

b) Potency

In-vitro antigen content test.

REFERENCES

1. BARLOW R.M. & PATTERSON D.S.P. (1982). Border disease of sheep: a virus-induced teratogenic disorder. *Adv. Vet. Med.* (Suppl. *J. Vet. Med.*), **36**, 1–87.

2. Becher P., Orlich M., Shannon A.D., Horner G., Konig M. & Thiel H-J. (1997). Phylogenetic analysis of pestiviruses from domestic and wild ruminants. *J. Gen. Virol.*, **78**, 1357–1366.

3. Becher P., Orlich M. & Thiel H-J. (1998). Complete genomic sequence of border disease virus, a pestivirus from sheep. *J. Virol.*, **72**, 5165–5173.

4. Brun A., Lacoste F., Reynaud G., Kato F. & Saint-Marc B. (1993). Evaluation of the potency of an inactivated vaccine against border disease pestivirus infection in sheep. *In:* Proceedings of the Second Symposium on Pestiviruses, Edwards S. ed. Fondation Marcel Merieux, Annecy, France, 1–3 October 1992, 257–259.

5. Carlsson U. (1991). Border disease in sheep caused by transmission of virus from cattle persistently infected with bovine virus diarrhoea virus. *Vet. Rec.*, **128**, 145–147.

6. Chappuis G., Brun A., Kato F., Dauvergne M., Reynaud G. & Duret C. (1986). Etudes serologiques et immunologiques realisées a la suite de l'isolement d'un pestivirus dans un foyer ovina chez des moutons de L'Aveyron. *In:* Pestiviroses des Ovins et des Bovins, Espinasse J. & Savey M., eds. Sté Francaise de Buiatrie, Paris, France, 55–66.

7. Dekker A., Wensvoort G. & Terpstra C. (1995). Six antigenic groups within the genus pestivirus as identified by cross-neutralisation assays. *Vet. Microbiol.*, **47**, 317–329.

8. Entrican G., Dand A. & Nettleton P.F. (1994). A double monoclonal-antibody ELISA for detecting pestivirus antigen in the blood of viraemic cattle and sheep. *Vet. Microbiol.*, **43**, 65–74.

9. Fenton A., Sinclair J.A., Entrican G., Herring J.A. & Nettleton P.F. (1991). A monoclonal antibody capture ELISA to detect antibody to border disease virus in sheep sera. *Vet. Microbiol.*, **28**, 327–333.

10. Laude H. & Gelfi J. (1979). Properties of border disease virus as studied in a sheep cell line. *Arch. Virol.*, **62**, 341–346.

11. Nettleton P.F., Gilmour J.S., Herring J.A. & Sinclair J.A. (1992). The production and survival of lambs persistently infected with border disease virus. *Comp. Immunol. Microbiol. infect. Dis.*, **15**, 179–188.

12. Nettleton P.F., Gilray J.A., Russo P. & Dlissi E. (1998). Border disease of sheep and goats. *Vet. Res.*, **29**, 327–340.

13. Paton D.J., Sands J.J., Lowings J.P., Smith J.E., Ibata G. & Edwards S. (1995). A proposed division of the pestivirus genus into subgroups using monoclonal antibodies, supported by cross-neutralization assays and genetic sequencing. *Vet. Res.*, **26**, 92–109.

14. Ridpath J.F. & Bolin S.R. (1997). Comparison of the complete genomic sequence of the border disease virus, BD31, to other pestiviruses. *Virus Res.*, **50**, 237–243.

15. Sandvik T., Paton D.J & Lowings P.J. (1997). Detection and identification of ruminant and porcine pestiviruses by nested amplification of the 5' untranslated cDNA region. *J. Virol. Methods*, **64**, 43–56.

16. Thiel H.-J., Plagemann P.G.W. & Moennig V. (1996). Pestiviruses. *In:* Field's Virology, Third Edition, Fields B.B., Knipe D.M., Howley P.M., eds. Lippiniott-Raven, Philadelphia, USA, 1059–1073.

17. Van Rijn P.A., Van Gennip H.G.P., Leenclerse C.H., Bruschke C.J.M., Paton D.J., Moormann R.J.M. & Van Oirschot J.T. (1997). Subdivision of the pestivirus genus based on envelope glycoprotein E2. *Virology*, **237**, 337–348.

18. Vantsis J.T., Barlow R.M., Fraser J. & Mould D.L. (1976). Experiments in border disease VIII. Propagation and properties of a cytopathic virus. *J. Comp. Pathol.*, **86**, 111–120.

19. Vantsis J.T., Rennie J.C., Gardiner A.C., Wells P.W., Barlow R.M. & Martin W.B. (1980). Immunisation against Border disease. *J. Comp. Path.*, **90**, 349–354.

20. Vilcek S., Herring A.J., Herring J.A., Nettleton P.F., Lowings J.P.L. & Paton D.J. (1994). Pestiviruses isolated from pigs, cattle and sheep can be allocated into three genogroups using polymerase chain reaction and restriction endonuclease analysis. *Arch. Virol.*, **136**, 309–323.

21. VILCEK S., NETTLETON P.F., PATON D.J. & BELAK S. (1997). Molecular characterisation of ovine pestiviruses. *J. Gen. Virol.*, **78**, 725–735.

22. WENSVOORT G. & TERPSTRA C. (1988). Bovine viral diarrhoea virus infection in piglets born to sows vaccinated against swine fever with contaminated virus. *Res. Vet. Sci.*, **45**, 143–148.

23. WENSVOORT G., TERPSTRA C. & DE KLUYVER E.P. (1989) Characterization of porcine and some ruminant pestiviruses by cross-neutralization. *Vet. Microbiol.*, **20**, 291–306.

*
* *

CHAPTER X.11.

SURRA (*Trypanosoma evansi*)

SUMMARY

Trypanosomosis[1] *caused by* Trypanosoma evansi *('surra') is the most widely distributed of the pathogenic animal trypanosomoses, affecting domesticated livestock in Asia, Africa and Central and South America. The principle host species affected varies geographically, but buffalo, cattle, camels and horses are particularly affected, although other animals are also susceptible. It is an arthropod-borne disease,* Tabanus *spp. being implicated as the main vectors. The diagnosis of surra is usually based on the demonstration of the parasites in the blood, supplemented by haematological, biochemical and serological tests.*

The disease in susceptible animals is manifested by pyrexia, directly associated with parasitaemia, together with a progressive anaemia, loss of condition and lassitude. Recurrent episodes of fever and parasitaemia occur during the course of the disease. Oedema, particularly of the lower parts of the body, urticarial plaques and petechial haemorrhages of the serous membranes are often observed. Abortions have been reported in buffaloes in Asia. There are indications that the disease causes immunodeficiencies. The clinical signs of surra, although indicative, are not pathognomonic, therefore diagnosis must be confirmed by laboratory methods.

Identification of the agent: *As the general clinical signs of the various forms of* T. evansi *infection are not pathognomonic, laboratory diagnosis is required. When there is a high parasitaemia, the examination of wet blood films, stained blood smears and lymph node material should reveal the trypanosomes. In other more chronic cases, such as the carrier state, the examination of thick blood smears, as well as methods of parasite concentration and the inoculation of laboratory animals, are recommended. An attractive complementary approach now being explored is the application of antigen-detection tests. Pilot versions of immunoenzyme and latex agglutination assays already exist. Using the polymerase chain reaction, minute amounts of well defined and highly specific trypanosomal DNA sequences can be detected in blood and other samples from infected hosts.*

Haematological and biochemical tests are not specific for T. evansi *infection, but they reveal the pathological consequences of infection. In areas where the disease is endemic, such tests help to monitor the results of chemotherapy. The tests include measurements of the packed blood cell volume and immunoglobulin levels.*

Serological tests: *Infection gives rise to specific antibody responses and a variety of antibody-detection tests have been introduced. These have been partially validated, but await large-scale evaluation and standardisation. In the laboratory, immunofluorescence and immunoenzyme assays can be employed. For field use, relatively simple tests have yet to be developed. Obvious candidates are direct agglutination tests with trypanosomes from the bloodstream, and indirect agglutination tests with antigen-coated red blood cells (indirect haemagglutination) or latex particles. Assays for detection of circulating antibodies have high measures of validity. Estimates of predictive values of different serological tests indicate that enzyme-linked immunosorbent assays (ELISAs) for detecting IgG antibodies are more likely to classify correctly uninfected animals and that card agglutination tests (CATT) are more likely to classify correctly truly infected animals. An IgG ELISA would thus be suitable to check that animals were free from infection, prior to movement or during quarantine. In situations where there is overt disease, CATT tests can be used to target individual animals for treatment with trypanocidal drugs. For declaring disease-free*

1 Nomenclature of parasitic diseases: see the note in Chapter X.6. Trypanosomosis (Tsetse-transmitted).

status, serial testing – ELISA followed by re-testing of suspect samples by CATT – is recommended. It must be stressed, however, that there are considerable antigenic similarities between the different species of pathogenic trypanosomes, hence in areas where tsetse-transmitted trypanosomoses occur, cross-reactions will occur with any serological test employed.

Requirements for vaccines and diagnostic biologicals: *No vaccines are available for the disease.*

A. DIAGNOSTIC TECHNIQUES

The diagnosis of *Trypanosoma evansi* infection, an arthropod-borne disease, is based on clinical signs and on the demonstration of the parasites by direct or indirect methods.

The clinical signs of surra, the disease caused by *T. evansi,* are indicative but are not sufficiently pathognomonic and diagnosis must be confirmed by laboratory methods. The disease in susceptible animals is manifested by pyrexia, directly associated with parasitaemia, together with a progressive anaemia, loss of condition and lassitude. Recurrent episodes of fever and parasitaemia occur during the course of the disease. Oedema, particularly of the lower parts of the body, urticarial plaques and petechial haemorrhages of the serous membranes are often observed. Abortions have been reported in buffaloes in Asia (13). There are indications that the disease causes immunodeficiency (24).

There is considerable variation in the pathogenicity of different strains and the susceptibility of different host species to disease. Disease may manifest as an acute or chronic condition, and in the latter case may persist for many months. The disease is often rapidly fatal in camels, buffaloes, horses, cattle, llama and dogs, but mild and subclinical infections can also occur in these species. Wild animals such as deer and capybara can become infected. Animals subjected to stress – malnutrition, pregnancy, work – are more susceptible to disease.

Biologically, *T. evansi* is very similar to *T. equiperdum,* the causative agent of dourine, and morphologically resembles the slender forms of the tsetse-transmitted trypanosomes *T. brucei, T. gambiense* and *T. rhodesiense.* Molecular characterisation indicates that various strains of *T. evansi* isolated from Asia, Africa and South America have a single origin; moreover, it is also likely that *T. evansi* and *T. equiperdum* belong to the same species. Like all pathogenic trypanosomes, *T. evansi* is covered by a dense protein layer consisting of a single protein called the variable surface glycoprotein. This acts as a major immunogen and elicits the formation of specific antibodies. The parasites are able to evade the consequences of these immune reactions by switching the variant surface glycoprotein, the phenomenon known as antigenic variation.

1. Identification of the agent

The classical direct method for the diagnosis of trypanosomosis led to the original discovery of the parasite. It is still employed for examining blood or lymph node material, but rarely with extracts of other tissues. In regions where *T. brucei* and *T. equiperdum* occur in addition to *T. evansi,* a specific identification on blood smears by microscopy is not possible. In the future, specific DNA probes may become available (18, 31) that allow the identification of trypanosome species by nonradioactive DNA hybridisation.

• Direct methods

a) Usual field methods

i) *Blood sampling*

As with all the other members of the subgenus *Trypanozoon, T. evansi* is a parasite of the blood and tissues; it particularly inhabits the deep blood vessels in cases of low parasitaemia. For this reason, it is recommended that blood for diagnosis be obtained from both the peripheral and deep blood vessels. However it should be realised that less than 50% of infected animals may be identified by examination of peripheral blood.

Peripheral blood is obtained by puncturing a small vein in the ear or tail. Deeper samples are taken from a larger vein by syringe. An area of the ear margin or tip of the tail is first cleansed with alcohol and, when dry, a vein is punctured with a suitable instrument. It is important to sterilise instruments or to use disposable instruments between individual animals, so that infection cannot be transmitted by residual blood.

ii) *Wet blood films*

A small drop of blood is placed on to a clean glass slide and covered with a cover-slip to spread the blood as a monolayer of cells. This is examined by light microscopy (×200) to detect any motile trypanosomes.

iii) *Stained thick smears*

A large drop of blood is placed on the centre of a microscope slide and spread with a toothpick or the corner of another slide so that an area of approximately 1.0–1.25 cm in diameter is covered. This is air-dried for 1 hour or longer, while protecting it from insects. The unfixed smear is stained with Giemsa (one drop of commercial Giemsa + 1 ml of phosphate buffered saline [PBS, 2.4 g $Na_2HPO_4.2H_2O$, 0.54 g $NaH_2PO4.2H_2O$, 0.34 g NaCl], pH 7.2), for 25 minutes. After washing, the slides are examined under a light microscope at high magnification (×500–1000). The advantage of the thick smear technique is that it concentrates the drop of blood into a small area, and thus less time is required to detect the parasites. The disadvantage is that the trypanosomes may be damaged in the process, and the method is therefore not suited for species identification in case of mixed infections.

iv) *Stained thin smears*

A drop of blood is placed 20 mm from one end of a clean microscope slide and a thin film is drawn out in the usual way. The film is air-dried briefly, fixed in methyl alcohol for 2 minutes and allowed to dry. The smears are then stained by Giemsa (one drop Giemsa + 1 ml PBS, pH 7.2) for 25 minutes. This preparation is poured off, the slide is washed in tap water and dried. Unfixed smears can be stained by covering them with May–Grünwald stain for 2 minutes, and then adding an equal volume of PBS, pH 7.2, and leaving the slides for a further 3 minutes. This preparation is poured off and diluted Giemsa is added for 25 minutes. This is again poured off, the slides are washed with tap water, and dried. Slides are examined at high magnification (×400–1000). This technique permits detailed morphological studies and identification of the trypanosome species. Rapid staining techniques also exist (Field's stain, Diff Quick®).

v) *Lymph node biopsies*

Samples are usually obtained from the prescapular or precrural (subiliac) lymph nodes. A suitable node is selected by palpation and the site is cleansed with alcohol. The node is punctured with a suitable gauge needle and lymph node material is aspirated into the syringe. This material is then expelled on to a slide, covered with a cover-slip and examined as for the fresh blood preparations. Fixed smears can also be stored for later examination.

b) Concentration methods

In most hosts *T. evansi* can induce mild clinical or subclinical carrier state infections with low parasitaemia in which it is difficult to demonstrate the parasites. Concentration methods become necessary.

i) *Haemotocrit centrifugation*

Blood is collected (70 µl) into heparinised capillary tubes (75 × 1.5 mm), which are then sealed at the dry end and centrifuged, sealed end down, at 3000 ***g*** for 10 minutes. Two pieces of glass (25 × 10 × 1.2 mm) are glued to a slide and the capillary tube is placed between them. A cover-slip is placed on top at the level of the buffy coat junction where the trypanosomes will be concentrated. The space around this part of the tube is flooded with water or immersion oil, and the buffy coat area is examined under the microscope (×100–200).

ii) *Dark-ground/phase-contrast buffy coat technique*

Blood is collected into heparinised capillary tubes and centrifuged as above. The tube is scratched and broken 1 mm below the buffy coat layer – the upper part thus contains the top layer of red blood cells (RBCs), the buffy coat (white blood cells) and some plasma. The contents of this piece are partially expelled on to a slide, covered with a cover-slip and examined under dark-ground, phase-contrast or ordinary illumination.

As an alternative to the electrically powered haematocrit centrifuge, hand-powered micro-centrifuges have been successfully used for detection of trypanosomosis in cattle and camels (9, 11).

iii) *Haemolysis techniques*

Sodium dodecyl sulphate (SDS) can be used as a reagent to haemolyse RBCs to facilitate detection of motile trypanosomes in parasitised blood samples. As SDS is toxic, contact with skin, inhalation and ingestion should be avoided (do not pipette out by mouth). SDS solution can be stored for several months at ambient temperature. Both the SDS solution and the blood samples should be used at a temperature above 15°C. At lower temperatures the trypanosomes may be destroyed.

This method, introduced by Van Meirvenne (29), might be applicable to a wide range of mammalian host species infected with either salivarian (trypanosome species that complete their cyclical development within the salivary glands or mouthparts of the insect hosts and where the infective metacyclic trypanosomes are introduced into the blood when the insects introduce saliva while feeding; this group also includes *T. evansi*) or stercorarian (trypanosomes that complete their life cycle within the posterior part of the insect gut and where metacyclic trypanosomes are introduced into the skin by contamination when the insect excretes during the feeding process). The haemolysis techniques are under evaluation with promising results for the diagnosis of human and animal trypanosomoses (3).

Two general procedures, namely wet blood film clarification and haemolysis centrifugation, can be applied[2].

- *Wet blood film clarification method*

  This method uses the partial lysis of RBCs to facilitate the detection of motile trypanosomes. The method requires an SDS solution (1% SDS dissolved in Tris/glucose/saline, pH 7.5), inoculating loops (10 µl), slides and cover-slips (24 × 24 mm), and a drop of fresh neat or heparinised blood. Dissolve 100 mg of SDS in 100 ml of isotonic Tris/NaCl/glucose buffer, pH 7.5 (Trizma base 14.0 g, NaCl 3.8 g, glucose 10.8 g; dissolve chemicals in 750 ml distilled H_2O, add 90–100 ml 1 N HCl and adjust pH to 7.5, then make up to final volume of 1000 ml with distilled H_2O). This buffer can be stored in small vials at ambient temperature for several months.

  The test does not give a significantly higher sensitivity than wet film technique. In addition, the SDS can cause problems in focusing the microscope and the movements of trypanosomes may be severely curtailed owing to the high viscosity of the SDS.

  Put approximately 10 µl of blood on a slide. Add 10 µl of SDS solution using a dip inoculation loop and mix gently. Apply a cover-slip. Read the entire preparation without delay at low magnification (×100 or ×200).

- *Haemolysis centrifugation technique*

  Nearly complete lysis of RBCs is required for this procedure. The materials needed include: SDS solution (0.1% SDS dissolved in Tris/glucose/saline, pH 7.5), conical centrifuge tubes, ordinary test tubes, large and fine plastic tapering pipettes with attached bulb, slides, cover-slips (24 × 24 mm or 24 × 32 mm), and heparinised blood.

  Using a pipette or syringe, transfer nine volumes (maximum 6.3 ml) of SDS solution into an ordinary test tube. Aspirate one volume (maximum 0.7 ml) of heparinised blood into a bulb pipette and expel it just above the surface of the SDS solution; mix quickly and thoroughly. Avoid foam formation, which may result in destruction of the trypanosomes. Wait for 10 minutes so as to achieve complete haemolysis.

  Pour the haemolysed suspension into a conical centrifuge tube and spin at approximately 500 ***g*** for 10 minutes. With a clean bulb pipette, remove as much supernatant as possible without disturbing the sediment. Again with a fine tapering bulb pipette, remove more supernatant, leaving 10–20 µl of undisturbed sediment at the bottom. Then very carefully collect the entire sediment and put on to a microscope slide. Apply a cover-slip and examine the entire preparation without delay at low magnification (×100 or ×200).

iv) *Mini-anion exchange centrifugation technique*

When a blood sample from humans or animals infected with salivarian trypanosomes is passed through an appropriate anion-exchange column, the host blood cells, being more negatively charged than trypanosomes, are adsorbed into the anion-exchanger, while the trypanosomes are eluted, retaining viability and infectivity. A simplified field method for detection of low parasitaemia has been developed (12, 15, 27).

2 All necessary materials and instructions can be obtained from the Institute of Tropical Medicine, Laboratory of Serology, Nationalestraat 155, B-2000 Antwerp, Belgium.

- *Preparation of phosphate buffered saline glucose, pH 8*

  Na_2HPO_4 (anhydrous) (13.48 g); $NaH_2PO_4.2H_2O$ (0.78 g); NaCl (4.25 g); distilled water (1 litre).

  Solutions of different ionic strength are made by diluting the stock PBS, pH 8, and adding glucose to maintain a suitable concentration. For blood of mice, domestic and wild ruminants and dog, add four parts of PBS to six parts of distilled water and adjust the final glucose concentration to 1%. For blood of pigs and rabbits, add three parts of PBS to seven parts distilled water and adjust final glucose concentration to 1.5%. The PBS–glucose solution (PSG) must be sterile.

- *Equilibration of DEAE-cellulose*

  Suspend 500 g of DEAE-cellulose (diethylamino-ethylcellulose) in 2 litres of distilled water. Adjust the pH to 8 with phosphoric acid. Allow to settle for 30 minutes. Discard the supernatant fluid containing the fine granules. Repeat the procedure three times. Store the equilibrated concentrated suspension of DEAE-cellulose (slurry) at 4°C or in small aliquots at –20°C.

- *Packing of equilibrated DEAE-cellulose*

  A syringe of 2 ml without the plunger is placed on a test-tube rack complete with needle (20 G × 1.5 inch). A disc of Whatman no. 41 filter paper is placed at the bottom of the syringe and moistened by adding a few drops of PSG. Pour 2–2.5 ml of the slurry of equilibrated cellulose into the syringe and allow to pack by elution of the buffer. The height of the sediment should be approximately 3 cm. Wash and equilibrate the column with 2 ml of PSG without disturbing the surface.

- *Adsorption of blood eluate of the trypanosomes*

  Gently place 100–300 µl of heparinised blood above the surface of the cellulose column and let it enter. Add ten drops of PSG and discard the first ten drops of the eluate. Progressively add 1.5 ml of PSG and start collecting the eluate into a finely tapered Pasteur pipette with a sealed end. Put the filled pipette, protected by a conical plastic pipette tip, in a tube and centrifuge at 525 ***g*** (or up to 1000 ***g***) for 10 minutes. Examine the bottom of the pipette under the microscope (×100 or ×200) using a special mounting device.

  The column should constantly remain wet throughout the procedure.

c) Animal inoculation

Laboratory animals may be used to reveal subclinical (nonpatent) infections in domesticated animals. *Trypanosoma evansi* has a broad spectrum of infectivity for small rodents, and so rats and mice are often used. In studies of *T. evansi* infections in camels, comparisons have been made between thick blood film examinations and rat or mouse inoculation methods; the latter animal inoculation gave 15.2% and 17%, respectively, more positive results than thick smears alone (8, 25). However, even mouse inoculation is not 100% sensitive (19).

Blood treated with the anticoagulant sodium heparin is inoculated intraperitoneally into rats (1–2 ml) or mice (0.25–0.5 ml). Inoculation of a minimum of two animals is recommended; these are bled from the tail three times a week to detect parasitaemia. The incubation period before appearance of the parasites and their virulence depends on the strain of trypanosomes, their concentration in the inoculum, and the strain of laboratory animal used. Sensitivity of this *in-vivo* culture system may perhaps be increased by use of immunosuppressed laboratory animals. Drugs such as cyclophosphamide or hydrocortisone acetate, or X-ray irradiation or splenectomy are used for this purpose.

d) Recombinant DNA probes

Specific DNA probes to detect trypanosomes in infected blood or tissue, are being evaluated (18, 31).

• Indirect methods

These methods involve haematological or biochemical tests that demonstrate the effects of the parasite on its host rather than directly detecting the parasite itself.

a) Haematology

Anaemia is usually a reliable indicator of trypanosome infection, although it is not in itself pathognomonic. However, animals with a mild subclinical infection can have parasitaemia without evidence of anaemia.

Anaemia can be estimated by measuring the packed cell volume and may be used in surveys of herds at risk. The technique is identical to that of haematocrit centrifugation. The capillary tube is examined and the results are expressed as a percentage of packed RBCs to total blood volume.

b) Biochemical tests

Biochemical tests include flocculation, formol-gel, mercuric chloride precipitation and thymol turbidity tests. Several older methods considered to be outdated still have some use in the field because they are simple to perform. The tests all depend on an increase in serum globulins as the result of infection, but this increase is not specific for *T. evansi* infection. The formol-gel and mercuric chloride tests are the tests of choice. These tests are mainly of use in camels and have rarely been used for other species. There are no data on the levels of globulins that are likely to produce a positive reaction.

For the formol-gel test, approximately 3–5 ml of blood is collected into a dry tube and allowed to clot. Approximately 1 ml of cell-free serum is transferred to a smaller tube and two drops of concentrated formalin solution (40% formaldehyde [w/v]) are added. The test is positive if the serum coagulates immediately and turns white. In negative reactions, the serum remains unchanged or coagulation may take up to 30 minutes to appear.

For the mercuric chloride test, approximately 1–2 ml of venous blood is collected into a dry tube and allowed to clot. To detect early cases of *T. evansi* infection, it is necessary to use the strongest concentration of mercuric chloride that would not precipitate normal serum, i.e. between 1/20,000 and 1/30,000. A solution of diluted mercuric chloride (1 ml) in distilled water is transferred to a small tube, and one drop of serum, free from RBCs, is added with gentle shaking.

A positive reaction consists of the appearance of opacity, whereas the test is negative if there is no change within 15 minutes. Some authorities claim that this test is only effective in the case of camels (7).

c) Antigen detection

Some enzyme-linked immunosorbent assay (ELISA) pilot methods for the detection of circulating trypanosomal invariable antigens have been introduced and evaluated on a relatively large scale (10). In principle, test systems designed for *T. brucei* spp. can be expected to work equally well for all representatives of the subgenus *Trypanozoon*, including *T. evansi* (5, 6, 20, 23, 32). Recently a commercial latex agglutination antigen test for diagnosis of surra has been developed (21), but requires further evaluation.

d) Detection of trypanosomal DNA

During the past few years, several research centres have been working on the development of polymerase chain reaction procedures for the detection of minute amounts of trypanosomal DNA sequences. A recent publication concerning possible applications for *T. evansi* is that of Wuyts *et al.* (33). Species-specific DNA probes for the identification of *Trypanozoon* organisms, however, are not available yet.

2. Serological tests

Methods to detect specific humoral antibodies to trypanosome antigens include complement fixation (CF), indirect haemagglutination and precipitation tests. These have not been applied in large-scale surveys. More recently, indirect fluorescent antibody (14, 16, 30), ELISA (2, 6, 14, 22, 26–28, 35) and card agglutination tests (CATT) (1, 34) have been employed. Extensive evaluation of ELISA and CATT has been carried out in buffaloes in Indonesia (4).

a) Indirect fluorescent antibody test

The antigen consists of dried blood smears containing from five to ten *T. evansi* trypanosomes per field at ×500 magnification, collected from a mouse or rat within 4 days post-infection. Smears are dried at room temperature for 1 hour and fixed in acetone for 15 minutes. When kept dry, the fixed smears may be stored at –20°C for several months.

On testing, the slides are first subdivided into several areas with nail varnish, then washed in PBS, pH 7.2, at room temperature for 10 minutes. Stock PBS contains $Na_2HPO_4.2H_2O$ (9.27 g); KH_2PO_4 (2.15 g); NaCl (36.00 g); NaN_3 (1.0 g); and distilled water (to 1 litre). This is stored at room temperature and replenished each month. It is diluted five-fold in distilled water before use.

After washing, a positive and a negative control serum and field sera to be tested (diluted from 1/50 to 1/100 or more in PBS), are added and allowed to react for 30 minutes. The slides are washed three successive times in PBS for 5 minutes each. A fluorescein-conjugated antiserum specific to the animal species tested is then added at a suitable dilution and left for 30 minutes. The slides are rewashed in PBS, mounted with 50% glycerol in PBS, and examined by fluorescence microscopy. The glycerol solution should be stored at 4°C and renewed every 2 weeks.

The fluorescein conjugate should be stored at –20°C in small aliquots to avoid repeated freezing and thawing. The tube should be shielded from light in some way, for example by wrapping in aluminium foil. The conjugate is diluted in PBS, pH 7.2, or in PBS containing Evans blue 1/1000 (w/v) as a counterstain to facilitate discrimination between positive (green) and negative (red) fluorescence.

In general, monospecific anti-IgG (gamma-chain) conjugates give the most specific results.

b) **Enzyme-linked immunosorbent assay**

The principle of this technique is that specific antibodies to trypanosomes can be detected by enzyme-linked anti-immunoglobulins using solid-phase polystyrene plates coated with soluble antigen. The enzyme may be peroxidase, alkaline phosphatase or any other suitable enzyme. The enzyme conjugate binds to the antigen/antibody complex and then reacts with a suitable substrate to yield a characteristic colour change either of the substrate itself or of an added indicator (the chromogen).

The antigen for coating the plates is derived from the blood of a heavily parasitaemic rat. The trypanosomes are separated on a DEAE-cellulose column and washed three times by centrifugation in cold PSG (PBS with 1% glucose, pH 8). The final pellet is suspended in cold PSG to a concentration of 3–5%, and briefly ultrasonicated on ice for 30–120 seconds until disintegration of the organisms is complete. This preparation is centrifuged at 4°C and 40,000 ***g*** for 60 minutes. The supernatant is diluted in water so as to obtain a protein concentration of 1 mg/ml. The reagent thus obtained can be stored in small aliquots at –70°C for several months. It can also be freeze-dried and stored at –20°C. Possible future developments in antigen preparation will include use of predominant 'variable' antigens in place of the crude, sonicated antigens. (See section on card agglutination tests below).

- **Test procedure**

i) Prior to use, the frozen or freeze-dried antigen is diluted or reconstituted with freshly prepared 0.01 M carbonate/bicarbonate buffer, pH 9.6. The reagent is added (100 µl) to each well of a microtitre plate and the plates are incubated overnight at 4°C or for 1 hour at 37°C.

ii) Excess antigen is removed, the plates are washed with 0.01 M PBS containing 0.05% Tween 20 (PBST), and serum dilutions in PBST are added (100 µl). Current screening dilutions are between 1/100 and 1/1000.

iii) The plates are incubated at 37°C for 30 minutes and washed three times with PBST.

iv) The specific conjugated anti-globulin (100 µl) appropriately diluted in PBST (usually between 1/1000 and 1/50,000) is added.

v) The plates are reincubated at 37°C for 30 minutes and washed three times with PBST.

vi) For peroxidase conjugates a number of substrate–chromogen solutions can be used, consisting of hydrogen peroxide with a chromogen such as tetramethylbenzidene (TMB), 2,2'-Azino-bis-(3-ethylbenzothiazoline-6-sulphonic acid) (ABTS) and ortho-diphenylenediamine (OPD). A possible substrate–chromogen solution for peroxidase conjugates is 30% hydrogen peroxide (0.167 ml and 35 mg) in citrate buffer (100 ml), pH 6.0. The citrate buffer is made up as follows: Solution A (38.85 ml): (0.1 M citric acid [21.01 g/litre]); Solution B (65.15 ml): (0.2 M, Na_2HPO_4 [35.59 g/litre]); and distilled water (100 ml). Dissolve 10 mg TMB in 1 ml dimethyl suphoxide and add to 99 ml of the citrate buffer. A number of these combinations are available commercially in ready-to-use formulations that remain stable at 4°C for up to 1 year.

vii) The substrate–chromogen solution is added (100 µl) and the plates are incubated at room temperature for 15–20 minutes.

viii) The reaction is stopped by the addition of 1 M sulphuric acid (50 µl). The absorbance of each well mixture is read at 450 nm for TMB chromogen. Other chromogens may require the use of a different wavelength. All tests should include known high and medium positive control sera, a negative control serum, and a buffer control.

A large variety of other test procedures exists. For closely related animal species, cross-reacting reagents may often be used (e.g. anti-bovine immunoglobulin for buffaloes). As with immunofluorescence, the use of monospecific anti-IgG conjugates is generally recommended. There are a number of methods that can be used to determine a cut-off point to discriminate between positive and negative results. The simplest method is to base the cut-off on visual inspection of the test results from known positive and negative populations. These results are likely to show some overlap. The operator can choose the most appropriate point to modify the false-negative or false-positive results depending on the required application of the assay. An alternative is to base the cut-off on the mean +2SD or +3SD values from a large sample of negative animals. Finally, if no suitable negative/positive samples are available, a cut-off can be based on the analysis of the data from animals in an endemic situation. If a bimodal distribution separates infected from uninfected animals, then an appropriate value can be selected. The ELISA is likely to identify correctly uninfected animals. Equivocal results can be re-tested using CATT. Currently there are no readily available defined antigens. The Institute for Tropical Medicine in Antwerp has a number of antigens that are still undergoing evaluation. CATT test kits are readily available from this institute.

c) Card agglutination tests

It is well known that certain predominant variable antigen types (VATs) are expressed in common in different strains of salivarian trypanosomes from different areas. On this basis, a field test for the diagnosis of Gambian sleeping sickness, the card agglutination test – CATT/*T. brucei gambiense* – was developed at the Laboratory of Serology, Institute of Tropical Medicine, Antwerp (17). The test makes use of fixed and stained trypanosomes of defined VAT. Both variable and invariable surface antigens take part in the agglutination reaction. For the diagnosis of *T. evansi* infections, a similar test system has been developed (1). CATT/*T. evansi* is based on the use of a widespread VAT of *T. evansi* – RoTat 1/2. This antigen is also currently being evaluated for its use in ELISAs. The CATT requires lyophilised antigen, PBS, pH 7.4, plastic-coated cards, heparinised blood or serum, and a rotator. The lyophilised antigen can be stored at 2–8°C for up to 1 year. Reconstituted antigen can be stored at 2–8°C for 2 days, but preferably should be used within 8 hours.

For screening, put 25 µl of diluted test serum (1/4 or 1/8) and one drop (45 µl) of antigen suspension on one of the circles of the test card. After mixing and spreading the reagents, the card is rotated for 5 minutes. A positive reaction is revealed by blue granular deposits visible to the naked eye[3].

B. REQUIREMENTS FOR VACCINES AND DIAGNOSTIC BIOLOGICALS

No vaccines are available for this disease.

REFERENCES

1. BAJYANA SONGA E. & HAMERS R. (1988). A card agglutination test (CATT) for veterinary use based on an early VAT RoTat 1–2 of *Trypanosoma evansi. Ann. Soc. Belg. Med. Trop.*, **68,** 233–240.

2. BOID R., EL AMIN E.A., MAHMOUD M.M. & LUCKINS A.G. (1981). *Trypanosoma evansi* infections and antibodies in goats, sheep and camels in the Sudan. *Trop. Anim. Health Prod.*, **13**, 141–146.

3. BOQUENTIN R., DUVALLET G. & BALTZ T. (1989). Une méthode sensible de détection de *Trypanosoma congolense*: lyse avec détergent/centrifugation. *In:* 20e réunion CSITRC, Mombassa, Kenya, 142–148.

4. DAVISON H.C., THRUSFIELD M.V., MUHARSINI S., HUSEIN A., PARTOUTOMO S., MASAKE R. & LUCKINS A.G. (1999). Evaluation of antigen-and antibody-detection tests for *Trypanosoma evansi* infections of buffaloes in Indonesia. *Epidemiol. Infect.*, **123,** 149–155.

5. DIALL O., NANTULYA V.M., LUCKINS A.G., DIARRA B. & KONYATE B. (1992). Evaluation of mono- and polyclonal antibody based antigen detection of *Trypanosoma evansi* infection in the dromedary camel. *Rev. Elev. Med. Vet. Pays Trop.*, **456**, 149–153.

6. FRANKE C.R., GREINER M. & MEHLITZ D. (1994). Investigations on naturally occurring *Trypanosoma evansi* infections in horses, cattle, dogs and capybaras *(Hydrochaeris hydrochaeris)* in Pantanal de Pocone (Mato Grosso, Brazil). *Acta Trop.*, **58**, 159–169.

3 Experimental CATT/*T. evansi* kits for evaluation purposes are available at the Laboratory of Serology, Institute of Tropical Medicine, Nationalestraat 155, B-2000 Antwerp, Belgium. They are being evaluated in collaboration with the Institute of Molecular Biology of the Free University of Brussels, with financial support from the International Laboratory for Research on Animal Diseases (ILRAD), Nairobi, Kenya.

7. GILL B.S. (1977). Trypanosomes and Trypanosomiasis of Indian Livestock. Indian Council of Agricultural Research, New Dehli, India.

8. GODFREY D.G. & KILLICK-KENDRICK R. (1962). *Trypanosoma evansi* of camels in Nigeria. A high incidence demonstrated by inoculation of blood into rats. *Ann. Trop. Med. Parasitol.*, **56**, 14–19.

9. HOLMSTEDT H. (1965). Simple microcentrifuge for use in the field. *Science*, **149**, 977–978.

10. INTERNATIONAL ATOMIC ENERGY AGENCY (IAEA) (1993). Improving the diagnosis and control of trypanosomiasis and other vector-borne diseases of African livestock using immunoassay methods. International Atomic Energy Agency, TECDOC 707, 171 pp.

11. KELLY S. & SCHILLINGER D. (1983). Improved field diagnostic technique for trypanosomiasis by use of a microcentrifuge. *Vet. Rec.*, **113**, 219.

12. LANHAM S.M. & GODFREY D.G. (1970). Isolation of salivarian trypanosomes from man and other mammals using DEAE-cellulose. *Exp. Parasitol.*, **28**, 521–534.

13. LOHR K.F., PHOLPARK S., SIRIWAN P., LEESIRIKUL N., SRIKITJAKARN & STAAK C. (1986). *Trypanosoma evansi* infection in buffaloes in North-East Thailand. II. Abortions. *Trop. Anim. Health Prod.*, **18**, 103–108.

14. LUCKINS A.G., BOID R., RAE P., MAHMOUD M.H., MALIK K.H. & GRAY A.R. (1979). Serodiagnosis of infection with *Trypanosoma evansi* in camels in the Sudan. *Trop. Anim. Health Prod.*, **11**, 1–12.

15. LUMSDEN W.H.R., KIMBER C.D., EVANS D.A. & DOIG S.J. (1979). *Trypanosoma brucei:* miniature anion – exchange centrifugation technique for detection of low parasitaemia: adaptation for field use. *Trans. R. Soc. Trop. Med. Hyg.*, **73**, 312–317.

16. MAGNUS E. (1988). Contribution à la standardisation du test d'immunofluorescence pour le serodiagnostic de la maladie du sommeil à *Trypanosoma brucei gambiense*. *Rev. Assoc. Belge Tech. Lab.*, **15**, 321–343.

17. MAGNUS E., VERVOORT T. & VAN MEIRVENNE N. (1978). A card agglutination test with stained trypanosomes (CATT) for serological diagnosis of *T. b. gambiense* trypanosomiasis. *Ann. Soc. Belg. Med. Trop.*, **58**., 169–176.

18. MASIGA D.K. & GIBSON W.C. (1990). Specific probes for *Trypanosoma (Trypanozoon) evansi* based on kinetoplast DNA minicircles. *Mol. Biochem. Parasitol.*, **40**, 279–284.

19. MONZON C.M., MANCEBO O.A. & ROUX J.P. (1990). Comparison between 6 parasitological methods for diagnosis of *Trypanosoma evansi* in the subtropical area of Argentina. *Vet. Parasitol.*, **36**, 141–146.

20. MONZON C.M., JARA A. & NANTULYA V.M. (1995). Sensitivity of antigen Elisa test for *detecting Trypanosoma evansi* in horses in the subtropical area of Argentina. *J. Parasitol.*, **81**, 806–808.

21. NANTULYA V. (1994). Suratex®: a simple latex agglutination test for diagnosis of *Trypanosoma evansi* infection (surra). *Trop. Med. Parasitol.*, **45**, 9–12.

22. NANTULYA V.M., BAJYANA SONGA E. & HAMERS R. (1989). Detection of circulating trypanosomal antigens in *Trypanosoma evansi* infected animals using a *T. brucei* group-specific monoclonal antibody. *Trop. Med. Parasitol.*, **40**, 263–266.

23. OLAHO-MUHANI W., MUNYUA W.K., MUTUGI M.W. & NJOGU A.R. (1994). Comparison of antibody and antigen detection enzyme immunoassay for the diagnosis of *Trypanosoma evansi* infections in camels. *Vet. Parasitol.*, **45**, 231–240.

24. ONAH D. N., HOPKINS J. A. & LUCKINS A.G. (1998) Increase in $CD5^+$ B cells and depression of immune responses in sheep infected with *Trypanosoma evansi. Vet. Immunol. Immunopathol.*, **63**, 209–222.

25. PEGRAM R.G. & SCOTT J.M. (1976). The prevalence and diagnosis of *Trypanosoma evansi* in Southern Ethiopia. *Trop. Anim. Health Prod.*, **8**, 20–27.

26. RAE P.F., THRUSFIELD M.V., HIGGINS A., AITKEN C.G.G., JONES T.W. & LUCKINS A.G. (1989). Evaluation of enzyme immunoassays in the diagnosis of camel *(Camelus dromedarius)* trypanosomiasis: a preliminary investigation. *Epidemiol. Infect.*, **102**, 297–307.

27. SACHS R. (1984). Improvements in the miniature anion exchange centrifugation technique for detecting trypanosomes in domestic pigs. *Trans. R. Soc. Trop. Med. Hyg.*, **78**, 561.

28. TUNTASUVAN D., CHOMPOOCHAN T., VONGPAKORN M. & MOHKAEW K. (1996). Detection of *Trypanosoma evansi* antibodies in pigs using an enzyme linked immunosorbent assay. *J. Thai Vet. Med. Assoc.*, **47**, 45–53

29. VAN MEIRVENNE N. (1988). A haemolytic detergent concentration method for detection of trypanosomes in blood. *In:* Minutes of the 9th meeting of the International Working Group on *Trypanosoma evansi.* Annex II, 1–5, OIE, Paris, France.

30. VERMA B.B. & GAUTAM O.P. (1977). Serological diagnosis of experimental bovine surra (*Trypanosoma evansi* infection). A comparison of passive haemagglutination, gel diffusion and indirect fluorescent antibody test. *Indian Vet. J.*, **54**, 809–813.

31. VISESHAKUL N. & PANYIM S. (1990). Specific DNA probe for the sensitive detection of *Trypanosoma evansi. Southeast Asian J. Trop. Med. Public Health,* **21**, 21–27.

32. WAITUMBI J.N. & NANTULYA V.M. (1993). A comparison of the antigen detection ELISA and parasite detection of *Trypanosoma evansi* infections in camels. *Vet. Parasitol.*, **49**, 159–178.

33. WUYTS N., CHODESAJJAWATEE N. & PANYIM S. (1994). A simplified and highly sensitive detection of *Trypanosoma evansi* by DNA amplification. *Southeast Asian J. Trop. Med. Public Health,* **25**, 266–271.

34. ZWEYGARTH E., SABWA E.C. & ROTTCHER D. (1984). Serodiagnosis of trypanosomiasis in dromedary camels using a card agglutination test (TESTRYP [R] CATT). *Ann. Soc. Belg. Med. Trop.*, **64**, 309–313.

35. ZWEYGARTH E., SABWA C. & ROTTCHER D. (1986). An enzyme linked-immunosorbent assay for the detection of antibodies to *Trypanosoma evansi* in camels *(Camelus dromedarius)* using peroxidase conjugated protein A. *Trop. Med. Parasitol.*, **37**, 105–106.

*

* *

CHAPTER X.12.

PORCINE REPRODUCTIVE AND RESPIRATORY SYNDROME

SUMMARY

Porcine reproductive and respiratory syndrome (PRRS) is characterised by reproductive failure of sows and respiratory problems of piglets and growing pigs. The disease is caused by the PRRS virus, a virus currently classified as a member of the newly established order of Nidovirales, family Arteriviridae, genus Arterivirus. *The primary target cell of the virus is the alveolar macrophage of the pig. Two major antigenic types of the virus exist, the European and the American type.*

PRRS occurs in most major pig-producing areas throughout the world. The reproductive failure is characterised by abortions, stillbirths, and the birth of weak piglets that often die soon after birth from respiratory disease and secondary infections. Older pigs may demonstrate mild signs of respiratory disease, sometimes complicated by secondary infections. Animals other than pigs do not seem to be affected by PRRS .

Identification of the agent: *Laboratory confirmation is principally based on isolation of the virus from serum, ascitic fluids, or organ samples, such as lungs, tonsil, lymph nodes and spleen of affected pigs. As porcine alveolar macrophages are the most susceptible culture system for virus of both antigenic types, these cells are recommended for virus isolation. MARC-145 (MA-104 clone) cells are also suitable. The virus is identified and characterised by immunostaining with specific antisera. Additional techniques, such as immunohistochemistry and* in situ *hybridisation on fixed tissues and reverse-transcription polymerase chain reaction, have been developed for laboratory confirmation of PRRS virus infection.*

Serological tests: *A wide range of serological tests is currently available. The immunoperoxidase monolayer assay uses alveolar macrophages and the indirect immunofluorescence assay uses MARC-145 cells that are usually infected using either the European or the American antigenic type of the virus, respectively. Both assays can however be designed with both PRRS virus types. Commercial or in-house enzyme linked immunosorbent assays (ELISA) are now often used. One commercial ELISA is specific for both the European and American types of the virus. An indirect ELISA, a blocking ELISA and a double ELISA that can distinguish between serological reactions to the European and the American types have been described.*

Requirements for vaccines and diagnostic biologicals: *Vaccines can be of value as an aid in the prevention of reproductive and respiratory forms of PRRS. Modified live vaccines are not suitable for use in pregnant sows and gilts and in boars. Vaccination may result in shedding of vaccine in semen. Modified live virus vaccines can persist in vaccinated animals, and potential transmission to nonvaccinated animals and subsequent vaccine-virus-induced disease have been reported.*

A. DIAGNOSTIC TECHNIQUES

Porcine reproductive and respiratory syndrome (PRRS) is characterised by reproductive failure of sows and respiratory distress of piglets and growing pigs (3, 17, 37). The disease was first recognised in 1987 in the United States of America (USA), where it was soon known as mystery swine disease because of the elusive nature of its causal agent, but later was called swine infertility and respiratory syndrome. During the winter of 1990–1991 the disease emerged in Western Europe, where it spread rapidly and acquired many more names, including Seuchenhafter Spätabort der Schweine,. Abortus blauw, blue-eared pig disease, syndrome dysgénésique et respiratoire du porc, and porcine epidemic abortion and respiratory syndrome (10, 13, 47). Throughout this chapter, the name PRRS will be used for the disease; this is the name most generally accepted by the international veterinary community.

The PRRS virus (PRRSV) is currently classified as a member of the newly established order of Nidovirales, family Arteriviridae, genus *Arterivirus* (7). It has a predilection to grow in porcine alveolar macrophages, both *in vivo* and *in vitro*. The virus is an enveloped positive-stranded RNA virus with a diameter of 50–70 nm. The genomic sequence of the virus has been determined (14, 34), the viral RNA is approximately 15 kb long and encodes eight open reading frames (ORF). Three major structural proteins have been identified: a nucleocapsid protein (N; ORF 7) of 14–15 kDa, a membrane protein (M; ORF 6) of 18–19 kDa, and an envelope glycoprotein (E; ORF 5) of 24–25 kDa. Three other less abundant structural glycoproteins are encoded by ORFs 4, 3, and 2 (38). Monoclonal antibodies have been prepared against these major and minor structural proteins (15, 19, 32, 35, 43, 45, 49). The European strains of the virus are antigenically closely related to each other, but distinct from American strains of the virus (4, 46). The American strains in themselves are also antigenically closely related. The presence of PRRS has been reported from various countries in Asia and a few countries in South America. Australia and Sweden are reported to be free from PRRSV infection.

Detailed clinical manifestations and lesions resulting from PRRSV infection of pigs of different age groups have been reviewed recently (3, 17, 37). Briefly, PRRSV-infected neonatal pigs show dyspnoea (thumping), but also a variety of other signs such as conjunctivitis, fever, rough hair coat, anorexia, diarrhoea, shaking, cutaneous erythema, eyelid oedema and mortality may be high. In weaned and grower pigs, fever, pneumonia, failure to thrive and an increase in mortality from concurrent bacterial infection are observed. Subclinical infections are more common in finishing pigs, boars and unbred replacement gilts and sows. Transient fever and inappetence may be common. In PRRSV infected and vaccinated boars, PRRSV can be shed in semen, and changes in sperm morphology and function have been described. Mortality associated with PRRSV infection of adult swine has been reported. More recently a virulent form of PRRS has been described: sow abortion and mortality syndrome (SAMS).The reproductive disease is fairly well understood. A causal relationship between PRRSV infection and reproductive failure in breeding herds has been shown repeatedly by various research groups, and the disease can be reproduced experimentally. Infections in the last third of the gestation period seem to cause the most problems, manifested by abortions late in gestation with mummified fetuses and by the birth of dead or weak piglets that die soon after birth (13, 47). It is not clear whether infections earlier in gestation may cause reproductive failure or repeat breeding problems. Limited evidence is available for the existence of various isolates with different reproductive virulence; some countries report the existence of strains that cause transplacental infection without detrimental effect to the fetuses.

The importance of the respiratory infection is less well understood. It has been difficult to constantly reproduce significant respiratory disease with the virus alone and the increase in susceptibility to bacterial infection attributed to PRRSV infection has also been difficult to reproduce experimentally in pigs. Some studies have reported differences in severity of clinical signs and in gross and microscopic lesions following experimental inoculation of pigs with different PRRSV isolates (22, 23). Such a predisposition by PRRSV to exacerbate other diseases is currently a topic of research by various groups, and although it seems that the virus may indeed cause some secondary infections to be more severe, the mechanisms are not yet fully understood.

Gross and microscopic lesions characteristic of PRRSV infection are mostly observed in neonatal and nursery pigs. In older pigs, lesions may be similar but less marked. Gross lesions associated with PRRSV vary. Lung lesions vary from none to diffuse consolidation, and are commonly complicated by concurrent bacterial infections. Affected lymph nodes, most commonly in young pigs, can be markedly enlarged. Light microscopic lesions most commonly involve lung and lymphoid tissue. Lung lesions are characterised by multifocal interstitial pneumonia showing alveolar septal infiltration by mononuclear cells, type 2 pneumocyte hypertrophy and hyperplasia, and marked accumulation of inflammatory and necrotic alveolar exudate. Lymph nodes demonstrate follicular hyperplasia, foci of follicular necrosis and debris within follicles. Vascular, heart and brain lesions have also been described. Inconsistently observed fetal lesions are characterised by vasculitis, myocarditis and encephalitis.

In general, antibodies seem to have limited protective value. Infected pigs can remain viraemic for 4–6 weeks after detectable antibody has been formed, and can transmit the virus to other pigs. It is not known whether maternal antibodies can protect against early infection, but viraemia in pigs born from seropositive females can be detected from week 4 onwards. However, some level of protection is seen in piglets with maternal antibody, and a rise in neutralising antibody titres often corresponds to a decline in virus titres in the blood. Furthermore, females that are infected for a second time do not show recurring reproductive failure. In short, the relationship between antibody titres and protection is not very well understood. Cell-mediated immunity has not been widely studied, but is thought to play a protective role. An intriguing aspect of PPRSV infection is the prolonged duration of viraemia and subsequent transmission of the virus to contact animals in comparison with other viral infections. However, it is generally agreed that lifelong persistence of the infection does not seem to occur.

1. Identification of the agent

Virological diagnosis of PRRS is difficult. This is mainly because the cell of choice for virus isolation is the porcine alveolar macrophage, which needs to be harvested from pigs (preferably specific pathogen free [SPF]) under 6–8 weeks of age (47, 50). Not all laboratories have a ready supply of such pigs available, and continuous cell lines cannot fully replace the alveolar macrophages because these cell lines are generally less susceptible to the virus. In addition, different batches of macrophages are not always equally susceptible to the virus; the reason for this is not yet known, but it necessitates the testing of each batch before use.

Certain monkey kidney cell lines (e.g. MA-104) can be a good replacement for macrophages (2, 26), but such cell lines do not support the growth of all isolates, particularly European strains. This chapter therefore only describes virus isolation with alveolar macrophages. Immunohistochemistry and immunofluorescence to detect PRRSV antigen in tissues have been reported. These tests are more rapid than virus isolation and do not necessitate cell culture infrastructure. In addition, immunohistochemistry (21, 28) performed on formalin-fixed tissues enables the visualisation of antigen together with histological lesions and permits retrospective analysis on archival specimens. *In situ* hybridisation capable of detecting and differentiating North American and European PRRSV genotypes in formalin-fixed tissues has also been reported (29, 41). Reverse-transcription polymerase chain reaction (RT-PCR) and nested PCR are highly sensitive tests for detecting viral RNA (12, 27, 30, 33, 44) and are now more commonly used on different tissues including serum. These tests are also useful when virus isolation is problematic, such as when testing semen (12) and when testing tissues partially degraded by autolysis or by heat during transport of specimens for virus isolation. A multiplex PCR assay has been designed to differentiate North American and European PRRSV isolates (20). More recently restriction fragment length polymorphism analysis of PCR-amplified products has been developed for the molecular epidemiology of field and vaccine PRRSV isolates (48).

a) Harvesting of alveolar macrophages from lungs

Lungs should preferably be obtained from SPF pigs or from a herd of pigs that is proven to be free from PRRSV infection. Best results are obtained with pigs that are under 8 weeks of age. The macrophages should be harvested from the lung on the same day that the pig is slaughtered. The lungs should be washed three or four times with a total volume of approximately 200 ml sterile phosphate buffered saline (PBS). The harvested wash fluid is then centrifuged for 10 minutes at 1000 ***g***. The resulting pellet of macrophages is resuspended in PBS and centrifuged (washed) twice more. The final pellet is resuspended in 50 ml PBS, and the number of macrophages is counted to determine the cell concentration. The macrophages can then be used fresh, or can be stored in liquid nitrogen according to standard procedures at a final concentration of 4×10^7 macrophages/1.5 ml. Macrophage batches should not be mixed.

b) Batch testing of alveolar macrophages

Before a batch of macrophages can be used it should be validated. This should be done by titrating a standard PRRSV with known titre in the new macrophages, and by performing an immunoperoxidase monolayer assay (IPMA) with known positive and negative sera on plates seeded with the new macrophages. The cells are suitable for use only if the standard PRRSV grows to its specified titre. It is recommended that alveolar macrophages and fetal bovine serum (FBS) to supplement culture medium be pestivirus free.

c) Virus isolation on alveolar macrophages

Alveolar macrophages are seeded in the wells of flat-bottomed tissue-culture grade microtitre plates. After attachment, the macrophages are infected with the sample. Samples can be sera or ascitic fluids, or 10% suspensions of tissues, such as tonsils, lung, lymph nodes, and spleen. In general, the PRRSV gives a cytopathic effect (CPE) in macrophages after 1–2 days of culture, but sometimes viruses are found that give little CPE or give a CPE only after repeat passage. Once a CPE has been observed, the PRRSV needs to be identified by immunostaining with a specific antiserum.

i) *Seeding macrophages in the microtitre plates*

Defrost one vial containing 6×10^7 macrophages/1.5 ml. Wash the cells once with 50 ml PBS and centrifuge the cell suspension for 10 minutes at 300 ***g*** (room temperature). Collect the cells in 40 ml RPMI 1640 medium supplemented with 5% FBS and 10% antibiotic mixture (growth medium). Dispense 100 µl of the cell suspension into each well of a microtitre plate (with one vial of cells, four plates can be seeded at a concentration of 10^5 cells in each well of the plates).

ii) *Preparation of sample (serum, ascitic fluid, 10% tissue suspension) dilutions in a dummy plate*

Dispense 90 µl of growth medium into each well of a microtitre plate. Add 10 µl samples to the wells of rows A and E (duplicate 1/10 dilution). Shake the plates and transfer 10 µl from rows A and E to rows B and F (1/100 dilution). Shake the plates and transfer 10 µl from rows B and F to rows C and G (1/1000 dilution). Shake the plates and transfer 10 µl from rows C and G to rows D and H (1/10,000 dilution). Shake the plates.

iii) *Incubation of samples*

Transfer 50 µl of the sample dilutions from the dummy plates to the corresponding wells of the plate with macrophages (first passage). Incubate for 2–5 days and observe daily for a CPE. At day 2, seed macrophages in new microtitre plates (see above). Transfer 25 µl of the supernatants from the plates of the first passage to the corresponding wells of the freshly seeded plates (second passage). Incubate for 2–5 days and observe daily for a CPE.

iv) *Reading and interpreting the results*

Wells in which macrophages show CPE in the first passage only are considered to be false positive because of the toxicity of the sample. Wells in which macrophages show CPE in both passages or in the second passage only are considered to be suspect positive. All wells with macrophage monolayers that do not show CPE need to be identified as PRRSV negative by immunostaining with a PRRSV-positive antiserum. CPE-positive samples need to be identified as PRRSV positive by culturing CPE-positive supernatant samples, or the original sample dilutions, for both 24 and 48 hours in macrophages, followed by immunostaining with a PRRSV-positive antiserum.

v) *Immunostaining with a PRRSV-positive antiserum*

Infect macrophages with 50 µl of supernatant or tissue sample as described in Section A.2.a., and grow the infected cells for 24 and 48 hours. Prepare an appropriate dilution of a PRRSV-positive serum in dilution buffer, and immunostain the macrophages as described in Section A.2.a. or A.2.b.

2. Serological tests

Serological diagnosis is, in general, easy to perform, with good specificity and sensitivity, especially on a herd basis. Sera of individual pigs sometimes cause difficulties because of nonspecific reactions, but this problem may be solved by resampling the pig after 2–3 weeks. Serology is generally performed with a binding assay, such as the IPMA, immunofluorescence assay, or the enzyme-linked immunosorbent assay (ELISA) – of which many varieties are described (1, 8, 9, 16, 24, 36, 39, 40, 47, 51). These tests are often performed with viral antigen of one antigenic type, which means that antibodies directed against the other, heterologous, antigenic type may be detected with less sensitivity. A blocking ELISA has been used extensively in Denmark (39) and has been described as a double ELISA set-up using both European and American virus as antigen and thus it can distinguish between serological reaction to the European and the American types (40). The first live attenuated vaccine for PRRS based on the American type virus has been observed to spread to nonvaccinated animals (6, 42), and subsequent development in herds of vaccine-virus-induced PRRS reproductive failures has been reported in Denmark (6, 31). Reaction to American-type vaccine-like PRRSV can be anticipated in countries using or having used this vaccine; European countries may therefore observe reactions and isolation of both antigenic types (6, 31). Until recently there has been no evidence, based on virus isolation and sequencing data, to demonstrate the existence of Lelystad-like (European type) strains circulating in North America. However, one such virus has now been isolated and characterised at the University of Minnesota, USA.

Antibodies to the virus can be detected by antibody-binding assays as early as 7–14 days after infection, and antibody levels reach maximal titres by 30–50 days. Some pigs may become seronegative within 3–6 months, but others remain seropositive for much longer. Neutralising antibodies develop slowly and do not reach high titres. They can be detected from 3 to 4 weeks after infection and they can persist for 1 year or more. The use of complement to make the serum virus neutralisation test more sensitive has been reported (25). Extensive research into the duration of antibody titres after infection has not yet been done, and the results probably depend on the test used. Maternal antibodies have a half-life of 12–14 days, and maternal antibody titre can, in general, be detected until 4–8 weeks after birth, depending on the antibody titre of the sow at birth and the test used. In an infected environment, pigs born from seropositive females seroconvert actively from the age of 3–6 weeks. This chapter describes the IPMA in detail as this test can easily be performed in laboratories where virus isolation procedures using macrophages have been established, and can be used with virus of both antigenic types. This assay can also be adapted to the MARC-145 cell line for both the European and American types (39, 40). An indirect immunofluorescence assay (IFA) using MARC-145 cells can also be performed for PRRSV serology and is included in the present chapter. Commercial ELISAs with good sensitivity and specificity are available and have been reviewed recently (18).

a) **Detection of antibodies with the immunoperoxidase monolayer assay**

Alveolar macrophages are seeded in the wells of microtitre plates. After attachment, the macrophages are infected with PRRSV. The object is to infect approximately 30–50% of the macrophages in a well so as to be able to distinguish nonspecific sera. After an incubation period, the macrophages are fixed and used as a cell substrate for serology. On each plate, 11 sera can be tested in duplicate. Test sera are diluted and incubated on the cell substrate. If antibodies are present in the test serum, they will bind to the antigen in the cytoplasm of the macrophages. In the next incubation step, the bound antibodies will be detected by an anti-species horseradish-peroxidase (HRPO) conjugate. Finally, the cell substrate is incubated with a chromogen/substrate[1] solution. Reading of the test is done with an inverted microscope.

- **Seeding macrophages in the microtitre plates**

i) Defrost one vial containing 6 × 10^7macrophages/1.5 ml.

ii) Wash the cells once with 50 ml of PBS and centrifuge the cell suspension for 10 minutes at 300 *g* (room temperature).

iii) Collect the cells in 40 ml RPMI 1640 medium supplemented with 5% FBS, 100 IU (International Units) penicillin and 100 µg streptomycin (growth medium).

iv) Dispense 100 µl of the cell suspension into each well of a microtitre plate (with one vial of cells, four plates can be seeded at a concentration of 10^5 cells in each well of the plates).

v) Incubate the plates for 18–24 hours at 37°C in a 5% CO_2 cabinet, under humid conditions. Alternatively, use HEPES buffer (N-2-hydroxyethylpiperazine, N-2-ethanesulphonic acid) in the medium.

- **Infection of cells with porcine reproductive and respiratory syndrome virus**

i) Add to each well 50 µl of a virus suspension containing 10^5 $TCID_{50}$ (50% tissue culture infective dose)/ml, but leave two wells uninfected to act as controls.

ii) Incubate the plates for 18–24 hours at 37°C in a 5% CO_2 cabinet.

- **Fixation of the cells**

i) Discard the growth medium and rinse the plates once in saline.

ii) Knock the plates dry gently on a towel and dry them (without lid) for 45 minutes at 37°C.

iii) Freeze the plates (without a lid) for 45 minutes at –20°C. (Plates that are not used immediately for testing must be sealed and stored at –20°C.)

iv) Incubate the cells for 10 minutes at room temperature with cold 4% paraformaldehyde (in PBS). Alternatively the cells could be fixed in ice-cold absolute ethanol for 45 minutes at 5°C (5).

v) Discard the paraformaldehyde and rinse the plates once in saline.

- **Preparation of serum dilutions in a dummy plate**

i) Dispense 180 µl of 0.5 M NaCl with 4% horse serum and 0.5% Tween 80, pH 7.2 (dilution buffer), to the wells of rows A and E of the dummy plate(s).

ii) Dispense 120 µl of dilution buffer to all other wells.

iii) Add 20 µl of the test serum or control sera to the wells of rows A and E (= 1/10 dilution), and shake.

iv) Dilute the sera four-fold by transferring 40 µl from rows A and E to rows B and F, and so on to provide further dilutions of 1/40, 1/160 and 1/640.

---

1 *Preparation of chromogen solution*
Stock solution of chromogen (3-amino-9-ethyl-carbazole [AEC]): (a) 4 mg AEC; (b) 1 ml N,N-dimethyl-formamide.
Dissolve (a) in (b) and store the AEC stock solution at 4°C in the dark.
Preparation of chromogen/substrate solution (prepare shortly before use)
Prepare 0.05 M sodium acetate buffer, pH 5.0, as follows: Dissolve 4.1 g sodium acetate in 1 litre distilled water. Adjust the pH to 5.00 with 100% acetic acid.
Add 1 ml AEC stock solution to 19 ml of 0.05 M sodium acetate buffer.
Add 10 µl 30% H_2O_2 for each 20 ml of chromogen/substrate solution.
Filter the solution through a 5 µm filter.

- **Incubation of sera in the plate with fixed macrophages**

i) Transfer 50 µl from each of the wells of the dummy plate(s) to the corresponding wells of the plate with the fixed macrophages. Seal the plate(s) and incubate 1 hour at 37°C.

ii) Discard the serum dilutions and rinse the plate(s) three times in 0.15 M NaCl + 0.5% Tween 80.

- **Incubation with conjugate**

i) Dilute the rabbit-anti-swine HRPO conjugate to a predetermined dilution in 0.15 M NaCl + 0.5% Tween 80. Add 50 µl of the conjugate dilution to all wells of the plate(s). Seal the plate(s) and incubate for 1 hour at 37°C. Rinse the plates three times.

- **Staining procedure**

i) Dispense 50 µl of the filtered chromogen/substrate (AEC) solution to all wells of the plate(s) (see footnote 1).

ii) Incubate the AEC for at least 30 minutes at room temperature.

iii) Replace the AEC with 50 µl of 0.05 M sodium acetate, pH 5.0 (see footnote 1).

- **Reading and interpreting the results**

If antibodies are present in the test serum, the cytoplasm of approximately 30–50% of the cells in a well are stained deeply red by the chromogen. A negative test serum is recognised by cytoplasm that remains unstained. A serum that reacts nonspecifically might stain all cells in a well (compared with a positive control serum). The titre of a serum is expressed as the reciprocal of the highest dilution that stains 50% or more of the wells. A serum with a titre of <10 is considered to be negative. A serum with a titre of 10 or 40 is considered to be a weak positive. Often nonspecific staining is detected in these dilutions. A serum with a titre of ≥160 is considered to be positive.

b) Detection of antibodies with the indirect immunofluorescence assay

Although there is no single standard accepted immuofluorescence assay in use at this time, several protocols have been developed and used by different laboratories in North America. The IFA can be performed in microtitre plates or eight-chamber slides using the MARC-145 cell line and a MARC-145 cell-line-adapted PRRSV isolate. After an incubation period, PRRSV-infected cells are fixed and used as a cell substrate for serology. Serum samples are tested at a single screening dilution of 1/20 and samples are reported as being negative or positive at this dilution. Each porcine serum to be tested is added to wells or chambers containing PRRSV-infected cells. Antibodies to PRRSV, if present in the serum, will bind to antigens in the cytoplasm of infected cells. Following this step, an anti-porcine-IgG conjugated to fluorescein is added and will bind to the porcine antibodies that have bound to PRRSV antigens in the infected cells. The results are read using a fluorescence microscope. Microtitre plates may also be prepared for serum titration purposes (see b.1. below).

- **Seeding and infection of MARC-145 cells in microtitre plates**

i) Add 50 µl of cell culture medium (e.g. Minimal Essential Medium [MEM] containing 2 mM L-glutamine, 1 mM sodium pyruvate, 100 IU penicillin and 100 µg streptomycin) without FBS to each well of columns 2, 4, 6, 8, 10 and 12 of a 96-well plate using a multichannel pipettor.

ii) Trypsinise confluent MARC-145 cells (grown in culture flasks) to be used for seeding 96-well microtitre plates and resuspend cells in cell culture medium containing 8% FBS at a concentration of 100,000–125,000 cells/ml. The MARC-145 cells are trypsinised from culture flasks for IFA once a week using trypsin/EDTA (ethylene diamine tetra-acetic acid) and are seeded in culture flasks at a concentration of 250,000 cells/ml. After 4 days in culture flasks, new cell culture medium containing 2% FBS is added for 3 additional days.

iii) Using a multichannel pipettor, add 150 µl of the cell suspension to each well of the 96-well plate.

iv) Dilute PRRSV preparation in MEM without FBS to $10^{2.2}$ $TCID_{50}$/50 µl and distribute 50 µl in each well of columns 1, 3, 5, 7, 9 and 11.

v) Incubate the plates for approximately 48–72 hours at 37°C in a humidified 5% CO_2 cabinet to obtain a monolayer with approximately 40–50% of the cells infected as determined by indirect immunofluorescence. Alternatively, microtitres plates may first be seeded with MARC-145 cell suspensions (e.g. concentration of 100,000 cells/ml in medium supplemented with 5–10% FBS) and incubated for up to 72 hours until they are confluent. Then volumes of 50 µl of PRRSV preparations (e.g. 10^5 $TCID_{50}$/ml) are added per well and the plates are incubated for an additional 48–72 hours prior to fixation. The use of organic buffers such as HEPES in medium has been suggested to stabilise the pH when CO_2 incubators are not available.

- **Seeding and infection of MARC-145 cells in eight-chamber glass slides**

i) Add 500 µl a MARC-145 cell suspension (e.g. in MEM supplemented with 10% FBS) at a concentration of 100,000 cells/ml to each chamber of eight-chamber glass slides.

ii) Incubate the cells for approximately 48–72 hours at 37°C in a humidified 5% CO_2 until they are confluent.

iii) Add to each chamber 50 µl of PRRSV suspension containing 10^5 $TCID_{50}$/ml and further incubate cells for approximately 18 hours at 37°C in a humidified 5% CO_2 cabinet. At this time 15–20 infected cells per field of view may be observed by indirect immunofluorescence.

- **Fixation of the cells**

i) Discard the medium, rinse once with PBS and discard PBS. For chamber slides, remove the plastic chamber walls, leaving the gasket intact.

ii) Add volumes of 150 µl cold (4°C) acetone (80% in water) to each well of the 96-well plate. Place the plates at 4°C for 30 minutes. For chamber slides, acetone (80–100%) at room temperature is used to fix the cells for 10–15 minutes at room temperature. Some manufactured brands of acetone will degrade the chamber slide gasket leaving a film on the slide. It is recommended to check the acetone before using for routine fixation.

iii) Discard the acetone and dry the plates and slides at room temperature.

iv) The plates can then be placed in a plastic bag, sealed and stored at –70°C until use. Chamber slides can be kept similarly in slide cases.

- **Preparation of serum dilutions**

i) Dilute serum samples to a 1/20 dilution in PBS (0.01 M; pH 7.2) in separate 96-well plates (e.g. add 190 µl of PBS using a multichannel pipettor followed by 10 µl of the sera to be tested).

ii) Include as controls reference PRRSV antibody positive and negative sera of known titre.

- **Incubation of sera with fixed MARC-145 cells**

i) Stored plates are removed from the –70°C freezer and when the plates reach room temperature rehydrate the cells with 150 µl PBS for a few minutes. Discard the PBS by inverting the plates and blotting dry on paper towels. Cells of eight-chamber slides are not rehydrated.

ii) Add volumes of 50 µl of each diluted serum to one well containing the fixed noninfected cells and to one well containing the fixed infected cells. Add similar volumes for each serum to a single chamber.

iii) Add volumes of 50 µl of the negative control serum and positive control serum dilutions in the same manner.

iv) Incubate the plates with their lids on at 37°C for 30 minutes in a humid atmosphere. Slides should be incubated similarly in boxes or slide trays with a cover.

v) Remove the serum samples and blot the plates dry on paper towels. A total of six washes using 200 µl of PBS are performed. The PBS is added to each well, followed by inversion of the plates to remove the PBS. After removing serum samples, slides are rinsed in PBS followed by a 10-minute wash.

- **Incubation with conjugate**

i) Add volumes of 50 µl of appropriately diluted (in freshly prepared PBS) rabbit or goat anti-swine IgG (heavy and light chains) conjugated with FITC (fluorescein isothiocyanate) to each well using a multichannel pipettor. Similar volumes are added to individual chambers.

ii) Incubate plates or slides with their lids on at 37°C for 30 minutes in a humid atmosphere.

iii) Remove the conjugate from the plates and blot the plates dry on paper towels. A total of four washes using PBS are performed as described above. Discard the conjugate from the slides, rinse in PBS, wash for 10 minutes in PBS and rinse in distilled water. Tap the slides on an absorbent pad to remove excessive water.

iv) The plates and the slides are read using a fluorescence microscope.

- **Reading and interpreting the results**

The presence of a green cytoplasmic fluorescence in infected cells combined with the absence of such a signal in noninfected cells is indicative of the presence of antibodies to PRRSV in the serum at the dilution tested. The degree of intensity of fluorescence may vary according to the amount of PRRSV-specific antibody present in the serum tested.

Absence of specific green fluorescence in both infected and noninfected cells is interpreted as absence of antibody to PRRSV in that serum at the dilution tested. The test should be repeated if the fluorescence is not seen with the use of the positive control sera on infected cells or if fluorescence is seen using the negative control serum on infected cells. No fluorescence should be seen on noninfected cells with any of the control sera. Any test serum giving suspicious results should be retested at a 1/20 dilution and if results are still unclear, a new serum sample of the same animal is requested for further testing.

b.1) Evaluation by IFA of sera for antibody titres

Microtitre plates and IFA may also be used for serum titration purposes. Up to 16 sera may be titred per 96-well microtitre plate.

i) Seed 96-well microtitre plates with MARC-145 cells and incubate at 37°C in a humidified 5% CO_2 cabinet until they are confluent.

ii) Inoculate all wells with the PRRSV preparation except the wells of columns 1, 6 and 11, and incubate the plates at 37°C in a humidified 5% CO_2 cabinet for 48–72 hours.

iii) Discard culture medium and rinse the monolayers once with PBS (0.01 M, pH 7.2). Fix the monolayers with cold acetone (80% aqueous solution) for 10 minutes at ambient temperature. Discard the acetone, air-dry the plates and keep the plates with lids at –20°C for short-term storage or –70°C for long-term storage, until use.

iv) Serially dilute sera including a PRRSV-positive control serum using a four-fold dilution in PBS, beginning at 1/16 or 1/20. Dilute a negative control serum at 1/16 or 1/20 dilution. Dispense 50 µl of each dilution (1/16, 1/64, 1/256, 1/1024 or 1/20, 1/80, 1/320, 1/1280) in wells containing viral antigen of columns 2, 3, 4, 5 or 7, 8, 9, 10. For each serum, also dispense 50 µl of dilution 1/16 or 1/20 in control wells of columns 1 and 6. Similarly dispense dilutions of positive and negative control sera in wells of columns 11 and 12.

v) Incubate the plates at 37°C for 30 minutes in a humid chamber. Discard the sera and rinse the plates three times using PBS.

vi) Add 50 µl of appropriately diluted anti-swine IgG conjugated with FITC and incubate plates at 37°C for 30 minutes in a humid chamber. Discard conjugate, rinse plates several times and tap the plates on absorbent material to remove excessive liquid.

- **Reading and interpreting the results**

Following examination with a fluorescence microscope, the titre of a serum is recorded as the reciprocal of the highest serum dilution in which typical cytoplasmic fluorescence is observed. For paired serum samples, a four-fold increase in titre with a 2-week interval is indicative of active infection in an individual animal. No specific fluorescence should be observed with test sera, positive and negative control sera on noninfected control cells. No fluorescence should be seen on infected cells with negative control serum. Specific fluorescence should be observed on infected cells with positive control serum at appropriate dilutions. The IFA end-point may vary among laboratories. Test results may also vary depending on the PRRSV isolate used in the test because of antigenic diversity.

c) Detection of antibodies with the enzyme-linked immunosorbent assay

ELISA kits are available commercially to determine the serological status of swine towards PRRSV. These kits use as antigens either the European or the American PRRSV types separately or as combined antigens. Their main advantage is the rapid handling of a large number of samples. Several laboratories have developed ELISAs (indirect or blocking) for serological testing (1, 8, 9, 16, 24, 39, 40). In addition, a double-blocking ELISA format that can distinguish between serological reactions to the European and the American antigenic type has been described (40).

B. REQUIREMENTS FOR VACCINES AND DIAGNOSTIC BIOLOGICALS

In the USA, a killed virus vaccine is licensed as an aid to the reduction of abortions and weak piglets caused by the reproductive form of PRRS. Also, modified live virus (MLV) vaccines are approved for the control of the respiratory and reproductive forms of PRRS. All PRRS vaccines currently licensed in the USA contain the American antigenic type. In Europe, two MLVs are licensed and available commercially.

As vaccination of pigs does not prevent PRRSV infection, vaccination may be helpful in herds experiencing problems with PRRS or herds at high risk of PRRSV infection. MLV vaccines are not intended to be used in naïve herds, pregnant sows or gilts or boars of breeding age. Vaccine virus can persist in boars and be disseminated through semen (11). MLV vaccine virus may be shed and transmitted to nonvaccinated contact pigs (42). MLV vaccines are intended to be used in sows and gilts 3–6 weeks prior to breeding and, for one MLV vaccine, in piglets from 3 weeks of age or older as aids for the reduction of PRRS.

1. Seed management

a) Characteristics of the seed

The isolate of PRRSV used for vaccine production must be accompanied by a history describing its origin and tissue culture passage. The isolate must be safe in swine at the intended age of vaccination and provide protection against challenge. Isolates for an MLV must be shown not to revert to a virulence after passage in animals.

b) Method of culture

The PRRSV is propagated in a continuous African green monkey kidney cell line, such as MA-104 or Vero. Viral propagation should not exceed five passages from the master seed virus (MSV).

c) Validation as a vaccine

The MSV should be free from bacteria, fungi and mycoplasma. The MSV must be tested for the detection of extraneous viruses, such as transmissible gastroenteritis virus, porcine adenovirus, porcine haemagglutinating encephalitis virus, porcine parvovirus, bovine viral diarrhoea virus, and rabies virus by the fluorescent antibody technique. The MSV must be free from extraneous virus by CPE and haemadsorption on the Vero cell line and an embryonic swine cell type.

Attenuated PRRSV isolates are known to cause viraemia and will transmit to susceptible animals. The MSV should be shown to be nonvirulent in piglets and pregnant animals by five serial passages of the MSV through susceptible swine using the most natural route of infection.

In an immunogenicity trial, the MSV must protect susceptible swine against a virulent challenge at the highest passage level intended for production. For the respiratory form, 3-week-old piglets are vaccinated with the highest passage level of MSV. The piglets are challenged with a virulent isolate of PRRSV 2–16 weeks later to determine protection. To determine protection from the losses caused by the reproductive form of PRRS, vaccinated animals are challenged at about 85 days' gestation. A significant number of the vaccinates must be protected from the clinical signs of mummification, stillborn, and weak piglets, when compared with the controls.

Field trial studies should be conducted to determine the safety of the vaccine. Nonvaccinated sentinel pigs should be included at each site for monitoring the shed of the attenuated virus.

2. Method of manufacture

The African green monkey kidney cell line is seeded into suitable vessels. MEM supplemented with FBS is used as the medium for production. Incubation is at 37°C.

Cell cultures are inoculated directly with PRRS working virus stock, which is generally from one to four passages from the MSV. Inoculated cultures are incubated for 1–8 days before harvesting the culture medium. During incubation, the cultures are observed daily for CPE and bacterial contamination.

Killed virus vaccines are chemically inactivated and mixed with a suitable adjuvant. MLV vaccines are generally mixed with a stabiliser before bottling and lyophilisation.

3. In-process control

Production lots of PRRSV must be titrated in tissue culture for standardisation of the product. Low titred lots may be concentrated or blended with higher titred lots to achieve the correct titre.

4. Batch control

Final container samples are tested for purity, safety and potency.

a) Purity

Samples are examined for bacterial and fungal contamination. Ten tubes containing 120 ml of soybean casein digest medium are inoculated with 0.2 ml from ten final-container samples. Incubation is at 30–35°C for 14 days.

b) Safety

Safety tests can be conducted in a combination of guinea-pigs, mice or pigs.

c) Potency

Final container samples of an MLV vaccine are titrated (log_{10}) in microtitre plates for determination of the release titre.

- **Test procedure**

i) Prepare tenfold dilutions from 10^{-1} through 10^{-5} by using 0.2 ml of rehydrated test vaccine and 1.8 ml of MEM. An internal positive control PRRSV should be titrated in the appropriate range.

ii) Inoculate 0.1 ml/well from each dilution into five wells of a 96-well plate containing African green monkey kidney monolayers.

iii) Incubate the plate at 37°C in a CO_2 atmosphere for 5–7 days.

iv) Read the plates microscopically for CPE. The internal positive control PRRSV should give a titre within 0.3 log_{10} $TCID_{50}$ from its predetermined mean.

v) Determine the $TCID_{50}$/dose by the Spearman–Kärber method. The release titre is 1.2 logs higher than the titre used in the immunogenicity trial. The 1.2 logs include 0.5 logs for stability throughout the shelf life of the product and 0.7 logs for potency test variability.

Killed virus vaccines may use host animal or laboratory animal vaccination/serology tests or challenge to determine potency of the final product. Parallel-line assays using ELISA antigen-quantifying techniques to compare a standard with the final product are acceptable in determining the relative potency of a product. The standard should be shown to be protective in the host animal.

d) Duration of immunity

Duration of immunity studies are conducted before the vaccine receives final approval. For the respiratory form of PRRS, duration should be shown up to the market age in pigs. Duration of immunity for the reproductive form should be shown through weaning of the piglets.

e) Stability

All vaccines are initially given 24 months before expiry. Real-time stability studies are conducted on MLV products to determine the actual half-life of the vaccine.

f) Preservatives

Antibiotics are added during production, generally gentamicin sulphate or neomycin.

g) Precautions (hazards)

Vaccination is only recommended in pigs in PRRSV-positive herds. MLV vaccines intended as an aid in the reduction of disease associated with the respiratory and reproductive form of PRRS are not recommended to be used in pregnant sows or gilts or boars of breeding age. Vaccination of breeding boars with an MLV is not recommended due to the shedding of the vaccine virus in semen (11). The first MLV vaccine for PRRS based on the American-type virus has been observed to spread to nonvaccinated animals (6, 42) and subsequent development in herds of vaccine-virus-induced PRRS reproductive failures have been reported (6, 31).

5. Tests on the final product

a) Safety

See Section B.4.b.

b) Potency

See Section B.4.c.

REFERENCES

1. ALBINA E., LEFORBAN Y., BARON T., PLANA DURAN J. & VANNIER P. (1992). An enzyme linked immunosorbent assay (ELISA) for the detection of antibodies to the porcine reproductive and respiratory syndrome (PRRS) virus. *Ann. Rech. Vet.*, **23**, 167–176.

2. BAUTISTA E.M., GOYAL S.M., YOON I.J., JOO H.S. & COLLINS J.E. (1993). Comparison of porcine alveolar macrophages and CL2621 for the detection of porcine reproductive and respiratory syndrome (PRRS) virus and anti-PRRS antibody. *J. Vet. Diagn. Invest.*, **5**, 163–165.

3. BENFIELD D.A., COLLINS J.E., DEE S.A., HALLBUR P.G., JOO H.S., LAGER K.M., MENGELING W.L., MURTAUGH M.P., ROSSOW K.D., STEVENSON G.W. & ZIMMERMAN J.J. (1999). Porcine reproductive and respiratory syndrome. *In:* Diseases of Swine, Eight Edition, Straw B.E., D'Allaire S., Mengeling W.L. & Taylor D.J., eds. Iowa State University Press. Ames, Iowa, USA, 201–232.

4. BENFIELD D.A., NELSON E., COLLINS J.E., HARRIS L., GOYAL S.M., ROBISON D., CHRISTIANSON W.T., MORRISON R.B., GORCYCA D. & CHLADEK D. (1992). Characterization of swine infertility and respiratory syndrome (SIRS) virus (isolate ATCC VR-2332). *J. Vet. Diagn. Invest.*, **4**, 127–133.

5. BOTNER A., NEILSEN J. & BILLE-HANSEN V. (1994). Isolation of porcine reproductive and respiratory syndrome (PRRS) virus in a Danish swine herd and experimental infection of pregnant gilts with the virus. *Vet. Microbiol.*, **40**, 351–360.

6. BOTNER A., STRANDBYGAARD B., SORENSEN K.J., HAVE P., MADSEN K.G., MADSEN E.S. & ALEXANDERSEN S. (1997). Appearance of acute PRRS-like symptoms in sow herds after vaccination with a modified live PRRS vaccine. *Vet. Rec.*, **141**, 497–499.

7. CAVANAGH D. (1997). Nidovirales: a new order comprising Coronaviridae and Arteriviridae. *Arch. Virol.*, **142**, 629–633.

8. CHO H.J., ENTZ S.C., MAGAR R. & JOO H.S. (1997). Performance of ELISA antigens prepared from 8 isolates of porcine reproductive and respiratory syndrome virus with homologous and heterologous antisera. *Can. J. Vet. Res.*, **61**, 299–304.

9. CHO H.J., MCNAB B., DUBUC C., JORDAN L., AFSHAR A., MAGAR R., PRINS S. & EERNISSE K. (1997). Comparative study of serological methods for the detection of antibodies to porcine reproductive and respiratory syndrome virus. *Can. J. Vet. Res.*, **61**, 161–166.

10. CHRISTIANSON W.T. & JOO H.S. (1994). Porcine reproductive and respiratory syndrome. *Swine Health Prod.* (AASP), **2**, 10–28.

11. CHRISTOPHER-HENNINGS J., NELSON E.A., NELSON J.K. & BENFIELD D.A. (1997). Effects of a modified-live virus vaccine against porcine reproductive and respiratory syndrome in boars. *Am. J. Vet. Res.*, **58**, 40–45.

12. CHRISTOPHER-HENNINGS J., NELSON E.A., NELSON J.K., HINES R.J., SWENSON S.L., HILL H.T., ZIMMERMAN J.J., KATZ J.B., YAEGER M.J., CHASE C.C.L. & BENFIELD D.A. (1995). Detection of porcine reproductive and respiratory syndrome virus in boar semen by PCR. *J. Clin. Microbiol.*, **33**, 1730–1734.

13. COLLINS J.E., BENFIELD D.A., CHRISTIANSON W.T., HARRIS L., HENNINGS J.C., SHAW D.P., GOYAL S.M., MCCULLOUGH S., MORRISON R.B., JOO H.S., GORCYCA D. & CHLADEK D. (1992). Isolation of swine infertility and respiratory syndrome virus (isolate ATCC VR-2332) in North America and experimental reproduction of the disease in gnotobiotic pigs. *J. Vet. Diagn. Invest.*, **4**, 117–126.

14. CONZELMANN K.-K., VISSER N., VAN WOENSEL P. & THIEL H.J. (1993). Molecular characterization of porcine reproductive and respiratory syndrome virus, a member of the arterivirus group. *Virology,* **193**, 329–339.

15. DEA S., GAGNON C.A., MARDASSI H. & MILANE G. (1996). Antigenic variability among North American and European strains of porcine reproductive and respiratory syndrome virus as defined by monoclonal antibodies to the matrix protein. *J. Clin. Microbiol.*, **34**, 1488–1493.

16. DENAC H., MOSER C., TRATSCHIN J.D. & HOFMANN M.A. (1997). An indirect ELISA for the detection of antibodies against porcine reproductive and respiratory syndrome virus using recombinant nucleocapsid protein as antigen. *J. Virol. Methods*, **65**, 169–181.

17. DONE S.H., PATON D.J. & WHITE M.E.C. (1996). Porcine reproductive and respiratory syndrome (PRRS): a review, with emphasis on pathological, virological and diagnostic aspects. *Br. Vet. J.*, **152**, 153–174.

18. DREW T.W. (1995). Comparative serology of porcine reproductive and respiratory syndrome in eight European laboratories, using immunoperoxidase monolayer assay and enzyme-linked immunosorbent assay. *Rev. sci. tech. Off. int. Epiz.*, **14**(3), 761–775.

19. DREW T.W., MEULENBERG J.J.M., SANDS J.J. & PATON D.J. (1995). Production, characterization and reactivity of monoclonal antibodies to porcine reproductive and respiratory syndrome virus. *J. Gen. Virol.*, **76**, 1361–1369.

20. GILBERT S.A., LAROCHELLE R., MAGAR R., CHO H. J. & DEREGT D. (1997). Typing of porcine reproductive and respiratory syndrome viruses by a multiplex PCR assay. *J. Clin. Microbiol.*, **35**, 264–267.

21. HALBUR P.G., ANDREWS J.J. HUFFMAN E.L., PAUL P.S., MENG X.-J. & NIYO Y. (1994). Development of a streptavidin-biotin immunoperoxidase procedure for the detection of porcine reproductive and respiratory syndrome virus antigen in porcine lung. *J. Vet. Diagn. Invest.*, **6**, 254–257.

22. HALBUR P.G., PAUL P.S., FREY M.L., LANDGRAF J., EERNISSE K., MENG X.-J., LUM M.A., ANDREWS J.J. & RATHJE J.A. (1995). Comparison of the pathogenicity of two US porcine reproductive and respiratory syndrome virus isolates with that of the Lelystad virus. *Vet. Pathol.*, **32**, 648–660.

23. HALBUR P.G., PAUL P.S., MENG X.-J., LUM M.A., ANDREWS J.J. & RATHJE J.A. (1996). Comparative pathogenicity of nine U.S. porcine reproductive and respiratory syndrome virus (PRRSV) isolates in a five-week-old cesarean-derived, colostrum-deprived pig model. J. *Vet. Diagn. Invest.*, **8**, 11–20.

24. HOUBEN S., CALLEBAUT P. & PENSAERT M.B. (1995). Comparative study of a blocking enzyme-linked immunosorbent assay and the immunoperoxidase monolayer assay for the detection of antibodies to the porcine reproductive and respiratory syndrome virus in pigs. *J. Virol. Methods*, **51**, 125–128.

25. JUSA E.R., INABA Y., KOUNO M., HIROSE O., SHIBATA I., KUBOTA M. & YASUHARA H. (1996). Slow-reacting and complement-requiring neutralizing antibody in swine infected with porcine reproductive and respiratory (PRRS) virus. *J. Vet. Med. Sci.*, **58**, 749–753.

26. KIM H.S., KWANG J., YOON I.J., JOO H.S. & FREY M.L. (1993). Enhanced replication of porcine reproductive and respiratory syndrome (PRRS) virus in a homogeneous subpopulation of MA-104 cell line. *Arch. Virol.*, **133**, 477–483.

27. KONO Y., KANNO T., SHIMZU M., YAMADA S., OHASHI S., NAKAMINE M. & SHIRAI J. (1996). Nested PCR for the detection and typing of porcine reproductive and respiratory syndrome (PRRS) virus in pigs. *J. Vet. Med. Sci.*, **58**, 941–946.

28. LAROCHELLE R. & MAGAR R. (1995). Comparison of immunogold silver staining (IGSS) with two immunoperoxidase staining systems for the detection of porcine reproductive and respiratory syndrome virus (PRRSV) antigens in formalin-fixed tissues. *J. Vet. Diagn. Invest.*, **7**, 540–543.

29. LAROCHELLE R. & MAGAR R. (1997). Differentiation of North American and European porcine reproductive and respiratory syndrome virus genotypes by in situ hybridization. *J. Virol. Methods,* **68**, 161–168.

30. LAROCHELLE R. & MAGAR R. (1997). Evaluation of the presence of porcine reproductive and respiratory syndrome virus in packaged pig meat using virus isolation and polymerase chain reaction (PCR) method. *Vet. Microbiol.*, **58**, 1–8.

31. MADSEN K.G., HANSEN C.M., MADSEN E.S., STRANDBYGAARD B., BOTNER A. & SORENSEN K.J. (1998). Sequence analysis of porcine reproductive and respiratory syndrome virus of the American type collected from Danish swine herds. *Arch. Virol.*, **143**, 1683–1700.

32. MAGAR R., LAROCHELLE R., NELSON E.A. & CHARREYRE C. (1997). Differential reactivity of a monoclonal antibody directed to the membrane protein of porcine reproductive and respiratory syndrome virus. *Can. J. Vet. Res.,* **61**, 69–71.

33. MARDASSI H., WILSON L., MOUNIR S. & DEA S. (1994). Detection of porcine reproductive and respiratory syndrome virus and efficient differentiation between Canadian and European strains by reverse transcription and PCR amplification. *J. Clin. Microbiol.*, **32**, 2197–2203.

34. MEULENBERG J.J.M., HULST M.M., DE MEIJER E.J., MOONEN P.J.L.M., DEN BESTEN A., DE KLUYVER E.P., WENSVOORT G. & MOORMANN R.J.M. (1993). Lelystad virus, the causative agent of porcine epidemic abortion and respiratory syndrome (PEARS), is related to LDV and EAV. *Virology,* **192**, 62–72.

35. NELSON E.A., CHRISTOPHER-HENNINGS J., DREW T., WENSVOORT G., COLLINS J.E. & BENFIELD D.A. (1993). Differentiation of U.S. and European. isolates of porcine reproductive and respiratory syndrome virus by monoclonal antibodies. *J. Clin. Microbiol.*, **31**, 3184–3189.

36. NODELIJK G., WENSVOORT G., KROESE B., VAN LEENGOED L., COLIJN E. & VERHEIJDEN J. (1996). Comparison of a commercial ELISA and an immunoperoxidase monolayer assay to detect antibodies directed against porcine respiratory and reproductive syndrome virus. *Vet. Microbiol.*, **49**, 285–295.

37. ROSSOW K.D. (1998). Porcine reproductive and respiratory syndrome. *Vet. Pathol.*, **35**, 1–20.

38. SNIJDER E.J. & MEULENBERG J.J.M. (1998). The molecular biology of arteriviruses. *J. Gen. Virol.,* **79**, 961–979.

39. SORENSEN K.J., BOTNER A., MADSEN E.S., STRANDBYGAARD B. & NIELSEN J. (1997). Evaluation of a blocking ELISA for screening of antibodies against porcine reproductive and respiratory syndrome (PRRS) virus. *Vet. Microbiol.*, **56**, 1–8.

40. SORENSEN K.J., STRANDBYGAARD B., BOTNER A., MADSEN E.S., NIELSEN J. & HAVE P. (1998). Blocking ELISAs for the distinction between antibodies against European and American strains of porcine reproductive and respiratory syndrome virus. *Vet. Microbiol.*, **60**, 169–177.

41. SUR J.-H., COOPER V.L., GALEOTA J.A., HESSE R.A., DOSTER A.R. & OSORIO F.A. (1996). *In vivo* detection of porcine reproductive and respiratory syndrome virus RNA by *in situ* hybridization at different times postinfection. *J. Clin. Microbiol.,* **34**, 2280–2286.

42. TORRISON J., KNOLL M. & WISEMAN B. (1996). Evidence of pig-to-pig transmission of a modified-live PRRS virus vaccine. *Proc. Am. Assoc. Swine Practitioners*, 89–91.

43. VAN NIEUWSTADT A.P., MEULENBERG J.J.M., VAN ESSEN-ZANDBERGEN A., PETERSEN-DEN BESTEN A., BENDE R.J., MOORMANN R.J.M. & WENSVOORT G. (1996). Proteins encoded by open reading frames 3 and 4 of the genome of Lelystad virus (Arteriviridae) are structural proteins of the virion. *J. Virol.,* **70**, 4767–4772.

44. VAN WOENSEL P., VAN DER MOUW J. & VISSER N. (1994). Detection of porcine reproductive and respiratory syndrome virus by polymerase chain reaction. *J. Virol. Methods.*, **47**, 273–278.

45. WEILAND E., WIECZOREK-KROHMER M., KOHL D., CONZELMANN K.K. & WEILAND F. (1999). Monoclonal antibodies to three GP5 of porcine reproductive and respiratory syndrome virus are more effective in virus neutralization than monoclonal antibodies to the GP4. *Vet. Microbiol.*, **66**, 171–186.

46. WENSVOORT G., DE KLUYVER E.P., LUIJTZE E.A., DEN BESTEN A., HARRIS L, COLLINS J.E., CHRISTIANSON W.T. &. CHLADEK D. (1992). Antigenic comparison of Lelystad virus and swine infertility and respiratory syndrome (SIRS) virus. *J. Vet. Diagn. Invest.*, **4**, 134–138.

47. WENSVOORT G., TERPSTRA C., POL J.M.A., TER LAAK E.A., BLOEMRAAD M., DE KLUYVER E.P., KRAGTEN C., VAN BUITEN L., DEN BESTEN A., WAGENAAR F., BROEKHUIJSEN J.M., MOONEN P.L.J.M., ZETSTRA T., DE BOER E.A., TIBBEN H.J., DE JONG M.F., VAN'T VELD P., GROENLAND G.J.R., VAN GENNEP J.A., VOETS M.TH., VERHEIJDEN J.H.M. & BRAAMSKAMP J. (1991). Mystery swine disease in the Netherlands: the isolation of Lelystad virus. *Vet. Q.*, **13**, 121–130.

48. WESLEY R.D., MENGELING W.L., LAGER K.M., CLOUSER D.F., LANDGRAF J.G. & FREY M.L. (1998). Differentiation of a porcine reproductive and respiratory syndrome virus vaccine strain from North American field strains by restriction fragment lenght polymorphism analysis of ORF 5. *J. Vet. Diagn. Invest.* **10**, 140–144.

49. YANG L., YOON K.-J., LI Y., LEE J.-H., ZIMMERMAN J.J., FREY M.L., HARMON K.M. & PLATT K.B. (1999). Antigenic and genetic variations of the 15 kD nucleocapsid protein of porcine reproductive and respiratory syndrome virus isolates. *Arch. Virol.*, **144**, 525–546.

50. YOON I.J., JOO H.S., CHRISTIANSON W.T., KIM H.S., COLLINS J.E., CARLSON J.H. & DEE S.A. (1992). Isolation of a cytopathic virus from weak pigs on farms with a history of swine infertility and respiratory syndrome. *J. Vet. Diagn. Invest.*, **4**, 139–143.

51. YOON I.J., JOO H.S., CHRISTIANSON W.T., KIM H.S., COLLINS J.E., MORRISON R.B. & DIAL G.D. (1992). An indirect fluorescent antibody test for the detection of antibody to swine infertility and respiratory syndrome virus in swine sera. *J. Vet. Diagn. Invest.*, **4**, 144–147.

*
* *

CHAPTER X. 13

FOWL POX

SUMMARY

Fowl pox is a disease of chickens and turkeys caused by a DNA virus of the genus Avipoxvirus *of the family Poxviridae. Its distribution is world-wide. It is slow-spreading and characterised by the formation of proliferative lesions and scabs on the skin, and diphtheritic lesions in the upper parts of the digestive and respiratory tracts. In the case of the cutaneous form the mortality rate is usually low, and affected birds are more likely to recover than those with the diphtheritic form. In the diphtheritic form, proliferative lesions involving the nasal passages, larynx or trachea can result in respiratory distress and death from suffocation.*

Fowl pox causes a transient drop in egg production and a reduced growth rate in young birds.

Identification of the agent: *Fowl pox should be suspected where skin eruptions occur on exposed areas. Histological examination of cutaneous or diphtheritic lesions reveals epithelial hyperplasia with intracytoplasmic inclusions in affected cells. Elementary bodies may be detected in smears from lesions by the use of the Gimenez method. Electron microscopy of lesions will detect virus particles with the characteristic poxvirus morphology by negative staining or in ultrathin sections of the lesion.*

The diphtheritic form of fowl pox involving the trachea must be differentiated from infectious laryngotracheitis, which is caused by a herpesvirus and is characterised by the presence of intranuclear inclusion bodies.

Virus isolation is done by inoculation of chorioallantoic membranes of 9–12-day-old developing chicken embryos or avian cell cultures.

Serological tests: *Immune responses to fowl pox virus may be demonstrated by the use of virus neutralisation, agar gel immunodiffusion, immunofluorescence, or passive hemagglutination tests, enzyme-linked immunosorbent assay and by immunoblotting.*

Requirements for vaccines and diagnostic biologicals: *Modified live fowl pox or pigeon pox virus vaccines of chicken embryo or avian cell culture origin are available commercially. The use of vaccines is indicated in areas where the disease is endemic, or on premises where infection has been diagnosed.*

A. DIAGNOSTIC TECHNIQUES

Fowl pox has a world-wide distribution and is caused by a DNA virus of the genus *Avipoxvirus* of the family Poxviridae (10, 14). Its incidence is variable in different areas because of differences in climate, management and hygiene or the practice of regular vaccination. It can cause drops in egg production, or retarded growth in younger birds.

Fowl pox is a slow-spreading virus disease of chickens and turkeys, characterised in the cutaneous form (dry pox) by the development of proliferative lesions, ranging from small nodules to spherical wart-like masses on the skin of the comb, wattle and other unfeathered areas. In the diphtheritic form (wet pox), slightly elevated white opaque nodules develop on the mucous membranes. They rapidly increase in size to become a yellowish diphtheritic membrane. Lesions occur on the mucous membranes of the mouth, oesophagus, larynx or trachea. The mortality rate is higher in the diphtheritic form than in the cutaneous form, sometimes nearing 50% (15), particularly in young birds. Recently, integration of reticuloendotheliosis virus (REV) sequences has been observed in the genome of fowl pox virus (8). While most field strains contain REV provirus, vaccine strains have only remnants of long terminal repeats.

1. Identification of the agent

Fowl pox virus multiplies in the cytoplasm of epithelial cells with the formation of large intracytoplasmic inclusion bodies (Bollinger bodies) that contain smaller elementary bodies (Borrel bodies). The inclusions can be demonstrated in sections of cutaneous and diphtheritic lesions by the use of haematoxylin and eosin (H&E), acridine orange or Giemsa stains (12). The elementary bodies can be detected in smears from lesions, for example by the Gimenez method (11), which is described below. Electron microscopy can be used to demonstrate viral particles of typical poxvirus morphology by negative staining or in ultrathin sections of infected tissues (2).

a) A smear technique for fowl pox

i) Place a drop of distilled water and the lesion (cutaneous or diphtheritic) on a clean slide. Prepare a thin smear by pressing the lesion with another clean slide and rotating the upper slide several times.

ii) Air dry and gently fix the smear over a flame.

iii) Stain the smear for 5–10 minutes with freshly prepared primary stain (8 ml stock solution[1] of basic fuchsin mixed with 10 ml of phosphate buffer[2], pH 7.5, and filtered through Whatman filter paper No. 1).

iv) Wash thoroughly with tap water.

v) Counterstain with malachite green (0.8% in distilled water) for 30–60 seconds.

vi) Wash the smear with tap water and then dry.

vii) Examine the smear under oil immersion. The elementary bodies appear red and are approximately 0.2–0.3 µm in size.

b) Virus isolation

Fowl pox virus can be isolated by the inoculation of suspected material into embryonated chicken eggs. Approximately 0.1 ml of tissue suspension of skin or diphtheritic lesions, with the appropriate concentration of antibiotics, is inoculated on to the chorioallantoic membranes (CAMs) of 9–12-day-old developing chicken embryos. These are incubated at 37°C for 5–7 days, and then examined for focal white pock lesions or generalised thickening of the CAMs. Histopathological examination of the CAM lesions will reveal eosinopilic intracytoplasmic inclusion bodies following staining with H&E (12, 14).

Primary chicken embryo fibroblasts, chicken embryo kidney cells, chicken embryo dermis cells, or the permanent quail cell line QT-35, can also be used to propagate fowl pox virus (4, 7). The adaptation of virus strains to cell cultures is an important requirement for plaque formation, as not all strains will form plaques initially.

c) Molecular methods

Restriction endonuclease analysis is a useful method for comparing closely related DNA genomes and can be used for comparison of field isolates and vaccine strains of fowl pox virus (4, 7).

Cloned genomic fragments of fowl pox virus can be used effectively as nucleic acid probes for diagnosis of fowl pox. Viral DNA isolated from lesions can be detected by hybridisation either with radioactively or nonradioactively labelled genomic probes. This method is especially useful for differentiation of fowl pox from infectious laryngotracheitis when tracheal lesions are present (3).

Genomic DNA sequences of various sizes can be amplified by the polymerase chain reaction (PCR) using specific primers (5). This technique is useful when there is only an extremely small amount of viral DNA in the sample.

1 Stock solution: A solution of basic fuchsin (5 g) in 95% ethanol (100 ml) is slowly added to a second solution of crystalline phenol (10 g) in distilled water (900 ml). This stock solution, kept in a tightly screw-capped glass bottle, is incubated for 48 hours at 37°C, and then stored at room temperature.

2 Phosphate buffer, pH 7.5: $NaH_2PO_4H_2O$ (2.47 g) and Na_2HPO_4 (11.65 g) are added to distilled water (1000 ml) and stored at 4°C.

2. Serological tests

Although both cell-mediated immunity (CMI) and humoral immunity play an important role in poxvirus infections, routine use of CMI test is not convenient. Therefore, serological tests, such as virus neutralisation (VN), agar gel immunodiffusion (AGID), passive haemagglutination, fluorescent antibody tests as well as enzyme-linked immunosorbent assay (ELISA) are used to measure specific humoral antibody responses.

a) Virus neutralisation

After virus/serum interaction, the residual virus activity may be assayed in embryonating chicken eggs or in cell cultures (6). This technically demanding test may not be convenient for routine diagnosis. Only some selected strains of the virus have plaque-forming ability in chicken embryo cells. Neutralising antibodies develop within 1–2 weeks of infection.

b) Agar gel immunodiffusion

Precipitating antibodies can be detected by reacting test sera against viral antigens. The antigen can be derived by sonication and homogenisation of infected skin or CAM lesions as well as treatment of infected cell cultures as described in Section A.2.f. below. The lysed suspension is centrifuged and the supernatant is used as antigen. Gel-diffusion medium is prepared with 1% agar, 8% sodium chloride and 0.01% thiomersol. The viral antigen is placed in the central well and the test sera are placed in the peripheral wells. It is important to include a positive and negative control serum. The plates are incubated at room temperature. Precipitation lines develop in 24–48 hours after incubation of the antigen with antibody to homologous or closely related strains. The test is less sensitive than the ELISA (1) or the passive haemagglutination test (13).

c) Passive haemagglutination

Tanned sheep or horse red blood cells are sensitised with a partially purified fowl pox viral antigen (13). The antigen is prepared from infected CAMs or cells as described in Section A.2.f. below. Passive haemagglutination is more sensitive than AGID. The test will give cross-reactions among avian pox viruses.

d) Fluorescent antibody tests

Direct or indirect immunofluorescence tests will reveal specific intracytoplasmic fluorescence in infected cells. The latter test is commonly used and involves two steps: the antibody against fowl pox virus is reacted with the antigen in the infected cells, followed by a secondary fluorescein-isothiocyanate-labelled antibody against chicken gamma globulin (e.g. goat anti-chicken). Such labelled antibodies are available commercially. In this regard, formalin-fixed tissue sections can be used effectively for fluorescent antibody tests.

e) Immunoperoxidase

Specific staining of cytoplasmic inclusions is achieved when horseradish-peroxidase-conjugated specific polyclonal antibody against fowl poxvirus is reacted with the hydrated sections of fowl pox-infected fixed tissues (CAM and skin) or cell culture. Similar results are obtained when either polyclonal or monoclonal antibodies are used in an indirect test. An advantage of the technique is that the sections can be examined with the light microscope and can be stored for an extended period without loss of colour (12).

f) Enzyme-linked immunosorbent assay

ELISAs have been developed to detect humoral antibodies to fowl pox virus. They are capable of detecting antibody 7–10 days after infection (1), but commercial kits for this test are not available.

Fowl pox virus antigens are prepared either from infected QT-35 cell monolayers or CAM lesions. Infected QT cells are pelleted (700 ***g*** for 10 minutes at 4°C), washed with isotonic buffer (10 mM Tris, pH 8.0, 150 mM NaCl, 5 mM ethylene diamine tetra-acetic acid [EDTA]) followed by lysis in hypotonic buffer (10 mM Tris, pH 8.0, 10 mM KCl, 5 mM EDTA) containing 0.1% Triton X-100 and 0.025% beta-mercaptoethanol. Nuclei and cellular debris are removed by slow speed centrifugation (500 ***g*** for 5 minutes at 4°C) and the resulting supernatant is used as a source of fowl pox virus antigens for ELISA or immunoblotting. To isolate viral antigen from CAM lesions, initial grinding of the lesions with subsequent detergent treatment as described earlier would be required.

Wells of microtitre plates are coated with 1 µg of soluble fowl pox virus antigen in 100 µl of coating buffer (15 mM Na_2CO_3, 35 mM $NaHCO_3$, pH 9.6) and incubated overnight at 4°C. Each well is then rinsed once with wash solution (0.29 M NaCl, 0.05% Tween 20) and then blocked with phosphate buffered saline (PBS, pH 7.4) containing 3% bovine serum albumin (BSA) for 1 hour at 37°C. After one wash, serial dilutions of the test sera in PBS containing 1% BSA are added to the wells. After rocking for 2 hours at 37°C, the wells are washed three times prior to the addition of 100 µl/well horseradish-peroxidase-conjugated goat anti-chicken IgG (H+L) antibodies[3] at a recommended dilution in PBS. After 2 hours' incubation at 37°C and three subsequent washes, 100 µl of the peroxidase substrate TMB[3] is added to each well. Reactions are terminated by the addition of 1 M phosphoric acid and absorbance at 450 nm is recorded using an ELISA plate reader[4].

g) Immunoblotting

Antigenic variations that occur between strains of fowl pox virus can be evaluated by means of immunoblotting. In this method, viral antigens separated by SDS/PAGE (sodium dodecyl sulphate/ polyacrylamide gel electrophoresis) are reacted either with polyclonal or monoclonal antibodies against fowl pox virus (4, 9).

B. REQUIREMENTS FOR VACCINES AND DIAGNOSTIC BIOLOGICALS

Early studies indicated the feasibility of protecting chickens from fowl pox by the use of pigeon pox or fowl pox viruses (16). Vaccination is indicated in areas where fowl pox is endemic or on premises where infection has been diagnosed previously. Live fowl and pigeon pox virus vaccines, and also fowl pox vectored vaccines that protect against pox, are available commercially. These vaccines are derived from chicken embryos or avian cell cultures.

Passively acquired immunity should be taken into consideration during vaccination of progeny from flocks that have either had a recent natural infection or been recently vaccinated. As passive immunity may interfere with vaccine virus multiplication, such progeny should be vaccinated only after the decline of passively acquired antibody. Fowl pox vaccine is applied by a wing web stab method.

1. Seed management

a) Characteristics of the seed

A master seed virus (MSV) must be established and used according to a seed-lot system. A record must be kept of its origin, passage history and characteristics. Viruses used may be either fowl pox or pigeon pox viruses. The MSV must be propagated in suitable premises with materials that meet approved standards, and must be tested for freedom from contamination as well as for identity and purity.

b) Method of culture

The MSV may be propagated in specific pathogen free (SPF) chicken embryos, using the CAMs, or in avian cell cultures, such as primary chicken embryo fibroblasts, chicken embryo kidney or chicken embryo dermis.

c) Validation as a vaccine

i) *Purity*

The MSV may be neutralised with a specific hyperimmune serum before testing for purity. Because of difficulty in neutralising avian pox virus, it is acceptable to treat the MSV by centrifugation at 1000 ***g*** for 20 minutes, followed by filtration through a 0.2 µm filter. The neutralised or filtered MSV is then used in tests to demonstrate freedom from extraneous agents. These tests should be done in: embryonating eggs or avian cell cultures, to demonstrate absence of extraneous virus replication, and SPF chickens, to demonstrate freedom from antibodies to extraneous agents.

3 Kirkegaard and Perry Laboratories, Gaithersberg, Maryland, United States of America.
4 Dynatech, Chantilly, Virginia, United States of America.

ii) *Safety*

Vaccines should be prepared only from virus that is a stable attenuated strain or a naturally occurring isolate of low virulence.

The vaccine must be shown to be safe by the recommended route of administration, which is wing web stab, in all ages of susceptible birds. A suitable test is to take ten SPF chickens and inoculate each by piercing the wing web with a needle dipped in the vaccine. The birds are observed for 7–10 days for evidence of 'takes' and for the absence of adverse effects attributable to the vaccine. A 'take' consists of swelling of the skin or a scab at the site where the vaccine was applied and is evidence of successful vaccination. The safety test should be repeated after at least six serial passages of the virus to show that there has been no reversion to virulence.

iii) *Efficacy*

Data should be obtained using the highest passage level and the lowest titre of virus to be used in the final product: 20 SPF chickens of the minimum age indicated for vaccination should receive one dose of vaccine by the recommended method. The chickens, together with 20 unvaccinated chickens of the same age and source, should be challenged 3 weeks later by scarification with a virulent strain of fowl pox virus. The birds should be observed for 3 weeks. All the control birds should develop lesions due to the challenge virus and at least 90% of the vaccinated birds should remain free of such lesions.

2. Method of manufacture

Vaccine is manufactured on a seed-lot system from the validated MSV. This must be done in approved premises designed to avoid the risk of contamination. All media and cell cultures must be tested to ensure freedom from contamination.

3. In-process control

During the process of validation as a vaccine, the efficacy data must be compared with the virus content of the vaccine. A suitable potency can thus be established. The vaccine should be filled into final containers to ensure that each container has sufficient virus to achieve the specified potency.

4. Batch control

a) Sterility

Tests for sterility and freedom from contamination of biological materials may be found in the Chapter I.4.

b) Safety

The test described in Section B.1.c.ii above should be used on each batch of vaccine.

c) Potency

Virus content tests should be carried out using each of at least three containers. The dilutions should span 0–100% infection range, using five-fold dilution steps and at least seven replicates per dilution. Tests should be done in parallel with a standard vaccine, if available. Each lot of vaccine should be titrated in the diluent provided for its use. The virus titre should not normally be higher than 1/10 of the dose at which the vaccine has been shown to be safe and must not be lower than the release titre determined in the test for efficacy. A suitable potency for an attenuated live fowl pox vaccine is likely to be in the region of 10^5 EID_{50} (50% embryo infective dose) per ml.

d) Duration of immunity

The efficacy test given in Section B.1.c.iii may be used to determine the duration of immunity by testing at intervals after vaccination, using separate groups of birds for each test.

e) Stability

Evidence of stability must be presented to justify the shelf life. This should be based on virus titrations carried out at intervals until 3 months beyond the requested shelf life on at least six batches of vaccine kept under recommended storage conditions.

f) **Preservatives**

Preservatives are not used in live vaccines.

g) **Precautions (hazards)**

It is usually recommended not to vaccinate birds that are in lay. Avoid human contact with the live vaccine. Fowl pox vaccine is not to be used in pigeons, though they can be vaccinated with pigeon pox vaccine.

5. Tests on the final product

a) **Safety**

The safety test described in Section B.1.c.ii above is used on each batch.

b) **Potency**

The potency test described in Section B.4.c. above is used on each batch.

REFERENCES

1. BUSCAGLIA C., BANKOWSKI R.A. & MIERS L. (1985). Cell-culture virus neutralization test and enzyme-linked immunosorbent assay for evaluation of immunity in chickens against fowl pox. *Avian Dis.*, **29**, 672–680.

2. DOANE F.W. & ANDERSON N. (1987). Electron Microscopy in Diagnostic Virology: A Practical Guide and Atlas. Cambridge University Press, Cambridge, UK.

3. FATUNMBI O.O., REED W.M., SCHWARTZ D.I. & TRIPATHY D.N. (1995). Dual infection of chickens with pox and infectious laryngotracheitis (ILT) confirmed with specific pox and ILT DNA dot-blot hybridization assays. *Avian Dis.*, **39**, 925–930.

4. GHILDYAL N., SCHNITZLEIN W.M. & TRIPATHY D.N. (1989). Genetic and antigenic differences between fowlpox and quailpox viruses. *Arch. Virol.*, **106**, 85–92.

5. LEE L.H. & LEE K.H. (1997). Application of the polymerase chain reaction for the diagnosis of fowl poxvirus infection. *J. Virol. Methods,* **63**, 113–119.

6. MORITA C. (1973). Studies on fowlpox viruses. II. Plaque neutralization test. *Avian Dis.*, **17**, 93–98.

7. SCHNITZLEIN W.M., GHILDYAL N. & TRIPATHY D.N. (1988). Genomic and antigenic characterisation of avipoxviruses. *Virus Res.*, **10**, 65–76.

8. SINGH P., KIM T.-J. & TRIPATHY D.N. (2000). Re-emerging fowlpox: evaluation of isolates from vaccinated flocks. *Avian Pathol.*, **29**, 449–455.

9. SINGH P. & TRIPATHY D.N. (2000). Characterization of monoclonal antibodies against fowl poxvirus. *Avian Dis.,* **44**, 365–371.

10. TRIPATHY D.N. (1993). Avipoxviruses. *In:* Virus Infections of Vertebrates – Virus Infections of Birds, Vol. 4, McFerran J.B. & McNulty M.S., eds. Elsevier Science Publishers, Amsterdam, the Netherlands, 5–15.

11. TRIPATHY D.N. & HANSON, L.E. (1976). A smear technique for staining elementary bodies of fowl pox. *Avian Dis.*, **20**, 609–610

12. TRIPATHY D.N., HANSON L.E. & KILLINGER A.H. (1973). Immunoperoxidase technique for detection of fowl pox antigen. *Avian Dis.*, **17**, 274–278.

13. TRIPATHY D.N., HANSON L.E. & MYERS W.L. (1970). Passive hemagglutination test with fowl pox virus. *Avian Dis.*, **14**, 29–38.

14. TRIPATHY D.N. & REED W.M. (1997). Pox. *In:* Diseases of Poultry, Tenth Edition, Calnek B.W., Barnes H.J., Beard C.W., McDougald L.R. & Saif Y.M., eds. Iowa State University Press, Ames, Iowa, USA, 643–659.

15. TRIPATHY D.N. & REED W.M. (1998). Pox. *In:* A Laboratory Manual for the Isolation and Identification of Avian Pathogens, Fourth Edition, Swayne D.E., Glisson J.R., Jackwood M W., Pearson J.E., & Reed W.M., eds. American Association of Avian Pathologists, University of Pennsylvania, New Bolton Center, Kennett Square, PA 19348-1692, USA, 137–140.

16. WINTERFIELD R.W. & HITCHNER S.B. (1965). The response of chickens to vaccination with different concentrations of pigeon pox and fowl pox viruses. *Avian Dis.*, **9**, 237–241.

*

* *

CHAPTER X.14.

MANGE

SUMMARY

Most types of mange (scabies) are forms of allergic dermatitis characterised by encrustation, alopecia, and pruritus of the skin, initiated by and maintained by a number of mite species. Mites and ticks are a subclass of the Arachnida divided into two superorders, dependent on the presence of a layer of optically active material, actinochitin, that exhibits birefringence in polarised light: the anactinotrichida (Parasitiformes. Mesostigmata) and the actinotrichida (Acariformes). The actinotrichida contains three orders: the Astigmata (Acaridida, not possessing stigmata), the prostigmata (Actinedida, possessing stigmata behind the gnathosoma), and the Oribatida (Cryptostigmata). All the major mange mite species are contained within the orders Astigmata and Prostigmata. The Astigmata are a well defined group of slow-moving, weakly sclerotised mites, including the medically or veterinary important families Sarcoptidae and Psoroptidae. The prostigmata are the most heterogeneous of acarine orders with adults ranging in size from 100 µm to 16 mm (15). Included in the Prostigmata are the Trombiculidae (harvest mites), parasitic as larvae but free-living predators in the nymphal and adult stages and the true mange mite families Cheletoidea (Psorobia [Psoreregates] *sp.*), *Demodicidae* (Demodex *sp.*) *and Cheyletiellidae* (Cheyletiella *sp.*).

***Identification of the agent:** All mange mites are classified by structure and are typically composed of an anterior gnathosoma or capitulum.(mouthparts) and a posterior 'body' (idiosoma). The mouthparts (gnathosoma) bear a pair of lateral palps either side of the chelicerae. The chelicerae are normally chelate with the third segment being movable, but are modified according to the feeding habits of the mite. The idiosoma is subdivided into the area of legs (the podosoma) and the area behind the last pair of legs, the opisthosoma. In most mange mites the four pairs of legs are arranged in anterior and posterior pairs and their relative areas are referred to as the propodosoma (containing leg pairs I and II) and the metapodosoma (containing leg pairs III and IV). The leg of a typical mite is seven jointed giving the coxa, trochanter, femur, genu, tibia, tarsus and pretarsus. The pedicel (pretarsus, pulvillus, ambulacral stalk) bears an 'ambulacrum' composed of a pair of claws, a median empodium and possibly a terminal membranous pulvillus. The pretarsi of* Cheyletiella *are comb-like. The empodium may be hair-like, pad-like or sucker-like. Most mange mites are globose or oval in outline, with the exception of the 'worm-like'* Demodex *sp. In the larger mesostigmatid mites, gaseous exchange is facilitated by a complex tracheal system, opening to the exterior at the stigmata. In mesostigmatid mites, there is one pair of stigmata located laterally. In the prostigmata, stigmata are located behind the mouthparts. Stigmata are absent in the Astigmata. The typical acarine life cycle consists of the egg, hexapod larva, octopod nymphs and octopod adult males and females. There may be two to three nymphal stages before the development of an adult mite. The three nymphal stages are referred to as the protonymph, the deuteronymph and the tritonymph. In the Astigmata, the deuteronymph may be fundementally different to the preceding or succeeding instars, both morphologically and behaviourally. Such heteromorphic nymphs (hypopus/hypopi) are adapted to survive environmental stress and are not present in the life cycles of the major mange species, with nymphal stages restricted to the protonymph and the tritonymph ('pubescent female'). Adult male and female mites may be morphologically different.*

***Serological tests:** An enzyme linked immunosorbent assay (ELISA) for the serological diagnosis of sarcoptic mange in dogs and pigs is used in Sweden and ELISA techniques have been developed to monitor* Psoroptes *infections in sheep, cattle and nondomesticated animals, but none is in routine use. Researchers routinely use ELISA to detect and quantify circulating antibody specific for* Sarcoptes scabiei.

Requirements for vaccines and diagnostic biologicals: *There are no commercial vaccines currently available.*

A. DIAGNOSTIC TECHNIQUES

The diagnosis of mange in domestic animals is based on clinical manifestations and the demonstration of mites or their developmental stages in skin scrapings (15). Specialist illustrated keys should be consulted in order to identify the causative organism (3).

1. Identification of the agent

Mange can be the result of infestation by the astigmatid mites, *Chorioptes, Knemidokoptes, Notoedres, Otodectes, Psoroptes* and *Sarcoptes* or the prostigmatid mites *Cheyletiella, Demodex* and *Psorobia.*

• The Astigmata

The astigmata are small thin-skinned mites, generally lacking obvious shields. The bases of the coxae are sunk into the body and referred to as epimeres (apodemes). The empodium is claw-like and the pedicel is stalked or sessile. True claws are absent. Fertilised eggs are extruded through an antero-ventral slit, the oviporus or genital opening. Most species of medical or veterinary importance are in the division Psoroptidia, comprising the Psoroptoidea (Sarcoptidae and Psoroptidae), the Analgoidea (Knemidokoptidae, Cytoditidae and Laminosoptidae) and the Pyroglyphoidea (Pyroglyphidae). The division Acaridae contains the stored product mites, which can cause transitory mange and can be an important source of allergens.

• Sarcoptidae

Sarcoptid (sarcoptiform) mites are obligate parasites, burrowing into the skin of mammals. They are globose mites with the ventral surface flattened and the cuticle finely striated. The chelicerae are adapted for cutting and paring.

a) *Sarcoptes scabiei*

Sarcoptes can be identified on the basis of size, shape and morphology. The body outline of adult mites is circular and approximately 250 µm in length, but as ovaries develop in the female she can increase in size to 300–500 µm in length. The cuticle (integument) is striated, bearing a central patch of raised tooth and peg-like structures on the dorsum, decreasing in density posterolaterally. Legs are weakly developed and in both sexes the pretarsi of legs I and II bear empodial claws, but the ambulacral suckers are on long unjointed pedicels (stalks). The epimeres (apodemes) of the first pair of legs are fused in a 'Y' shape. Legs III and IV in the female (identified by the transverse egg-laying slit [oviporus] in the middle of the ventral surface) end in long setae and lack a stalked pedicel. They are located on the ventral surface and are not visible in dorsal view. Males are smaller and distinguished by the presence of a stalked pedicel on legs IV, between which there is an obvious sclerotised genital apparatus. Nymphs are similar to the female, but smaller and without an oviporus. Larvae resemble nymphs, but have only three pairs of legs. A similar mite, *Trixicara caviae,* occurs on guinea-pigs, but is smaller and the anus is terminal. Secondary immune reactions may produce a rash at sites away from the infested area. Humans are easily infested, particularly in crowded or poor living conditions (25).

The itch mite *(Sarcoptes scabiei)* is the cause of scabies in humans and mange in a wide range of domestic and wild mammals (both carnivorous and herbivorous) throughout the world, generally affecting the sparsely haired parts of the body. The numbers of species within the genus is still open to debate. Studies of populations of *Sarcoptes* mites from a wide range of hosts have suggested that there is only one type species *(Sarcoptes scabiei)* with a number of variants infesting a wide range of mammalian hosts (11). Recent investigations based on molecular analysis of the ITS-2 of the mRNA gene suggest that the genus *Sarcoptes* is monospecific (27).

b) *Notoedres* sp.

Notoedres also burrows into the host epidermis and is similar to *Sarcoptes,* but can be distinguished by the dorsal anus. Over 20 species of *Notoedres* have been described of which the cat mange mite, *N. cati,* is of veterinary interest, producing a highly contagious and intensely pruritic mange on cats (and sometimes dogs and rabbits). Infestation usually starts on the head of the cat, from where it may spread. *Notoedres muris* occurs on rats and *N. musculi* on house mice. *Notoedres cati* is similar to *S. scabiei,* having unjointed stalked pedicels with terminal suckers on legs I and II in all stages, and on leg IV in the male. *Notoedres cati* is considerably smaller, the female being 225 µm and the male 150 µm. The anus is located on the dorsal surface and there are no projecting scales, but mid-dorsally the striae are broken into a scale-like pattern and stout setae replace the lanceolate spines of *S. scabiei.*

• Analgoidea

The analgoidea include 12 species of the mange mites: *Knemidokoptes (*Knemidokoptidae), the air sac mite of poultry (*Cytodites nudus*: Cytoditidae) and the Laminosoptidae, represented by *Laminosoptes cysticola,* infesting the subcutaneous cellular tissue of turkeys and chickens.

a) *Knemidocoptes* sp.

Three species of *Knemidokoptes* are of veterinary importance: *K. mutans* infesting the epidermis of the legs of poultry (causing 'scaly leg'), *K. gallinae (Neoknemidokoptes gallinae, Mesoknemidokoptes laevis gallinae),* the 'depluming mite' infesting the skin of poultry near the base of the feathers and *K. pilae* infesting the cere of cage and aviary birds (causing 'scaly face'). Female *Knemidokoptes* are 400 µm long, and scales, if present, are feint and irregular. *Knemidokoptes gallinae (Mesoknemidokoptes)* do not have any scales (3). Two sclerotised, almost parallel, longitudinal bands are present on the anterior mid-dorsal surface, connected posteriorly by a less well developed transverse band. In the male, the epimeres (apodemes) of the first pair of legs are joined in a 'Y' shape, and in the female, the epimeres (apodemes) are joined in a 'U' shape. Stalked pulvilli are present on all legs in the male and larvae, but are absent in the nymphal stages and the female. The anus is situated terminally. The female is viviparous and there are one larval and two nymphal stages.

• Psoroptidae

The family Psoroptidae are oval, nonburrowing mites, parasitic on mammalian skin. The cuticle (integument) is striated and legs III and IV are usually visible from above. The epimeres (apodemes) of leg I are not fused and there are no vertical setae on the propodosoma. The male has prominent adanal suckers that engage with the copulatory tubercles of the female tritonymph ('pubescent female'). The inverted U-shaped oviporus is prominent on the venter (ventral surface of the body) of the ovigerous female, posterior to leg II. Three genera, *Psoroptes, Chorioptes* and *Otodectes* are of veterinary importance.

a) *Psoroptes* sp.

Psoroptes sp. have strongly developed legs bearing, in all stages, funnel-shaped suckers on long three segmented pedicels. The ovigerous mite is pearly white and 750 µm in length. The male has a pair of opisthsomal lobes and a pair of copulatory suckers. *Psoroptes* mites cause a debilitating dermatitis involving wool/hair loss and a pruritic scab formation. Five species of *Psoroptes* are recognised (23): *P. ovis,* a body mite causing mange in sheep, cattle and horses, *P. equi*, a body mite of equids, *P. natalensis,* a body mite of cattle and horses, *P. cuniculi,* the ear mite of rabbits, goats, horses and sheep, and *P. cervinus,* an ear mite of bighorn sheep, elk and wapiti. A sixth, unvalidated, species is *P. auchinae*, an ear mite of New World camelids. *Psoroptes natalensis* and *P. equi* can be distinguished morphologically by the length of the fourth outer opisthosomal seta (L_4OOS) of the male (23). In *P. natalensis,* the seta is also spatulate, as is the shorter L_4OOS of male *P. cervinus* (23). It is difficult to separate *P. ovis* and *P. cuniculi* on morphological grounds. Like the genus *Sarcoptes*, the numbers of species in the genus *Psoroptes* is open to debate, *P. ovis* and *P. cuniculi* may be variants of the same species (4).

b) *Chorioptes*

Chorioptes mites have broad bowl-shaped suckers borne on very short unsegmented pedicels, except legs III of the female, which terminate in two long setae. Ovigerous *C. bovis* are smaller than *Psoroptes*, being 300 µm in length. The male *C. bovis* has pedicels on all four pairs of legs, a pair of squarish to rectangular opisthsomal lobes and a pair of copulatory suckers anteriorly. The opisthosomal lobes have two spatulate (paddle-like) hairs, together with three normal setae of varying length. The mouthparts are broad and rounded, adapted for chewing. Two species of *Chorioptes* are recognised: *C. bovis*, infesting cattle, goats, horses, sheep and rabbits, and *C. texanus,* recorded on goats, reindeer and cattle (20, 22). The opisthosomal lobes of *C. texanus* are more triangular in outline than those of *C. bovis* and the pair of spatulate opisthosomal setae are much longer. In goats, horses and camels, the mite generally inhabits the lower parts of the leg, similarly on sheep but the scrotum may also be infested. In cattle, chorioptic mange commonly occurs on the base of the tail, the perineum and the back of the udder. The mite feeds on the external surface of the skin causing inflammation, exudation and scab formation. Heavy infestations can cause loss of condition, which can lead to emaciation and damage to hides (25).

c) *Otodectes*

Otodectes is similar to *Chorioptes* except that the male opisthosomal lobes are much less distinct, though copulatory suckers are present and the hairs are less spatulate. The epimeres (apodemes) extending from the coxae of legs I and II are joined. The male has broad bowl-shaped suckers borne on very short unsegmented pedicels on all the legs, but only legs I and II of the female have pedicels and suckers. Legs III of the female terminate in two long setae and legs IV are reduced (3). *Otodectes cynotis* occurs in the ears of domestic dogs, cats, foxes and ferrets and a number of wild carnivores, causing parasitic otitis (and occasionally the body) (24). *Otodectes cynotis* feeds on the external surface of the skin causing inflammation and exudation. Excessive exudation may lead to wet eczema on adjacent skin surfaces. The tympanic membrane may be perforated and otitis media and nervous signs (e.g. convulsions) can develop.

- **Free-living astigmatid mites**

Free-living astigmatid ('forage') mites can occur in large numbers in stored food, spilled grain, poultry feed, etc. Their ingestion can lead to gastrointestinal disturbance. Mites may also be the cause of incidental mange of mammals through contact with antigenic material present in infested feed or the environment. Workers handling infested stored food can develop allergic reactions to the mites manifested as pruritus, dermatitis, rhinitis or asthma (25). The most obvious characteristic of the more common forage mites *(Tyroglyphidae)* is the possession of many 'hairs', which are much longer than the parasitic forms, and may be simple, branched or spatulate. In some genera (e.g. *Glycyphagus*), the posterior hairs often become entangled in debris. *Acarus siro*, probably the commonest of these mites, has shorter hairs.

- **Prostigmata**

Prostigmatid mites are weakly sclerotised and, where there is a respiratory system, the stigmata open on the gnathosoma or anterior part of the propodosoma. The palpi are usually free and highly developed, either as pincer-like clasping or sensory organs. The chelicerae are usually modified for piercing (3, 25). Included in the Prostigmata are the Trombiculidae (harvest or chigger mites), parasitic as larvae, but free-living predators in the nymphal and adult stages, and the true mange mite families Cheletoidea (*Psorobia* [*Psoreregates*] sp.), Demodicidae (*Demodex* sp.) and Cheyletiellidae (*Cheyletiella* sp.).

a) ***Psorobia (Psorergates)* sp.**

Two species of *Psorobia* have been isolated from domestic animals: the benign 'parasite' *P. bos* from cattle, and the more important *P. ovis* occurring in Merino sheep. Larval *Psorobia* hatch with reduced legs, becoming progressively larger at each of three nymphal moults, and by the adult stage the legs are well developed and the mites are motile. Adults of both sexes are very small (200 µm) and can be recognised by the radially arranged legs around a more or less circular body. Each leg has an inward-curving spine on each femur. Most mites are found under the stratum corneum in the superficial layers of the skin of the sides, flanks and thighs, feeding on the exuding fluid. The infested area is dry and scurfy, wool fibres break easily, with the remaining wool comes together as ragged tufts. Irritation causes the sheep to rub and kick the affected area and chew its' fleece, resulting in 'fleece derangement' and down-grading of the wool clip.

b) ***Cheyletiella* sp.**

Cheyletiella (fur mites) are large mites (385 µm) with large curved palpal claws and an obvious 'M'-shaped respiratory peritreme or stomata at the base of the chelicerae. *Cheyletiella* is an obligate parasite, inhabiting the keratin layer of the epidermis. The mites develop rapidly, giving rise to the term 'walking dandruff'. Three species are of veterinary importance causing mild, nonsuppurative dermatitis in mammals and transitory dermatitis in humans: *C. parasitovorax* occurring on the scapular region of rabbits, *C. yasguri* causing a highly infectious infestation of puppies (adult dogs as carriers), and *C. blakei*, causing a mild dermatitis in cats. *Cheyletiella parasitovorax* has an ovate (spade-shaped) sensory organ or seta (solenidion) on the genu of the first leg, whereas that of *C. yasguri* is apically cleaved (heart-shaped) (3).

c) ***Demodex* sp.**

Demodex are easily recognised by their annulate, vermiform ('worm-like') shape, but may be overlooked on account of their small size. Demodex inhabit the hair follicles and the sebaceous and meibomian glands of the skin of a number of wild and domesticated mammals, including humans. Male *Demodex* live at or near the skin surface and females live in the follicles. Different species occur on different hosts, and more than one species may occur on the same host, e.g. *D. folliculorum* and *D. brevis* on humans (9). Demodectic mange is of great importance in dogs (especially short-haired breeds), goats and pigs, and of lesser importance in cattle, horses, sheep and cats. There is usually no irritation or pathological conditions, but in some individuals the numbers and spread of mites on the hosts increases to form clinical demodecosis. On cattle this occurs as flat nodules in the skin with a massive enlargement of the sebaceous glands, which contain vast numbers of *Demodex* mites. In dogs, infestations may become generalised as a squamous form, with associated hair loss and thickening of the skin. Pustular demodecosis is a more severe form in dogs and is complicated by secondary bacterial infection. However, demodecosis does not cause pruritus (25). Diagnosis of demodecidosis is dependant on the recovery of mites from deep skin scrapings. Mites can easily be identified as *Demodex*, but specialist keys are required for specific identification (19).

2. Diagnosis of scabies or mange

A firm diagnosis of scabies or mange must be made on the recovery and identification of the mite from the affected hosts. Visual examination of a suspect mange lesion may reveal the larger mites (e.g. *Psoroptes*), but in most cases it is necessary to take skin scrapings from the edge of visible lesions. Specialist illustrated keys should be consulted in order to identify the causative organism (3).

An indication of the presence of *Psoroptes* mites is the reaction of the host to scratching or rubbing of the affected skin by the operator, where it responds by a nibbling mouth reflex and/or scratching itself. Forced exercise followed by close penning will increase body heat and the associated percutaneous absorption of mite antigens/irritants, inducing the presentation of clinical signs. Skin scrapings are taken from the affected area. In diagnosing scabies it must be borne in mind that the distribution of rash on the body bears no relation to the distribution of mites. Wool or hair should be clipped (and stored for the differential diagnosis of other ectoparasites or mycoses). The area selected for scraping should be the moist part or the edge of the lesion. If sarcoptic mange is suspected, the scraping should be taken from the hairless area or where pruritus or pimples are seen. In psoroptic mange of sheep (sheep scab) the area selected is the edge of the progressing lesion, but scrapings can be taken from any part of the lesion for *Psoroptes* infestations of rabbits or cattle. In general, for mites living on the skin surface (i.e. *Psoroptes* or *Chorioptes*) scrapings should be taken with the scalpel blade held at an acute angle, shaving rather than scraping off the outer epidermis. *Demodex, Psorobia* or *Sarcoptes* are found burrowing into the skin and the scalpel blade should be held at right angles and the skin scraped until it oozes blood. A drop of glycerine or liquid paraffin put on the skin or scalpel blade before the skin is scraped will aid in the collection of mites (21). In pustular demodectic mange, mites are usually abundant and can be demonstrated on examination of the cheesy contents of an expressed or incised pustule. In the case of squamous lesions, a deep scraping may be necessary. In cases of ear mange (canker) in cats, dogs or rabbits, the scabby material within the external ear may be detached with blunt-ended forceps. A vacuum cleaner technique for collecting mange mites has been found to be useful and more sensitive than skin scraping (17). These authors found *Cheyletiella, Sarcoptes, Psoroptes, Otodectes, Demodex* and forage mites from infested dogs, sheep or swine, using 10% KOH treatment of the collected material before microscopic examination.

In suspected cases of otoacariasis (*Otodectes* or *Psoroptes*), in the ears of cats, dogs, rabbits, sheep and goats, live mites can be observed through auroscopic examination of the external ear canal (EAC), but this technique may be difficult if applied to larger animals or large numbers of animals. In this situation, it may be necessary to swab the EAC. Suitable sized swabs are inserted into the EAC until resistance is met, then gently twisted and removed. Care must be taken that the swabs enter the EAC and not the blind pouches of the tragus. Care should also be taken with young animals.

Skin scrapings or ear swabs should be immediately transferred into small tubes that can be securely stoppered or into 'self sealing' envelopes. Live *Chorioptes, Otodectes, Psoroptes* and *Sarcoptes* can easily be seen during direct examination of the original skin scraping or ear swab under a dissecting microscope (×40) with overhead lighting. Mites will be active after incubation of the sample at 37°C for 30 minutes and can easily be transferred to microscope slides using a mounted needle.

Mites can be mounted in either Berlese's fluid (gum chloral), Vitzhums' fluid, Hoyer's medium or Heinze's modified PVA medium (10). Put a drop of medium on the centre of the slide and transfer the specimen into it by means of a fine brush or mounted needle, and remove air bubbles with a needle. Put the cover-slip on its' edge to the side of the medium and let it down slowly using a needle and then press slightly with the needle. If there is too much medium the pressure will force some of it out. If there is too little medium, add small drops at a time, letting it flow under the cover-slip. After mounting allow the slides to dry at room temperature for 5–7 days before ringing with nail varnish or another nonsoluble sealant. The drying time can be decreased by placing the slides in an oven (40–45°C) for at least 2 days.

To locate dead mites and live mites of smaller mite species (e.g. *Demodex*), the scraping will have to be processed in hot potassium hydroxide. Large amounts of material (up to 5.0 g) can be placed in a glass boiling tube and covered with 10% potassium hydroxide. The tube is then placed in a beaker of water, which is gradually brought to the boil. After boiling for 5–10 minutes the digest is allowed to cool and then centrifuged at 600 ***g*** (2000 rpm) for 10 minutes. Prolonged boiling should be avoided as the mites may eventually disintegrate. Faster centrifugation may be required for smaller species. The supernatant is quickly decanted and the deposit examined microscopically. Alternatively, small numbers of specimens can be placed in lactic acid on a glass cavity (indented) slide. The slide is then passed constantly over a bunsen burner or spirit lamp flame. Care must be taken that the slide does not get too hot, as escaping body gases in the mite may cause the mites to 'jump'. If smoke appears on the surface of the fluid, the process is too hot. These methods are necessary to clear out the opaque body contents in order to prepare the mites for microscopic examination. It is advisable to carry out both these methods in a cabinet with an extractor fan due to the caustic fumes released.

Potential zoonotic problems may occur when handling infested animals or diagnostic material containing *Cheyletiella*, *Sarcoptes*, *Notoedres* or *Trixacara*. Faeces or cuticular debris from any mite species may be a hazard to those prone to house dust mite *(Dermatophagoides pteronyssinus)* allergy.

3. Serological tests

An enzyme linked immunosorbent assay (ELISA) for the serological diagnosis of sarcoptic mange in dogs and pigs is used in Sweden (5, 6) and is currently used in the porcine scabies eradication campaigns in Sweden (14) and Switzerland (16). ELISA techniques have been developed to monitor *Psoroptes* infestations of sheep, cattle and nondomesticated animals (7, 8, 12, 13, 18, 26), but none is in routine use. However, ELISAs are in routine use by researchers for detection of specific antibodies to *S. scabiei* (1, 2).

B. REQUIREMENTS FOR VACCINES AND DIAGNOSTIC BIOLOGICALS

There are no commercial vaccines available to protect animals against mange mites.

REFERENCES

1. Arlian L.G., Morgan M.S., Rapp C.M. & Vyszenski-Moher D.L. (1996). The development of protective immunity in canine scabies. *Vet. Parasitol.*, **62**, 133–142.

2. Arlian L.G., Morgan M.S., Vyszenski-Moher D.L. & Stemmer B.L. (1994). *Sarcoptes scabiei*: The circulating antibody response and induced immunity to scabies. *Exp. Parasitol.*, **78**, 37–50.

3. Baker A.S. (1999). Mites and Ticks of Domestic Animals. An Identification Guide and Information Source. The Natural History Museum, London. Her Majesty's Stationery Office, UK.

4. Bates P.G. (1999). Inter- and intra-specific variation within the genus *Psoroptes* (Acari: Psoroptidae). *Vet. Parasitol.*, **83**, 201–217.

5. Bornstein S. & Zakrisson G. (1993). Humoral antibody response to experimental *Sarcoptes scabiei* var *vulpes* infection in the dog. *Vet. Dermatol.*, **4**, 107–110.

6. Bornstein S. & Zakrisson G. (1993). Clinical picture and antibody response in pigs infected by *Sarcoptes scabiei* var *suis*. *Vet. Dermatol.*, **4**, 123–131.

7. Boyce W.M., Jessup D.A. & Clark R.K. (1991). Serodiagnostic antibody responses to *Psoroptes* spp. Infestations in bighorn sheep. *J. Wildl. Dis.*, **27**, 10–15.

8. Boyce W.M., Mazet J.A.K., Mellies J., Gardner I., Clark R.K. & Jessup D.A. (1991). Kinetic ELISA for the detection of antibodies to *Psoroptes* sp. (Acari. Psoroptidae) in bighorn sheep *(Ovis canadensis)*. *J. Parasitol.*, **27**, 692–696.

9. Desch C.E. & Nutting W.B. (1972). *Demodex folliculorum* (Simon) and *D. brevis* Akbulatova of man. redescription and reevaluation. *J. Parasitol.*, **58**, 169–177.

10. Evans G.O. (1992). Principles of Acarology. CAB International, Wallingford, Oxon OX10 8DE, UK.

11. Fain A. (1968). Etude de la variabilite de *Sarcoptes scabiei* avec une revision des Sarcoptidae. *Acta Zool. Pathol. Antverp.*, **47**, 1–196.

12. Fisher W.F. (1983). Development of serum antibody activity as determined by Enzyme linked Immunosorbent assay in *Psoroptes ovis* (Acarina: Psoroptidae) antigens in cattle infested with *P. ovis*. *Vet. Parasitol.*, **13**, 1218–1219.

13. FISHER W.R., GUILLOT F.S. & COLE N.A. (1986). Development and decline of serum antibody activity to *Psoroptes ovis* antigens and infested cattle in an endemic and non-endemic scabies area of Texas. *Exp. Appl. Acarol.*, **2**, 239–248.

14. JACOBSON M., BORNSTEIN S. & WALLGREN P. (1999). The efficacy of simplified eradication strategies against sarcoptic mange mite infections in swine herds monitored by an ELISA. *Vet. Parasitol.*, **81**, 249–258.

15. KETTLE D.S. (1995). Medical and Veterinary Entomology, Second Edition. CAB International, Wallingford, Oxon OX10 8DE, UK.

16. KIRCHER P. & ZIMMERMANN W. (1999). Serologische Bestandesuntersuchung und Sanierungsuberwachung der *Sarcoptes scabiei* var *suis* Infektion: eine seroepidemiologische Studie in raudefreien und chronisch infizierten Betrieben. *Schweiz. Arch. Tierheil.*, **144**, 567–573.

17. KLAYMAN E. & SCHILLHORN VAN VEEN T.W. (1981). Diagnosis of Ectoparasitism. *Mod. Vet. Pract.*, **62**, 767–771.

18. LONNEUX J.F., NGUYEN T.Q., DELHEZ M. & LOSSON B.J. (1997). Antibody response after treatment in cattle affected with *Psoroptes ovis*. *Res. Vet. Sci.*, **63**, 57–60.

19. NUTTING W.B. (1967). Hair follicle mites (*Demodex* spp.) of medical and veterinary concern. *Cornell Vet.*, **66**, 214–231.

20. ROSEN S., YERUHAM I. & HADANI A. (1989). *Chorioptes texanus* (Hirst 1924), Psoroptidae on cattle in Israel. *Acarologia*, **30**, 373–376.

21. SMITH E.K. (1988). How to detect common skin mites through skin scrapings. *Vet. Med.*, 165–170.

22. SWEATMAN G.K. (1957). Life history, non-specificity and revision of the genus *Chorioptes*, a parasitic mite of herbivores. *Can. J. Zool.*, **35**, 641–689.

23. SWEATMAN G.K. (1958). On the life history and validity of the species in *Psoroptes*, a genus of mange mites. *Can. J. Zool.*, **36**, 905–929.

24. SWEATMAN G.K. (1958). The biology of *Otodectes cynotis*, the ear canker mite of carnivores. *Can. J. Zool.*, **36**, 849–862.

25. WALKER A. (1994). Arthropods of Humans and Domestic Animals. A Guide to Preliminary Identification. Chapman and Hall, London, UK.

26. WASSALL D.A., KIRKWOOD A.C., BATES P.G. & SINCLAIR I.J. (1978). Enzyme linked immunosorbent assay for the detection of antibodies to the sheep scab mite *Psoroptes ovis*. *Res. Vet. Sci.*, **43**, 34–35.

27. ZAHLER M., ESSIG A., GOTHE H. & RINDER H. (1999). Molecular analyses suggests monospecificity of the genus *Sarcoptes* (Acari: Sarcoptidae). *Int. J. Parasitol.*, **29**, 759–766.

*

* *

CHAPTER X.15.

TROPILAELAPS INFESTATION OF HONEY BEES (*Tropilaelaps clareae, T. koenigerum*)

SUMMARY

The mites Tropilaelaps clareae *Delfinado and Baker and* T. koenigerum *Delfinado-Baker and Baker (Mesostigmata: Laelapidae), are parasites of the honey bee brood. Feeding on bee larvae and pupae causes brood malformation, death of bees and subsequent colony decline or absconding. Development requires about 1 week, and the mites are dispersed on bees.*

Identification of the agent: *An infestation by* Tropilaelaps *can be recognised either visually or by examining bee debris. Irregular brood pattern, dead or malformed immatures, bees with malformed wings that crawl at the hive's entrance, and especially the presence of fast-running, large, red-brown, elongated mites on the combs, are diagnostic for the presence of* T. clareae. *An early diagnosis can be made after opening brood cells and finding immature and adult mites therein. The hive (colony) may be treated with various chemicals that cause the mites to drop off combs and bees. The debris can then be examined visually or by using a flotation procedure.*

Serological tests: *No serological tests are applicable.*

Requirements for vaccines and diagnostic biologicals: *No biological products are available.*

A. DIAGNOSTIC TECHNIQUES

Tropilaelaps clareae occurs in Asia, from Iran in the north-west to Papua New Guinea in the south-east (9), whereas *T. koenigerum* is known only from Sri Lanka and Nepal (5). *Tropilaelaps clareae* can easily be distributed by *A. mellifera*. There has been a single report of *T. clareae* from Africa (9), but this record has not been subsequently substantiated (10).

The colonising *Tropilaelaps* female (or females; as many as a dozen may occur in individual cells) places from one to four eggs on mature bee larvae shortly before capping. The drone brood is preferred by *Tropilaelaps* and may be almost 100% parasitised (2). The mite progeny, usually one male and several females, feed and seriously damage the bee brood. Development of the mite requires about 1 week. The adults, including the initial female, emerge with the adult bee and search for new hosts. The short life-cycle, as well as a very brief stay on adult bees, explains why populations of *T. clareae* increase faster than those of *Varroa* mite. When both *T. clareae* and *Varroa destructor* infest the same colony, the former may out-compete the *Varroa* mite (2). The natural host of both species of *Tropilaelaps* is the giant Asian bee *Apis dorsata*, but in addition *T. clareae* was collected from *A. cerana*, *A. florea*, *A. mellifera* and *A. laboriosa*, whereas *T. koenigerum* occurs on A. *laboriosa* and *A. dorsata* (5).

Infestation by *Tropilaelaps* is accompanied by irregular brood pattern and death of many bee larvae (up to 50%), of which the cadavers may partially protrude from the cells. Many malformed bees occur, with distorted abdomens, stubby wings and deformed or missing legs. Some of the affected bees crawl at the hive's entrance (1). In addition, perforated cappings are seen, the result of sanitation activities of the workers, which evict the infested bee pupae or young adults. In some cases the colony absconds, carrying the mites to a new location.

Phoretic survival on bees is quite short (only 1–2 days) because *Tropilaelaps* cannot pierce the integument of adult bees. Gravid mite females will die within 2 days unless they deposit their eggs (11).

1. Identification of the agent

a) Colony and brood examination

The first sign of an infestation by *T. clareae* is often the occurrence of large (almost 1 mm in length), red-brown, elongated mites on the combs or on adult bees. *Tropilaelaps koenigerum* is slightly smaller, only about 0.7 mm in length (4). Both species of *Tropilaelaps* can easily be recognised and separated from the *Varroa* mite using a ×10 magnifying glass. The body of the *Varroa* mite is wider than it is long and it moves slowly, whereas the body of *Tropilaelaps* is elongated, with a heavily sclerotised epigynial (or holoventral) shield, and it is a fast-running mite. When monitoring honey bee colonies for its presence, an examination of both drone and worker brood may provide an early indication of attack. The younger mite stages are whitish and may be almost motionless while feeding on their hosts' bodies. Extent of parasitisation can be estimated by opening a predetermined number of brood cells; infestation rates are then calculated as per cent of capped brood containing live mites (3).

b) Debris examination

A precise diagnosis can be made by using an acaricide and knocking off mites on to a sticky board. A white board, coated with white grease, is placed underneath the combs in the colony to catch fallen mites. Strips of plastic-impregnated fluvalinate (Apistan™) or cimiazol trickled on to bees will knock off *T. clareae.* Alternatively, strips of filter paper for fumigation are prepared by soaking in an aqueous solution of 15% potassium nitrate to which two drops of amitraz (usually 12.5%) are added (8). After the paper dries, the strip is ignited and inserted into the hive. The smoke causes many mites to drop off their host bees. Another method is to use plates soaked with 20 ml of 65% formic acid, which are placed in the colonies, near the top (7). The knocked off mites can then be identified visually and may be counted if necessary. Alternatively, the debris can be examined by using a flotation procedure.

2. Serological tests

No serological tests are available for diagnosis.

3. Treatment

In countries with infestations of *T. clareae*, fluvalinate in slow-release formulations controls *T. clareae* (8), as do monthly dustings with sulphur (1) and treatments with formic acid (6). The inability of this mite to feed on adult bees, or to survive outside sealed brood for more than a few days, is being used as a nonchemical control method (11).

B. REQUIREMENTS FOR VACCINES AND DIAGNOSTIC BIOLOGICALS

There are no biological products available.

REFERENCES

1. ATWAL A.S. & GOYAL N.P. (1971). Infestations of honeybee colonies with *Tropilaelaps*, and its control. *J. Apic. Res.*, **10**, 137–142.

2. BURGETT M., AKRATANAKUL P. & MORSE R.A. (1983). *Tropilaelaps clareae*: a parasite of honeybees in south-east Asia. *Bee World*, **64**, 25–28.

3. BURGETT D.M. & KITPRASERT C. (1990). Evaluation of Apistan™ as a control for *Tropilaelaps clareae* (Acari: Laelapidae), an Asian honey bee brood mite parasite. *Am. Bee J.*, **130**, 51–53.

4. DELFINADO-BAKER M. & BAKER E.W. (1982). A new species of *Tropilaelaps* parasitic on honey bees. *Am. Bee J.*, **122**, 416–417.

5. DELFINADO-BAKER M., BAKER E.W. & PHOON A.C.G. (1989). Mites (Acari) associated with bees (Apidae) in Asia, with description of a new species. *Am. Bee. J.*, **122**, 416–17.

6. GARG R., SHARMA O.P. & DOGRA G.S. (1984). Formic acid: an effective acaricide against *Tropilaelaps clareae* Delfinado & Baker (Laelapidae: Acarina) and its effect on the brood and longevity of honey bees. *Am. Bee J.*, **124**, 736–738.

7. HOPPE H., RITTER W. & STEPHEN E. (1989). The control of parasitic bee mites: *Varroa jacobsoni* and *Tropilaelaps clareae* with formic acid. *Am. Bee J.*, **129**, 739–742.

8. LUBINEVSKI Y., STERN Y., SLABEZKI Y., LENSKI Y. ,BEN YOSSEF H. & GERSON U. (1988). Control of *Varroa jacobsoni* and *Tropilaelaps clareae* mites using Mavrik under subtropical and tropical climates. *Am. Bee J.*, **128**, 48–52.

9. MATHESON A. (1993). World bee health report. *Bee World*, **74**, 176–212.

10. MATTHESON A. (1997). Country records for honey bee diseases, parasites and pests. *In:* Honey Bee Pests, Predators, and Diseases, Third Edition, 2, 13–31, Morse R.M. & Flottum P.K., eds. Medina OH, A.I. Root, USA, 587–602.

11. WOYKE J. (1987). Length of stay of the parasitic mite *Tropilaelaps clareae* outside sealed honeybee brood cells as a basis for its effective control. *J. Apic. Res.*, **26**, 104–109.

*

* *

PART 4

OIE REFERENCE EXPERTS

AND DISEASE INDEX

LIST OF OIE REFERENCE LABORATORIES IN 2000*

List A diseases

2.1.1. Foot and mouth disease – Fièvre aphteuse – Fiebre aftosa

Dr R.P. Kitching
Institute for Animal Health, Pirbright Laboratory, Ash Road
Pirbright, Woking, Surrey GU24 ONF
UNITED KINGDOM
Tel: (44.1483) 23.24.41, Fax: (44.1483) 23.24.48
E-mail: paul.kitching@bbsrc.ac.uk

Dr R. Allende
Centro Panamericano de Fiebre Aftosa - OPS/OMS
Av. President Kennedy 7778
Sao Bento, Duque de Caxias
ZC 20054-40 Rio de Janeiro
BRAZIL
Tel: (55.21) 671.31.28
Fax: (55.21) 671.23.87
E-mail: rallende@panafoftosa.ops-oms.org

Dr M. Proteau
Botswana Vaccine Institute, Department of Animal Health
and Production, Broadhurst Industrial Site, Lejara Road
Private Bag 0031, Gaborone
BOTSWANA
Tel: (267) 31.27.11, Fax: (267) 35.67.98, Telex: 2535 BD
E-mail: tmbvi@mega.bw

Dr V.M. Zakharov
Deputy Director
All-Russian Research Institute for Animal Health
600900 Yur'evets, Vladimir
RUSSIA
Tel: (7.0922) 26.06.14/26.19.14, Fax: (7.0922) 24.36.75/23.72.61
Telex: 218124 URAL RUS, E-mail: sinko@arriah.elcom.ru

2.1.2. Vesicular stomatitis – Stomatite vésiculeuse – Estomatitis vesicular

Dr S.L. Swenson
National Veterinary Services Laboratories, P.O. Box 844
Ames, IA 50010
UNITED STATES OF AMERICA
Tel: (1.515) 663.75.51, Fax: (1.515) 663.73.48
E-mail: sabrina.l.swenson@aphis.usda.gov

Dr R. Allende
Centro Panamericano de Fiebre Aftosa - OPS/OMS
Av. President Kennedy 7778
Sao Bento, Duque de Caxias
ZC 20054-40 Rio de Janeiro
BRAZIL
Tel: (55.21) 671.31.28
Fax: (55.21) 671.23.87
E-mail: rallende@panafoftosa.ops-oms.org

2.1.3. Swine vesicular disease – Maladie vésiculeuse du porc – Enfermedad vesicular porcina

Dr E. Brocchi
Istituto Zooprofilattico Sperimentale della Lombardia e dell'Emilia
Romagna 'B. Ubertini', Via A. Bianchi n° 9, 25124 Brescia
ITALY
Tel: (39.030) 229.03.10, Fax: (39.030) 229.03.77
E-mail: ebrocchi@bs.izs.it

Dr R.P. Kitching
Institute for Animal Health, Pirbright Laboratory, Ash Road
Pirbright, Woking, Surrey GU24 ONF
UNITED KINGDOM
Tel: (44.1483) 23.24.41, Fax: (44.1483) 23.24.48
E-mail: paul.kitching@bbsrc.ac.uk

* For certain diseases, two institutions have been jointly designated as OIE Reference Laboratory or Collaborating Centre. Where this occurs, the superscript (1) or (2) will be placed after the name of the designated Reference Expert.

2.1.4. Rinderpest – Peste bovine – Peste bovina
2.1.5. Peste des petits ruminants – Peste des petits ruminants – Peste de pequeños rumiantes

Dr J. Anderson
Institute for Animal Health, Pirbright Laboratory, Ash Road
Pirbright, Woking, Surrey GU24 ONF
UNITED KINGDOM
Tel: (44.1483) 23.24.41, Fax: (44.1483) 23.24.48
E-mail: john.anderson@bbsrc.ac.uk

Dr J.S. Wafula & Dr H.M. Wamwayi
Kenya Agricultural Research Institute, National Veterinary
Research Centre, Muguga, P.O. Box 32, Kikuyu
KENYA
Tel: (254.154) 32.450/33.412/32.106/32.107,
Fax: (254.154) 32.450

Dr G. Libeau
CIRAD/EMVT, Campus international de Baillarguet
Montferriez-sur-Lez, B.P. 5035, 34032 Montpellier Cedex 01
FRANCE
Tel: 33 (0)4 67.59.38.50, Fax: 33 (0)4 67.59.37.98
E-mail: genevieve.libeau@cirad.fr

2.1.6. Contagious bovine pleuropneumonia – Péripneumonie contagieuse bovine – Perineumonía contagiosa bovina

Dr J.L. Martel
AFSSA Lyon, Laboratoire de pathologie bovine
31 avenue Tony Garnier, BP 7033, 69342 Lyon Cedex 07
FRANCE
Tel: 33 (0)4 78.72.65.43, Fax: 33 (0)4 78.61.91.45
E-mail: jl.martel@lyon.afssa.fr

Dr J. Regalla
Laboratório Nacional de Investigação Veterinária (LNIV),
Estrada de Benfica 701, 1500 Lisboa
PORTUGAL
Tel: (351.21) 711.53.39, Fax: (351.21) 711.52.36
E-mail: bib.lniv@mail.telepac.pt

Dr El Haji Tall
Organisation for African Unity/Interafrican Bureau for Animal
Resources, P.O. Box 30786, Nairobi
KENYA
Tel: (254.2) 33.85.44/33.20.46, Fax: (254.2) 33.20.46
E-mail: alhaji.tall@oau-ibar.org

Dr F.G. Santini
CESME, Istituto Zooprofilattico Sperimentale dell'Abruzzo
e del Molise 'G. Caporale', Via Campo Boario, 64100 Teramo
ITALY
Tel: (39.0861) 33.22.31, Fax: (39.0861) 33.22.51

2.1.7. Lumpy skin disease – Dermatose nodulaire contagieuse – Dermatosis nodular contagiosa

Dr R.P. Kitching
Institute for Animal Health, Pirbright Laboratory, Ash Road
Pirbright, Woking, Surrey GU24 ONF
UNITED KINGDOM
Tel: (44.1483) 23.24.41, Fax: (44.1483) 23.24.48
E-mail: paul.kitching@bbsrc.ac.uk

Dr G.H. Gerdes
Onderstepoort Veterinary Institute, Private Bag X05
Onderstepoort 0110
SOUTH AFRICA
Tel: (27.12) 529.91.14, Fax: (27.12) 529.94.18
E-mail: magda@moon.ovi.ac.za

2.1.8. Rift Valley fever – Fièvre de la Vallée du Rift – Fiebre del Valle del Rift

Dr G.H. Gerdes
Onderstepoort Veterinary Institute, Private Bag X05
Onderstepoort 0110
SOUTH AFRICA
Tel: (27.12) 529.91.14, Fax: (27.12) 529.94.18
E-mail: magda@moon.ovi.ac.za

2.1.9. Bluetongue – Fievre catarrhale du mouton – Lengua azul

Dr J.T. Paweska
Onderstepoort Veterinary Institute, Private Bag X05
Onderstepoort 0110
SOUTH AFRICA
Tel: (27.12) 529.91.17, Fax: (27.12) 529.94.18 or 565.65.73
E-mail : janusz@moon.ovi.ac.za

Dr E.N. Ostlund
Diagnostic Virology Laboratory, National Veterinary Services Laboratories, P.O. Box 844, Ames, IA 50010
UNITED STATES OF AMERICA
Tel: (1.515) 663.75.51, Fax: (1.515) 663.73.48
E-mail: eileen.n.ostlund@aphis.usda.gov

Dr J. Anderson
Institute for Animal Health, Pirbright Laboratory, Ash Road
Pirbright, Woking, Surrey GU24 ONF
UNITED KINGDOM
Tel: (44.1483) 23.24.41, Fax: (44.1483) 23.24.48
E-mail: john.anderson@bbsrc.ac.uk

Dr B.T. Eaton
CSIRO, Australian Animal Health Laboratory, Division of Animal Health, Institute of Animal Production and Processing, Ryrie Street
P.O. Bag 24, Geelong, Victoria 3220
AUSTRALIA
Tel: (61.3) 52.27.50.00, Fax: (61.3) 52.27.55.55
E-mail: bryan.eaton@dah.csiro.au

2.1.10. Sheep pox and goat pox – Clavelée et variole caprine – Viruela ovina y viruela caprina

Dr R.P. Kitching
Institute for Animal Health, Pirbright Laboratory, Ash Road
Pirbright, Woking, Surrey GU24 ONF
UNITED KINGDOM
Tel: (44.1483) 23.24.41, Fax: (44.1483) 23.24.48
E-mail: paul.kitching@bbsrc.ac.uk

Dr M. Hessami
RAZI Vaccine and Serum Research Institute, P.O. Box 11365
1558 Tehran
IRAN
Tel: (98.261) 452.005/452.009/311.97.08,
Fax: (98.261) 452 194/454 658,
E-mail: rirc@neda.net.ir

2.1.11. African horse sickness – Peste équine – Peste equina

Dr J.T. Paweska
Onderstepoort Veterinary Institute, Private Bag X05
Onderstepoort 0110
SOUTH AFRICA
Tel: (27.12) 529.91.17, Fax: (27.12) 529.94.18 or 565.65.73
E-mail : janusz@moon.ovi.ac.za

Dr P.S. Mellor
Institute for Animal Health, Pirbright Laboratory, Ash Road
Pirbright, Woking, Surrey GU24 ONF
UNITED KINGDOM
Tel: (44.1483) 23.24.41, Fax: (44.1483) 23.24.48
E-mail: philip.mellor@bbsrc.ac.uk

Dr J.M. Sánchez-Vizcaíno[1]
Centro de Investigación en Sanidad Animal, Instituto Nacional de Investigación y Tecnología Agraria y Alimentaria (CISA-INIA)
28130 Valdeolmos, (Madrid)
SPAIN
Tel: (34.91) 620.23.00, Fax: (34.91) 620.22.47

Dr C. Rubio[2]
Laboratorio de Sanidad y Producción Animal de Madrid
Carretera de Madrid-Irún, Desviación Algete, km 5,4
28110 Algete, (Madrid)
SPAIN
Tel: (34.91) 629.03.00, Fax: (34.91) 629.05.98

2.1.12. African swine fever – Peste porcine africaine – Peste porcina africana

Dr D.A. Gregg
National Veterinary Services Laboratories, APHIS
Foreign Animal Disease Diagnostic Laboratory (Plum Island)
USDA, P.O. Box 848, Greenport, NY 11944
UNITED STATES OF AMERICA
Tel: (1.631) 323.33.79, Fax: (1.631) 323.33.66
E-mail: douglas.a.gregg@aphis.usda.gov

Dr P.J. Wilkinson
Institute for Animal Health, Pirbright Laboratory, Ash Road
Pirbright, Woking, Surrey GU24 ONF
UNITED KINGDOM
Tel: (44.1483) 23.24.41, Fax: (44.1483) 23.24.48

Dr J.M. Sánchez-Vizcaíno
Centro de Investigación en Sanidad Animal, Instituto Nacional de Investigación y Tecnología Agraria y Alimentaria (CISA-INIA)
28130 Valdeolmos, (Madrid)
SPAIN
Tel: (34.91) 620.23.00, Fax: (34.91) 620.22.47

Dr M.L. Penrith
Onderstepoort Veterinary Institute, Agricultural Research Council, Private Bag X6, Onderstepoort 0110
SOUTH AFRICA
Tel: (27.12) 529.91.01, Fax: (27.12) 565.46.67

2.1.13. Classical swine fever – Peste porcine classique – Peste porcina clásica

Dr J. Pasick
Canadian Food Inspection Agency, National Centre for Foreign Animal Disease, 1015 Arlington Street
Winnipeg, Manitoba R3E 3M4
CANADA
Tel: (1.204) 789.20.01/20.47, Fax: (1.204) 789.20.38
E-mail: jpasick@em.agr.ca

Prof. V. Moennig
Institute of Virology, Hannover Veterinary School
Bünteweg 17, 30539 Hannover
GERMANY
Tel: (49.511) 953.88.40, Fax: (49.511) 953.88.98
E-mail: moennig@viro.tiho-hannover.de

Prof. Dr Z. Pejsak
National Veterinary Research Institute, Partyzantow str. 57
24–100 Pulawy
POLAND
Tel: (48.81) 886.30.51, Fax (48.81) 886.25.95, Telex: 0642401
E-mail: zpejsak@piwet.pulawy.pl

Dr A. Fukusho
Director, Kyushu Research Station, National Veterinary Assay Laboratory
2702 Chuzan, Kagoshima 891-0105, JAPAN
Tel: (81.99) 268.20.78, Fax: (81.99) 268.30.88
E-mail: akifuku@sat.affrc.go.jp

Dr D.J. Paton
Department of Virology
VLA Weybridge, New Haw, Addlestone, Surrey KT15 3NB
UNITED KINGDOM
Tel: (44.1932) 35.72.85, Fax: (44.1932) 35.72.39
E-mail: d.paton@vla.maff.gsi.gov.uk

2.1.14. Highly pathogenic avian influenza – Influenza aviaire hautement pathogène – Influenza aviar altamente patógena
2.1.15. Newcastle disease – Maladie de Newcastle – Enfermedad de Newcastle

Dr D.J. Alexander
VLA Weybridge, New Haw, Addlestone, Surrey KT15 3NB
UNITED KINGDOM
Tel: (44.1932) 34.11.11, Fax: (44.1932) 34.70.46
E-mail: d.alexander@vla.maff.gsi.gov.uk

Prof. E.F. Kaleta
Institut für Geflügelkrankheiten der Justus-Liebig-Universität
Giessen, Frankfurter Strasse 91, 35392 Giessen
GERMANY
Tel: (49.641) 993.84.30, Fax: (49.641) 20.15.48
E-mail: erhard.f.kaleta@vetmed.uni-giessen.de

Dr I. Capua
Istituto Zooprofilattico Sperimentale delle Venezie, Virology Department, Via Romea 14/1, 35020 Legnaro, Padova
ITALY
Tel: (39.049) 808.43.69 Fax: (39.049) 808.43.60
Email: icapua.izs@interbusiness.it

Dr A.J. Della-Porta
CSIRO, Australian Animal Health Laboratory, Division of Animal Health, Institute of Animal Production and Processing
Ryrie Street Private Bag 24, Geelong, Victoria 3220
AUSTRALIA
Tel: (61.3) 5227.5000, Fax: (61.3) 5227.5555
E-mail: tony.della-porta@dah.csiro.au

Dr B. Panigrahy
National Veterinary Services Laboratories, P.O. Box 844
Ames, IA 50010
UNITED STATES OF AMERICA
Tel: (1.515) 663.75.51, Fax: (1.515) 663.73.48
E-mail: brundaban.panigrahy@aphis.usda.gov

List B diseases

Multiple species diseases/Maladies communes à plusieurs espèces/Enfermedades comunes a varias especies

2.2.2. Aujeszky's disease – Maladie d'Aujeszky – Enfermedad de Aujeszky

Prof. B. Toma(1)
Services des maladies contagieuses, Ecole Nationale Vétérinaire d'Alfort, 7 avenue du Général de Gaulle
94704 Maisons-Alfort Cedex
FRANCE
Tel: 33 (0)1 43.68.73.34, Fax: 33 (0)1 43.96.71.31
E-mail: toma@vet-alfort.fr

Dr P. Vannier(2)
AFSSA Ploufragan, Laboratoire d'études et de recherches avicoles et porcines, Zoopôle Beaucemaine-Les Croix
BP 53, 22440 Ploufragan
FRANCE
Tel: 33 (0)2 96.01.62.50, Fax: 33 (0)2 96.01.62.53
E-mail: p.vannier@ploufragan.afssa.fr

Dr R.V. Pálfi
Central Veterinary Institute, Tábornok u. 2., 1149 Budapest
HUNGARY
Tel: (36.1) 252.75.33, Fax: (36.1) 222.60.69, Telex: 22.4430

Dr A.T.J. Bianchi
Institute for Animal Science and Health (ID Lelystad)
Research Branch Houtribweg, P.O. Box 65
8200 AB Lelystad
THE NETHERLANDS
Tel: (31.320) 236.808, Fax: (31.320) 23.668
E-mail: a.t.j.bianchi@id.wag-ur.nl

Dr S.L. Swenson
National Veterinary Services Laboratories, P.O. Box 844
Ames, IA 50010
UNITED STATES OF AMERICA
Tel: (1.515) 663.75.51, Fax: (1.515) 663.73.48
E-mail: sabrina.l.swenson@aphis.usda.gov

2.2.3. Echinococcosis/hydatidosis – Echinococcose/hydatidose – Equinococosis/hidatidosis

Prof. M. Kamiya
Parasitology Laboratory, Graduate School of Veterinary Medicine
Hokkaido University, Kita-18, Nishi-9, Kita-ku, Sapporo 060-0818
JAPAN
Tel: (81.11) 706.51.98, Fax: (81.11) 706.51.90
E-mail: kamiya@vetmed.hokudai.ac.jp

Dr P.S. Craig
Department of Biological Sciences, University of Salford
Salford M5 4WT
UNITED KINGDOM
Tel: (44.161) 295.55.48, Fax: (44.161) 295.52.10
E-mail: p.s.craig@salford.ac.uk

Prof. A. Dakkak & Prof. H. Ouhelli
Département de Parasitologie, Institut Agronomique et Vétérinaire
Hassan II, BP 6202, Rabat-Instituts
MOROCCO
Tel/Fax: (212.37) 77.64.32, E-mail: dakkak@maghrebnet.net.ma

Dr P. Economides
Director Veterinary Services, Ministry of Agriculture, Natural Resources and Environment, 1417 Nicosia
CYPRUS
Tel: (357.2) 80.52.00/80.52.01, Fax: (357.2) 33.28.03
E-mail: vet.services@cytanet.com.cy

2.2.4. Leptospirosis – Leptospirose – Leptospirosis

Dr R.A. Hartskeerl
Royal Tropical Institute, N.H. Swellengrebel Laboratory of Tropical Hygiene, Division of Health, Department of Biomedical Research, Meibergdreef 39, 1105 AZ Amsterdam
THE NETHERLANDS
Tel: (31.20) 566.54.54, Fax: (31.20) 697.18.41
E-mail: r.hartskeerl@kit.nl

Dr L. Samartino(1)
Instituto de Bacteriología, Centro de Investigaciones en Ciencias Veterinarias (CICV), Instituto Nacional de Tecnología Agropecuaria (INTA), Castelar, Casilla de Correo 77
1708 Morón, Pcia. de Buenos Aires
ARGENTINA
Tel: (54.11) 46.21.12.89, Fax: (54.11) 46.21.17.12
E-mail: lsanma@inta.gov.ar

Dr Gleyre T.D. de Mazzonelli(2)
Gerencia de Laboratorios (GELAB), Servicio Nacional de Sanidad y Calidad Agroalimentaria (SENASA), Av. Alexander Fleming 1653, 1640 Martínez, Pcia. de Buenos Aires
ARGENTINA
Tel/Fax: (54.11) 48.36.19.92
Email: dilab@inea.com.ar

Dr W.A. Ellis
Department of Agriculture, Veterinary Sciences Division
Stoney Road, Stormont, Belfast BT4 3SD, Northern Ireland
UNITED KINGDOM
Tel: (44.1232) 52.00.11, Fax: (44.1232) 52.57.73
E-mail: bill.ellis@dardni.gov.uk

Dr D. Miller
National Veterinary Services Laboratories, P.O. Box 844
Ames, IA 50010
UNITED STATES OF AMERICA
Tel: (1.515) 663.75.68, Fax: (1.515) 663.75.69
E-mail: david.a.miller@aphis.usda.gov

Dr L.D. Smythe
WHO Collaborating Centre for Leptospirosis, Queensland Health Scientific Services, 39 Kessels Road, Coopers Plains, P.O. Box 594, Archerfield, QUeensland 4108
AUSTRALIA
Tel: (61.7) 32.74.90.01 Fax: (61.7) 32.74.90.03
Email: lee_smythe@health.qld.gov.au

2.2.5. Rabies – Rage – Rabia

Dr A. Wandeler
Centre of Expertise for Rabies, Animal Diseases Research Institute, 3851 Fallowfield Road, P.O. Box 11300, Station H
Nepean, Ontario K2H 8P9
CANADA
Tel: (1.613) 228.66.98, Fax: (1.613) 228.66.69
E-mail: wandelera@em.agr.ca

Dr J. Barrat & Dr F. Cliquet
AFSSA Nancy, Laboratoire d'études sur la rage et la pathologie des animaux sauvages, Domaine de Pixérécourt
BP 9, 54220 Malzéville
FRANCE
Tel: 33 (0)3 83.29.89.50, Fax: 33 (0)3 83.29.89.59
E-mail: jbarrat@nancy.afssa.fr; fcliquet@nancy.afssa.fr

Dr J.H. Cox
Bundesforschungsanstalt für Viruskrankheiten der Tiere
Paul-Ehrlich-Str. 28, P.O. Box 1149, 72001 Tübingen
GERMANY
Tel: (49.7071) 967.206/226, Fax: (49.7071) 967.105
E-mail: james.cox@tue.bfav.de

Dr J. Bingham
Onderstepoort Veterinary Institute, Private Bag X05
Onderstepoort 0110
SOUTH AFRICA
Tel: (27.12) 529.94.20, Fax: (27.12) 529.93.90
E-mail: johnb@moon.ovi.ac.za

2.2.6. Paratuberculosis – Paratuberculose – Paratuberculosis

Dr R. Condron
Division of Animal Health, Victorian Institute of Animal Science
475-485 Mickleham Road, Attwood, Victoria 3049
AUSTRALIA
Tel: (61.3) 92.17.42.00, Fax: (61.3) 92.17.42.99
E-mail: condronr@woody.agvic.gov.au

Mme M.-F. Thorel
AFSSA Alfort, Laboratoire central de recherches vétérinaires
22 rue Pierre Curie, BP 67, 94703 Maisons-Alfort Cedex
FRANCE
Tel: 33 (0)1 49.77.13.00, Fax: 33 (0)1 43.68.97.62
E-mail: mf.thorel@alfort.afssa.fr

Dr A. Bernardelli
Gerencia de Laboratorios (GELAB), Servicio Nacional de Sanidad y Calidad Agroalimentaria (SENASA), Av. Alexander Fleming 1653, (1640) Martínez, Pcia. de Buenos Aires
ARGENTINA
Tel/Fax: (54.11) 48.36.19.92

Brucellosis – Brucellose – Brucellosis†

Dr K. Noeckler
Federal Institute of Consumers Health Protection
and Veterinary Medicine, Diedersdorfer Weg 1, 12277
P.O. Box 330013, 14191 Berlin
GERMANY
Tel: (49.188) 84.12.20.53 Fax: (49.188) 84.12.20.00
E-mail: k.noeckler@bgvv.de

Dr A.P. MacMillan
VLA Weybridge, New Haw, Addlestone, Surrey KT15 3NB
UNITED KINGDOM
Tel: (44.1932) 34.11.11, Fax: (44.1932) 34.70.46
E-mail: a.p.macmillan@vla.maff.gsi.gov.uk

Dr B. Garin-Bastuji
AFSSA Alfort, Unité Zoonoses Bactériennes
22 rue Pierre Curie, BP 67, 94703 Maisons-Alfort Cedex
FRANCE
Tel: 33 (0)1 49.77.13.00, Fax: 33 (0)1 49.77.13.44
E-mail: b.garin@afssa.fr

Dr D. Nannini
CESME, Istituto Zooprofilattico Sperimentale dell'Abruzzo
e del Molise 'G. Caporale', Via Campo Boario, 64100 Teramo
ITALY
Tel: (39.0861) 33.22.41, Fax: (39.0861) 33.22.51
E-mail: dnannini@izs.it

Dr K. Nielsen
Canadian Food Inspection Agency, Animal Diseases Research
Institute, 3851 Fallowfield Road, PO Box 11300, Station H
Nepean, Ontario K2H 8P9
CANADA
Tel: (1.613) 228.66.98, Fax: (1.613) 228.66.68
E-mail: nielsenk@em.agr.ca

Dr M. Banai
Department of Bacteriology, Kimron Veterinary Institute
P.O. Box 12, Beit Dagan 50250
ISRAEL
Tel: (972.3) 968.16.98, Fax: (972.3) 968.17.53
E-mail: mbana_vs@netvision.net.il

2.2.9. Trichinellosis – Trichinellose – Triquinelosis

Dr E. Pozio
Istituto Superiore di Sanità, Laboratorio di Parassitologia
Viale Regina Elena 299, 00161 Roma
ITALY
Tel: (39.06) 49.90.23.04, Fax: (39.06) 49.38.70.65
E-mail: pozio@iss.it

Dr A. Gajadhar
Canadian Food Inspection Agency, Centre for Animal Parasitology
116 Veterinary Road, Saskatoon, Saskatchewan S7N 2R3
CANADA
Tel: (1.306) 975.40.71 Fax: (1.306) 975.57.11
Email: agajadhar@em.agr.ca:

2.3.13. Bovine spongiform encephalopathy – Encéphalopathie spongiforme bovine – Encefalopatía espongiforme bovina
X.9. Scrapie – Tremblante – Prurigo lumbar

Dr M. Jeffrey
VLA Weybridge, New Haw, Addlestone, Surrey KT15 3NB
UNITED KINGDOM
Tel: (44.1932) 35.73.06, Fax: (44.1932) 34.70.46
E-mail: m.jeffrey@vla.maff.gsi.gov.uk

Prof. M. Vandevelde
Institute of Animal Neurology, University of Bern
Bremgartenstrasse 109A, 3012 Bern
SWITZERLAND
Tel: (41.31) 631.23.70, Fax: (41.31) 631.25.38
E-mail: vandevelde@itn.unibe.ch

† There are currently four diseases on OIE List B that are included under the umbrella term 'Brucellosis'. These are: 3.2.1.Bovine brucellosis – Brucellose bovine – Brucellosis bovina; 3.3.1. Ovine epididymitis – Epididymite ovine – Epididimitis ovina (*Brucella ovis*); 3.3.2. Caprine and ovine brucellosis – Brucellose caprine et ovine – Brucelosis ovina y caprina (excluding *B. ovis*); and 3.5.2. Porcine brucellosis – Brucellose porcine – Brucelosis porcina.

Cattle diseases/Maladies des bovins/Enfermedades de los bovinos

2.3.3. Bovine tuberculosis – Tuberculose bovine – Tuberculosis bovina

Dr A. Reniero
c/o Dr J. Estupiñán, Director, Instituto Panamericano de Protección de Alimentos y Zoonosis (INPPAZ)
Talcahuano 1660, 1640 Martínez, Pcia. de Buenos Aires
ARGENTINA
Tel: (54.11) 48.36.10.00, Fax: (54.11) 48.36.09.27
E-mail: inppaz@inppaz.ops-oms.org

Dr N.M.A. Palmer
VLA Weybridge, New Haw, Addlestone, Surrey KT15 3NB
UNITED KINGDOM
Tel: (44.1932) 34.11.11 Fax: (44.1932) 34.70.46
Email: n.palmer@vla.maff.gsi.gov.uk

Dr D.V. Cousins
Australian Reference Laboratory for Bovine Tuberculosis
Agriculture Western Australia, Locked Bag N° 4, Bentley Delivery Centre, Bentley WA 6983
AUSTRALIA
Tel: (61.8) 93.68.34.29 Fax: (61.8) 94.74.18.81
E-mail: dcousins@agric.wa.gov.au

Mme M.-F. Thorel‡
AFSSA Alfort, Laboratoire central de recherches vétérinaires
22 rue Pierre Curie, BP 67, 94703 Maisons-Alfort Cedex
FRANCE
Tel: 33 (0)1 49.77.13.00, Fax: 33 (0)1 43.68.97.62
E-mail: mf.thorel@alfort.afssa.fr

2.3.4. Enzootic bovine leukosis – Leucose bovine enzootique – Leucosis bovina enzoótica

Dr L.M.H. Renström
The National Veterinary Institute, Department of Virology
P.O. Box 7073, SVA, S-750 07 Uppsala
SWEDEN
Tel: (46.18) 67.40.00, Fax: (46.18) 67.46.44
E-mail: lena.renstrom@sva.se

Mrs R.E. Lysons
VLA Weybridge, New Haw, Addlestone, Surrey KT15 3NB
UNITED KINGDOM
Tel: (44.1932) 34.11.11, Fax: (44.1932) 34.70.46
E-mail: r.lysons@vla.maff.gsi.gov.uk

Dr D. Beier
Bundesforschungsanstalt für Viruskrankheiten der Tiere
Institute für epidemiologische Diagnostik, Seestraße 55
16868 Wusterhausen/Dosse
GERMANY
Tel: (49.33979) 80.190, Fax: (49.33979) 80.222
E-mail: dagmar.beier@wus.bfav.de

2.3.5. Infectious bovine rhinotracheitis/infectious pustular vulvovaginitis – Rhinotrachéite infectieuse bovine/vulvovaginite pustuleuse infectieuse – Rinotraqueítis infecciosa bovina/vulvovaginitis pustular infecciosa

Dr J.T. van Oirschot
Institute of Animal Science and Health (ID Lelystad), Virology Department, Edelhertweg 15, P.O. Box 65, 8200 AB Lelystad
THE NETHERLANDS
Tel: (31.320) 23.82.13/217, Fax: (31.320) 23.82.25
E-mail: j.t.vanoirschot@id.wag-ur.nl

Dr A. Moussa
AFSSA Lyon, Laboratoire de pathologie bovine
31 avenue Tony Garnier, BP 7033, 69342 Lyon Cedex 07
FRANCE
Tel 33 (0)4 78.72.65.43, Fax: 33 (0)4 78.61.91.45
Email: a.moussa@lyon.afssa.fr

Dr M. Banks
VLA Weybridge, New Haw, Addlestone, Surrey KT15 3NB
UNITED KINGDOM
Tel: (44.1932) 34.11.11, Fax: (44.1932) 34.70.46
E-mail: m.banks@vla.maff.gsi.gov.uk

Dr D. Deregt(1)
Animal Diseases Research Institute, Canadian Food Inspection Agency, P.O. Box 640, Lethbridge, Alberta T1J 3Z4
CANADA
Tel: (1.403) 382.55.20, Fax: (1.403) 381.12.02
E-mail: deregtd@em.agr.ca

Dr L.A. Babiuk(2)
Veterinary Infectious Disease Organisation, 120 Veterinary Road
Saskatoon, Saskatchewan S7N 5E3
CANADA
Tel: (1.306) 966.74.65, Fax: (1.306) 966.74.78

‡ Also a reference laboratory for paratuberculosis.

Sheep and goat diseases/Maladies des ovins et des caprins/Enfermedades de los ovinos y caprinos

2.4.4. Caprine arthritis/encephalitis – Arthrite/encéphalite caprine – Artritis/encefalitis caprina
2.4.5. Maedi-visna – Maedi-visna – Maedi-visna

Dr C. Vitu
AFSSA Sophia Antipolis, Laboratoire de pathologie des petits ruminants et des abeilles, Unité de pathologie des petits ruminants, 'Les Templiers', 105 route des Chappes
BP 111, 06902 Sophia Antipolis Cedex
FRANCE
Tel: 33 (0)4 92.94.37.00, Fax: 33 (0)4 92.94.37.01
E-mail: c.vitu@sophia.afssa.fr

Dr D.P. Knowles, Jr
Animal Diseases Research Unit, USDA, ARS, Washington State University, Pullman, Washington 99164–7030
UNITED STATES OF AMERICA
Tel: (1.509) 335.60.29, Fax: (1.509) 335.83.28
E-mail: dknowles@vetmed.wsu.edu

2.4.6. Contagious caprine pleuropneumonia – Pleuropneumonie contagieuse caprine – Pleuroneumonía contagiosa caprina

Dr G. Bölske
The National Veterinary Institute (SVA)
P.O. Box 7073, S-750 07 Uppsala
SWEDEN
Tel: (46.18) 67.40.00, Fax: (46.18) 30.91.62
E-mail: goran.bolske@sva.se

Dr F. Thiaucourt
CIRAD/EMVT, Campus international de Baillarguet
Montferriez-sur-Lez, B.P. 5035, 34032 Montpellier Cedex 01
FRANCE
Tel: 33 (0)4 67.59.37.11, Fax: 33 (0)4 67.59.37.98
E-mail: thiaucourt@cirad.fr

Equine diseases/Maladies des équidés/Enfermedades de los équidos

2.5.1. Contagious equine metritis – Métrite contagieuse équine – Metritis contagiosa equina

Dr P. Heath
VLA Bury St Edmunds, Rougham Hill, Bury St Edmunds IP33 2RX
UNITED KINGDOM
Tel: (44.1284) 72.44.99, Fax: (44.1284) 72.45.00
E-mail: p.heath@vla.maff.gsi.gov.uk

Dr D. Miller
National Veterinary Services Laboratories, P.O. Box 844
Ames, IA 50010
UNITED STATES OF AMERICA
Tel: (1.515) 663.75.68, Fax: (1.515) 663.75.69
E-mail: david.a.miller@aphis.usda.gov

Dr J.H. Bongers
Institute for Animal Science and Health (ID Lelystad)
Bacteriology Department, P.O. Box 65, 8200 AB Lelystad
THE NETHERLANDS
Tel: (31.320) 23.82.38, Fax: (31.320) 23.80.50
E-mail: j.h.bongers@id.wag-ur.nl

2.5.2. Dourine – Dourine – Durina

Prof. V.T. Zablotskij
All-Russian Research Institute for Experimental Veterinary Medicine (VIEV), Veterinary Department, Ministry of Agriculture & Food, Kuzminki, 109472 Moscow
RUSSIA
Tel: (7.095) 377.94.42, Fax: (7.095) 377.80.84
E-mail: efzabegina@mtu-net.ru

2.5.3. Equine encephalomyelitis (Eastern and Western) – Encéphalomyélite équine de l'Est ou de l'Ouest – Encefalomielitis equina del Este o del Oeste

2.5.12. Venezuelan equine encephalomyelitis – Encéphalomyélite équine vénézuélienne – Encefalomielitis equina venezolana

Dr E.N. Ostlund
Diagnostic Virology Laboratory, National Veterinary Services Laboratories, P.O. Box 844, Ames, IA 50010
UNITED STATES OF AMERICA
Tel: (1.515) 663.75.51, Fax: (1.515) 663.73.48
E-mail: eileen.n.ostlund@aphis.usda.gov

2.5.4. Equine infectious anaemia – Anémie infectieuse des équidés – Anemia infecciosa equina

Dr E.N. Ostlund
National Veterinary Services Laboratories, APHIS/USDA
P.O. Box 844, Ames, IA 50010
UNITED STATES OF AMERICA
Tel: (1.515) 663.75.51, Fax: (1.515) 663.73.48
E-mail: eileen.n.ostlund@aphis.usda.gov

Dr H. Sentsui
National Institute of Animal Health, 3-1-1 Kannondai
Tsukuba, Ibaraki 305-0856
JAPAN
Tel: (81.298) 38.78.41, Fax: (81.298) 38.79.07
E-mail: sentsui@niah.affrc.go.jp

Prof. B. Toma
Services des maladies contagieuses, Ecole Nationale Vétérinaire d'Alfort, 7 avenue du Général de Gaulle
94704 Maisons-Alfort Cedex
FRANCE
Tel: 33 (0)1 43.68.73.34, Fax: 33 (0)1 43.96.71.31
E-mail: toma@vet-alfort.fr

2.5.5. Equine influenza – Grippe équine – Gripe equina

Dr W. Eichhorn
Institute for Medical Microbiology, Infectious and Epidemic Diseases, Veterinary Faculty, Ludwig-Maximilians-University
Veterinärstrasse 13, 80539 München
GERMANY
Tel: (49.89) 21.80.25.31, Fax: (49.89) 21.80.25.97
E-mail: werner.eichhorn@micro.vetmed.uni-muenchen.de

Dr J.A. Mumford
Animal Health Trust, Lanwades Park, Kentford, Newmarket
Suffolk CB8 7UU
UNITED KINGDOM
Tel: (44.1638) 75.06.59, Fax: (44.1638) 75.07.94
E-mail: jenny.mumford@aht.org.uk

Dr T.M. Chambers
Maxwell H. Gluck Equine Research Center, Dept of Veterinary Science, University of Kentucky, Lexington, Kentucky 40546-0099
UNITED STATES OF AMERICA
Tel: (1.859) 257.34.07, Fax: (1.859) 257.85.42
E-mail: tmcham1@pop.uky.edu

2.5.7. Equine rhinopneumonitis – Rhinopneumonie équine – Rinoneumonía equina

Dr J.A. Mumford
Animal Health Trust, Lanwades Park, Kentford, Newmarket
Suffolk CB8 7UU
UNITED KINGDOM
Tel: (44.1638) 75.06.59, Fax: (44.1638) 75.07.94
E-mail: jenny.mumford@aht.org.uk

Dr G. Allen
Maxwell H. Gluck Equine Research Center, Dept of Veterinary Science, University of Kentucky, Lexington, Kentucky 40546-0099
UNITED STATES OF AMERICA
Tel: (1.859) 257.36.63, Fax: (1.859) 257.85.42
E-mail: gallen@ca.uky.edu

Prof. K.P. Yurov
All-Russian Research Institute for Experimental Veterinary Medicine (VIEV), Veterinary Department, Ministry of Agriculture & Food, Kuzminki, 109472 Moscow
RUSSIA
Tel: (7.095) 377.79.93, Fax: (7.095) 377.80.84
E-mail: efzabegina@mtu-net.ru

2.5.10. Equine viral arteritis – Artérite virale équine – Arteritis viral equina

Dr P.J. Timoney
Maxwell H. Gluck Equine Research Center, Dept of Veterinary Science, University of Kentucky, Lexington, Kentucky 40546-0099
UNITED STATES OF AMERICA
Tel: (1.859) 257.15.31, Fax: (1.859) 257.85.42
E-mail: ptimoney@ca.uky.edu

Dr Y. Fukunaga
Epizootic Research Station, Equine Research Institute, The Japan Racing Association, Kokubunji-machi, Shimotsuga-gun, Tochigi 329-0412
JAPAN
Tel: (81.285) 44.00.90, Fax: (81.285) 44.56.76
E-mail: yoshiof@epizoo.equinst.go.jp

Dr D.J. Paton
Department of Virology
VLA Weybridge, New Haw, Addlestone, Surrey KT15 3NB
UNITED KINGDOM
Tel: (44.1932) 35.72.85, Fax: (44.1932) 35.72.39
E-mail: d.paton@vla.maff.gsi.gov.uk

Swine diseases/Maladies des suidés/Enfermedades de los suidos

2.6.4. Transmissible gastroenteritis – Gastro-entérite transmissible – Gastroenteritis transmisible

Dr D.J. Paton
Department of Virology
VLA Weybridge, New Haw, Addlestone, Surrey KT15 3NB
UNITED KINGDOM
Tel: (44.1932) 35.72.85, Fax: (44.1932) 35.72.39
E-mail: d.paton@vla.maff.gsi.gov.uk

Dr L.J. Saif
Food Animal Health Research Program, Ohio Agricultural Research and Development Center, The Ohio State University
1680 Madison Avenue, Wooster, OH 44691-4096
UNITED STATES OF AMERICA
Tel: (1.330) 263.37.44, Fax: (1.330) 263.36.77
E-mail: saif.2@osu.edu

Avian diseases/Maladies des oiseaux/Enfermedades de las aves

2.7.1. Infectious bursal disease (Gumboro disease) – Bursite infectieuse (Maladie de Gumboro) – Bursitis infecciosa (Enfermedad de Gumboro)

Dr Y.M. Saif
Food Animal Health Research Program, Ohio Agricultural Research and Development Center, The Ohio State University
1680 Madison Avenue, Wooster, OH 44691-4096
UNITED STATES OF AMERICA
Tel: (1.330) 263.37.43, Fax: (1.330) 263.36.77
E-mail: saif.1@osu.edu

Dr N. Eterradossi
AFSSA Ploufragan, Unité de virologie, immunologie et parasitologie aviaires et cunicoles (VIPAC), BP 53, 22440 Ploufragan
FRANCE
Tel: 33 (0)2 96.01.62.88, Fax: 33 (0)2 96.01.62.63
E-mail: n.eterradossi@ploufragan.afssa.fr

2.7.2. Marek's disease – Maladie de Marek – Enfermedad de Marek

Dr K. Venugopal
Institute for Animal Health, Compton Laboratory, Compton
Newbury, Berkshire RG20 7NN
UNITED KINGDOM
Tel: (44.1635) 57.84.11, Fax: (44.1635) 57.72.37
E-mail:venu.gopal@bbsrc.ac.uk

Dr J.L. Spencer
Animal Diseases Research Institute, 3851 Fallowfield Road
P.O. Box 11300, Station H, Nepean, Ontario K2H 8P9
CANADA
Tel: (1.613) 228.66.98, Fax: (1.613) 228.66.69
E-mail: spencerl@em.agr.ca

2.7.3. Avian mycoplasmosis – Mycoplasmose aviaire – Micoplasmosis aviar *(M. gallisepticum)*

Dr S.H. Kleven
The University of Georgia, College of Veterinary Medicine
Department of Avian Medicine, 953 College Station Road
Athens, Georgia 30602-4875
UNITED STATES OF AMERICA
Tel: (1.706) 542.56.44, Fax: (1.706) 542.56.30
E-mail: skleven@arches.uga.edu

Dr I. Kempf
AFSSA Ploufragan, UR Mycoplasmologie-Bactériologie
Unité de pathologie aviaire, Zoopôle Beaucemaine-Les Croix
BP 53, 22440 Ploufragan
FRANCE
Tel: 33 (0)2 96.01.62.81, Fax: 33 (0)2 96.01.62.73
E-mail: i.kempf@ploufragan.afssa.fr

Lagomorph diseases/Maladies des lagomorphes/Enfermedades de los lagomorfos

2.8.2. Tularemia – Tularémie – Tularemia

Dr T. Mörner
National Veterinary Institute, Department of Wildlife
751 89 Uppsala
SWEDEN
Tel: (46.18) 67.42.14 Fax: (46.18) 30.91.62
Email: torsten.morner@sva.se

2.8.3. Rabbit haemorrhagic disease – Maladie hémorragique du lapin – Enfermedad hemorrágica del conejo

Dr D. Gregg
National Veterinary Services Laboratories, APHIS
Foreign Animal Disease Diagnostic Laboratory (Plum Island)
USDA, P.O. Box 848, Greenport, NY 11944
UNITED STATES OF AMERICA
Tel: (1.613) 323.33.79, Fax: (1.613) 323.33.66
E-mail: douglas.a.gregg@aphis.usda.gov

Dr L. Capucci
Istituto Zooprofilattico Sperimentale della Lombardia e dell'Emilia
Romagna 'B. Ubertini', Via A. Bianchi n° 7/9, 25124 Brescia
ITALY
Tel: (39.30) 229.03.66, Fax: (39.30) 229.03.11
E-mail: capucci@bs.izs.it

Bee diseases/Maladies des abeilles/Enfermedades de las abejas

2.9.1.–2.9.5. Bee diseases – Maladies des abeilles – Enfermedades de las abejas

Mr J.-P. Faucon
AFSSA Sophia Antipolis, Laboratoire de pathologie des petits
ruminants et des abeilles, Unité Pathologie de l'abeille
'Les Templiers', 105 Route des Chappes, BP 111
06902 Sophia Antipolis
FRANCE
Tel: 33 (0)4 92.94.37.13, Fax: 33 (0)4 92.94.37.01
E-mail: jp.faucon@sophia.afssa.fr

Dr W. Ritter
Tierhygienisches Institut Freiburg, Am Moosweiher 2
Postfach 5140, 79108 Freiburg
GERMANY
Tel: (49.761) 150.21.41, Fax: (49.761) 150.22.99
E-mail: ritter@thi.cvuafr.bwl.de

Diseases not covered in the *International Animal Health Code*

X.4. Salmonellosis – Salmonellose – Salmonelosis

Dr R. Davies
VLA Weybridge, New Haw, Addlestone, Surrey KT15 3NB
UNITED KINGDOM
Tel: (44.1932) 35.73.61, Fax: (44.1932) 35.75.95
E-mail: r.h.davies@vla.maff.gsi.gov.uk

Dr C. Poppe
Health Canada, Guelph Laboratory, 110 Stone Road West
Guelph, Ontario N1G 3W4
CANADA
Tel: (1.519) 822.33.00, Fax: (1.519) 822.22.80
E-mail: cornelius_poppe@hc-sc.gc.ca

Dr M. Hartung
Bundesinstitut für gesundheitliche Verbraucherschutz und
Veterinärmedizin, P.O. Box 330013, 14191 Berlin
GERMANY
Tel: (49.1888) 412.22.12 Fax: (49.1888) 412.47.41
E-mail: m.hartung@bgvv.de

X.5. Bovine viral diarrhoea – Diarrhée virale des bovins – Diarrea viral bovina

Dr T.W. Drew
VLA Weybridge, New Haw, Addlestone, Surrey KT15 3NB
UNITED KINGDOM
Tel: (44.1932) 34.11.11, Fax: (44.1932) 34.70.46
E-mail: t.w.drew@vla.maff.gsi.gov.uk

Dr D. Deregt
Animal Diseases Research Institute, Canadian Food Inspection
Agency, Government of Canada, P.O. Box 640, Lethbridge
Alberta T1J 3Z4
CANADA
Tel: (1.403) 382.55.20, Fax: (1.403) 381.12.02
E-mail: deregtd@em.agr.ca

X.12. Porcine reproductive and respiratory syndrome – Syndrome dysgénésique et respiratoire du porc – Síndrome disgenésico y respiratorio porcino

Dr R. Magar
Laboratoire d'hygiène vétérinaire et alimentaire
Agence canadienne d'inspection des aliments
3400 Casavant ouest, Saint-Hyacinthe, Québec J2S 8E3
CANADA
Tel: (1.450) 773.77.30, Fax: (1.450) 773.81.52
E-mail: magarr@em.agr.ca

LIST OF OIE COLLABORATING CENTRES

Veterinary Medicinal Products/Médicaments vétérinaires/Medicamentos veterinarios

AFSSA Fougères, Agence nationale du médicament vétérinaire
B.P. 203, 35302 Fougères Cedex
FRANCE
Tel: 33 (0)2 99.94.78.72
Fax: 33 (0)2 99.94.78.99
E-mail: j.boisseau@anmv.afssa.fr

ELISA and Molecular Techniques in Animal Disease Diagnosis
Diagnostic des maladies animales par l'ELISA et les techniques moléculaires
Diagnóstico de enfermedades animales por el método ELISA y las técnicas moleculares

FAO/IAEA Centre for ELISA and Molecular Techniques in Animal Disease Diagnosis
International Atomic Energy Agency, Wagramerstrasse 5, P.O. Box 100
A-1400 Vienna
AUSTRIA
Tel: (43.1) 2600.283.55
Fax: (43.1) 2600.282.22
E-mail: m.h.jeggo@iaea.org

Diagnosis and Control of Animal Diseases in Tropical Regions
Diagnostic et contrôle des maladies animales en régions tropicales
Diagnóstico y control de las enfermedades animales en las regiones tropicales

CIRAD/EMVT, Campus international de Baillarguet, Montferriez-sur-Lez
B.P. 5035, 34032 Montpellier Cedex 01
FRANCE
Tel: 33 (0)4 67.59.37.11
Fax: 33 (0)4 67.59.37.98
E-mail: domenech@cirad.fr

Surveillance and Control of Animal Diseases in Africa
Surveillance et contrôle des maladies animales en Afrique
Vigilancia y control de enfermedades animales en África

Onderstepoort Veterinary Institute, Private Bag X05, Onderstepoort 0110
SOUTH AFRICA
Tel: (27.12) 529.91.01
Fax: (27.12) 565.46.67
E-mail: fred@moon.ovi.ac.za

Animal Disease Surveillance Systems and Risk Analysis
Systèmes de surveillance des maladies animales et analyse des risques
Sistemas de vigilancia de enfermedades animales y análisis de riesgos

Centers for Epidemiology and Animal Health
USDA/APHIS-VS
555 South Howes, Suite 300
Fort Collins, Colorado 80521
UNITED STATES OF AMERICA
Tel: (1.970) 490.80.00
Fax: (1.970) 490.80.99
E-mail: steve.weber@aphis.usda.gov

Diagnosis and Control of Animal Diseases in Eastern Europe, Central Asia and Transcaucasia
Diagnostic et contrôle des maladies animales en Europe de l'Est, en Asie centrale et en Transcaucasie
Diagnóstico y control de las enfermedades animales en Europa oriental, Asia central y Transcaucasia

All-Russian Research Institute for[1]
Animal Health (ARRIAH)
600900 Yur'evets, Vladimir
RUSSIA
Tel: (7.0922) 26.06.14/26.19.14
Fax: (7.0922) 24.36.75/23.72.61
E-mail: sinko@arriah.elcom.ru
Telex: 218124 URAL RUS

All-Russia State Research Institute for Control[2]
Standardisation and Certification of Veterinary Preparations
Ministry of Agriculture and Food, 5 Zvenigorodskoye
shosse, 123022 Moscow, RUSSIA
Tel/Fax: (7.095) 253.14.91
E-mail: vgnki_vet@mtu-net.ru

Epidemiology and Organisation of Veterinary Services in Developing Countries
Épidémiologie et organisation des Services vétérinaires dans les pays en développement
Epidemiología y organización de los Servicios Veterinarios en los países en desarrollo

Istituto Zooprofilattico Sperimentale dell'Abruzzo e del Molise 'G. Caporale'
Via Campo Boario, 64100 Teramo
ITALY
Tel: (39.0861) 33.22.33
Fax: (39.0861) 33.22.51
E-mail: caporale@izs.it

Diagnosis of Animal Diseases and Vaccine Evaluation in the Americas
Diagnostic des maladies animales et évaluation des vaccins dans les Amériques
Diagnóstico de las enfermedades animales y evaluación de las vacunas en las Américas

National Veterinary Services Laboratory[1]
APHIS/USDA
P.O. Box 844
Ames
Iowa 50010
UNITED STATES OF AMERICA
Tel: (1.515) 663.72.66
Fax: (1.515) 663.73.97
E-mail: director.nvsl@aphis.usda.gov

Institute for International Cooperation in Animal Biologics[2]
College of Veterinary Medicine
Iowa State University
Ames
Iowa 50011
UNITED STATES OF AMERICA
Tel: (1.515) 294.18.50
Fax: (1.515) 294.82.59
E-mail: iicab@iastate.edu

OIE COLLABORATING CENTRE FOR AQUATIC ANIMAL DISEASES

Information on Aquatic Animal Diseases
Information sur les maladies des animaux aquatiques
Información sobre las enfermedades de los animales acuáticos

The Centre for Environment, Fisheries and Aquaculture Sciences (CEFAS)
Weymouth Laboratory, Barrack Road, The Nothe, Weymouth, Dorset, DT4 8UB
UNITED KINGDOM
Tel: (44.1305) 20.66.26
Fax: (44.1305) 20.66.27
E-mail: b.j.hill@cefas.co.uk

OIE Reference Laboratories for fish, mollusc and crustacean diseases*

2.1.1. Epizootic haematopoietic necrosis – Nécrose hématopoïétique épizootique – Necrosis hematopoyética epizoótica

Dr A. Hyatt(1)
Australian Fish Health Reference Laboratory, c/o CSIRO
Australian Animal Health Laboratory, Private Bag 24
Geelong, Victoria 3213
AUSTRALIA
Tel: (61.3) 52.27.50.00, Fax (61.3) 52.27.55.55
E-mail: alex.hyatt@li.csiro.au

Dr R. Whittington(2)
Elizabeth Macarthur Agricultural Institute, NSW Agriculture
PMB 8, Camden NSW 2570
AUSTRALIA
Tel: (61.2) 46.293.333, Fax (61.2) 46.293.343
E-mail: richard.whittington@agric.nsw.gov.au

2.1.2 Infectious haematopoietic necrosis – Nécrose hématopoïétique infectieuse – Necrosis hematopoyética infecciosa (Rhabdoviruses)

Dr J.-A. Leong
Oregon State University, Center for Salmon Disease Research,
Department of Microbiology
Nash Hall 220,Corvallis, Oregon 93331-3804
UNITED STATES OF AMERICA
Tel: (1.541) 737.18.34 (1.541) 737.04.96
E-mail: leongj@orst.edu

Dr J. Winton
U.S. Geological Survey, Western Fisheries Research Center,
Biological Resources Division, 6505 N.E. 65th Street
Seattle, Washington 98115
UNITED STATES OF AMERICA
Tel: (1.206) 526.65.87, Fax: (1.206) 526.66.54
E-mail: jim_winton@usgs.gov

2.1.3. *Oncorhynchus masou* virus disease – Herpèsvirose du saumon *masou* – Herpesvirosis del salmón *masou*

Dr M. Yoshimizu
Hokkaido University, Faculty of Fisheries, Laboratory of
Microbiology, 3-1-1 Minato-cho, Hakodate, Hokkaido 041-0821
JAPAN
Tel/Fax: (81.138) 40.00.10
E-mail: yosimizu@pop.fish.hokudai.ac.jp

2.1.4. Spring viraemia of carp – Virémie printanière de la carpe – Viremia primaveral de la carpa

Prof. B.J. Hill
The Centre for Environment, Fisheries and Aquaculture Sciences
(CEFAS), Weymouth Laboratory, Barrack Road, The Nothe
Weymouth, Dorset, DT4 8UB
UNITED KINGDOM
Tel: (44.1305) 20.66.26, Fax: (44.1305) 20.66.27
E-mail: b.j.hill@cefas.co.uk

* The numbers correspond to the chapters in the *International Aquatic Animal Health Code*
Les références correspondent aux chapitres dans le *Code sanitaire international pour les animaux aquatiques*
Las referencias corresponden a los capítulos en el *Código internacional para las enfermedades de los animales acuáticos*

2.1.5. Viral haemorrhagic septicaemia – Septicémie hémorragique virale – Septicemia hemorrágica viral

Dr N.J. Olesen
Danish Veterinary Laboratory, Hangøvej 2, DK-8200 Aarhus N
DENMARK
Tel: (45) 89.37.24.31, Fax: (45) 89.37.24.70
E-mail: njo@svs.dk

2.2.1. Channel catfish virus disease – Herpèsvirose du poisson-chat – Virosis del bagre de canal

Dr L.A. Hanson
College of Veterinary Medicine, Fish Diagnostic Laboratory,
Mississippi State University, Box 9825, Spring Street
Mississippi 39762
UNITED STATES OF AMERICA
Tel: (1.662) 325.12.02, Fax: (1.662) 325.10.31
E-mail: hanson@cvm.msstate.edu

2.2.2. Viral encephalopathy and retinopathy – Encéphalopathie et rétinopathie virales – Encefalopatía y retinopatía virales

Dr G. Bovo
Istituto Zooprofilattico Sperimentale delle Venezie, Dipartimento di Ittiovirologia, Via Romea 14/A, 35020 Legnaro PD
ITALY
Tel: (39.049) 88.30.380, Fax: (39.049) 88.30.046
E-mail: bovo.izs@interbusiness.it

Dr T. Nakai
Hiroshima University, Fish Pathology Laboratory, Faculty of Applied Biological Science, Higashihiroshima 739-8528
JAPAN
Tel: (81.824) 24.79.47, Fax: (81.824) 22.70.59
E-mail: nakaitt@hiroshima-u.ac.jp

2.2.3. Infectious pancreatic necrosis – Nécrose pancréatique infectieuse – Necrosis pancreática infecciosa

Prof. B.J. Hill
The Centre for Environment, Fisheries and Aquaculture Sciences (CEFAS), Weymouth Laboratory, Barrack Road, The Nothe
Weymouth, Dorset, DT4 8UB
UNITED KINGDOM
Tel: (44.1305) 20.66.26, Fax: (44.1305) 20.66.27
E-mail: b.j.hill@cefas.co.uk

2.2.4. Infectious salmon anaemia – Anémie infectieuse du saumon – Anemia infecciosa del salmón

Dr B. Dannevig
National Veterinary Institute, Ullevålsveien 68
P.O. Box 8156 Dep., 0033 Oslo
NORWAY
Tel: (47.22) 96.46.63, Fax: (47.22) 60.09.81
E-mail: birgit.dannevig@vetinst.no

2.2.5 Epizootic ulcerative syndrome – Syndrome ulcératif épizootique – Síndrome ulcerante epizoótico

Dr K. Tonguthai
Aquatic Animal Health Research Institute (AAHRI)
Department of Fisheries, Kasetsart University Campus
Chatuchak, Bangkok 10900
THAILAND
Tel: (66.2) 579.41.22, Fax: (66.2) 561.39.93
E-mail: kamonpot@fisheries.go.th

2.2.6. Bacterial kidney disease (*Renibacterium salmoninarum*) – Rénibactériose – Renibacteriosis

Dr R.J. Pascho
U.S. Geological Survey, Western Fisheries Research Center,
Biological Resources Division, 6505 N.E. 65th Street
Seattle, Washington 98115
UNITED STATES OF AMERICA
Tel: (1.206) 526.65.88, Fax: (1.206) 526.66.54
E-mail: ron_pascho@usgs.gov

2.2.7. Enteric septicaemia of catfish – Entérosepticémie du poission-chat – Septicemia entérica del bagre

Dr L.A. Hanson
College of Veterinary Medicine, Fish Diagnostic Laboratory,
Mississippi State University, Box 9825, Spring Street
Mississippi 39762
UNITED STATES OF AMERICA
Tel: (1.662) 325.12.02, Fax: (1.662) 325.10.31
E-mail: hanson@cvm.msstate.edu

2.2.8. Piscirickettsiosis (*Piscirickettsia salmonis*) – Piscirickettsiose – Piscirickettsiosis

Dr J.L. Fryer
Oregon State University, Distinguished Professor Emeritus,
Department of Microbiology, 220 Nash Hall, Corvallis,
Oregon 97331-3804
UNITED STATES OF AMERICA
Tel: (1.541) 737.47.53, Fax: (1.541) 737.21.66
E-mail: fryerj@orst.edu

2.2.9 Gyrodactylosis *(Gyrodactylus salaris)* – Gyrodactylose – Girodactilosis

Dr T.A. Mo
National Veterinary Institute, Fish Health Section
Ullevålsveien 68, P.O. Box 8156 Dep., 0033 Oslo
NORWAY
Tel: (47.22) 96.47.22, Fax: (47.22) 46.38.77
E-mail: tor-atle.mo@vetinst.no

2.2.10. Red sea bream iridoviral disease – Iridovirose de la daurade japonaise – Iridovirosis de la dorada japonesa

Dr K. Nakajima
Virology Section, Fish-Pathology Division, National Research
Institute of Aquaculture, Fisheries Agency, 422-1 Nakatsuhama
Nansei-cho, Watarai-gun, Mie 516-0193
JAPAN
Tel: (81.5996) 618.30, Fax: (81.5996) 619.62
E-mail: kazuhiro@ss.nria.affrc.go.jp

3.1.1.–3.1.5. Mollusc pathogens – Agents pathogènes des mollusques – Agentes patógenos de los moluscos

Dr F. Berthe
Laboratoire de Génétique Aquaculture et Pathologie, IFREMER
Station de La Tremblade, Ronce les bains, BP 133
17390 La Tremblade
FRANCE
Tel: 33 (0)5 46.36.98.36, Fax: 33 (0)5 46.36.37.51
E-mail: fberthe@ifremer.fr

4.1.1.–4.1.3 & 4.2.1.–4.2.5 Crustacean pathogens – Agents pathogènes des crustacés – Agentes patógenos de los crustáceos

Prof. D.V. Lightner
Aquaculture Pathology Laboratory, Department of Veterinary
Science and Microbiology, University of Arizona, Building 90
Room 202 Pharmacy/Microbiology, Tucson, AZ 85721
UNITED STATES OF AMERICA
Tel: (1.520) 621.84.14, Fax: (1.520) 621.48.99
E-mail: dvl@u.arizona.edu

Prof. S.N. Chen
Department of Zoology and Fishery Research, National Taiwan
University, No. 1, Roosevelt Road, Section 4, Taipei, Taiwan
10764
TAIPEI CHINA
Tel: (886.2) 368.71.01/02, Fax: (886.2) 368.71.22
E-mail: snchen@cc.ntu.edu.tw

ALPHABETICAL LIST OF DISEASES COVERED IN THIS *MANUAL*